Ocular Disease: Mechanisms and Management

Commissioning Editor: *Russell Gabbedy*
Development Editor: *Ben Davie*
Editorial Assistant: *Kirsten Lowson*
Project Manager: *Srikumar Narayanan*
Design: *Charles Gray*
Illustration Manager: *Bruce Hogarth*
Marketing Managers (UK/USA): *Richard Jones / Radha Mawrie*

Ocular Disease: Mechanisms and Management

Leonard A. Levin, MD, PhD
Canada Research Chair of Ophthalmology and Visual Sciences
University of Montreal
Montreal, Quebec, Canada
Professor of Ophthalmology and Visual Sciences
University of Wisconsin
Madison, WI, USA

Daniel M. Albert, MD, MS
RRF Emmett A. Humble Distinguished Director of
the UW Eye Research Institute
F.A. Davis Professor, Department of Ophthalmology
and Visual Sciences
School of Medicine and Public Health
University of Wisconsin-Madison
University of Wisconsin
Madison, WI, USA

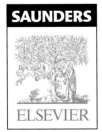

SAUNDERS

ELSEVIER

SAUNDERS
ELSEVIER

SAUNDERS an imprint of Elsevier Inc

First published 2010

The right of Leonard A. Levin and Daniel M. Albert to be identified as authors of this work has been asserted by them in accordance with the Copyright, Designs and Patents Act 1988.

13 digit ISBN: 978-0-7020-2983-7

British Library Cataloguing in Publication Data
A catalogue record for this book is available from the British Library

Library of Congress Cataloging in Publication Data
A catalog record for this book is available from the Library of Congress

Notice
Medical knowledge is constantly changing. Standard safety precautions must be followed, but as new research and clinical experience broaden our knowledge, changes in treatment and drug therapy may become necessary or appropriate. Readers are advised to check the most current product information provided by the manufacturer of each drug to be administered to verify the recommended dose, the method and duration of administration, and contraindications. It is the responsibility of the practitioner, relying on experience and knowledge of the patient, to determine dosages and the best treatment for each individual patient. Neither the Publisher nor the author assume any liability for any injury and/or damage to persons or property arising from this publication.

The Publisher

ELSEVIER
your source for books,
journals and multimedia
in the health sciences

www.elsevierhealth.com

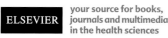

Working together to grow
libraries in developing countries

www.elsevier.com | www.bookaid.org | www.sabre.org

ELSEVIER   BOOK AID International   Sabre Foundation

The publisher's policy is to use paper manufactured from sustainable forests

Printed in China
Last digit is the print number: 9 8 7 6 5 4 3 2 1

Contents

SECTION 9 Retina

SECTION 10 Uveitis

List of Contributors

Anthony P Adamis MD
Adjunct Professor
Division of Ophthalmology and
Visual Sciences
University of Illinois College of Medicine
Bronxville, NY, USA

Grazyna Adamus PhD
Professor of Ophthalmology and
Graduate Neuroscience
Ocular Immunology Laboratory
Casey Eye Institute
Department of Ophthalmology
Oregon Health and Science University
Portland, OR, USA

Daniel M Albert MD MS
Emmett A Humble Distinguished Director
Eye Research Institute,
Professor and Chair Emeritus,
F A Davis Professor,
Lorenz E Zimmerman Professor
Ophthalmology & Visual Sciences
School of Medicine and Public Health
Clinical Sciences Center
University of Wisconsin
Madison, WI, USA

Ann-Christin Albertsmeyer Can Med
Research Assistant (Predoctoral)
Department of Ophthalmology
Schepens Eye Research Institute
Boston, MA, USA

Nishani Amerasinghe BSc MBBS MRCOphth
Specialist Registrar
Southampton Eye Unit
Southampton University Hospitals
NHS Trust
Southampton, UK

Michael G Anderson PhD
Assistant Professor of Molecular Physiology
and Biophysics
Department of Molecular Physiology
and Biophysics
University of Iowa
Iowa City, IA, USA

Sally S Atherton PhD
Regents Professor and Chair
Department of Cellular Biology
and Anatomy
Medical College of Georgia
Augusta, GA, USA

Tin Aung MBBS MMed(Ophth)
FRCS(Ed) FRCOphth
Senior Consultant and Head
Glaucoma Service
Singapore National Eye Centre,
Deputy Director, Singapore Eye
Research Institute,
Associate Professor
National University of Singapore
Singapore

Rebecca S Bahn MD
Professor of Medicine
Division of Endocrinology
Mayo Clinic
Rochester, MN, USA

David Sander Bardenstein MD
Professor
Departments of Ophthamology and Visual
Sciences, and Pathology
Case Western Reserve University School
of Medicine
Cleveland, OH, USA

Neal P Barney MD
Associate Professor of Ophthalmology
Department of Ophthalmology and
Visual Sciences
University of Wisconsin School of Medicine
Madison, WI, USA

David C Beebe PhD FARVO
The Janet and Bernard Becker Professor of
Ophthalmology and Visual Sciences,
Professor of Cell Biology and Physiology
Department of Ophthalmology and
Visual Sciences
Washington University
St Louis, MO, USA

Adrienne Berman MD
Clinical Assistant Professor
Department of Ophthalmology and
Visual Sciences
University of Illinois Eye and Ear Infirmary
Chicago, IL, USA

Audrey M Bernstein PhD
Assistant Professor of Ophthalmology
Department of Ophthalmology
Mount Sinai School of Medicine
New York, NY, USA

Pooja Bhat MD
Fellow
Massachusetts Eye Research &
Surgery Institute
Cambridge, MA, USA

Douglas Borchman PhD
Professor
Department of Ophthalmology and
Visual Sciences
Kentucky Lions Eye Center
University of Louisville
Louisville, KY, USA

Stephen Brocchini
Professor of Chemical Pharmaceutics
Department of Pharmaceutics
The School of Pharmacy
University of London
London, UK

Claude Burgoyne MD
Research Director
Optic Nerve Head Research Laboratory
Devers Eye Institute
Portland, OR, USA

Michelle Trager Cabrera MD
Clinical Associate
Department of Opthalmology
Duke University
Durham, NC, USA

Richard J Cenedella
Professor
Department of Biochemistry
A T Still University of Health Sciences,
Kirksville College of Osteopathic Medicine
Kirksville, MO, USA

Jin-Hong Chang PhD
Assistant Professor of Ophthalmology
Department of Opthalmology and
Visual Sciences
University of Illinois at Chicago
Chicago, IL, USA

Aimee Chappelow MD
Cole Eye Institute
The Cleveland Clinic Foundation
Cleveland, OH, USA

Anuj Chauhan PhD
Associate Professor and Director of
the Graduate Programs
Department of Chemical Engineering
University of Florida
Gainesville, FL, USA

Abbot F Clark PhD
Professor of Cell Biology and Anatomy
and Director
North Texas Eye Research Institute
University of North Texas Health
Science Center
Fort Worth, TX, USA

Ellen B Cook PhD
Associate Scientist
Department of Medicine
University of Wisconsin School of Medicine
and Public Health
Madison, WI, USA

Zélia M Corrêa MD PhD
Assistant Professor of Ophthalmology
Department of Ophthalmology
University of Cincinnati College
of Medicine
Cincinnati, OH, USA

Scott Cousins MD
The Robert Machemer Professor of
Ophthalmology and Immunology,
Vice Chair for Research
Department of Ophthalmology
Duke University School of Medicine
Durham, NC, USA

Gerald Cox MD PhD FACMG
Staff Physician in Genetics, Children's
Hospital Boston
Instructor of Pediatrics, Harvard
Medical School
Vice President of Clinical Research
Genzyme Corporation
Cambridge, MA, USA

Scott Adam Croes MS PhD
Professor of Human Anatomy
and Physiology
Department of Biology
Shasta College
Redding, CA, USA

Karl G Csaky MD PhD
Associate Professor
Department of Ophthalmology
Duke University
Durham, NC, USA

Annegret Hella Dahlmann-Noor
Dr med PhD FRCOphth FRCS(Ed) DipMedEd
Senior Clinical Research Associate
Ocular Biology and Therapeutics
UCL Institute of Ophthalmology
London, UK

Reza Dana MD MPH MSc
Professor and Director of Cornea Service
Massachusetts Eye & Ear Infirmary
Harvard Medical School
Boston, MA, USA

Helen Danesh-Meyer MBChB FRANZCO
Sir William & Lady Stevenson Associate
Professor of Ophthalmology
Department of Ophthalmology
University of Auckland
Auckland, New Zealand

Julie T Daniels BSc(Hons) PhD
Reader in Stem Cell Biology and
Transplantation
UCL Institute of Ophthalmology
London, UK

Darlene A Dartt PhD
Senior Scientist, Harold F. Johnson
Research Scholar
Schepens Eye Research Institute,
Associate Professor
Harvard Medical School
Schepens Eye Research Institute
Boston, MA, USA

Mohammad H Dastjerdi MD
Postdoctoral Fellow
Schepens Eye Research Institute
Boston, MA, USA

Nigel W Daw PhD
Professor Emeritus of Ophthalmology and
Visual Science
Departments of Ophthalmology and
Visual Science
University of Yale
New Haven, CT, USA

Daniel G Dawson MD
Visiting Assistant Professor of
Ophthalmology
Emory University Eye Center
Atlanta, GA, USA

Alejandra de Alba Campomanes
MD MPH
Director of Pediatric Ophthalmology
San Francisco General Hospital
San Francisco, CA, USA

Joseph L Demer MD PhD
The Leonard Apt Professor of
Ophthalmology,
Professor of Neurology
Jules Stein Eye Institute
David Geffen School of Medicine
University of California, Los Angeles
Los Angeles, CA, USA

Suzanne M Dintzis MD PhD
Assistant Professor
Department of Pathology
University of Washington School of
Medicine
Seattle, WA, USA

J Crawford Downs PhD
Associate Scientist and Research Director
Ocular Biomechanics Laboratory
Devers Eye Institute
Portland, OR, USA

Henry Edelhauser PhD
Ferst Professor and Director of
Ophthalmology Research
Department of Ophthalmology
Emory University Eye Center
Atlanta, GA, USA

David Ellenberg MD
Research Fellow
Department of Ophthalmology and
Visual Sciences
University of Illinois at Chicago
Chicago, IL, USA

Victor Elner MD PhD
The Ravitz Foundation Professor of
Ophthlamology and Visual Sciences
Professor, Department of Pathology
Kellogg Eye Center
University of Michigan
Ann Arbor, MI, USA

Steven K Fisher PhD
Professor, Molecular Cellular and
Developmental Biology
Neuroscience Research Institute
University of California, Santa Barbara
Santa Barbara, CA, USA

Robert Folberg MD
Dean, Oakland University William
Beaumont School of Medicine,
Professor of Biomedical Sciences, Pathology,
and Ophthalmology
Oakland University William Beaumont
School of Medicine
Rochester, MI, USA

C Stephen Foster MD FACS FACR
*Founder and President, Ocular Immunology
and Uveitis Foundation,
Clinical Professor of Ophthalmology
Harvard Medical School,
Founder and President
Massachusetts Eye Research and
Surgery Institution
Cambridge, MA, USA*

Gary N Foulks MD FACS
*The Arthur and Virginia Keeney Professor
of Ophthalmology and Vision Science
Division of Ophthalmology
University of Louisville School of Medicine
Louisville, KY, USA*

Frederick T Fraunfelder MD
*Professor of Ophthalmology
Casey Eye Institute
Portland, OR, USA*

Frederick W Fraunfelder MD
*Associate Professor of Ophthalmology
Casey Eye Institute
Portland, OR, USA*

Anne Fulton MD
*Senior Associate in Ophthalmology
Department of Ophthalmology
Children's Hospital Boston
Boston, MA, USA*

Ronald Gaster MD
*Professor of Ophthalmology
Department of Opthalmology
University of California
Irvine, CA, USA*

Stylianos Georgoulas MD
*Ocular Repair and Regeneration
Biology Unit
UCL Institute of Ophthalmology
London, UK*

Michael S Gilmore PhD
*The C L Schepens Professor of
Ophthalmology
Harvard Medical School,
Senior Scientist
Schepens Eye Research Institute
Boston, MA, USA*

Ilene K Gipson PhD
*Senior Scientist and Professor of
Ophthalmology
Department of Ophthalmology
Schepens Eye Research Institute
Boston, MA, USA*

Michaël J A Girard PhD
*Ocular Biomechanics Laboratory
Devers Eye Institute, Legacy Health System
Portland, OR, USA*

Lynn K Gordon MD PhD
*Associate Professor Ophthalmology
Jules Stein Eye Institute
UCLA School of Medicine
Los Angeles, CA, USA*

Irene Gottlob MD
*Professor of Ophthalmology
Department of Cardiovascular Sciences
Ophthalmology Group
University of Leicester
Leicester Royal Infirmary
Leicester, UK*

John D Gottsch MD
*The Margaret C Mosher Professor of
Ophthalmology
Johns Hopkins School of Medicine
Wilmer Eye Institute
Baltimore, MD, USA*

Frank M Graziano MD PhD
*Professor of Medicine
Department of Medicine
University of Wisconsin School of Medicine
and Public Health
Madison, WI, USA*

Hans E Grossniklaus MD MBA
*Professor of Medicine
Emory Eye Center
Emory University School of Medicine
Atlanta, GA, USA*

Deborah Grzybowski PhD
*Professor of Ophthalmology and
Biomedical Engineering
The Ohio State University
College of Medicine
Columbus, OH, USA*

Clyde Guidry PhD
*Associate Professor of Ophthalmology
Department of Ophthalmology
University of Alabama School of Medicine
Birmingham, AB, USA*

Neeru Gupta MD PhD FRCSC DABO
*Professor of Ophthalmology and Vision
Sciences, Laboratory Medicine and
Pathobiology, University of Toronto,
Director
Glaucoma & Nerve Protection Unit
Keenan Research Centre at the Li Ka Shing
Knowledge Institute
St Michael's Hospital
Toronto, ON, Canada*

David H Gutmann MD PhD
*The Donald O Schnuck Family Professor
Department of Neurology,
Director, Neurofibromatosis Center
Washington University School of Medicine
St Louis, MO, USA*

Vinay Gutti MD
*Private Practice
Cornea, External Disease and
Refractive Surgery
La Mirada Eye and Laser Center
La Mirada, CA, USA*

John R Guy MD
*Bascom Palmer Eye Institute
Miami, FL, USA*

J William Harbour MD
*The Paul A Cibis Distinguished Professor
of Ophthalmology
Department of Ophthalmology and
Visual Sciences
Washington University School of Medicine
St Louis, MO, USA*

Mary Elizabeth Hartnett MD
*Professor of Ophthalmology
Department of Ophthalmology
University of North Carolina
Chapel Hill, NC, USA*

Sohan S Hayreh MD MS PhD DSc FRCS(Edin)
FRCS(Eng) FRCOphth(Hon)
*Professor Emeritus of Ophthalmology
Department of Ophthalmology & Director
Ocular Vascular Clinic
University of Iowa Hospitals and Clinics
Iowa City, IA, USA*

Susan Heimer PhD
*Postdoctoral Research Fellow
Schepens Eye Research Institute and
Department of Ophthalmology
Harvard Medical School
Boston, MA, USA*

Robert Hess DSc
*Professor and Director of Research
Department of Ophthalmology
McGill University
Montreal, QC, Canada*

Nancy M Holekamp MD
*Partner, Barnes Retina Institute,
Professor of Clinical Ophthalmology
Department of Ophthalmology and
Visual Sciences
Washington University School of Medicine
St Louis, MO, USA*

Suber S Huang MD MBA
*The Philip F. and Elizabeth G. Searle
Professor of Ophthalmology,
Vice-Chair, Department of Ophthalmology
& Visual Sciences
Case Western Reserve University School
of Medicine,
Director, Center for Retina and
Macular Disease
University Hospitals Eye Institute
Cleveland, OH, USA*

Sudha K Iyengar PhD
Professor
Departments of Epidemiology & Biostatistics
and Department of Ophthalmology
Case Western Reserve University
Cleveland, OH, USA

Allen T Jackson
Massachusetts Eye Research and
Surgery Institute
Harvard Medical School
Cambridge, MA, USA

L Alan Johnson MD
Private Practice
Sierra Eye Associates
Reno, NV, USA

Peter F Kador PhD
Professor
Departments of Ophthalmology and
Pharmaceutical Sciences
University of Nebraska Medical Center
Omaha, NE, USA

Alon Kahana MD PhD
Full Member, University of Michigan
Comprehensive Cancer Center,
Attending Surgeon, C S Mott
Children's Hospital,
Assistant Professor
Department of Ophthalmology and
Visual Sciences
Kellogg Eye Center
University of Michigan
Ann Arbor, MI, USA

Randy Kardon MD PhD
Professor and Director of
Neuro-ophthalmology,
Pomerantz Family Chair in Ophthalmology,
Director for Iowa City VA Center for
Prevention and Treatment of Vision Loss
Department of Ophthalmology and
Visual Sciences
University of Iowa and Department of
Veterans Affairs
Iowa City, IA, USA

Maria Cristina Kenney MD PhD
Professor of Ophthalmology
The Gavin Herbert Eye Institute
Orange, CA, USA

Timothy Scott Kern PhD
Professor of Medicine
Department of Medicine
Division of Clinical and Molecular
Endocrinology
Center for Diabetes Research
Case Western Reserve University
Cleveland, OH, USA

Peng Tee Khaw PhD FRCP FRCS FRCOphth
FIBiol FRCPath FMedSci
Professor of Ocular Healing and Glaucoma
and Consultant Ophthalmic Surgeon,
Director of Research and Development,
Moorfields Eye Hospital NHS
Foundation Trust,
Director, National Institute for Health
Biomedical Research Centre,
Programme Director, Eyes & Vision, UCL
Partners Academic Health Science Centre
London, UK

Alice S Kim MD
Division of Ophthalmology
Maimonides Medical Center
Brooklyn, NY, USA

Henry Klassen MD PhD
Assistant Professor
Department of Ophthalmology
University of California, Irvine,
School of Medicine
Orange, CA, USA

Paul Knepper MD PhD
Research Scientist
University of Illinois at Chicago
Department of Opthalmology &
Visual Science
Chicago, IL, USA

Jane F Koretz PhD
Professor of Biophysics
Biochemistry and Biophysics Program
Rensselaer Polytechnic Institute,
Science Center
Troy, NY, USA

Mirunalini Kumaradas MD Opth(SL)
FRCS (UK)
Lecturer
Faculty of Medicine
University of Colombo
Colombo, Sri Lanka

Jonathan H Lass MD
The Charles I Thomas Professor and
Chairman
Department of Ophthalmology and
Visual Sciences
Case Western Reserve University,
Director, University Hospitals Eye Institute
Cleveland, OH, USA

David Lederer MD
Fellow
Department of Ophthalmology
Duke University
Durham, NC, USA

Mark Lesk MSc MD FRCS(C) CM DABO
Director of Vision Health Research
University of Montreal
Montreal, QC, Canada

Leonard A Levin MD PhD
Canada Research Chair of Ophthalmology
and Visual Sciences
Department of Ophthalmology
University of Montreal,
Professor, Department of Ophthalmology
and Visual Sciences
University of Wisconsin
Madison, WI, USA

Geoffrey P Lewis PhD
Research Biologist, Neurobiology
Neuroscience Research Institute
University of California, Santa Barbara
Santa Barbara, CA, USA

Zhuqing Li MD PhD
Staff Scientist
Laboratory of Immunology
National Eye Institute
National Institutes of Health
Bethesda, MD, USA

Amy Lin MD
Assistant Professor of Ophthalmology
Department of Ophthalmology
Loyola University
Maywood, IL, USA

Robert A Linsenmeier PhD
Professor of Biomedical Engineering,
Neurobiology & Physiology, and
Ophthalmology
Biomedical Engineering Department
Northwestern University
Evanston, IL, USA

Robert Listernick MD
Professor of Pediatrics, Feinberg School of
Medicine, Northwestern University,
Attending Physician
Division of General Academic Pediatrics
Children's Memorial Hospital
Chicago, IL, USA

Martin Lubow MD
Associate Professor of Ophthalmology
Department of Ophthalmology
The Ohio State University Eye and
Ear Institute
Columbus, OH, USA

Andrew Maniotis PhD
Visiting Associate Professor of
Bioengineering
Division of Science and Engineering
University of Illinois at Chicago
Chicago, IL, USA

Pascale Massin MD PhD
Professor of Ophthalmology
Ophthalmology Department
Lariboisiere Hospital
Paris, France

Katie Matatall BS
*Department of Ophthalmology &
Visual Sciences
Washington University School of Medicine
St Louis, MO, USA*

Russell L McCally PhD
*Associate Professor of Ophthalmology,
The Wilmer Eye Institute, Johns Hopkins
Medical Institutions
Principal Professional Staff
Applied Physics Laboratory
Johns Hopkins University
Laurel, MD, USA*

Stephen D McLeod MD
*Professor of Ophthalmology
Department of Ophthalmology
University of California San Francisco
San Francisco, CA, USA*

Muhammad Memon MD
*Visiting Academic
Department of Neuroscience
Imperial College London
London, UK*

Joan W Miller MD
*The Henry Willard Williams Professor of
Ophthalmology and Chair, Harvard
Medical School,
Chief, Department of Ophthalmology
Massachusetts Eye and Ear Infirmary
Boston, MA, USA*

Austin K Mircheff PhD
*Professor of Physiology & Biophysics and
Professor of Ophthalmology
Department of Physiology & Biophysics
Keck School of Medicine
University of Southern California
Los Angeles, CA, USA*

Jay Neitz PhD
*The Bishop Professor
Department of Ophthalmology
University of Washington
Seattle, WA, USA*

Maureen Neitz PhD
*The Ray H Hill Professor
Department of Ophthalmology
University of Washington
Seattle, WA, USA*

Christine C Nelson MD FACS
*Professor of Ophthalmology and Surgery
Kellog Eye Center
University of Michigan
Ann Arbor, MI, USA*

Robert Nickells BSc PhD
*Professor of Ophthalmology and
Visual Sciences
Department of Ophthalmology and
Visual Sciences
University of Wisconsin
Madison, WI, USA*

Robert B Nussenblatt MD MPH
*Department of Pathology and
Cancer Center
University of Illinois
Chicago, IL, USA*

Joan M O'Brien MD
*Professor of Ophthalmology and Pediatrics
Comprehensive Cancer Center
University of California San Francisco
San Francisco, CA, USA*

Daniel T Organisciak PhD
*Professor of Biochemistry and
Molecular Biology,
Director, Petticrew Research Laboratory
Department of Biochemistry and
Molecular Biology
Boonshoft School of Medicine
Wright State University
Dayton, OH, USA*

Michel Paques MD PhD
*Professor of Ophthalmology
Clinical Investigation Center
XV-XX Hospital and University of Paris VI
Paris, France*

Heather R Pelzel BSc
*Research Assistant
Department of Ophthalmology and
Visual Sciences
University of Wisconsin
Madison, WI, USA*

Shamira Perera MBBS BSc FRCOphth
*Research Fellow, Singapore Eye
Research Institute,
Consultant
Glaucoma Service
Singapore National Eye Centre
Singapore*

Eric A Pierce MD PhD
*Associate Professor of Ophthalmology
F M Kirby Center for Molecular
Ophthalmology
University of Pennsylvania School of
Medicine
Philadelphia, PA, USA*

Jean Pournaras MD
*Research Fellow
Service d'ophtalmologie
Hôpital Lariboisière
Paris, France*

Jonathan T Pribila MD, PhD
*Pediatric Ophthalmology and Adult
Strabismus Fellow
Department of Ophthalmology
University of Minnesota
Minneapolis, MN, USA*

Frank A Proudlock PhD
*Lecturer in Ophthalmology
Ophthalmology Group
University of Leicester
Robert Kilpatrick Clinical Sciences Building
Leicester Royal Infirmary
Leicester, UK*

Xiaoping Qi MD
*Associate Scientist of Ophthalmology
College of Medicine
University of Florida
Gainesville, FL, USA*

Narsing A Rao MD
*Professor of Ophthalmology and Pathology,
Keck School of Medicine, University of
Southern California,
Director of Experimental Ophthalmic
Pathology and Ocular Inflammations
Doheny Eye Institute
Los Angeles, CA, USA*

Robert Ritch MD
*Professor of Ophthalmology, New York
Medical College, Valhalla, NY,
The Shelley and Steven Einhorn
Distinguished Chair in Ophthalmology,
Chief, Glaucoma Services
Surgeon Director
New York Eye and Ear Infirmary
New York, NY, USA*

Joseph F Rizzo III
*Associate Professor of Ophthalmology
Massachusetts Eye and Ear Infirmary
Harvard Medical School
Boston, MA, USA*

Michael D Roberts PhD
*Post Doctoral Research Fellow
Ocular Biomechanics Laboratory
Devers Eye Institute
Portland, OR, USA*

James T Rosenbaum MD
*Professor of Ophthalmology, Medicine and
Cell Biology
The Edward E Rosenbaum Professor of
Inflammation Research
Oregon Health & Science University
Portland, OR, USA*

Barry Rouse PhD DSc
*Distinguished Professor
Department of Pathobiology
University of Tennessee
Knoxville, TN, USA*

Daniel R Saban PhD
Postdoctoral Fellow in Ophthalmology
Division of Ophthalmology
Schepens Eye Research Institute
Boston, MA, USA

Alfredo A Sadun MD PhD
Thornton Professor of Ophthalmology
and Neurosurgery
Department of Ophthalmology
USC Keck School of Medicine
Los Angeles, CA, USA

Abbas K Samadi PhD
Assistant Professor of Surgery and
Biochemistry
Department of Biochemistry
University of Kansas Medical Center
Kansas City, KS, USA

Pranita Sarangi BVSc&AH PhD
Postdoctoral Research Associate
David H Smith Center for Vaccine Biology
and Immunology
University of Rochester Medical Center
Rochester, NY, USA

Andrew P Schachat MD
Professor of Ophthalmology, Lerner College
of Medicine
Vice Chairman
Cole Eye Institute
Cleveland Clinic Foundation
Cleveland, OH, USA

Joel E Schechter PhD
Professor of Cell and Neurobiology
Keck School of Medicine
University of Southern California
Los Angeles, CA, USA

A Reagan Schiefer MD
Trainee in Endocrinology
Division of Endocrinology
Mayo Clinic
Rochester, MN, USA

Ursula Schlötzer-Schrehardt ProfDr
Professor
Department of Ophthalmology
University of Erlangen-Nürnberg
Erlangen, Germany

Ingo Schmack MD
Attending Physician
University of Bochum
Department of Ophthalmology
Bochum, Germany

Leopold Schmetterer PhD
Professor
Departments of Clinical Pharmacology and
Biomedical Engineering and Physics
Medical University of Vienna
Vienna, Austria

Genevieve Aleta Secker PhD BSc
Post-Doctoral Fellow
SA Pathology
Centre for Cancer Biology
Department of Haematology
Adelaide, SA, Australia

Srilakshmi M Sharma MRCP MRCOphth
Uveitis Fellow
Bristol Eye Hospital
University of Bristol NHS Trust
Bristol, UK

James A Sharpe MD FRCPC
Professor of Neurology, Medicine,
Ophthalmology and Visual Sciences, and
Otolaryngology, University of Toronto,
Director
Neuro-ophthalmology Center
University Health Network
Toronto, ON, Canada

Heather Sheardown BEng PhD
Professor
Department of Chemical Engineering and
School of Biomedical Engineering
McMaster University
Hamilton, ON, Canada

Alex Shortt MD PhD MRCOphth
Clinical Lecturer in Ophthalmic
Translational Research
Biomedical Research Centre for
Ophthalmology
Moorfields Eye Hospital
London, UK

Ying-Bo Shui MD PhD
Senior Scientist
Department of Ophthalmology and
Visual Sciences
Washington University in St Louis
St Louis, MO, USA

Ian Sigal PhD
Research Associate
Devers Eye Institute
Ocular Biomechanics Laboratory
Portland, OR, USA

James L Stahl PhD
Associate Scientist
Department of Medicine
University of Wisconsin School of Medicine
and Public Health
Madison, WI, USA

Roger F Steinert MD
Professor and Chair of Ophthalmology,
Professor of Biomedical Engineering,
Director, Gavin Herbert Eye Institute
University of California Irvine
Irvine, CA, USA

Arun N E Sundaram MBBS FRCPC
Fellow, Division of Neurology and Vision
Sciences Research Program, University of
Toronto,
Consultant
Neuro-ophthalmology Center
University Health Network
Toronto, ON, Canada

Janet S Sunness MD
Medical Director
Richard E Hoover Rehabilitation Services
for Low Vision and Blindness
Greater Baltimore Medical Center
Baltimore, MD, USA

Nathan T Tagg MD
Neurologist and Neuro-ophthalmologist
Walter Reed Army Medical Center
National Naval Medical Center
Bethesda, MD, USA

Daniela Toffoli MD
Ophthalmology Resident, PGY-5
Department of Ophthalmology
Université de Montréal
Montréal, QC, Canada

Cynthia A Toth MD
Professor of Ophthalmology and
Biomedical Engineering
Department of Biomedical Engineering
Duke University
Durham, NC, USA

Elias I Traboulsi MD
Professor of Ophthalmology
Cleveland Clinic Lerner College of Medicine
Case University
The Cole Eye Institute
Cleveland, OH, USA

James C Tsai MD
The Robert R Young Professor and
Chairman
Department of Ophthalmology and
Visual Science
Yale University School of Medicine,
Chief of Ophthalmology, Yale-New
Haven Hospital
Yale Eye Center
New Haven, CT, USA

Budd Tucker PhD
Investigator
Department of Ophthalmology
Schepens Eye Research Institute, Harvard
Medical School
Boston, MA, USA

Russell N Van Gelder MD PhD
Boyd K Bucey Memorial Chair,
Professor and Chair
Department of Ophthalmology,
Adjunct Professor
Department of Biological Structure
University of Washington School
of Medicine
Seattle, WA, USA

Hans Eberhard Völcker MD
Professor of Medicine
Department of Ophthalmology
University of Heidelberg
Heidelberg, Germany

Christopher S von Bartheld MD
Professor of Physiology and Cell Biology
Department of Physiology and Cell Biology
University of Nevada School of Medicine
Reno, NV, USA

Jianhua Wang MD PhD
Assistant Professor, Bascom Palmer
Eye Institute
Department of Ophthalmology
University of Miami, Miller School of
Medicine
Miami, FL, USA

Judith West-Mays PhD
Professor of Pathology and
Molecular Medicine
Division of Pathology
McMaster University
Hamilton, ON, Canada

Corey B Westerfeld MD
Vitreoretinal Surgeon
Private Practice
Eye Health Vision Center
Dartmouth, MA, USA

Steven E Wilson MD
Professor of Ophthalmology
Staff Cornea and Refractive Surgeon,
Director, Cornea Research
Cole Eye Institute
Cleveland Clinic Foundation
Cleveland, OH, USA

Fabricio Witzel de Medeiros MD
Department of Ophthalmology
University of São Paulo
São Paulo, Brazil

Chih-Wei Wu MD
Fellow, Cornea and External Eye Diseases
Department of Ophthalmology and
Visual Sciences
University of Illinois at Chicago
Chicago, IL, USA

Ai Yamada MD
Postdoctoral Research Fellow
Schepens Eye Research Institute and
Department of
Ophthalmology
Harvard Medical School
Boston, MA, USA

Steven Yeh MD
Vitreoretinal Fellow
Casey Eye Institute
Oregon Health and Sciences University
Casey Eye Institute, OHSU
Portland, OR, USA

Thomas Yorio PhD FARVO
Professor of Pharmacology and
Neuroscience,
Provost and Executive Vice President for
Academic Affairs
University of North Texas Health
Science Center
Fort Worth, TX, USA

Michael J Young PhD
Director, deGunzburg Research Center for
Retinal Transplantation,
Associate Scientist, Schepens Eye
Research Institute,
Associate Professor
Department of Ophthalmology
Harvard Medical School
Boston, MA, USA

Terri L Young MD FAAO FAOS FARVO
Professor of Neuroscience, Duke University,
National University of Singapore Graduate
Medical School,
Professor of Ophthalmology, Pediatrics
and Medicine
Duke University Medical Center
Durham, NC, USA

Yeni H Yücel MD PhD FRCPC
Professor and Director, Ophthalmic
Pathology
Division of Ophthalmology &
Vision Sciences
Laboratory Medicine & Pathobiology,
University of Toronto
Keenan Research Centre at the Li Ka Shing
Knowledge Institute
St Michael's Hospital
Toronto, ON, Canada

Beatrice Y J T Yue PhD
The Thanis A Field Professor of
Ophthalmology and Visual Sciences
Department of Ophthalmology and
Visual Sciences
University of Illinois at Chicago College
of Medicine
Chicago, IL, USA

Marco A Zarbin MD PhD FACS
The Alfonse A Cinotti MD/Lions Eye
Research Professor and Chair
Institute of Ophthalmology and
Visual Science
New Jersey Medical School
Newark, NJ, USA

Xinyu Zhang PhD
Senior Scientist II
BioTherapeutic
Alcon Research Ltd
Fort Worth, TX, USA

Mei Zheng MD
Resident
Department of Pathology
Medical College of Georgia
Augusta, GA, USA

Dedication

To our children: Emily, Eric, Eva, Rachel, and Eli (LAL)

Steven and Michael (DMA)

Foreword

Translational research offers both the opportunity and the challenge for medical research in the decades ahead, as physicians and clinician-scientists work to understand disease by utilizing the vast storehouse of detailed biological information that has been uncovered about the eye and visual system. Ultimately, the practice of medicine, and delivery of care to ameliorate disease, advances best and most effectively upon understanding the causative pathophysiology, as is addressed in this book.

I am delighted to see the advances represented in the chapters of this book. While no one volume can encompass the entirety of the clinical medicine of ophthalmology, the editors have assembled a broad and expert group of clinician-scientists who have written thoughtfully and cogently on many topics of modern ophthalmic disease research. These chapters are multidisciplinary and provide a good source of current knowledge. Clearly much work lies ahead of us to fully understand the causes, biological mechanisms and treatments of ocular and vision diseases. This book, *Ocular Disease: Mechanisms and Management*, provides a substantial starting point to launch insightful studies that will move our field even closer to rational therapeutics.

One of the drivers of this new understanding of disease comes from the vigorous work of the vision research community over the past two decades, which has led to identifying more than 500 genes that cause Mendelian ocular diseases. These genes encompass a wide assortment of conditions that clinicians diagnose and treat, and no tissues are spared. We have identified genes that cause retinal and macular degenerations, glaucoma, uveitis, cataract and corneal dystrophies, optic neuropathies, and amblyopia, strabismus and ocular motility disorders.

Disease gene discovery recently advanced into the previously intractable realm of the more common and widespread conditions that have genetically complex etiology. In 2005 several groups independently identified the first gene that conveys substantial risk for developing age-related macular degeneration, the complement factor H gene. Shortly thereafter several additional AMD risk genes were identified in the immune pathways, including complement modulatory factors, using the new and powerful techniques of haplotype mapping and genome-wide association studies. This new basic knowledge forced our attention toward the immune cascade as harboring mechanisms that culminate in vision loss from macular degeneration in as many as one in seven of the elderly.

As disease gene identification rocketed ahead, attention turned to genomics and studies of the expression, cellular localization and biological function of the aberrant gene products. It is these considerations that the present book addresses, for ultimately a true understanding of disease mechanisms, in many cases, lies buried within the genomic biology of these diseases.

Studying any one of these genes requires major effort to piece together an understanding of the relationship between gene and disease. Consider, for example, the TIGR/MYOC gene that encodes the protein myocillin that is expressed in the trabecular meshwork. Mutations in this gene result in early onset or even congenital dysregulation of intraocular pressure and leads to severe glaucoma in humans. Yet laboratory-created mice carrying the myocilin gene knockout show only a minimal phenotype. Two lessons are immediately apparent: first, we have a long path ahead to translate genetic discoveries into identifiable mechanisms of disease and pathophysiology that will support rationally designed therapeutic interventions. Second, although our field of eye disease research is amazingly rich in mouse models that generally mimic the human condition with good fidelity across a variety of ocular conditions, the fullest understanding of human disease mechanisms ultimately will require that we turn our attention directly to careful and detailed analysis of disease in human patients, as is considered in this textbook.

The future for treating diseases of the eye and visual system will require novel insight into disease biology. But already we can see major areas of opportunity to employ a new range of therapeutic interventions, from gene therapy to stem cells for regenerative medicine. This new book is the medical companion to the basic textbook *Adler's Physiology of the Eye*. This companion volume by Levin and Albert tackles the translation of basic knowledge into the realm of medical understanding and practice and thereby highlights that the best of basic and clinical knowledge increasingly have an interdependent existence and future.

Paul A. Sieving MD, PhD
Director, National Eye Institute, NIH
Bethesda, MD
September 2009

Preface

The eye is a microcosm for the world of disease. Its synonym, "the globe," has profound implications because, in addition to the geometric meaning, within its tablespoon of contents there is a world of physiology and pathophysiology. Autoimmune diseases, neoplasms, infections, neurodegenerations, infarcts: these all occur within the eye and the eye's transit stations within the central nervous system. Almost all of the same pathophysiological principles that apply to the eye apply equally to the body.

This book is a guide to the world of ocular disease. Each chapter is written by scientists who carry out exciting research in the corresponding field. Like tour guides who are native to a region or country, these experienced authors can help the reader travel through a scientific landscape, pointing out new features of familiar territory and blazing trails through areas of wilderness. We believe this familiarity with the mechanics of the disease lend each chapter an immediacy and relevance that will inform the reader for and serve as a map or GPS for his or her subsequent visits. The chapters themselves are deliberately succinct, a Baedeker somewhere between a gazetteer and a comprehensive travelogue, but with all the critical details that make understanding of a specific pathological mechanism possible.

This book arose from a long-running a series named "Mechanisms of Ophthalmic Disease" in the *Archives of Ophthalmology*. Similar goals to those enunciated above were followed in soliciting chapters from internationally recognized experts in specific areas of ophthalmic pathophysiology, targeted to readers of the *Archives* who had curiosity about current advances in diagnosing and treating eye disease. The concept – focused reviews by working scientists describing up-to-date research in a clinically relevant area – has been carried through to "Ocular Disease: Mechanisms and Management." The world of disease is covered from pole to pole, and the book is organized by "continent", i.e. area of disease. A short publication cycle has been used so that the information contained within is as current today as is possible with contemporary publishing technology. Critical references are at the end of each chapter, and more extensive references are available online.

We hope that this book will be as instructive for the readership as it has been for its editors and the authors in its planning and writing. Its successful production would not have been possible without the contributions of Laura Cruz, who did the administrative organizing for the authors, and the helpful involvement of the publisher, particularly Russell Gabbedy and Ben Davie.

LAL
DMA

Loss of corneal transparency

Russell L McCally

Overview

Loss or reduction in corneal transparency occurs from a variety of causes, including edema resulting from diseases such as Fuchs' dystrophy and bullous keratopathy, scarring resulting from wound healing, haze following photorefractive keratectomy, and certain metabolic diseases such as corneal macular dystrophy. The intent of this chapter is to review the present understanding of mechanisms or structural alterations that cause loss of corneal transparency. Transparency loss resulting from edema, scarring, and photorefractive keratectomy will be emphasized.

Understanding the mechanisms of transparency loss requires understanding the structural bases of corneal transparency itself. Because the cornea does not absorb light in the visible portion of the electromagnetic spectrum, its transparency is the result of minimal light scattering.[1,2] Visible light is an electromagnetic wave with wavelengths between 400 and 700 nm. Light scattering results when an incident light wave encounters fluctuations in the refractive index of a material. These fluctuations cause some of the light to be redirected from the incident direction, thus reducing the irradiance in the forward direction. The transmissivity, F_T, is defined as:

$$F_T = \frac{I(t)}{I_0} = \exp(-\alpha_{scat}t) \qquad (1)$$

where $I(t)$ is the irradiance of the light transmitted through a scattering material of thickness t (e.g., the cornea), I_0 is the irradiance of the incident light, and α_{scat} is the extinction coefficient due to scattering.[3,4] As will be shown in the remainder of this chapter, the quantity α_{scat} provides significant information on the nature of the structural features responsible for the scattering.

Collagen fibrils, which lie parallel to one another within the lamellae of the corneal stroma, have a somewhat larger refractive index than the optically homogeneous ground substance surrounding them. Thus they scatter light. In fact, because they are so numerous they would scatter approximately 60% of an incident beam of light having a wavelength of 500 nm if they were randomly arranged like gas molecules and therefore scattered independently of one another (i.e., F_T would be 0.40).[1,5] A normal cornea scatters only about 5% of 500 nm light[1]; thus transparency theories

seek to explain why the scattering is so small (Box 1.1). The key is that destructive interference among the scattered fields, which arises because the fibrils possess a certain degree of spatial ordering about one another, reduces the scattering that would otherwise occur. Indeed, Maurice's lattice theory of transparency postulated that the fibrils within the stromal lamellae are arranged in a perfect hexagonal lattice. Because their spacing (which is approximately 60 nm) is less than the wavelength of visible light, Bragg scattering cannot occur and such an arrangement leads to perfect transparency.[5] Obviously the corneal stroma is not perfectly transparent. If it were, it could not be visualized in the slit-lamp microscope. Although scattering from keratocytes could be used to explain visibility in the slit lamp, all present evidence suggests that they are not a significant source of scattering in normal cornea except under the specialized condition of specular scattering that occurs in confocal images or in the slit lamp when the incident and viewing directions are configured to make equal angles with the surface normal.[1,2,6,7] Additionally, transmission electron micrographs (TEM) of the normal stroma do not depict a perfect lattice arrangement (Figure 1.1). Thus, as described in the remainder of this section, investigators have built on the Maurice model by relaxing the condition of perfect crystalline order.

Scattering from an array of parallel cylindrical collagen fibrils is characterized by a quantity $\sigma_t(\lambda)$, called the total scattering cross-section. It is equal to $\sigma_{0t}(\lambda)\sigma_{tN}(\lambda)$, where $\sigma_{0t}(\lambda)$ is the total scattering cross-section per unit length of an isolated fibril, $\sigma_{tN}(\lambda)$ is the interference factor, and λ is the wavelength of light in the stroma.[8] The total scattering cross-section per unit length of an isolated fibril, $\sigma_{0t}(\lambda)$, depends on the fourth power of fibril radius and the ratio of the fibril index of refraction to that of its surroundings and its wavelength dependence is inverse cubic (i.e., $\sigma_{0t}(\lambda) \sim 1/\lambda^3$).[3,4] The interference factor, $\sigma_{tN}(\lambda)$, is the subject of all modern transparency theories.[5,9–12] These have been reviewed extensively elsewhere and will not be discussed in detail here.[1,2,13] The value of the interference factor varies between zero (for Maurice's perfect lattice theory) and one (for fibrils with random positions – the independent scattering result discussed above). In order to agree with experimental values of transmissivity, its value is about 0.1 at a wavelength of 500 nm (Box 1.2).

Measurements of how the total scattering cross-section depends on light wavelength can be used both to distinguish

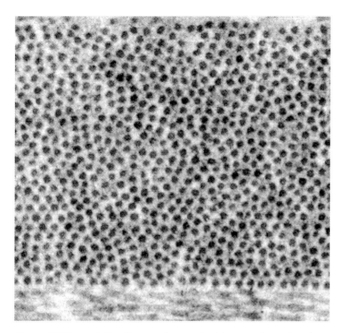

Figure 1.1 Transmission electron micrograph of the posterior region of a human cornea. The fibrils are shown in cross-section.

Box 1.1 Characteristics of light scattering in normal cornea

- The matrix of collagen fibrils is the major source of light scattering in normal cornea
- Keratocytes are not a significant source of scattering in normal cornea except under the specialized condition of specular scattering
- Measurements of how the total scattering cross-section depends on light wavelength can be used to distinguish between the various transparency theories

---

Box 1.2 Factors underlying corneal transparency

Corneal transparency is due to three major factors:[1,2,13]

- Individual fibrils are ineffective scatterers because of their small diameter and their refractive index is relatively close to the surrounding ground substance (the ratio is ~ 1.04)
- Destructive interference among the scattered fields reduces the scattering by a factor of ~10 over that which would occur if the fibrils scattered independently of one another
- The cornea is thin

Box 1.3 Factors underlying transparency loss in edematous cornea

- Edematous corneas appear cloudy due to increased light scattering
- Transmission electron micrographs of edematous corneas show mildly disordered fibrillar distributions and regions called "lakes" where fibrils are missing
- Lakes would cause large fluctuations in the refractive index, which would increase light scattering
- Lakes alter the form of the total scattering cross-section in a manner that can be tested by light-scattering measurements
- Measurements of the wavelength dependence of the total scattering cross-section are consistent with the presence of lakes, confirming that they are not fixation artifact

---

between the various transparency theories,[1,2,13] and to distinguish between types of structural alterations that reduce transparency.[14–16] The total scattering cross-section can be determined by measuring transmissivity as a function of light wavelength and noting that the extinction coefficient α_{scat} for cornea (cf., Equation 1) is given by $\rho\sigma_t(\lambda)$, where ρ is the number of fibrils per unit area in a cross-section of a corneal lamella (usually called the fibril number density). Details have been discussed elsewhere.[2,15] The results of such measurements indicate that $\rho\sigma_t(\lambda)$ (where ρ is simply a number) is proportional to $1/\lambda^3$ (i.e., the total scattering cross-section has the form A/λ^3, where A is a constant that depends on the fibril radius and the fibril refractive index

relative to that of the ground substance). Because the scattering cross-section of an isolated fibril, $\sigma_{0t}(\lambda)$, has this same dependence, the structure factor of normal corneal stroma must be essentially independent of wavelength. This is in accordance with the short-ranged order theory of Hart and Farrell,[11] which is based on the structures shown in TEM (Figure 1.1), as well as with the correlation area theory of Benedek[9] and the hard-core coating theory of Twersky.[12] It is in disagreement with theories based on long-range order in fibril positions (e.g., Feuk's disturbed lattice theory), which predict that the total scattering cross-section would vary as $1/\lambda^5$.[10]

Transparency loss from corneal edema

It has been known for well over a century that swollen corneas become cloudy, thus reducing their transparency.[17] Corneal swelling is induced by causes such as endothelial or epithelial damage, bullous keratopathy, and Fuchs' corneal dystrophy.[13,18–20] In this section, the structural alterations underlying the loss of transparency in edematous corneas are discussed (Box 1.3).

When corneas imbibe water and swell, X-ray diffraction methods show that the distance between fibrils increases, but that the fibril radii are unchanged.[21,22] Because more volume would be available per fibril, transparency loss could result from a homogeneous disruption in the short-range order in fibril positions, as proposed by Twersky.[12] Or, based on considerations discussed in the previous section, it could be the result of another mechanism that causes large-scale fluctuations in refractive index. Figure 1.2 shows a TEM of a rabbit cornea swollen to approximately 1.6 times its in vivo thickness. It shows moderately disrupted fibrillar order compared to that in normal corneas (Figure 1.1) and it also shows regions where fibrils are missing. Such regions have been observed previously in edematous corneas,[15,23,24] as well as in corneas with bullous keratopathy and in Fuchs' dystrophy corneas.[13,18] The presence of voids has also been inferred from X-ray diffraction measurement of swollen cornea.[22,25] Electron micrographs show that the voids become larger and more numerous as corneas become more swollen. Goldman et al called these regions "lakes" and suggested that they were responsible for the increased scattering because they would be expected to introduce large-scale fluctuations in the refractive index.[24] Subsequently, Benedek developed a method of explicitly accounting for the presence of lakes.[9] Benedek's lake theory was extended by Farrell et al, who showed that the presence of lakes would add a term to the total scattering cross-section that was proportional to the inverse square of the light wavelength.[15] Thus if lakes are present (and are not a preparation artifact), the total scattering cross-section would be given by:

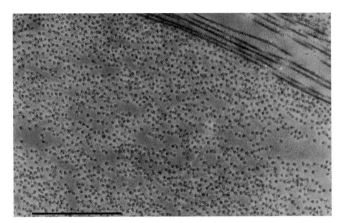

Figure 1.2 Transmission electron micrograph of the anterior region of a rabbit cornea swollen to 1.6 times its in vivo thickness. The fibrils are disordered compared to normal and there are large regions, often called lakes, where fibrils are missing. The scale bar is 1 μm.

$$\sigma_t(\lambda) = \frac{A}{\lambda^3} + \frac{B}{\lambda^2} \qquad (2)$$

where A and B are constants. The constant B depends on the sizes and number of lakes.

The result in Equation 2 allows one to test the structural basis of increased scattering in edematous corneas and to determine if features such as lakes are real or are the result of preparation artifact. If the increased scattering were due to a homogeneous disordering of fibril positions as proposed by Twersky,[12] the scattering cross-section would have the same dependence on light wavelength as normal cornea (i.e., it would have the form A/λ^3 and B would be zero). On the other hand, if lakes are an important factor causing the increased scattering, the cross-section would be given by Equation 2. Figure 1.3A shows the transmissivity of normal and cold-swollen rabbit corneas for swelling ratios up to 2.25 times normal thickness. The total scattering cross-sections obtained from these measurements using Equation 1 are shown in Figure 1.3B.[15] In the figure the cross-sections were multiplied by λ^3 in order to remove the $1/\lambda^3$ dependence of the first term in Equation 2. Thus, if lakes were present, plots of $\lambda^3\sigma_t(\lambda)$ would be straight lines of slope B. This is indeed observed. Moreover, calculations of the scattering cross-section from fibril distributions depicted in TEM of swollen corneas using the direct summation of fields (DSF) method have the same dependence on wavelength and are in close agreement with the measured scattering cross-sections.[26,27] These results suggest that lakes are an important factor causing increased scattering in edematous

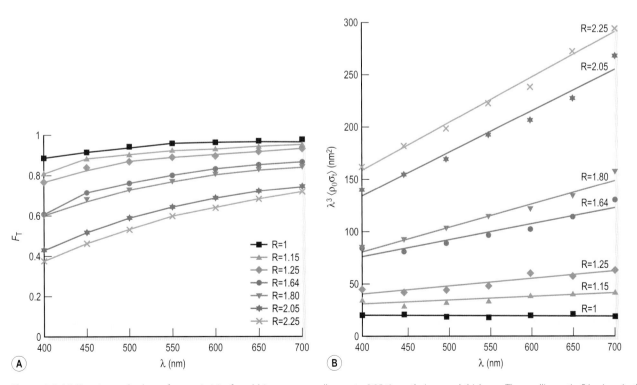

Figure 1.3 (A) Experimental values of transmissivity for rabbit corneas swollen up to 2.25 times their normal thickness. The swelling ratio R is given in the key. (B) The wavelength dependence of the total scattering cross-sections per fibril obtained from the transmissivities in (A). As discussed in McCally & Farrell,[2] the data were normalized to a standard thickness of 380 μm to account for animal-to-animal variations in corneal thickness. The data have a linear dependence on wavelength as predicted by the lake theory (i.e., they have the functional form $A + B\lambda$). The slope B increases with swelling, suggesting that lakes become larger and more numerous as the swelling increases.

corneas and that the lakes depicted in TEM of edematous corneas are not caused by preparation artifacts.

Transparency loss in scarred corneas

It is well known that linear incisions or penetrating wounds cause scarring as the corneal heals. Typically the scars are highly scattering and are often opaque. Although one can speculate on the cause or causes of the increased scattering, few studies have been conducted to determine the relative importance of various structural alterations that are observed in contributing to the increased scattering.

Farrell et al analyzed TEM taken from the literature[28] of a scar that formed from a linear incision in a human cornea.[29,30] Unlike normal cornea, where the collagen fibrils have mean diameters near 30 nm with a small standard deviation of approximately 2 nm,[31] the fibril diameters in the scar were widely distributed between 30 and 120 nm. Moreover the spatial ordering of fibrils appeared to be disrupted. Assuming the increased diameters were due to the fibrils in the scar having more collagen (and therefore the same refractive index as those in normal cornea) and not to their being hydrated, they would be expected to contribute significantly to the increased scattering. Based on considerations discussed in the first section, disruptions in fibrillar ordering would also be expected to contribute. However, an analysis using the DSF method showed that the spatial ordering is actually comparable to that in micrographs of normal human tissue.[27,29,30] It also showed that, with the variable fibril diameters, fluctuation in the area fraction occupied by fibrils is an important factor in determining the scattering. Based on several simplifying assumptions regarding the compositions of the fibrils and ground substance (viz., that they are the same as in normal cornea), the analysis showed that the enlarged fibril diameters would lead to a 200–250-fold increase in scattering.[29,30]

Charles Cintron[32-35] conducted extensive studies of corneal wounds resulting from the removal of a 2-mm diameter full-thickness button in the central cornea. These penetrating wounds ultimately healed to form an avascular network of collagen fibrils. It was first reported that the initially opaque scars became "transparent" after about a year of healing, but in subsequent investigations this was qualified to state that they became less opaque and sometimes transparent.[32]

In a recent study, penetrating wounds produced in Cintron's laboratory were allowed to heal for periods up to 4.5 years, after which they were studied using light scattering and detailed analyses of TEM (Box 1.4).[16] Figure 1.4 shows examples of these scars. An analysis of the total scattering cross-sections obtained from transmissivity measurements showed that the scars could be grouped into three categories: moderately transparent, less transparent, and nearly opaque, as indicated in the figure. Figure 1.5A shows the average transmissivities obtained by using the averages of $\rho\sigma_t(\lambda)$ that were obtained for the three scar categories. Figure 1.5B shows that $\lambda^3\rho\sigma_t(\lambda)$ depends linearly on wavelength. As discussed in the previous section, this dependence suggests that lakes are present in the fibril distribution in the scars. Moreover, the fact that the slopes become greater for the

---

> **Box 1.4 Factors underlying transparency loss in penetrating wounds**
>
> - Measurements of the wavelength dependence of the total scattering cross-section in healed penetrating corneal wounds are consistent with the presence of lakes
> - Transmission electron micrographs (TEMs) of the scars confirmed that lakes were present
> - TEM revealed some regions with ordered lamellar structures with parallel arrays of fibrils and other more prevalent regions with highly disorganized lamellar structures and with disordered fibrils
> - Quantitative analyses of the TEM showed that the increased scattering could be explained by the existence of lakes, disordered fibril distributions, and enlarged fibrils

groups having greater scattering suggests that lakes are more abundant in these scars.[16]

TEMs of the scars showed that lakes were indeed present. They also showed that there were regions with varying degrees of order, ranging from areas having a lamellar structure in which there were parallel arrays of fibrils and lakes (Figure 1.6A and B) to areas having disorganized lamellar structures in which the fibrils were highly disordered and which contained lakes and deposits of granular material (Figure 1.6C and D). The highly disorganized regions were more typical.[16] TEMs from the more ordered regions were analyzed to determine fibril positions and diameter distributions, which were then used in DSF calculations. The fibrils were larger and much more widely distributed than in normal rabbit cornea. Moreover some micrographs showed bimodal distributions of diameters. Calculated scattering was consistent with that from regions containing lakes. The values of the structure factor, $\sigma_{tN}(\lambda)$, for the three categories were respectively 0.18 ± 0.13, 0.38 ± 0.22, and 0.80 ± 0.33 compared to ~0.11 in the anterior stroma and ~0.085 in the posterior stroma of normal rabbit cornea.[16] The values of $\sigma_{tN}(\lambda)$ for the scars indicate a significant degree of fibrillar disorder that increases as the density of the scars increases. This investigation, which is the only quantitative study of scattering from scars, showed that the increased scattering could be explained by the existence of lakes, disordered fibril distributions, and enlarged fibrils. A contribution from cells could not be ruled out; however, it was noted that it was unlikely that cellular scattering would have the same dependence on wavelength as that observed for the scars.[16]

Haze following photorefractive keratectomy

Corneas frequently develop anterior light scattering that gives them a hazy appearance following photorefractive keratectomy (PRK) performed with the argon fluoride laser (Box 1.5).[36-39] In humans, haze usually peaks 2–6 months postsurgery, after which it diminishes.[38,40,41] In rabbits, it peaks 3–4 weeks postsurgery and then diminishes.[42,43] Corneas having greater corrections (i.e., deeper treatments) tend to develop higher levels of haze.[44,45] It has been suggested that patients undergoing photorefractive keratectomy

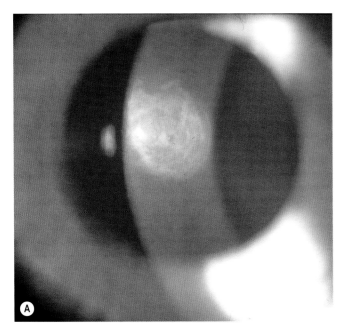

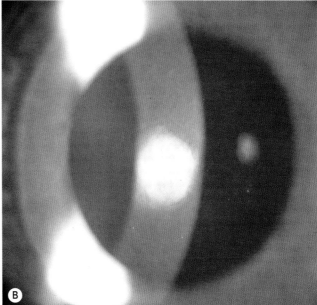

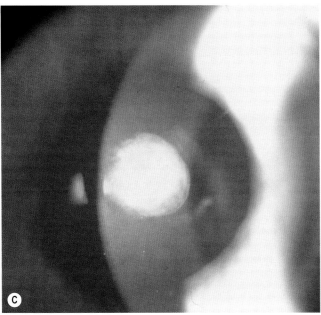

Figure 1.4 Slit-lamp photographs of scars resulting from 2-mm diameter penetrating wounds in rabbit corneas. As discussed by McCally et al,[16] the healed wounds could be grouped into three categories based on the level of light scattering (lowest, intermediate, and greatest). (A) Cornea from the lowest scattering group 4.5 years after wounding. (B) Cornea from the intermediate scattering group. This cornea is from the pair eye of that shown in (A). (C) Cornea from the highest scattering group 3.6 years after wounding. All scars show considerable variation in scattering intensity across the wound.

Box 1.5 Characteristics of PRK-induced haze

- Corneas frequently develop anterior light scattering that causes a hazy appearance following photorefractive keratectomy (PRK)
- Haze peaks 2–6 months postsurgery in humans and 3–4 weeks postsurgery in rabbits, after which it diminishes
- Objective measurements of haze showed that rabbits have two distinct haze responses following identical phototherapeutic treatments
- The cause of different haze responses is not known

can be divided into three groups: normal responders, whose initial hyperopic overcorrection regresses to normal after 6 months; inadequate responders, whose hyperopic overcorrection does not adequately regress; and aggressive responders, whose overcorrection rapidly regresses, but who develop higher levels of haze than the other groups.[36,46] A recent study done using a scatterometer to make objective measurements of haze showed that rabbits developed distinct low and high levels of haze after receiving identical phototherapeutic treatments (Figure 1.7).[42] The cause for different haze responses is not known, but several factors may be involved either individually or collectively.[42] These include: behavior

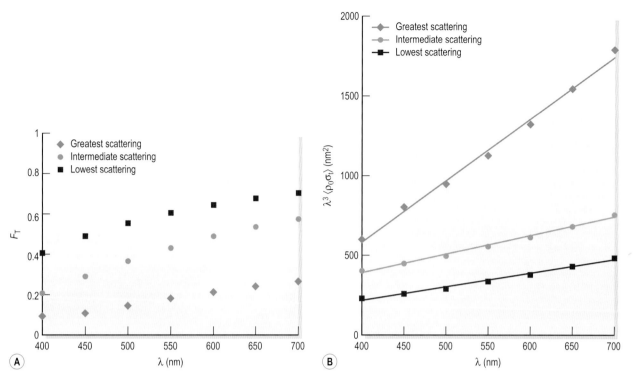

Figure 1.5 (A) Experimental values of the average transmissivity of scars resulting from 2-mm diameter penetrating wounds in rabbit corneas. As discussed by McCally et al,[16] the data were normalized to a thickness of 260 μm, which was the average thickness of the wounds. The data clearly show the distinction between the three scattering groups. (B) Wavelength dependence of the total scattering cross-sections per fibril for the three scattering categories in (A). The lines are least squares fits to a function of the form $A + B\lambda$, which suggests a strong contribution of scattering from lakes.

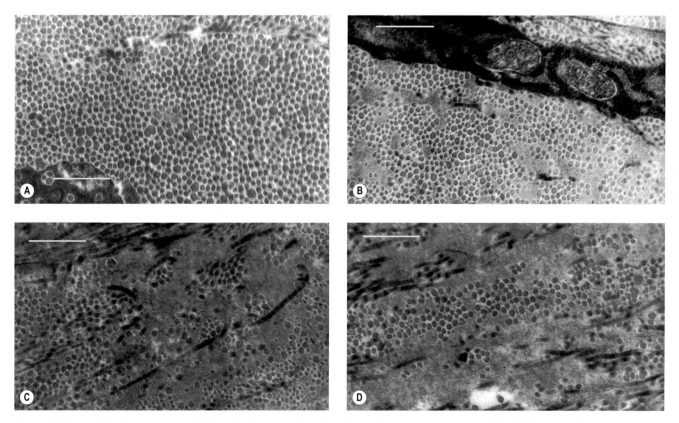

Figure 1.6 Transmission electron micrograph of regions in scars resulting from 2-mm diameter penetrating wounds in rabbit corneas. The scale bars are 500 nm. (A) A midstromal region of the scar shown in Figure 1.4b. In this region the fibrils are parallel, but have a wide distribution of diameters. There are several lakes. (B) An anterior region of the scar shown in Figure 1.4c. The fibrils are parallel in this region and they have a wide distribution of diameters. Several large lakes are present. (C) Another region in the midstroma of the scar shown in Figure 1.4b. The fibrils in this region are much less orderly than those in (A) and the lakes are much larger. (D) A posterior region of the scar shown in Figure 1.4c. The fibrils have significant disorder compared to those in (B). There are also large lakes and regions containing granular material.

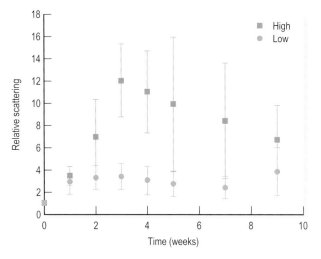

Figure 1.7 The relative scattering levels measured with a scatterometer following identical phototherapeutic treatments (6 mm diameter, 100 μm stromal depth) in rabbits. As discussed by McCally et al,[42] the mean scattering levels split into two statistically distinct groups 2 weeks after treatment and remained so up to 7 weeks (*P* < 0.005).

of the plasminogen activator-plasmin system[47–51]; variable levels of collagen IV after surgery[47–52]; rate of re-epithelialization[53–55]; keratocyte apoptosis[56–59]; and the relationship between transforming growth factor-β and myofibroblast transformation.[57,60,61]

There has been considerable speculation regarding the underlying cause(s) of haze.[1,42] Among them are: disorganized fibrillar and lamellar structures[62–66]; increased numbers of keratocytes[64,66–68]; vacuoles within and around keratocytes[64,66]; convolutions and discontinuities in the basement membrane[63,66,69]; and transforming growth factor-β-moderated transformation of keratocytes to highly reflective migrating myofibroblasts.[43,57,61,70,71]

Connon et al analyzed TEM of the anterior stroma of rabbit corneas 8 months after receiving a 100-μm deep photorefractive keratectomy treatment.[62] They used the DSF method to calculate scattering and concluded that, although the extension coefficient for scattering in the mildly disorganized regions was twice that of the untreated controls, the increase was not sufficient to explain the level of haze. However, one should exercise caution before discounting fibrillar scattering as a significant contributor to haze because the scars Connon et al analyzed had healed for 8 months, whereas haze in rabbits peaks at 3–4 weeks. It also is noteworthy that light scattered from different fibrils in disordered lamellae where the fibrils lack their normal parallel arrangement cannot interfere (and cannot be analyzed using the DSF method). Fibrils from these locations would therefore act as independent scatterers (Box 1.6).

Møller-Pederson et al investigated haze using the method of confocal microscopy through focusing (CMTF) and found that the greatly enhanced reflectivity associated with haze appeared to originate primarily from high numbers of brightly reflecting wound-healing keratocytes (myofibroblasts).[72] Moreover the appearance of myofibroblasts correlates temporally with increased haze as determined from CMTF measurements.[71,73] These observations led Møller-Pederson et al to suggest that haze is caused by the enhanced reflection from cells and not extracellular matrix deposi-

tion.[72] There is evidence that the levels of certain crystalline proteins contained within keratocytes are markedly reduced in the highly reflective wound-healing keratocytes.[74] This reduction might cause the refractive index of the wound-healing keratocytes to differ markedly from that of normal keratocytes, thus turning them into highly effective scatterers. At this time, however, not even the refractive index of normal keratocytes is known; nor is there a comprehensive theory describing cellular scattering.[7,16] Such a theory would lead to a deeper understanding of light scattering from both wounded and normal cornea and would allow one to evaluate the relative importance of fibrillar and putative cellular scattering.[16]

Summary

This chapter has dealt with the ultrastructural basis of the normal cornea's transparency and how alterations in ultrastructure or other mechanisms lead to transparency loss or opacity in edematous corneas and corneal scars, and in haze following photorefractive corneal surgery. Transparency is the result of minimal light scattering from the collagen fibrils in the corneal stroma, which occurs because the fibrils are weak scatterers, and because short-ranged correlations in their positions about one another cause sufficient destructive interference in their scattered electromagnetic fields to reduce scattering by a factor of 10 over that which would occur if they were arranged randomly. Lakes or voids in the fibril distribution, which would cause large-scale fluctuations in refractive index, were shown to be a major factor leading to transparency loss in edematous corneas. Lakes were also shown to be an important factor causing loss of transparency in scars caused by penetrating wounds; however, disordered fibril distributions and enlarged fibrils were shown to be other important factors. Several speculative causes of corneal haze were noted, including disorganized fibrillar and lamellar structures; increased numbers of keratocytes; vacuoles within and around keratocytes; convolutions and discontinuities in the basement membrane; and the transformation of keratocytes to highly reflective migrating myofibroblasts. Two of these for which some data exist, namely disorganized fibrillar structures and highly reflective myofibroblasts, were discussed. Although both may indeed be factors, it was noted that a comprehensive theory of cellular scattering will be required before their relative importance can be assessed.

Key references

A complete list of chapter references is available online at www.expertconsult.com. See inside cover for registration details.

2. McCally RL, Farrell RA. Light scattering from cornea and corneal transparency. In: Masters BR (ed.) Noninvasive Diagnostic Techniques in Ophthalmology. New York: Springer-Verlag, 1990:189–210.

5. Maurice DM. The structure and transparency of the corneal stroma. J Physiol (Lond) 1957;136:263–285.

15. Farrell RA, McCally RL, Tatham PER. Wavelength dependencies of light scattering in normal and cold swollen rabbit corneas and their structural implications. J Physiol (Lond) 1973;233:589–612.

16. McCally RL, Freund DE, Zorn A, et al. Light scattering and ultrastructure of healed penetrating corneal wounds. Invest Ophthalmol Vis Sci 2007;48:157–165.

18. Kanai A, Kaufman HE. Electron microscopic studies of swollen corneal stroma. Ann Ophthalmol 1973;5:178–190.

24. Goldman JN, Benedek GB, Dohlman CH, et al. Structural alterations affecting transparency in swollen human corneas. Invest Ophthalmol 1968;7:501–519.

31. Freund DE, McCally RL, Farrell RA, et al. Comparison of the ultrastructure in anterior and posterior stroma of normal human and rabbit corneas, and its relation to transparency. Invest Ophthalmol Vis Sci 1992;33(Suppl.):1411.

35. Cintron C, Schneider H, Kublin C. Corneal scar formation. Exp Eye Res 1973;17:251–259.

40. Lohmann CP, Garrtry DS, Muir MK, et al. Corneal haze after laser refractive surgery: objective measurements and functional implications. Eur J Ophthalmol 1991;1:173–180.

41. Møller-Pedersen T. On the structural origin of refractive instability and corneal haze after excimer laser keratectomy for myopia. Acta Ophthalmol Scand Suppl 2003;81:6–20.

42. McCally RL, Connolly PJ, Stark WJ, et al. Identical excimer laser PTK treatments in rabbits result in two distinct haze responses. Invest Ophthalmol Vis Sci 2006;47:4288–4294.

49. Csutak A, Tözsér J, Békési L, et al. Plasminogen activator activity in tears after excimer laser photorefractive keratectomy. Invest Ophthalmol Vis Sci 2000;41:3743–3747.

58. Wilson SE. Analysis of keratocyte apoptosis, keratocyte proliferation, and myofibroblast transformation responses after photorefractive keratectomy and laser in situ keratomileusis. Trans Am Ophthalmol Soc 2002;100:411–433.

72. Møller-Pederson T, Cavanagh HD, Petroll WM. Stromal wound healiing explains refractive instability and haze development after photorefractive keratectomy. Opthalmology 2000;107:1235–1245.

74. Jester JV, Møller-Pederson T, Huang J, et al. The cellular basis of corneal transparency: evidence for corneal crystallins. J Cell Sci 1999;112:612–622.

CHAPTER 2

Abnormalities of corneal wound healing

Audrey M Bernstein

Overview

The human cornea consists of an outer stratified epithelium, and an inner monolayer of epithelial cells referred to as the corneal endothelium. The middle layer, or stroma, constitutes 90% of the thickness of the cornea and is primarily a structural matrix of collagen fibrils embedded with transparent cells (keratocytes). The structural integrity of the stroma is essential for maintaining corneal shape, strength, and transparency. All of these features are attributed to the precise alignment and spacing of the stromal collagen fibrils and associated proteoglycans, which provide a clear, undistorted optical path for vision. If the cornea is damaged by trauma, surgery, or disease, a wound-healing response rapidly begins in order to prevent infection and restore vision. In other tissues it is sufficient for wounds to heal with replacement connective tissue, in which the collagen structural organization appears to be random, resulting in scarring. Since wound healing in the cornea has the additional requirement for transparency in order to maintain clear vision, precise repair of the matrix by the corneal cells must occur while maintaining the organization of the stromal connective tissue.

Stromal keratocytes (Figure 2.1) are quiescent, mesenchymal-derived cells that form a network connected by gap junctions.[1] Keratocytes appear transparent because they have a refractive index similar to that of the surrounding extracellular matrix (ECM). This has been attributed to the presence of high concentrations of soluble proteins (corneal crystallines) in the cytoplasm of the keratocytes.[2] The first step in corneal repair is apoptosis of keratocytes immediately surrounding the site of trauma. Following that, keratocytes bordering the acellular zone are activated and become visible corneal fibroblasts.[3] The fibroblasts proliferate and migrate to the margin of the wound in response to a number of growth factors and cytokines derived from the epithelial cells, the adjacent basement membrane, or tears.[4] In response to transforming growth factor-β (TGF-β) some of the fibroblasts differentiate into nonmotile myofibroblasts containing α-smooth-muscle actin (α-SMA) and large focal adhesions, which promote a strong adherence to the ECM (Figure 2.2).[5,6] After attachment, alpha-SMA stress fibers (a defining characteristic of the myofibroblast phenotype) are formed (Figure 2.3). These are required for myofibroblasts

to exert tension on the matrix and close the wound.[7] The fibroblasts and myofibroblasts secrete new ECM that initially appears opaque, resulting in a visual haze experienced by individuals during the corneal repair process.[8] If the wound heals correctly, the myofibroblasts and fibroblasts gradually disappear, leaving a properly organized, transparent network of collagen fibrils once again embedded with a quiescent network of keratocytes.[9] Conversely, if normal wound healing is compromised, for example if myofibroblasts persist or the source of the trauma remains, corneal fibrosis may develop due to the presence of excessive repair cells and consequently an excessive build-up of ECM in the stroma (Box 2.1).

Clinical manifestations of wound healing

The key sign of corneal fibrosis is the presence of haze in the cornea that impairs an individual's ability to see clearly. A variety of conditions lead to fibrosis including corneal ulcers that can result from genetic factors such as hereditary keratitis, which is passed on through autosomal dominant inheritance[10]; a secondary response to an autoimmune disease; infectious keratitis due to fungi, bacteria, or viruses; persistent inflammation; or a change in neurotrophic factor related to a decrease in corneal innervation.[11,12] If the ulcer extends into the stroma, corneal fibrosis may occur as the tissue attempts to repair the breach. Symptoms of corneal ulcers are red, watery eyes, pain, colored discharge, and light sensitivity. A deficiency in vitamin A increases the chances of developing a corneal ulcer, consistent with increased prevalence of corneal ulcers and fibrosis in developing countries.[13] Corneal ulcers are one of the leading causes of blindness in the world, estimated to account for 1.5–2 million new cases of monocular blindness per year.[14]

If a patient displays signs of corneal haze, a diagnosis of corneal fibrosis is likely. Wounds or ulcers are detected using a slit-lamp microscope in conjunction with a fluorescent dye. If detected early enough, most ulcers can be reversed before irreversible damage occurs. Advances in treating neurotrophic and autoimmune ulcers with topical nerve growth factor drops have recently been successful for previously incurable conditions.[15,16] Currently, there are no pharmaceutical solutions for fibrosis, but surgical procedures such as photothreapeutic keratectomy have proven effective in treating subepithelial corneal scars.[17] The procedure uses an excimer laser to vaporize corneal scars while minimizing damage to the surrounding tissue (Figure 2.4). If the haze is advanced enough to impair vision severely, a corneal transplant may be required. Although considered a highly successful procedure, about 15% of corneal grafts are rejected due to either a buildup of corneal edema from an immune response or a recurrence of opacification (Box 2.2).[18,19]

Clinical studies show that maintaining an intact basement membrane prevents fibrosis, presumably because it prevents epithelial–stromal cross-talk (see below).[20] For example, debridement of the corneal epithelium without removing the basement membrane leads to apoptosis of the underlying stromal keratocytes. This is followed by proliferation of neighboring keratocytes, but they remain quiescent and do not differentiate into a repair phenotype, thus maintaining corneal clarity.[21] Conversely, when the basement membrane is penetrated or removed, the epithelial cytokines

---

Box 2.1 Stages of stromal wound healing

- After wounding, transparent keratocytes differentiate into migratory fibroblasts
- Fibroblasts migrate into the wound margin
- At the wound margin fibroblasts differentiate into nonmotile, contractile myofibroblasts
- After wound closure, myofibroblasts disappear
- The persistence of myofibroblasts in a wound correlates with fibrotic healing

---

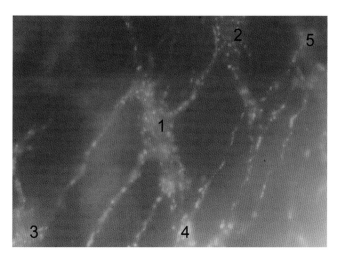

Figure 2.1 Visualization of keratocytes in the rabbit cornea. Each keratocyte (1–5) extends cytoplasmic projections that connect to other keratocytes and communicate with one another via gap junctions. Keratocytes in the rabbit cornea were viewed en face by fluorescence microscopy. The intact cornea had been incubated in phosphate-buffered saline containing acridine orange (AO). AO accumulated in acidic vesicles visualizes the keratocytes embedded in the collagen-rich matrix. (Courtesy of Dr. Sandra K. Masur.)

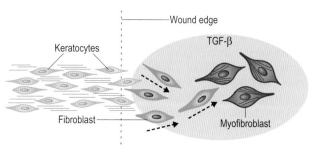

Figure 2.2 Illustration of activated keratocytes moving into the wound margin. Keratocytes bordering the acellular zone are activated to become corneal fibroblasts. The fibroblasts proliferate and migrate into the margin of the wound in response to growth factors and cytokines, which are released from the basement membrane, from the epithelium, or from tears. The presence of transforming growth factor-β (TGF-β) within the wound causes some of the fibroblasts to transform into nonmotile myofibroblasts expressing alpha-smooth-muscle actin stress fibers, which contributes to wound closure. (Redrawn from sketch courtesy of Dr. Edward Tall.)

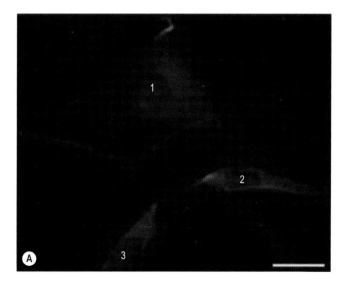
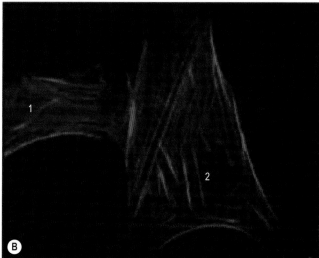

Figure 2.3 Imaging of fibroblasts and myofibroblasts in cell culture. Human corneal fibroblasts were grown for 72 hours in supplemented serum-free media (SSFM) with fibroblast growth factor-2 and heparin (fibroblasts 1–3) (A) or SSFM with transforming growth factor-β_1 (myofibroblasts 1, 2) (B). α-Smooth-muscle actin was detected by immunocytochemistry. Only the myofibroblasts have incorporated α-smooth-muscle actin into stress fibers. Bar = 40 μm.

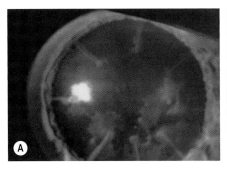
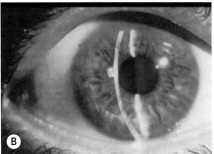

Figure 2.4 Fibrotic scar in the cornea. Significant corneal subepithelial fibrosis before excision and phototherapeutic keratectomy (PTK) in the right eye (A). The cornea was much clearer after excision and PTK (B). (From Fong YC, Chuck RS, Stark WJ, et al. Phototherapeutic keratectomy for superficial corneal fibrosis after radial keratotomy. J Cataract Refract Surg 2000;26:616–619, reproduced with permission of Elsevier Science Inc.)

Box 2.2 Basics of corneal fibrosis

- Key sign of corneal fibrosis is corneal haze
- In many cases corneal ulcers lead to corneal scarring
- Currently, no pharmaceutical intervention is available for fibrosis
- If haze is advanced enough, corneal transplant may be required

---

Box 2.3 Cytokines in stromal wound healing

- Interleukin-1 is a master regulator that stimulates keratocytes to secrete secondary cytokines
- Maintaining an intact epithelial basement membrane is the key to preventing epithelial–stromal interactions
- Transforming growth factor-β crossing the basement membrane is a primary factor in fibrotic wound healing

---

reach the stroma, leading to formation of fibroblasts and myofibroblasts and at least a temporary loss of vision due to stromal haze,[22] such as is observed after photorefractive keratectomy (PRK) to correct refractive errors.[23]

Several techniques have been developed to prevent or minimize haze. Applying an amniotic membrane to the eye after PRK has been shown to limit inflammation, apoptosis, and TGF-β effects, resulting in a decrease of postoperative haze in cases of severe fibrosis.[24] In addition, adding mitomycin C, a reagent that acts to limit cellular proliferation, after PRK for severe nearsightedness has been shown to reduce haze by limiting myofibroblast formation.[25] Conversely, in refractive surgery using laser in situ keratomileusis (LASIK), an epithelial–stromal hinged flap is cut with a microkeratome or laser and then the underlying stroma is ablated with a laser to modify corneal curvature. Because the epithelium and basement membrane are penetrated only at the edges of the flap, the stromal wound-healing response is limited and myofibroblasts have been found only at the flap margin (see below).[6]

The science of fibrosis

The immune response and angiogenesis

The cornea is considered an immune-privileged tissue.[26] Normally, few inflammatory cells are detectable in the stroma. A full-blown immune response, such as observed in the skin, would disrupt corneal transparency. Nevertheless, there are circumstances when immune cells from the surrounding limbic vessels, such as T cells and macrophages, are attracted into the stroma by the cytokines released from epithelial cells and keratocytes.[27] Severe trauma or persistent infection leading to the enhanced immunological reaction appears to coincide with the growth of new blood vessels (neovascularization) into the normally avascular cornea, consistent with the observed secretion of proangiogenic chemical mediators by the invading leukocytes.[28] Extensive

neovascularization causes severe corneal opacity, sometimes leading to blindness. In the USA, neovascularization is observed in about 1.4 million patients annually, and blinds about 7 million people worldwide.[29]

Epithelial–stromal interactions

In vascularized tissues platelets secrete many factors that recruit inflammatory cells and fibroblasts to the wound site. However, since the cornea is normally avascular, during wound repair, the source of cytokines such as interleukin-1 and TGF-β is the corneal epithelium and its basement membrane. A penetrating wound to these layers permits diffusion of released cytokines that are quickly sensed by keratocyte receptors. Interleukin-1 is a master regulator that stimulates keratocytes to secrete secondary cytokines such as hepatocyte growth factor, keratinocyte growth factor, and platelet-derived growth factor.[30] A wound that penetrates the basement membrane also permits epithelial TGF-β to diffuse into the stroma, which is considered one of the primary factors in fibrotic healing. This epithelial–stroma communication promotes the proliferation, migration, and differentiation of the underlying stromal cells and initiates a cascade of keratocyte cytokine expression (Box 2.3).[30,31]

The importance of TGF-β

Decades of research have focused on the role of TGF-β during wound healing. To date, three TGF-β isoforms have been identified. Normally in most ocular tissues TGF-β_2 is the dominantly expressed isoform.[20] Low levels of TGF-β_1 and TGF-β_2 promote fibroblast proliferation and migration but do not promote the differentiation to the myofibroblast phenotype.[32,33] Cell migration and proliferation to the wound site are critical because fibroblasts secrete matrix molecules that act as "glue" to seal the wound. When fibroblast migration is inhibited, the wound never heals properly. Fibroblasts must produce properly oriented collagen fibers to generate the transparency and strength of a properly healed wound. This process is not currently understood but is critical to regenerative healing.

After wounding, all three isoforms are expressed in the cornea.[20,34] High levels of TGF-β_1 and TGF-β_2 result in the persistence of the myofibroblast phenotype and overproduction of ECM molecules, including collagen, fibronectin, vitronectin, and their cell surface receptors (integrins).[35,36] When expression of TGF-β_1 and TGF-β_2 is exaggerated and sustained, an imbalance between: (1) proteases that degrade the matrix (metalloproteases, plasmin); (2) protease inhibitors (tissue inhibitors of metalloproteases (TIMPs) and plasminogen activator inhibitor-1 (PAI-1)); and (3) secretion of ECM components results in improper degradation and buildup of unorganized collagen fibrils. Studies show that administering a therapeutic dose of a pan-TGF-β antibody prevents myofibroblast differentiation and corneal haze after wounding,[37] but other functions of TGF-β, such as cell migration and cell proliferation into the wound margin, were also reduced.[33] Thus, targeting TGF-β signaling pathways instead of TGF-β isoforms may be a more selective approach to fighting corneal fibrosis.

TGF-β_3 appears to have a different function than that of TGF-β_1 and TGF-β_2. No fibrosis is observed during embryonic wound healing in mice before day 16, which coincides with elevated levels of TGF-β_3 and reduced expression of TGF-β_1 and TGF-β_2. However, from day 17 until birth (day 21), the formation of a scar is evident.[38] This suggests that increasing TGF-β_3 expression in a wound may be a useful approach to reducing fibrosis. Fibrotic healing probably developed as an important evolutionary adaptation to prevent infection, because a quickly healed scar, even if accompanied by a partial loss of function, yielded better chances of survival than the possible deadly consequences of infection.[38] These ideas are consistent with the observation that dermal wounds treated with TGF-β_3 have reduced scarring.[39] Thus, treating corneal wounds with TGF-β_3 may be a useful therapeutic tool. More research is needed to understand the significance of the tissue-specific and temporally regulated TGF-β isoform expression during wound healing.

Unhealed wounds

Some wounds in the cornea never heal because keratocytes do not repopulate the wound and the stroma remains hypocellular. This occurs after refractive surgery with LASIK. In the hinged flap, the majority of the epithelial–stromal interface is not disrupted. Only in the area where the laser has made the cut, around the edge of the flap, is there the potential for a fibrotic response. Consequently, since after laser ablation of the stroma the keratocytes do not proliferate and repopulate the anterior stromal tissue under the flap, there is no challenge to the transparency, there is little trauma to the corneal nerves, and millions of patients enjoy the restoration of visual acuity. However, the structural integrity of the flap is compromised because new stromal connections are not created and thus the flap never heals completely, resulting in a dramatic decrease in tensile strength.[40] For this reason, eye banks do not accept corneal donors who have had LASIK refractive surgery.[41] In vivo confocal studies have shown a progressive decrease in keratocyte density in the anterior stroma each year after treat-

Box 2.4 Consequence of unhealed wounds

- If the stromal fibroblasts do not repopulate a wound, the wound is "hypocellular" and remains unhealed
- This occurs after laser-assisted intrastromal keratoplasty (LASIK)
- Lack of healing results in a loss of tensile strength and the creation of a molecular space for fluid to accumulate
- Fluid accumulation in the cornea (interface fluid syndrome) can result in obstructed vision

ment, and after 5 years the keratocytes in the posterior stroma also begin to decrease in number.[42]

Another consequence of hypocellularity in the anterior stroma is an increase in the potential for corneal edema because the unhealed wound creates a space where fluid may accumulate.[43] This is critical because the stroma is normally maintained in a deturgescent state. Fluid is constantly removed by active transport of salt and water out of the stroma by the underlying corneal endothelial cells. Disturbed endothelial cell function and/or sustained high intraocular pressure increase the fluid load in the stroma which rapidly accumulates in the interface between the flap and ablated stromal ECM, leading to edema or interface fluid syndrome and blurry vision (Figure 2.5).[43] Endothelial cell density and function decrease with age, suggesting that post-LASIK, a rise in stromal edema due to LASIK is likely to increase (Box 2.4).

Altered corneal wound healing in diabetes mellitus

Corneal abnormalities associated with diabetes mellitus (diabetic keratopathy) occur in over 70% of diabetic patients.[44] The dramatic rise in diabetes has resulted in more research, leading to a better understanding of corneal dystrophies that arise from this disease. Many of the underlying problems in these corneas are exacerbated when surgeries to combat diabetic retinopathy are performed, thus compounding the already serious problems facing diabetic patients. The abnormalities are characterized by epithelial fragility, thickening of the basement membrane, tear dysfunction, and a slowed healing rate.[45,46] As a result, affected individuals are more prone to infectious ulcers and fibrotically healed wounds.[45,47] Although the exact mechanisms through which diabetic keratopathy affects the corneal epithelium are not fully understood, recent data suggest that abnormal levels of growth factors, glycoproteins, and proteinases are responsible for the irregular cell migration and slowed wound healing observed in patients.[48] Topical application of insulin and fibronectin in eye drops has shown promise in restoring epithelial integrity and hastening wound closure.[47,49]

Future treatments for corneal dystrophies

Gene therapy

The cornea is an obvious target for gene therapy given its immune privilege, transparency, and opportunity for

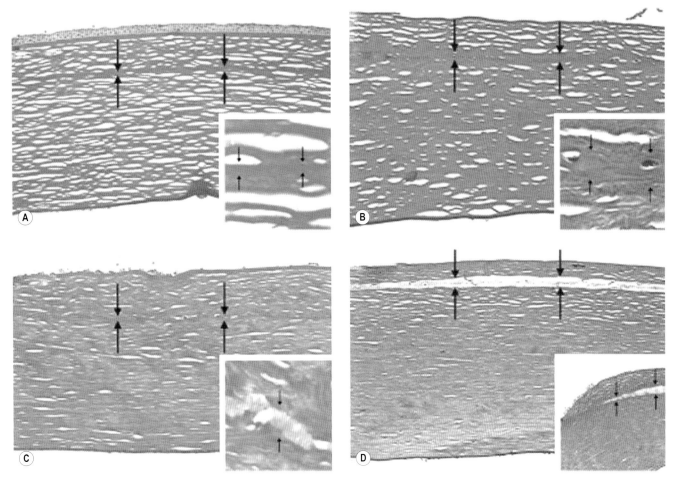

Figure 2.5 Unhealed wound. Edema in a cornea after laser in situ keratomileusis (LASIK). Representative light microscopy cross-sections of human corneoscleral specimens demonstrating findings seen at the LASIK interface wound at the end of the corneal endothelial perfusion period. (A) A normal control LASIK cornea shows a normal hypocellular primitive LASIK interface scar. (B) Mild or stage 1 interface fluid syndrome (IFS) shows mild to moderate thickening of the LASIK interface scar. (C) Moderate or stage 2 IFS shows even more thickening of the LASIK interface scar with swollen adjacent keratocytes. (D) Severe or stage 3 IFS shows a marked diffuse interface fluid pocket formation. Arrows, hypocellular primitive LASIK interface scar. Stain, periodic acid–Schiff; original magnification, ×25 insets, higher magnification views ×100 to ×400. (From Dawson DG, Schmack I, Holley GP, et al. Interface fluid syndrome in human eye bank corneas after LASIK: causes and pathogenesis. Ophthalmology 2007;114:1848–1859, reproduced with permission of Elsevier Science Inc.)

easy-access, noninvasive treatment. In treating corneal disorders, locally administered gene therapy has the potential advantage of continuously providing the necessary cytokines and growth factors to the affected area at consistently localized and safe levels. Several gene delivery methods have been tested successfully, including biological vectors such as viruses and liposomes and physical processes such as electro- and sonoporation.[50] But, despite the many studies testing its efficacy in addressing issues such as graft rejection, neovascularization, corneal haze, and herpetic keratitis, gene therapy in the cornea has produced mixed results and remains largely confined to animal studies.[50]

In vitro wound-healing models and biomimetic corneas

In vitro wound-healing models have been actively utilized to study stromal wound healing. For cell culture, human keratocytes are isolated from donated corneas. The epithe-lium and endothelium are chemically removed and the collagen is degraded, thus releasing the keratocytes,[51] which, when grown in serum, are activated and become fibroblasts. Further treatment with TGF-β_1 or TGF-β_2 stimulates the conversion of fibroblasts into myofibroblasts.[20,52] This primary cell culture model is used to study the regulation of these phenotypic variations: keratocyte, fibroblast, and myofibroblasts. A more complex model for the study of the cornea uses organ culture, in which the corneal button is mounted on an agar base and bathed in media.[53] Studies on a whole human corneal organ culture can be performed over the course of 6 weeks. Similarly, using various combinations of tethered and floating fibroblast-containing three-dimensional collagenous "gels," researchers have obtained data about cell behavior in a three-dimensional environment, including the relationship of mechanical stress (tensegrity) and ECM components to cell phenotype. Furthermore, data from these studies become the basis for building an artificial cornea (biomimetic cornea). The primary challenge to biomimetic corneas to date has been

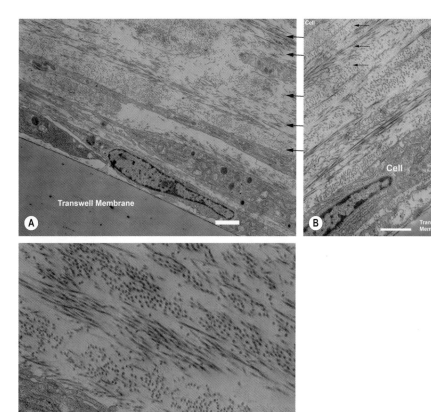

Figure 2.6 Corneal stromal construct. Transmission electron micrographs of lamellar-like architecture of the constructs. (A) Low-magnification view of the cells and synthesized arrays of fibrils. Arrows, putative "lamellae" where fibril orientation appears to change direction. Of note is the fact that the lamellae can extend over significant (tens of micrometers) distances. (B) Higher-magnification view of the organization of fibrils and their apparent change in direction within the lamellae. Again, arrows indicate the location of changes in fibril orientation. (C) High-magnification view of alternating fibril arrays in the construct. Scale bar: (A, B) 2 μm; (C) 1 μm. (From Guo X, Hutcheon AE, Melotti SA, et al. Morphologic characterization of organized extracellular matrix deposition by ascorbic acid-stimulated human corneal fibroblasts. Invest Ophthalmol Vis Sci 2007;48:4050–4060, reproduced with permission of Association for Research in Vision and Ophthalmology.)

that the tensile strength is significantly less than that of a human cornea.[54] However, recently, a transparent cornea constructed with increased strength was generated when human stromal fibroblasts were cultured in a stabilized vitamin C derivative with collagen. This protocol produced a collagen matrix composed of fibroblast-secreted factors and collagen fibrils aligned in an orthogonal array (Figure 2.6).[55] This approach is promising since this stromal construct could act as the scaffold for in vitro cultured epithelial and endothelial cells. It is likely that current advances in the identification, isolation, and in vitro growth of the corneal stem cells for each of the corneal cellular components,[56] together with a biomimetic stroma, will eventually generate a clinically viable corneal equivalent. This has the potential to reduce the need for tissue donation significantly and remove the risk of infection from donor tissue and of tissue rejection (Box 2.5).

Conclusion

To date, there are no effective pharmaceutical therapies for treating a fibrotically healed corneal scar. Thus, understanding the molecular pathways that guide corneal wound healing is critical to finding novel therapeutic strategies for combating corneal diseases and promoting regenerative repair. Current research that addresses issues of wound healing include understanding the biochemical mechanisms that control the regulation of fibroblast to myofibroblast differentiation so that the persistence of myofibroblasts in a healing wound can be modulated; understanding the signals

---

Box 2.5 Methodologies for the study of wound healing

To study wound healing in vitro:

- Cells are released from the collagenous matrix and modulated in culture
- Corneal organ culture can be sustained for 6 weeks
- Isolated fibroblasts can be embedded in a three-dimensional "gel" of different matrices
- Synthetic stroma could be used as a base to manufacture a biomimetic cornea

---

that maintain the quiescent keratocyte in hopes of dedifferentiating fibroblasts into transparent keratocytes; investigating ways to promote existing fibroblasts to migrate into an unhealed wound; and isolating new populations of stem cells that can be promoted to repopulate a wounded cornea or to populate a synthetic cornea. Understanding the molecular mechanisms of corneal wound healing is particularly exciting because the tissue is easily accessed for therapy. Molecular manipulation with new technologies may lead to prevention or cure of corneal fibrosis without surgical manipulation or transplantation.

Acknowledgments

I am grateful to Alex Imas and Ben Pedroja for their assistance in preparing this chapter.

Key references

A complete list of chapter references is available online at www.expertconsult.com. See inside cover for registration details.

3. Zieske JD, Guimaraes SR, Hutcheon AE. Kinetics of keratocyte proliferation in response to epithelial debridement. Exp Eye Res 2001;72:33–39.

4. Wilson SE, Schultz GS, Chegini N, et al. Epidermal growth factor, transforming growth factor alpha, transforming growth factor beta, acidic fibroblast growth factor, basic fibroblast growth factor, and interleukin-1 proteins in the cornea. Exp Eye Res 1994;59:63–71.

5. Jester JV, Petroll WM, Barry PA, et al. Expression of alpha-smooth muscle (alpha-SM) actin during corneal stromal wound healing. Invest Ophthalmol Vis Sci 1995;36:809–819.

7. Tomasek JJ, Gabbiani G, Hinz B, et al. Myofibroblasts and mechano-regulation of connective tissue remodelling. Nat Rev Mol Cell Biol 2002;3:349–363.

18. Kirkness CM, Ficker LA, Steele AD, et al. The success of penetrating keratoplasty for keratoconus. Eye 1990;4:673–688.

20. Stramer BM, Zieske JD, Jung JC, et al. Molecular mechanisms controlling the fibrotic repair phenotype in cornea: implications for surgical outcomes. Invest Ophthalmol Vis Sci 2003;44: 4237–4246.

21. Wilson SE, He YG, Weng J, et al. Epithelial injury induces keratocyte apoptosis: hypothesized role for the interleukin-1 system in the modulation of corneal tissue organization and wound healing. Exp Eye Res 1996;62:325–327.

22. Møller-Pedersen T. Keratocyte reflectivity and corneal haze. Exp Eye Res 2004;78: 553–560.

36. Fini ME, Stramer BM. How the cornea heals: cornea-specific repair mechanisms affecting surgical outcomes. Cornea 2005;24(Suppl.):S2–S11.

37. Møller-Pedersen T, Cavanagh HD, Petroll WM, et al. Neutralizing antibody to TGFbeta modulates stromal fibrosis but not regression of photoablative effect following PRK. Curr Eye Res 1998;17: 736–747.

40. Schmack I, Dawson DG, McCarey BE, et al. Cohesive tensile strength of human LASIK wounds with histologic, ultrastructural, and clinical correlations. J Refract Surg 2005;21:433–445.

43. Dawson DG, Schmack I, Holley GP, et al. Interface fluid syndrome in human eye bank corneas after LASIK: causes and pathogenesis. Ophthalmology 2007;114:1848–1859.

CHAPTER 3

Wound healing after laser in situ keratomileusis and photorefractive keratectomy

Fabricio Witzel de Medeiros and Steven E Wilson

Clinical background

The safety and predictability of laser in situ keratomileusis (LASIK) and photorefractive keratectomy (PRK) have improved since these procedures were introduced, but the corneal wound-healing response remains a major contributor to variability of results following these procedures. Corneal wound healing entails the complex interactions of different cellular types, including corneal epithelial cells, keratocytes, and, possibly, endothelial cells, in addition to corneal fibroblasts, myofibroblasts, inflammatory cells, lacrimal gland cells, and others. In large part, this communication is mediated by soluble growth factors, cytokines, and chemokines via membrane-bound and soluble receptors.[1,2]

The unwounded adult cornea is a transparent and avascular structure, providing not only the major refractive surface involved in visual image transmission, but also a protective barrier against external injuries, including microbial infections that are potentially vision-threatening. Activation of these systems during refractive surgery can result in the deposition of opaque fibrotic repair tissue and, possibly, scarring. In order to understand and control these complex interactions better and improve the results and safety of LASIK and PRK, it is important to have a basic understanding of normal and abnormal corneal wound-healing responses. This chapter provides a framework that will allow the clinician not only to understand these interactions, but also at least partially to control them through surgical technique and rational application of medications.

Pathophysiology and pathology

The normal wound-healing response

Corneal stromal fibrils and other matrix components are precisely organized to provide transparency essential to corneal function. However, cellular repair processes during corneal healing can disturb this architecture and lead to visual impairment. The corneal wound-healing response involves a complicated balance of cellular changes, including cell death (apoptosis and necrosis), cell proliferation, cell motility, cell differentiation, expression of cytokines, growth factors, chemokines and their receptors, influx of inflammatory cells, and production of matrix materials (Box 3.1). In large part, communications between corneal cells, nerves, inflammatory cells, bone marrow-derived cells, and other cells are the critical determinants of normal and abnormal corneal wound-healing responses. Although many of these interactions occur simultaneously, for discussion purposes it is convenient to describe the wound-healing response as a pathway, similar to glycolysis or the Kreb's cycle.

Corneal epithelial injury is a common initiator of the corneal wound-healing response to refractive surgical procedures, as well as in trauma and some diseases. Here we will concern ourselves only with surgical injury associated with LASIK and PRK. Corneal epithelial injury triggers the release of a variety of cytokines, such as interleukin-1 (IL-1)-α and -β, transforming growth factor (TGF)-β, tumor necrosis factor (TNF)-α, platelet-derived growth factor (PDGF), and epithelial growth factor (EGF), that regulate keratocyte apoptosis, proliferation, motility, differentiation, and other functions during the minutes to months after surgical insult.[1,2] In turn, once stimulated by these epithelial-derived soluble factors via membrane-bound receptors, keratocytes not only alter cellular functions, but also produce other soluble modulators that regulate corneal epithelial proliferation and migration (hepatocyte growth factor (HGF) and keratinocyte growth factor (KGF)), attract inflammatory cells (granulocyte chemotactic and stimulating factor (G-CSF), monocyte chemotactic and activating factor (MCAF), neutrophil-activating peptide (ENA-78)), and other corneal changes.[3-7] Collagenases, metalloproteinases, and other enzymes are activated and released in the stroma during the wound-healing response and function to degrade, remove, and regenerate damaged tissue.[8] The expression of these collagenases and metalloproteinases by keratocytes and corneal fibroblasts is also regulated by IL-1 and fibroblast growth factor-2 derived from the injured corneal epithelial cells.[9]

A recurring theme that must be appreciated to understand corneal wound healing is ongoing communication between epithelial cells and stromal cells mediated by soluble cytokines and chemokines. These interactions occur immediately after injury and continue for weeks, months, or occasionally even years, for example with persistence of haze following PRK.

Many growth factors released during the corneal wound-healing response can be derived from more than one cell type and regulate more than one process. EGF can be used to illustrate this principle. EGF is produced by epithelial cells, keratocytes, corneal fibroblasts, lacrimal cells, and, possibly, other cells. EGF regulates corneal epithelial cell proliferation, motility, and differentiation.[1,2] EGF also triggers the formation of new hemidemosomes on epithelial cells after injury.[6,7,10] EGF also has influence on the proliferation of limbal cells that migrate toward the injury site to seal the wound and to reform a normal stratified epithelial layer.[11,12] In addition, different growth factors may regulate a single function. For example, EGF, HGF, and KGF all regulate corneal epithelial proliferation.[1,2] The effect that predominates at a particular point in the wound-healing response likely depends on factors such as receptor expression, cellular localization, cellular differentiation, and the influences of interacting networks of soluble and intracellular factors.

Box 3.1 Key processes in the corneal wound-healing response

- Epithelial injury
- Stromal cell death (apoptosis and necrosis)
- Influx of inflammatory cells
- Cell proliferation
- Cell motility
- Cell differentiation
- Release of cytokines, growth factors, chemokines, and expression of their receptors
- Production of extracellular matrix materials
- Epithelium healing

Epithelial injury is typically the initiator of the wound-healing response associated with corneal surgery or injury. For example, epithelial scrape or epithelial ethanol exposure associated with PRK or laser epithelial keratomileusis (LASEK), respectively, epithelial blade penetration associated with Epi-LASEK or LASIK are initiators of corneal wound healing that result in the release of IL-1α, IL-1β, TNF-α, and a host of other modulators that alter the functions of keratocytes, inflammatory cells, and the epithelial cells themselves. Similarly, damage to the epithelium at the edge of the flap in femtosecond LASIK flap formation triggers the wound-healing cascades, although the femtosecond laser has direct stromal necrotic effects that influence the overall wound-healing response of surgery performed with this procedure,[13] as will be covered later.

Apoptosis and necrosis in initiation, modulation, and termination of wound healing (Box 3.2)

The first stromal change that is noted following epithelial injury is apoptosis of the underlying keratocyte cells (Figure 3.1). Apoptosis, or programmed cell death, is a gentle, regulated form of cell death that occurs with the release of only limited intracellular components such as lysosomal enzymes that would potentially damage surrounding tissue.[14] Keratocytes undergoing apoptosis are found to have chromatin

---

Box 3.2 Apoptosis and necrosis in initiation, modulation, and termination of wound healing

- Apoptosis of the underlying keratocyte cells
- Modulation by eliminating excess inflammatory, fibroblast, and other cells
- Elimination of myofibroblasts

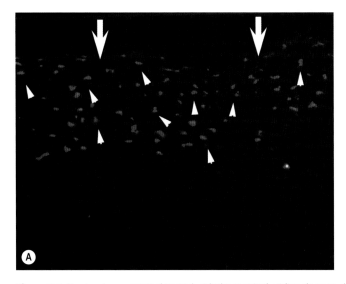
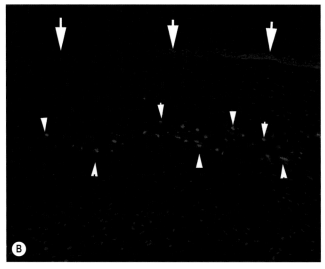

Figure 3.1 Keratocyte apoptosis detected with the terminal uridine deoxynucleotidyl transferase dUTP nick end labeling (TUNEL) assay at 4 hours after photorefractive keratectomy (PRK) or laser in situ keratomileusis (LASIK). Note that after PRK (A, 600× magnification) keratocytes undergoing apoptosis (arrowheads) are located in the anterior stroma. Arrows in (A) indicate the anterior stromal surface. After LASIK (B, 200× magnification) keratocytes undergoing apoptosis (arrowheads) are localized in the deeper stroma anterior and posterior to the lamellar cut. The epithelium in (B) is indicated by arrows.

condensation, DNA fragmentation, cell shrinkage, and formation of membrane-bound vesicles called apoptotic bodies that contain intracellular contents. The localization of the apoptosis response is related to the type of injury, and in large part determines the localization of the subsequent wound-healing events. For example, in PRK, LASEK, and Epi-LASEK, keratocyte apoptosis occurs in the anterior stroma beneath the site of epithelial injury (Figure 3.1A). In contrast, keratocyte apoptosis associated with microkeratome LASIK occurs at the site of blade penetration at the edge of the flap and along the lamellar cut in the central stroma (Figure 3.1B).

The apoptosis process is likely regulated by soluble cytokines such as IL-1 and TNF-α released from injured epithelial cells and the Fas-Fas ligand system expressed in keratocytes.[1,2] Apoptosis is an extremely rare event in unwounded normal cornea. Once an injury to the epithelium occurs, however, keratocytes undergoing apoptosis can be detected within moments.[14,15] This early wave of relatively pure apoptosis makes a transition into a later phase in which both apoptosis and necrosis occur in many stromal cells, including keratocytes, corneal fibroblasts, and invading inflammatory cells. Although all of these cells are typically labeled with the terminal uridine deoxynucleotidyl transferase dUTP nick end labeling (TUNEL) assay, careful analysis with transmission electron microscopy demonstrates that cellular necrosis, a more random death associated with release of intracellular enzymes and other components, also makes a major contribution.[15] It is unknown whether necrosis that occurs during corneal wound healing is a regulated event or merely a result of cells being killed by inflammation or other contributors to healing. A much later low-level phase of apoptosis occurring in myofibroblasts is also noted in corneas that develop haze.

Precise regulation of the apoptosis processes that occur during corneal wound healing implies an important function besides a merely reactionary response to the injury.[16] Studies have suggested that the earliest apoptosis response is likely a defense mechanism designed to limit the extension of viral pathogens, such as herpes simplex and adenovirus, into the stroma and eye after initial infection of the corneal epithelium.[17] The second phase of stromal apoptosis extending from hours to a week after injury likely functions to modulate the corneal wound-healing response by eliminating excess inflammatory, fibroblast, and other cells. The latest phase of stromal apoptosis that occurs in corneas with haze serves to rid the stroma of myofibroblasts that are no longer needed.[17]

Mitosis and migration of stromal cells

Mitosis and migration of stromal cells are noted approximately 8–12 hours after the initial corneal injury.[13] Initially, most cells undergoing mitosis appear to be keratocytes, but corneal fibroblasts and other cells may make subsequent contributions to this response. This cellular mitosis response provides corneal fibroblasts and other cells that participate in corneal wound healing and replenish the stroma. Once again, localization of the stromal mitosis response is related to the type of injury. Thus, in PRK stromal mitosis tends to occur in the anterior stroma, as well as in the peripheral and posterior stroma outside the zone of apoptosis (Figure 3.2).

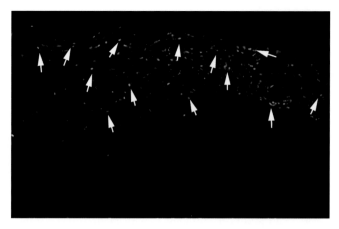

Figure 3.2 Stromal cell mitosis at 24 hours after photorefractive keratectomy. Arrows indicate cells in the stroma that stain for Ki-67, a marker for mitosis. Blue is the 4′,6-diamidino-2-phenylindole (DAPI) stain for the nucleus that stains all cells. 500× magnification.

In LASIK, stromal mitosis occurs at the periphery of the flap where the epithelium was injured, and anterior and posterior to the lamellar cut.

Mitosis and migration of stromal cells are regulated by cytokines released from the epithelium and its basement membrane. For example, PDGF is produced by corneal epithelium and bound to basement membrane due to heparin-binding properties of the cytokine. It is released from the epithelial basement membrane after injury and stimulates mitosis of corneal fibroblasts. It is also highly chemotactic to corneal fibroblasts, tending to attract them to the source of the cytokine. Thus, in PRK, for example, PDGF released from the injured epithelium and basement membrane stimulates surviving keratocytes in the peripheral and posterior stroma to undergo mitosis and the daughter cells are attracted to the ongoing PDGF release and repopulate the anterior stroma. Other cytokines such as TGF-β also likely contribute to this keratocyte/corneal fibroblast mitosis and migration.[2]

Corneal fibroblasts derived from keratocytes produce collagen, glycosaminoglycans, collagenases, gelatinases, and metalloproteinases[18] used to restore corneal stromal integrity and function. These cells also produce cytokines such as EGF, HGF, and KGF that direct mitosis, migration, and differentiation of the overlying healing epithelium.[1,2,19] After total epithelialization, the fibronectin clot disappears and the nonkeratinized stratified epithelium is re-established.[11,12,20–22]

Inflammatory cell influx (Box 3.3)

Beginning approximately 8–12 hours after the initial epithelial injury, and lasting for several days, a wave of inflammatory cells migrates into the cornea (Figure 3.3) from the limbal blood vessels and tear film.[23,24] These cells function to clear cellular and other debris from the injury and to respond to pathogens that could be associated with injuries such as viral or bacterial infections.

The inflammatory cells that sweep into the cornea are chemotactically attracted into the stroma by cytokines and chemokines released directly by the injured epithelium and induced in keratocytes and corneal fibroblasts by cytokines

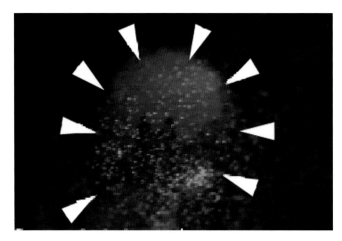

Figure 3.3 At 24 hours after epithelial scrape, as performed in photorefractive keratectomy, thousands of bone marrow-derived cells invade the cornea in a chimeric mouse with fluorescent green protein-labeled, bone marrow-derived cells. Magnification 10×.

Box 3.4 Completion of healing response

- Elimination of excess cells by apoptosis and necrosis
- Replenishment by mitosis and migration of keratocytes
- Healing time in 1–2 weeks of epithelium re-established
- Perform enhancement procedures after refractive stability

Box 3.5 Altered healing in corneas that develop haze

- Development of haze in the cornea correlates with the appearance of myofibroblast cells
- Sustained exposure of transforming growth factor-β, and possibly other cytokines required for development and persistence of myofibroblasts
- Defective regeneration of the basement membrane commonly associated with surface irregularity, possibly genetic influences, and other factors

---

Box 3.3 Inflammatory cell influx

- Inflammatory cell migration
- Clear cellular and other debris
- Varies with type of injury

released from the epithelium. IL-1 appears to be the master regulator of this response since corneal fibroblasts produce dozens of proinflammatory chemokines in response to IL-1 binding to IL-1 receptors on the stromal cells.[23]

The pattern of entry of the inflammatory cells into the central cornea may differ depending on the type of injury. In PRK and other surface ablation procedures the cells tend to be fairly equally distributed across the anterior to mid stroma. In LASIK, however, many of the cells enter along the lamellar cut since this is the path of least resistance. In the LASIK procedure, augmented release of epithelial IL-1, for example, with epithelial slough caused by a microkeratome, triggers massive influx of cells along the lamellar cut and produces the disorder diffuse lamellar keratitis.[25] Since the potential space produced by the lamellar cut persists for years following LASIK, epithelial trauma even many years later may precipitate diffuse lamellar keratitis.

Completion of the healing response (Box 3.4)

As the corneal wound-healing response is completed, excess cells are eliminated by apoptosis and necrosis, and the keratocyte cells that were lost are replenished by mitosis and migration of keratocytes that did not undergo apoptosis. In the normal cornea that does not develop haze, most of these stromal processes appear to be completed within 1–2 weeks after injury, as long as the integrity of the epithelium is re-established. In eyes with persistent epithelial defects, cytokine triggers from the epithelium continue, along with stromal apoptosis, necrosis, and mitosis, eventually leading to destruction of the stroma and perforation if the epithelium does not heal.

In corneas where the epithelium heals normally, there may be persistent epithelial hyperplasia and/or hypertrophy that may mask the full refractive correction.[15] Thus, a cornea that appears to be undercorrected after PRK or LASIK for myopia may have a portion of the attempted correction masked by a temporary thickening of the epithelium. At the molecular level, this could result from excess penetration and binding of EGF, HGF, KGF, and other cytokines to the epithelial receptors. The higher levels of epithelium-modulating cytokines are likely derived from fibroblasts "activated" during the wound-healing response in the stroma. Once the wound-healing response subsides and the stromal cells return to their normal metabolic activity, the levels of these cytokines diminish and the epithelial architecture is restored. This points out the importance of waiting to perform enhancement procedures until there is refractive stability. The length of time required likely varies with the individual patient.

Etiology and treatment of wound healing-associated corneal abnormalities

Altered healing in corneas that develop haze (Box 3.5)

After surface ablation, including PRK, LASEK, and Epi-LASEK, depending on the level of attempted correction, a proportion of corneas develop trace to severe stromal opacity, termed haze.[26,27] The higher the attempted correction, the greater the percentage of corneas that develop haze and the greater the incidence of severe haze associated with regression of the refractive correction and decreased vision (Figure 3.4A). Rarely, central haze can also occur in LASIK, typically associated with severe diffuse lamellar keratitis, buttonhole, or other abnormal flaps. Marginal haze at the flap margin, where the microkeratome or femtosecond laser penetrated the epithelium, is common.

The development of haze in the cornea correlates with the appearance of myofibroblast cells in the anterior stroma (Figure 3.4B) beneath the epithelial basement membrane.[15]

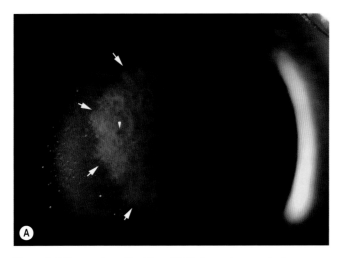 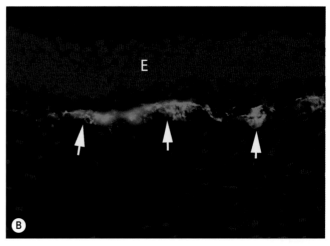

Figure 3.4 Haze and myofibroblasts. (A) Slit-lamp photograph of severe corneal haze in an eye that had photorefractive keratectomy (PRK) for −9 D of myopia at 12 months after surgery. Arrows indicate the border of haze at the edge of the ablation. Small arrowhead indicates an area of early clearing of haze, termed a lacuna. (B) In a rabbit eye that had PRK for −9 D of myopia there are large numbers of myofibroblasts (arrows) that stain green for α-smooth-muscle actin. The myofibroblasts are located immediately beneath the epithelium (E). Magnification 600×.

Myofibroblasts are themselves opaque, due to diminished production of corneal crystallins.[28–30] In addition, these cells are active factories that produce collagen and other matrix materials that do not have the normal organization associated with corneal stromal transparency.

The earliest appearance of myofibroblasts after PRK, detected with the α-smooth muscle actin marker, is noted approximately 1 week after surgery.[15,31] Sustained exposure to TGF-β, and possibly other cytokines, derived primarily from the epithelium, is required for development and persistence of myofibroblasts.[15,31–33] If the basement membrane of the healing epithelium is regenerated with normal structure and function, penetration of TGF-β into the stroma is limited and only small numbers of myofibroblasts are generated and persist.[31] Defective regeneration of the basement membrane, however, commonly associated with surface irregularity, possibly genetic influences, and other factors, leads to ongoing penetration of TGF-β and development of large numbers of persistent myofibroblasts and haze, typically immediately below the epithelium.[31]

The identity of the progenitor cell(s) for the myofibroblast in the corneal stroma remains uncertain. Myofibroblasts can be generated from corneal fibroblasts in vitro under proper culture conditions, including availability of TGF-β.[18,32,33] However, in other tissues, myofibroblasts have also been shown to develop from bone marrow-derived cells.[34,35] A dual origin for myofibroblasts could provide an explanation for haze being corticosteroid-responsive in some corneas and corticosteroid-unresponsive in others.

Haze typically persists for 1–2 years after surgery and then slowly disappears over a period of months or years. This time course, however, may be significantly prolonged in corneas treated with mitomycin C, which subsequently develop "breakthrough haze." When haze finally disappears, it is likely that the slow repair of the epithelial basement membrane, and restoration of basement membrane barrier function, eventually results in diminished penetration of TGF-β into the stroma to a level insufficient to maintain myofibroblast viability, and the cells undergo apoptosis.[31] This is followed by reabsorption and/or reorganization of

myofibroblast-produced collagens and other matrix materials by keratocytes. Thus, there is a slow restoration of stromal transparency.

Mitomycin C treatment to prevent haze

Mitomycin C is a chemotherapeutic agent with cytostatic effects that is applied topically to the stromal surface to prevent haze after PRK. Mitomycin C blocks RNA/DNA production and protein synthesis. This results in inhibition of the cell proliferation, and presumably reduces the formation of progenitor cells to myofibroblasts.[36] The resulting effect in diminishing haze has been confirmed in clinical studies.[37] Although mitomycin C at the lower concentrations of 0.002% decreases haze formation in animal studies,[36] there tends to be a higher incidence of "breakthrough haze" and, therefore, the higher concentration of 0.02% for 30–60 seconds has once again become the most commonly used.

Some surgeons restrict mitomycin C use to corrections greater than 5–6 D of myopia. Although rare, haze is seen in lower corrections that are not treated with mitomycin C. In addition, most refractive surgeons use mitomycin C for any eye that has PRK after previous surgery, including PRK, LASIK, radial keratotomy, and corneal transplantation.

Corneas treated with mitomycin C have a lower anterior stromal keratocyte density than corneas that are not treated with mitomycin C.[36] This effect persists for at least 6 months after treatment in animal models. It is not known whether there will be long-term effects from diminished keratocyte maintenance of the stroma decades after surgery.

Altered wound healing in femtosecond LASIK

Recent studies have demonstrated that the femtosecond laser directly triggers necrosis of keratocytes anterior and posterior to the lamellar cut.[13] This results in greater inflammatory cell infiltration into the stroma during the early wound-healing response and, therefore, greater inflammation. Stromal necrosis is proportional to the amount of femtosecond laser energy used to generate the cut, especially with earlier models

Box 3.6 Nerves and corneal wound-healing response

- Damage to corneal nerves diminishes epithelial viability
- Neurotrophic factors needed for epithelial homeostasis
- Laser-induced neurotrophic epitheliopathy continues until nerves regenerate into the flap
- Photorefractive keratectomy damage to nerve terminals resolves more quickly than laser-assisted intrastromal keratoplasty (LASIK)
- Ciclosporin A may be of benefit

of the femtosecond laser, such as the 15 kHz Intralase (Irvine, CA). This effect is diminished with more recent models, including the 30 kHz and 60 kHz Intralase models. However, even with these more efficient lasers, it is prudent to use the minimum energy level that yields a flap that is easy to lift. In our experience, 1.0 µJ settings with the 60 kHz Intralase for both the lamellar and side cuts yield similar inflammation to LASIK performed with a microkeratome.

Nerves and the corneal wound-healing response (Box 3.6)

Disorders that damage the corneal nerves may diminish corneal epithelial viability and lead to neurotrophic ulceration. Corneal nerves have important influences on corneal epithelial homeostasis through the effects of neurotrophic factors like nerve growth factor and substance P. These neurotrophic factors have been shown to accelerate epithelial healing in vivo.[38] After LASIK corneas often develop a neurotrophic epitheliopathy characterized by punctate epithelial erosions on the flap with only marginal decreases in tear production.[39] This condition has been termed LASIK-induced neurotrophic epitheliopathy (LINE).[39] The condition typically presents from 1 day to 1 month following LASIK and

continues for 6–8 months, until the nerves regenerate into the flap. Many patients who develop severe LINE probably have an underlying tendency towards chronic dry eye and often benefit from treatment with topical ciclosporin. In our experience, LINE is less common and less severe after femtosecond LASIK with 100-µm thick flaps, presumably because thinner flaps result in less corneal nerve damage (Medeiros and Wilson, unpublished data, 2007).

PRK also damages the corneal nerve terminals. Neurotrophic epithelial after PRK may occasionally be problematic, but tends to resolve more quickly than after LASIK. Topical ciclosporin A may also be of benefit in these patients.

Conclusions

The corneal wound-healing response, and the complex cellular interactions associated with it, are major determinates of the response of corneas to surgical procedures, including LASIK and PRK. An understanding of these interactions is important to optimize surgical outcomes and limit complications.

Acknowledgment

This work was supported in part by US Public Health Service grants EY10056 and EY15638 from National Eye Institute, National Institutes of Health, Bethesda, Maryland and Research to Prevent Blindness, New York, NY. Dr. Wilson is the recipient of a Research to Prevent Blindness Physician-Scientist Award.

Declaration of interest
Dr. Medeiros has no proprietary or financial interest in any materials or methods described in this chapter. Dr. Wilson is a consultant to Allergan, Irvine, CA.

Key references

A complete list of chapter references is available online at www.expertconsult.com. See inside cover for registration details.

1. Wilson SE, Liu JJ, Mohan RR. Stromal–epithelium interactions in the cornea. Prog Retin Eye Res 1999;18:293–309.
14. Wilson SE, He Y-G, Weng J, et al. Epithelial injury induces keratocyte apoptosis: hypothesized role for the interleukin-1 system in the modulation of corneal tissue organization and wound healing. Exp Eye Res 1996;62:325–328.
15. Mohan RR, Hutcheon AE, Choi R, et al. Apoptosis, necrosis, proliferation, and myofibroblast generation in the stroma following LASIK and PRK. Exp Eye Res 2003;76:71–87.
18. Funderburgh JL, Mann MM, Funderburgh ML. Keratocyte phenotype mediates

proteoglycan structure: a role for fibroblasts in corneal fibrosis. J Biol Chem 2003;278:45629–45637.
28. Jester JV, Møller-Pedersen T, Huang J, et al. The cellular basis of corneal transparency: evidence for 'corneal crystallins'. J Cell Sci 1999;112:613–622.
31. Netto MV, Mohan RR, Sinha S, et al. Stromal haze, myofibroblasts, and surface irregularity after PRK. Exp Eye Res 2006;82:788–797.
32. Jester JV, Petroll WM, Cavanagh HD. Corneal stromal wound healing in refractive surgery: the role of myofibroblasts. Prog Retin Eye Res 1999;18:311–356.

33. Mansur SK, Dewal HS, Dinh TT, et al. Myofibroblasts differentiate from fibroblasts when plated at low density. Proc Natl Acad Sci USA 1996;93:4219–4223.
36. Netto MV, Mohan RR, Sinha S, et al. Effect of prophylactic and therapeutic mitomycin C on corneal apoptosis, cellular proliferation, haze, and long-term keratocyte density in rabbits. J Refract Surg 2006;22:562–574.
39. Wilson SE. Laser in situ keratomileusis-induced (presumed) neurotrophic epitheliopathy. Ophthalmology 2001;108:1082–1087.

CHAPTER 4

Genetics and mechanisms of hereditary corneal dystrophies

John D Gottsch

Overview

Over the past century, a number of corneal diseases have been documented with detailed family histories suggesting autosomal-dominant, autosomal-recessive, and X-linked recessive hereditary patterns. Modern genetic techniques such as whole-genome linkage analysis and gene sequencing have led to the discovery of specific gene mutations (genotypes) which correlate with specific disease presentations of clinical signs (phenotypes). For many of these clearly defined hereditary corneal dystrophies, the discovery of the underlying genetic mechanism has led to an understanding at the molecular level of the disease pathophysiology.

The hereditary corneal dystrophies subsequently described are, in order of the primary corneal layer most affected, epithelium, Bowman layer, stroma, Descemet's membrane, and endothelium. Fuchs' dystrophy is covered in another chapter. Some designations of the hereditary corneal dystrophies have recently been changed because of new histopathologic and genetic data suggesting distinct disease categories, such as corneal dystrophies of the Bowman layer type I and II, and this has clarified the differences between Reis–Bücklers and Thiel–Behnke dystrophies. Some dystrophies appear to have the same gene involved with slight differences in the clinical presentation. These similar hereditary corneal dystrophies have been grouped together with a mention of the historical reporting and similarities in clinical presentations, such as with Meesmann's and Stocker–Holt dystrophies. Gene names are italicized. Where mutations are known to be causative of certain hereditary corneal dystrophies and result in amino acid changes at particular codons, the substitution of the wild type for the mutant amino acid will be given in full. In subsequent references, the mutation will be given as standard abbreviated designations. As an example, in the 124 codon of keratoepithelin (KE), a cysteine is substituted for arginine in lattice corneal dystrophy I (LCDI). Thereafter this mutation would be referred to as Arg124Cys.

Epithelial dystrophies

Meesmann corneal dystrophy (MCD) MIM 122100 (Stocker–Holt dystrophy)

Clinical background

MCD is characterized by numerous epithelial microcysts which can be noted in early childhood.[1] The discrete, round cysts usually become more numerous with age. If in later years the microcysts erode the surface, affected individuals can become symptomatic with foreign-body sensation, photophobia, and decreased vision. Pameijer[2] made the first clinical description of the disease in 1935, with Meesmann and Wilke[3] describing the histologic features in 1939. In 1964, Kuwabara and Ciccarelli[1] found aggregates of electron-dense material in corneal epithelial sheets studied by electron microscopy, termed "peculiar substance." Stocker and Holt[4] in 1955 reported families from Moravia who had microcysts apparent early in life, leading to decrease in vision, light sensitivity, and tearing. Irvine et al[5,6] in 1997 reported mutations in the KRT3 and KRT12 genes cause MCD. Klintworth et al[7] later identified a mutation in the KRT12 gene in a family with microcysts described by Stocker and Holt.

Pathology

Epithelial cells contain an intermediate filament cytoskeleton which protects against trauma. Keratins are expressed in pairs and keratin 3 and 12 are produced in the corneal anterior epithelium. Aggregation of the abnormal keratins occurs within the epithelium, resulting in microcysts. Environmental factors, such as wearing contact lenses, may contribute to epithelial fragility, worsening the disease and contributing to symptoms.

Pathophysiology

Mutations in keratin KRT3 and KRT12 genes have been demonstrated to be causative of MCD.[5,6,8,9] Mutations have been reported as missense substitutions in the conserved helix initiation motif of KRT12 or in the helix termination

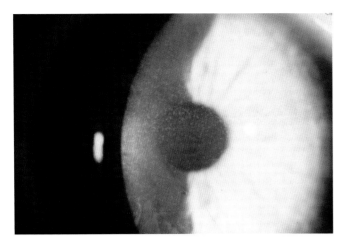

Figure 4.1 Meesmann corneal dystrophy: microcysts representing aggregation of abnormal keratins.

motifs in *KRT12* and *KRT3*. These motifs are involved in the assembly of intermediate filaments. Mutations which occur in the helix boundary motifs of *KRT5* and *KRT14* are associated with the severe Dowling–Meara form of hereditary epidermolysis bullosa simplex.[8] Interestingly, a thickened corneal epithelial basement membrane has been reported in epidermolysis bullosa disease (Figure 4.1).[10]

Epithelial basement membrane corneal dystrophy (Cogan's microcystic dystrophy; map-dot-fingerprint dystrophy) (EBMD) MIM 121820

Clinical background

In EBMD, reduplicated basement membrane is noted bilaterally in patterns of microcystic dots, map-like sheets, and fingerprint or horsetail lines. The map pattern is often described as grayish-white patches. The majority of patients are asymptomatic but some have painful recurrent erosions.

Vogt,[11] in 1930, first described the condition which Cogan et al[12,13] further characterized with a histopathological examination that clarified the microcystic nature of the dystrophy. Guerry[14] noted in 1950 the fingerprint lines which later became associated with the dystrophy and also made the observation in 1965 of the map-like changes characteristic of the disease.[15] In 1974 Krachmer and Laibson[16] noted the hereditary pattern of the disease as autosomal dominant and most commonly affecting middle-aged and older adults. In 2006, Boutboul et al[17] reported mutations in the *TGFB1/BIGH3* gene in patients with EBMD.

Pathology

The different manifestations of EBMD, map, dot, and fingerprint, are all characterized by abnormal deposition of multilaminar basement membrane.[13,16,18,19] Inverted basal cell layers, which continue to proliferate, cause the formation of the characteristic microcysts. The multilaminar basement lacks the adhesive strength of normal basement membrane and thus contributes to epithelial sloughing and the development of recurrent erosions.

Pathophysiology

Two point mutations in the *TGFB1/BIGH3* gene were noted in patients with EBMD, resulting in a leucine to arginine shift at codon 509 in one pedigree, and arginine to serine at codon 666 in another pedigree.[17] Mutations in *TGFB1/BIGH3* cause a number of corneal dystrophies and are believed to result from alterations in the *TGFB1/BIGH3*-encoded protein, keratoepithelin (KE). KE is secreted in the extracellular matrix and is believed to bind various collagens. The Leu509Arg and the Arg666Ser mutations have not been associated with other *TGFB1/BIGH3*-associated dystrophies. The Leu509Arg and the Arg666Ser mutations could result in a misfolding of the protein, loss of function, and an increase in the epithelial extracellular matrix.

Band-shaped, whorled microcystic corneal dystrophy (Lisch corneal dystrophy)

Clinical background

Unilateral or bilateral gray intraepithelial opacities that are band-shaped and feathery, sometimes in a whorled pattern, characterize the disease.[20,21] The microcysts are in a dense pattern as opposed to those noted in Meesmann's dystrophy. No symptoms are associated with the condition.

The condition was first noted by Lisch et al[20] in 1992. Linkage of the dystrophy to Xp22.3 was noted by Lisch et al[21] in 2000, confirming that the disease is likely unrelated to Meesmann's dystrophy, which has been associated with mutations of the *KRT3* and *KRT12* genes.

Pathology

The pathological mechanism involved in the disease remains unknown. However, histopathology demonstrates vacuolization of basal epithelial cells as opposed to the fibrillogranular or peculiar substance noted in Meesmann's dystrophy.[20,22–24] As yet the underlying genetic mechanism of the disease remains undetermined.

Bowman membrane dystrophies

Corneal dystrophy of the Bowman layer type I (CDBI) MIM 608470 (Reis–Bücklers dystrophy)

Clinical background

Corneal dystrophy of the Bowman layer type I (CDBI) is an extremely rare autosomal-dominant disease characterized by confluent geographic opacities in the Bowman layer. Patients typically have recurrent corneal erosions which can be quite painful. Vision loss can occur early and can be severe.

Reis[25] described the disease in 1917 and Bücklers[26] in 1949 provided further follow-up of Reis' pedigree. Küchle et al,[27] in 1995, proposed distinguishing Reis–Bücklers dystrophy from another anterior stromal dystrophy (Thiel–Behnke) with similar signs and symptoms by referring to them as CDBI and CDBII. Okada et al,[28] in 1998, described a mutation in the *TGFB1/BIGH3* gene encoding the protein keratoepithelin (KE), with an amino acid change of leucine for arginine at codon 124.

Pathology

CDBI is characterized by the destruction of Bowman's layer with the deposition of granular band-shaped material and irregular epithelium. The deposits and irregular epithelia can be noted by light microscopy[29] and electron microscopy.[27] The staining patterns are similar to granular corneal dystrophy.

Pathophysiology

Mutations in the *TGFB1/BIGH3* gene have been associated with a number of corneal dystrophies with varied pheno-types. The *TGFB1/BIGH3* gene encodes the KE protein with position 124 as a "hot spot" for mutations.[30] The increased severity of the disease in CDBI is believed to be related to the amino acid replaced at codon 124 with a leucine for an arginine. Leucine is hydrophobic and arginine is charged polar, a change which would result in a severe alteration in the KE protein. The Arg124Leu mutation is characterized by a nonamyloid-type deposition and appears not to affect abnormal proteolysis of KE.[31] A summary of the genetics and pathogenesis of CDBI and CDBII and several other hereditary corneal dystrophies is given in Box 4.1.

Box 4.1 Summary of genetics and pathogenesis of selected hereditary corneal dystrophies

TGFBI (5q31)-associated dystrophies	Exon	Amino acid change	Histopathology/deposit type
Corneal dystrophy of Bowman's layer type I (CDB I) Reis–Bücklers dystrophy	4	Arg124Leu	Deposits of granular band-shaped materials into Bowman's layer Opacities stain red with Masson trichrome
Corneal dystrophy of Bowman's layer type II (CDB II) Thiel–Behnke dystrophy Honeycomb-shaped dystrophy	12	Arg555Gln	Irregular epithelium due to iron deposits Bowman layer is mostly or totally absent Fibrous tissue is interposed between the epithelium and stroma in a "sawtooth" pattern Peculiar collagen filaments or "curly fibers" are noted
Granular dystrophy type I (GCD I) Groenouw type I	12	Arg555Trp	Rod-shaped bodies with discrete borders are noted in the stroma These opacities stain red with Masson trichome
Lattice corneal dystrophy I (LCD I) Biber–Habb–Dimmer dystrophy	4	Arg124Cys	Stromal deposits and amyloid stain positive with Congo red and periodic acid–Schiff On electron microscopy, deposits are irregularly shaped and are noted to be interspersed among the collagen lamellae
Combined granular lattice corneal dystrophy (CGLCD) Avellino corneal dystrophy Epithelial basement membrane corneal dystrophy (EBMD)	4	Arg124His	Granular deposits are noted in the anterior third of the stroma Amyloid may be detected in some granular deposits Typical fusiform deposits identified as amyloid are noted deep to the granular deposits
Cogan's microcystic dystrophy Map-dot-fingerprint dystrophy	11 15	Leu509Arg Arg666Ser	Grayish map, dot (microcysts), and fingerprint lines characterized by abnormal deposition of multilaminar basement membrane Basement membrane lacks normal adhesive strength so it may slough off periodically, causing recurrent erosions

Corneal dystrophy of the Bowman layer type II (CBDII) MIM 602082 (Thiel–Behnke or honeycomb dystrophy)

Clinical background

CDBII (Thiel–Behnke) dystrophy is an autosomal-dominant disease that is more common than CDBI (Reis–Bücklers).[27] The dystrophy is characterized clinically by honeycomb-shaped opacities occurring at the level of Bowman's membrane. Vision is not usually as severely affected as it is in CDBI; however, patients often have recurrent erosions.

Thiel and Behnke[32] described the condition in 1967 as an anterior stromal dystrophy distinct from Reis–Bücklers. Küchle et al[27] proposed that Thiel–Behnke was indeed distinct from Reis–Bücklers, was more common, and had distinct histopathological features. They proposed that this disease be referred to as CDBII. Okada et al,[28] in 1998, described a mutation in the *TGFBI/BIGH3* gene resulting in an amino acid change in the KE protein, glycine for arginine at codon 555.

Pathology

In CDBII, the epithelium is usually irregular due to iron deposition.[27] Bowman layer is either mostly or totally absent. Interposed fibrous tissue between the epithelium and the stroma is noted in an undulating or "sawtooth" pattern. On transmission electron microscopy, peculiar collagen filaments or "curly fibers" are found.[29]

Pathophysiology

CDBII has been reported to be caused by mutations in *TGFBI/BIGH3*, resulting in substitution of glycine for arginine at codon 555 in the KE protein. This Arg555Gln mutation would be expected to alter the secondary structure of the KE protein and could result in the precipitation of the protein and the honeycomb pattern characteristic of the disease (Figure 4.2).[28]

Stromal dystrophies

Granular dystrophy type I (GCD1) MIM 1219000 (Groenouw type I)

Clinical background

The breadcrumb-type lesions of the dystrophy can become apparent in the first decade of life, and, as the disease progresses, the lesions become discrete corneal opacities, mostly in the central anterior cornea. With further progression the opacities coalesce but the peripheral cornea usually remains clear. Visual acuity is usually mildly affected, but patients who are homozygous for the Arg555Trp mutation are more likely to be more severely affected with symptoms at an earlier age. Epithelial erosions are common.

Groenouw described a corneal dystrophy with autosomal-dominant inheritance that had large numbers of small, irregular discrete opacities in the central cornea.[33] The larger opacities appear nodular, raise the epithelium, and give the corneal surface an irregular appearance – thus his designation of a "nodular degeneration."[33] Groenouw studied a small biopsy specimen from one of his patients and noted the material was positive with an acidophilic stain and was likely hyaline in nature.[34] As opposed to the lattice dystrophies, which occur commonly in the Japanese population, GCD1 and the Arg555Trp mutation in the *TGFB1* are rare in Japan.[35]

Pathology

The distinct corneal opacities stain red with Masson trichrome and the noted rod-shaped bodies with discrete borders can be detected by electron microscopy.[36]

Pathophysiology

A mutation in the *TGFB1/BIGH3* gene that results in the substitution of tryptophan for arginine at codon 555, Arg555Trp, in the KE protein is responsible for the disease.[30,37–39] The deposits in GCD1 are believed to be accumulations of mutant KE protein.[38,39] The Arg555Trp mutant is associated with nonamyloid phenotypes as well as the other Arg555 mutant CDBII (Arg555Gln) (Figure 4.3).[31,38]

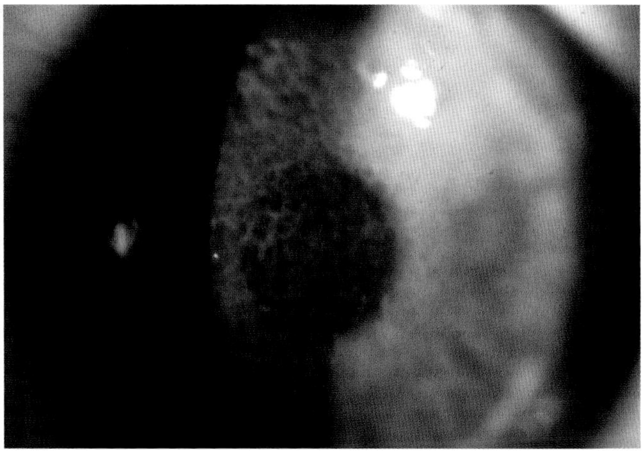

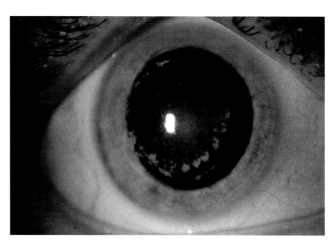

Figure 4.2 Corneal dystrophy of the Bowman layer type II (Thiel–Behnke or honeycomb dystrophy): honeycomb-shaped opacities; altered secondary structure of keratoepithelin.

Figure 4.3 Granular type I (Groenouw type I): breadcrumb lesions and corneal opacities.

Lattice corneal dystrophy I MIM 122200 (Biber–Habb–Dimmer dystrophy)

Clinical background

The dystrophy, which is bilateral but can be asymmetric, usually begins late in the first or early in the second decade with progressive branching linear opacities. These linear arrays are mostly in the central cornea. As the dystrophy progresses, a generalized haziness develops in the central cornea while the peripheral cornea remains clear. Recurrent erosions occur early in the course of the disease. As the disease progresses the opacities can coalesce, with resultant declining vision, usually in the fourth to sixth decade.

Biber,[40] in 1890, described this dystrophy as *gitterige Keratitis*, noting branching twig-like patterns with a clear peripheral cornea. Haab[41] further described a lattice-like appearance and, along with Dimmer[42] in 1889, recognized that the disease appeared inheritable. Seitelberger and Nemetz[43] determined that lattice dystrophy was a localized amyloid degeneration. Munier et al[30] in 1997 noted mutations in *TGFB1/BIGH3*, resulting in the substitution of cysteine for arginine at codon 124 in the encoded protein KE in patients with lattice dystrophy.

Pathology

Amyloid deposits, which stain positive with Congo red and periodic acid–Schiff, are found throughout the stroma. On electron microscopy, irregular deposits are noted interspersed among the collagen lamellae.[36]

Pathophysiology

Mutations in *TGFB1/BIGH3* gene, which encode KE proteins, are responsible for the protein amyloid deposits noted in the disease.[30] Mutation "hot spots" have been found at the 124 codon position of the protein as multiple families with this mutation have been screened and identified.[37] Haplotype analysis of these families demonstrates that these mutations have arisen independently and do not share a common ancestor.[37] Amyloidogenesis in LCDI with the Arg124Cys mutation occurs with the accumulation of N-terminal fragments of KE. It is believed that amyloidogenesis in the Arg-124Cys mutated cornea is associated with abnormal proteolysis of the protein.[44] Because there is no other evidence of systemic amyloid deposition in patients with the Arg124Cys mutation, there are likely tissue-specific factors that lead to KE fragment aggregation. Evidence suggests that the Arg124Cys mutation in KE affects protein structure, resulting in increased beta sheet content. Korvatska et al have proposed that the Arg124Cys mutation abolishes a critical site of proteolysis of the KE protein that is essential for normal turnover of the protein (Figure 4.4).[31]

Lattice corneal dystrophy type II MIM 105120 (familial amyloid polyneuropathy type IV (Finnish or Meretoja type))

Clinical background

In this hereditary systemic amyloidosis, in the third decade lattice-type lines appear which are fewer in number than LCDI and begin in the periphery.[45–47] The central cornea is

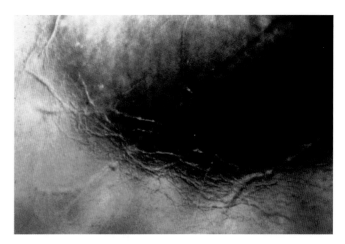

Figure 4.4 Lattice corneal dystrophy type I (Biber–Habb–Dimmer dystrophy): lattice lines and haziness in central cornea.

spared until later when vision can be affected, usually mildly. If the disease is homozygous for the mutant gelsolin protein, disease onset is earlier.[48] The corneal findings are part of a systemic amyloidosis which involves cranial nerves, causing nerve palsies and affecting the skin with lichen amyloidosis and cutis laxa, leading to frozen facial features. Corneal nerves may be affected, leading to an anesthetic cornea.

Meretoja[45] described in 1969 a family with systemic amyloidosis and a lattice type dystrophy. Klintworth[47] recognized the corneal clinical findings as different from LCDI and termed this lattice dystrophy LCDII. Paunio et al[48] described a mutation in the *GSN* gene, which encodes the protein gelsolin, in affected patients with Finnish-type familial amyloidosis. Most cases have a Finnish origin but families with the disease have been identified in Japan, Portugal, Czech Republic, and Denmark.[48,49] Amyloid positivity for antigelsolin antibody, along with genetic testing, can confirm the diagnosis. The associated systemic findings for LCDII and several other hereditary corneal dystrophies are given in Box 4.2.

Pathology

Gelsolin is an actin-modulating protein that is expressed in most tissues.[48] The amyloid deposits in LCDII consist of gelsolin fragments which coalesce underneath the corneal epithelium and the anterior stroma.[50] There is a mostly continuous deposition of this amyloid beneath Bowman's layer. Less amyloid deposition occurs in LCDII than in LCDI.[51]

Pathophysiology

A substitution of asparagine for aspartic acid at codon 187 in the *GSN* gene encodes a mutated gelsolin protein. The accumulated gelsolin protein fragments are responsible for the amyloid deposits (Figure 4.5).[48]

Combined granular-lattice dystrophy (CGLCD) OMIM 607541 (Avellino corneal dystrophy)

Clinical background

The dystrophy becomes manifest in the second decade. By biomicroscopy, it has discrete gray-white opacities in the superficial to anterior one-third of the stroma. Intervening

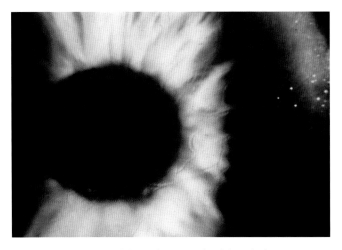

Figure 4.5 Lattice corneal dystrophy type II (familial amyloid polyneuropathy type IV Finnish or Meretoja type): lattice-like lines represent amyloid deposits of gelsolin fragments.

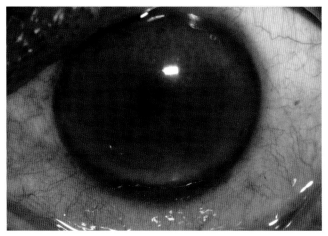

Figure 4.6 Combined granular lattice dystrophy (Avellino corneal dystrophy): discrete gray-white opacities, intervening stroma hazy with linear opacities.

Box 4.2 Associated systemic findings in the hereditary corneal dystrophies

Corneal dystrophies	Associated systemic diseases/symptoms
Lattice corneal dystrophy type II (LCDII) Familial amyloid polyneuropathy type IV: Finnish or Meretoja type	Cranial neuropathy, primarily in the facial nerves Peripheral polyneuropathy, mainly affecting vibrations and sense of touch Minor autonomic dysfunction Nephrotic syndrome and eventual renal failure associated with homozygous patients
Schnyder crystalline corneal dystrophy (SCCD)	Increased risk of hypercholesterolemia or dyslipoproteinemia Genu valgum is reported in some patients
Pre-Descemet dystrophy with ichthyosis (XLRI)	Scaly skin with hyperpigmentation and large scales prominently on the flexor and extensor surfaces, trunk, neck, and scalp Eyelids and conjunctiva may also be affected
Harboyan syndrome congenital dystrophy and perceptive deafness (CDPPD)	Sensorineural deafness
Posterior polymorphous dystrophy (PPCD, PPMD)	Alport syndrome: a genetic disease characterized by glomerulonephritis, end-stage kidney disease, and nerve-related hearing loss Blood in the urine is a common symptom PPCD3 is also linked to inguinal hernias and hydroceles

stroma can be hazy and linear opacities can be observed, while the periphery is clear. The disease progression is slower than in GCD or LCDI and vision is usually not severely affected. Corneal erosions are less common than with GCD.

In 1988, Folberg et al[52] presented four patients from three families with clinical features similar to granular dystrophy but with histopathologic features similar to lattice dystrophy (LCDI) with fusiform stromal deposits of amyloid. In addition, deposits that appear morphologically similar to what is noted in GCD did not react with the usual histochemical stains. Folberg et al traced the ancestry of these families to Avellino, Italy; hence in some literature the disease is referred to as Avellino corneal dystrophy. The disease has been noted in many countries, particularly in Japan.[53]

Pathology

In CGLCD granular deposits are noted in the anterior third of the stroma. Amyloid can be detected in some granular deposits. Typical fusiform deposits, identified as amyloid, are noted deep to granular deposits.[52] CGLCD is associated with a mutation in the *TGFB1/BIGH3* gene resulting in a substitution of histidine for arginine at codon 124, Arg124His, in the KE protein.[30] Patients homozygous for the Arg124His mutation have much more severe disease.[53]

Pathophysiology

The Arg124His mutation in the KE protein had mostly non-amyloid inclusions. The accumulation of the pathologic KE also occurred with abnormal proteolysis of the protein. A unique 66-kDa KE protein was noted in CGLCD and could be responsible for the deposits found in the disease (Figure 4.6).[31]

Gelatinous drop-like corneal dystrophy (GDLD) MIM 204870 (primary familial subepithelial corneal amyloidosis)

Clinical background

This dystrophy is characterized by severe corneal amyloidosis which can lead to marked visual impairment.[54–57] At an early stage of the disease, whitish-yellow subepithelial and nodular lesions are noted centrally. As the lesions coalesce, a "mulberry" appearance with a whitish-yellow color occupies the central cornea. Ide et al have classified these different clinical presentations as band keratopathy type, stromal opacity type, kumquat-like type, and typical mulberry type.[55]

Nakaizumi[54] first reported this rare dystrophy in a Japanese patient in 1914. The disease occurs in about one in 300,000 of the general population in Japan with scattered reports in other countries and is inherited as an autosomal-recessive disorder.[55] Tsujikawa et al[58] in 1999 found GDLD to be a result of a mutation in the *M1S1* gene.

Pathology

GDLD is an autosomal-recessive disorder with mutations in the *M1S1* gene localized to chromosome 1p.[58] The commonest mutation resulted in a glutamine replaced with a stop at codon 118. Sixteen of 20 members of the families studied were homozygous for the Q118X mutation. All alleles studied carried the disease haplotype which strongly suggested that the Q118X mutation is the major mutation in the Japanese GDLD patients. Other nonsense and frameshift mutations have been noted in the *M1S1* gene.

Pathophysiology

The function of the M1S1 protein is not understood. The *M1S1* Q118X mutation and other mutations predict a truncated protein with loss of function or aggregation of the M1S1 protein.[58] Cells transfected with the truncated M1S1 protein demonstrate aggregate perinuclear cytoplasmic bodies, supporting the possibility that an aggregation of protein leads to the formation of amyloid deposits and is responsible for the disease (Figure 4.7).

Macular corneal dystrophy (MCD) MIM 217800 (Groenouw type II)

Clinical background

MCD is characterized by progressive bilateral corneal clouding beginning in the first decade with grayish opacities and

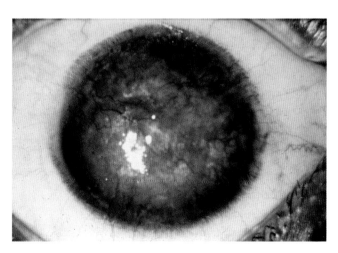

Figure 4.7 Primary familial subepithelial corneal amyloidosis (gelatinous drop-like corneal dystrophy): nodular yellow-white mulberry-like lesions.

poorly defined borders. The opacities start centrally and can extend throughout the stroma, leading in most cases to corneal thinning.[34,59,60] The diffuse opaque spotty clouding is initially noted in the superficial central cornea and spreads peripherally and into deeper stroma with age. The endothelium and Descemet's membrane can be affected with the development of guttae. Severe visual impairment can occur as early as the age of 40. The disease is rare except in Iceland.

Groenouw described the characteristics of MCD in his original report of corneal nodular dystrophies along with the clinical findings of granular corneal dystrophy.[34] The two diseases have been referred to as Groenouw type II and Groenouw type I, respectively. Jones and Zimmerman[59] demonstrated accumulation of acid mucopolysaccharide and Klintworth and Vogel[60] found that MCD is an inherited storage disorder of mucopolysaccharide in corneal fibroblasts in 1964. Hassell et al,[61] in 1980, found that failure to synthesize a mature keratan sulfate proteoglycan was responsible for the disease. Akama et al,[62] in 2000, found that the carbohydrate sulfotransferase gene (*CHST6*), encoding an enzyme designated corneal *N*-acetylglucosamine-6-sulfotransferase, was responsible for MCD I and II.

Studies of mutations in this gene in multiple populations have demonstrated marked heterogeneity with many different missense mutations, deletions, and insertions.[63–68]

In the diagnostic workup of MCD, the dystrophy has been divided into three subtypes (MCD type I, IA, and II) based on the immunoreactivity of the patient's serum and cornea to an antibody to sulfated keratan sulfate.[69] MCD I has no reactivity of the antibody to serum or the cornea. In MCD IA, antigenicity is missing in the serum and cornea but can be detected in keratocytes. MCD II has reactivity in the cornea and in the serum.[69]

Pathology

Sulfation of polylactosamine, the nonsulfated precursor to keratan sulfate, is critical to obtaining proper hydration of the stroma and maintaining corneal clarity. The *CHST6* gene encodes the enzyme *N*-acetyl glucosamine-6-sulfotransferase which catalyzes the sulfation of polylactosamine of the keratan sulfate containing proteoglycans in the cornea.[62]

Pathophysiology

It is yet unknown how the various mutations in the *CHST6* gene cause disease. However, due to the high degree of mutational heterogeneity found in patients with this disease and this gene, it is believed that loss of function with deficient enzyme activity is responsible for the dystrophy (Figure 4.8).[62–68]

Schnyder crystalline corneal dystrophy (SCCD) MIM 121800

Clinical background

SCCD is a rare autosomal disease with slow progressive corneal clouding due to deposition of cholesterol and phospholipids.[70,71] The lipid deposition occurs in the stroma, often with a discoid pattern. There can be an accompanying prominent arcus. Affected patients have a higher likelihood of developing hypercholesterolemia.

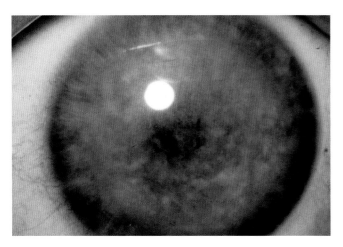

Figure 4.8 Macular corneal dystrophy (Groenouw type II): corneal clouding with grayish opacities and poorly defined borders.

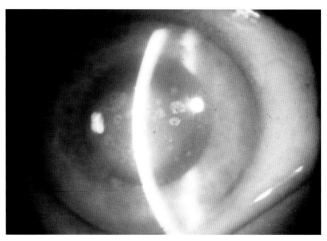

Figure 4.9 Schnyder crystalline corneal dystrophy: deposits representing phospholipids and cholesterol in discoid pattern; corneal clouding.

The first description of SCCD was in 1924 by Van Went and Wibaut[72] with later detailed descriptions of the disease by Schnyder in 1929[73] and 1939.[74] Bron and others reported the association of SCCD with hyperlipoproteinemia.[70] In 1996 Shearman et al reported the mapping of the gene for SCCD to chromosome 1[75] and in 2007 multiple investigators reported that mutations with the *UBIAD1* gene were associated with SCCD.[76–79] Although the disease is rare, multiple families have been reported with the disease, strongly suggesting autosomal-dominant inheritance.

Pathology

The etiology of SCCD is as yet unclear but appears to be associated with mutations in the *UBIAD1* gene[76–79] and the resultant changes that occur in lipid metabolism locally in corneal keratocytes and fibroblasts in skin.[71] There can be high cholesterol levels in some patients with SCCD, and the cornea has been shown to have nonesterified cholesterol, cholesterol esters, and phospholipids.

Pathophysiology

As yet, it is unclear how missense mutations identified thus far for *UBIAD1* lead to lipid deposition in the cornea. However, *UBIAD1* encodes a potential prenyltransferase and may interact with apolipoprotein E.[76–79] Cholesterol metabolism may be affected directly or other alterations in cellular structural elements could lead to abnormal lipid metabolism (Figure 4.9).

Congenital hereditary stromal dystrophy (CHSD)

Clinical background

The disease is usually characterized by stationary flaky or feathery clouding of the corneal stroma without abnormalities of the epithelium or endothelium.[80]

Turpin et al[81] described the original family in 1939. The condition was named and distinguished from congenital hereditary endothelial dystrophy (CHED) by Witschel et al[80] in 1978.

Pathology

The histopathologic findings in CHSD are confined to the stroma where normal tightly packed lamellae alternate with layers of loosely arranged collagen fibrils of half the normal diameter.[80,82]

Pathophysiology

Linkage to chromosome 12q22 with a frameshift mutation in the *DCN* gene that encodes the stromal protein, decorin, has been found in patients with CHSD.[83] The mutation predicts a truncation of the decorin protein. It is believed that the truncated decorin protein would bind to collagen in a suboptimal way, leading to a disruption in the regularity of collagen fibril formation and loss of corneal transparency.

Fleck corneal dystrophy (CFD) MIM 121850 (François–Neetens Mouchetée)

Clinical background

The condition is characterized by small white flecks at all levels in the corneal stroma. The intervening stroma is clear and there is no involvement with the epithelium or endothelium. Vision is not usually affected and patients are asymptomatic.[84,85]

François and Neetens,[84] in 1956, described *dystrophie mouchetée* (speckled) as characterized by white flecks throughout the stroma. Li et al[86] in 2005 found mutations in the *PIP5K3* gene associated with the dystrophy.

The disease is rare and thought to be nonprogressive and has been noted in patients as young as 2 years. Confocal microscopy in vivo reveals bright-appearing deposits that are found around keratocyte nuclei.[87]

Pathology

The corneal speckled flecks found throughout the stroma are believed to be pathologically affected keratocytes which are inspissated with membrane-bound intracytoplasmic vesicles with lipids and mucopolysaccharides.[85]

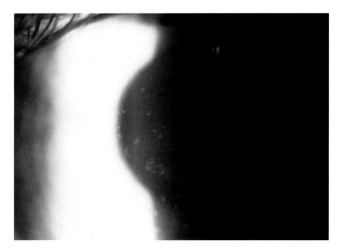

Figure 4.10 Fleck corneal dystrophy (François–Neetens mouchetée): small white flecks in stromal layer.

Pathophysiology

Missense, frameshift, and protein-truncating mutations in *PIP5K3* were found in multiple families studied with Fleck corneal dystrophy.[86] These predicted truncated proteins would result in loss of function of the PIP5K3 protein. The histological and clinical characteristics of patients with CFD are consistent with biochemical studies of PIP5K3 protein indicating that it plays a role in endosomal sorting and that its dysfunction is related to the abnormal storage of lipids and glycosaminoglycans noted in stromal keratocytes (Figure 4.10).

Bietti crystalline corneoretinal dystrophy (BCD) MIM 210370

Clinical background

This rare corneoretinal dystrophy is characterized in some patients with peripheral, glistening yellow-white crystals at the limbus and peripheral cornea.[88] The disease, however, can lead to marked loss of vision due to involvement of the retina. The same yellow-white crystals are noted in the posterior pole with retinal pigment epithelial atrophy, choroidal sclerosis, and pigment clumping. The disease is progressive with loss of vision, night blindness, and peripheral visual field loss.

The disease was described by Bietti[89] in 1937. Li et al[90] described mutations in the *CYP4V2* gene in 2004.

The disease has a pattern of autosomal-recessive inheritance and has been reported as more common in Asiatic populations. Diagnosis can be confirmed by the presence of crystalline lysosomal inclusions in lymphocytes and fibroblasts from skin biopsies.[88]

Pathology

Abnormal lipid metabolism is thought to be involved in Bietti crystalline dystrophy. Histopathology demonstrates crystals and lipid inclusions in choroidal fibroblasts, corneal keratocytes, and lymphocytes. *CYP4V2* is as yet an unknown gene but has sequence homology to other CYP450 proteins which are involved in fatty acid and corticosteroid metabo-

lism which would be functions consistent with the lipid pathology associated with the disease.[90,91]

Pre-Descemet dystrophy associated with X-linked recessive ichthyosis (XLRI)

Clinical background

The disease is characterized by scaly skin with hyperpigmentation and large scales prominently on the flexor and extensor surfaces, trunk, neck, and scalp.[92–94] Eyelids can be involved as well as the conjunctiva. The cornea is involved in about 50% of affected individuals with fine, filiform corneal opacities located in the posterior stroma. Female carriers may only have the corneal opacities as a sign of the disease.

The association of deep corneal opacities associated with ichthyosis was made in 1954 by Franceschetti and Maeder,[95] who termed the biomicroscopic appearance as dystrophia punctiformis profunda. Shapiro et al[96] identified deletions in the *STS* gene as responsible for XLRI in 1989. The X-linked recessive disease affects men in a ratio of 1:6000. The diagnosis of XLRI is confirmed by an assay of STS.

Pathology

Deficiency of STS produces X chromosome-linked ichthyosis, one of the most common inborn errors of metabolism in humans.[96] Most XLRI-affected individuals have deletions in *STS*. The function of STS is the desulfation of cholesterol sulfate, which leads to an increase in plasma levels of cholesterol sulfate. Ocular opacities may result from the accumulation of cholesterol sulfate, but this has not yet been confirmed.

Endothelial dystrophies

Congenital hereditary endothelial dystrophy I (CHED I) MIM 121700

Congenital hereditary endothelial dystrophy II (CHED II) MIM 217700

Harboyan syndrome congenital dystrophy and perceptive deafness (CDPD) MIM 217400

Clinical background

Both CHED I and II are rare bilateral congenital dystrophies resulting in diffuse stromal edema.[97–102] With the recessive form of the disease, gross stromal edema is noted at birth or shortly thereafter, while the dominant form is usually less severe with a clear cornea at birth and stromal edema slowly progressing later in childhood.[99,103] Although mild photophobia and epiphora can be noted early in the disease, these symptoms usually ameliorate with progression. Corneal clouding in CHED has been reported from birth to 8 years of age. Progression can be seen in both the recessive and dominant forms of the disease with the increase in stromal edema, the development of stromal fibrosis, and plaques. The Harboyan syndrome or CDPD presents with the clinical picture of CHED at birth and with the development of sensorineural hearing loss most commonly during the second decade of life.[104] With the findings of a genetic cause of CHED II in the *SLC4A11* gene and the association of hearing loss with mutations in this gene, it is thought advisable to obtain screenings for hearing loss regularly in patients with CHED.[105]

Congenital hereditary corneal edema was described by Komoto[106] in 1909. In 1960, Maumenee[97] postulated that the disease could occur as a result of primary endothelial dysfunction. This was confirmed by Pearce et al[98] in their electron microscopic study of the endothelium of patients with hereditary congenital edema reported in 1969. Pearce et al also postulated that the dystrophy was caused by a gene or point mutation. Judisch and Maumenee[99] distinguished the clinical signs and confirmed the two forms of inheritance of the condition, autosomal recessive and autosomal dominant. CHED was mapped to chromosome 20 and later homozygosity mapping and linkage analysis demonstrated that CHED I and CHED II were at different loci on chromosome 20.[103] In 2006, Vithana et al[105] demonstrated that mutations in *SLC4A11* cause CHED II. Harboyan et al[104] reported the syndrome of CDPD in 1971 and Desir et al[107] reported that mutations in *SLC4A11* were also responsible for CDPD.

Pathology

Mutations in *SLC4A11*, the gene that encodes the sodium borate transporter protein termed NaBC1, can cause CHED II.[108] Initially the sequence homology of the protein suggested that it functioned as a bicarbonate transporter and was termed bicarbonate transporter protein or BTR1, but in fact, the NaBC1 protein is a borate transporter in the cell membrane.

Pathophysiology

The *SLC4A11* gene encodes the boron-concentrating membrane transporter.[105] The large number of mutations that have been reported in *SLC4A11* associated with CHED II suggest the disease is genetically heterogenous.[108,109] In transfected cells with mutant and wild-type *SLC4A11*, a decrease in transporter proteins was noted in cells with the mutant gene. Cell-surfacing processing assays demonstrated that mutated protein was not membrane-bound, which indicates that when mutated, the protein likely loses its function. Exactly how these mutations in *SLC4A11* lead to CHED and Harboyan syndrome with hearing loss is not understood, but some loss of ion transport is believed to be essential in maintaining fluid transport across the endothelium and maintaining the endolymph in the inner ear (Figure 4.11).[107]

Fuchs' dystrophies

This group of hereditary endothelial dystrophies (early- and late-onset Fuchs' dystrophies) are covered in Chapter 5.

Posterior polymorphous dystrophy (PPCD, PPMD) MIM 122000

Clinical background

PPMD can affect both corneas, usually in the second or third decade of life. There is a wide variation in the signs of the disease: some individuals are slightly affected whereas others have severe corneal decompensation requiring penetrating

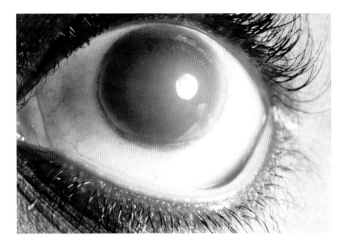

Figure 4.11 Congenital hereditary endothelial dystrophies (CHED) type II: diffuse stromal edema with stromal fibrosis.

keratoplasty.[110-114] Posterior vesicles often characterize the disease, with bands and retrocorneal membranes appearing as glass-like structures extending across the angle on to the iris, forming peripheral anterior synechiae.

The disease was first described by Koeppe[110] in 1916: he termed the disease keratitis bullosa interna. In 1953 McGee and Falls[111] reported that the disease was autosomal dominantly inherited. Iris synechiae were reported by Soukup[112] in 1964. The association of PPMD with glaucoma was made by Rubenstein and Silverman[113] in 1968. The discovery of the epithelial-like nature of the endothelium in PPCD was made through electron microscopic findings by Krachmer[114] and Boruchoff and Kuwabara.[115] The association of PPCD with Alport's disease was made by Colville and Savige.[116]

With or without posterior polymorphous corneal dystrophy, a diagnosis of anterior lenticonus requires that a medical history be taken and a workup for Alport syndrome should be done. PPCD3 has been associated with inguinal hernias and hydroceles.

Pathology

PPCD has been associated with the *VSX1* gene (PPCD1),[117] *COL8A2* (PPCD2),[118] and *TCF8* or *ZEB1* (PPCD3),[119,120] and has been linked to 20p11.2 (PPCD4).[121] Subsequent studies have not confirmed mutations in the *VSX1* or *COL8A2* as associated with PPCD[120,121]; however, mutations of the *TCF8* gene have been confirmed by others[120,122] to be associated with PPCD.

Pathophysiology

The disease is characterized by endothelial cellular proliferation with an abnormal regulation of protein expression resulting in an altered structure of Descemet's membrane, with the endothelium taking on epithelial-like characteristics.[114,115]

In PPCD3, *TCF8* heterozygous frameshift mutations segregate in families with PPCD3.[119] Five of 11 probands were found to have *TCF8* mutations, suggesting that 45% of PPCD is caused by this gene. There may be an age-related aspect to the penetrance of the gene mutation, especially in PPCD3 families.

Immunohistochemical evidence demonstrates that, in the presence of a familial proband's heterozygous *TCF8* muta-

Box 4.3 Summary of the genetics of the hereditary corneal dystrophies

Disease	MIM number	Inheritance pattern	Genes involved
Epithelial dystrophies			
Meesmann corneal dystrophy (MCD) Stocker–Holt dystrophy	122100	AD	*KRT3* and *KRT12*
Epithelial basement membrane corneal dystrophy (EBMD) Cogan's microcystic dystrophy Map-dot-fingerprint dystrophy	121820	AD	*TGFBI*
Band-shaped, whorled microcystic corneal dystrophy Lisch corneal dystrophy		XL	Locus = Xp22.3, gene unknown
Bowman membrane dystrophies			
Corneal dystrophy of Bowman's layer type I (CDB I) Reis–Bücklers dystrophy	608470	AD	*TGFBI*
Corneal dystrophy of Bowman's layer type II (CDB II) Thiel–Behnke dystrophy Honeycomb-shaped dystrophy	602082	AD	*TGFBI*
Stromal dystrophies			
Granular dystrophy type I (GCDI) Groenouw type I	121900	AD	*TGFBI*
Lattice corneal dystrophy (LCDI) Biber–Habb–Dimmer dystrophy	122200	AD	*TGFBI*
Lattice corneal dystrophy type II (LCDII) Familial amyloid polyneuropathy type IV: Finnish or Meretoja type	105120	AD	*GSN*
Combined granular–lattice corneal dystrophy (CGLCD) Avellino corneal dystrophy	607541	AD	*TGFBI*
Gelatinous drop-like corneal dystrophy (GDLD) Primary familial subepithelial corneal amyloidosis	204870	AR	*M1S1*
Macular corneal dystrophy Groenouw type II	217800	AR	*CHST6*
Schnyder crystalline corneal dystrophy (SCCD)	121800	AD	*UBIAD1*
Congenital hereditary stromal dystrophy (CHSD)		AD	*DCN*
Fleck corneal dystrophy (CFD) François–Neetens mouchetée	121850	AD	*PIP5K3*
Bietti crystalline corneoretinal dystrophy (BCD)	210370	AR	*CYP4V2*
Pre-Descemet dystrophy with ichthyosis (XLRI)		XL	*STS*
Endothelial dystrophies			
Congenital hereditary endothelial dystrophy I (CHED I)	121700	AD	Locus = 20p13, gene unknown
Congenital hereditary endothelial dystrophy II (CHED II)	217700	AR	*SLC4A11*
Harboyan syndrome congenital dystrophy and perceptive deafness (CDPD)	217400	AR	*SLC4A11*
Posterior polymorphous dystrophy (PPCD, PPMD)	122000	AD	*TCF8*
X-linked endothelial dystrophy (XCED)		XL	Locus = Xq25, gene unknown

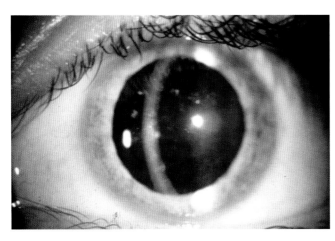

Figure 4.12 Posterior polymorphous dystrophy: posterior vesicles with bands.

tion, there is aberrant expression of *COL4A3*, which is a regulatory target of *TCF8*. Krafchak et al[119] demonstrated the overexpression of *COL4A3* in the corneal endothelium of a proband. Interestingly, *COL4A3* mutations are also associated with Alport's syndrome with coexisting PPCD (Figure 4.12).

X-linked endothelial dystrophy (XCED)

Clinical background

Schmid et al[123] in 2006 described a new X-linked endothelial dystrophy. With slit-lamp direct biomicroscopy, all patients were observed to have endothelial changes suggestive of pits resembling irregular cornea guttae. On retroillumination, these irregularities appeared as "moon craters." Two of 13 affected males had a milky ground-glass appearance at birth suggestive of CHED. Seven other patients developed subepithelial band keratopathy, which reduced vision and required penetrating keratoplasties to restore vision. Thirty-five of 60 members of the four-generational pedigree were found to be affected and males were found to be more severely affected than females. The endothelial changes are irregular.

Pathology

This endothelial dystrophy has been linked to the X chromosome with the interval defined between markers DXS8057 and DXS1047.[123]

The disease was found to be transmitted from all affected males to all of their female offspring, but not to their male offspring. Marked thickening of Descemet's membrane is characteristic of this dystrophy, especially in the anterior banded zone, suggesting that the alterations in this dystrophy occur in utero.

Summary

As detailed above, a number of hereditary corneal dystrophies have been linked to specific gene mutations (Box 4.3), opening lines of inquiry into the molecular pathogenesis and therapeutic options for alleviating or curing each dystrophy. Because of our unique access to the cornea as the external tissue of the eye and our ability to note in exquisite detail the layers of the cornea with biomicroscopy, hopefully in the near future we will be able to apply gene therapy techniques locally or apply topical agents to modify aberrant gene expression and observe a therapeutic effect.

Key references

A complete list of chapter references is available online at www.expertconsult.com. See inside cover for registration details.

5. Irvine AD, Corden LD, Swensson O, et al. Mutations in cornea-specific keratin K3 of K12 genes cause Meesmann's corneal dystrophy. Nature Genetics 1997;16:184–187.

27. Küchle M, Green WR, Volcker HE, et al. Reevaluation of corneal dystrophies of Bowman's layer and anterior stroma (Reis–Bücklers and Thiel–Behnke types): a light and electron microscopic study of eight corneas and a review of the literature. Cornea 1995;14:333–354.

28. Okada M, Yamamoto S, Tsujikawa M, et al. Two distinct kerato-epithelin mutations in Reis–Bücklers corneal dystrophy. Am J Ophthalmol 1998;126:535–542.

30. Munier FL, Korvatska E, Djemaï A, et al. Kerato-epithelin mutations in four 5q31-linked corneal dystrophies. Nat Genet 1997;15:247–251.

45. Meretoja J. Familial systemic paramyloidosis with lattice dystrophy of the cornea, progressive cranial neuropathy, skin changes and various internal symptoms: a previously unrecognized heritable syndrome. Ann Clin Res 1969;1:314–324.

52. Folberg R, Alfonso E, Croxatto JO, et al. Clinically atypical granular corneal dystrophy with pathological features of lattice-like amyloid deposits. A study of three families. Ophthalmology 1988;95:46–52.

60. Klintworth GK, Vogel FS. Macular corneal dystrophy: an inherited acid mucopolysaccharide storage disease of the corneal fibroblast. Am J Pathol 1964;45:565–586.

62. Akama TO, Nishida K, Nakayama J, et al. Macular corneal dystrophy type I and type II are caused by distinct mutations in a new sulphotransferase gene. Nat Genet 2000;26:237–241.

86. Li S, Tiab L, Jiao X, et al. Mutations in PIP5K3 are associated with François–Neetens mouchetée fleck corneal dystrophy. Am J Hum Genet 2005;77:54–63.

105. Vithana EN, Morgan P, Sundaresan P, et al. Mutations in sodium-borate cotransporter SLC4A11 cause recessive congenital hereditary endothelial dystrophy (CHED2). Nat Genet 2006;38:755–757.

107. Desir J, Moya G, Reish O, et al. Borate transporter SLC4A11 mutations cause both Harboyan syndrome and non-syndromic corneal endothelial dystrophy. J Med Genet 2007;44:322–326.

119. Krafchak CM, Pawar H, Moroi SE, et al. Mutations in TCF8 cause posterior polymorphous corneal dystrophy and ectopic expression of COL4A3 by corneal endothelial cells. Am J Hum Genet 2005;77:694–708.

CHAPTER 5

Fuchs' endothelial corneal dystrophy

Vinay Gutti, David S Bardenstein, Sudha Iyengar, and Jonathan H Lass

Clinical background

Fuchs' endothelial corneal dystrophy (FECD) is a bilateral, asymmetric, slowly progressive disorder specific to the corneal endothelium, resulting in decreased visual function and in some cases pain, secondary microbial infection, and corneal neovascularization (Figure 5.1A). The disease was first described in 1910 by Ernst Fuchs, an Austrian ophthalmologist. FECD is an age-related disorder that affects 4% of the population over 40 years of age and its typical symptomatic onset is in the fifth or sixth decade of life[1]; however, an early form of the disease does exist.[2,3] Women are predominantly affected and familial clustering is commonly seen with this disease, which suggests an autosomal-dominant inheritance with incomplete penetrance.[4-6]

The two different forms of FECD are mainly distinguished by the time of onset of disease. The more typical form presents in the fourth or fifth decade[1] and is known as late-onset FECD. Rare cases have been reported of early-onset FECD that demonstrate disease as early as the first decade with diffuse corneal edema by the third or fourth decades without prior guttae formation.[3,5] The two forms of FECD also vary in terms of histopathology (Figure 5.2), Descemet's membrane electron micrography, immunohistochemistry, distribution of various proteins in Descemet's membrane, corneal slit-lamp photography, specular microscopy, and genetic inheritance. These differences will be discussed further in the following sections of this chapter.

The underlying defect in FECD is believed to be a programmed decline in the number of functional endothelial cells. This causes a dysfunction of this layer which leads to a progressive sequence of stromal and epithelial edema, eventually resulting in structural alterations to the other corneal layers.[7] The endothelial dysfunction is thought to lead to a thickening of Descemet's membrane along with stromal and epithelial edema which, if extensive enough, can produce subepithelial bullae. The edema results in decreased vision and the bullae cause the pain associated with FECD.[8]

FECD overlaps with other conditions sharing endothelial attenuation, such as pseudophakic corneal edema (PCE), but is typically distinguished from these other corneal disorders by the presence of refractile endothelial excrescences called guttae. A nonguttate form of FECD does exist and is thought to be a variant.[9] In addition several other conditions can cause pseudoguttae in the setting of inflammation and infection (e.g., luetic keratitis).

Pathology and pathophysiology

Overview of the structure and function of the cornea

To understand the functional impact of FECD on the cornea, a brief discussion of normal corneal physiology is important, in particular understanding the function of each layer and comparing normal cornea to corneas affected by FECD, beginning with the endothelium and progressing anteriorly. The cornea is a thin, highly specialized tissue that faces the challenge of being an interface between the outside environment and the inside of the body while maintaining tissue clarity at a level which allows sharp visual acuity. This is achieved via the efficacy of specialized layers as thin as monolayers, in maintaining corneal health. The two main functions of the cornea are maintaining the structural integrity of the eye and clarity. Corneal clarity is most universally related to it, being maintained in a state of deturgescence. The endothelial monolayer function, supplemented by epithelial evaporation and augmented by the cornea's avascularity, is responsible for corneal deturgescence. Endothelial deturgescence is accomplished in two ways: (1) by acting as a barrier to the movement of salt and metabolites into the stroma; and (2) by actively pumping bicarbonate ions from the stroma to the aqueous humor.[10] Active transport is achieved as a result of the gradient of the Na-K-ATPase pump in the lateral cell membrane of endothelial cells. Endothelial dysfunction has been observed in corneas where ATPase inhibitors such as ouabain and carbonic anhydrase inhibitors such as acetazolamide have been used topically or intracamerally.[9,11]

The endothelium

The endothelial monolayer is composed of cells with hexagonal plate-like shape with nuclei that are round and spaced roughly 2–4 nuclear diameters from their neighbors.[12] Cell thickness equals that of the nuclei. With endothe-

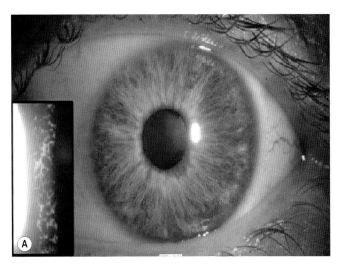
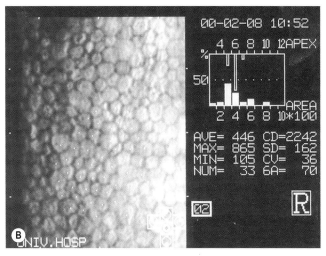

Figure 5.1 (A) Fuchs' endothelial corneal dystrophy showing stromal edema. Corner image displays a specular reflection photomicrograph showing endothelial cells that are large and disrupted by numerous guttata. (B) Specular microscopy image of corneal endothelium in Fuchs' endothelial corneal dystrophy demonstrating polymegethism and pleomorphism as a result of decreased endothelial cell density.

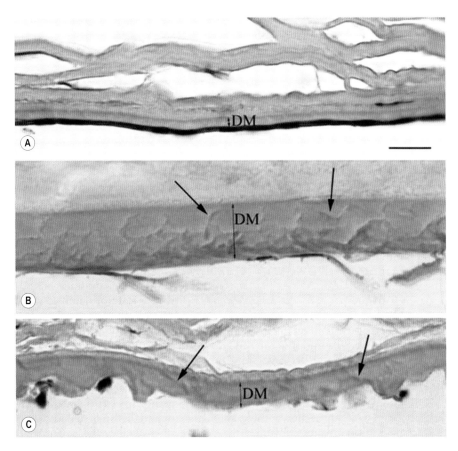

Figure 5.2 Morphologic changes in control and Fuchs' endothelial corneal dystrophy (FECD) corneas. Hematoxylin and eosin staining with bright-field microscopy. (A) Control cornea from a 30-year-old patient with keratoconus who had a healthy, normal Descemet's membrane (DM). Corneal endothelial cells were darkly stained and well aligned. (B) Early-onset FECD *COL8A2* L450W mutant, showing prominent network of wrinkle-like structures (arrows). Remaining endothelium on the posterior face (bottom) shows cytoplasmic degenerative changes. No posterior excrescences were visible in this or other sections. (C) Late-onset FECD cornea, showing refractile structures in the anterior and central portion of the DM (arrows). Prominent focal excrescences were present on the posterior surface of the DM. A few degenerated endothelial cells were present between the excrescences. Bar, 20 µm. (Reproduced with permission from Gottsch JD, Zhang C, Sundin O, et al. Fuchs corneal dystrophy: aberrant collagen distribution in an L450W mutant of the *COL8A2* gene. Invest Ophthalmol Vis Sci 2005;46:4504–4511.)

lial attenuation, the number of cells first decreases, then the cytoplasm thins, and finally the nuclei thin to adopt a progressively flattened shape.[12]

In FECD, several factors may contribute to corneal edema, though the primary cause of this endothelial dysfunction is unknown. Homeostasis of fluid across the posterior surface of the cornea is thought to occur as a result of the pump leak model.[10,13] A decreased number of endothelial cells may result in fewer sites of pump action. In addition, the attenu-ation of cell cytoplasm as cells spread and enlarge horizontally to cover Descemet's membrane may decrease the barrier function of the endothelium. Decreased pump activity within the endothelium has been identified (Figure 5.3).[14,15] Recent studies have shown advanced glycation end products (AGEs) in corneal endothelium, suggesting a possible role for oxidative stress and AGEs in FECD pathogenesis.[16] Keratin expression not normally seen in endothelium has been noted in patients with FECD as well as other conditions of

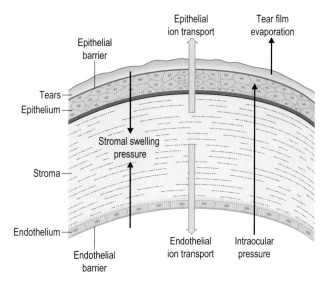

Figure 5.3 Diagram of Fuchs' endothelial corneal dystrophy pathophysiology, demonstrating increased stromal swelling pressure, resulting in corneal edema as a result of decreased pump activity in diseased corneal endothelium.

endothelial stress, though this may represent an epiphenomenon of the endothelial pathology.[17] Studies of aquaporins, a family of transport molecules, show a decreased expression of aquaporin 1 in both FECD and PCE corneas but increased aquaporin 3 and 4 in PCE alone, suggesting a role for these molecules in FECD which differs from that in PCE.[18] Similar findings occurred in thermally induced endothelial dysfunction in mice.[19] Most recently, ultrastructural studies of three cases of early-onset FECD showed swollen mitochondria, a sign of cell stress.[20]

Guttae formation and progression can be identified with slit-lamp biomicroscopy, specular microscopy, and confocal microscopy (Box 5.1; stage 1). Pachymetry can document the increased corneal thickness due to edema and fluorophotometry can demonstrate the loss of barrier and pump function.[21] Histopathologically, the edema fluid separates the corneal lamellae and forms "fluid lakes." The separation of collagen fibrils leads to loss of corneal transparency. As the disease progresses, the edema fluid enters the epithelium, resulting in an irregular epithelial surface. The edema varies from slight bedewing to frank bullae formation (Box 5.1; stage 2). Mild-to-moderate corneal guttae can remain as such for years without affecting vision. As the disease advances, vascular connective tissue is formed under and in the epithelium (Box 5.1; stage 3). This condition is followed by extremely limited visual acuity (Box 5.1; stage 4) and secondary complications (e.g., epithelial erosions, microbial keratitis, corneal vascularization).

Descemet's membrane in FECD

Descemet's membrane is divided into two layers: an anterior banded layer (ABL) laid down during embryogenesis, and a posterior nonbanded layer (PNBL) which represents the progressively thickening basement membrane of the endothelium throughout life.[22-24] At birth, the thickness of the ABL averages 3 μm and stays relatively constant throughout life. It acquires an intricate laminar structure formed from the

extracellular matrix secreted by endothelial cells. The ABL contains large, regularly spaced bands of collagen VIII. In contrast to the ABL, the PNBL continues to thicken throughout life, averaging 2 μm at 10 years and 10 μm at 80 years.[21] In prenatal development, the expression of short filaments is observed perpendicular to the plane of the anterior layer of Descemet's membrane. Transmission electron microscopy has shown these filaments to have a striated or banded pattern forming the ABL. The deposition of nonstriated material continues with age and forms the PNBL.[13,25]

The structure of Descemet's membrane is adversely affected by the FECD disease process (Figure 5.4). The ABL thickness in both normal corneas and those affected by late-onset FECD ranges from 3 to 4 μm. However, in early-onset FECD, the ABL can be as thick as 38 μm.[20] The PBNL of Descemet's membrane is the most prominent structure affected in late-onset FECD, accounting for the majority of the increase in thickness along with the corneal guttae. Unlike late-onset FECD, the PNBL in early-onset disease is similar to normal corneas, except for the presence of rare

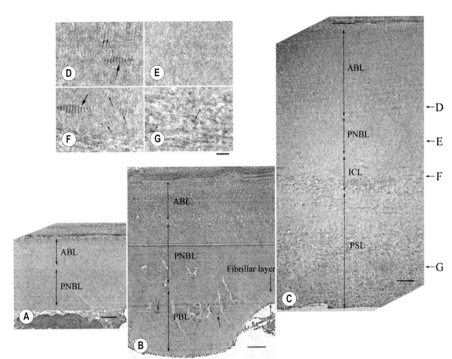

Figure 5.4 Ultrastructure of Descemet's membrane of normal, late-onset Fuchs' endothelial corneal dystrophy (FECD), and early-onset FECD as represented by the L450W mutant. Transverse sections of Descemet's membrane from (A) normal control; (B) late-onset FECD; and (C) early-onset FECD. Arrows and letters, to the right of (c) indicate layers of origin for the higher-magnification images (D–G). (D) Anterior banded layer (ABL), at its bottom edge. (E) Detail of posterior nonbanded layer (PNBL). (F) Internal collagenous layer (ICL) showing disorganized wide-banded collagen (arrows), and adjacent electron-dense fibrous material (bottom). (G) Posterior striated layer (PSL). (Reproduced with permission from Gottsch JD, Zhang C, Sundin O, et al. Fuchs corneal dystrophy: aberrant collagen distribution in an L450W mutant of the *COL8A2* gene. Invest Ophthalmol Vis Sci 2005;46:4504–4511.)

strips of widely spaced collagen. This layer is accompanied by a unique 2-µm internal collagenous layer (ICL) characterized by widely spaced collagen strips and a 12-µm posterior striated layer. Wide-spaced type VIII collagen was found to be the major structural component to Descemet's membrane in both the ABL and PBNL of normal, early-onset FECD, and late-onset FECD corneas.[26] A loose fibrillar layer can also be found between the PNBL and the endothelial cells.[8,27] The fibrillar layer seems to be thicker in corneas with more decompensation as there is presumably more fluid accumulation through diseased endothelial tight junctions.

Immunohistochemical analysis of the expression of collagen and associated proteins in FECD has been an important area of study. Collagen IV, fibronectin, and laminin are key components of the basal lamina of many different tissues, including Descemet's membrane.[28–32] Disparities with respect to the distribution of collagen, laminin, and fibronectin between normal corneas and those affected by FECD have also been identified.[20] In the normal cornea, highly periodic structures in Descemet's membrane contain both alpha-1 and alpha-2 subunits of collagen VIII.[20] Both subunits remain constant throughout normal corneas, suggesting that they were co-assembled in a structure with a well-defined composition. In both early-onset and late-onset FECD, this regular distribution is adversely affected. In early-onset FECD, the L450W mutant of *COL8A2* loses its periodic structure in Descemet's membrane. Furthermore, co-assembly of *COL8A1* and *COL8A2* does not occur in an organized fashion, as certain areas contain more of one subtype than another. In late-onset FECD, differences in the distribution of *COL8A1* and *COL8A2* in the PNBL of Descemet's membrane can also be detected immunohistochemically via increased expression of *COL8A1* and a less intense expression of *COL8A2*.[20] *COL8A2* was also identified in the abnormal ribosomes of endothelial cells in early-onset FECD patients, suggesting these cells as its source and thus the primary cause of FECD. Both forms of FECD are

probably associated with abnormal assembly and turnover of collagen VIII within the specialized extracellular matrix.[20]

Stroma, Bowman's layer, and epithelium

A variety of findings have been reported in the tissue anterior to Descemet's membrane/endothelium of FECD corneas. With associated endothelial dysfunction in FECD diffuse edema occurs with swelling in the interlamellar spaces of stromal collagen. As the dysfunction worsens edema fluid interposes below the epithelium, causing bullae and raising the epithelium off Bowman's layer and even intercellular epithelial edema. More recently, evidence for apoptosis has been identified using terminal uridine deoxynucleotidyl transferase dUTP nick end labeling (TUNEL) methodology in the epithelium, stroma, and endothelium of FECD corneas. The significance of these findings as primary or consequent to an underlying abnormality remains to be determined.[33] Similarly, nonspecific alteration of extracellular matrix proteins has been suggested; however, its role is not completely understood.[33]

Etiology

Recently a molecular basis for FECD has begun to be understood. There appear to be distinct pathogenic mutations resulting in the respective phenotypes of early-onset and late-onset FECD. Both disease types vary in the specific genes that are affected. Pathogenic mutations in *COL8A2* gene[2,3] which encodes the alpha2 subtype of collagen VIII, a major component of Descemet's membrane,[26,28,34] have been identified as the cause of early-onset FECD.[20] Mutations in these genes have not been implicated in late-onset disease. For late-onset FECD, other genetic, physiological, and environmental factors may play a role in pathogenesis as there is a consistent ratio of 2.5:1.0 of affected females to males.

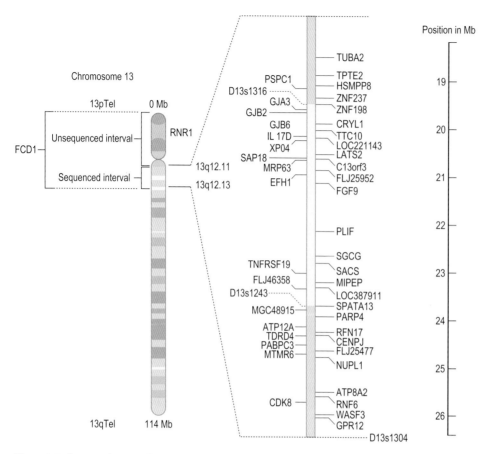

Figure 5.5 Genes in the *FCD1* disease interval. Ideogram of human chromosome 13, with *FCD1* interval indicated by vertical bracket. 13pTel, 13qTel indicate p and q telomeres, with nucleotide positions of 0–114 million basepairs. *FCD1* is represented by the first 7.6 million basepairs of chromosome 13. (Modified from Sundin OH, Jun AS, Broman KW, et al. Linkage of late-onset Fuchs corneal dystrophy to a novel locus at 13pTel-13q12.13. Invest Ophthalmol Vis Sci 2006;47:140–145.)

Approximately 50% of clinical patients with FECD have siblings, parents, or offspring who are also affected.[2,35] *FCD1* gene at 13pTel-13q12.13 (Figure 5.5) was the first genetic locus identified for late-onset FECD.[36] The defect in the gene may be a noncoding region promoter mutation that causes changes in mRNA levels. It has followed mendelian inheritance as a single autosomal-dominant trait. *FCD2* at 18q21 (Figure 5.6) was the second genetic locus identified for late-onset FECD.[37] This locus was found in three large families, indicating its potential widespread involvement in late-onset FECD. There was incomplete penetrance with a high phenocopy rate, indicating that other environmental and/or genetic factors may play a role for the inherited disease trait.[37] The defect in the *FCD2* genetic locus leading to late-onset FECD has not yet been identified. Mutations in the *SLC4A11* gene, recently found in patients with recessive congenital hereditary endothelial dystrophy (CHED II), may also be implicated in late-onset FECD. Four heterozygous mutations, three missense mutations (E399K, G709E, and T754M), and one deletion mutation (c.99–100delTC) were recognized in a screen of 89 FECD patients. Missense proteins encoded by the mutants were defective in localization to the cell surface and may play a role in FECD pathology.[38] Late-onset FECD is now recognized as a multifactorial disease with a complex genetic etiology. In an effort to find genetic loci causing susceptibility to disease, several groups have initiated compilations of large data sets of families and case-control sets.

Most ongoing investigations have used the Krachmer grading system or a modified version to classify disease into a semi-quantitative scale.[35,39,40]

Clinical diagnosis and evaluation of FECD

Clinical diagnosis of FECD is initially made by the presence of central corneal guttae. As the disease progresses, corneal haziness due to stromal thickening, subepithelial bullae, and Descemet's folds may be seen. Further analysis with specular or confocal microscopy characterizes the baseline state and progression of guttae formation, decrease in endothelial cell density, and increase in endothelial pleomorphism and polymegethism (Figure 5.1B). Corneal pachymetry, as measured ultrasonically or optically, with specular, confocal microscopy, or optical coherence tomography, is an effective method of measuring an increase in corneal edema and the progression of the disease.[41] Presence of Descemet's folds, epithelial edema, and thickness greater than 0.62 mm indicates potential corneal decompensation.[42] However, with our greater appreciation of the varying thickness in normal corneas without stromal edema, the clinician must correlate pachymetric changes with patient symptoms and slit-lamp findings as regards worsening of the disease.

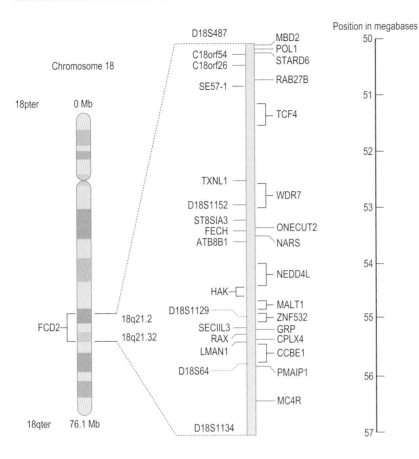

Figure 5.6 Gene interval of the chromosome 18 *FCD2* locus based on haplotypes of a kindred as identified by Sundin et al (Sundin OH, Broman K, Chang H, et al. A common locus for late-onset Fuchs corneal dystrophy maps to 18q21.2-q21.32. Invest Ophthalmol Vis Sci 2006;47:3919–3926.) *FCD2* is represented by approximately 7 million basepairs between 18q21.2 and 18q21.32. (Modified from Sundin OH, Broman K, Chang H, et al. A common locus for late-onset Fuchs corneal dystrophy maps to 18q21.2-q21.32. Invest Ophthalmol Vis Sci 2006;47:3919–3926.)

Until recently the pathologic diagnosis of FECD was based on evaluation of full-thickness corneal buttons which demonstrated overall thickening, endothelial attenuation, central guttae formation, thickening of Descemet's membrane (Figure 5.7), varying degrees of diffuse or focal stromal edema, and varying degrees of epithelial edema with or without subepithelial bullae. With the advent of endothelial keratoplasty procedures, pathologic diagnosis is typically limited to examination of the central portion of Descemet's membrane and the endothelium.[43] Nonetheless, the ability to diagnose FECD and to distinguish it reliably from similar conditions such as pseudophakic corneal edema remains, if appropriate techniques are utilized.[44]

Management

There is no current preventive treatment for the advancement of FECD. As we gain further understanding of the pathophysiology of the disorder based on ongoing genetic, biochemical, and immunohistochemical studies, future treatments will become available, obviating the need for keratoplasty in advanced disease. Early symptomatic relief due to epithelial edema is aimed at increasing the osmolality of the tear film by using hypertonic solutions such as 5% sodium chloride.[45] Hypertonic ointments such as 5% sodium chloride used prior to sleeping can also increase tear film osmolality and decrease morning symptoms of blurred vision. In patients with more advanced corneal edema and bullous keratopathy, a bandage contact lens can be used to decrease irregular astigmatism and alleviate the pain caused by the bullae.[46] In patients with increased intraocular pressure, treatment with topical ß-blockers or α-agonists may be of benefit, as a temporary reduction in corneal edema can be achieved by lowering intraocular pressure[47]; topical carbonic anhydrase inhibitors should be avoided since they potentially contribute to the endothelial dysfunction in the disorder.[48] In cases of advanced corneal edema and scar formation associated with pain or corneal infection in which extenuating medical or social reasons for keratoplasty are not feasible, a total conjunctival flap is an option for pain relief and prevention of infection. However, visual restoration requires corneal transplantation.

Corneal transplantation is indicated when either corneal edema causes an unacceptable level of visual impairment or epithelial bullae cause incapacitating discomfort.[47] In patients with full-thickness corneal edema, a penetrating keratoplasty has been the gold standard to replace diseased endothelium, stroma, and epithelium. This procedure remains an important modality, particularly in more advanced cases where there is structural and irreversible damage to the stroma and subepithelial areas of the cornea. However, delayed healing, postoperative astigmatism, and risk for traumatic wound rupture have led to increasing interest in the use of endothelial keratoplasty procedures, most recently Descemet stripping endothelial keratoplasty (DSEK) or its automated method (DSAEK) as a surgical alternative. Early results are promising as the absence of corneal surface incisions and sutures preserves normal corneal topography, minimizing astigmatism, providing more rapid visual recovery, and preventing traumatic wound and suture-related infection problems.[49] The incidence of graft rejection may

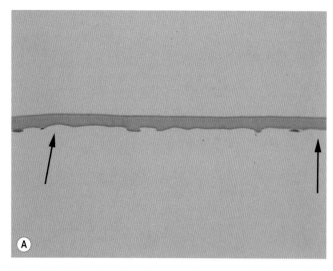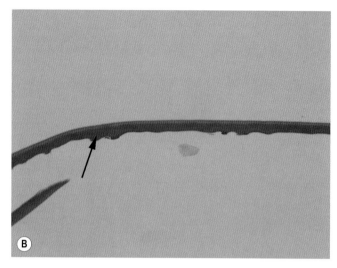

Figure 5.7 (A) Specimen from Descemet stripping endothelial keratoplasty (DSEK) procedure, showing guttae and loss and attenuation of endothelial cell nucleus. Anterior banded layer is seen along upper surface. Hematoxylin and eosin × 400. (B) Specimen from DSEK procedure, showing guttae and attenuated endothelial cell nucleus. Anterior banded layer is seen along upper surface. PAS × 400.

also be lower with DSEK,[50] but further long-term large-scale studies are indicated to address this question. Concerns about higher primary donor failure rates and greater long-term endothelial cell loss compared to penetrating keratoplasty also exist. Nevertheless, the initial recognized benefits, particularly for less advanced disease prior to permanent structural changes to the stroma and subepithelial area, make these endothelial keratoplasty procedures most appealing.

The management of patients with both FECD and cataract requires an assessment of the contribution of each condition to the visual loss, dictating what procedure(s) are to be performed.

Conclusion

There is still relatively little known about the pathophysiology and genetic basis for FECD. Recent discoveries have yielded novel theories as to its disease process. A pathogenic mutation in COL8A2 has been identified as the cause of early-onset FECD.[2,3] Late-onset FECD is a multifactorial disease with potential genetic and environmental factors playing a role in the disease process. Current ongoing investigations have been encouraging, with several genetic loci being identified among large sets of families.[36–38] We are currently conducting a large multisite study characterizing the phenotype, obtaining blood samples for DNA, and pathological specimens to confirm the phenotype in the index case in FECD families. We also have a case control group in order to conduct a dense genome-wide search for disease genes using high-density single nucleotide polymorphism marker sets coupled with modern statistical genetic methodology. Discovery of susceptibility genes will inform the biology, enable early detection of mutation carriers, and spawn the possibility of genetic therapy as a preventive treatment modality for the disease.

Acknowledgments

The authors wish to thank Stefan Trocme, MD, for his careful review and contributions to this manuscript; John Gottsch, MD, for allowing publication of previously published figures; and the use of the core facilities of the Visual Sciences Research Center, supported by P30 EY11373.

Key references

A complete list of chapter references is available online at www.expertconsult.com. See inside cover for registration details.

1. Fuchs E. Dystrophia epithelialis corneae. Graefes Arch Clin Exp Ophthalmol 1910;76:468–478.

2. Gottsch JD, Sundin OH, Liu S, et al. Inheritance of a novel COL8A2 mutation defines a distinct early-onset subtype of Fuchs' corneal dystrophy. Invest Ophthalmol Vis Sci 2005;46:1934–1939.

3. Biswas S, Munier FL, Yardley J, et al. Missense mutations in COL8A2, the gene encoding the alpha2 chain of type VIII collagen, cause two forms of corneal endothelial dystrophy. Hum Mol Genet 2001;10:2415–2423.

7. Wilson SE, Bourne WM, O'Brien PC, et al. Endothelial function and aqueous humor flow rate in patients with Fuchs' dystrophy. Am J Ophthalmol 1988;106:270–278.

11. Geroski DH, Matsuda M, Yee RW, et al. Pump function of the human corneal endothelium. Ophthalmology 1985;92:1–6.

13. Waring GO, Bourne WM, Edelhauser HF, et al. The corneal endothelium; normal and pathologic structure and

function. Ophthalmology 1982;89:531–590.

20. Gottsch JD, Zhang C, Sundin O, et al. Fuchs' corneal dystrophy: aberrant collagen distribution in an L450W mutant of the *COL8A2* gene. Invest Ophthalmol Vis Sci 2005;46:4504–4511.

35. Krachmer JH, Purcell JJ Jr, Young CW, et al. Corneal endothelial dystrophy: a study of 64 families. Arch Ophthalmol 1978;96:2036–2039.

36. Sundin OH, Broman K, Chang H, et al. A common locus for late-onset Fuchs' corneal dystrophy maps to 18q21.2-q21.32. Invest Ophthalmol Vis Sci 2006; 47:3919–3926.

37. Sundin OH, Jun AS, Broman KW, et al. Linkage of late-onset Fuchs' corneal dystrophy to a novel locus at 13pTel-13q12.13. Invest Ophthalmol Vis Sci 2006;47:140–145.

39. Iyengar SK, Shaffer S, Kluge A, et al. Analysis of mutations in the gene for the alpha 2 chain of type VIII collagen. (*COL8A2*) in families and cases with Fuchs' endothelial corneal dystrophy. Available online at: www.ARVO.org, 2005.

40. Afshari NA, Li YJ, Pericak-Vance MA, et al. Genome wide linkage scan in Fuchs' endothelial corneal dystrophy. Invest Ophthalmol Vis Sci 2009;50(3):1093–1097.

46. Wilson SE, Bourne WM. Fuchs' dystrophy. Cornea 1988;7:2–18.

49. Terry MA, Shamie N, Chen ES, et al. Precut tissue for Descemet's stripping automated endothelial keratoplasty: vision, astigmatism, and endothelial survival. Ophthalmology 2009;116(2): 248–256.

50. Price MO, Jordon CS, Moore G, et al. Graft rejection episodes after Descemet stripping with endothelial keratoplasty: part two: the statistical analysis of probability and risk factors. Br J Ophthalm 2009;93(3):391–395.

CHAPTER 6

Keratoconus

M Cristina Kenney and Ronald N Gaster

Clinical background

Key symptoms and signs

Keratoconus (KC) is a slowly progressive, noninflammatory condition in which there is central thinning of the cornea, changing it from dome-shaped to cone-shaped. KC comes from the Greek words *kerato*, meaning cornea, and *conus*, meaning cone. KC causes the cornea to become thinner centrally or inferiorly with resultant gradual bulging outward (Figure 6.1).

Patients with KC initially notice blurring and distortion of vision (Box 6.1). They may also complain about photophobia, glare, disturbed night vision, and headaches from eyestrain. As KC progresses, patients are increasingly myopic and astigmatism can become more irregular. KC is a bilateral condition, though usually asymmetric in severity and progression. In the early stages of the disease, KC is not visible to the naked eye. However, in the later stages of progression, the cone-shaped cornea can be visible to an observer when the patient looks down while the upper lid is raised. The pointed cornea will push the lower lid out in the area of the cone like a V-shaped dent in the lower lid. This anterior protrusion seen in the lower lid is called Munson's sign (Figure 6.2). Fleischer's ring is a partial or complete iron deposition ring in the deep epithelium encircling the base of the KC cone. It appears yellow to dark brown in color and is best seen with the cobalt blue light at the slit lamp. Rizutti's sign is a conical reflection on the nasal cornea when light is shined from the temporal side. Vogt's striae may be seen in the deep stroma of the apex of the cone.

Historical development

KC has been recognized since the 1750s and was first carefully described and differentiated from other ectatic conditions in the 1850s. Diagnosis of KC, especially in its early forms (forme fruste KC), has been greatly improved with the development of videokeratography and algorithms which allow quantification of the topographical surface and identification of the KC phenotypes.

Epidemiology

KC is the commonest corneal dystrophy in the USA, affecting approximately 1 in 2000 people. Although KC occurs spo-radically in most individuals, approximately 6–10% have a hereditary component since it is reported in multiple generations of families and identical twins.[1-6] If a first-degree relative has KC then the prevalence of other family members developing KC is approximately 3.34%, which is significantly higher than the general population.[7] It affects people of all races and both sexes, though there is a slight female preponderance.

Diagnostic workup

Corneal distortion with KC is seen on retinoscopy, keratometry, keratoscopy, and computed corneal topography (Figure 6.3). There is often localized, abnormal inferior or central corneal steepening. This results in asymmetry with a large refractive power difference across the surface of the cornea. Some ophthalmologists use the inferior–superior (I-S) value when determining if KC is present on corneal topography. This measurement determines differences in corneal refractive power between inferior and superior points on the cornea and may aid in determining if KC is present or may develop in the future.

Gene array analyses of KC corneas have demonstrated altered levels of alpha-enolase, beta-actin, aquaporin 5, and desmoglein 3,[8-10] some of which have been proposed as molecular markers for KC. However, at the present time markers are not used routinely in clinical practice for diagnosis.

Treatment

Management of KC usually begins with spectacle correction, if possible. When eye glasses can no longer correct the condition as the astigmatism worsens, specially fitted contact lenses can often reduce the distortion from the irregular shape of the cornea (Box 6.2). Finding a KC contact lens specialist is important as frequent contact lens changes and checkups are usually required for good visual results. In advanced KC, when good vision can no longer be attained with contact lenses and/or the patient is intolerant of contact lens wear, penetrating keratoplasty is usually recommended. Approximately 10–20% of KC patients eventually require penetrating keratoplasty, and the success rate is greater than 90%, one of the highest for corneal transplantation. A new, major advancement in penetrating keratoplasty involves the use of the femtosecond laser to make the cuts in the donor and recipient corneas so that the fit between the two is more

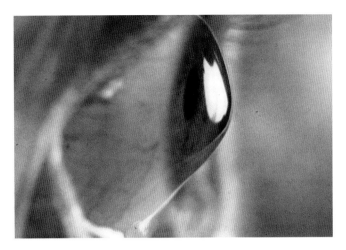

Figure 6.1 Keratoconus cornea showing cone-like protrusion.

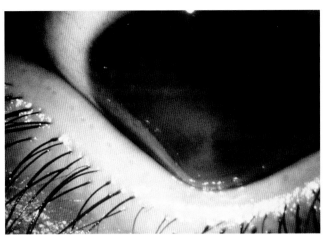

Figure 6.2 Munson's sign in keratoconus cornea showing V-shaped protrusion of lower lid when the patient looks down.

Box 6.1 Key symptoms and signs

- Keratoconus is a slowly progressive, noninflammatory condition that involves central or inferior thinning of the cornea, changing it from dome-shaped to cone-shaped
- Keratoconus affects approximately 1 in 2000 people in the USA. Most cases are sporadic but approximately 6–10% have a hereditary component for this ocular disorder[1-6]
- Keratoconus can be diagnosed by retinoscopy, keratometry, keratoscopy, and computed corneal topography
- Munson's sign, Fleischer's ring, Rizutti's sign, and Vogt's striae are signs of keratoconus

---

precise. This new development has shown great promise for penetrating keratoplasty for KC where there is improved wound healing, faster visual recovery, and quicker removal of sutures postoperatively. Another relatively new treatment option is the placement of intracorneal polymethyl methacrylate (PMMA) segments (Intacs, Addition Technology) inserted into the mid-stroma of the more peripheral cornea in an attempt to flatten the cone. Some patients still require contact lenses in order to attain functional vision after placement of Intacs.

Corneal collagen cross-linking is a new treatment concept which involves applying photosensitizing riboflavin (vitamin B$_2$) eye drops to the de-epithelialized cornea and then exposing the eye to ultraviolet A light. Researchers have found a significant increase in corneal rigidity in animal eyes following this treatment regimen. Early studies in KC patients have shown that progression of KC was halted after this cross-linking treatment. Randomized controlled trials to investigate the safety and efficacy of this treatment are under way at this time.

Prognosis and complications

KC usually has its onset during puberty, with a gradual and irregular progression over approximately 20 years. The rate of progression and severity of the condition are quite variable, ranging from mild astigmatism to severe corneal thinning, protrusion, and scarring. In advanced KC, there may be a rupture in Descemet's membrane, causing sudden

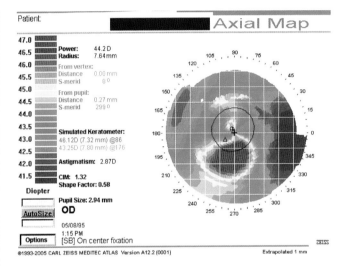

Figure 6.3 Corneal topography showing steepening and distortion of keratoconus cornea.

Box 6.2 Treatments

- Treatment for most patients includes specially fitted contact lenses
- Approximately 10–20% of keratoconus patients eventually require penetrating keratoplasty and the success rate is greater than 90%
- Recent advancements in penetrating keratoplasty involve the use of the femtosecond laser to make precise cuts in the donor and recipient corneas to improve their fit
- Another new treatment option is the placement of intracorneal polymethyl methacrylate (PMMA) segments (Intacs, Addition Technology) into the midstroma of the peripheral cornea in an attempt to flatten the cone
- Corneal collagen cross-linking is a new treatment concept which involves applying photosensitizing riboflavin (vitamin B$_2$) eye drops to the de-epithelialized cornea and then exposing the eye to ultraviolet A light
- Controlled trials are under way to investigate the safety and efficacy of this ultraviolet cross-linking procedure

---

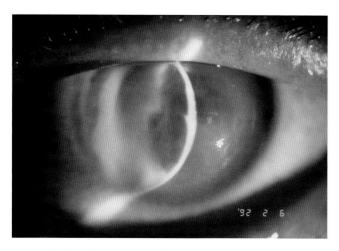

Figure 6.4 Acute hydrops in acute keratoconus cornea.

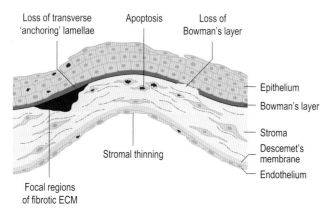

Figure 6.5 Schematic of the pathology of keratoconus corneas. ECM, extracellular matrix.

clouding of vision due to acute stromal or epithelial edema, called acute corneal hydrops (Figure 6.4). Topical corticosteroid and 5% NaCl drops are usually used to treat the acute hydrops episode. This condition often resolves over weeks to months and may result in central corneal scarring or flattening.

Pathology

Loss of Bowman's layer and stromal thinning

A hallmark histological feature of the KC cornea is focal regions where the Bowman's layer is absent and the epithelial cells are in direct contact with the underlying stroma (Figure 6.5). These sites also show decreased levels of fibronectin, laminin, entactin, type IV collagen, and type XII collagen (Box 6.3).[11-13] In areas of active disease, the stromal extracellular matrix (ECM) demonstrates elevated levels of type III collagen, tenascin-C, fibrillin-1, and keratocan,[11,12,14,15] but many of these changes are nonspecific and can also be found in general wound-healing processes. Most interestingly, the ECM abnormalities in KC corneas are not uniform. The corneal stroma can lose more than half its normal thickness and have deposits of fibrotic ECM while in an adjacent,

thicker region the matrix patterns are normal. In addition, there is variability in the epithelial thickness, with some areas having only 1–3 cell layers and other regions appearing completely normal.

KC corneas are unusually thin and pliable. Biochemical studies reported decreased total protein and sulfated proteoglycan levels, normal collagen cross-linking, and variable total collagen content.[16-19] Recent studies showed that stromal lamellar slippage may contribute to the thinning and anterior protrusion of KC corneas.[20-22]

Apoptosis in keratoconus

Apoptosis is the process by which cells undergo an organized, programmed cell death. KC corneas have increased levels of apoptosis associated with the anterior stromal keratocytes,[23-25] epithelial cells, and endothelial cells[24] (Figure 6.5). Erie and coworkers[26] showed an even greater decline in keratocyte density in KC patients using contact lenses. The KC corneas have elevated levels of leukocyte common antigen-related protein (LAR),[27] a transmembrane phosphotyrosine phosphatase that stimulates apoptosis, and cathepsins G, B, and V/L2,[28-31] which represent a caspase-independent pathway for apoptosis. Cathepsins mediate apoptosis by triggering mitochondrial dysfunction, cleaving Bid and releasing cytochrome c.[32-35] Furthermore, KC corneas have decreased levels of tissue inhibitors of metalloproteases, TIMP-1 and TIMP-3, which can modulate apoptosis.[36-38] Finally, the moderate to severe atopy and vigorous eye rubbing often found in KC patients may contribute to apoptosis since studies showed that chronic, repetitive injury to the corneal epithelium stimulates anterior stromal cell apoptosis.[39-41]

Enzyme activities in human corneas

It is generally accepted that KC stromal thinning is associated with increased activities in ECM-degrading enzymes. In the early 1960s it was noted that KC corneas had degraded epithelial basement membranes and increased gelatinase activities.[42-44] It was subsequently demonstrated that KC corneas have increased levels of lysosomal enzymes (acid esterase, acid phosphatase, acidic lipase), cathepsins G, B, and VL2, matrix metalloproteinase-2 (MMP-2) and MT1-MMP (MMP-14) which can degrade many forms of ECM.[28-31,45-50] Moreover, many of the naturally occurring inhibitors for those enzyme families are found in lower levels.[28,38,47,51-53] In addition to corneal involvement, the conjunctiva of KC patients shows increased lysosomal enzyme activities.[54]

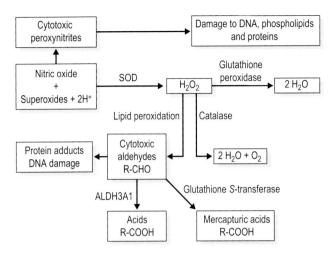

Figure 6.6 Schematic of the antioxidant corneal enzymes. SOD, superoxide dismutase; H_2O_2, hydrogen peroxide; ALDH$_3$, aldehyde dehydrogenase.

Box 6.4 Etiology

- Associations between keratoconus and atopy, which includes asthma, eczema, and hayfever, have been described
- Vigorous eye rubbing may contribute to the development of keratoconus
- Patients with trisomy 21 (Down syndrome) have a high incidence of keratoconus
- Keratoconus has an autosomal-dominant inheritance with variable penetration[94,95]
- At least 10 different chromosomes are linked to keratoconus[96-102]
- The genetics of keratoconus are complex and involve multiple genes

---

A major corneal function is to eliminate the reactive oxygen/nitrogen species (ROS/RNS) and aldehydes that are generated by ultraviolet light. For this purpose, the cornea possesses numerous antioxidant enzymes such as superoxide dismutases (SODs), catalase, aldehyde dehydrogenases (ALDH$_3$A1), glutathione reductase, glutathione S-transferase, and glutathione peroxidase (Figure 6.6).[31,55-60] When ROS/RNS are not eliminated, they can react with other molecules and form cytotoxic aldehydes and peroxynitrites. These antioxidant enzyme activities change with aging[61] and in response to cytokines and growth factors[58] and this can increase the susceptibility to oxidative damage. Many of the antioxidant enzymes of the lipid peroxidation and nitric oxide pathways are abnormal, suggesting their involvement in KC pathology.

Etiology

Environmental risk factors for keratoconus

Numerous studies report an association between KC and atopy, which includes asthma, eczema, and hayfever (Box 6.4).[62-67] Recently Kaya and coworkers provided evidence that KC patients with full or partial atopy have unique topo-graphical and pachymetric characteristics compared to KC patients without atopy.[68] However, some suggest that it is not so much that atopy per se leads to KC but it is the associated vigorous eye rubbing which contributes to the development of KC. Many case reports exist in the literature describing persistent, vigorous eye rubbing and development of KC in children, patients with Down syndrome, and even adults with unilateral KC.[67,69-73] The Collaborative Longitudinal Evaluation of Keratoconus (CLEK) study also suggests that asymmetry in corneal curvature may be related to vigorous, unilateral eye rubbing that occurs in some KC patients.[74] It is likely that KC is influenced by both environmental factors and some genetic component.[75]

Genetic risk factors for keratoconus

KC can be found in 0.5–15% of trisomy 21 (Down syndrome) patients[76-78] and is less frequently associated with Ehlers–Danlos syndrome[79,80] and osteogenesis imperfecta.[81-83] Case reports show KC patients also having other ocular diseases such as Leber's congenital amaurosis, cataracts, granular corneal dystrophy, Avellino corneal dystrophy, and posterior polymorphous dystrophy.[84-93] However, the vast majority of KC patients do not have other ocular or systemic diseases.

Rabinowitz et al showed that KC has an autosomal-dominant inheritance with variable penetration.[94,95] At the present time, 10 different chromosomes have been linked to KC (21, 20q12, 20p11-q11, 18p, 17, 16q, 15q, 13, 5q14.3-q21.1, 3p14-q13, 2p24)[96-102] but at least 50 candidate genes have been excluded as playing a role in development of KC.[101,103,104] A Japanese study showed that three human leukocyte antigens (HLA-A26, B40, and DR9) were associated with early-onset KC.[105] A defect in the *SOD1* gene on chromosome 21 has also been linked to KC.[106] It is controversial as to whether the homeobox gene *VSX1* is associated with KC. Novel mutations of *VSX1* were reported in a patient with both KC and posterior polymorphism dystrophy[90] and in a series of individual KC patients.[107] However, another study reported a single nondisease-causing polymorphism of Asp144Glu and concluded that the *VSX1* gene lacked association with KC.[108] The expression of *VSX1* occurs during wound healing as myofibroblasts differentiate[109] and may play a role in abnormal stromal repair processes.

The genetics of KC are complex and involve multiple genes. As seen in other diseases, the general KC phenotype may result from defects in a variety of genes that are all related to a final common pathway. Further investigations will be required to clarify the contributions of the genetic and environmental components to the development and progression of KC.

Pathophysiology

The biological basis of oxidative damage in keratoconus corneas

KC corneas have numerous signs of oxidative damage (Table 6.1 and Box 6.5) with increased levels of cytotoxic aldehydes from the lipid peroxidation pathway, ROS (superoxides, hydrogen peroxide, and hydroxyl radicals) and RNS (nitric

Table 6.1 Oxidative stress elements in keratoconus corneas (data from references[31,55–57,106,110,111,118])

Decreased
 Aldehyde dehydrogenase
 Extracellular superoxide dismutase activity

Altered
 Superoxide dismutase 1 gene

Increased
 Glutathione *S*-transferase
 Catalase
 Inducible nitric oxide synthase
 Peroxynitrites
 Damage to mtDNA
 Reactive oxygen/nitrogen species production

Box 6.5 Oxidative damage in keratoconus

- Keratoconus corneas are defective in their ability to process and eliminate reactive oxygen/nitrogen species, which causes oxidative damage[55–57,110]
- A number of antioxidant enzymes are abnormal in keratoconus corneas
- Oxidative elements can alter cellular structure and function by reacting with the proteins, DNA, and lipids
- The cultured keratoconus fibroblasts demonstrate inherent, hypersensitive responses to oxidative stressors[118]
- Keratoconus involves multiple molecular and biochemical events, all related to a "final common pathway" that yields the keratoconus phenotype

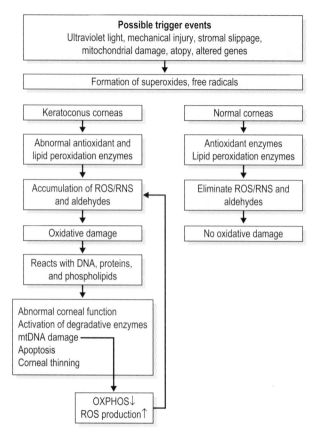

Figure 6.7 The elimination of reactive oxygen/nitrogen species (ROS/RNS) and aldehydes in keratoconus corneas compared to normal corneas.

---

oxide and peroxynitrite) (Figure 6.6).[55–57,110] These elements can alter cellular structure and function by reacting with the proteins, DNA, and lipids (Figure 6.7).

Mitochondria are specialized organelles that provide energy for the cells through oxidative phosphorylation (OXPHOS) and possess their own unique, circular DNA (mtDNA) which is maternally inherited. In KC corneas the mtDNA is extensively damaged.[111] The mtDNA codes for 13 OXPHOS proteins, 22 tRNAs, and 2 rRNAs[112] and its damage can lead to mitochondrial dysfunction, altered gene expression, oxidative damage, and apoptosis.[113–115] An important relationship exists between mitochondria, ROS/RNS production, and oxidative stress. During OXPHOS some electrons can "leak" from the electron transport chain, form superoxides, and subsequently large levels of endogenous ROS/RNS are produced that cause further damage to the mitochondria. This "vicious cycle" of mitochondrial damage and ROS/RNS production feeds back to damage the cells further (Figure 6.7).[116,117] This damaging cycle may be at play since these same components (mtDNA damage, ROS/RNS production, and apoptosis) are present in the KC cells.

Cultured KC fibroblasts demonstrate inherent, hypersensitive responses to oxidative stressors that include mtDNA damage, increased ROS production, mitochondrial dysfunction, and apoptosis.[118] If the KC cells are innately hypersensitive then increased environmental stress such as matrix substrate instability, vigorous eye rubbing, and/or atopy may trigger the hypersensitive cells to undergo exaggerated oxida-

tive response and cause oxidative damage. This may initiate a downstream cascade of events that include enzyme activation, rupture of lysosomes, induction of transcription factors, and cytokines along with altered regulation of genes that can play a role in KC.

The literature has multiple seemingly unrelated biochemical, molecular, and genetic alterations associated with KC. Therefore, it is unlikely that a single, primary defect causes KC but rather an involvement of multiple events all related to a "final common pathway" that yields the KC phenotype. A working hypothesis is that the oxidative stress pathway is the "final pathway" that ties together the multiple genes and biochemical events (Figure 6.7). The initial "trigger" event is unknown and may be a genetic defect(s) exacerbated by environmental factors. In any case KC corneas are defective in the ability to process and eliminate ROS/RNS and thereby undergo oxidative damage which cascades into "downstream" events, leading to corneal thinning and loss of vision.

The biological basis of corneal thinning in keratoconus

KC corneas exhibit extensive stromal thinning representing degradation of the normal ECM (Box 6.6). These corneas have multiple enzyme families which are activated and have a wide range of matrix substrates.[29,45–50,119] The triggers for

---

Box 6.6 Corneal thinning in keratoconus

- Increased activities in extracellular matrix-degrading enzymes and decreased levels of inhibitors play a role in the stromal thinning of keratoconus[28–31,38,45–53]
- Uneven distribution of the stromal lamellae and lack of "anchoring" fibrils may also play a role in keratoconus thinning and anterior protrusion[20–22,123,124]

Box 6.7 Prominent corneal nerves in keratoconus

- Clinically many keratoconus patients report significant ocular discomfort
- The nerves in keratoconus corneas show a lower density but have increased diameters and pathology[30,125–127]
- Transcription factors and signal transduction pathways may play a role in nerve abnormalities[128]

---

enzyme activation are not known but KC corneas have increased oxidative damage and abnormal cytokines and growth factors, some of which may activate these enzymes.

Normally a variety of inhibitors in the cornea regulate the enzyme activities. In KC corneas, the levels of α_2-macroglobulin, α_1-proteinase inhibitor, and TIMPs are decreased.[28,38,47,51–53] The α_2-macroglobulin inhibits trypsin, chymotrypsin, papain, collagenase, elastase, thrombin, plasmin, and kallikrein while the α_1-proteinase inhibitor can block the activities of trypsin, chymotrypsin, elastase, and plasmin and the TIMPs inhibit matrix metalloproteinases. KC corneas have elevated levels of Sp1 and Krüppel-like factor 6 (KLF6), transcription factors that can repress the promoter activity of the α_1-proteinase inhibitor.[120–122] However, the regulating mechanisms for the other inhibitors or degradative enzymes are still unclear.

It is proposed that stromal lamellar slippage may play a role in KC thinning and anterior protrusion. Confocal microscopy and X-ray scattering techniques revealed additional changes in the ECM structure of KC corneas.[20,21] Meek and coworkers showed that KC corneas have uneven distribution of the stromal lamellae, which may cause slippage of the interlamellar and intralamellar layers.[22] The KC corneas also lack "anchoring" lamellae that insert transversely for 120 μm into the Bowman's layer.[20] These interweaving anterior lamellae may help maintain the corneal shape and their loss could contribute to corneal lamellar slippage, stretching, and warpage.[123,124] Furthermore, lamellar slippage could cause biomechanical instability, leading to molecular stress of the cells.

The biological basis of prominent corneal nerves: role of the transcription factors and signal transduction pathways

By slit-lamp examination, a clinical feature of KC is enlarged, prominent corneal nerves which show specific pathologies (Box 6.7). Confocal microscopy demonstrated significantly lower density but increased diameter for corneal nerves in KC corneas.[125–127] KC corneas have elevated levels of the Sp3 repressor short proteins[128] which can decrease levels of nerve growth factor receptor, TrkA[NGFR], a critical protein for corneal sensitivity.[128] Furthermore, high levels of the cathepsins B

and G are intimately associated with nerves as they cross the Bowman's layer towards the epithelium, possibly contributing to the anterior stromal destruction.[30] Clinically many KC patients report significant ocular discomfort and these corneal nerve abnormalities may be contributing factors. However, further investigations are needed to determine if the nerve abnormalities are causative or a biological response to other factors.

Conclusions

KC is a slowly progressive, noninflammatory condition which causes the cornea to become thinner centrally or inferiorly, resulting in a "cone-like" shape. The onset is usually during puberty and the progression and severity are quite variable, ranging from mild astigmatism to severe corneal thinning, protrusion, and scarring. Traditional treatments include the use of specially fitted contact lenses, intracorneal PMMA segments (Intacs), and penetrating keratoplasty. Pathologic features of KC include loss of Bowman's layer, stromal thinning, corneal nerve abnormalities, apoptosis, and evidence of extensive oxidative damage. The development and progression of KC are likely influenced by both environmental and genetics factors. To date over 10 genes have been associated with KC and many diverse, seemingly unrelated biochemical and molecular events are abnormal. Therefore, it is likely that unknown "trigger" events in different molecular pathways finally converge into a "final common pathway" that yields the KC phenotype. Future studies should be aimed at identifying the initial "trigger" event, developing treatments to block the "final common pathway," and protect the cornea from oxidative damage that plays a role in the corneal thinning and loss of vision.

Acknowledgments

We gratefully acknowledge support from Discovery Eye Foundation, Schoellerman Charitable Foundation, Guenther Foundation, Iris and B. Gerald Cantor Foundation, Research to Prevent Blindness Foundation, and the National Keratoconus Foundation.

Key references

A complete list of chapter references is available online at www.expertconsult.com. See inside cover for registration details.

7. Wang Y, Rabinowitz YS, Rotter JI, et al. Genetic epidemiological study of keratoconus: evidence for major gene determination. Am J Med Genet 2000;93:403–409.

13. Cheng EL, Maruyama I, SundarRaj N, et al. Expression of type XII collagen and hemidesmosome-associated proteins in keratoconus corneas. Curr Eye Res 2001;22:333–340.

20. Morishige N, Wahlert AJ, Kenney MC, et al. Second-harmonic imaging microscopy of normal human and keratoconus cornea. Invest Ophthalmol Vis Sci 2007;48:1087–1094.

22. Meek KM, Tuft SJ, Huang Y, et al. Changes in collagen orientation and distribution in keratoconus corneas. Invest Ophthalmol Vis Sci 2005;46: 1948–1956.

48. Smith VA, Hoh HB, Littleton M, et al. Over-expression of a gelatinase A activity in keratoconus. Eye 1995;9:429–433.

53. Smith VA, Matthews FJ, Majid MA, et al. Keratoconus: matrix metalloproteinase-2 activation and TIMP modulation. Biochim Biophys Acta 2006;1762:431–439.

58. Olofsson EM, Marklund SL, Pedrosa-Domellof F, et al. Interleukin-1alpha downregulates extracellular-superoxide dismutase in human corneal keratoconus stromal cells. Mol Vis 2007;13:1285–1290.

68. Kaya V, Karakaya M, Utine CA, et al. Evaluation of the corneal topographic characteristics of keratoconus with orbscan II in patients with and without atopy. Cornea 2007;26:945–948.

74. Zadnik K, Steger-May K, Fink BA, et al. Between-eye asymmetry in keratoconus. Cornea 2002;21:671–679.

94. Rabinowitz YS, Maumenee IH, Lundergan MK, et al. Molecular genetic analysis in autosomal dominant keratoconus. Cornea 1992;11:302–308.

99. Tyynismaa H, Sistonen P, Tuupanen S, et al. A locus for autosomal dominant keratoconus: linkage to 16q22.3-q23.1 in Finnish families. Invest Ophthalmol Vis Sci 2002;43:3160–3164.

100. Brancati F, Valente EM, Sarkozy A, et al. A locus for autosomal dominant keratoconus maps to human chromosome 3p14-q13. J Med Genet 2004;41:188–192.

106. Udar N, Atilano SR, Brown DJ, et al. SOD1: a candidate gene for keratoconus. Invest Ophthalmol Vis Sci 2006;47:3345–3351.

111. Atilano SR, Coskun P, Chwa M, et al. Accumulation of mitochondrial DNA damage in keratoconus corneas. Invest Ophthalmol Vis Sci 2005;46:1256–1263.

128. de Castro F, Silos-Santiago I, Lopez de Armentia M, et al. Corneal innervation and sensitivity to noxious stimuli in trkA knockout mice. Eur J Neurosci 1998;10:146–152.

CHAPTER 7

Infectious keratitis

Michael S Gilmore, Susan R Heimer, and Ai Yamada

Infectious keratitis is characterized by corneal inflammation and defects caused by replicating bacteria, fungi, or protozoa. These infections can progress rapidly with devastating consequences, including corneal scarring and loss of vision. Thus, it is imperative to identify this condition promptly and begin an aggressive course of therapy to limit tissue damage. This chapter summarizes the current understanding of various clinical and pathophysiological aspects of infectious keratitis.

Clinical background

Key symptoms and signs

Clinical features of infectious keratitis include redness, tearing, edema, discharges, decreased vision, pain, and photophobia. The hallmark of keratitis is the appearance of diffuse or localized infiltrates within the corneal epithelium, stroma, and often the anterior chamber. Severe cases are denoted by necrotic ulceration of the epithelium and stroma.

Some clinical signs may be indicative of a particular infectious organism (Table 7.1).[1,2] Bacterial keratitis is often identified by the absence of epithelium and suppurative stromal infiltrates. Gram-negative bacterial infections are associated with hazy corneal rings and soup ulcerations, whereas Gram-positive infections tend to produce well-defined grayish-white infiltrates and localized ulcerations (Figures 7.1 and 7.2). Fungal keratitis generally exhibits a slow progression, satellite lesions, and elevated infiltrates with undefined, feathery edges (Figure 7.3). Some parasitic infections, like Acanthamoeba, are frequently misdiagnosed as fungal or viral because of the pseudodendritic appearance. In many cases, patients infected with parasites report disproportionate pain, which is characteristic of radial keratoneuritis (Figure 7.4).

Epidemiology and risk factors

Incidence rates, risk factors, and causative agents of keratitis vary geographically and socioeconomically. Incidence in the USA is estimated to be 11 in 100 000, whereas rates in South-East Asia are near 800 in 100 000.[3] The principal risk factors include trauma, contact or orthokeratology lens wear, ocular surface disease, ocular surgery, and systemic disease.

In Europe, Japan, and USA, contact lens wear constitutes the major risk factor for infectious keratitis.[4-6] Ocular trauma is the main predisposing factor in developing countries.[7]

Among contact lens-related infections, Staphylococcus spp., Streptococcus spp., and Pseudomonas aeruginosa are the leading causes in temperate climates.[4,6] In subtropical climates, like northern India, fungal keratitis has been strongly linked to contact lens wear, representing 20–30% of total isolates.[8] Although rare in temperate climates, there has been a recent increase in fungal and parasitic keratitis associated with contact lens wear involving Fusarium and Acanthamoeba.[9] These appear to be associated with specific contact lens care solutions and storage hygiene.

Infections due to ocular trauma are often attributed to fungal and mixed infections (fungi and bacteria).[7,10] Candida and other yeasts are commonly reported in temperate climates[10] and filamentous fungi, i.e., Aspergillus and Fusarium, in warmer climates.[8]

Diagnostic workup

Preliminary diagnoses are based on clinical signs, symptoms, and patient history. Noninvasive techniques, such as slit-lamp microscopy, confocal microscopy, and histological examination of impression cytology, are often used. If bacterial keratitis is suspected, empirically based therapies are started immediately without definitive information about the organism. It is always advisable to confirm the presence and identity of an infectious agent. This can be accomplished by examining corneal scrapings using standard diagnostic staining, culturing, immunochemistry, and polymerase chain reaction techniques (Table 7.2). Biopsies may be necessary if the disease is contained within the stroma. If the infectious agent is culturable, susceptibility profiles should be determined for optimizing treatment strategies.

Treatment, prognosis, and complications

Bacterial keratitis

If bacterial keratitis is suspected, therapies are often started before confirming the identity of the causative agent. For this reason, broad-spectrum antibiotics are used in single or combination therapies, such as: (1) fluoroquinolones; (2) fluoroquinolone with a cephalosporin; or (3) an aminogly-

Table 7.1 Clinical features of infectious keratitis

	Common pathogens	Distinguishing clinical features	Therapeutic strategies
Bacteria			
Gram-positive	*Staphylococcus* CNS (coagulase negative staphylococcus)	Localized ulcers: round or oval	
		Stromal infiltrates: discrete grayish-white	Fluoroquinolones
	Staphylococcus aureus	Stromal haze: minimal, distinct borders	Fluoroquinolones with cephalosporin
	Streptococcus pneumoniae		
Gram-negative	*Pseudomonas aeruginosa*	Undefined ulcers: soupy	
	Neisseria gonorrhoeae	Stromal infiltrates: dense and suppurative	Aminoglycosides with cephalosporin
		Stromal haze: intense immune rings	
Fungi			
Yeast	*Candida albicans*	Ulcers, epithelial defects	Polyenes
	Cryptococcus spp.	Stromal infiltrates: discrete grayish-white	
		Slow progression	Imidazoles
Filamentous	*Fusarium*	Slough: dry, elevated	Fluorinated pyrimidines
	Aspergillus	Stromal infiltrates: feathery margins	
		Satellite lesions	Imidazoles with fluorinated pyrimidine
Parasitic			
	Acanthamoeba spp.	Severe pain, radial keratoneuritis	Cationic antiseptics
	Microsporidia spp.	Stromal infiltrates: pseudodendritic	Aromatic diamidines
		Stromal haze: intense immune rings	Azoles

Data from Matsumoto[45] and Szliter et al.[42]

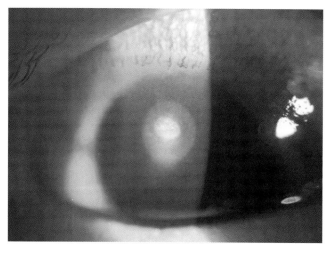

Figure 7.1 Contact lens-associated bacterial keratitis caused by *Staphylococcus aureus*. Note discrete infiltrates and minimal corneal haze. (Reprinted with permission of Macmillan Publishers from Whiting MAN, Raynor MK, Morgan PB et al. Continuous wear silicone hydrogel contact lenses and microbial keratitis. Eye 2004;18:935–937, copyright ©.)

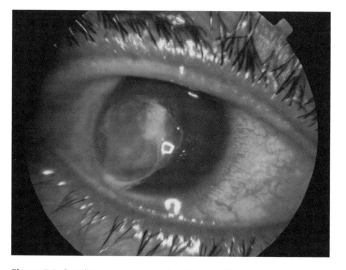

Figure 7.2 *Pseudomonas aeruginosa* keratitis in a silicone hydrogel contact lens wearer. Note the undefined soup ulceration. (Reprinted with permission of Macmillan Publishers from Whiting MAN, Raynor MK, Morgan PB et al. Continuous wear silicone hydrogel contact lenses and microbial keratitis. Eye 2004;18:935–937, copyright ©.)

coside combined with a cephalosporin (Table 7.1).[1] With the emergence of fluoroquinolone resistance among ocular isolates, progress on monotherapies should be monitored.[11] Regimens should be modified if improvement is not observed after 48 hours. To achieve optimal drug levels within the lesion, topical administration is highly recommended. Systemic administration should be considered if there is a risk of perforation, endophthalmitis, or evidence of scleritis. Topical corticosteroids can be used to modulate the inflammatory response; however, concern remains for the potentiation of bacterial growth.[1] In addition to antimicrobials, cycloplegic agents are used to inhibit synechia and pain as

needed. Penetrating keratoplasty should be considered in cases with extensive perforation.

As antibiotic resistance increases among infectious microorganisms, there is growing interest in adjunctive treatment strategies, such as antivirulence therapies or prophylactic immunization prior to ocular surgery. For example, salicyclic acid has been shown to reduce the expression of proteases produced by *P. aeruginosa*.[12] Passive immunization with antiserum, derived from a live-attenuated *P. aeruginosa* vaccination, was demonstrated to reduce bacterial loads and pathology in animals when administered therapeutically 24 hours postinfection.[13] Although not widely used to treat bacterial keratitis, studies have also shown that macrolides limit expression of virulence traits in *Staphylococcus aureus* and *P. aeruginosa* in addition to inhibiting bacterial growth.[14,15]

The prognosis for bacterial keratitis is highly variable. Minimal infiltration can result in subtle corneal scarring which has no impact on visual outcome; however, extensive ulceration can cause significant scarring, leading to irregular astigmatisms. In some cases, synechia and cataract formation may occur.

Fungal keratitis

Fungal keratitis is often difficult to eradicate, requiring a prolonged course of treatment. Most antifungal therapies involve one or more of the following: (1) polyenes; (2) imidazoles; or (3) fluorinated pyrimidines (Table 7.1).[1] Topical polyenes vary in their effectiveness against yeast and filamentous fungi. For example, amphotericin B is highly effective against yeast, including *Candida*, but is less effective on filamentous fungi.[16] Similarly, pyrimidine therapies are highly effective against yeasts; however, some reports indicate growing resistance among *Candida*.[1] Imidazoles have broad-spectrum activity and are often used in combination with a pyrimidine. Polyenes and imidazoles are antagonistic

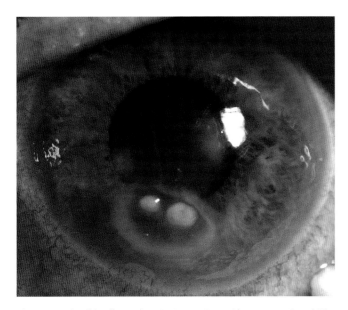

Figure 7.3 *Candida albicans* keratitis in a patient with severe conjunctivitis. (Reproduced with permission from O'Day D. Fungal keratitis. In: Albert DM, Miller JW, Azar DT, et al (eds) Principles and Practice of Opthalmology, 3rd edn. Amsterdam: Elsevier, 2008.)

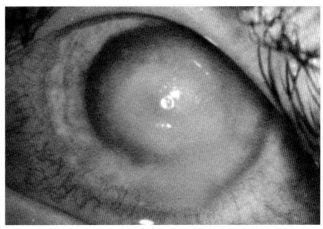

Figure 7.4 Advanced keratitis caused by *Acanthamoeba*. Note classic ring infiltrate. (Reproduced with permission from Parmar DN, Awwad ST, Petroll WM, et al. Tandem scanning confocal microscopy in the diagnosis of suspected acanthamoeba keratitis. Ophthalmology 2006;113:538–547.)

Table 7.2 Diagnostic stains and standard culture media

Type of stain	Organisms visualized/cultured	Comments
Gram stain	Bacteria, fungi, *Acanthamoeba*	Peptidoglycan, teichoic acids – violet
Giemsa stain	Bacteria, fungi, *Acanthamoeba*	Acidophilic/basophilic – contrast
Acridine orange	Bacteria, fungi, *Acanthamoeba*	DNA – fluorescent orange
Calcoflur white	Fungi, *Acanthamoeba*	Cellulose/chitin – fluorescent blue
Gomori methenamine silver	Fungi, *Acanthamoeba*	Uric/urate particles – dark blue
Periodic acid–Schiff	Fungi, *Acanthamoeba*	Cell wall – pink
Hematoxylin and eosin	*Acanthamoeba*	Intracellular structures – contrast
Standard agar culture media		
Blood agar*	Bacteria, fungi,[†] *Acanthamoeba*	General purpose, including fastidious agents
Chocolate agar	Bacteria, fungi[†]	General purpose, including fastidious agents
Brain–heart infusion agar	Bacteria, fungi[†]	General purpose
Sabouraud dextrose agar	Fungi	
Escherichia coli overlay on non-nutrient agar	*Acanthamoeba*	
Standard liquid culture media		
Brain–heart infusion broth	Bacteria, fungi[†]	
Thioglycollate broth	Bacteria	Good for small inocula
Glucose neopeptone broth	Fungi	

*Ideal for culturing bacteria such as *Staphylococcus*, *Streptococcus*, and *Pseudomonas*.
[†]Fungi can be recovered from standard bacterial media in the presence of antibiotics.
Data from Matsumoto[45] and Szliter et al.[42]

and should not be used simultaneously. Like bacterial keratitis, the use of corticosteroids is discouraged.

Treatment outcome depends greatly on the extent of fungus penetration. Nearly 30% of fungal keratitis cases do not respond to antifungal therapy and require penetrating keratoplasty.[17]

Parasitic keratitis

With *Acanthamoeba* or microsporidia keratitis, the preferred treatment is single or combinational therapies with: (1) cationic antiseptics, i.e., polyhexamethylene biguanide or chlorhexidine; (2) aromatic diamidines, i.e., propamidine isothionate; or (3) azoles (Table 7.1).[1] *Acanthamoeba* and microsporidia have varying susceptibilities to different azoles, which may require testing. In *Acanthamoeba* infections, prolonged and aggressive treatment is often required since therapeutic conditions can induce encystment. Some data indicate that povidone-iodine at high concentrations acts on both trophozoites and cysts.[18]

Preliminary studies have demonstrated that oral immunization with an *Acanthamoeba* surface antigen following infection can ameliorate disease in animals; however, this strategy was not effective against stromal infections.[19] Further investigation is needed to assess whether this strategy has therapeutic value.

Deep stromal infections with microsporidia and *Acanthamoeba* are prone to recrudescence. Therapeutic penetrating keratoplasty is usually required for cases involving advanced disease, drug resistance organisms, and recurring infections.[1]

Pathophysiology

The ocular surface is protected from infectious organisms by an array of antimicrobial factors and blink shear forces which together limit access to the corneal epithelium. These antimicrobial factors include lactoferrin, lysozyme, immunoglobulin A (IgA), and cationic peptides in the tear film. Microorganisms can also become entrapped in secreted mucins that are removed through blinking and tear drainage. Overcoming these defenses is crucial for disease progression. Epidemiological data suggest defects in the ocular surface increase the likelihood of colonization by infectious microorganisms. Subsequent pathology is mediated by the innate immune response and toxic effectors produced by the infectious agent. The following sections describe various models of keratitis pathophysiology, focusing on organisms that are exemplary of bacterial, fungal, and parasitic keratitis.

Gram-positive bacterial keratitis

Staphylococcus aureus model (Box 7.1)

Colonization of the cornea

Bacterial adhesion to the corneal surface is the first step in infection. Corneal scarification and/or intrastromal injection are generally required to establish *S. aureus* keratitis in animal models.[20,21] These manipulations bypass some of the natural processes involved in colonization. For this reason, keratitis models have extrapolated the early steps of disease from other infection models. Many *S. aureus* surface adhes-

---

> **Box 7.1 Pathophysiology of *Staphylococcus aureus* infections**
>
> - Extracellular matrix proteins serve as the primary ligands for bacterial adherence
> - Pore-forming and leukocidin toxins contribute to the severity of keratitis
> - The role of Toll-like receptor 2 in sensing bacterial cell wall components is still controversial

ins, known as MSCRAMMs (microbial surface components recognizing adhesive matrix molecules), have been identified based on their activities and sequence relationships inferred from genome data. These adhesins mediate bacterial interaction with host extracellular matrix (ECM) components, including collagen, fibronectin, fibrinogen, laminin, and elastin. Fibronectin-binding protein A and B (FnBP A, B) were found to be key factors mediating adherence and facilitating invasion of human corneal epithelial cells in vitro.[22] Binding and internalization of an isogenic FnBP-deficient strain were reduced 100-fold compared to wild type. An independent study found that *S. aureus*, deficient in the collagen-binding adhesion (Cna), was also attenuated in rabbit models.[23] However, relatively few keratitis isolates were found to express this adhesin.

Role of S. aureus *toxins in keratitis*

S. aureus produces a variety of virulence traits that contribute to pathogenesis, i.e., coagulase, staphylolysins, leukocidins, and protein A. Staphylolysins are further divided into alpha-, beta-, delta-, and gamma-toxins.[24] A majority of clinical staphylococcal isolates produce alpha- and/or delta-toxins.[24] Alpha-toxin is a pore-forming toxin that inserts into host cell membranes and disrupts membrane integrity. This may lead to cell death by rupture or the induction of apoptosis. Exposure to sublytic concentrations of pore-forming toxins can induce proinflammatory host cell responses and lipid mediator production.[24] Leukocidins, like gamma-toxin, increase the permeability of leukocytes to cations, which can also lead to rupture. Protein A interferes with bacterial opsonization by binding to the Fc portion of immunoglobulin. The impact of alpha-toxin, gamma-toxin, and protein A in keratitis has been assessed with *S. aureus* isogenic mutants in a rabbit model of infection.[25,26] Rabbits, injected intrastromally with alpha-toxin or gamma-toxin-deficient strains, developed keratitis with reduced severity. In the same model, the absence of protein A does not affect virulence, which contradicts the observation that protein A can induce a proinflammatory response in cultured corneal epithelial cells.[27]

Immune response

The role of Toll-like receptors (TLRs) in corneal innate defense against *S. aureus* is the subject of some debate. It was shown that peptidoglycan, a cell wall component recognized by TLR2 in other cell types, failed to induce secretion of proinflammatory cytokines and human ß-defensin 2 (hBD2, inducible antimicrobial peptide) in transformed and primary human corneal epithelial cells.[28] The poor responsiveness was due to atopic expression of TLR2 within intracellular pools. Other reports support a role for TLR2 in the innate defense of the cornea. *S. aureus* exoproducts and an alternative TLR2 agonist, Pam3Cys, were shown to induce hBD2 secretion from human corneal limbal epithelial cells and primary corneal epithelial cells.[29] In this case, TLR2 was identified on the surface of corneal epithelial cells in vitro. Preliminary studies in C57BL/6 mice challenged with Pam3Cys demonstrate neutrophil recruitment into the corneal stroma. Conversely, neutrophil recruitment was not observed in isogenic TLR2[-/-] and Myd88[-/-] mice.[30] These findings indicate that a cell population within the cornea expresses functional TLR2 and is involved in ocular defense; however, it is unclear which cell types are most important. Knockout mice experiments have also illustrated the importance of interleukin (IL)-4 and IL6 in mediating the host response to *S. aureus* keratitis.[31,32]

Gram-negative bacterial keratitis

Pseudomonas aeruginosa model (Box 7.2)

Colonization of the cornea

In *P. aeruginosa* infections, adherence is primarily driven by a host protein called the cystic fibrosis transmembrane conductance regulator (CFTR) and bacterial lipopolysaccharide (LPS). In animal models, the absence of CFTR was shown to reduce bacterial loads and overall keratitis severity.[33] Bacterial internalization mediated by CFTR was demonstrated to occur more readily in rabbits fitted with contact lenses,[34] which may relate to the observation that CFTR expression is enhanced in corneal epithelium under hypoxic conditions.[35] These findings implied that contact lens wear increases susceptibility to infection through hypoxia-driven changes in corneal cell membrane receptor composition. However, infection rates for highly gas-permeable silicone hydrogel contact lens are not fundamentally different from earlier designs,[36] casting some doubt on the relationship between hypoxia and contact lens-associated keratitis.

The primary ligand for CFTR was identified as LPS by its ability to block competitively *P. aeruginosa* adherence to epithelium and scratch-injured corneas.[37] Evidence suggests that LPS also serves as a ligand for the glycolipid, sialo-GM1, which localizes to wounded regions within damaged corneas.[38] Other *P. aeruginosa* factors that have been implicated in corneal invasion are flagellum and pili.[39]

Immune response

The recruitment of neutrophils into *P. aeruginosa*-infected corneas is mediated primarily by IL-8 secreted from corneal epithelial cells and resident immune cells.[40] Several mechanisms have been proposed for triggering IL-8 production. LPS from *P. aeruginosa* have been shown to activate TLR4-dependent responses (i.e., IL8) by corneal cells in vivo and

in vitro.[29,30] Similar effects have been reported for flagellin-stimulated TLR5, and TLR9 stimulated with *P. aeruginosa* DNA.[29] Mice with defects in expression of TLR4, TLR9, and IL6 are predisposed to severe *P. aeruginosa* infection, which stems from limited neutrophil recruitment into the central cornea.[29,30,40]

Balancing pro- and anti-inflammatory signals is critical for clearing *P. aeruginosa* infections with minimal corneal destruction. Prolonged IL-1, IL-6, and IL-8 expression results in sustained neutrophil infiltration and susceptibility to corneal perforation.[40] Several negative-feedback mechanisms have been shown to enhance the effectiveness of the inflammatory response in controlling *P. aeruginosa* infections. For example, transmembrane proteins SIGIRR and ST2 competitively inhibit TLR4- and IL1-dependent signaling pathways,[29,41] limiting the severity of keratitis. Similarly, the neuropeptide vasoactive intestinal peptide (VIP) has been shown to downregulate corneal inflammation and protect against ulcerations during infection.[42]

Evasion of immune response

P. aeruginosa can interfere with immune competency by manipulating neutrophil and macrophage functions. This ability is linked to the *P. aeruginosa* type III secretion system which injects effector proteins directly into host cells via a needle-like apparatus. In keratitis, the most potent type III effectors are ExoU and ExoT.[39] ExoU was shown to kill macrophages and epithelial cells in vitro through its phospholipase activity. It also represses polymorphonucleocyte migration into the central cornea, which may explain the peripheral ring opacities seen in *P. aeruginosa* keratitis.[43] ExoT is an adenosine diphosphate ribosyltransferase that interferes with actin cytoskeletonal rearrangements. Its negative impact on phagocytosis promotes *P. aeruginosa* survival.[39] Similar antiphagocytic activities have been ascribed to exotoxinA in keratitis models.[44] Elastase also plays a role in immune evasion. It has been reported to degrade immunoglobulin G, lysozyme, interferon-γ, and tumor necrosis factor-α in vitro and inhibit monocyte chemotaxis towards bacterial formylated peptides.[45]

Altered tissue integrity

Corneal ulcerations are often observed in severe *P. aeruginosa* infections and result from destruction of the stromal architecture. Both the elastase and alkaline protease contribute to this pathology by degrading ECM components, i.e., collagen and laminin.[45] Furthermore, elastase cleaves and activates host membrane metalloproteinases (MMP2, MM9) and kallikrein. MMPs also rapidly degrade stromal ECM, leading to pathological destruction. Stimulation of the kallikrein-killin system promotes vascular permeability, which contributes to the edema present in some infections. Thus, elastase contributes to pathogenesis by eliciting structural damage and compromising innate immunity.[45]

Fungal keratitis

Candida albicans model (Box 7.3)

Role of hyphae in C. albicans *keratitis*

Several factors contribute to *C. albicans* pathogenicity, such as surface adhesins, protease secretions, and morphological

---

Box 7.2 Pathophysiology of *Pseudomonas aeruginosa* infections

- Adherence is mediated by both host cystic fibrosis transmembrane conductance regulator (CFTR) and sialo-GM1
- Bacterial elastase contributes to tissue destruction directly and indirectly by activating host proteases
- Type III system effector proteins facilitate immune evasion and are involved in immune ring formation

---

> **Box 7.3 Pathophysiology of *Candida albicans* infections**
>
> - Morphologically transformable strains produce more severe keratitis
> - Biofilm growth can adhere to contact lens and is resistant to contact lens care solutions

> **Box 7.4 Pathophysiology of *Acanthamoeba* infections**
>
> - Cysts are resistant to many stresses, including contact lens care solutions, and facilitate immune evasion
> - Glycoproteins and glycolipids serve as the primary ligands for trophozoite adherence
> - Trophozoites secrete destructive proteases in the presence of mannose
> - Neurons are susceptible to parasitic cytotoxin which contributes to radial keratoneuritis

transformations from yeast to the hyphal form.[46] In studying *Candida* virulence, Ura-blaster methodology has been used to generate mutants for testing the relationship between gene structure and function. However, this methodology can produce transcriptional artifacts that confound interpretation.[47] This has led to the re-evaluation of various genes previously ascribed a role in virulence. To date, mostly genes related to hyphal formation, i.e., rim13,[48] sap6,[49] and rbt 4,[50] have a confirmed role in keratitis severity in mice models. Rim13p is a protease which mediates activation of the transcription factor Rim101p via C-terminal cleavage. This pathway is required for hyphal formation induced at alkaline pH. The sap6 gene product is involved in filamentation, and rbt4 encodes a hyphal protein. A comparison of nonisogenic wild-type *C. albicans* strains revealed that failure to form true hyphae results in less pathology in rabbits fitted with contact lens.[51] To date, *C. albicans* adhesins have not been shown to be essential in animal models of keratitis. However, these models required corneal scarification, which may bypass some naturally occurring events; thus, the importance of adhesins in virulence cannot be excluded. Other studies suggest that adherence related to biofilm formation plays a role in infection. *Candida* biofilms bind more tightly to the contact lens compared to *Fusarium* biofilms. Moreover, *Candida* biofilms are more resistant to contact lens care solutions than planktonic organisms.[52]

Immune reponse

The pathogenesis of *C. albicans* keratitis depends on alterations in several environmental factors, such as host immunity, competition from other saprophytes, and physical perturbation of the niche. In mice challenged with *C. albicans* after corneal scarification, treatments with an intramuscular injection of cyclophosphamide or methylprednisolone exacerbated fungal invasion and disease progression.[53]

Parasitic keratitis

Acanthamoeba model (Box 7.4)

Life cycle

There are two stages to the *Acanthamoeba* life cycle: a vegetative, motile trophozoite and a dormant cyst. The cyst stage is resistant to many stresses, including desiccation, ultraviolet irradiation, detergents, and chlorine.[54] Of chief concern, cysts can persist in the biocidal agents of contact lens care solutions.[55]

Colonization of the cornea

The principal adhesin of *Acanthamoeba* is the mannose-binding protein (MBP), which is expressed exclusively by the trophozoite.[56] MBP binds mannosylated glycoproteins and glycolipids expressed on the host cell. The importance of MBP has been demonstrated by the competitive inhibition of trophozoite adherence to corneal epithelium with mannose.[56,57] Mild abrasions or trauma to the corneal epithelium have been correlated with localized production of mannosylated glycoproteins and subsequent trophozoite attachment.[58]

Contact lens wear has been identified as the principal risk factor for *Acanthamoeba* keratitis, accounting for >80% of infections.[54] Both trophozoites and cysts have been shown to adhere to soft and rigid, gas-permeable contact lenses.[59] Recent studies indicate that *Acanthamoeba* binds the newer generation of silicone hydrogel lenses with greater affinity than the conventional hydrogel lenses[60]; moreover, worn or spoiled contact lens bind *Acanthamoeba* more avidly. Presumably, contact lens spoilage increases ligand availability on the synthetic material.

Immune response

Macrophages and neutrophils are critical components of the immune response to *Acanthamoeba*. Depletion of conjunctival macrophages or neutrophils in hamsters increases susceptibility and severity of keratitis.[54] Unlike trophozoites, cysts evoke weak chemotactic responses in phagocystic cells. This contributes to the immune-evasiveness of cysts and the recrudescence of *Acanthamoeba* infections. Cysts have been shown to be partly susceptible to phagocytic killing in vitro, with neutrophils being more effective than macrophages.[54]

Serological studies indicate >50% of healthy individuals secrete *Acanthamoeba*-reactive IgA, which is consistent with its ubiquitous nature. Interestingly, patients diagnosed with *Acanthamoeba* keratitis have significantly lower parasite-specific IgA titers in their tears compared to asymptomatic individuals.[54] Studies have shown that mucosal IgA does not affect trophozoite viability in hamster models, but decreases adherence to corneal epithelium.[54]

Altered tissue physiology

Trophozoites produce several factors that allow them to penetrate the corneal epithelium and stroma. Many of these factors are induced by mannose or mannosylated glycoproteins, thereby linking colonization with subsequent pathology.[57,61] The mannose-inducible protein (MIP133) mediates cytolysis and apoptosis of corneal epithelial cells in animal models and organ cultures.[19] Similarly, mannose-regulated ecto-ATPases can signal through purinergic receptors to induce apoptosis in epithelial cells.[62]

Following epithelial desquamation, trophozoites disrupt the stromal architecture with secreted proteases, i.e., a cysteine protease, a metalloprotease, elastase, MP133, and serine proteases.[57,61] Evidence suggests these proteases contribute to the ring-like stromal infiltrates which are characteristic of *Acanthamoeba* infections; however, the precise mechanism is not understood (Figure 7.4). *Acanthamoeba* can also activate host MMPs through a constitutively expressed plasminogen activator.[63] Elevated MMPs activity results in pathological destruction similar to bacterial keratitis.

A hallmark of *Acanthamoeba* keratitis is a radial keratoneuritis, which has been correlated with clusters of trophozoites around the corneal nerves. In vitro studies have demonstrated a chemotactic attraction of trophozoites to neural crest-derived cells, and an overall susceptibility of neurons to the parasitic cytotoxins.[64] These observations offer a possible explanation for the severe pain often associated with *Acanthamoeba* keratitis.

Key references

A complete list of chapter references is available online at www.expertconsult.com. See inside cover for registration details.

1. McLeod S. Infectious keratitis. In: Yanoff M, Duker J (eds) Ophthalmology. St. Louis: Mosby, 2004:466–491.

2. Thomas PA, Geraldine P. Infectious keratitis. Curr Opin Infect Dis 2007;20: 129–141.

4. Bourcier T, Thomas F, Borderie V, et al. Bacterial keratitis: predisposing factors, clinical and microbiological review of 300 cases. Br J Ophthalmol 2003;87: 834–838.

22. Jett BD, Gilmore MS. Internalization of *Staphylococcus aureus* by human corneal epithelial cells: role of bacterial fibronectin-binding protein and host cell factors. Infect Immun 2002;70:4697– 4700.

25. Callegan MC, Engel LS, Hill JM, et al. Corneal virulence of *Staphylococcus aureus*: roles of alpha-toxin and protein A in pathogenesis. Infect Immun 1994;62: 2478–2482.

29. Yu FS, Hazlett LD. Toll-like receptors and the eye. Invest Ophthalmol Vis Sci 2006; 47:1255–1263.

32. Hume EB, Cole N, Garthwaite LL, et al. A protective role for IL-6 in staphylococcal microbial keratitis. Invest Ophthalmol Vis Sci 2006;47:4926–4930.

33. Zaidi TS, Lyczak J, Preston M, et al. Cystic fibrosis transmembrane conductance regulator-mediated corneal epithelial cell ingestion of *Pseudomonas aeruginosa* is a key component in the pathogenesis of experimental murine keratitis. Infect Immun 1999;67:1481– 1492.

39. Evans DJ, McNamara NA, Fleiszig SM. Life at the front: dissecting bacterial–host interactions at the ocular surface. Ocul Safety 2007;5:213–227.

40. Hazlett LD. Corneal response to *Pseudomonas aeruginosa* infection. Prog Retin Eye Res 2004;23:1–30.

45. Matsumoto K. Role of bacterial proteases in pseudomonal and serratial keratitis. Biol Chem 2004;385:1007–1016.

48. Jackson BE, Wilhelmus KR, Mitchell BM. Genetically regulated filamentation contributes to *Candida albicans* virulence during corneal infection. Microb Pathog 2007;42:88–93.

49. Jackson BE, Wilhelmus KR, Hube B. The role of secreted aspartyl proteinases in *Candida albicans* keratitis. Invest Ophthalmol Vis Sci 2007;48:3559– 3565.

54. Clarke DW, Niederkorn JY. The immunobiology of *Acanthamoeba* keratitis. Microbes Infect 2006;8:1400– 1405.

56. Yang Z, Cao Z, Panjwani N. Pathogenesis of *Acanthamoeba* keratitis: carbohydrate-mediated host–parasite interactions. Infect Immun 1997;65:439–445.

61. Leher H, Silvany R, Alizadeh H, et al. 1998. Mannose induces the release of cytopathic factors from *Acanthamoeba castellanii*. Infect Immun 66:5–10.

CHAPTER 8

Corneal graft rejection

Daniel R Saban, Mohammad H Dastjerdi, and Reza Dana

Clinical background

Corneal transplantation is the most common and successful form of human solid-tissue transplantation, which is widely practiced as a sight-restorative therapy for patients with congenital or acquired corneal opacification, infection, or damage (Box 8.1). The major indications for this procedure include keratoconus (corneal thinning and warping which cause visual distortion), bullous keratopathy (corneal edema, which is both painful and reduces visual acuity), failed previous grafts, corneal scarring, corneal dystrophy, and infection.[1] Currently, the most common form of corneal transplantation is "penetrating," which is the engraftment of a full-thickness corneal button. However, partial-thickness grafts or "lamellar" transplantation is also performed in a significant number of patients. Outcomes of corneal transplantation are typically excellent; 2-year graft rejection rates are approximately 10% in uncomplicated first grafts.[2] However, this preponderance has led to the common misconception that immune rejection is not a significant clinical problem. Indeed, immune rejection is the leading cause of corneal graft failure, and, as reported in the 2006 Eye Banking Statistical Report, the number of regrafts due to previous failure is increasing.[3]

Historical development

Several early studies have been formative in our current understanding of corneal immune rejection and instrumental in stimulating the rapid progress made during the past two decades. Just over 100 years ago, Zirm[4] reported the first successful human corneal transplantation, and subsequently corneal immune rejection was described by Paufique et al[5] in 1948 and further confirmed by Maumenee[6] in 1951. Arguably one of the most important studies in corneal immune rejection was carried out by Khodadoust and Silverstein[7] in 1969. They demonstrated, by transplanting individual layers of the cornea in rabbits, that the epithelium, stroma, and endothelium could separately undergo immunologic rejection – important observations which are seminal in the diagnosis, prevention, and treatment of corneal immune rejection even today.

Key symptoms and signs

While symptoms are by no means universal, patients undergoing or in the very early stages of a graft rejection episode may experience irritation or pain, redness of the eye, decreased vision, and photophobia. Such symptoms may occur as early as 1 month or as late as 20 years after transplantation.[8] Signs of rejection include circumcorneal injection, which is the dilation and engorgement of blood vessels around the circumference of the cornea and conjunctiva. A mild-to-moderate form of anterior-chamber reaction (cellular) and flare (acellular) may also be associated. In addition, edema and presence of keratic precipitates on the donor endothelium, either diffusely scattered precipitates or in an irregular line (commonly referred to as a "Khodadoust line"), are key signs of graft rejection (Box 8.2).

Clinical features

There are potentially three distinct forms of corneal graft rejection, which may occur singly or in combination. They include: (1) epithelial rejection; (2) stromal rejection; and (3) endothelial rejection.[7] Endothelial rejection, however, is the most common and profound form. It can be identified by endothelial surface precipitates in scattered clumps or in a classic linear form (Khodadoust line) (Figure 8.1) that usually begins at a vascularized portion of the peripheral graft–host junction and progresses, if untreated, across the endothelial surface over several days. A mild-to-moderate anterior-chamber cellular and flare reaction may be associated with the process. Damage to the endothelium results in compromised regulation of corneal hydration and thereby is associated with edema, in addition to inflammation.

Other forms of corneal graft rejection, including epithelial, subepithelial, and stromal rejection, occur less frequently (10–15% of all rejected cases; Box 8.3).[8,9] These forms of rejection are not problematic per se; however, they often serve as harbingers of a more serious endothelial rejection.

Epidemiology

The number of corneal transplants carried out worldwide is thought to exceed 70 000 per year. Eye Bank Association of

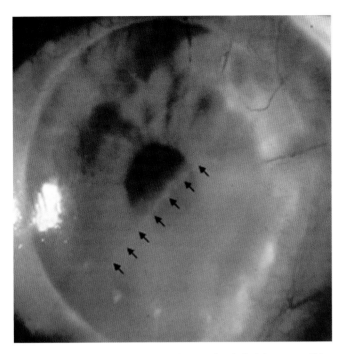

Figure 8.1 Khodadoust line: A clinical feature of endothelial rejection. This is a rejection line (arrows) formed by adherent macrophages and T cells, referred to as keratic precipitates, which traverse across the donor endothelium leaving behind a zone of graft destruction. The presence of a Khodadoust line is associated with graft edema since damage to the endothelium results in compromised regulation of corneal hydration.

Box 8.1 Clinical significance

- Corneal transplantation is the most common and successful form of solid-tissue transplantation
- Immune rejection is the leading cause of corneal graft failure

---

Box 8.2 Signs and symptoms of corneal allograft rejection

- Signs and symptoms of corneal graft rejection can occur as early as 1 month or as late as 20 years after transplantation
- Edema and presence of keratic precipitates on the donor endothelium (Khodadoust line) are key signs of corneal graft rejection

---

America (EBAA) alone provided 45 000 donor corneas in 2006.[3] Of corneal transplants placed in uncomplicated or "normal-risk" graft beds (i.e., absence of inflammation and neovessels), approximately 20–40% experience at least one bout of immune rejection. In spite of this, only 10% of grafts fail due to immune rejection by 1 year postsurgery in the normal-risk setting, since rejection is often reversible with intensive steroid treatment. By 15 years postsurgery, graft failure due to immune rejection nearly doubles to 17%, according to the Australian Corneal Graft Registry.[10]

In high-risk graft beds (i.e., presence of inflammation and neovessels), which make up approximately one-third of all transplants, 50–90% of grafts fail even with maximal topical and systemic immune suppression.[11] Indeed, these rates in

---

Box 8.3 Graft endothelial rejection

- Endothelial rejection is the most common and profound form of corneal graft rejection

---

Box 8.4 Risk factors for corneal allograft rejection

- The two most important risk factors in corneal graft rejection are stromal neovascularization and host bed inflammation

---

high-risk transplantation are far worse than those experienced in vascularized solid-organ transplantation (e.g., heart, liver, or kidney).[12] Moreover, data reported in the 2006 Statistical Report from the EBAA[3] show a significant increase in the proportion of patients needing second and third grafts, by definition also considered high-risk.

Risk factors

There are several important risk factors which are used universally to determine if a patient is at high risk for corneal graft rejection and these factors have been established by large, multicenter, prospective studies such as the Corneal Transplant Follow-Up Study[13] in the UK, the Collaborative Corneal Transplantation Studies (CCTS)[14] in the USA, and the Australian Corneal Graft Registry.[10] While numerous risk factors for immune rejection have been considered and studied extensively (e.g., gender-matching, age of donor, circumference of graft tissue), the two most important prognostic factors are stromal neovascularization (Figure 8.2A) and host bed inflammation (Figure 8.2B; Box 8.4).

Corneal neovascularization (Figure 8.3C) is almost invariably associated with high graft rejection and the level of blood vessels at the time of transplantation is significantly correlated with graft survival.[10] Khodadoust[15] reported that endothelial rejection occurred in 3.5% of avascular cases, 13.3% of mildly vascular cases, 28% of moderately vascular cases, and 65% of heavily vascularized cases. As per the CCTS definition, graft bed vascularization in two or more quadrants is classified as "high-risk."[14]

Corneal inflammation is another important risk factor. Even previous inflammation in graft beds which are quiet at the time of transplantation (e.g., herpetic eye disease) has substantially diminished chances of graft survival (Figure 8.2B). This could be due to a subclinical presence of inflammatory cells and persistence of vascular channels. Transplantation in inflamed graft beds at the time of surgery (e.g., active microbial keratitis) and similarly in inflamed graft beds triggered postoperatively (i.e., in the case of suture abscess or recurrent herpes simplex virus infection) also has a substantially increased risk for graft rejection.[16] In addition, previous ipsilateral rejection is an important risk factor, which is thought to be due to corneal inflammation or presensitization to donor tissue via previous engraftment.

Other noteworthy risk factors involve poor ocular surface function, usually found in conjunction with inflammation and corneal neovascularization. Hence, ocular surface diseases (e.g., severe dry eye, ocular pemphigoid, Stevens–

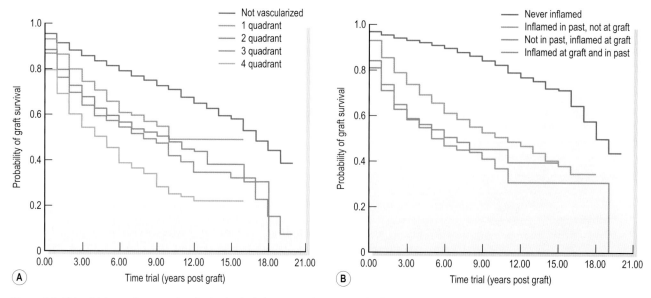

Figure 8.2 Major risk factors for corneal graft rejection include neovascularization and inflammation of host graft bed. Corneal neovascularization is almost invariably associated with high graft rejection and the level of blood vessel ingrowth at the time of transplantation is directly correlated with graft survival (A). Corneal inflammation is another important risk factor and, even in previously inflamed graft beds which are quiet at the time of transplantation (e.g., herpetic eye disease), substantially diminishes the chance of graft survival (B). (Redrawn with permission from Williams KA, Lowe MT, Barlett CM, et al (eds) The Australian Corneal Graft Registry: 2007 Report. Flinders: Flinders University Press, 2007.)

Johnson syndrome, and neuroparalytic disease) or injury (e.g., severe chemical or radiation burns) is associated with poor prognosis for corneal transplantation.

Differential diagnosis

Several clinical situations exist which make the diagnosis of corneal allograft rejection difficult; the largest confounder is recurrent ocular inflammation in herpetic keratouveitis. The occurrence of corneal allograft rejection is very common in herpetic patients, and repeated bouts of inflammation carry a more dismal prognosis for the graft. Indicators for herpetic inflammation include the presence of typical dendriform epithelial lesions, unusually intensive anterior-chamber reaction, or endothelial keratic precipitates not confined to the graft.

Another significant confounder in diagnosing immune rejection includes graft endothelial decompensation, since this condition also leads to corneal graft edema. However, any questionable presence of edema in a corneal graft is nonetheless treated with corticosteroids as rejection.

Prevention and treatment of corneal allograft rejection

Postoperative prophylactic immunosuppressive regimens can be devised according to the degree of risk of rejection. In low-risk cases, low-frequency use of topical steroids is adequate initially, and tapered off to 6–12 months. High-risk corneal grafts require more intensive treatment. Topical and systemic corticosteroids in conjunction with topical and/or systemic ciclosporin are used for prevention of corneal rejection.

Corticosteroid therapy is also the treatment of choice for acute corneal immune rejection, and can be administrated topically, periocularly, and/or systemically. Most episodes of corneal graft rejection can be reversed if therapy is initiated early and aggressively; thus, it is imperative for the patient to identify and report any onset of symptoms associated with immune rejection (i.e., decreased vision, pain, and redness). In mild episodes of graft rejection topical steroids are preferred and can be applied as often as every 15 minutes to 2 hours. For severe episodes of rejection, such as those experienced by high-risk recipients, intensive steroid therapy administered via frequent topical eye drops, periocular injection, and/or systemically (oral or intravenous) may be given.

Pathology

There is little information in this regard since human cornea grafts are not typically biopsied and clinical examination relies heavily on biomicroscopic or "slit-lamp" evaluation. Moreover, because rejection is treatable, donor tissue is only replaced once the graft has irrevocably failed, not before or at the time of a rejection episode. Hence, clinical use of pathology in corneal transplantation is not common practice.

Etiology

Graft rejection is triggered by genetically nonidentical (allogeneic) donor peptides known as histocompatibility antigens, or "alloantigens." Alloantigens which pose the greatest barrier to graft survival in transplantation en bloc are

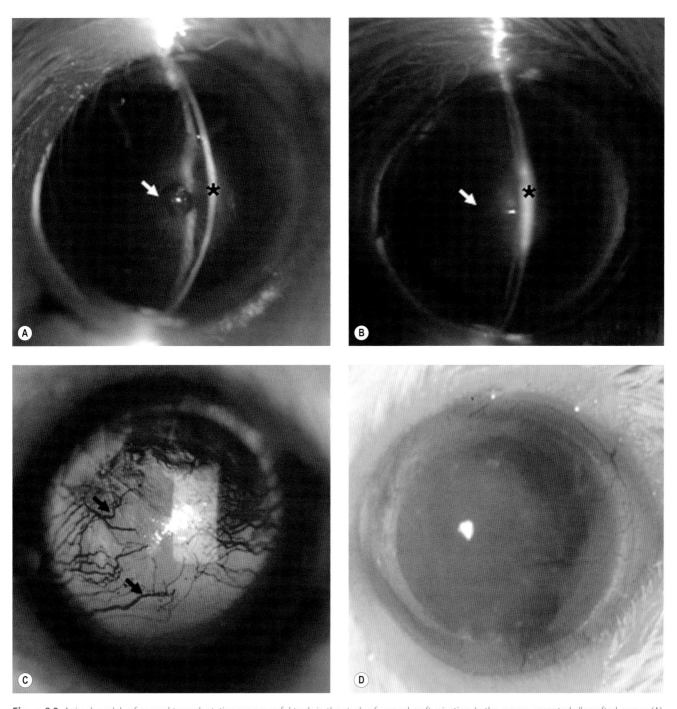

Figure 8.3 Animal models of corneal transplantation are powerful tools in the study of corneal graft rejection. In the mouse, accepted allografted cornea (A) is indicated by a clear and readily visible pupillary margin (arrow) and iris vasculature via slit-lamp observation. In contrast, for an allograft undergoing immunologic rejection (B), the pupillary margin is not readily visible (arrow). Grafts undergoing immunologic rejection are associated with graft edema, as indicated by corneal thickness observed via obtuse angle slit-lamp illumination in rejecting grafts (B* versus A*). As in humans, graft rejection in the murine model is associated with pathologic neovascularization (C, arrow) of graft bed and donor tissue. Graft failure due to immunologic rejection results in a severely opaque donor tissue (D).

encoded by the major histocompatibility complex (MHC), also referred to as human leukocyte antigen (HLA), system in humans. Class I MHC antigens (or HLA-A, -B, and -C) are constitutively expressed by all nucleated cells and platelets, while class II MHC antigens (or HLA-DR, -DQ, and -DW) are constitutively expressed on leukocytes.

Unlike in other forms of solid-tissue/organ transplantation, histocompatibility-matching donor tissue to the intended recipient for promotion of graft survival is variably performed in the cornea. This is in part because the normal cornea expresses very low levels of HLA antigens.[17] However, during inflammation and in graft rejection the expression levels of these antigens are strongly upregulated and can trigger immune rejection.[18] The role of histocompatibility-matching has been studied extensively in the clinic and while CCTS reported no overall beneficial effect of this practice,[19] a myriad of other independent studies have indicated the contrary by showing that histocompatibility-matching (particularly at HLA-A and HLA-B loci) does significantly reduce the risk of rejection.[20] Moreover, in the murine model of corneal transplantation, it has been clearly demonstrated that MHC alloantigens per se trigger immune rejection, particularly in the high-risk setting.[21]

Interestingly, unlike in other forms of solid-tissue/organ transplantation, minor histocompatibility antigens (minor H) have been shown to play a significant role in triggering immune rejection (Box 8.5). These alloantigens are encoded throughout the genome and include ABO blood antigens and Lewis antigens in humans, and H3 antigens in mice. Studies conducted in mice have indicated that minor H alloantigens are a critical barrier to graft survival (particularly in the normal-risk setting).[22] Moreover, it has also been reported that ABO-matching is a relatively feasible and inexpensive clinical practice which can be effective in reducing the risk of graft failure.[19]

Pathophysiology

Rodent models of corneal transplantation, particularly the mouse, are powerful tools in study of corneal graft rejection (Figure 8.3). While the pathophysiology is a highly complex multistep process which is not fully understood, many critical steps have been defined. These include the following, which are further reviewed below (Figure 8.4):

1. Alterations in the local microenvironment: factors which maintain the microenvironment in the cornea and anterior segment constitutively immunosuppressive, referred to as "immune privilege," begin to erode.
2. Capture of graft alloantigen: specialized immune cells called antigen-presenting cells (APC) capture and process alloantigen for subsequent presentation to T cells.
3. Homing to regional lymph nodes: alloantigen-bearing APC traffic from the cornea to T-cell reservoirs located in the ipsilateral regional lymph nodes and prime T cells.
4. T-cell-mediated graft destruction: primed (or effector) T cells peripheralize via circulation seeking to target and destroy the graft via various mechanisms.

Alterations in the local microenvironment

The eye is known as an immunologically privileged site, which means that specific branches of immunity such as inflammation are inhibited within the intraocular compartments, and similar inhibitory mechanisms are also found in

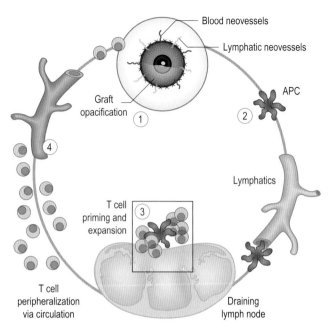

Figure 8.4 Pathophysiology of corneal allograft rejection. The critical steps involved in the pathophysiology of corneal graft rejection that have been defined include: (1) alterations in the local microenvironment; (2) capture of graft alloantigen; (3) homing to regional lymph nodes; (4) T-cell-mediated graft destruction. APC, antigen-presenting cell.

the brain, testis, and pregnant uterus. Ocular immune privilege protects visual acuity from inflammation, and involves numerous distinct mechanisms. These include: blood–ocular barrier due to endothelial cell tight junctions; avascularity and angiostatic mechanisms of the cornea (vascular endothelial growth factor receptor "sink"[23]); low expression of MHC molecules; expression of immunomodulatory molecules (e.g., Fas-FasL, TRAIL, and PDL-1);[24–26] and presence of immunoregulatory factors/cytokines (e.g., α-melanocyte-stimulating hormone, thrombospondin, and transforming growth factor-ß).[27–29]

A series of changes to the normal local microenvironment ensues during episodes of rejection and similarly in high-risk graft beds, leading to the erosion of immune privilege and possible graft failure (Table 8.1). These changes include: secretion of proinflammatory cytokines (e.g., interleukin (IL)-1, tumor necrosis factor-α, interferon-γ)[30] and chemokines (e.g., MIP-1α, MIP-2, RANTES);[31] expression of cellular adhesion molecules (e.g., intercellular adhesion molecule-1 (ICAM-1), VLA-1);[32,33] and angiogenic factors (e.g., vascular endothelial growth factor (VEGF)).[34] In addition, another component of immune privilege similarly lost is anterior chamber-associated immune deviation (ACAID), a form of peripheral immune tolerance which was first described by Kaplan and Streilein (Box 8.6).[35] ACAID is mediated by regulatory T cells (Treg) induced in response to intraocular antigens which selectively impair delayed-type hypersensitivity (DTH) in an antigen-specific fashion. Sonoda et al[36] and Sano et al[37] demonstrated that mice with longstanding accepted allografts are unable to mount donor-specific DTH, indicating that the allograft of itself induces ACAID and this affords protection from host immunity.

Capture of graft alloantigen and antigen-presenting cells APC are sentinel mediators of graft rejection in that they are

Table 8.1 Functional changes to the normal corneal microenvironment that ensue during immunologic rejection

Factors promoting immune privilege	Mechanism	Factors abrogating immune privilege
Blood–ocular barrier	Vascular endothelial cell tight junctions	Cellular extravasation into cornea
Cornea avascularity	VEGFR "sink"	Heme/lymphangiogenic invasion of graft/donor tissue
Antigen presentation	Low expression of MHC I/II moluecules	Upregulation of donor MHC and CD 80/86
Immunomodulatory molecules	Fas-FasL, TRAIL, and PDL-1	ICAM-1, VLA-1
Cytokines and neuropeptides	α-MSH, TSP, and TGF-β	IL-1, TNF-α, IFN-γ, MIP-1α, MIP-2, CCL5
Immunological tolerance	Donor-specific ACAID	Donor-specific DTH

VEGFR, vascular endothelial growth factor receptor; MHC, major histocompatibility complex; TRAIL, tumor necrosis factor-related apoptosis-inducing ligand; PDL-1, programmed death ligand-1; α-MSH, α-melanocyte-stimulating hormone, TSP, thrombospondin; TGF-β, transforming growth factor-ß, ACAID, anterior chamber-associated immune deviation; ICAM-1, intercellular adhesion molecule 1; VLA-1, very late antigen-1; IL-1, interleukin-1; TNF-α, tumor necrosis factor-α; IFN-γ, interferon-γ; MIP-1α, macrophage inflammatory protein-1α; CCL5, chemokine C-C motif ligand-5; DTH, delayed-type hypersensitivity.

Box 8.6 Local microenvironment

- Alteration in the local immunosuppressive microenvironment is an important factor that leads to rejection
- This alteration includes erosion of ocular immune privilege and loss of anterior chamber-associated immune deviation

Box 8.7 Antigen-presenting cells

- Antigen-presenting cells are sentinel mediators of graft rejection
- These immune cells are responsible for alloantigen capture and presentation to prime T cells

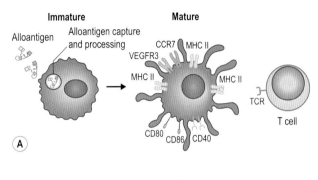

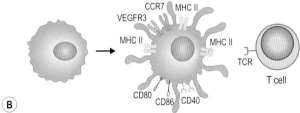

Figure 8.5 Phenotypic maturation of antigen-presenting cell (APC) maturation and subsequent T-cell priming. APCs are sentinel mediators of graft rejection because they are responsible for alloantigen capture and subsequent presentation of processed alloantigen to prime naïve T cells. Maturation, which renders alloantigen-bearing APC more potent in stimulating T cells, includes upregulation of major histocompatibity complex (MHC) II (a peptide complex that loads and presents alloantigen to T cells) and costimulatory molecules (CD80, CD86, CD40). Homing receptors (CCR7, vascular endothelial growth factor receptor (VEGFR)-3) are upregulated to facilitate APC trafficking to regional lymph nodes. T cells are primed by (A) host-derived APC, and in some cases by (B) donor-derived APC; the latter is referred to as direct priming.

---

responsible: (1) for alloantigen capture; and (2) for presentation of processed alloantigen to prime naïve T cells (Box 8.7). Regarding the former, APC are recruited into the corneal matrix from the vascular compartment by way of the limbal vasculature, and also from the peripheral cornea (which houses various subpopulations of APC, including Langerhans cells, dendritic cells, and macrophages[38]). With the aid of adhesion molecules, cytokines and a chemokine gradient, APC traverse centrally towards the graft and their ultimate proximity to the donor tissue and increased presence allow for effective alloantigen capture. A series of phenotypic and functional changes, referred to as "maturation," also take place in the APC. These include acquisition of MHC class II (a peptide complex that loads and presents alloantigen to T cells) and acquisition of costimulatory molecules (secondary signals required to prime T cells) that render alloantigen-bearing APC more potent in stimulating T cells (Figure 8.5).

In addition to host APC, it is known that donor APCs prime T cells as well, as demonstrated in other forms of solid-tissue/organ transplantation and, more recently, in cornea transplantation (Figure 8.5). Referred to as "direct priming," this process occurs because grafts carry over APC from the donor and stimulate T cells in recipient regional lymph nodes. Interestingly, it was long believed that direct priming was not functionally relevant in corneal transplan-

tation. This was based on the tenet that corneal APC reside exclusively in the peripheral cornea and cornea grafts (which are harvested from the central cornea) are therefore devoid of donor APC. However, a series of studies had demonstrated the contrary; specifically, (1) it was first shown that APC reside in the central cornea in the normal condition, albeit at lower densities and at an immature state[38]; and (2) these donor APC play a significant role in priming host T cells under certain conditions, such as pre-existing inflammation and neovascularization present in high-risk graft beds.[39] Such levels of inflammation are associated with the presence of mature donor APC, which are absent in the normal-risk setting despite lower-grade surgically induced inflammation.

Homing to regional lymph nodes

Regional draining lymph nodes are key sites for T-cell priming following corneal transplantation, although there is some debate as to whether this is focused in the cervical or submandibular lymph nodes. The discovery that regional lymphadenectomy in mice results in complete immunological ignorance of the corneal graft and indefinite graft survival strongly supported this concept.[40] However, it was unclear at the time how mature APC reached these lymph nodes since the cornea was thought to be alymphatic. Recent evidence has helped explain this phenomenon with the discovery that pathologic corneal neovascularization following transplantation, which has long been known to stimulate viable blood neovessels (i.e., vessels that are CD36^{high} LYVE-1$^-$), also stimulates parallel ingrowth of lymphatic neovessels (i.e., vessels that are CD36^{low} LYVE-1+; Box 8.8).[41,42] Moreover, it was demonstrated that mature APC in the cornea express VEGF receptor-3, which guides their trafficking along a VEGF-C ligand gradient into lymphatic neovessels and to the regional lymph nodes.[43] Other chemokines such CCR7 have also been implicated in this process.[44]

T cells and effector mechanisms of graft destruction

As in most forms of solid allograft rejection, one of the principal mechanisms for rejection in the corneal graft rejection is DTH – a CD4+-mediated T helper (Th)-1 response involving interferon-γ cytokine secretion and macrophage recruitment. A series of convergent studies have supported this theory, particularly by the use of CD4-deficient hosts, which results in significant impairment in graft rejection.[45] In addition, studies focused on cytokine profiles of rejected cornea, aqueous humor, and draining lymph node have indicated a bias towards Th1 activity.[46] Likewise, local depletion of macrophages was shown to promote corneal allograft survival.[47] Recent work has also demonstrated that, in addition to functioning as helper T cells, CD4+ cells can directly execute graft destruction, although this mechanism is not completely understood.[48] It was also recently demonstrated that another subtype termed double-negative (CD4−CD8−) T cells, which were shown to be involved in DTH elicitation,

are also implicated in graft rejection via apoptosis of graft corneal endothelium.[49]

Other studies have indicated, however, that DTH is not the sole mechanism of cornea rejection (Box 8.9). Th1-deficient mice (via genetic deletion of interferon-γ), for example, can still reject corneal allografts.[50] It has also been demonstrated in a transplant model of allergic atopic conjunctivitis that heightened graft rejection can be associated with a Th2 phenotype (IL-4 and IL-5 secretion) – another branch of immunity responsible for humoral responses.[51] Despite these findings, however, there is substantial evidence that alloantibodies and complement-mediated mechanisms are not relevant in corneal rejection, as demonstrated by B-cell-deficient and complement-deficient (C3, and C5) engrafted mice.[52] An alternate branch of immunity also distinguished from DTH yet shown to be relevant in cornea transplantation involves CD8+ T lymphocytes. While the CD8+ compartment is deemed unnecessary for corneal rejection, demonstrated by graft rejection in CD8-defieicnt or perforin-deficient recipients, priming of CD8+ T cells does take place.[53] Furthermore, adoptive transfer of CD8+ T cells alone into engrafted severe combined immunodeficiency (SCID: T-cell-deficient) mice proved that these cells can mediate graft rejection, albeit in a significantly delayed fashion.[54]

Conclusion

The practice of corneal transplantation is increasing worldwide and yet even now the demand exceeds the supply of donor corneas. Hence, as the most prominent cause for corneal graft failure, the need to abrogate corneal graft rejection in the clinic is paramount. To this end, basic science research is a fundamental vista to elucidate key mechanisms of immune rejection and identify important targets for effective promotion of allograft survival. While technologies in instrumentation, surgical techniques, and tissue storage have greatly increased, the current mainstay for prevention and treatment of graft rejection is corticosteroids – a broad-spectrum drug which is variably effective in high-risk patients and is fraught with various systemic and ocular side-effects (e.g., glaucoma, and cataract). Rather than broad-spectrum immunosuppression, the next great stride in treating immunological conditions such as allograft rejection involves antigen-specific immune therapies. Indeed, the development of monoclonal antibodies for blockade of novel molecular pathways, and cellular therapies capable of specifically suppressing alloimmunity (i.e., autologous expansion of alloantigen-specific Tregs) is currently under way.

Key references

A complete list of chapter references is available online at www.expertconsult.com. See inside cover for registration details.

7. Khodadoust AA, Silverstein AM. Transplantation and rejection of individual cell layers of the cornea. Invest Ophthalmol 1969;8:180–195.

10. The Australian Corneal Graft Registry 2007 report. Available online at: http://hdl.handle.net/2328/1723.

14. Maguire MG, Stark WJ, Gottsch JD, et al. Risk factors for corneal graft failure and rejection in the collaborative corneal transplantation studies. Collaborative Corneal Transplantation Studies Research Group. Ophthalmology 1994;101:1536–1547.

19. [No authors listed] The collaborative corneal transplantation studies (CCTS). Effectiveness of histocompatibility matching in high-risk corneal transplantation. The Collaborative Corneal Transplantation Studies Research Group. Arch Ophthalmol 1992;110:1392–1403.

23. Cursiefen C, Chen L, Saint-Geniez M, et al. Nonvascular VEGF receptor 3 expression by corneal epithelium maintains avascularity and vision. Proc Natl Acad Sci USA 2006;103:11405–11410.

29. Masli S, Turpie B, Hecker KH, et al. Expression of thrombospondin in TGFbeta-treated APCs and its relevance to their immune deviation-promoting properties. J Immunol 2002;168:2264–2273.

35. Kaplan HJ, Streilein JW. Immune response to immunization via the anterior chamber of the eye. I. F1 lymphocyte-induced immune deviation. J Immunol 1977;118:809–814.

38. Hamrah P, Dana MR. Corneal antigen-presenting cells. Chem Immunol Allergy 2007;92:58–70.

39. Huq S, Liu Y, Benichou G, et al. Relevance of the direct pathway of sensitization in corneal transplantation is dictated by the graft bed microenvironment. J Immunol 2004;173:4464–4469.

40. Yamagami S, Dana MR. The critical role of lymph nodes in corneal alloimmunization and graft rejection. Invest Ophthalmol Vis Sci 2001;42:1293–1298.

43. Chen L, Hamrah P, Cursiefen C, et al. Vascular endothelial growth factor receptor-3 mediates induction of corneal alloimmunity. Nat Med 2004;10:813–815.

45. Yamada J, Kurimoto I, Streilein JW. Role of CD4+ T cells in immunobiology of orthotopic corneal transplants in mice. Invest Ophthalmol Vis Sci 1999;40:2614–2621.

48. Hegde S, Beauregard C, Mayhew E, et al. CD4(+) T-cell-mediated mechanisms of corneal allograft rejection: role of Fas-induced apoptosis. Transplantation 2005;79:23–31.

51. Beauregard C, Stevens C, Mayhew E, Niederkorn JY. Cutting edge: atopy promotes Th2 responses to alloantigens and increases the incidence and tempo of corneal allograft rejection. J Immunol 2005;174:6577–6581.

52. Goslings WR, Yamada J, Dana MR, et al. Corneal transplantation in antibody-deficient hosts. Invest Ophthalmol Vis Sci 1999;40:250–253.

CHAPTER 9

Corneal edema

Daniel G Dawson and Henry F Edelhauser

Overview

The corneal stroma accounts for 90% of the corneal thickness. The corneal stroma is predominantly composed of water (78% water or 3.5 g H_2O/g dry weight). Its dry weight is organized into a structural network of insoluble and soluble cellular and extracellular proteins: collagen (68%), keratocyte constituents (10%), proteoglycans (9%), and salts, glycoproteins, or other substances.[1] It is optically clear or transparent due to its lattice-like arrangement of small-diameter collagen fibrils and the near invisibility of its cells.

Although other cell types do exist in the cornea (e.g., Langerhans and dendritic bone marrow-derived immune cells, trigeminal nerve dendrites, Schwann cells, and histiocytes), the human cornea is primarily composed of three cell types: epithelial cells, stromal keratocytes, and endothelial cells.[1] They can all replicate through mitosis, but they vary significantly in their in vivo self-mitotic capacity (proliferative capacity), with epithelial cells being the most renewable, stromal keratocytes in the middle, and endothelial cells the least renewable. The limited proliferative capacity of human corneal endothelial cells is apparently only an in vivo phenomenon as endothelial cells can proliferate quite well in ex vivo cell culture conditions.[2–4] The in vivo mitotic quiescence of human corneal endothelium has been found to be predominantly due to cell contact inhibition, in part through the activity of p27.[3] This results in corneal endothelial cells being arrested in the G_1-phase of the cell cycle.[3] High aqueous humor concentrations of transforming growth factor (TGF)-$ß_2$, age-related cellular senescence, and lack of an injury-inducible cytokine-stimulating pathway are also secondary failsafe mechanisms that keep in vivo endothelial cell proliferation in check, if cell-to-cell contact is compromised.[2,3] These facts about corneal cellular proliferative capacity can be seen clinically since epithelial cells can completely regenerate after injury (e.g., corneal abrasions) or can develop into cancer (e.g., squamous cell cancers that originate from limbal progenitor cells, or stem cells, at the palisades of Vogt). On the other hand, age-related (e.g., Fuchs' dystrophy) or injury-related (e.g., pseudophakic bullous keratopathy) disease most commonly affects the corneal endothelium since it has little in vivo proliferative capacity.

The purpose of this chapter is to describe the pathophysiology of corneal edema.

Clinical background

Corneal edema is a term often used loosely and sometimes nonspecifically by clinicians, but literally refers to a cornea that is more hydrated than the normal 78% water content (Box 9.1).[1] With minor (<5%) hydration changes, the corneal thickness changes with minimal effect on the retractive, transparency, and biomechanical functions of the cornea. Only when the cornea become hydrated >5% above its physiologic level of 78% does it begin to scatter significant amounts of light and gradually loses transparency. Some loss of retractive function may also occur, particularly if the epithelial surface becomes irregular. The topic of corneal edema is important for clinicians to understand because it affects the architecture and function of the entire cornea.[1,5,6] Epithelial edema clinically causes a hazy microcystic appearance to occur in the epithelium in mild-to-moderate cases of corneal edema (Figure 9.1A), significantly decreasing vision, and increasing glare. It can also cause the development of large painful, subepithelial bullae in severe cases of corneal edema (Figure 9.1B). Stromal edema clinically appears as a painless, cloudy, thickening of the corneal stroma (Figure 9.1B), resulting in a mild-to-moderate reduction in visual acuity and an increase in glare. At the same time, Descemet's membrane folds commonly appear on the posterior surface of the cornea, particularly in severe cases of corneal edema (Figure 9.1B).

The exact incidence of corneal edema is unknown and is difficult to quantify since it is due to many causes and can fluctuate during the day or be transient or permanent in nature.

Clinically, the diagnostic workup includes slit-lamp examination and, commonly, pachymetry and/or specular or confocal microscopy to confirm whether corneal edema is present and to measure to what degree (Box 9.2).

The differential diagnosis of corneal edema includes corneal scarring, corneal inflammation, corneal infection, and corneal dystrophies.

The treatment options include limited temporary medical options, such as topical salt drops (e.g., Muro) to remove the excess water from the cornea via osmosis, hair drier blowing on the cornea to induce increased evaporation, or topical steroids to increase endothelial cell tight junctions temporarily, and surgery (Descemet's membrane-stripping

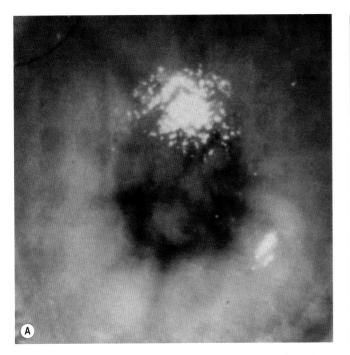 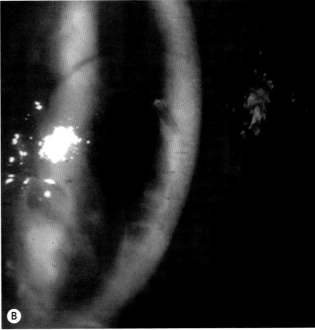

Figure 9.1 (A) Diffuse illumination view of a patient's cornea with moderate corneal edema from Fuchs' dystrophy. Notice the irregular corneal surface and focal areas of cloudy epithelium from microcystic epithelial edema. (B) Slit illumination view of a patient's cornea with a severe case of pseudophakic bullous keratopathy. Notice the diffuse cloudiness of the stroma and the Descemet's membrane folds. On the left side of the photo, a large epithelial bulla is also seen.

Box 9.1 Clinical background: corneal edema

- Hydration > 78%
- Epithelial edema
  - Microcystic appearance (reduces vision and increases glare)
  - Bullae (sometimes very painful and causes epithelial erosions)
- Stromal edema
  - Cloudy thickening (reduces vision and increases glare)
  - Descemet's membrane folds (reduces vision)

Box 9.2 Clinical background: diagnosis of corneal edema

Diagnosis

- Slit-lamp examination of cornea
- Confirmatory: pachymetry or specular microscopy

Box 9.3 Clinical background: treatment options

Treatment

- Medical adjuncts
  - Increase evaporation (hair drier)
  - Remove excess water with hyperosmotic agents (Muro eye drops)
  - Enhance tight junctions (topical steroids)
- Surgery
  - Full-thickness replacement (penetrating keratoplasty)
  - Component replacement (Descemet's membrane-stripping endothelial keratoplasty)

---

endothelial keratoplasty, penetrating keratoplasty) to replace the damaged or deficient number of remaining endothelial cells (Box 9.3). The main complications of surgery are graft rejection (endothelial cell allograft rejection), graft failure (transplanted endothelial cells are damaged by surgery or decrease to below optimal cell densities, usually because of chronic ongoing cell loss that is higher than normal unoperated eyes), decreased vision (irregular astigmatism, high astigmatism, or interface irregularity), infection (suture infections, ocular surface disease), and wound-healing issues (graft dehiscence, graft neovascularization, graft haze, neurotrophic epitheliopathy).

Pathology

Epithelial edema is seen histopathologically as hydropic basal epithelial cell degenerative changes and the development of extra-epithelial cellular fluid-filled spaces (e.g., cysts and bullae: Figure 9.2A).[7] Interestingly, if bullae are chronically present, a fibrocollagenous degenerative pannus oftentimes will grow into the subepithelial space, decreasing vision further, while reducing the pain. Histopathologically, the signs of stromal edema are seen on the light microscope as thickening of the corneal stroma in the posterior cross-sectional direction with loss of artifact stromal clefting (Figure 9.2A) and Descemet's membrane folds (Figure 9.2B).[6–8] Ultrastructural and biochemical studies have further

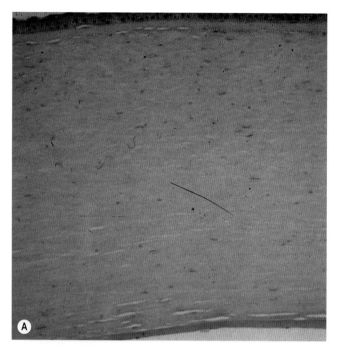

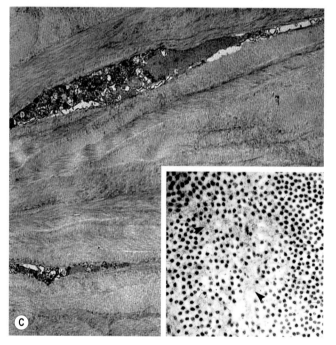

Figure 9.2 (A) Light microscopic photomicrograph (20×; hematoxylin and eosin stain) of a moderately edematous cornea due to pseudophakic bullous keratopathy. The basal epithelial cells display the signs of hydropic degeneration-enlarged cells with a pale washed-out-appearing cytoplasm. Normal artifacteous cleftings are only slightly found in this case because the corneal stroma is so edematous. There are few endothelial cells present on this cornea (1 endothelial cell/high-power field). (B) Light microscopic photomicrograph (20×; toluidene blue stain) of a severely edematous cornea due to acute endothelial cell damage. The keratocytes display signs of hydropic degeneration and the posterior corneal surface displays wavy folds in Descemet's membrane. (C) Transmission electron micrograph (12 000×) of the same severely edematous cornea as in (B). Notice the hydropic degenerative changes of the corneal stromal keratocytes: keratocytes exhibit loss of intracellular organelles, dissolution of cytoplasm, presence of intracellular spaces, and vacuoles. Inset: higher-magnification view (90 000×) of the collagen fibrils showing how corneal edema forms lakes between fibrils (arrowheads) and causes the normal lattice-like arrangement of fibrils to become quite irregular.

shown that stromal edema causes hydropic degenerative changes or cell lysis to occur in the resident keratocyte population (Figure 9.2B and C),[8] an increase in the distance and disruption of spatial order between collagen fibrils (Figure 9.2C inset),[9,10] a decrease in the refractive index of the extracellular matrix,[11] and a loss of proteoglycans.[12] The hydropic degenerative changes of the keratocyte and possibly the intrafibrillar lakes of fluid are the main correlates for the stromal cloudiness resulting from corneal edema. Although different proportions of the two types of negatively charged proteoglycan may account for the higher hydration levels in the posterior stroma compared to the anterior stroma (anterior cornea: 1.59 ratio of keratin sulfate to dermatan sulfate,

3.04 g H_2O/g dry weight; posterior cornea: 2.23 ratio of keratin sulfate to dermatan sulfate, 3.85 g H_2O/g dry weight), it appears that the directional orientation of the collagen fibrils and stromal lamellae probably have the greatest influence on how much each region thickens, or swells, as a result of increased hydration levels.[1,13 15] Because the collagenous architecture of the stroma (i.e., limbus-to-limbus directional orientation of collagen fibrils) highly resists circumferential expansion, only anterior–posterior expansion occurs in the human cornea, predominantly in the posterior direction. This latter fact occurs because extensive lamellar interweaving occurs in the anterior third of the corneal stroma, while weaker bridging filaments (i.e., type VI and fibril-associated collagens with interrupted terminals collagens) occur diffusely throughout the entire corneal stroma. Furthermore, this lamellar interweaving also explains why the anterior third of the cornea mildly swells, whereas the remaining corneal stroma can swell to up three times its normal thickness.[10] This anisotropic elasticity characteristic of the human cornea in swelling is important since the anterior corneal surface accounts for two-thirds of the refractive power of the eye. Because fibrotic corneal scars have random directionally oriented interweaving collagen fibrils, they have also been found to resist swelling under edematous conditions.[16]

Therefore, although it is commonly stated that corneal thickness and interfibrillar spacing increase in a linear fashion to the hydration level of the corneal stroma,[1,8] one needs to be aware that this relationship mainly applies to the mid and posterior stromal regions.

Etiology

Corneal edema is usually caused by one of two pathogenic mechanisms: endothelial cell dysfunction or high intraocular pressure (IOP). Common causes of endothelial dysfunction include Fuchs' endothelial dystrophy, pseudophakic bullous keratopathy (i.e., from cataract surgery), trauma, other ophthalmic surgery (corneal transplantation, trabeculectomy/tube shunt glaucoma surgery), infections, and toxic anterior-segment surgery (Box 9.4).[17–20] Common causes of high IOP include uncontrolled glaucoma (acute angle closure glaucoma, neovascular glaucoma, pseudoexfoliation glaucoma), postoperative pressure spikes from retained viscoelastics, and medications (topical steroids).

Pathophysiology

Embryology to birth

During embryogenesis, the corneal endothelium forms during the 5th week of gestation as the first wave of neural crest-derived mesodermal cells form a two-cell layered primitive endothelium. By 8 weeks of gestation, a monolayer of cells is formed. The epithelium and endothelium remain closely opposed until 7 weeks of gestation (49 days) when a second wave of neural crest-derived mesodermal cells begins to grow centrally from the limbus between the epithelium and endothelium, producing the corneal stroma. By the 3rd month of gestation, Descemet's membrane can be clearly recognized on histologic sections. Studies have inferred that during the 5th month of gestation the tight junctions completely form and the endothelial barrier is established; similarly, by 5–7 months' gestation, the density of Na^+/K^+-ATPase pump sites eventually reaches adult levels so that the cornea becomes dehydrated and transparent.[21,22] By the 7th month of gestation, the cornea resembles that of the adult in most structural characteristics other than size. At birth in the full-term infant, the horizontal diameter of the cornea is only around 9.8 mm (surface area 102 mm^2), or approximately 75–80% the size of an adult human cornea (note at birth, that the posterior segment is <50% the size of an adult human cornea).

Infancy to adulthood

The endothelium of a newborn infant cornea is composed of a single layer of approximately 500 000 neural crest-derived endothelial cells, each measuring around 5 μm in thickness by 20 μm in diameter, and covering a surface area of 250 μm^2.[5,20,23–25] The cells lie on the posterior surface of the cornea and form an irregular polygonal mosaic. The tangential appearance of each corneal endothelial cell is uniquely irregular, usually uniform in size to one another, and typically six-sided hexagons (which is the most energy-efficient and optimal shape to cover a surface area without leaving gaps).[1] They abut one another in an interdigitating fashion with a 20 nm wide intercellular space between each other (Figure 9.3A and B). The intercellular space is known to contain discontinuous apical tight junctions (Figure 9.3C), or macula occludens tight junctions, and lateral gap junctions (Figure 9.3D). Thus, intercellular space of the corneal endothelium represents an incomplete diffusion barrier to small molecules. As corneal endothelial cells have numerous cytoplasmic organelles, particularly mitochondria, they have been studied and are presumed to have the second highest aerobic metabolic rate of all cells in the eye next to retinal photoreceptors.[7] At birth, the central endothelial cell density of the human cornea is around 5000 cells/mm^2.[5] Because the corneal endothelium has very limited in vivo regenerative capacity (endothelial cells are currently hypothesized to proliferate at too low a rate in vivo to replace dying cells) and because aging results in progressive cellular senescence, particularly in the central regions of the cornea in part through the activity of the cyclin-dependent kinase inhibitor p21, there is a well-documented decline in central endothelial cell density with age that typically involves two phases: a rapid and slow component (Figure 9.4).[2–4,5,20,23–25] During infancy, the cornea continues to grow over the first 2 years of life, reaching adult size at 2 years of age with an average horizontal diameter of 11.7 mm (surface area 138 mm^2). Thereafter, it changes very little in size, shape, and optical properties. However, the only significant structure in the cornea that continues to grow after age 2 is the Descemet's membrane as it gradually increases an additional 6–11 μm in thickness from birth to death. Due to corneal growth and age-related or developmentally selec-

---

Box 9.4 Etiology

Endothelial cell dysfunction

- Fuchs' endothelial cell dystrophy
- Pseudophakic bullous keratopathy (cataract surgery)
- Trauma
- Other intraocular surgeries (glaucoma shunts, corneal transplantation)
- Infections (corneal ulcers or endophthalmitis)
- Toxic anterior-segment syndrome (toxic substances in anterior chamber)

High intraocular pressure

- Uncontrolled glaucoma (acute angle closure glaucoma, neovascular glaucoma, pseudoexfoliation glaucoma)
- Postoperative pressure spikes (retained viscoelastics)
- Medications (topical steroids)

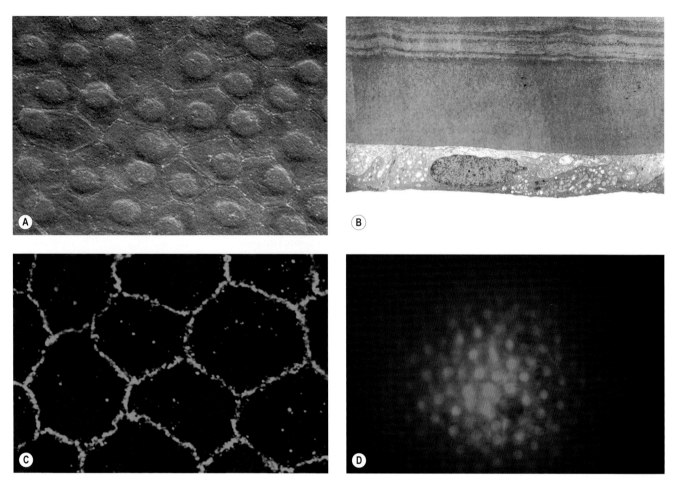

Figure 9.3 (A) Scanning electron micrograph (1000×) on the posterior surface of the corneal endothelium from a 65-year-old patient with healthy eyes. Note how the hexagonal endothelial cells form a uniform monolayer with small 20 nm intercellular spaces between adjacent endothelial cells. E, endothelial cells; IS, intercellular space. (B) Transmission electron micrograph (4750×) of the posterior corneal stroma, Descemet's membrane, and corneal endothelium from a 65-year-old patient with healthy eyes. PS, posterior stroma; BDM, banded portion of Descemet's membrane; NBDM, nonbanded portion of Descemet's membrane; E, endothelial cells; IS, intercellular space. (C) Immunoflourescence confocal microscopy photomicrograph (2000×) of human corneal endothelial tight junctional complexes stained with immunolabeled monoclonal antibodies to junctional adhesion molecule-A (green). Nuclei are counterstained with TO-PRO (blue). (Courtesy of Kenneth J. Mandell, MD, PhD) (D) Photomicrograph (400×) of fluorescein dye spreading between many adjacent endothelial cells in a human cornea, demonstrating the intimate importance of gap junctions in how endothelial cells communicate with one another. (Courtesy of Mitchell A. Watsky, PhD.)

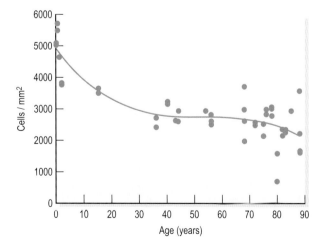

Figure 9.4 Scatterplot with best-fit curve showing the average central corneal endothelial cell density for normal, healthy eyes of different ages. (Redrawn with permission from Williams KK, Noe RL, Grossniklaus HE, et al. Correlation of histologic corneal endothelial cells counts with specular microscopic cell density. Arch Ophthalmol 1992;110:1146–1149).

tive cell death, during the fast component of cell loss, the central endothelial cell density decreases exponentially to about 3500 cells/mm^2 by age 5 and 3000 cells/mm^2 by age 14–20.[5,20,23–25] Thereafter, a slow component of cell loss occurs where central endothelial cell density decreases to a linear steady rate between 0.3 and 0.6% per year, resulting in cell density measurements around 2500 cell/mm^2 in late adulthood.[5,20,23–25] Because the corneal endothelium essentially maintains its continuity by migration and expansion of surviving cells, it is not surprising that the percentage of hexagonal cells decreases (pleomorphism) and the coefficient of variation of cell area increases (polymegathism) with age.[23]

When reviewing this information it is important to realize that these are average central corneal endothelial cell counts from predominantly Caucasian US populations. Several studies reveal that important racial and geographic differences exist as Japanese, Filipino, and Chinese corneas have been found to have higher central cell density measurements than Caucasians, while Indian corneas have lower central

Table 9.1 Comparison of central endothelial cell density in Indian, American, Chinese, Filipino, and Japanese populations

Age groups (years)	Indian* No. of eyes	Indian* Cell density (cells/mm²)	American† No. of eyes	American† Cell density (cells/mm²)	Chinese‡ No. of eyes	Chinese‡ Cell density (cells/mm²)	Filipino§ No. of eyes	Filipino§ Cell density (cells/mm²)	Japanese† No. of eyes	Japanese† Cell density (cells/mm²)
20–30	104	2782 ± 250	11	2977 ± 324	100	2988 ± 243	114	2949 ± 270	18	3893 ± 259
31–40	96	2634 ± 288	6	2739 ± 208	100	2920 ± 325	112	2946 ± 296	10	3688 ± 245
41–50	97	2408 ± 274	11	2619 ± 321	97	2935 ± 285	112	2761 ± 333	10	3749 ± 407
51–60	98	2438 ± 309	13	2625 ± 172	97	2810 ± 321	102	2555 ± 178	10	3386 ± 455
61–70	88	2431 ± 357	8	2684 ± 384	90	2739 ± 316	114	2731 ± 299	6	3307 ± 330
>70	54	2360 ± 357	15	2431 ± 339	83	2778 ± 365	86	2846 ± 467	15	3289 ± 313

*Rao SK, Sen PR, Fogla R, et al. Corneal endothelial cell density and morphology in normal Indian eyes. Cornea 2000;19: 820–823.
†Matsuda M, Yee RW, Edelhauser HF. Comparison of the corneal endothelium in an American and a Japanese Population. Arch Ophthalmol 1985;103: 68–70.
‡Yunliang S, Yuqiang H, Ying-peng L, et al. Corneal endothelial cell density and morphology in healthy Chinese eyes. Cornea 2007;26: 130–132.
§Padilla MDB, Sibayan SAB, Gonzales CSA. Corneal endothelial cell density and morphology in normal Filipino eyes. Cornea 2004;23: 129–135.

cell densities (Table 9.1).[26-29] It is hypothesized that this range of central cell densities may be predominantly due to racial differences in corneal diameter and endothelial surface area between these groups (e.g., Japanese, Caucasian, and Indian horizontal corneal diameters averaged 11.2, 11.7, and 12.0 mm, respectively), but genetic and environmental factors are also possible. Additionally, these data only apply to central corneal endothelial counts since recent work has shown that higher endothelial cell densities can typically be found in more peripheral aspects of the cornea, where a potential "stem-like" endothelial cell population or storage zone may reside (Figure 9.5).[30-32] Therefore, overall it appears that corneal endothelial cell numbers decrease on average about 50% from birth to death in normal subjects. As corneal decompensation or overt corneal edema typically does not occur until the central endothelial cell density approaches values around 500 cells/mm² (90% decreased from infant values), there appears to be plenty of cellular reserve remaining after an average human life span of 75–80 years.[5,20,23-25] In fact, estimates suggest that normal human corneal endothelium should maintain corneal clarity up to a minimum of 224–277 years of life, if humans lived that long.[25]

The primary function of the corneal endothelium is to maintain the deturgescence (i.e., it keeps the cornea near 78% water) and clarity of the cornea through both barrier and a pump leak mechanism first described by David Maurice.[33] Secondarily, it is also known to secrete an anteriorly located basement membrane called Descemet's membrane and a posteriorly located glycocalyx layer.[1]

Barrier function

The barrier function of the endothelium is dependent upon having a sufficient number of corneal endothelial cells to cover the posterior surface of the cornea and having integrity of endothelial cellular tight junctions, which are present in the intercellular spaces between endothelial cells (Figure 9.6). Macula occludens tight junctions are characterized by

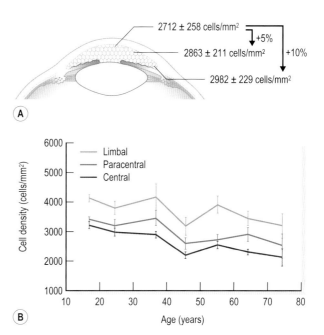

Figure 9.5 Diagram (A) and graph (B) illustrating the central, paracentral, and peripheral corneal endothelial cell densities in healthy, normal subjects. ((A) Modified from Edelhauser HF. The resiliency of the corneal endothelium to refractive and intraocular surgery. Cornea 2000;19:263–273; (B) redrawn with permission from Edelhauser HF. The Proctor lecture: the balance between corneal transparency and edema. Invest Ophthalmol Vis Sci 2006;47:1755–1767.)

partial total obliteration of the 20 nm wide intercellular space and partial sub-total retention so that 10 nm intercellular spaces remain. Clinically, the barrier function of the cornea can be assessed by the use of the specular microscope or the confocal microscope (endothelial cell density), and fluorophotometry (permeability). In healthy human corneas, this barrier prevents the bulk flow of fluid from the aqueous humor to the corneal stroma, but does allow moderate diffusion of some nutrients, water, and other metabolites to cross into the stroma through the 20 nm wide intercellular

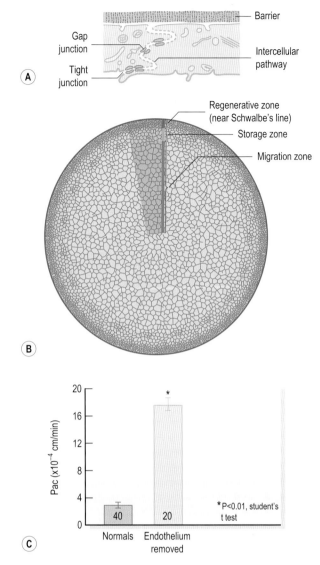

Figure 9.6 Diagrams (A and B) illustrating the normal barrier function of corneal endothelium, which is due to endothelial cells covering the posterior corneal surface with gap and the focal, tight junctions (macula occludens). The bar graph (C) shows the normal permeability of the human endothelial monolayer to carboxyfluorescein compared to that without endothelium, which resulted in a sixfold increase in permeability. (Modified from Watsky MA, McDermott ML, Edelhauser HF. In vitro corneal endothelial permeability in rabbit and human: the effects of age, cataract surgery, and diabetes. Exp Eye Res 1989;49:751–767.)

spaces. The leaky endothelial barrier may initially seem inefficient, but when one considers that most nutrients of the cornea come from the aqueous humor, some leakiness of the monolayer is reasonable. Additionally, despite the normal loss of endothelial cells that occurs with age, there appears to be no appreciable increase in the permeability of normal aged corneas to diffusion across the corneal endothelium.[34] Only when the endothelium is severely reduced in cell density (central endothelial cell density < 2000 cells/mm^2), is acutely damaged, and/or has disrupted cell junctions, does its permeability increase (up to a maximum sixfold increase in permeability to carboxyfluorescein (12.85×10^{-4} cm/min) compared to normal (2.26×10^{-4} cm/min)).[34]

Pump leak mechanism

The classic temperature reversal studies provided the first evidence that the maintenance of corneal hydration and transparency was metabolically dependent.[35] Corneal thickness and corneal cloudiness were found to increase when intact eyes were refrigerated. This effect was observed to reverse (i.e., the tissue thinned and regained transparency) when the tissue was rewarmed (temperature reversal). Subsequent in vitro corneal perfusion studies demonstrated that temperature reversal still occurred in the absence of the corneal epithelium, implicating active metabolically dependent processes on the corneal endothelium as mediating corneal deturgescence.[1] These studies also demonstrated that transporters, located primarily on a corneal endothelial cell's lateral cell membrane, affected the transport of ions – principally sodium (Na^+) and bicarbonate (HCO_3^-) – out of the stroma and into the aqueous humor. An osmotic gradient is created and water is osmotically drawn from the stroma into the aqueous humor.[36] It is important to note that this osmotic gradient only occurs if the endothelial barrier is maintained. The transport protein essential for endothelial "pump function" was later identified as Na^+/K^+-ATPase (Figure 9.7A).[37,38] Subsequently, the number and density of Na^+/K^+-ATPase sites have also been quantified using [^{3}H]-ouabain.[39] These studies have shown that approximately 2.1 million Na^+/K^+-ATPase sites are present on the lateral membrane of a single human corneal endothelial cell. This corresponds to an average pump site density of 4.4 trillion ATPase sites/mm^2 along the lateral plasma membrane wall of an intact corneal endothelial cell.[39] Clinically, the metabolic pump of the corneal endothelium can be assessed in vivo by measuring how quickly the corneal thickness (pachymetry) recovers after being purposefully swollen by wearing oxygen-impermeable contact lens or by measuring the diurnal change in corneal thickness (normal = $6 \pm 3\%$; eyelid closure during sleep induces hypoxia and decreased evaporation loss).

A number of factors are known to alter endothelial pump function. Fortunately, physiologic compensatory mechanisms prevent corneal edema from occurring to a certain degree when central endothelial cell densities are between 2000 and 750 cells/mm^2. This occurs by either increasing the activity of pump sites already present, which requires more ATP production by the cell, and/or by increasing the density of pump sites on the lateral membranes of endothelial cells (Figure 9.7B and C).[39] A similar phenomenon occurs in the proximal tubule cells of the human kidney to adjust for an increased salt load. For example, in Fuchs' endothelial dystrophy, the cornea has been found to remain clear and of normal thickness despite having very low endothelial cell densities and increased endothelial monolayer permeability to fluorescein (5.30×10^{-4} cm/min).[39] Apparently, this occurs because the metabolic activity and density of the Na^+/K^+ pump sites increase to compensate for the increased permeability.[40] The point at which compensatory mechanisms appear to fail is when the central endothelial cell density reaches around 500 cells/mm^2 (range of 750–250 cells/mm^2) (Figure 9.7B and C).[5,41] At this low cell count, the permeability has greatly increased to such a point that the endothelial cells – which are spread so thin – do not have enough room on their lateral cell membranes for more metabolic pump sites and all the current pumps are maximally active. Therefore, the metabolic pump fails to balance the leak and corneal edema results. A summary of the entire corneal endothelial cell transport system was most recently reviewed by Bonanno.[42]

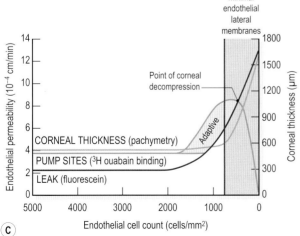

When the corneal endothelial barrier and metabolic pump are functioning normally, the corneal stroma has a total Na+ concentration of 179 mEq/L (134.4 mEq/L free and 44.6 mEq/L bound to stromal proteoglycans), while the aqueous humor has a total Na+ concentration of 142.9 mEq/L (all free).[43] Therefore, after accounting for chloride activity and stromal imbibition pressure, an osmotic gradient of +30.4 mmHg exists, causing water to diffuse from the stroma to the aqueous humor (Figure 9.8A). When the corneal endothelium is damaged, there is a loss of both the corneal barrier and pump function, followed by a loss of the ionic gradients, ultimately resulting in corneal edema and stromal swelling (Figure 9.8B).

Pathophysiology of corneal edema

The Donnan effect states that the swelling pressure in a charged gel (e.g., the corneal stroma) results from ionic imbalances. The fixed negative or anionic charges on corneal stromal proteoglycan glycosaminoglycan (GAG) side-chains – one carboxylic acid and one sulfate ester side chain per disaccharide repeat on a dermatan sulfate GAG polymer, and one or two sulfate ester side-chains per disaccharide repeat on a keratan sulfate GAG polymer – have a central role in this effect. The antiparallel GAG duplexes (tertiary structure) produce long-range electrostatic repulsive forces that induce an expansive force termed swelling pressure. Because the corneal stroma also has cohesive and tensile strengths that resist expansion, the normal swelling pressure of the non-edematous corneal stroma is around 55 mmHg.[44,45] If the stroma is further compressed (e.g., increasing IOP or mechanical applanation) or expanded (e.g., corneal edema), the swelling pressure will correspondingly increase or decrease. Conversely, the negatively charged GAG side-chains also form a double-folded helix in aqueous solution (secondary structure) that attracts and binds Na+ cations, which results in an osmotic effect, leading to the diffusion and subsequent absorption of water. Thus, the central corneal thickness is maintained with an average value of

Figure 9.7 Diagram (A) illustrates the corneal endothelial cell pump, which is due to many Na+/K+-ATPase pump sites on the lateral membrane of each corneal endothelial cell. (Modified from Dawson DG, Watsky MA, Geroski DH, et al. Physiology of the eye and visual system: cornea and sclera. In: Tasman W, Jaeger EA (eds) Duane's Foundation of Clinical Ophthalmology on CD-ROM. Philadelphia: Lippincott Williams & Wilkins, 2006:v. 2 c. 4:1–76.) Diagram (B) and graph (C) illustrate the relationship between central endothelial cell density, barrier function, pump sites, and pachymetry. Note that the number pump sites are not all maximally used in the normal state (5000–2000 cells/mm²). With increased leaking (2000–750 cells/mm²), there is an adaptive phase in which the endothelial cells can maximally use all their pump sites and/or can form more pump sites to offset the leak up to a point. When the surface area of the lateral membranes of endothelial cells progressively becomes too small (750–0 cells/mm²), these adaptations reach a maximum and eventually decline. The point where endothelial cell pump site adaptations cross permeability (500 cells/mm²) is typically when corneal decompensation occurs. ((B) Modified from Chandler JW, Sugar J, Edelhauser HF. External diseases: cornea, conjunctiva, sclera, eyelids, lacrimal system, vol. 8. London: Mosby, 1994; (C) redrawn with permission from Dawson DG, Watsky MA, Geroski DH, et al. Physiology of the eye and visual system: cornea and sclera. In: Tasman W, Jaeger EA (eds) Duane's Foundation of Clinical Ophthalmology on CD-ROM. Philadelphia: Lippincott Williams & Wilkins, 2006:v. 2 c. 4:1–76.)

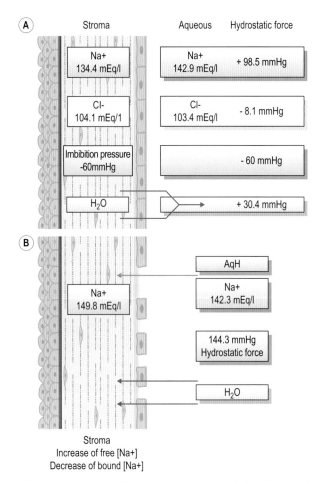

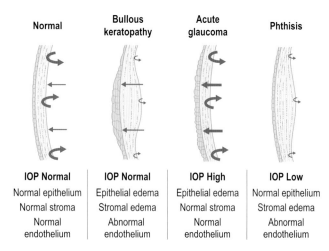

Figure 9.9 Diagram demonstrating the delicate balance between stromal swelling pressure, endothelial pump function, and intraocular pressure (IOP). Usually if endothelial cell pump function fails and IOP remains normal, both stromal and epithelial edema occurs (B). Only when IOP increases above the swelling pressure of the stroma and the endothelium functions normally do we see epithelial cell edema alone (C) and only when IOP is near zero and the endothelium functions abnormally do we see stromal edema alone (D). (Modified from Hatton MP, Perez VL, Dohlman CH. Corneal oedema in ocular hypotony. Exp Eye Res 2004;78:549–552.).

Figure 9.8 Diagram (A) illustrates the total transendothelial osmotic force due to Na+ activity, Cl− activity, and imbibition pressure. Although the Na+ activity within the aqueous humor is greater than that within the stroma (142.9 versus 134.4 mEq/L; $P < 0.05$.), using a reflection coefficient of 0.6, the calculated osmotic force due to Na+ is 98.5 mmHg. Similar calculations for Cl− and imbibition pressure result in osmotic forces of −8.1 and −60 mmHg, respectively. The sum of these forces results in a total osmotic force of +30.4 mmHg, which ultimately results in deturgescence of the cornea. Diagram (B) illustrates what happens to the ionic gradients and osmotic forces when the corneal endothelium is damaged and corneal edema and swelling set in. (Modified from Stiemke MM, Roman RJ, Palmer M, et al. Na+ activity in the aqueous humor and corneal stroma of the rabbit. J Exp Eye Res 1992;55:425–433.)

520 µm (based on optical pachymetry) or 540 µm (based on ultrasound pachymetry) because the fixed negatively charged proteoglycans induce a constant swelling pressure through anionic repulsive forces, and because the hydration level of corneal stroma is constantly maintained at around 78% water because corneal stromal proteoglycans imbibe water through cationic attractive forces.[46] Interestingly, there is a difference in the water-absorbing characteristics between the anterior and posterior cornea from differences in the distribution of proteoglycans made in these two regions (anterior: more dermatan sulfate, low free water-binding capacity, high retentive water-binding capacity; posterior: more keratin sulfate, high free water-binding capacity, low retentive water-binding capacity).[14] Under normal circumstances, the negative pressure drawing fluid into the cornea, called the imbibition pressure of the corneal stroma, is approximately −40 mmHg.[47] This implies that the negative

charges on corneal proteoglycans are only about one-quarter (~27%) saturated, or bound, with Na+ and water, and that the remaining unbound proportion is still available to bind more Na+ and absorb more water if given either a compromised endothelium or epithelium, or both. Normally, the highly impermeable epithelium and mildly impermeable endothelium keep the diffusion of electrolytes and fluid flow in the stroma to such a low level (resistance to diffusion of electrolytes and fluid flow = epithelium (2000) >> endothelium (10) > stroma (1)) that the aqueous humor ionic gradient created by the endothelial cell metabolic pump can maintain stromal hydration in the normal range of 78%.

Although imbibitions pressure (IP) = swelling pressure (SP) when corneas are in the ex vivo state, IP is actually lower than SP in the in vivo state because of the hydrostatic pressure induced by IOP, which must now be accounted for. This is best represented by the equation IP = IOP − SP[1] and explains why the hydration level of a patient's cornea is not only dependent on having normal barrier functions, but also on having a normal IOP. Therefore, a loss of corneal barrier function, an IOP ≥ 55 mmHg, or a combination of the two results in corneal edema.[48]

Finally, while both epithelial and stromal edema commonly coexist, there are two notable exceptions (Figure 9.9). As the epithelium lacks fixed negatively charged proteoglycans and has much weaker cohesive and tensile strength values than the corneal stroma, its state of hydration is mainly dictated by IOP levels.[49] Conversely, because collagen fibrils in the corneal stroma are anchored at the limbus for 360°, they exert increasing or decreasing cohesive strength on the corneal stroma as the IOP elevates above or decreases below normal, respectively. This results in the transmission of stromal edema to the epithelial surface in cases of high IOP or to the stroma in cases of low IOP. Therefore, if IOP is ≥ 55 mmHg with normal endothelial barrier and pump function, epithelial edema usually occurs by itself, or if endothelial cell dysfunction and hypotony (IOP ~0 mmHg) occur together, then stromal edema occurs alone.

Summary

In summary, although born with a substantial reserve of extra corneal endothelial cells for maintenance of normal corneal hydration and function, normal wear and tear on the human cornea from growth, development, and aging to an average human life span of 75–80 years of age reduce an individual's central endothelial cell density on average by 50% (5000 cells/mm^2 to 2500 cells/mm^2). Compounding this normal decline are other potential exogenous stressors (trauma, infections, corneal transplant procedures, and intraocular surgery at a very young age) that could potentially damage the endothelial monolayer further so that it reaches a 90% reduction in cell density (~500 cells/mm^2) from intent values. It is typically only around a central endothelial cell density of 500 cells/mm^2 that corneal edema manifests clinically and corneal function drops precipitously.

Acknowledgment

This work was supported in part by NEI grants EY-00933, P30-EY06360, and an unrestricted departmental grant from Research to Prevent Blindness.

Key references

A complete list of chapter references is available online at www.expertconsult.com. See inside cover for registration details.

1. Dawson DG, Watsky MA, Geroski DH, et al. Physiology of the eye and visual system: cornea and sclera. In: Tasman W, Jaeger EA (eds) Duane's Foundation of Clinical Ophthalmology on CD-ROM. Philadelphia: Lippincott Williams & Wilkins, 2006:v. 2 c. 4:1–76.

5. Edelhauser HF. Castroviejo lecture: the resiliency of the corneal endothelium to refractive and intraocular surgery. Cornea 2000;19:263–273.

6. Edelhauser HF. The balance between corneal transparency and edema. The Proctor lecture. Invest Ophthalmol Vis Sci 2006;47:755–767.

7. Hogan MJ, Alavarado JA, Weddell E. Histology of the Human Eye. Philadelphia: WB Saunders, 1971:55–180.

8. Dawson DG, Holley GP, Schmack I, et al. Hydropic degenerative keratocytes contribute to corneal haze in edematous human corneas. IOVS 2006;47:ARVO e-abstract B93.

20. Bourne WM. Biology of the corneal endothelium in health and disease. Eye 2003;17:912–918.

25. Armitage WJ, Dick AD, Bourne WM. Predicting endothelial cell loss and long-term corneal graft survival. Invest Ophthalmol Vis Sci 2003;44:326–331.

31. Amann J, Holley GP, Lee S, et al. Increased endothelial cell density in the paracentral and peripheral regions of the human cornea. Am J Ophthalmol 2003; 135:584–590.

32. Whikehart DR, Parikh CH, Vaugh AV, et al. Evidence suggesting the existence of stem cells for the human corneal endothelium. Mol Vis 2005;11:816–824.

33. Maurice DM. The cornea and sclera. In: Davson H (ed.) The Eye, vol. IB, 3rd edn. Orlando: Academic Press, 1984:1–158.

35. Harris JE. Symposium on the cornea. Introduction: factors influencing corneal hydration. Invest Ophthalmol 1962;1: 151–157.

38. Lim JJ, Ussing HH. Analysis of presteady-state Na$^+$ fluxes across the rabbit corneal endothelium. J Membrane Biol 1982;65: 197–204.

39. Geroski DH, Matsuda M, Yee RW, et al. Pump function of the human corneal endothelium. Effects of age and corneal guttata. Ophthalmology 1985;92:759–763.

42. Bonanno JA. Identity and regulation of ion transport mechanisms in the corneal endothelium. Prog Retin Eye Res 2003; 22:69–94.

48. Ytteborg J, Dohlman CH. Corneal edema and intraocular pressure. II. Clinical results. Arch Ophthalmol 1965;74:477–484.

CHAPTER 10

Corneal angiogenesis and lymphangiogenesis

Chih-Wei Wu, David Ellenberg, and Jin-Hong Chang

Overview

Corneal neovascularization (NV) and lymphangiogenesis are sight-threatening conditions that introduce vascular conditions into the normally avascular cornea (Box 10.1). Corneal NV is induced by various stimuli and is mainly associated with inflammation, trauma, transplantation, and infection of the ocular surface[1,2]; lymphangiogenesis is usually concurrent with hemangiogenesis in the human cornea.[3] Both corneal NV and lymphangiogenesis are promoted or inhibited by a balance of factors, including the dynamics between vascular endothelial growth factor (VEGF), VEGF-C, VEGF-D, sFlt, VEGFR3, endostatin, and thrombospondin-1 and -2 contained in the cornea (Box 10.2). Recently, evidence has shown that soluble VEGF receptor (VEGFR-1) and ectopic VEGFR-3 are expressed in corneal epithelial cells, and act as decoy receptors for VEGF-A and VEGF-C/-D, respectively.[4–7] These decoy receptors function to maintain corneal clarity and prevent corneal NV and lymphangiogenesis. In corneas that are diseased by inflammation, infection, degeneration, transplantation, or trauma, the normal balance of pro- and antiangiogenic factors is shifted toward proangiogenic status, leading to corneal NV and/or lymphangiogenesis. The pathogenesis of corneal NV and lymphangiogenesis may be influenced by growth factors, cytokines, matrix components, and matrix metalloproteinases (MMPs). New medical and surgical treatments that have been effective in corneal NV/lymphangiogenesis in animals and humans include immunosuppressant agents, angiostatic steroids, nonsteroidal anti-inflammatory drugs (NSAIDs), argon laser photocoagulation, and both photodynamic and antiangiogenic therapies.

The main purpose of this chapter is to describe the pathophysiology of corneal NV and lymphangiogenesis. The current treatments and potential antiangiogenic and/or antilymphangiogenic therapies will also be addressed at the end of this chapter.

Clinical background

Corneal NV and lymphangiogenesis together represent major public health burdens in the USA, affecting an estimated 1.4 million patients in any given year.[1] These conditions are caused by a wide range of inflammatory, infectious, degenerative, toxic, and traumatic disorders; major ocular complications include corneal scarring, edema, lipid deposition, and inflammation (Box 10.3). Corneal NV and lymphangiogenesis not only significantly alter visual acuity, but also worsen the prognosis of subsequent penetrating keratoplasty.

Corneal NV originates from the perilimbal plexus of conjunctival venules and capillaries and may invade the cornea at any level. Two types of corneal NV can be clinically discerned: pannus and stromal NV. In pannus NV, the proliferation of blood vessels spreads between the epithelium and Bowman's layer and is usually associated with ocular surface disorders such as infection, trauma, or metabolic dysfunction. In stromal NV, the vessels are usually in a straight line, following the anatomical divisions of the corneal lamellae and branching in a brushlike manner. This is most common in inflammatory status of the cornea, like stromal keratitis.

Clinically, patients with corneal NV may complain of a decrease in visual acuity. The diagnostic workup should include slit-lamp examination, which will identify the origin of the NV, as well as the depth of its invasion in the cornea. If corneal edema is presented at the same time, employment of pachymetry, specular microscopy, or confocal microscopy can aid in confirmation of the diagnosis.

Treatment of corneal NV has been widely investigated both medically and surgically. Current treatments for corneal NV in humans include steroids, NSAIDs, ciclosporin A, anti-VEGF-A antibody, argon laser, electrocoagulation, limbal transplantation, amniotic membrane transplantation, and conjunctival transplantation.

Pathology

In corneal pannus, a fibrous tissue with a significant vascular component is seen between the epithelium and Bowman's layer; this is called "subepithelial fibrovascular pannus." There are two types of corneal pannus: inflammatory pannus and degenerative pannus. Inflammatory pannus is associated with prominent leukocytic infiltration and includes polymorphonuclear leukocytes in the active stages. However, by the time the pathologist detects the inflammatory pannus, it is commonly constituted by overwhelming numbers of lymphocytes and plasma cells. Frequently, the Bowman's layer is disrupted, and the vessels wander haphazardly through the anterior stroma. In degenerative pannus, there are fewer inflammatory cells. The vascular component has never been prominent and is liable to regress, leaving a

Box 10.1 Corneal neovascularization (NV) and lymphangiogenesis

- Corneal NV and lymphangiogenesis are sight-threatening conditions that introduce vascular conditions into the normally avascular cornea
- Corneal NV and lymphangiogenesis are derived from:
  - Inflammatory disorders
  - Infection
  - Degenerative congenital disorders
  - Trauma and other causes

Box 10.2 Balance of angiogenic/antiangiogenic and lymphangiogenic/antilymphangiogenic factors dictates corneal neovascularization and lymphangiogenesis

Both corneal neovascularization and lymphangiogenesis are promoted or inhibited by a balance of proangiogenic, antiangiogenic, prolymphangiogenic, and antilymphangiogenic factors:

- Basic fibroblast growth factor, vascular endothelial growth factor (VEGF), VEGF-C, VEGF-D
- sFlt, VEGFR3, endostatin, thrombospondin-1, -2, and others

hyalinized, relatively acellular layer of fibrous tissue. This type of pannus is especially common in conditions that give rise to chronic epithelial edema, such as glaucoma.

Stromal NV differs from its superficial counterparts and is located beneath the Bowman's layer. Although it can occur anywhere in the stroma, it is usually identified at the upper and middle third of this layer.

Etiology

The clinical situations precluding corneal NV are replete; however, they can be grouped into four categories (Table 10.1 and Figures 10.1–10.3):

Box 10.3 Corneal neovascularization and lymphangiogenesis may cause ocular complications

Corneal neovascularization and lymphangiogenesis together represent major public health burdens and can cause many ocular complications, including:

- Corneal scarring
- Edema
- Lipid deposition
- Inflammation
- Transplantation rejection

Table 10.1 Diseases associated with corneal neovascularization and lymphangiogenesis

Disease	Corneal neovascularization	Lymphangiogenesis	Figures	References
Inflammatory disorders				
Ocular pemphigoid	Yes	NA	Figure 10.1	45
Atopic conjunctivitis	Yes	NA	Figure 10.2	46, 47
Rosacea	Yes	NA		48
Graft rejection	Yes	Yes		49
Stevens–Johnson syndrome	Yes	NA	Figure 10.1	45
Graft-versus-host disease	Yes	NA		50
Infection				
Herpes simplex	Yes	NA		
Herpes zoster	Yes	NA		51
Pseudomonas	Yes	NA		52
Chlamydia trachomatis	Yes	NA		53
Candida	Yes	NA		54
Onchocerciasis	Yes	NA		55
Degenerative congenital disorders				
Pterygium	Yes	NA		56
Terrien's marginal degeneration	Yes	NA		57
Aniridia	Yes	NA		58, 59
Traumatic and others				
Contact lens	Yes	NA		60
Chemical burn	Yes	Yes	Figures 10.1 and 10.2	47, 61
Ulceration	Yes	NA		62
Stem cell deficiency	Yes	Yes	Figure 10.3	34, 47, 63

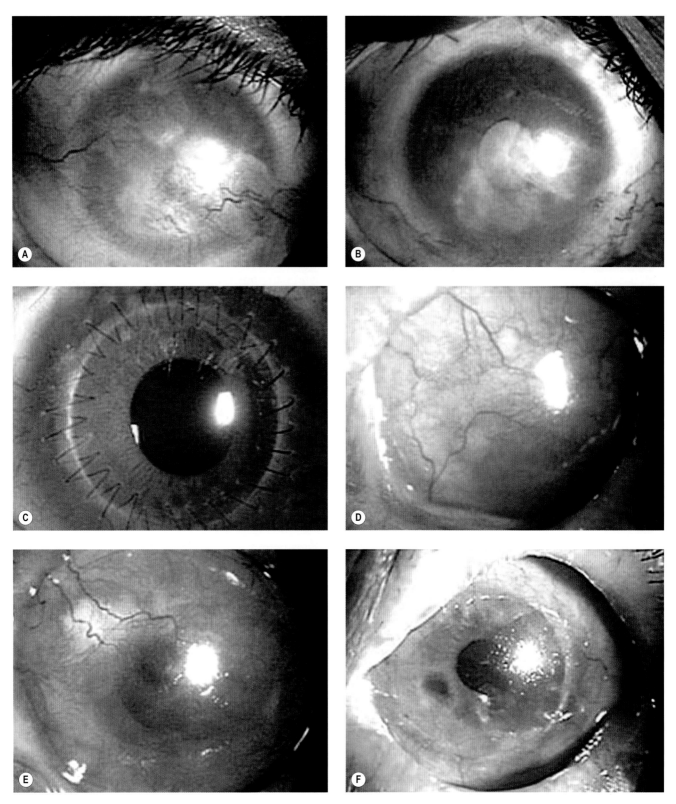

Figure 10.1 Clinical outcome of patients 1 (A–C) and 5 (D–F). The clinical appearance of patient 1 (a 24-year-old man) is shown: preoperatively (A); 2 months after autologous cultivated limbal epithelial transplantation (CLET) for chemical burns, showing appropriately resurfaced cornea and residual stromal opacity (B); and 8 months after keratoplasty, extracapsular lens extraction, and intraocular lens implantation, showing clear graft with reduced vascularization and inflammation (C). The clinical appearance of patient 5 (an 82-year-old woman) is also shown: preoperatively (D), 8 months after allogeneic (living relative) CLET for Stevens–Johnson syndrome and subsequent phacoemulsification and aspiration (E), and 12 months after keratoplasty (F). (Reproduced with permission from Kawashima M, Kawakita T, Satake Y, et al. Phenotypic study after cultivated limbal epithelial transplantation for limbal stem cell deficiency. Arch Ophthalmol 2007;125:1337–1344.)

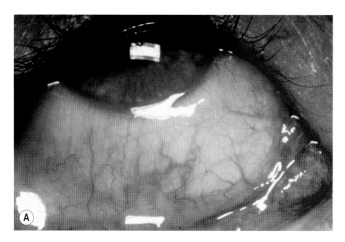
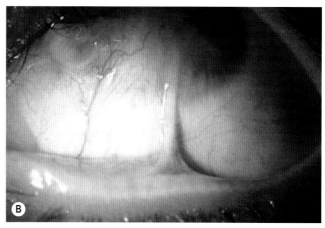

Figure 10.2 Stage 1 partial limbal stem cell deficiency. (A) Conjunctival epithelium with extensive blood vessels covering one-third of the corneal surface in a 32-year-old patient with atopic keratoconjunctivitis. A clear demarcation line at the border of invading conjunctival tissue is seen. The remaining two-thirds are covered by corneal epithelium, which is "sustained" by remaining intact limbus. (Reproduced with permission from Ono SJ, Abelson MB. Allergic conjunctivitis: update on pathophysiology and prospects for future treatment. J Allergy Clin Immunol 2005;115:118–122.) (B) Localized inferior vascularization with scarring secondary to an alkali injury in a 65-year-old patient. (Reproduced with permission from Al-Swailem SA. Graft failure: II. Ocular surface complications. Int Ophthalmol 2008;28:175–189.)

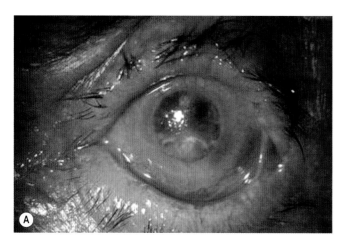
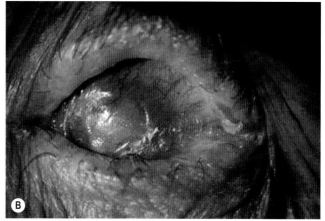

Figure 10.3 Stage 2 complete limbal stem cell deficiency. (A) A conjunctival fibrosis, 360° vascularized corneal scarring, and severe dry eye secondary to trachoma in an 85-year-old patient. (B) Chronic conjunctival inflammation is persistent in a 70-year-old patient with total limbal stem cell deficiency secondary to ocular cicatricial pemphigoid. (Reproduced with permission from Al-Swailem SA. Graft failure: II. Ocular surface complications. Int Ophthalmol 2008;28:175–189.)

1. Inflammatory disorders: ocular pemphigoid, atopic keratoconjunctivitis, rosacea, graft rejection, Lyell's syndrome, Stevens–Johnson syndrome, and graft-versus-host disease.
2. Infectious diseases: viral keratitis (i.e., herpes simplex keratitis, herpes zoster keratitis), bacterial keratitis (i.e., *Pseudomonas* infection, syphilis), fungal keratitis (i.e., *Candida, Fusarium, Aspergillus*), and parasitic infection (i.e., onchocerciasis).
3. Degenerative: congenital disorders: pterygium, Terrien marginal degeneration, and aniridia.
4. Traumatic: iatrogenic disorders and miscellaneous: contact lens wear, chemical burns, iatrogenic injury, and stem cell deficiency.

Pathophysiology

Multiple steps involved in corneal NV and lymphangiogenesis

Corneal NV consists of the formation of new vascular structures in previously avascular areas. In an in vivo experimental corneal model, the growth of a capillary involves an ordered sequence of events: the release of angiogenic factors, vascular endothelial cell activation, lysis of the basement membrane of a parent venule, vascular endothelial cell proliferation, directional migration of capillary endothelial cells towards the angiogenic stimulus, lumen formation, development of branches, and anastomosis of the tip of one tube with another to form a loop. Similarly, lymphangiogenesis consists of the growth of new lymphatic vessels that are derived from pre-existing lymphatic endothelial cells.[8] In adulthood, lymphangiogenesis is primarily associated with pathological processes, such as chronic inflammation, tissue injury, lymphedema, and tumor metastasis. Lymphatic vessels differ from blood vessels in that they do not have a continuous basement membrane. Moreover, the initial lymphatics display an irregular shape, intercellular openings, intracellular channels, and phagocytotic power, which constitute major paths for transport of matrix components in inflammatory diseases.

Localization of corneal vascular and lymphatic vessels

Under normal conditions, the cornea is transparent and without vascular and lymphatic vessels. Recent findings suggest that maintenance of the cornea devoid of corneal vascular and lymphatic vessels is an active process for preventing and modulating angiogenic and lymphangiogenic reactions.[2,7] The active mechanism for maintaining the corneal avascularity has been termed "corneal angiogenic privilege".[2,9] The onset of corneal NV is characterized by blood supply that arises from the ciliary arteries branching off from the ophthalmic artery, which subsequently divide and end in the pericorneal plexus within the limbus.[10] Corneal NV can be derived from stroma, which is mainly associated with stromal keratitis. Corneal NV can also develop from the superficial corneal periphery, which is mainly associated with ocular surface disorders, such as Stevens–Johnson syndrome, ocular pemphigoid, and thermal or chemical burns.[11–13] Although NV may involve several corneal layers, a study has demonstrated that the main locations of vascularized corneal buttons are in the upper and middle third areas of the anterior stroma.[14] Similarly, induced lymphatic vessels are localized to the corneal subepithelium and stroma layers in the wounded cornea.

Matrix involvement in corneal NV and lymphangiogenesis

The extracellular matrix, an active regulator of cellular proliferation, migration, adhesion, and invasion, can influence corneal NV and lymphangiogenesis. The MMPs comprise a large family of proteolytic enzymes that are responsible for matrix degradation. These MMPs may also modulate vascular and lymphatic endothelial cell sprouting and extension.

Cornea provides a tool for evaluating angiogenic/lymphangiogenic and antiangiogenic/lymphangiogenic factors

The "corneal angiogenic and immunogenic privileged" site has been used to assay the molecular basis of angiogenesis and lymphangiogenesis both in vivo and in vitro. The cornea is a good model for evaluating proangiogenic/lymphangiogenic and antiangiogenic/lymphangiogenic factors, due to the absence of blood and lymphatic vessels.[2,7,9] Corneal avas-

---

Box 10.4 Modulation of corneal angiogenic/ lymphangiogenic factors regulates corneal neovascularization and lymphangiogenesis

Modulation of corneal angiogenic/lymphangiogenic factors regulates corneal neovascularization. For example:

Limbal stem cell deficiency (loss of limbal stem cells)

Defects in renewal and repair of ocular surface caused by:
- Pterygium
- Herpes simplex virus infection
- Stevens–Johnson syndrome
- Aniridia
- Cicatricial pemphigoid
- Chemical injury

Treatment
- Surgical modality to replenish or repopulate the ocular surface epithelium

---

cularity requires low levels of angiogenic factors and high levels of antiangiogenic factors under basal conditions. Shifting of the balance towards higher levels of angiogenic and lymphangiogenic factors in the cornea is associated with pathological processes (Box 10.4). Here we review certain corneal disorders associated with NV and lymphangiogenesis, the molecular basis of such complications, and current potential therapeutics.

Function of vascular and lymphatic vessels

During development, vascular vessels function to foster new tissue growth, but they become tightly regulated during adulthood.[15] The major role of lymphatic vessels, on the other hand, is to maintain tissue fluid homeostasis by transporting lymph fluid from tissues to the circulatory system. Tissue fluid may readily be transported in the lymph to the nearest lymph node. During corneal inflammation, a rapid upregulation of proinflammatory cytokines takes place, attracting the migration of inflammatory cells into the cornea. Interactions between resident or infiltrated cells with extracellular matrices may induce cytokine productions in a paracrine fashion. These cytokines are beneficial to the cornea because they protect against the invasion of bacteria and other microorganisms. While inflammation is part of a physiological process for repairing damage, uncontrolled inflammation may actually cause damage. Therefore, understanding the lymphatic status in structure and function is an important step towards the control of unwanted corneal inflammation, edema, and transplant rejection.

Corneal NV and lymphangiogenesis-related disorders

Immunologic and infectious disorders of the cornea and conjunctiva, including ocular pemphigoid, graft rejection, viral and bacterial infection, pterygium, and aniridia, may involve the production of angiogenic and lymphangiogenic molecules responsible for corneal NV and lymphangiogenesis. Accordingly, a long-term follow-up of patients with inflammatory disorders, such as atopic keratoconjunctivitis, has revealed that the percentage of corneal NV may be as high as 60% during the course of their diseases. Corneal transplant rejection has been correlated with alloantigen-specific delayed-type hypersensitivity, infiltration of CD4+ T cells, and an increased amount of interferon-γ.[16,17] Additionally, corneal lymphangiogenesis may play a role in explaining why certain patients (particularly younger ones) have increased corneal transplant rejection.[18] Among different infectious agents, the herpes virus family (mostly herpes simplex virus (HSV) and herpes zoster) appears to be the primary cause of keratitis-induced NV in penetrating keratoplasty buttons. This complication occurs after interstitial, necrotizing, or recurrent keratitis and is not solely dependent on the host reaction. HSV-1 virus-infected cells can also produce interleukin-6 to stimulate noninfected resident corneal cells and other inflammatory cells to secrete VEGF, a potent angiogenic factor, in a paracrine manner. Following ocular HSV-1 infection, the NV of the avascular cornea is a critical event in the pathogenesis of herpetic stromal keratitis. There are approximately 300 000 cases of ocular HSV-1 infection diagnosed annually in the USA. The initial infection involves the corneal epithelium, and the neovascularized cornea lacks stromal NV. Repeated episodes of recurrent disease can lead to the involvement of the underlying stroma.[19]

Corneal NV may occur in degenerative disorders, such as pterygium and Terrien's marginal degeneration, as well as in congenital disorders such as aniridia. Recently, Ambati et al[7] have shown that patients with aniridia have mutated *PAX6* genes and deficiencies in corneal sFlt-1 expression. This study demonstrates that antiangiogenic factors are involved in the pathogenesis of corneal NV.

Corneal NV and lymphangiogenesis: molecular basis and factors involved

NV and lymphangiogenesis occur in a tissue when the balance between angiogenic and antiangiogenic factors is tilted towards angiogenic molecules.[1,2] In animal models, corneal NV and lymphangiogenesis are induced not only by the upregulation of angiogenic and/or lymphangiogenic factors (such as VEGF, VEGF-C, or -D), but also by the downregulation of antiangiogenic or lymphangiogenic factors (sFlt-1, ectopic expressed VEGFR3).

While many factors have been characterized and published, only a few of these factors have reached clinical trials. Here we discuss the potential benefits of using anti-VEGF antibodies, MMP inhibitors, and proteolytic fragments of extracellular matrix (endostatin and angiostatin).

Vascular endothelial growth factors

The VEGF family is structurally related to four other members: placenta growth factor, VEGF-B, -C, and -D. VEGF-A and VEGF-C are highly specific mitogens for vascular and lymphatic endothelial cells, in vitro and in vivo, respectively.[20] This VEGF family of proteins binds selectively with varying affinities to distinct VEGF receptors. The binding of VEGF to endothelial-specific receptor tyrosine kinases, VEGFR1 and VEGFR2 (expressed primarily on vascular endothelial cells), mediates angiogenic responses. In one case, VEGF-C bound

to VEGFR3 (flt-4, which is predominantly expressed in lymphatic endothelial cells in adult tissues) induced corneal lymphangiogenesis.[21,22]

During corneal NV and lymphangiogenesis, an upregulation of angiogenic and lymphangiogenic factors is usually present. For example, it has recently been shown that the vascular endothelial growth factor (VEGF, VEGF-C or VEGF-D) was upregulated in inflamed and vascularized human and animal corneal models.[6,23] VEGFs are secreted growth factor peptides generated by alternative splicing in five isoforms (VEGF115, VEGF121, VEGF 165, VEGF 189, and VEGF 206). VEGF is produced by macrophages, T cells, astrocytes, and smooth-muscle cells in corneal hypoxia and inflammatory conditions. The requirement of VEGF and VEGF-C in corneal NV and lymphangiogenesis has been demonstrated by the inhibition of NV or lymphangiogenesis after stromal implantation of anti-VEGF neutralizing antibodies: the soluble recombinant molecules VEGFR1 or VEGFR3.[6,7]

Matrix metalloproteinases

Corneal extracellular matrix turnover by MMPs is usually associated with wound healing during corneal NV and lymphangiogenesis. MMPs are a group of zinc-binding proteolytic enzymes that participate in extracellular matrix remodeling, NV, and lymphangiogenesis. They are produced as proenzymes and are activated by a variety of proteinases, including MMPs and serine proteases. Among the 25 MMPs already described, at least 11 have been identified in the cornea, including collagenases (MMP-1, -8, and -13), gelatinases A and B (MMP-2 and -9), stromelysins (MMP-3, -10, -11), matrilysin (MMP-7), and membrane-type (MT)-MMP (MMP-14).[24,25] Their upregulation during corneal NV has been published, and their roles in the regulation of NV are gradually being demonstrated. Individual MMPs may have more distinct roles in corneal NV. For example, MMP-2 and MT1-MMP possess proangiogenic potential because experiments demonstrated that MMP-2 and MT1-MMP knockout mice displayed a diminished basic fibroblast growth factor (bFGF)-induced corneal NV.[26,27] However, MMP-7 has been shown to have antiangiogenic functions, since: (1) MMP-7 knockout mice displayed enhanced keratectomy-induced corneal NV; and (2) MMP-7 may cleave corneal extracelluar matrix to generate antiangiogenic fragments.[28] The roles of MMPs in corneal lymphangiogenesis are under current investigation. Understanding the functions of MMPs in corneal NV and lymphangiogenesis may lead to new venues for the development of therapeutic interventions, in conjunction with anti-VEGF therapy for disorders related to corneal NV and lymphangiogenesis.

Endostatin

Endostatin, a putative antiangiogenic factor, is a 20-kDa proteolytic fragment of collagen XVIII.[29] Recombinant endostatin and its related fragments have been shown to inhibit bFGF-induced corneal NV in vivo and bFGF- and VEGF-induced vascular endothelial cell migration and proliferation in vitro.[30] Specifically, endostatin implanted in the cornea demonstrated an inhibition of the bFGF-induced NV. Collagen XVIII is a nonfibrillar collagen localized mainly to the corneal vascular and epithelial basement membrane. Cleavage of collagen XVIII by proteases (including MMPs, cathepsin L, and elastase) generates endostatin-like fragments that may display antiangiogenic properties. Local production of endostatin may occur during corneal wound healing, as both the cleaving enzymes (MMPs) and the substrate (collagen XVIII) are present in the basement membrane area to prevent corneal NV. Endostatin has been approved by the US Food and Drug Administration (FDA) for the treatment of NV-related cancer; thus, it may be an additional drug that can be added to anti-VEGF therapy to treat corneal NV- and lymphangiogenesis-related disorders.

Corneal NV and lymphangiogenesis management

Current therapy of the vascularized corneas includes using antiangiogenic/lymphangiogenic factors for the blocking of chemokines and cytokines produced by the inflammatory, vascular, and lymphatic cells. Specifically, inhibitors for the vascular endothelial growth factors (VEGF-A, VEGF-C, VEGF-D), bFGF, ang1, insulin-like growth factor, platelet-derived growth factor-BB, CCL21, interleukin-6, and CD4+ T cells have been shown to be effective in preventing and regressing corneal NV and lymphangiogenesis, based on animal models and clinical trials. Additionally, clinical experience with angiogenesis signaling inhibitors has focused on VEGF blockers. Anti-VEGF therapies have been extensively applied to corneal NV and lymphangiogenesis-related disorders. Several antiangiogenic factors derived from collagens or the extracellular matrix (endostatin, angiostatin, arrestin, thrombospondins) have also been discovered, but their roles in corneal NV have not been fully characterized. Recently, ectopic expression of VEGFR3 in corneal epithelial cells has been shown to have a direct inhibitory effect on corneal lymphangiogenesis. Administration of anti-VEGFR3 neutralizing antibodies in the cornea diminishes the epithelium's ability to dampen injury-induced corneal lymphangiogenesis. In addition, the application of chimeric VEGFR3 in the cornea can prevent cautery-induced corneal lymphangiogenesis. Thus, modulation of VEGFR3 function may be able to provide a therapeutic intervention for the treatment of lymphangiogenesis-related corneal disorders.

Neostatin-7, a 28-kDa fragment, is generated by MMP-7 cleavage of type XVIII collagen. Neostatin-7 is one of several naturally occurring endostatin-spanning fragments.[31] Neostatin-7 possesses antilymphangiogenic activity and may provide therapeutic interventions to treat lymphangiogenesis-related disorders, such as lymphedema, transplantation rejection, and cancer (Box 10.5).

Examples

Bevacizumab (Avastin; a recombinant, humanized, monoclonal antibody against VEGF-A) was the first antibody that the FDA approved to inhibit the formation of new blood vessels in tumors. In the corneal NV and lymphangiogenesis models, several studies were designed and performed to show that eyedrop application, and subconjunctival and intraperitoneal injection of bevacizumab all have effects on the suture-induced or alkali burn-induced corneal NV and/

> **Box 10.5 Corneal neovascularization and lymphangiogenesis treatment**
>
> - Surgical treatment/laser treatment
> - Recombinant neutralizing antibody to angiogenic factors
> - Competitive or noncompetitive antagonists to angiogenic factors
> - Kinase inhibitors
> - Combined treatment of corneal angiogenesis/lymphangiogenesis-associated diseases with various Food and Drug Administration-approved treatments (photodynamic therapy and antiangiogenic/lymphangiogenic factor therapy) is promising in achieving optimal effectiveness

or lymphangiogenesis.[32–37] In rabbit models, Hosseini et al[32] showed that administration of bevacizumab (2.5 mg) to the rabbits' eyes by a subconjunctival injection immediately after the chemical cauterization of the corneal surface inhibited chemical cauterization-induced corneal NV. In another experiment, Manzano et al[35] treated silver nitrate-injured rat corneas with topical eyedrops of bevacizumab solution (4 mg/ml) twice daily. These researchers showed that bevacizumab could inhibit silver nitrate-induced corneal NV. Finally, in a mouse suture-induced inflammatory corneal NV model, systemic (5 mg/kg injected intraperitoneally) and topical (5 mg/ml bevacizumab as eye drops (0.25 ml/drop) five times daily) applications of bevacizumab were applied after scraping away the central 2 mm of corneal epithelium and suture placement. Again, bevacizumab inhibited suture-induced corneal NV and lymphangiogenesis.[34] In conclusion, the administration of bevacizumab reduced corneal NV and/or lymphangiogenesis up to 40% when compared to that of untreated control in these injured corneas.

In the clinical setting, the results of administration of bevacizumab to the diseased corneas were varied.[38–43] For example, patients who experienced corneal NV following keratoplasty were treated with a single dose of subconjunctival injection of 2.5 mg bevacizumab. The results showed an immediate regression of the corneal vessels after bevacizumab injection. However, corneal vessels began to progress at week 2, followed by eventual failure of the corneal graft.[41] Harooni et al[38] reported one corneal transplanted patient with stromal vascularization crossing the host–graft interface; this patient received one subconjunctival injection of bevacizumab (1.25 mg/0.05 ml) adjacent to the base of NV, a 10 mg subconjunctival injection of triamcinolone, prednisolone acetate 1% drops every hour, and Protopic 0.03% ointment four times daily. In this investigation, the cornea remained stable for 5 months.

These and other studies suggest that therapy is promising for the anti-VEGF-targeted corneal NV in patients manifesting the initial stages of corneal NV and lymphangiogenesis. In the animal models, there was no total blockage of corneal NV with the use of bevacizumab, which suggests that factors other than VEGF control NV. Additionally, bevacizumab is more effective in preventing corneal NV if it is administered soon after wounding. These findings suggest that bevacizumab may work on new, active vessels but not on mature,

Table 10.2 Current treatments and potential antiangiogenic and/or lymphangiogenic therapies in corneal disorders

Target molecules/ treatment	Inhibit corneal neovascularization	Inhibit corneal lymphangiogenesis	Corneal clinical application	Animal model	References
mAb to VEGF (bevacizumab)	Yes	Yes	HSV infection Graft rejection	Suture-induced	32–35
Integrin a5b1	Yes	ND	ND	Alkali injury	64
flt-1/intraceptor	Yes	ND	ND	Alkali injury	65,66
Photodynamic therapy	Yes	ND	Yes	Suture-induced	67
Rapamycin	Yes	ND	ND	Corneal graft	68
Topical plasminogen k5 administration	Yes	Yes	ND	Alkali injury	69
Endostatin	Yes	ND	ND	bFGF corneal pellet	70,71
12-methyl tetradecanoic acid (12-MTA)	Yes	ND	ND	Alkali injury	53
mAb to VEGFR3	No	Yes	ND	Suture-induced	63
Thymoquinone	Yes	ND	ND	Silver nitrate	72
PAF antagonist LAU8080	Yes	ND	ND	PAF-induced	73
Ciclosporin A	Yes	ND	Yes	Wound or VEGF-induced	74
Thalidomide	Yes	ND	ND	VEGF-induced	75
Vasohibin	Yes	ND	ND	bFGF-induced	76
Curcumin	Yes	ND	ND	bFGF-induced	77,78
COX inhibitor	Yes	ND	ND	Alkali injury	79
Laser argon	Yes	ND	Yes		80
Limbal transplantation	Yes	ND	Yes	Alkali injury	81
Conjunctival /amniotic membrane transplantation	Yes	ND	Bacterial keratitis	Limbal stem cell deficiency	52,82
Vasostatin	Yes	ND	ND	bFGF-induced	83
IL-12	Yes	ND	ND	Tumor-induced	84
IL-18	Yes	ND	ND	bFGF-induced	85,86
Thrombospondin	Yes	ND	ND	bFGF-induced	87
Brain-specific angiogenesis inhibitor 1	Yes	ND	ND	Heptanol injury model	88
PDGF/PDGF receptor inhibitor	Yes	ND	ND	Limbal epithelium removal	89

mAB, monoclonal antibody; VEGF, vascular endothelial growth factor; HSV, herpes simplex virus; bFGF, basic fibroblast growth factor; VEGFR3, vascular endothelial growth factor receptor 3; PAF, platelet-activating factor; COX, cyclooxygenase; IL, interleukin; PDGF, platelet-derived growth factor.

established vessels. These results are similar to those of Jo et al,[44] who showed that anti-VEGF treatment alone is not sufficient to cause vessel regression in the advanced stages of aberrant and mature (established and inactive) vessels. In addition, Jo et al demonstrated that, in comparison to the application of single antiangiogenic therapy, the combination of anti-VEGF and anti-PDGFR antibodies to treat the corneal epithelial debridement wound is more effective in preventing and regressing corneal vessels. Thus, a combination of angiogenic and lymphangiogenic inhibitors may be required in order to achieve the maximum effect in the aversion and reversal of NV and lymphangiogenesis-related corneal disorders.

As listed in Table 10.2, all of these specific inhibitors are designed and targeted to dampen vascular or lymphatic endothelial cell proliferation, migration, and/or tube formation and to minimize adverse effects in their designed animal models. These molecules and treatments include monoclonal antibodies to VEGFs, proteolytic fragments of matrix components (endostatin, angiostatin), interleukin, steroid, ciclosporin A, argon laser treatment, and others. Improving the efficacy of antiangiogenic and antilymphangiogenic molecules, together with surgical interventions to reduce their side-effects, will be instrumental in the future treatment of corneal angiogenic- and lymphangiogenic-related disorders.

Advantages, limitations, and precautions for use of antiangiogenic and/or antilymphangiogenic therapy

The following criteria should be taken into consideration in order to achieve the greatest success in treating corneal NV and lymphangiogenesis, bearing in mind that individual intervention may target a specific step of corneal NV or lymphangiogenesis:

1. Age of the patient: antiangiogenic/lymphangiogenic therapies may affect normal angiogenesis/lymphangiogenesis during child development.
2. Status of the corneal vessels: whether they are new or established.
3. Purpose of the vascular/lymphangiogenic therapy: whether it is preventive or regressive.
4. Single versus cocktail drug (single/combination therapy).
5. Half-life of antiangiogenic/lymphangiogenic drugs.
6. Route of administration: topical eye drops, subconjunctiva injection or systematic administration.
7. Side-effects of combined cocktail therapy.

Summary

Corneal NV and lymphangiogenesis are usually caused by inflammatory disorders, infectious diseases, degenerative conditions, and mechanical or iatrogenic injury of the cornea. These may result in a decrease of visual acuity and may also worsen the prognosis of subsequent penetrating keratoplasty. Several factors, including VEGF, VEGF-C, VEGF-D, sFlt, endostatin, and thrombospondin-1 and -2, have been proposed to be involved in corneal NV and lymphangiogenesis. New modalities of treatment have also been investigated to reduce corneal NV and lymphangiogenesis.

Acknowledgment

This work was supported by NIH EY14048 (JHC).

Key references

A complete list of chapter references is available online at www.expertconsult.com. See inside cover for registration details.

1. Chang JH, Gabison EE, Kato T, et al. Corneal neovascularization. Curr Opin Ophthalmol 2001;12:242–249.
2. Azar DT. Corneal angiogenic privilege: angiogenic and antiangiogenic factors in corneal avascularity, vasculogenesis, and wound healing (an American Ophthalmological Society thesis). Trans Am Ophthalmol Soc 2006;104:264–302.
4. Tammela T, Zarkada G, Wallgard E, et al. Blocking VEGFR-3 suppresses angiogenic sprouting and vascular network formation. Nature 2008;454:656–660.
6. Cursiefen C, Chen L, Saint-Geniez M, et al. Nonvascular VEGF receptor 3 expression by corneal epithelium maintains avascularity and vision. Proc Natl Acad Sci USA 2006;103:11405–11410.
7. Ambati BK, Nozaki M, Singh N,et al. Corneal avascularity is due to soluble VEGF receptor-1. Nature 2006;443:993–997.
16. Hori J, Niederkorn JY. Immunogenicity and immune privilege of corneal allografts. Chem Immunol Allergy 2007;92:290–299.
21. Kubo H, Cao R, Brakenhielm E, et al. Blockade of vascular endothelial growth factor receptor-3 signaling inhibits fibroblast growth factor-2-induced lymphangiogenesis in mouse cornea.
Proc Natl Acad Sci USA 2002;99:8868–8873.
22. Chang LK, Garcia-Cardena G, Farnebo F, et al. Dose-dependent response of FGF-2 for lymphangiogenesis. Proc Natl Acad Sci USA 2004;101:11658–11663.
29. O'Reilly MS, Chang JH, Kato T, et al. Endostatin: an endogenous inhibitor of angiogenesis and tumor growth. Cell 1997;88:277–285.
31. Kojima T, Azar DT, Chang JH. Neostatin-7 regulates bFGF-induced corneal lymphangiogenesis. FEBS Lett 2008;582:2515–2520.

CHAPTER 11

Ocular surface restoration

Julie T Daniels, Genevieve A Secker, and Alex J Shortt

Clinical background

The ocular surface comprises the entire and continuous mucosal outer epithelial lining of the eye lids, conjunctiva, and cornea. This chapter will focus upon ocular surface failure caused by insult to the corneal epithelium and discuss current therapeutic strategies and the underlying pathophysiology.

The cornea on the front surface of the eye is comprised of five layers: the outermost multilayered epithelium, Bowman's layer (which is acellular), the keratocyte (corneal fibroblast)-populated collagen stroma, and Descemet's membrane on the inner corneal surface, upon which lies a monolayer of endothelial cells (Figure 11.1). Transparency of the cornea, and therefore vision, is dependent upon the coordinated functionality of all layers.

Integrity of the epithelium is essential for corneal clarity and light refraction. Corneal epithelial cells are constantly lost from the ocular surface during blinking.[1] These desquamated cells are replenished from a population of limbal epithelial stem cells (LESCs) which reside in the basal epithelial layer of the corneoscleral junction, known as the limbus.[2,3] The specific location of LESCs remains unclear; however, they are likely to reside in or on structures known as the palisades of Vogt at the periphery of the cornea (Figure 11.2).[4] When the LESCs divide asymmetrically they produce daughter transient amplifying cells which migrate, proliferate, and differentiate to maintain the corneal epithelium (Figure 11.3). Hence, LESCs are responsible for homeostatic and posttraumatic regeneration of the corneal epithelium and loss of their function causes ocular surface failure.

Key symptoms and signs

The key symptoms of ocular surface failure include: loss of corneal epithelial transparency, superficial subepithelial corneal neovascularization, epithelial irregularity, history of recurrent epithelial breakdown, stromal inflammation, corneal melting and perforation, loss of limbal palisades of Vogt, and reduction of visual acuity. An example of ocular surface failure caused by a chemical burn injury is shown in Figure 11.4.

Epidemiology

The diseases and injuries which can cause LESC deficiency can affect either gender.

Chemical/thermal injuries are most prevalent in countries with poor health and safety records, although domestic accidents do occur. Stevens–Johnson syndrome (SJS) has high morbidity and mortality, with an incidence of 1 per million per year. Advanced ocular cicatricial pemphigoid occurs more frequently in females and LESC deficiency associated with this disease can result from inflammatory cytokine damage. Inappropriate overwearing of contact lenses, multiple surgeries, exposure to ultraviolet or ionizing radiation and antimetabolites and extensive microbial infection may also cause LESC deficiency and ocular surface failure. Loss of LESC function due to the inherited eye disease aniridia is associated with vision loss during the early teens.

Diagnostic workup and differential diagnosis

Accurate diagnosis of LESC deficiency is important as patients suffering from these conditions are unlikely to respond well to conventional treatment, including corneal transplantation. LESC deficiency is diagnosed on the basis of the key signs and symptoms described above and by using a technique called impression cytology. This involves placing a filter paper on the front surface of the eye which, when removed, takes with it a sample of the surface layer cells. Immunohistochemical staining and microscopy are then used to detect the profile of cytokeratin expression in the harvested cells. The presence of cytokeratins 3 and 12, identified using monoclonal antibodies, would indicate cells of the correct corneal phenotype. However, cytokeratin 19 positivity together with the presence of mucin-producing goblet cells (following staining with periodic acid–Schiff reagent) is indicative of conjunctivalization of the corneal surface and hence LESC deficiency (Figure 11.5). It is also possible to observe a mixed population of cells which may indicate partial rather than total LESC failure. When fluorescein dye is placed on the eyes of patients with LESC failure, the corneal surface viewed through a slit lamp is often abnormally stained. Areas of the epithelium may be thin with signs of erosion.

Treatment

Previous conservative attempts to correct LESC deficiency have included harvesting healthy autologous limbal tissue from the contralateral eye for transplantion to the diseased eye (keratolimbal autograft). Whilst potentially successful in terms of vision recovery, there is a risk of creating LESC deficiency in the donor eye if too much tissue is harvested.[5] Alternatively, allogeneic tissue from a living related or cadaveric donor may be used in conjunction with long-term systemic immunosuppression (Box 11.1). In 1997, the first description of the successful use of ex vivo expanded autologous LESCs to treat LESC deficiency in chemical burn injury patients was published by Pellegrini et al.[6] For this technique, just a 1–2 mm² limbal biopsy is harvested, posing little risk to the donor eye. The isolated epithelial cells are then cultured on a growth-arrested feeder layer of murine 3T3 fibroblasts. Upon formation of a multilayered cell sheet the epithelial cells are released from the culture dish and transferred to a carrier for patient grafting. A number of techniques for ex vivo expansion of autologous and allogeneic limbal epithelial cells have since been developed, including the use of human amniotic membrane,[7] as a surrogate stem cell niche. An example of therapeutic LESC culture methodology and clinical outcome is shown in Figures 11.6 and 11.7 respectively.

Prognosis and complications

With no standard protocol for assessing clinical outcome, prognosis following cultured LESC therapy can be difficult to predict since patients are of mixed etiological background and have usually undergone a variety of surgical procedures. Nonetheless, the majority of reports agree that LESC cultures may be a useful addition to the management protocols for LESC deficiency since improved visual acuity has been reported in approximately 70% of cases (extensively reviewed by Shortt et al.[8]). Complications associated with cultured LESC therapy have included graft loss due to recurrence of residual infection and corneal neovascularization.

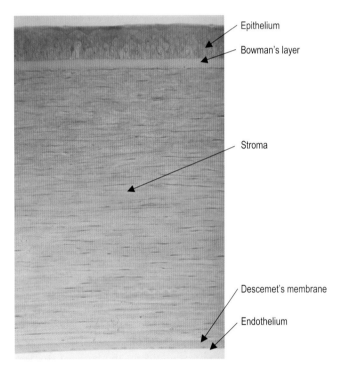

Figure 11.1 The human cornea in histological cross section.

Epithelium

Bowman's layer

Stroma

Descemet's membrane

Endothelium

Box 11.1

- Integrity and functionality of the cornea are essential for vision
- The cornea is comprised of five layers: epithelium, Bowman's layer, stroma, Descemet's membrane, and endothelium
- Epithelium is regenerated by stem cells in the limbus at the edge of the cornea
- Limbal epithelial stem cell (LESC) deficiency can result from a variety of inherited or acquired conditions causing blinding ocular surface failure
- LESC deficiency is diagnosed by epithelial cell cytokeratin profile and clinical appearance
- Treatment includes transplantation of cultured autologous or allogeneic LESCs

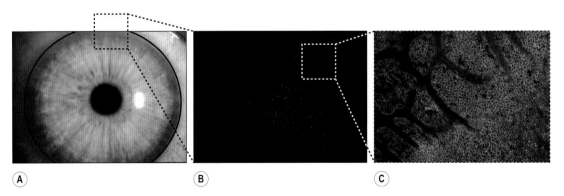

Ⓐ   Ⓑ   Ⓒ

Figure 11.2 The location of limbal epithelial stem cells (LESCs). LESCs reside in the corneoscleral limbus (A, solid black line) in the palisades of Vogt. The finger-like palisades are shown (B) by 4',6-diamidino-2-phenylindole (DAPI) staining of a cadaveric human cornea. The confocal image (C) shows the actin cytoskeleton stained with fluorescein isothiocyanate-phallodin (green) and the nuclei labeled with propidium iodide (orange) of limbal epithelial cells in the palisades.

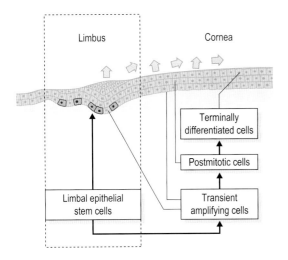

Figure 11.3 The limbal and corneal epithelial junction in diagrammatic cross-section. Limbal epithelial stem cells (shaded in black) give rise to daughter transient amplifying cells which migrate towards the center of the cornea, proliferate, and differentiate to replenish the corneal epithelial continuously throughout life.

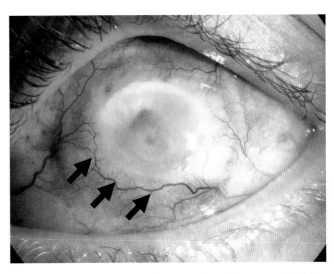

Figure 11.4 Ocular surface failure following chemical burn injury. Limbal epithelial stem cell deficiency has developed in this eye as a result of a chemical burn injury. Typically, neovascularization (arrowed), epithelial surface breakdown, and corneal opacity due to scarring have occurred.

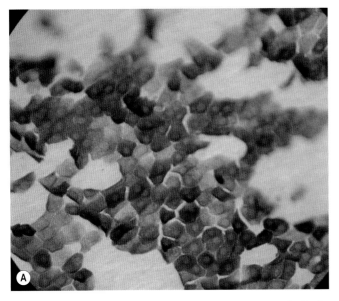

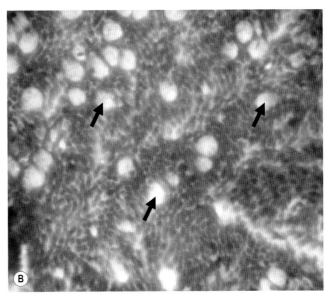

Figure 11.5 Diagnostic ocular surface impression cytology. Superficial cells removed from the normal ocular surface by impression cytology were immunostained for cytokeratin 3 (brown stain) (A). Following limbal epithelial stem cell deficiency-induced conjunctivalization of the ocular surface the cytokeratin profile is changed to cytokeratin 19 (purple stain in B). The presence of mucin-producing goblet cells (arrowed in B) is also characteristic of conjunctivalization of the ocular surface.

Etiology

Primary causes of LESC deficiency

Genetic risk factors

A variety of primary disorders can lead to a deficiency of LESCs as a result of inadequate stem cell support by the stromal microenvironment. These include heritable genetic disorders such as aniridia which is caused by a mutation in the eye development gene *Pax6*.[9] Multiple endocrine deficiencies can also lead to keratitis and LESC failure.[10]

Secondary causes of LESC deficiency

Environmental risk factors

LESC deficiency occurs more commonly as a result of acquired factors which destroy the stem cells, such as chemical or thermal injury. In heavily industrialized areas it is common for manual workers to sustain chemical or thermal burn injuries to the eyes, resulting in partial or complete physical destruction of the limbal palisades of Vogt, causing LESC deficiency and ocular surface failure, particularly where health and safety practices are not optimal or are not strictly

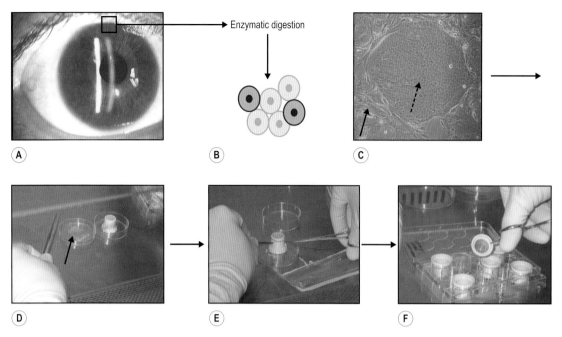

Figure 11.6 Cultured limbal epithelial stem cell (LESC) therapy methodology. A limbal tissue biopsy is harvested from the patient (A) or a cadaveric donor. The epithelial cells are isolated with a series of enzymatic digestions to release a mixed population, a proportion of which are LESCs (red cells in B). The epithelial cells (dashed arrow) may be cultured in the presence of a growth-arrested 3T3 feeder fibroblasts (solid arrow, C). Upon reaching confluence, the epithelial cells may be transferred to a substrate for further culture prior to transfer to the patient. In this example, human amniotic membrane (solid arrow, D) is sutured on to a tissue culture insert (E) to make a well for the seeding of limbal epithelial cells (F). Following further culture, the composite graft is packed and delivered to theater.

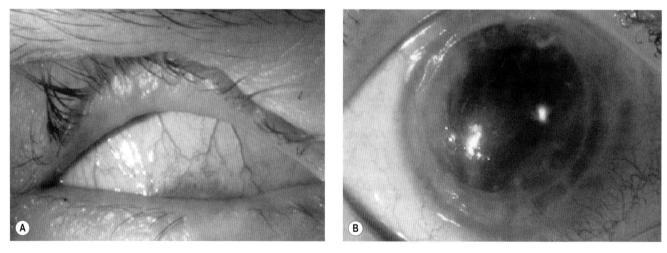

Figure 11.7 Cultured limbal epithelial stem cell (LESC) therapy outcome. This patient (A) has the inherited eye disease aniridia. The cornea is vascularized and the ocular surface unstable. The patient found it too painful to be examined fully, hence the obscured cornea. Nine months following transplantation of cultured allogeneic LESCs the central cornea now maintains a transparent epithelium, the patient is able to tolerate examination, and has improved visual acuity (B).

adhered to. LESC deficiency has occurred in some patients as the result of soft contact lens wear, the effects of which have included ulceration, stromal scarring, neovascularization and decreased visual acuity (Box 11.2). Occasionally surgical or medical intervention may cause temporary or permanent loss of LESC function. Examples include the use of antimetabolite drugs, cryotherapy, and radiation therapy. Multiple ocular surgery procedures can also increase the risk, as can extensive microbial infection. The onset of inflammatory disorders and autoimmune diseases, including SJS and advanced cicatricial pemphigoid, have also been linked with LESC failure. If the neighbouring conjunctival cells are also depleted, the cornea surface becomes heavily keratinized.[10]

Usually, when LESC deficiency occurs, the neighboring conjunctival epithelial cells and blood vessels migrate over the corneal surface.[11] This conjunctivalization process causes persistent epithelial breakdown and superficial vascularization of the cornea. Patients experience impaired vision and chronic discomfort. LESC deficiency may be partial or total depending upon the insult.

Box 11.2

- Genetic risk factors such as *Pax6* gene haploinsufficiency cause limbal epithelial stem cell (LESC) failure
- More commonly, LESC deficiency occurs due to physical insult such as chemical burn
- LESC deficiency can also occur following inappropriate contact lens wear, ocular surgery, infection, and inflammation
- The cornea undergoes "conjunctivalization" with neovascularization, ulceration, and/or scarring

Box 11.3

- Chemical and thermal injury can destroy the stem cell niche (microenvironment)
- Cultured autologous limbal epithelial stem cells (LESCs) can restore functionality of the ocular surface
- Cultured allogeneic LESCs can also restore function but the mechanism of efficacy is unknown as the transplanted cells do not seem to survive several months

Pathophysiology

The pathophysiology of three examples of LESC deficiency involved in ocular surface failure is described below.

Chemical/thermal injury

LESCs reside in a specialized niche environment at the palisades of Vogt[12] which regulates self-renewal and cell fate decisions. Properties of this niche have recently been described and include specific tissue architecture, the presence of a vascular and neural network, and close proximity of stromal cells.[13] Physical destruction of this niche can occur with chemical/thermal injury with subsequent ocular surface failure. However, transplantation of cultured autologous LESCs can restore a normal corneal epithelial phenotype (Box 11.3).[6,14] Allogeneic cells can also produce a similar clinical outcome, which is very interesting since the transplanted cells do not appear to survive on the cornea for longer than 28 weeks, as determined by polymerase chain reaction genotyping of sampled cells.[15] It is possible that the cultured transplanted cells create a permissive environment for any remaining host LESCs to resume function or that bone marrow stem cells are recruited. It is also not clear whether surviving transplanted cells are able to regenerate the niche to any extent.

Stevens–Johnson syndrome

Clinical features

SJS, also known as erythema multiforme (EM) major, is a complex immunological syndrome involving blistering of at least two mucous membranes and the skin.[16] Toxic epidermal necrolysis (TEN) is the most severe form of EM. Both SJS and TEN can be fatal due to systemic visceral involvement or extensive skin exfoliation. The acute stage of the disease can cause corneal damage but often this occurs as a result of chronic complications[17] and is the most common long-term problem for survivors of SJS.[18] LESC failure is a major cause of chronic disease and is associated with keratinization and opacity of the cornea. Conjunctival scarring can also occur.[19] Severe inflammation can cause ocular surface failure acutely or as late as 4 years after the onset of SJS.[17] This delay may be the result of limbus destruction during the acute phase, which leaves sufficient transient amplifying cells to maintain a normal corneal epithelium for several years.[17] Late LESC failure may be caused by prolonged inflammation of the limbus.[17]

Box 11.4

- Stevens–Johnson syndrome (SJS) is a potentially fatal complex immunological syndrome which can result from hypersensitivity to drugs, including antibiotics and nonsteroidal anti-inflammatory agents
- Corneal damage is the most common complication for survivors of SJS
- Limbal epithelial stem cell deficiency correlating with inflammation can occur as late as 4 years postinsult
- Epithelial cell apoptosis is a hallmark of SJS

Pathophysiology

The exact mechanisms of pathogenesis of EM are unclear; however, infective, autoimmune, and allergic factors may be involved. Hypersensitivity to microbes and drugs is thought to be important.[20] These include bacterial, viral, protozoan, and mycotic infections and drugs such as antibiotics, nonsteroidal anti-inflammatory agents and several vaccines. Herpes simplex virus is also a relatively common cause of EM (Box 11.4).[21] It has been shown that episodic showers of circulating immune complexes may result in deposition of immune complexes in predisposed, previously damaged vessels with resultant immune complex vasculitis/perivasculitis with lymphocytes and neutrophil participation causing vessel damage and hence conjunctival inflammation.[22]

SJS is almost always associated with drug intake. The hallmark of SJS is epithelial cell apoptosis.[23] Overexpression of Fas antigen, a mediator of apoptosis, has been found in the keratinocytes of patients with SJS.[24] Strong expression of the apoptosis-blocking protein Bcl-2 has also been detected in the epithelial basal layer and in the dermal infiltrate in SJS patients. This suggests that Fas-dependent keratinocyte apoptosis may play a role in the pathogenesis of SJS.[24] Alternatively, cytotoxic T-cell release of perforin and granzyme may trigger apoptosis.[23] T-cell proinflammatory cytokines including tumor necrosis factor-α (TNF-α) are found in significantly higher concentrations in the sera of patients with SJS and are thought to regulate pathogenesis as well as Fas, caspase activity, and M30.[25]

Aniridia

One of the causes of blindness in children with aniridia is progressive ocular surface failure (Box 11.5). The disease is caused by *PAX6* heterozygosity, which leads to a panocular, bilateral condition most prominently characterized by iris hypoplasia. Aniridia is often associated with cataracts, corneal vascularization, and glaucoma, with a significant number of cases of visual morbidity being due to corneal abnormalities. The underlying process of these abnormalities is poorly understood and is thought to be due to stem cell failure[9,26,27]; however, it has recently been proposed that it may be due to a deficiency in the stem cell niche and adjacent corneal stroma.[28] Treatment usually involves replacement of LESC using limbal allografts and/or corneal grafts or, more recently, ex vivo cultured LESC grafts.[8,29]

Clinical features

Aniridia represents a spectrum of disease, with iris anatomy defects ranging from the total absence of the iris to mild stromal hypoplasia with a pupil of normal appearance. Other associated defects include foveal hypoplasia, optic nerve hypoplasia, nystagmus, glaucoma, and cataracts, which may develop with age, causing progressive visual loss. Another important factor leading to progressive loss of vision is aniridic-related keratopathy (ARK),[26,30] which occurs in 90% of patients. Initially the cornea of patients appears normal during childhood.[9,31] Changes occur in patients in their early teenage years, with the disease manifesting as a thickened irregular peripheral epithelium. This is followed by superficial neovascularization and, if left untreated, it may result in subepithelial fibrosis and stromal scarring. Furthermore patients develop recurrent erosions, ulcerations, chronic pain, and eventual blindness.[29] Histologically, stromal neovascularization and infiltration of inflammatory cells are seen with the destruction of Bowman's layer. Additionally, the presence of goblet and conjunctival cells is seen on the corneal surface.[30]

Pathogenesis of aniridic-related keratopathy

Based on the clinical and histological manifestation of aniridia, LESC deficiency has been presumed to be the pathogenesis behind ARK.[9,30,32] As a LESC marker has yet to be definitively identified, a true demonstration of LESC deficiency cannot be assumed. Furthermore treatment for these patients involving replacement of LESC, either by keratolimbal allografts[29,33] or, more recently, ex vivo expanded LESC grafts, provides a variable long-term outcome.[8] Alternatively, ARK may be a consequence of abnormal corneal epithelial/stromal healing response as there is insufficient evidence to indicate that the proliferative potential of LESC is impaired.[34,35] Recently, studies looking at the regulation of genes downstream of PAX6 in the *Pax6* mutant mouse, suggest the pathogenesis of ARK is due to a number of mechanisms and not solely due to LESC deficiency.[28] Further studies are needed to elucidate the exact mechanism of ARK progression to allow the use of appropriate treatments.

Pathophysiology

The *PAX6* gene is a highly conserved hierarchical transcriptional factor regulating a multitude of genes involved in eye development and adult homeostasis. In humans *PAX6* is located on chromosome 11p13 and encodes two products due to alternative splicing of exon 5a, *PAX6*, and *PAX6(5a)*.[36,37] The PAX6 protein is a 422-amino-acid transcriptional regulator consisting of 14 exons contained within a 22 kb genomic region. It contains two DNA-binding domains, a paired-type domain (PD) and a homeodomain (HD), which are separated by a linker region in the N-terminal region. There is also a C-terminal proline, serine, and threonine-rich transregulatory domain (PST), which has been implicated in modulation of DNA binding to the homeodomain.[38] Mutations in the *PAX6* gene are archived in the Human *PAX6* Allelic Variant Database (www.pax6.hgu.mrc.ac.uk), which currently contains 408 records, with 307 of these being linked to patients with eye malformations. The most recent analysis of this database found that mutations that introduce a premature stop codon in the open reading frame are usually associated with aniridia, with most of these mutations being nonsense mutations.[39]

The PAX6 protein has been found to be expressed in the adult eye, cerebellum, and pancreas, suggesting it has an important role in maintenance and remodeling of adult tissues.[40–42] Identification of the downstream effects of PAX6 has been greatly helped through the use of animal models, especially the heterozygous *Pax6*[+/−] mouse or small eye (sey) mouse, which provides an excellent model for aniridia and the progressive nature of associated corneal abnormalities.[34,43] As the name suggests, mice with semidominant mutations develop small eyes and other ocular deformities (Figure 11.8). Homozygotes generate an ultimately lethal phenotype with no eyes and nasal primordial.[44] A number of *sey* mice arose independently, all of which are semidominant and, by examining comparative mapping studies and phenotypic similarities to aniridia, it was suggested to be the mouse homolog of the human disease.[45] This research led to the discovery that the *Pax6* gene was responsible for the *Sey* phenotype and suggested that it was also responsible for the human disease, aniridia.[44]

Using mouse models it has been found that upregulation of Pax6 in mice has been found during the proliferative phase of wound healing, being necessary to restore the stratified structure of the corneal epithelium following injury.[46] Recent studies have found that overexpression of Pax6 protein in rabbit corneal epithelial (RCE) cells suppresses

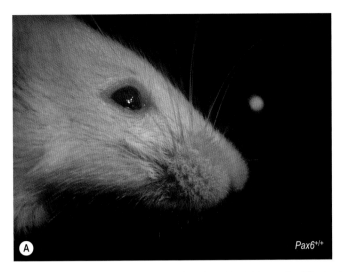 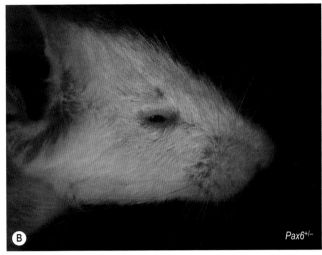

Figure 11.8 The small-eyed mouse model of aniridia. Wild-type Pax6$^{+/+}$ mice have normal eyes. Whereas Pax6$^{-/-}$ mice do not survive, their heterozygous Pax6$^{+/-}$ littermates have small eyes. The phenotypic and genotypic characteristics of the Pax6$^{+/-}$ small-eyed (sey) mouse are similar to the human inherited eye disease aniridia and hence can be used as a model of this disease.

proliferation and retards cell cycle progression.[47] *Pax6* is involved in a number of regulatory roles in the adult mouse cornea and is essential for the expression of cytokeratin 12, gelatinase B (matrix metalloproteinase-9: MMP-9), and cell adhesion molecules (CAM)[35,43,48] and, more recently, it has been suggested that knockdown of Pax6 expression promotes epidermal growth factor-induced cell proliferation.[49]

The various ECM in the cornea provide structural support and undergo slow constant remodeling during homeostasis or rapid remodeling during wound healing.[28] Corneal stromal remodeling is mediated by zinc-containing MMPs, which are produced by both corneal epithelial cells and fibroblasts.[50] MMP9 is upregulated during corneal wound healing, which has been found to be dependent on Pax6 expression, also being upregulated during wound healing.[51] MMP9 deficiency leads to a buildup of fibrin and infiltration of inflammatory cells' together with the accumulation of ECM, this disturbs the normally ordered collagen structure of the corneal stroma, thus impairing transparency. This and other factors have been proposed to lead to the ingrowth of blood vessels and corneal opacities commonly seen in patients with ARK, with mutations in *PAX6* being responsible.[28]

Cytokeratins (CK) are structural proteins expressed by epithelial cells, with CK12 being a specific for differentiated corneal epithelial cells. It has been found that CK12 expression is Pax6-dependent,[51] with CK12-deficient mice producing a fragile superficial corneal epithelium, which often detaches.[52] This phenotype is also seen in the *Pax6*$^{+/-}$ mice[53] and, when comparing them to *Pax6*$^{+/+}$ mice, there is a decrease in CK12 staining. Further to this, aniridic patients also have a decrease in CK12 staining.[27] This suggests that corneal fragility, seen in both *Pax6*$^{+/-}$ mice and aniridic patients, is due to a lack of CK12, being a downstream consequence of altered *PAX6/Pax6* expression.

Maintenance of the corneal epithelium in both homeostasis and corneal wound healing is mediated through intracellular junctions, including tight, gap, and adherent junctions and desmosomes. Additionally, other nonjunctional proteins such as integrins and cadherins play an important role in the prevention of epithelial loss through

shearing.[43] The *Pax6*$^{+/-}$ mouse model has reduced levels of desmoglein and ß-catenins; also there are large spaces separating epithelial cells and the appearance of desmosomes is unusual.[43] Further to this, the integrin subunit α_4 and Pax6 are coexpressed in rabbit corneal epithelial cells (RCEC), suggesting that Pax6 directly regulates the expression of the α_4 gene during corneal wound healing.[54] This implies reduced levels of Pax6 lead to compromised cellular adhesion in the corneal epithelium, which has also been suggested to contribute to the ARK phenotype.

Ex vivo studies in mice showed that the wound-healing rate for heterozygous mice was faster when compared to wild-type.[55] This observation was attributed to reduced levels of epithelial cell adhesion and increased rates of proliferation. Further to this, they demonstrated an increase in stromal cell apoptosis with *Pax6*$^{+/-}$ mouse corneas following epithelial removal, suggesting it could contribute to the corneal phenotype associated with ARK. Increased apoptosis may lead to tissue damage and activation of adjacent keratocytes with the generation of associated repair-activated fibroblasts or myofibroblasts resulting in fibrotic wound healing and scar formation. Interestingly, Leiper et al[56] found there to be a delay in the wound-healing response in the *Pax6*$^{+/-}$ mouse epithelial cultures, suggesting the stroma plays an important role in disease progress.

As *PAX6/Pax6* expression controls a multitude of downstream genes, it is difficult to differentiate the exact etiology of the corneal changes seen with the disease. It seems the combination of altered downstream gene expression leads to phenotype; however, more studies are needed to elucidate the exact mechanisms.

Conclusion

Transparency of the cornea depends upon the integrity and functionality of all its layers, including the outermost corneal epithelium. If the LESCs, which replenish this epithelium throughout life, are compromised, blinding ocular surface failure will occur. The causes of LESC failure are diverse and may be inherited or acquired. Precise diagnosis of LESC deficiency can be challenging due to the lack of specific markers for identification. Therapeutic strategies, including transplantation of cultured LESCs, have shown promise in the treatment of these difficult conditions. The transparency and ready accessibility of the cornea make it an ideal model system in which to study disease and develop novel therapeutic strategies. Hence, it is anticipated that in the future the cornea will help to advance science and medicine in relation to tissues beyond the ocular surface.

Acknowledgments

The authors gratefully acknowledge the funding support of the Medical Research Council (AJS), the ERANDA Foundation (GAS), and the Special Trustees of Moorfields Eye Hospital (JTD). JTD is a faculty member of the Moorfields Eye Hospital/UCL Institute of Ophthalmology Biomedical Research Centre, National Institutes for Health Research, UK.

Key references

A complete list of chapter references is available online at www.expertconsult.com. See inside cover for registration details.

2. Davanger M, Evenson A. Role of the pericorneal structure in renewal of corneal epithelium. Nature 1971;229: 560–561.

3. Cotsarelis G, Cheng G, Dong G, et al. Existence of slow-cycling limbal epithelial basal cells that can be preferentially stimulated to proliferate: implications on epithelial stem cells. Cell 1989;57:201–209.

6. Pellegrini G, Traverso CE, Franzi AT, et al. Long-term restoration of damaged corneal surfaces with autologous cultivated human epithelium. Lancet 1997;349:990–993.

7. Tsai RJ-F, Li L-M, Chen J-K. Reconstruction of damaged corneas by transplantation of autologous limbal epithelial cells. N Engl J Med 2000; 343:86–93.

8. Shortt AJ, Secker GA, Notara MD, et al. Transplantation of ex-vivo cultured limbal epithelial stem cells – a review of current techniques and clinical results. Surv Ophthalmol 2007;52:483–502.

13. Shortt AJ, Secker GA, Munro PM, et al. Characterisation of the limbal epithelial stem cell niche: novel imaging techniques permit in-vivo observation and targeted biopsy of limbal epithelial stem cells. Stem Cells 2007;5:1402–1409.

14. Rama P, Bonini S, Lambiase A, et al. Autologous fibrin-cultured limbal stem cells permanently restore the corneal surface of patients with total limbal stem cell deficiency. Transplantation 2001;72: 1478–1485.

15. Sharpe JR, Daya SM, Dimitriadi M, et al. Survival of cultured allogeneic limbal epithelial cells following corneal repair. Tissue Eng 2007;13:123–132.

34. Ramaesh T, Collinson JM, Ramaesh K, et al. Corneal abnormalities in Pax6 +/− small eye mice mimic human aniridia-related keratopathy. Invest Ophthalmol Vis Sci 2003;44:1871–1878.

35. Sivak JM, Mohan R, Rinehart WB, et al. Pax-6 expression and activity are induced in the reepithelialising cornea and control activity of the transcriptional promotor for matrix metalloproteinase gelatinase B. Dev Biol 2000;222:41–54.

CHAPTER 12

Herpetic keratitis

Pranita P Sarangi and Barry T Rouse

Clinical background

Herpetic keratitis usually results from infection with herpes simplex virus type 1 (HSV-1) in adults and by HSV-2 in neonates. Occasionally the cause is varicella-zoster virus (VZV), either during primary infection or more commonly, as a site during an outbreak of shingles. The epidemiology of HSV-1 and HSV-2 infection is being changed as a consequence of different patterns of human sexual behavior. Persons are seroconverting to HSV-1 later in life and many are now first exposed to the virus as a genital infection.[1] HSV-2 infection is on the increase and more frequently than before may be the cause of keratitis.

Primary infection, especially with HSV-1, may be subclinical or mild and misdiagnosed. However, it can cause a painful lesion that mainly affects the corneal epithelium, lasting for several days or even weeks, but which eventually resolves without permanent damage to the cornea. This event occurs more quickly if antivirals are administered topically or even systemically. However this ancient disease, first described by the Romans, is never cured since the virus ensconces itself in nerve ganglia where it can persist indefinitely in a dormant state, termed latency.[2] Unfortunately, the virus can reactivate from latency, giving rise to recurrent lesions, which are often those of most clinical consequence. Repeated recurrences may develop into a chronic immunoinflammatory event which can markedly impair vision (Figure 12.1). This later form is called stromal keratitis (SK) and accounts for about 20% of cases. SK is only rarely the consequence of primary infection.[2] The clinical aspects of herpetic keratitis are summarized in Table 12.1.

Overall, herpetic keratitis is the most frequent infectious cause of impaired vision in the developed world, with an estimated 20 000 new cases occurring annually in the USA and an incidence of 20.7 cases per 100 000 patient years (Box 12.1).[2] The disease shows no gender bias and any genetic factors that affect susceptibility are poorly understood. Virus strains could vary in virulence, as has been well documented to occur in studies with animal models.[2] Immunosuppressed patients, including the human neonate, however, are more likely to have severe clinical disease. Prolonged and severe lesions may also occur in patients with acquired immunodeficiency syndrome (AIDS).[3]

Primary and recurrent HSV-induced keratitis can be confused with abrasions as well as with infectious causes of keratitis by bacterial, chlamydial, parasitic, and fungal agents. Additionally, recurrent herpetic lesions need to be distinguished from graft rejection following keratoplasty and with zoster caused by VZV.[2] Accurate diagnosis can be made by demonstrating HSV in the corneal tissue samples or ocular secretions by cell culture, immunofluorescence staining, or by detecting the viral genome by polymerase chain reaction.[2] The appropriate response to therapy may also provide a clue. Serological diagnosis is unreliable except to confirm a primary infection since the majority of the population are seropositive, as will be all of those who experience recurrent lesions.

The acute and epithelial forms of herpetic keratitis respond to treatment with several types of antiviral drugs which are usually given topically. The most commonly administered drugs are various nucleoside analogs, such as vidarabin, trifluorothymidine, aciclovir, ganciclovir, and cidofovir.[2] Chronic forms of keratitis such as disciform and SK may not respond to antivirals since replicating virus may no longer be present in the cornea in later stages of disease. Treatment focuses on the use of anti-inflammatory drugs, particularly steroids. Typically treatment starts with a high dose given daily, tapering off to a very low dose that may be continued for weeks or even months. There is a place for future therapies aimed at essential steps in the pathogenesis of the disease, which modern research is revealing. Some of these are listed in Table 12.2, along with the event they target.

Conceptually, the best way to deal with herpetic keratitis is to develop effective prophylactic, or better still, therapeutic vaccines. The mission to develop such vaccines has been vigorously pursued but so far with no real success. Currently, the target HSV-induced diseases are genital infections caused mainly by HSV-2, since these are far more common than ocular problems. If success is achieved in the HSV-2 vaccine field, this could help reduce the incidence of neonatal ocular herpes. As mentioned, the most serious consequence of ocular HSV in adults results from recurrences and these often have an immunopathological component. Conceivably, therapeutic vaccines could make matters worse rather than better – an issue that will need to be examined carefully.

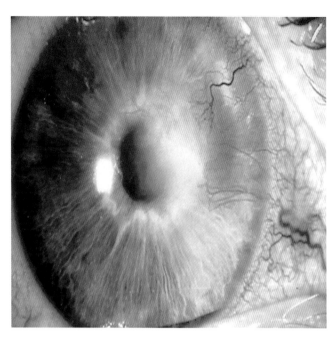

Figure 12.1 Human eye showing stromal keratitis.

Box 12.1 A typical case of stromal keratitis

- Herpetic keratitis is the commonest infectious cause of blindness in the USA
- Usual cause is herpes simplex virus (HSV)-1 or HSV-2 and, more rarely, varicella-zoster virus
- Virus remains dormant (latent) after infection

Pathology

Herpes simplex virus infection of the eye has two major consequences: firstly, direct lysis, the fate of all cells in which the virus completes a replication cycle. The second effect is the induction of an inflammatory reaction that itself may lead to tissue damage. The latter can ultimately become chronic, mainly because components of the virus become targets for an immunopathological reaction.

The commonest causes of pathologic lesions with HSV ocular infection are the lytic effects of viral replication (Box 12.2). Such lesions may be confined to the corneal epithelium or additionally affect the nearby tissues such as the conjunctiva, uveal tract, corneal endothelium, and even the retina, as occurs most often in HSV-2-infected neonates.[2] The lytic cells are shed, giving rise to ulcers, and an inflammatory reaction occurs. Frequently the ulcers are irregular in outline and are described as dendritic. Figure 12.2 shows such an ulcer in a recently infected rabbit. Lytic infection of the corneal endothelium usually results in edema, swelling of the stroma, and perhaps entrance of viral antigen into this tissue. This form of keratitis is called disciform keratitis. The viral antigens that enter the stroma react with antibody and may form ring-shaped opacities called Wessely rings.[4] Immune complexes can also fix complement, resulting in a necrotizing lesion which may represent one form of SK in humans as well as in the rabbit model.[2]

As already mentioned, herpes infections always result in latency. Such virus in the ophthalmic branch of the trigeminal ganglion can reactivate in response to a diverse array of stimuli that affect the physiology of the infected neurons and/or alter the function of the host response that prevents

---

Table 12.1 Clinical manifestation of ocular herpes and its management

Primary	Recurrent		
	Epithelial keratitis	Stromal keratitis	Disciform keratitis
Symptoms	**Symptoms**	**Symptoms**	**Symptoms**
• Mild malaise and fever with redness, irritation, and watery discharge from the eye (typically unilateral)	• Painful eye, corneal hypothesis, tearing, and photophobia	• Painful eye; both inflammatory and reparative events could be visible by slit lamp	• Blurred vision with photophobia, tearing, and mild orbital pain
• Follicular conjunctivitis associated with enlargement of the ipsilateral preauricular lymph node	• Ciliary injection	• Cellular infiltration, neovascularization, and scarring	• Unlike stromal keratitis, lesions are uniform. Intact epithelium with a central or eccentric zone of edema that surrounds a solid disc of edematous stroma
• Swollen lid and grouped vesicles or ulcers	• Dendritic ulcers on the epithelial surface and epithelial erosion	• Stratified opacities and presence of corneal lamellae	
• Similar lesions may be present near mouth	• Vesicles or ulcers may develop on the lids, face, mouth, and nose	• Corneal necrosis and ground-glass appearance of the stroma	• Wessely ring might appear
• Edematous or injected conjunctiva	**Management**	• Corneal scarring, facet formation, and perforation	• White keratitic precipitates on the endothelial surface
• Grittiness, photophobia, blurred vision mostly evident with 2 weeks of infection	• Similar to primary herpes	**Management**	**Management**
Management	• Analgesics can be used to relieve pain	• Steroid therapy to control inflammation (lowest effective dose to be used to minimize the side-effects)	• Similar to stromal keratitis
• Application of antiviral ointment	• Discontinue or reduce the dose of steroids in case of steroid-enhanced ulcers	• Administration of antivirals to reduce the chances of recurrence	• Application of steroid
• Debridement of the corneal epithelium vescicles on the lid		• Steroid dose can be reduced slowly but if inflammation recurs it needs to be increased	
• Appropriate antibiotics or antifungal if secondary bacterial infection is involved			

Table 12.2 Potential future approaches to control herpetic keratitis

Target	Approach
Inflammation	Anti-inflammatory molecules such as COX-1 and -2 inhibitors[30]
	Blocking critical cytokines and chemokines[31]
	Ciclosporin A[32]
Targeting angiogenic factors and their receptors	VEGF: anti-VEGF antibody[33] and siRNA[21]
	Inhibiting metalloproteinase with siRNA or TIMP-1[34]
Immunomodulation	Changing the balance from Th1 to Th2[35,36]
	Affecting T-cell activation: CTLA4 Ig,[37] anti-BB[38]
	Adoptive transfer of regulatory T cells[39]
	Nonmitogenic anti-CD3 antibody[40]
	Anti-CD200 Fc
	Sequestering T cells in lymph nodes using FTY720[41]
	Inducing regulatory T cells by administration of rapamycin,[42] FTY720,[41] retinoic acid,[43] and blocking histone deacetylase[44]
Tissue-repairing therapy	Application of FGF[45]

COX-1, cyclooxygenase-1; VEGF, vascular endothelial growth factor; TIMP-1, tissue inhibitor of metalloproteinase 1; CTLA4, cytotoxic T-lymphocyte antigen 4; Ig, immunoglobulin; FGF, fibroblast growth factor.

Box 12.2 General features

- Acute herpetic keratitis is mainly caused by herpes simplex virus (HSV)-1, but changing sexual behavior is making HSV-2 a more common cause
- Neonatal keratitis is usually caused by HSV-2 infection of seronegative infants
- Acute infections respond well to antiviral therapy
- Control of chronic lesions requires anti-inflammatory drugs

---

the virus from replicating.[5] The exact mechanisms involved in the establishment, maintenance, and breakdown of latency are currently poorly understood and this is an active topic of research. Reactivating virus passes back to the eye where it causes a recurrent lesion. Most often this mainly involves the epithelium but ultimately, especially after repeated recurrences, the stroma becomes a principal site for an inflammatory reaction, new blood vessel development, and tissue scarring (Figure 12.1). This SK impairs vision and can result in blindness. Corneal ulceration and perforation can also be a consequence. SK is considered to represent an immunopathological reaction, although the cellular and molecular mechanisms are still poorly understood, especially in the natural disease. Supporting the immunopathol-

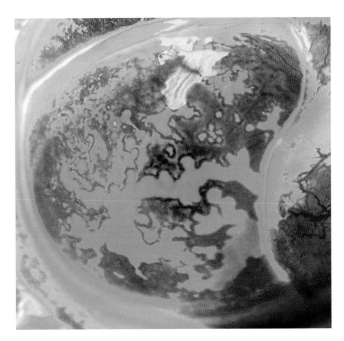

Figure 12.2 Rabbit eye showing dendritic ulcers. (Courtesy of Oscar Perng, Emory University.)

ogy hypothesis is that infectious virus and viral antigens may be difficult or impossible to demonstrate in eyes showing SK and that antiviral treatment may be ineffective. Therapeutic control requires anti-inflammatory drug administration which, as mentioned before, may be needed for months.

Etiology

Herpetic keratitis in adults is usually caused by HSV-1 but changing sexual behavior patterns are making HSV-2 an increasingly more common cause.[1] Primary keratitis either results from exposure to active lesions or virus-laden secretions of close contacts, or perhaps more commonly as a secondary site of recurrence. In this latter situation, primary clinical or subclinical infection affects other sites innervated by the facial nerve, but when the virus reactivates in the trigeminal ganglion, spread to the ophthalmic division can occur, setting the stage for ocular recurrence. Some cases of ocular HSV infection have resulted from the receipt of infected transplanted tissue.[6] In neonates, primary infection occasionally occurs in utero but, more commonly, infection of the seronegative neonate occurs when exposed to the virus-secreting mother.

Occasionally primary infection with VZV involves the cornea, but the disease has become very rare with the widespread use of an effective vaccine. Zoster lesions, however, occurring during shingles can also affect the eye. Such lesions may be severe, painful, and prolonged and often leave behind a scarred and damaged cornea (Box 12.3).

Pathophysiology

Most of our understanding of the pathogenesis of HSV-induced keratitis comes from experimental studies in animal

> **Box 12.3 Keratitis in human**
>
> - Acute lesions result from lytic effects of viral replication that usually involves the epithelium
> - Recurrences are common, usually resulting from reactivated dormant infection
> - Repeated recurrences often result in chronic inflammatory reactions in the stroma and the recurrences are probably wholly or in part immunopathological

> **Box 12.4 Pathogenesis**
>
> - Studies in animal models reveal that multiple key events are involved during the pathogenesis of the blinding stromal lesions
> - These events include viral replication, the induction of corneal neovascularization, the induction of multiple cytokines and chemokines, and invasion of the stroma by multiple types of inflammatory cells
> - The main orchestrators of stromal lesions are T lymphocytes that recognize viral antigens, and perhaps other antigens such as self-components derived from the cornea

models where HSV is not a natural infection. These models have proven most useful in constructing the likely series of events that culminate in the chronic vision-damaging stromal form of the disease. In humans, the tissue damage and scarring of SK are thought to be the consequence of immunological reactions to viral components and perhaps eventually to unmasked self-antigens derived from the cornea. It seems likely that T-cell-mediated immunopathology mainly explains how tissue damage occurs but additional roles for antibody-mediated immunopathology cannot be ruled out.[2,4] In support of T cells, both major subsets can be isolated from corneal lesions and some are reactive with peptides derived from a variety of HSV proteins.[7] Some suspect that chronic SK ultimately become autoinflammatory but to date autoreactive T cells have not been identified. The autoimmune hypothesis is supported by the usual failure to demonstrate viral components in SK samples and that SK usually responds to treatment with anti-inflammatory, but not antiviral, drugs.[8] A viable hypothesis is that lesions may be initiated by antiviral T-cell reactions but sustained by autoreactivity.

Experimental studies to understand the pathophysiology of keratitis are usually performed in the rabbit or mouse. The former has the advantage of a large eye and the fact that recurrent lesions, the main clinical problem in human keratitis, can occur or be induced in this model when infected with appropriate strains of virus.[7] However, rabbits are not suitable to unravel immunological phenomena, especially those that involve T cells. The reagent-rich mouse model, with its abundance of transgenic and knockout strains, is the better system to construct likely pathophysiological events that comprise human SK. Furthermore, using appropriate mouse and viral strains, SK can regularly be induced in mice following primary infection. In contrast, recurrent lesions are difficult to induce, but when this heroic model has been established the findings have largely confirmed those noted in the primary infection model.[8] The account that follows describes principal events noted in the mouse primary infection model using mainly Balb/c and C57Bl/6 mouse strains infected with HSV-1 RE.

Initial phase of infection

Experimental infection of the mouse cornea induces a cascade of events. These result in clearing the infection, setting the stage for a chronic immunoinflammatory reaction in the underlying stroma, as well as establishing and maintaining latency in the trigeminal ganglion. Viral replication, at least in immunocompetent animals, occurs mainly in the corneal epithelium, although spread to the conjunctiva and other nearby tissues is common in the mouse. Rep-

lication usually lasts for no more than 1 week and seldom involves the underlying stroma or the corneal endothelium. The infection triggers a wide range of cellular and molecular events, although how this is orchestrated at a molecular level is poorly understood. Numerous cytokines, chemokines as well as molecules that cause new blood vessels to sprout from the limbal vasculature, are expressed. Most of these do not derive from the infected epithelial cells since a consequence of HSV replication is that host cells quickly shut down their own synthetic machinery.[9] Some cytokines however are produced from the infected cell, such as the cytokines interleukin (IL)-1 and IL-6.[10] Adjacent epithelial cells, some underlying stromal keratocytes, as well as vascular and other cell types in limbal tissues probably produce most of the newly synthesized molecules. These paracrine reactions could occur in at least two ways. Firstly, HSV virions contain at least two ligands for receptors that trigger innate immune reactions.[11,12] These are ligands for Toll-like receptor (TLR) 2 and 9 but most likely other TLR ligands will be demonstrated as well as ligands for other sensing receptors of innate immunity. Recently, for example, children with TLR3 deficiency were shown to be apt to suffer herpes encephalitis.[13] Triggering via TLRs induces a wide range of cytokines and chemokines that participate in inflammatory reactions.[14] Animals lacking a critical TLR may be more resistant to develop SK, as has been shown with TLR knockout mice.[15]

The second paracrine means by which HSV-infected cells trigger other cells to make proinflammatory mediators is by their release of signaling molecules such as some cytokines, stress molecules, and cell breakdown products (Box 12.4). Both IL-6 and IL-1, made briefly by infected cells, can induce other cells to synthesize several cytokines and chemokines as well as some angiogenic factors such as vascular endothelial growth factor (VEGF).[10] They may also induce small peptides such as ß-defensins, as well as enzymes needed for the generation of lipid proinflammatory mediators such as prostaglandins and leukotrienes. Stress proteins, such as heat shock protein (HSP) 70, produced by infected cells, can act as a ligand for the TLR4 receptor and so induce the production of inflammatory mediators.[15]

Quite rapidly after infection, an abundance of new molecules are made but few have been investigated for the role they play in the pathogenesis of SK. Those that have been studied include the cytokines IL-1, IL-6, IL-12, tumor necrosis factor-α, interferon-α and interferon-γ.[10] One suspects that IL-23 and IL-21 as well as inhibitory cytokines such as IL-10, IL-27, and transforming growth factor-ß will also

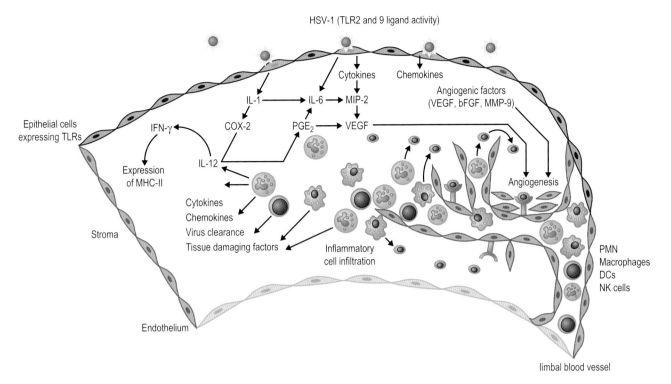

Figure 12.3 Schematic representation of early events occurring after herpes simplex virus ocular infection in mouse. TLR, Toll-like receptor; IFN-γ, interferon-γ; MHC, major histocompatibility complex; IL, interleukin; COX-2, cyclooxygenase-2; PGE₂, prostaglandin E₂; VEGF, vascular endothelial growth factor; HSV-1, herpes simplex virus-1; MIP-2, macrophage inflammatory protein-2; bFGF, basic fibroblast growth factor; MMP-9, MMP-9, matrix metalloproteinase 9.

prove to play relevant roles, but this requires further evaluation. Several chemokines are also rapidly produced.[10] Some are responsible for attracting several types of inflammatory cells that become evident in the stroma as early as 24 hours postinfection. These cells include natural killer (NK) cells, Langerhans dendritic cells, some macrophages but, most prominently of all, neutrophils. Neutrophils are probably attracted by chemokines such as macrophage inflammatory protein-2 (MIP-2) since mice unable to respond to this chemokine have diminished polymorphonuclear leukocyte infiltration.[16] Serial events that occur during the early phase of murine keratitis are summarized in Figure 12.3.

The infiltrating inflammatory cells also become a source of several molecules involved in the pathogenesis of lesions. For example, neutrophils may be a source of interferon-γ (IFN-γ) and tumor necrosis factor-α (TNF-α) as well as molecules responsible for angiogenesis such as VEGF and matrix metalloproteinase 9 (MMP-9).[10] Neutrophils, macrophages, and NK cells, along with the interferons and ß-defensins, probably contribute to clearing the infection.[17–19] For example, depleting neutrophils results in prolonged viral infection and often dissemination of virus to other sites such as the brain.[20]

Another event that begins early after infection is new blood vessel development. These gradually invade into the stroma, with this becoming an extensive event in murine disease (Figure 12.4). Angiogenesis is also evident in human SK (Figure 12.1). Several angiogenic factors are produced as a consequence of HSV infection. Most prominent of these are VEGF, fibroblast growth factor, MMP-9, and some angiogenic chemokines.[10] Their primary cell source has not been

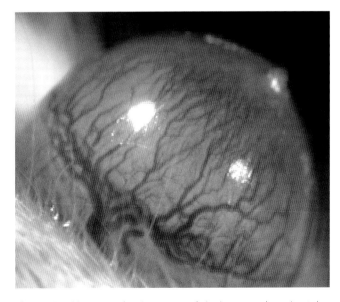

Figure 12.4 Mouse eye showing neovascularization, corneal opacity at day 12 postinfection.

established but it is unlikely to be the infected epithelial cells. Angiogenesis contributes to vision problems but this may also be a necessary process to facilitate the invasion of some types of inflammatory cells into the corneal stroma, particularly lymphocytes. Inhibition of angiogenesis results in a significant diminution of SK lesions which may represent a future therapy for SK.[21]

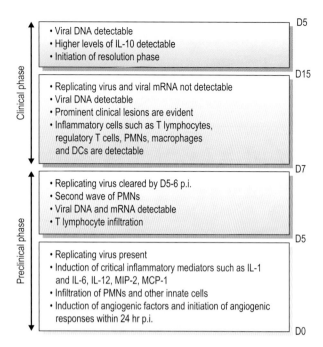

Figure 12.5 Key events during the pathogenesis of murine stromal keratitis. IL-10, interleukin-10; PMNs, polymorphonuclear leukocytes; DCs, dendritic cells; MIP-2, macrophage inflammatory protein-2; MCP-1, monocyte chemotactic protein-1; p.i., postinfection.

Currently the role of many molecules and cells that are rapidly produced after HSV infection is not fully understood. Some of the known key events in the pathogenesis of SK are illustrated in Figure 12.5.

The development of SK

The chronic tissue-damaging lesion begins once the antiviral immune response has been induced. This takes a few days. Lymphocytes become readily evident in the stroma infiltrates by 6–7 days postinfection. A few lymphocytes can be found as early as day 3,[22] but these are unlikely to be HSV-specific. Invasion by lymphocytes is probably facilitated by the leaky new blood vessels now present in the stroma by signals generated by the T cells. Without T cells, SK does not occur so it is assumed that such cells are the primary orchestrators of lesion.[23] Lymphocytes themselves may not participate directly in tissue damage. This is more likely to be performed by the more abundant neutrophils and macrophages that are recruited to the stroma. Curiously, CD4+ T cells far outnumber CD8+ T cells in murine SK and such CD4+ T cells are likely the main mediators of the inflammatory response. Many questions remain, however, as to how the CD4+ T cells function. One assumes that at least initially the critical cells are viral antigen-specific but this has not been formally shown. Moreover, demonstrating native or processed antigens in stromal tissues at the time when peak lymphocyte invasion is occurring (day 10–14) has not been achieved. One idea is that the infection results in the unmasking of corneal autoantigens which then act as the main targets for the CD4+ T cells.[24] Another suggestion is that T cells entering the damaged cornea are nonspecifically (bystander) activated to participate in the immunopathological process.[25,26] More studies are needed to resolve these issues.

Another unresolved issue is the identity of the types of T cells that are either pro- or anti-inflammatory in SK lesions. Earlier work had advocated that CD4+ T cells that produce type 1 cytokines (such as IFN-γ, TNF-α, and IL-2) were the principal orchestrators,[23,27] but T cells that produce IL-17 likely also participate. In human SK recent studies imply a role for IL-17-producing cells in stromal tissues.[28] From a future therapeutic control perspective, it will be important to understand how the host resolves lesion and perhaps assist this process in some way. For example, recent research is revealing that upregulation of cytokines such as IL-10 and TGF-ß or activating cells that express regulatory function serve to suppress lesion severity.[29] One anticipates that studies of the cellular and molecular events occurring at different stages of SK should reveal additional mechanisms that can be manipulated by novel therapies.

Summary

Herpetic ocular infections are the commonest causes of vision impairment in the western world. The virus most often involved in adults is HSV-1 but HSV-2, the usual cause in neonates, is becoming more common. Recurrent lesions usually occur, mainly resulting from activation of dormant virus following exposure of patients to various forms of stress. Acute lesions are the direct result of viral replication and these respond well to treatment with several antiviral drugs. Chronic lesions, the main cause of vision damage, are more difficult to control and require the prolonged use of anti-inflammatory drugs, especially steroids. Ongoing studies in animal models of herpetic keratitis should reveal novel means of improved treatment.

Acknowledgment

The authors' work has been supported by grant EY05093.

Key references

A complete list of chapter references is available online at www.expertconsult.com. See inside cover for registration details.

1. Pepose JS, Keadle TL, Morrison LA. Ocular herpes simplex: changing epidemiology, emerging disease patterns, and the potential of vaccine prevention and therapy. Am J Ophthalmol 2006;141:547–557.

2. Pepose JS, Leib DA, Stuart PM, et al. Herpes simplex virus diseases: anterior segment of the eye. In: Pepose JS, Holland GN, Wilhelmus KR (eds) Ocular Infections and Immunity. St. Louis: Mosby; 1996:905–932.

4. Streilein JW, Dana MR, Ksander BR. Immunity causing blindness: five different paths to herpes stromal keratitis. Immunol Today 1997;18:443–449.

5. Sheridan BS, Knickelbein JE, Hendricks RL. CD8 T cells and latent herpes simplex virus type 1: keeping the peace in sensory ganglia. Exp Opin Biol Ther 2007;7:1323–1331.

7. Maertzdorf J, Verjans GM, Remeijer L, et al. Restricted T cell receptor beta-chain variable region protein use by cornea-derived CD4+ and CD8+ herpes simplex virus-specific T cells in patients with herpetic stromal keratitis. J Infect Dis 2003;187:550–558.

8. Deshpande S, Banerjee K, Biswas PS, et al. Herpetic eye disease: immunopathogenesis and therapeutic measures. Exp Rev Mol Med 2004;6:1–14.

10. Biswas PS, Rouse BT. Early events in HSV keratitis – setting the stage for a blinding disease. Microbes Infect 2005;7:799–810.

15. Sarangi PP, Kim B, Kurt-Jones E, et al. Innate recognition network driving herpes simplex virus-induced corneal immunopathology: role of the toll pathway in early inflammatory events in stromal keratitis. J Virol 2007;81:11128–11138.

16. Yan XT, Tumpey TM, Kunkel SL, et al. Role of MIP-2 in neutrophil migration and tissue injury in the herpes simplex virus-1-infected cornea. Invest Ophthalmol Vis Sci 1998;39:1854–1862.

21. Kim B, Tang Q, Biswas PS, et al. Inhibition of ocular angiogenesis by siRNA targeting vascular endothelial growth factor pathway genes: therapeutic strategy for herpetic stromal keratitis. Am J Pathol 2004;165:2177–2185.

23. Mercadal CM, Bouley DM, DeStephano D, et al. Herpetic stromal keratitis in the reconstituted scid mouse model. J Virol 1993;67:3404–3408.

24. Zhao ZS, Granucci F, Yeh L, et al. Molecular mimicry by herpes simplex virus-type 1: autoimmune disease after viral infection. Science 1998;279:1344–1347.

26. Banerjee K, Deshpande S, Zheng M, et al. Herpetic stromal keratitis in the absence of viral antigen recognition. Cell Immunol 2002;219:108–118.

27. Niemialtowski MG, Rouse BT. Predominance of Th1 cells in ocular tissues during herpetic stromal keratitis. J Immunol 1992;149:3035–3039.

34. Lee S, Zheng M, Kim B, et al. Role of matrix metalloproteinase-9 in angiogenesis caused by ocular infection with herpes simplex virus. J Clin Invest 2002;110:1105–1111.

39. Sehrawat S, Suvas S, Rouse BT, et al. In vitro-generated antigen-specific CD4+ CD25+ Foxp3+ regulatory T cells control the severity of herpes simplex virus-induced ocular immunoinflammatory lesions. J Virol 2008;82:6838–6851.

CHAPTER 13

Ocular allergy

Neal P Barney, Ellen B Cook, James L Stahl,
and Frank M Graziano

Allergic diseases of the eye

Allergic eye disease is typically divided into four distinct types: allergic conjunctivitis, subdivided into seasonal and perennial allergic conjunctivitis (SAC and PAC, respectively), atopic keratoconjunctivitis (AKC), and vernal keratoconjunctivitis (VKC). Giant papillary conjunctivitis (GPC) is increasingly considered a result of microtrauma rather than an immunologically driven disease entity. In the discussion that follows, clinical, pathophysiological, and diagnostic aspects of each ocular process will be discussed in detail.

Allergic conjunctivitis – seasonal/perennial (Box 13.1)

Allergic conjunctivitis is a bilateral, self-limiting conjunctival inflammatory process. It occurs in sensitized individuals (no gender difference) and is initiated by allergen binding to immunoglobulin E (IgE) antibody on resident mast cells. The importance of this process is related more to its frequency rather than its severity of symptoms. The two forms of allergic conjunctivitis are defined by whether the inflammation occurs seasonally, SAC (spring, fall) or perennially, PAC. Both SAC and PAC must be differentiated from the sight-threatening allergic diseases of the eye, namely AKC and VKC.

Clinical background

The key symptom reported in allergic conjunctivitis is ocular itching. Symptoms, signs, and differential diagnosis are listed in Table 13.1. A survey conducted by the American College of Allergy, Asthma, and Immunology (ACAAI) found that 35% of families interviewed experience allergies, and at least 50% of these individuals describe associated eye symptoms. Most reports agree that allergic conjunctivitis affects up to 20% of the population.[1] Importantly, 60% of all allergic rhinitis sufferers have associated allergic conjunctivitis. The distribution of SAC depends largely on the climate. There are no racial or gender difference noted for allergic conjunctivitis. Onset of disease tends to be during infancy and is typically accompanied by the development of other allergic diseases such as atopic dermatitis or asthma.

There is little reason beyond the history and examination to investigate further the patient with allergic conjunctivitis. The commonest treatment for allergic conjunctivitis is once- or twice-daily topical administration of a dual-acting drop with mast cell-stabilizing and antihistamine activity. The self-limiting nature of the disease means there is quite a good prognosis for retention of good vision and no ocular surface scar formation.

Pathology

Histopathologic and laboratory manifestation of allergic ocular diseases is shown in Table 13.2. Granule-associated neutral proteases (tryptase and chymase) unique to mast cells are generally accepted as the most appropriate phenotypic markers to categorize human mast cells into subsets. Mast cells on this basis have been divided into MC_T (tryptase) and MC_{TC} (tryptase/chymase) phenotypes.[2] The phenotype of normal human conjunctival mast cells has been well documented using immunostaining of conjunctival biopsy specimens.[3] Mast cells are rarely present in the normal human conjunctival epithelium, but when they are found, they appear to be limited to the MC_T phenotype. Mast cells (MC_T phenotype) and eosinophils are increased in the conjunctival epithelium of individuals with SAC and PAC (Table 13.2). In the substantia propria of the normal human conjunctiva, mast cells are found and 95% are of the MC_{TC} phenotype.[3-5] The total number of mast cells (MC_{TC} phenotype) is also increased in the substantia propria of individuals with allergic conjunctivitis.[3]

Etiology

The etiology of the allergic conjunctivitis is the same as allergic disease in general. Genetic studies to date point to multiple genes. Strachan is credited with the theory that exposure to infection and unhygienic environments in general prevented allergic disease development.[6] Intitially based on the observation that allergies were less prevalent in the country compared to the inner city, this has been further refined as differences in cytokine environment, with Th-2 cytokines favoring an allergic phenotype and Th-1 cytokines favoring an autoimmune phenotype. Conserved pathogen-associated molecular patterns (PAMP) are found in different microbes, and interact with the pattern recognition receptors of surface cells to influence the adaptive immune response.

Pathophysiology

It has been understood for some time that antigen cross-linking of IgE antibody bound to the high-affinity IgE receptor (FcεRI) on mast cells induces release of both preformed (granule-associated, e.g., histamine and tryptase) and newly synthesized mediators (e.g., arachidonic acid metabolites, cytokines, chemokines) which have diverse and overlapping biological effects. Both tissue staining and tear film data have implicated the mast cell and IgE-mediated release of its mediators in the pathophysiology of the ocular allergic inflammatory response. Additionally, a number of clinical studies examining topical antihistamine, mast cell-stabilizing and dual-acting drugs have demonstrated relief of allergic conjunctivitis symptoms.

Clinical evidence for mast cell activation (with subsequent recruitment and activation of other cells such as eosinophils) is found in SAC and PAC (Table 13.2). Tear film analysis of patients consistently reveals the presence of IgE antibody, histamine,[7,8] tryptase,[9] eotaxin,[10] and eosinophil cationic protein (ECP).[11] The contributions of granule-associated, preformed (histamine, tryptase, bradykinin) and arachidonic acid-derived, newly formed (leukotrienes, prostaglandins) mast cell-derived mediators present in ocular inflammation have been well documented. Preformed mediators are released immediately upon allergen exposure, while minutes to hours are required for release of newly formed mediators. These mediators are known to have overlapping biological effects that contribute to the characteristic ocular itching, redness, and watery discharge associated with allergic eye disease. Mast cells also synthesize cytokines and chemokines. Less well documented and defined are the effects of these mediators in the ocular allergic inflammatory process. Cytokines stored in mast cells are likely the first signals initiating infiltration of inflammatory leukocytes, such as eosinophils. Once these cells arrive, they gain access to the conjunctival surface by moving through the already dilated capillaries. Recently, the tear film of patients with

---

Box 13.1 Acute allergic eye disease

- Seasonal allergic conjunctivitis is the commonest form of ocular allergy and is a self-limiting allergic process
- No conjunctiva scar formation is noted
- Treatment with topical combination mast cell stabilizer/antihistamine drops is usually sufficient for relief of symptoms
- Allergic disease of the eye is underreported by patients and often self-medicated with over-the-counter preparations
- Patients may not report the use of over-the-counter medication

---

Table 13.1 Allergic diseases of the eye

Disease	Clinical parameters	Signs/symptoms	Differential diagnosis
Seasonal allergic conjunctivitis (SAC)	Sensitized individuals Both females and males Bilateral involvement Seasonal allergies Self-limiting	Ocular itching Tearing (watery discharge) Ocular chemosis, redness Often associated with rhinitis Not sight-threatening	Infective conjunctivitis Preservative toxicity Medicamentosa Dry eye PAC/AKC/VKC
Perennial allergic conjunctivitis (PAC)	Sensitized individuals Both females and males Bilateral involvement Year-round allergies Self-limiting	Ocular itching Tearing (watery discharge) Ocular chemosis, redness Often associated with rhinitis Not sight-threatening	Infective conjunctivitis Preservative toxicity Medicamentosa Dry eye SAC/AKC/VKC
Atopic keratoconjunctivitis (AKC)	Sensitized individuals Peak incidence 20–50 years of age Both females and males Bilateral involvement Seasonal/perennial allergies Atopic dermatitis Chronic symptoms	Severe ocular itching Red flaking periocular skin Mucoid discharge, photophobia Corneal erosions Scarring of conjunctiva Cataract (anterior subcapsular) Sight-threatening	Contact dermatitis Infective conjunctivitis Blepharitis Pemphigoid VKC/SAC/PAC/GPC
Vernal keratoconjunctivitis (VKC)	Sensitized individuals Peak incidence 3–20 years old Males predominate 3:1 Bilateral involvement Warm, dry climate Seasonal/perennial allergies Chronic symptoms	Severe ocular itching Severe photophobia Thick, ropy discharge Cobblestone papillae Corneal ulceration and scarring Sight-threatening	Infective conjunctivitis Blepharitis AKC/SAC/PAC/GPC
Giant papillary conjunctivitis (GPC)	Sensitization not necessary Both females and males Bilateral involvement Prosthetic exposure Occurs any time Chronic symptoms	Mild ocular itching Mild mucoid discharge Giant papillae Contact lens intolerance Foreign-body sensation Protein build-up on contact lens Not sight-threatening	Infective conjunctivitis Preservative toxicity SAC/PAC/AKC/VKC

Table 13.2 Histopathology and laboratory manifestations of allergic ocular disease

Disease	Histopathology	Laboratory manifestations
Seasonal/perennial allergic conjunctivitis	Mast cell/eosinophil infiltration in conjunctival epithelium and substantia propia Mast cell activation Upregulation of ICAM-1 on epithelial cells	Increased tears Specific IgE antibody Histamine Tryptase TNF-α
Atopic keratoconjunctivitis	Increased mast cells, eosinophils in conjunctival epithelium and substantia propria Epithelial cell/goblet cell hypertrophy Increased CD4/CD8 ratio in conjunctival epithelium and substantia propria Increased collagen and fibroblasts Chemokines and chemokine receptor staining	Increased specific IgE antibody in tears Depressed cell-mediated immunity Increased IgE antibody and eosinophils in blood Eosinophils found in conjunctival scrapings
Vernal keratoconjunctivitis	Increased mast cells, eosinophils in conjunctival epithelium and substantia propria Eosinophil major basic protein deposition in conjunctiva CD4+clones from conjunctiva found to have helper function for local production of IgE antibody Increased collagen Increased ICAM-1 on corneal epithelium	Increased specific IgE/IgG antibody in tears Elevated histamine and tryptase in tears Reduced serum histaminase activity Increased serum levels of nerve growth factor and substance P
Giant papillary conjunctivitis	Giant papillae Conjunctival thickening Mast cells in epithelium	No increased histamine in tears Increased tryptase in tears

Ig, immunoglobulin; ICAM-1, intercellular adhesion molecule 1; TNF-α, tumor necrosis factor-α.

allergic conjunctivitis has been found to have a more rapid break-up time and to be thicker than the tear film of control patients.[12]

Immunohistochemical staining of human conjunctival tissue biopsies shows that inflammatory cytokines interleukin (IL)-4, IL-5, IL-6, and tumor necrosis factor-α (TNF-α) are localized to mast cells in normal and allergic conjunctivitis.[13] Inflammatory cytokines (e.g., TNF-α) have also been measured in human tears.[14–18] While it is difficult in vivo to determine the cellular source of cytokines in tears, recent studies comparing allergic and nonallergic subjects indicate that cytokine levels may be important indicators of ocular allergy.[18] It has been demonstrated that tears from allergic donors (when compared to nonallergic donors) contained significantly less of the anti-inflammatory cytokine IL-10 and a trend toward decreased levels of the Th1 cytokine, interferon-γ.[18] Differences in biological activity between allergic and nonallergic tears have also been demonstrated in vitro. Tears from allergic patients enhanced eosinophil adhesion to primary human conjunctival epithelial cells compared to tears from nonallergic patients.[19] Finally, IgE-mediated release of histamine and cytokines from mast cells can initiate secondary effects on conjunctival epithelial cells. The activation and participation of epithelial cells in allergic inflammation is an active field of research. Human conjunctival epithelial cells express H_1 receptors coupled to phosphatidylinositol turnover and calcium mobilization.[20] Mast cell-mediated activation of conjunctival epithelial cells has also been demonstrated in multiple in vitro studies in which primary cultures of conjunctival epithelial cells were stimulated with supernates from IgE-activated conjunctival mast cells.[18,19,21] These studies demonstrated that TNF-α released from mast cells upregulates intercellular adhesion molecule 1 (ICAM-1) expression on conjunctival epithelial cells.[21] ICAM-1 expression on the conjunctival epithelium in vivo has become a marker of allergic inflammation.[22] Fibroblasts stimulated during allergic conjunctivitis reactions of the ocular surface may be a further source of cytokines and chemokines, to include RANTES and eotaxin.[23]

The ratio of cytokines present in the tissues and tear film strongly influences the allergic reactions of the ocular surface. The Th2 cytokines TNF-α, IL-5, and IL-4 are all elevated in the tears of SAC patients compared to Th1 cytokine levels.[18] CD25+ T regulatory cells have been shown to inhibit T-cell proliferation and effector function. Depletion of CD25+ T cells during immunization in a mouse model of allergic conjunctivitis did not potentiate the disease development.[24] These same authors also noted that natural killer T cells can play a downregulatory role in the development of mouse experimental allergic conjunctivitis.[25] Suppressor of cytokine signaling 3 (SOCS3), mainly from naïve T cells, will result in increased Th2 development and suppressed Th1 development. In a mouse model of allergic conjunctivitis, inhibition of SOSC3 reduced the severity of the allergic reaction.[26]

Atopic keratoconjunctivitis (Box 13.2)

AKC is a bilateral, sight-threatening, chronic allergic inflammation occurring in the conjunctiva and eyelids of sensitized individuals with atopic dermatitis (Table 13.1, Figure 13.1).

Clinical background

Severe ocular itching is the major symptom of AKC. This may be more pronounced in certain seasons or be perennial. Details of symptoms, signs, and differential diagnosis are given in Table 13.1. Significant vision loss, the major and most critical outcome of this disease, is usually due to corneal pathology. Superficial punctate keratopathy is the most common corneal finding. Neovascularization, persist-

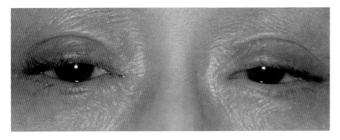

Figure 13.1 Reddened skin and severe conjunctival redness and chemosis of atopic keratoconjunctivitis.

Box 13.2 Chronic allergic eye disease

- Atopic keratoconjunctivitis and vernal keratoconjunctivitis are chronic allergic processes and sight-threatening diseases
- Vernal keratoconjunctivitis occurs in young males in hot dry climates
- Vernal keratoconjunctivitis tends to resolve following onset of puberty
- Atopic keratoconjunctivitis occurs in the second to fifth decade of life, although the onset of atopic dermatitis is typically before the age of 5 years
- The use of topical steroids to treat ocular allergic diseases should only be initiated in conjunction with an ophthalmologist
- Many potent antihistamines are available to treat the signs and symptoms of allergic disease
- Steroid use in a chronic ocular surface disease needs to be monitored carefully to allow early detection of cataract or increased intraocular pressure

---

ent epithelial defects, scarring, and microbial ulceration are the main corneal causes of decreased vision. Penetrating keratoplasty typically results in similar surface problems but has been shown to improve vision in some.[27] Herpetic keratitis is reported to occur in 14–18% of patients.[28,29] Keratoconus (noninflammatory progressive thinning of the cornea) occurs in 7–16% of patients.[28,29] Anterior uveitis and iris abnormalities are not reported. The prevalence of cataract associated with AKC is difficult to determine because steroids are so frequently used in treatment of the disease. The typical lens opacity associated with AKC is an anterior or posterior subcapsular cataract. The anterior cataract frequently has a "milk splash" appearance. Retinal detachment with or without previous cataract surgery is the principal posterior manifestation reported in AKC.[30–32]

The findings of chronic conjunctivitis and keratitis in patients with atopic dermatitis were first described by Hogan in 1953.[33] In all, 3–9% of the population has atopic dermatitis[34–36] and 15–67.5% of these individuals have ocular symptoms, most prominently as AKC.[34,36,37] In general, the chronicity of this disease is the most critical aspect of the history. The patient typically describes severe, persistent, periocular itching associated with findings of atopic dermatitis. There is usually a family history of atopic disease in one or both parents and other atopic manifestations in the patient (asthma or rhinitis).[38] Treatment of this vision-threatening disease requires the use of topical steroids with rapid taper and maintenance of quiescence with calcineurin inhibitors such as ciclosporin A or tacrolimus. Vision-threatening complications include cornea ulceration and plaque formation, lid scar, and lid malposition. Additionally, cataract and glaucoma are potential complications of long-term treatment with topical steroids.

Pathology

Whereas allergic conjunctivitis is a self-limiting allergic process, AKC is chronic and potentially sight-threatening. The exact mechanisms leading to this outcome are not completely understood. The involvement of mast cells, IgE antibodies, eosinophils and other inflammatory cells is similar to allergic conjunctivitis. The chronicity of the disease and sight threat are likely due to lymphocyte involvement in the pathogenesis (Table 13.2). The increase in CD4+ T cells and chemokine receptors likely serves to amplify the immune response occurring in the disease process.[39,40] The substantia propria in AKC has an increased number of mast cells compared to normal tissue as well as increased fibroblasts and collagen.[39] In vivo confocal microscope evaluation of the conjunctiva demonstrated an inverse relationship of the number of inflammatory cells to both cornea sensitivity and tear stability.[41]

Etiology

Known environmental risk factors are reported as exposure to animals and winter months as exacerbating factors. The genetic risk factors are those of allergy in general with multiple loci suggested as important.

Pathophysiology

Giemsa stain of scrapings from the upper tarsal conjunctiva will reveal eosinophils. Eosinophils (which are never found in normal tissue) as well as a large number of mononuclear cells are present in the substantia propria in AKC. These eosinophils are found to have increased numbers of activation markers on their surface.[42] Fibroblast number is increased and there is an increased amount of collagen compared to normal tissue. This finding is likely critical to the sight-threatening nature of the disease. The substantia propria also demonstrates an increased ratio of CD4+ to CD8+ T cells, B cells, human leukocyte antigen (HLA)-DR staining, and Langerhans cells.[39] The T-cell receptor on lymphocytes in the substantia propria is predominantly of the α or β subtype.[39] The T-cell population of the substantia propria includes CD4+ memory cells.[43] Th2 cytokines predominate in allergic disease yet lymphocytes with Th1 cytokines have been found in the substantia propria of AKC patients.[44]

Laboratory manifestations in AKC are shown in Table 13.2. The tears of patients with AKC contain increased amounts of IgE antibody, ECP, T cells, activated B cells, eotaxin, eosinophil-derived neurotoxin (EDN), soluble IL-2 receptor, IL-4, IL-5, osteopontin, macrophage inhibitory factor (MIF), and decreased Schirmer's values (56% less than 5 mm).[44–47] A dysfunctional systemic cellular immune response is demonstrated by reduction or abrogation of the cell-mediated response to *Candida*, and an inability of some patients to become sensitized to dinitrochlorobenzene.[48] Additionally, aberrations of the innate immune response are suggested by increased incidence of colonization with *Staphylococcus aureus*. Isolation of *S. aureus* from the eyes (conjunctiva, cilia, lid margin) of 80% of AKC patients (but not from control patients) has been reported.[49] While it is not known to what extent this contributes to the ocular surface inflammation, specific IgE antibodies to *S. aureus* enterotoxins have been detected in tears from AKC patients.[50] Furthermore, the potential of *S. aureus* cell wall products to activate the conjunctival epithelium has been suggested in vitro in studies reporting expression and activation of the innate immune receptor, Toll-like receptor-2 via an extract from *S. aureus* cell wall.[51] Immunostaining demonstrated that conjunctival epithelial cells from AKC patients expressed significantly more Toll-like receptor-2 than nonallergic patients. Despite these in vivo findings, AKC patients who improve with treatment are not found to have change in the rate of colonization with *S. aureus* bacteria.[52] Serum of AKC patients has been found to contain increased levels of IgE,[29] IgE to staphylococcal B toxin,[52] ECP,[53] EDN,[54] and IL-2 receptor.[55]

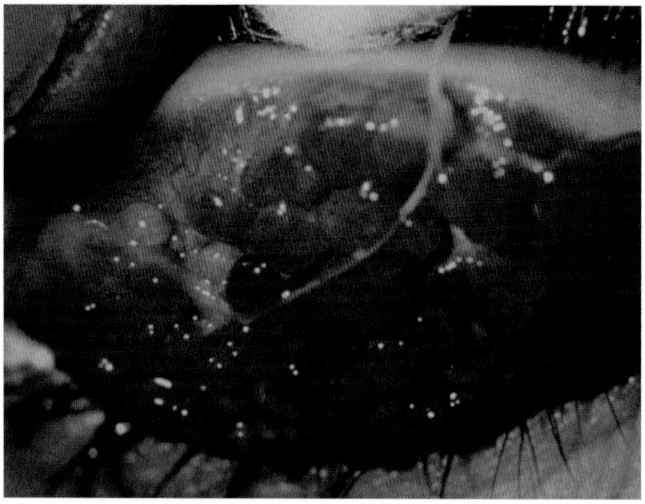

Vernal keratoconjuctivitis (Box 13.2)

Clinical background

VKC is a sight-threatening, bilateral, chronic conjunctival inflammatory process found in individuals predisposed due to their atopic background. An excellent review of the history and description of this disease was published by Buckley[56] in 1988. Beigelman's 1950 monograph *Vernal Conjunctivitis* continues to be the most exhaustive compilation of this disease and is unmatched in current times.[57]

Clinical background

Severe photophobia and ocular itching are the primary symptoms. Table 13.1 lists other symptoms, signs, and differential diagnosis. Foreign-body sensation, ptosis, and blepharospasm are also common. Signs of this inflammatory process are mostly confined to the conjunctiva and cornea. The skin of the eyelids and eyelid margin is relatively uninvolved compared to AKC. Characteristic of this ocular disease is the development of a papillary response. This papillary response is principally found in the tarsal conjunctiva and limbus (Figure 13.2).

The corneal findings may be sight-threatening. Buckley describes in detail the sequence of occurrence of corneal findings.[56,58] Mediators from the inflamed tarsal conjunctiva cause a punctate epithelial keratitis. Coalescence of these areas leads to frank epithelial erosion, leaving Bowman's membrane intact. If, at this point, inadequate or no treatment is rendered, a plaque containing fibrin and mucus deposits may develop over the epithelial defect.[59] Epithelial healing is then impaired, and new vessel growth is encouraged. This so-called shield ulcer usually has its lower border in the upper half of the visual axis. With resolution, the ulcerated area leaves a subepithelial ringlike scar. The peripheral cornea may show a waxing and waning, superficial stromal, gray-white deposition termed pseudogerontoxon. Iritis is not reported to occur in VKC. Treatment generally requires the use of topical steroids to control the allergic inflammation. Many strategies, both medical and surgical, have been used to reduce or rid patients of the severe papillary reaction under the upper lid. Numerous other classes of medication have been used in an effort to spare the amount of steroid used. The complications of the disease are cornea

Figure 13.2 Large, flat-topped papillae with stringy mucus of the underside of the upper lid.

scar and lid malposition and cataract and glaucoma from steroid use.

Pathology

VKC is chronic and sight-threatening, but the exact mechanism leading to this outcome is not completely understood. Evidence for the pathophysiological process in VKC comes from immunohistochemistry studies of the conjunctiva and cornea, and the cellular and mediator content of tear fluid. These are summarized in Table 13.2. A unique profile of lymphocytes is found in VKC tissue. CD4+ T-cell clones can be isolated from VKC biopsy specimens of tarsal conjunctiva and have been shown to have helper function for IgE synthesis in vitro and produce IL-4.[60] Calder et al,[61] in a separate work, found IL-5 expressed in T-cell lines from VKC biopsy specimens. These data support the concept of local production of IgE antibody in this tissue. The substantia propria also has an increased amount of collagen. Fibroblasts isolated from the tarsal conjunctiva of patients with VKC can be induced to proliferate by histamine[62] and tryptase.[63] This finding is likely critical to the sight-threatening nature of this ocular disease. Toll-like receptors were detected immunohistochemically in the epithelial cells, CD4+ T cells, mast cells, and eosinophils.[64] These findings may implicate the commensal flora in the pathophysiology.

Etiology

The disease is likely caused by environmental influences on the predisposed genetic background. Although a hygiene hypothesis regarding the development of allergy in general proposes less allergic disease in those with more siblings and less sterile environment, a recent paper suggests increased VKC in patients with intestinal worm infestations.[65]

Pathophysiology

The corneal epithelium of patients with VKC has been shown to express ICAM-1.[66] Eosinophil peroxidase, in contact with human corneal epithelial cells, causes disruption of cell adhesion.[67] major basic protein (MBP) and ECP are proinflammatory and MBP has been shown to damage monolayers of corneal epithelium but not stratified epithelial cells in culture.[68]

Analysis of tear film collected from VKC patients demonstrated elevated levels of histamine[69] and tryptase,[70] as well as allergen-specific IgE and IgG antibodies.[71,72] Tears from VKC patients contained up to four times the levels of eotaxin, IL-11, monocyte chemoattractant protein (MCP)-1 and macrophage colony-stimulating factor (M-CSF) and up to eight times the levels of eotaxin-2, IL-4, IL-6, IL-6-soluble receptor (IL-6sR), IL-7, macrophage inflammatory protein (MIP)-1delta, and tissue inhibitor of metalloproteinases (TIMP)-2, compared to tears from control patients.[50] In another study, Leonardi et al[73] examined a panel of cytokines and chemokines found in tears of patients with SAC, VKC, and AKC. While tears from allergic patients, in general, showed increased concentrations of cytokines and chemokines compared to nonallergic controls, only tears from VKC patients showed significantly increased concentrations of eotaxin and TNF-α. Additionally, tears from VKC patients had greater concentrations of IL-5, RANTES, and eotaxin, when compared with tears from SAC patients. They further found increased tear levels of urokinase plasminogen activator, and tissue plasminogen activator (tPA) in the tears of VKC patients.[74] Proteomic evaluation of tears from VKC patients reveals the presence of increased eotaxin and IL-6sR.[50] The serum of VKC patients contains decreased levels of histaminase[71] and increased levels of nerve growth factor. VKC is reported to occur in patients with the hyper-IgE syndrome.[75]

Giant papillary conjunctivitis

Diagnosis

GPC is a chronic inflammatory process leading to the production of giant papillae on the tarsal conjunctiva lining of the upper eyelids (Figure 13.2). The findings are most often associated with soft contact lens wear (Table 13.1).[76]

Clinical background

Symptoms of GPC include ocular itching after lens removal, redness, burning, increased mucus discharge in the morning, photophobia, and decreased contact lens tolerance. Blurred vision can result from deposits on the contact lens, or from displacement of the contact lens secondary to the superior eyelid papillary hypertrophy. Initial presentation may occur months or even years after the patient has begun wearing contact lenses. GPC has been reported in patients wearing soft, hard, and rigid gas-permeable contact lenses, as well as in patients with ocular prostheses and exposed sutures in contact with the conjunctiva. GPC may affect as many as 20% of soft contact lens wearers.[77] Patients wearing regular (as opposed to disposable) soft contact lenses are at least 10 times more susceptible to GPC than rigid (gas-permeable) contact lens wearers. Those patients wearing daily-wear disposable contact lenses and those wearing rigid contact lenses are about equally affected. Patients who wear disposable contact lenses during sleep are probably three times more likely to have GPC symptoms than if the lenses are removed daily. Patients with asthma, hayfever, or animal allergies may be at greater risk for GPC. Examination of the underside of the upper eyelid, in severe cases, will reveal large papillae with red, inflamed tissue. In milder cases of GPC, smaller papillae may occur. These papillae are thought to be caused by the contact lens riding high on the surface of the eye with each blink. In very mild cases, this tendency of the contact lens to ride up on the eye may contribute to the diagnosis in the absence of visible papillae. In cases of chronic GPC, tear deficiency may be a contributing factor. Redness of the upper eyelid on ocular examination is one of the earliest signs of GPC and this observation can facilitate early diagnosis. Abnormal thickening of the conjunctiva may progress to opacification as inflammatory cells enter the tissue. The diagnosis is made through a careful history and significant findings under the lid. Treatment consists of temporary cessation of lens wear and topical application of either anti-inflammatory or antiallergy drops. Lens wear may be resumed after 1 month. If symptoms recur, the lens style or type may need to be changed.

Etiology/pathology/pathophysiology

The onset of GPC may be the result of mechanical trauma secondary to contact lens fit or a lens edge causing chronic irritation of the upper eyelid with each blink. It is more likely, however, that a build-up of "protein" on the surface of the contact lens causes an allergic reaction in the eyelid tissue.[78,79] Tear clearance from the ocular surface of GPC patients is decreased compared to normal patients and this may allow the protein in the tear film longer contact time with the contact lens.[80] As with AKC and VKC, tissue biopsies are the primary source of data on the pathophysiology of this GPC, which is summarized in Table 13.2. Many of the published studies concerning mast cell involvement in GPC contrast the disease with VKC. Like VKC, conjunctival biopsies in GPC are found to have mast cells of the MC_T type in the conjunctival epithelium. However, there is no significant increase in mast cells in the substantia propria, and thus no overall increases in number of mast cells present in the conjunctival tissue.[2] Interestingly, while increased histamine is measured in tears in patients with VKC, patients with GPC have normal tear histamine levels.[7,77] This can be partially explained from electron microscopy data on biopsies from patients with GPC which have revealed less mast cell degranulation (30%) than is observed in patients with VKC (80%).[81] Tryptase has also been found in the tears from patients with GPC. This is not surprising considering the fact that rubbing, alone, can result in significant increases of tryptase in tears.[9] Eotaxin is not elevated in the tears of GPC patients.[82] As in SAC and PAC, release of mediators from mast cells results in increased capillary permeability and inflammatory cell infiltration of eyelid tissue. Cytologic scrapings from the conjunctiva of patients with GPC exhibit an infiltrate containing lymphocytes, plasma cells, mast cells, eosinophils, and basophils. All of these factors contribute to discomfort and formation of the papillae. The differentiating pathophysiologic characteristics between GPC and VKC are important because they could be considered as possible clues to the differences in pathogenesis between these two ocular diseases.

Ocular allergy encompasses a spectrum of disease from the self-limiting to the vision-threatening. A common pathologic finding is activation of mast cells of the conjunctiva. The sustained immunopathologic reaction with lymphocytes is most likely responsible for the risk of ocular surface sight-threatening changes.

Key references

A complete list of chapter references is available online at www.expertconsult.com. See inside cover for registration details.

1. Bielory L. Allergic and immunologic disorders of the eye. Part II: ocular allergy. J Allergy Clin Immunol 2000;106:1019–1032.

7. Abelson MB, Baird RS, Allansmith MR. Tear histamine levels in vernal conjunctivitis and other ocular inflammations. Ophthalmology 1980;87: 812–814.

16. Nakamura Y, Sotozona C, Kinoshita S. Inflammatory cytokines in normal human tears. Curr Eye Res 1998;17:673–676.

18. Cook EB, Stahl JL, Lowe L, et al. Simultaneous measurement of six cytokines in a single sample of human tears using microparticle-based flow cytometry: allergics vs. non-allergics. J Immunol Methods 2001;254:109–118.

19. Cook EB, Stahl JL, Brooks AM, et al. Allergic tears promote upregulation of eosinophil adhesion to conjunctival epithelial cells in an ex vivo model: inhibition with olopatadine treatment. Invest Ophthalmol Vis Sci 2006;47: 3423–3429.

20. Sharif NA, Xu SX, Magnino PE, et al. Human conjunctival epithelial cells express histamine-1 receptors coupled to phosphoinositide turnover and intracellular calcium mobilization: role in ocular allergic and inflammatory diseases. Exp Eye Res 1996;63:169–178.

43. Metz DP, Bacon AS, Holgate S, et al. Phenotypic characterization of T cells infiltrating the conjunctiva in chronic allergic eye disease. J Allergy Clin Immunol 1996;98:686–696.

44. Metz DP, Hingorani M, Calder VL, et al. T-cell cytokines in chronic allergic eye disease. J Allergy Clin Immunol 1997;100:817–824.

51. Cook EB, Stahl JL, Esnault S, et al. Toll-like receptor 2 expression on human conjunctival epithelial cells: a pathway for Staphylococcus aureus involvement in chronic ocular proinflammatory responses. Ann Allergy Asthma Immunol 2005;94:486-497.

73. Leonardi A, Curnow SJ, Zhan H, et al. Multiple cytokines in human tear specimens in seasonal and chronic allergic eye disease and in conjunctival fibroblast cultures. Clin Exp Allergy 2006;36:777–784.

79. Tan ME, Demirci G, Pearce D, et al. Contact lens-induced papillary conjunctivitis is associated with increased albumin deposits on extended wear hydrogel lenses. Adv Exp Med Biol 2002;506:951–955.

The lacrimal gland and dry-eye disease

Darlene A Dartt

Overview

A consensus from the recent International Dry Eye Workshop revised the definition of dry-eye disease to: "Dry eye is a multifactorial disease of the tears and ocular surface that results in symptoms of discomfort, visual disturbance, and tear film instability with potential damage to the ocular surface. It is accompanied by increased osmolarity of the tear film and inflammation of the ocular surface."[1] The tear film, which is altered in dry-eye disease, is produced by multiple types of ocular surface epithelia and the ocular adnexa (Figure 14.1). The meibomian glands that line the eyelid secrete the outer lipid layer of the tear film. The lacrimal gland, accessory lacrimal glands, conjunctival epithelium, and corneal epithelium secrete the aqueous component. The conjunctival goblet cells and stratified squamous cells of the conjunctiva and cornea secrete the mucous component. The lacrimal glands, lids, ocular surface (including the meibomian glands, corneal epithelium, and conjunctival epithelium), and the nerves that innervate these tissues function together to produce and maintain the tear film. These structures have been termed the lacrimal gland functional unit[1,2] or ocular surface system[3,4] and together represent the targets of dry-eye disease. The present chapter, however, will focus on the lacrimal gland and its role in dry-eye disease with the following caveats: (1) the lacrimal gland is part of a functional unit and is rarely the only target of dysfunction in dry-eye disease and (2) alteration in lacrimal gland secretion can alter the homeostasis of the ocular surface, causing secondary disease in this tissue that in turn can affect neural stimulation of lacrimal gland secretion.

Clinical background

Overview

Dry-eye disease can be divided into two major groups: aqueous-deficient and evaporative (Figure 14.2).[1] The lacrimal gland is the target of aqueous-deficient disease, which is usually classified into Sjögren syndrome dry eye (autoimmune) or non-Sjögren dry eye. The present chapter will focus predominantly on non-Sjögren dry eye, as Sjögren syndrome dry eye will be discussed in Chapter 15.

Key symptoms and signs

Dry eye can be graded according to severity using the symptoms and signs listed in Table 14.1. Symptoms are those derived from activation of the sensory nerves in the cornea and conjunctiva and result in feelings of ocular surface discomfort, including irritation, dryness, grittiness, burning, itching, and photophobia.[5-8] Validated questionnaires that can be used to evaluate the symptoms of dry-eye disease can be found in Smith et al.[9] The signs of dry eye include: visual symptoms; conjunctival injection; conjunctival staining with lissamine green or rose Bengal; corneal staining with fluorescein; evaluation of the cornea and tears for debris, mucus, or keratitis; evaluation of the lids and meibomian glands (evaporative dry eye), tear film break-up time (usually indicates evaporative dry eye); and Schirmer score.[1] These tests are described in detail in Bron et al.[10] Detailed descriptions of a standardized method for using these tests is provided in the index to the article by Bron et al.[10] New tests are being developed; potentially the most influential one that could become the gold standard is the measurement of tear film osmolarity. In the absence of osmolarity measurements, better performance of the tests for dry eye can be achieved by using selected tests in series or in parallel.[10,11]

Epidemiology

There have been eight large, population-based epidemiologic studies of dry eye in the USA, Australia, and Asia.[9] In these studies the prevalence of dry eye varied from 5% to 35% including all age categories. The two largest studies estimated that in the USA about 3.32 million women and 1.68 million men 50 years old and over have severe dry eye.[12] Many more individuals have less severe dry eye, i.e., occurring in adverse environments or during contact lens wear. The risk for dry eye is greater in women and with increasing age.[12] There are limited data indicating that the prevalence of severe dry eye may be greater in Hispanic and Asian compared to Caucasian women.[9]

Based on data repositories and a variety of databases, the incidence of dry eye cases per 100 fee-for-service beneficiaries increased from 1.22 in 1991 to 1.92 in 1998.[9,13] An excellent summary of the epidemiology of dry-eye disease can be found in Smith et al.[9]

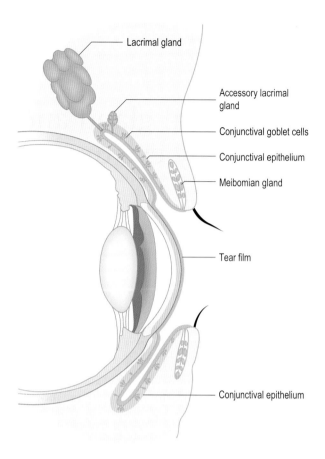

Figure 14.1 Schematic of glands and epithelia that secrete the tear film. Epithelia are shown in beige and tear film in green.

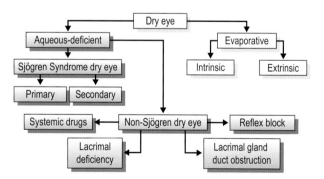

Figure 14.2 Etiology of dry eye. Dry eye can be divided into two major classifications: aqueous-deficient and evaporative. Aqueous deficiency can be further divided into Sjögren syndrome dry eye and non-Sjögren syndrome dry eye. The focus of the current chapter is non-Sjögren aqueous-deficient dry eye. Evaporative dry eye can be divided into additional classifications not shown here. (Modified from: The definition and classification of dry eye disease: report of the Definition and Classification Subcommittee of the International Dry Eye WorkShop (2007). Ocul Surf 2007;5:75–92.)

Diagnostic workup

The Dry Eye Workshop recommends the following diagnostic tests for dry eye[1] which do not depend on tests only available in specialty clinics or tests subject to bias:

1. Use of a validated dry-eye questionnaire. Seven are available and one can be chosen and used routinely. They can be found in Smith et al.[9]
2. Diagnosis of Sjögren syndrome dry eye. The international criteria that require one ocular symptom and one ocular sign be satisfied can be used. These are described in Vitali et al[14] or in Bron et al.[10]
3. Evaluation of tears. Measurement of noninvasive tear film breakup time following the template in Bron et al[10] and the use of the tear function index (TFI) should be used. The TFI is the quotient of the Schirmer value and the tear clearance rate. Methodology for both tests is described in Bron et al.[10] An alternative evaluation is the workup described in Table 14.1 that can also be used to evaluate the severity of dry-eye disease.
4. Better performance can be achieved when tests are used in parallel or in series, as described in Bron et al.[10]

Differential diagnosis

Dry-eye disease is symptom-based, varying in severity from mild (nuisance) to severely disabling. Tests described in Table 14.1 are necessary to distinguish its severity and type to allow directed treatment. It is also important to distinguish between other symptomatic ocular surface diseases such as meibomian gland disease, allergic eye disease, chronic conjunctivitis, and keratoconjunctivitis. More detailed information can be found in Gulati et al[8] and Bron et al.[10]

Treatment

In the past several years, treatment has shifted from lubricating and hydrating the ocular surface providing symptomatic relief to developing compounds that stimulate the natural production of tears.[15] The few current treatments that target the lacrimal gland include the following systemically administered drugs: anti-inflammatory agents (omega-3 fatty acids), secretagogues (muscarinic acetylcholine receptor 3 agonists), immunosuppressive drugs (ciclosporin), and sex hormones (androgens, estrogens, and combinations).

Treatments of aqueous deficiency that directly target lacrimal gland disease have been difficult to develop because of drug delivery problems. Topical treatments rarely penetrate to the lacrimal gland unless they are lipid-soluble, whereas systemic treatments have substantial side-effects in other tissues that possess the same receptors as the lacrimal gland. The lacrimal gland has not yet been shown to have any unique receptors or signaling pathways that would allow systemic use of drugs at effective levels that do not affect other tissues. A treatment that potentially could be successful is systemic omega-3 fatty acids that are currently marketed as dietary supplements. An epidemiologic study suggests that women with high intake of omega-3 fatty acids have a decreased incidence of dry-eye syndrome.[16] Experimentally, lacrimal gland secretion from aging mice appears to be susceptible to oxidative damage. Finally evidence in abstract form (Sicard P et al IOVS 2007;e-abstract 1906) suggested that the lacrimal gland can take up 100-fold more omega-3 fatty acids than the retina. A large clinical trial would be necessary to determine the effectiveness of omega-3 fatty acids.

Table 14.1 Dry-eye severity grading scheme

Symptom	Dry-eye severity level			
	1	2	3	4*
Discomfort, severity and frequency	Mild and/or episodic; occurs under environmental stress	Moderate, episodic or chronic, stress or no stress	Severe, frequent or constant without stress	Severe and/or disabling, constant
Visual symptoms	None or episodic mild fatigue	Annoying and/or activity-limiting episodic	Annoying, chronic and/or constant, limiting activity	Constant and/or possibly disabling
Conjunctival injection	None to mild	None to mild	+/−	+/++
Conjunctival staining	None to mild	Variable	Moderate to marked	Marked
Corneal staining (severity/location)	None to mild	Variable	Marked central	Severe punctate erosions
Corneal/tear signs	None to mild	Mild debris, ↓ meniscus	Filamentary keratitis, mucus clumping, ↑ tear debris	Filamentary keratitis, mucus clumping, ↑ tear debris, ulceration
Lid/meibomian glands	MGD variably present	MGD variably present	Frequent	Trichiasis, keratinization, symblepharon
TFBUT (seconds)	Variable	≤ 10	≤ 5	Immediate
Schirmer score (mm/5 minutes)	Variable	≤ 10	≤ 5	≤ 2

*Must have signs and symptoms.
(Reproduced with permission from: The definition and classification of dry eye disease: report of the Definition and Classification Subcommittee of the International Dry Eye WorkShop (2007). Ocul Surf 2007;5:75–92.)

Prognosis and complications

Complications from the decrease in lacrimal gland secretion in aqueous-deficient dry eye are infections, blepharitis, and conjunctivitis.[8] Dry-eye patients who wear contact lens are particularly susceptible to these complications.[17] Keratinization is a second complication that comes from a loss of conjunctival goblet cells that produce the gel-forming mucins in the mucous layer of the tear film. Other complications that can be the result of severe aqueous deficiency such as occurs in Sjögren syndrome dry eye are band keratopathy, limbal stem cell deficiency, sterile stromal ulcers and corneal perforation, and keratoconus-like changes.[8] Lacrimal gland deficiency is not the only contributor to these complications. Finally chronic aqueous tear-deficient dry eye, especially Sjögren syndrome, can have debilitating psychological effects, because of the lack of definitive treatments and cures, and can have substantial implications for quality of life.[8]

Pathology

The difficulty in removing biopsy samples from the human lacrimal gland makes pathological studies of the lacrimal gland difficult, although postmortem samples can be obtained. Available evidence indicates that there is an age-dependent lymphocytic infiltration of the lacrimal gland in dry eye similar to that which occurs in Sjögren syndrome.[18–20] The indirect effects of aqueous deficiency on the conjunctiva can be measured by impression cytology and conjunctival biopsy and include loss of goblet cells, squamous cell metaplasia, increased desquamation, and eventually keratinization.

Etiology

The etiology of aqueous deficiency dry eye can be divided into Sjögren and non-Sjögren dry eye (Figure 14.2). Non-Sjögren dry eye can result from a variety of causes that include alteration of tear secretion, destruction of the lacrimal gland, or closure of the lacrimal gland secretory ducts (Figure 14.3).[8] Obstruction of the tear drainage system or an alteration in its drainage properties can also affect the amount of tears in the tear film.[21] Two important mechanisms for the alteration or loss of lacrimal gland secretion are changes in the sensory nerves in the cornea that drive lacrimal gland secretion and systemic medications. Laser in situ keratomileusis (LASIK) surgery and contact lens wear cause dry eye from the alteration in corneal activity. For a complete listing of etiology of aqueous-deficiency dry eye, see Gulati and Dana.[8]

Pathophysiology

Mechanisms of aqueous-deficiency dry eye

As proposed by the 2007 International Dry Eye Workshop[10] and the Cullen Symposium,[22] the core mechanisms of dry eye can be divided into tear hyperosmolarity and tear film

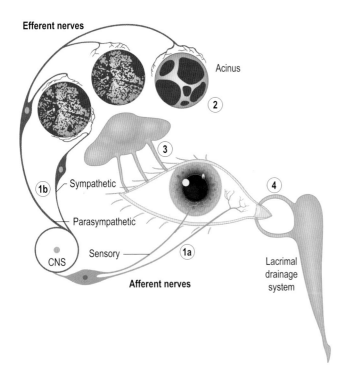

Efferent nerves

Acinus

②

①b — Sympathetic

Parasympathetic

③

④

CNS · Sensory — ①a

Afferent nerves

Lacrimal drainage system

Figure 14.3 Schematic of the neural regulation of lacrimal gland electrolyte, water, and protein secretion illustrating the components that can be affected causing aqueous-deficient dry-eye disease. A decrease in lacrimal gland secretion (lacrimal gland deficiency) contributes to tear hyperosmolarity and dry eye by four major mechanisms: (1) interruption in the activation of (a) sensory nerves in the cornea or conjunctiva and (b) efferent parasympathetic and sympathetic nerves that innervate the lacrimal gland; (2) destruction of the lacrimal gland by apoptosis; (3) mechanical damage to the lacrimal gland excretory ducts; and (4) alteration in the lacrimal drainage system. CNS, central nervous system.

Box 14.1 Multiple signaling pathways control lacrimal gland secretion

Neuronal

- Cholinergic agonists stimulate secretion using the phospholipase C/Ca^{2+}/protein kinase C pathways, but attenuate secretion using phospholipase D and p44/p42 mitogen-activated protein kinase (MAPK) pathways
- α_{1D}-Adrenergic agonists stimulate secretion using the nitric oxide/cyclic guanosine monophosphate and Ca^{2+}/protein kinase C pathways, but attenuate secretion using the endothelial growth factor (EGF)/EGF receptor/ p44/p42 MAPK pathway
- Vasoactive intestinal peptide stimulates secretion using the cyclic adenosine monophosphate and Ca^{2+} pathways

Hormonal

- Androgens regulate secretory immunoglobulin A production
- Prolactins regulate cellular trafficking of secretory proteins

---

Box 14.2 Mechanisms responsible for aqueous-deficiency dry eye

Alterations in stimulation of lacrimal gland secretion

- Blockage of afferent sensory nerves from the ocular surface
- Blockage of efferent parasympathetic and sympathetic nerves in the lacrimal gland
- Inhibition of lacrimal gland cellular signaling pathways

Destruction of the lacrimal gland

- Congenital absence or functional alteration
- Injured by trauma
- Injured by disease

Occlusion of lacrimal gland secretory ducts by disease

---

instability. Lacrimal gland deficiency primarily contributes to tear hyperosmolarity resulting from a decrease in fluid secretion. The causes of lacrimal gland deficiency can be divided into three categories: (1) alteration in stimulation of secretion; (2) destruction of the lacrimal gland; and (3) occlusion of lacrimal secretory ducts (Figure 14.3 and Box 14.1).[8]

Alteration in stimulation of secretion

Lacrimal gland secretion is predominantly under neural control. Stimuli from the external environment activate sensory nerves in the cornea and conjunctiva. By a neural reflex these nerves activate the parasympathetic and sympathetic nerves that surround the lacrimal gland secretory cells, the acinar and ductal cells (Figure 14.3 and Box 14.2). In humans it is well known that lacrimal gland secretion of both protein and electrolytes/water is stimulated by acetylcholine released from the parasympathetic nerves interacting with M_3 cholinergic receptors (M_3AChR) on the secretory cells (Figure 14.4).[23] The signaling pathways activated by these receptors have been investigated in the rat lacrimal gland and include activation of phospholipase C (PLC) to produce 1,3,4-inositol trisphosphate. This compound releases Ca^{2+} from intracellular stores to increase the intracellular [Ca^{2+}] and causes an increase in Ca^{2+} influx to maintain

elevated Ca^{2+} levels. An increase in PLC activity also produces diacylglycerol that activates protein kinase C isoforms. Both an increase in intracellular Ca^{2+} and activation of protein kinase C stimulate lacrimal gland secretion. Parasympathetic nerves also release the neuropeptide vasoactive intestinal peptide (VIP) that stimulates secretion of both protein and electrolytes/water (Figure 14.5).[23] That this is an important mechanism in humans was demonstrated in a patient with a VIP-secreting tumor in whom the tear volume was increased and the osmolarity decreased compared to normal age- and sex-matched controls.[24] In the rat and rabbit lacrimal gland VIP stimulates protein and fluid secretion by binding to its receptors (VPAC and II) that activate adenylyl cyclase to produce cyclic adenosine monophosphate (cAMP). Increased cellular levels of cAMP activate protein kinase A (PKA) to induce secretion. β-Adrenergic agonists released from sympathetic nerves are minor stimuli of the cAMP-dependent pathway (Figure 14.5). The third signaling pathway that, in the rat, has been shown to activate protein secretion, is an α_{1D}-adrenergic pathway activated by release of norepinephrine from the sympathetic nerves

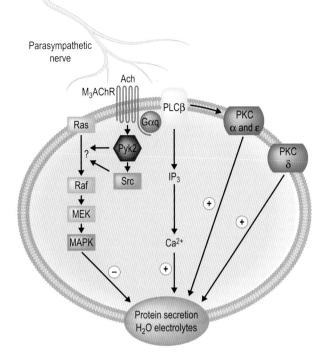

Figure 14.4 Schematic of the parasympathetic, cholinergic signaling pathway used to stimulate lacrimal gland protein, electrolyte, and water secretion. Stimulation of parasympathetic nerves releases their neurotransmitter acetylcholine (ACh) that binds to and activates muscarinic type 3 ACh receptors (M₃AChR) in the cell membrane. This interaction induces a stimulatory pathway involving phospholipase Cβ (PLCβ), Ca²⁺, and the protein kinase C (PKC) isoforms α, δ, and ε. ACh also induces an inhibitory pathway through the nonreceptor tyrosine kinases Pyk2 and Src that activate the p44/p42 mitogen-activated protein kinasae (MAPK) cascade (Ras, Raf, and MEK). Activation of the inhibitory pathway attenuates stimulated secretion. Gαq, a stimulatory subtype of guanine nucleotide-binding protein; IP₃, 1,4,5-inositol trisphosphate. (Reproduced with permission from Dartt DA. Exp Eye Res 2001;73:741–752.)

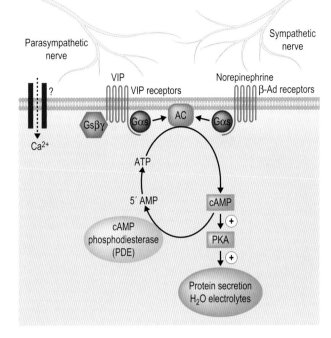

Figure 14.5 Schematic of cyclic adenosine monophosphate (cAMP)-dependent signaling pathways leading to production of lacrimal gland proteins, electrolytes, and water. Stimulation of the parasympathetic and sympathetic nerves releases their neurotransmitters vasoactive intestinal peptide (VIP) and norepinephrine, respectively. Both neurotransmitters bind to their receptors, VIP receptors I and II for VIP and β-adrenegic receptors for norepinephrine and increase the cellular levels of cAMP. cAMP is synthesized from adenosine triphosphate (ATP) by activating the guanine-binding proteins Gas to stimulate adenylyl cyclase (AC). The cAMP produced activates protein kinase A (PKA). cAMP is broken down by cAMP phosphodiesterases (PDE) to produce 5'adenosine monophosphate (AMP). VIP also increases intracellular Ca²⁺. (Modified with permission from Dartt DA. Regulation of lacrimal gland secretion by neurotransmitters and the EGF family of growth factors. Exp Eye Res 2001;73:741–752.)

(Figure 14.6). Activation of α₁D-adrenergic receptors stimulates protein secretion by inducing endothelial nitric oxide synthase to produce nitric oxide. Nitric oxide activates guanylyl cyclase to produce cGMP that in turn activates protein kinase G to stimulate protein secretion.[25] Electrophysiology experiments in rats and mice suggest that this pathway could also cause electrolyte and water secretion.

Surprisingly, in rat lacrimal gland, cholinergic and α₁D-adrenergic agonists also activate inhibitory pathways that can attenuate stimulated secretion. Cholinergic agonists activate the nonreceptor tyrosine kinases Pyk2 and Src to stimulate p44/p42 mitogen-activated protein kinase (MAPK) or ERK1/2 that decreases secretion (Figure 14.4).[26] α₁D-Adrenergic agonists activate the matrix metalloproteinase ADAM 17 that releases the active site of membrane-spanning epidermal growth factor (EGF). The active site interacts with the EGF receptor, causing it to be phosphorylated (Figure 14.6).[27] The phosphorylated receptor attracts adapter proteins that stimulate a cascade of kinases to activate MAPK that decreases secretion.

Neurotransmitters released from activated nerves stimulate acinar and duct cells to secrete proteins. A list of pro-

teins secreted by the lacrimal gland has been compiled.[23,28] Multiple secretory proteins are antibacterial as the tears function in the innate defense system. Other proteins are growth factors that sustain and maintain the health of the ocular surface. At least three different secretory processes are used for protein secretion, exocytosis, ectodomain shedding, and transcytotic secretion (secretory IgA). Additionally, electrolytes and water are secreted transcellularly and paracellularly. All these secretory processes are under neural control, with additional hormonal control of secretory IgA production.

Fluid (electrolytes and water) secretion occurs by activation of ion channels, Na/K-ATPase, and other ion transport mechanisms described in detail elsewhere.[23] The net result is the secretion of a plasma-like primary fluid containing Na⁺, K⁺, and Cl⁻ into the lumen. The primary fluid is modified by secretion of proteins, electrolytes, and water by the duct cells. In particular the duct cells secrete K⁺ so that the final lacrimal gland fluid is higher in potassium than plasma. The mechanism of ductal electrolyte secretion is described by Ubels et al.[29] With low flow rates lacrimal gland fluid is hypertonic, but with stimulation causing higher flow rates, lacrimal gland fluid is isotonic.[30]

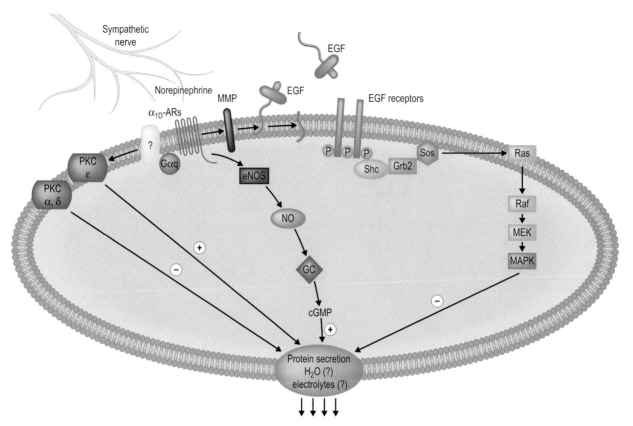

Figure 14.6 Schematic of the sympathetic, α_{1D}-adrenergic signaling pathway used to stimulate lacrimal gland protein and perhaps electrolyte and water secretion. Stimulation of sympathetic nerves releases their neurotransmitter norepinephrine that binds to and activates α_{1D}-adrenergic receptors (α_{1D}-AR) in the cell membrane. This interaction induces two stimulatory pathways. One pathway involves the activation of endothelial nitric oxide synthase (eNOS) to release nitric oxide (NO) activating guanylyl cyclase (GC) and increasing cyclic GMP (cGMP). The other pathway causes the activation of protein kinase C (PKC)ε by an as yet unidentified effector. Activation of the α_{1D}-AR also induces two inhibitory pathways that attenuate stimulated secretion. One pathway is activation of the PKC isoforms α and δ by an unknown effector. The second pathway is activation of a matrix metalloproteinase (MMP) that cleaves the precursor form of epidermal growth factor (EGF) located in the cell membrane. This releases the active EGF-like domain that interacts with EGF receptors causing them to be activated by autophosphorylation (P) that attracts the adaptor proteins Shc and Grb2. The adapter proteins activate SOS, Ras, Raf, Mek and p44/p42 mitogen-activated protein kinasae (MAPK). Gαq, a stimulatory subtype of guanine nucleotide-binding protein. (Modified with permission from Dartt DA. Regulation of lacrimal gland secretion by neurotransmitters and the EGF family of growth factors. Exp Eye Res 2001;73:741–752.)

While nerves acutely stimulate protein and fluid secretion, systemic hormones can regulate expression of key components of these processes. Androgens stimulate the synthesis of secretory component and hence the production of secretory IgA, a slower process than mediated by nerves. In addition androgens can influence the synthesis of Na/K-ATPase, the driving force for neurally mediated fluid secretion.[31] The peptide hormone prolactin can also function as a systemic hormone and a paracrine mediator of secretion by altering the cellular trafficking of the enzymes used in synthesis and storage of secretory proteins.[32,33]

Neural and hormonal stimulation of secretion can be interrupted at several points by different processes (Figure 14.3).

1. Activation of sensory nerves in the cornea and conjunctiva can be blocked. This can be the result of overuse of topical anesthetics, contact lens wear, refractive surgery, infection, neurotrophic keratitis, herpetic keratitis, diabetes mellitus, and aging.[8] If ocular surface sensory nerves are blocked, secretion is either decreased or completely prevented. In either case tear osmolarity increases (becoming hyperosmolar) from decreased lacrimal gland flow rate and the amount of lacrimal gland secretory proteins released by exocytosis is decreased.

2. Activation of efferent nerves to the lacrimal gland can be blocked (Figure 14.3). In familial dysautonomia, there is dysfunction of the sensory nerves of the cornea as well as the sympathetic and parasympathetic nerves to the lacrimal gland.[10] This defect blocks both afferent and efferent innervation to the gland and prevents secretion of protein, electrolytes, and water. Defects in both afferent and efferent nerves can lead to age-dependent lacrimal gland hyposecretion. Finally, dysfunction of the efferent nerves has been suggested to play a role in the pathology of Sjögren syndrome based on an animal model, the MRL/Mp-Fas^{lpr} mouse. In Sjögren syndrome T lymphocytes (CD4$^+$ and smaller amount of CD8$^+$ cells) infiltrate the lacrimal gland, forming foci and producing inflammatory cytokines such as interleukin-1β (IL-1β), interferon-γ (IFN-γ), and tumor necrosis factor-α (TNF-α).[34–37] Androgens play a role here as well, as androgens normally produce

anti-inflammatory cytokines such as transforming growth factor β (TGF-β). In androgen deficiency anti-inflammatory cytokine production is decreased, leading to production of proinflammatory cytokines from lymphocytes.[38] Production of proinflammatory cytokines by the lymphocytes, in a positive-feedforward mechanism, stimulates the lacrimal gland acinar cells to produce these destructive cytokines.[39] IL-1β can prevent release of neurotransmitters from efferent nerve endings, blocking stimulation of lacrimal gland secretion in both Sjögren syndrome and aging.[34,39–41]

3. Alteration in signaling pathways: systemic medications can induce aqueous-deficiency dry eye by altering the signaling pathways that induce lacrimal gland secretion (Figure 14.3). Antimuscarinics block the M_3AChR that is necessary for the stimulation of secretion. Antihistamines, as a side-effect, can also block the M_3AChR.[42] Multiple other systemic medications have antimuscarinic effects that would cause aqueous-deficiency dry eye. Beta-adrenergic blockers can cause vasoconstriction and would decrease lacrimal gland fluid secretion stimulated by parasympathetic nerve release of acetylchline and VIP.[43] Diuretics such as furosemide can decrease lacrimal gland secretion by blocking the ion transport processes that are vital for electrolyte and water secretion.[41] The signaling pathways are also altered in aging when not only does the release of neurotransmitters with age fail to stimulate secretion, the neurotransmitter agonists fail as well.[40]

Destruction of the lacrimal gland

The lacrimal gland can be absent in congenital alacrima, injured by trauma, or injured by disease (Figure 14.3). Diseases that injure the lacrimal gland include aging, graft-versus-host-disease, and Sjögren syndrome. In rat and mouse models of aging there are increased numbers of mast cells and lymphocyte foci along with increased lipofuscin accumulation, fibrosis, and acinar atrophy in the lacrimal gland.[40,44,45] In graft-versus-host disease there is uncontrolled fibrosis and excessive accumulation of extracellular matrix proteins in the lacrimal gland of patients with this disease.[46] Another hypothesis for lacrimal gland deficiency is that acinar cells are lost due to apoptosis. In mouse lacrimal gland injection of IL-1β can induce massive apoptosis that is reversed within days, suggesting that the proinflammatory cytokines can destroy the acinar cells.[47] The evidence that apoptotic cell death leads to lacrimal gland hyposecretion in Sjögren syndrome or other dry-eye diseases has not yet been substantiated.

Occlusion of lacrimal secretory ducts

Lacrimal gland fluid stimulated by nerves is secreted on to the ocular surface through a number of ducts (Figure 14.3). Dry eye occurs when this duct system is blocked by diseases such as trachoma, cicatricial pemphigoid, erythema multiforme, and chemical and thermal burns.[8,10] The dry eye that occurs is a mechanical consequence of secreted lacrimal gland fluid failing to reach the ocular surface.

Suggested mechanism of role of lacrimal gland deficiency in dry-eye disease

The following hypothetical mechanism for the role of the lacrimal gland in dry-eye disease has been suggested.[1,22,48] Under normal conditions, stimuli from the external environment activate sensory nerves in the cornea and conjunctiva that in turn stimulate efferent parasympathetic and sympathetic nerves to cause secretion of proteins, electrolytes, and water from the lacrimal gland on to the ocular surface in an isotonic fluid (Figure 14.3). Lacrimal gland secretions, combined with those of the other glands and epithelia that secrete tears, nourish and maintain a healthy, painfree ocular surface and a transparent cornea. As shown in Figure 14.7, dry eye can be caused by blocking: (1) afferent sensory nerves in the ocular surface by refractive surgery, contact lens wear, neurotrophic keratitis, or topical anesthesia; (2) efferent parasympathetic and sympathetic nerves that innervate the lacrimal gland that occurs in Sjögren syndrome and aging; (3) lacrimal gland cellular signaling pathways by systemic drugs, aging, androgen deficiency, and Sjögren syndrome, some of which produce inflammatory damage to the lacrimal gland; and (4) release of lacrimal gland fluid due to mechanical damage to the ducts occurring in scarring diseases of the ocular surface. The decreased lacrimal gland flow leads to tear hyperosmolarity that induces inflammation in the cornea and conjunctiva. This inflammation is a vicious circle that produces proinflammatory cytokines in the ocular surface epithelial cells. The cytokines can irritate the sensory nerves in the ocular surface and cause: (5) increased reflex drive to the lacrimal gland (not illustrated) or (6) neurogenic inflammation and the release of sensory neurotransmitters from the ocular surface sensory nerves. The released sensory neurotransmitters further exacerbate the disease by affecting the mucins of the goblet cells and stratified squamous cells of the cornea and conjunctiva. The meibomian gland also enters the picture as its dysfunction causes tear instability and increased evaporation, further exacerbating the dry eye. The role of ocular surface inflammation, mucins, and meibomian glands in dry eye will be presented in detail in Chapter 15.

Conclusion

The lacrimal gland is the major producer of the aqueous layer of the tear film and the primary target of aqueous deficiency, in contrast to evaporative, dry-eye disease. Diagnosing aqueous-deficiency dry-eye disease and distinguishing this form from other types of dry-eye disease is problematic because: (1) there is no gold-standard sign or symptom for aqueous-deficiency dry eye; and (2) many individuals have overlapping types of dry-eye disease. These problems lead to inaccuracy in diagnosing the disease, calculating incidence and prevalence, and treating the disease. In spite of this inadequacy, research has elucidated substantial information on the normal regulation and mechanism of lacrimal gland electrolyte, water, and protein secretion. This research can be used to describe the pathophysiology of the lacrimal gland in dry eye, identify potential targets for drug treatments of aqueous-deficiency dry eye, and unravel potential sites of disease vulnerability in the regulation and mechanism of lacrimal gland secretion.

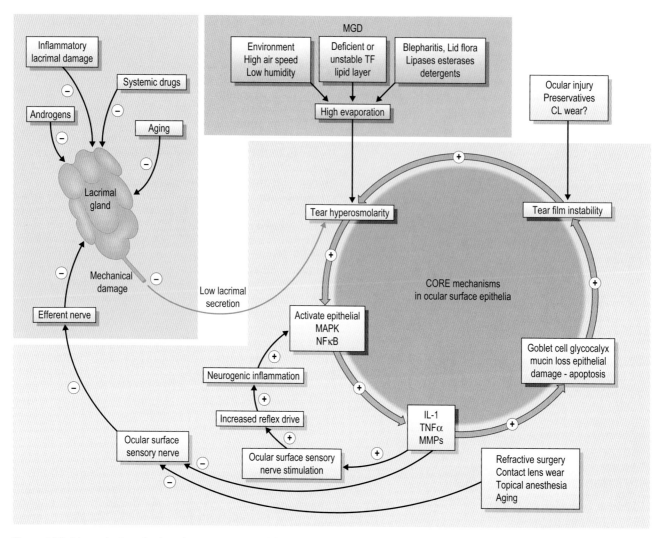

Figure 14.7 Schematic of mechanisms that cause aqueous-deficiency dry eye and damage the ocular surface. Refractive surgery, contact lens wear, topical anesthesia, and aging injure the sensory nerves in the cornea and conjunctiva (ocular surface), blocking their activation. A decrease in sensory nerve activity then fails to activate the efferent nerves that innervate the lacrimal gland, ultimately leading to decreased lacrimal gland secretion of proteins, electrolytes, and water into the tear film. Low androgens, inflammatory lacrimal damage, systemic drugs that inhibit secretion, and aging prevent activation of the stimulatory signaling pathways that increase lacrimal gland secretion, resulting in low lacrimal gland secretion. Mechanical damage to the lacrimal gland excretory ducts also decreases lacrimal gland secretion. Low lacrimal gland secretion causes tear film hyperosmolarity. In addition to lacrimal gland deficiency, meibomian gland disease (MGD), not discussed in the present chapter, leads to high evaporation of the tear film and tear hyperosmolarity. Ocular injury, preservatives, and perhaps contact lens wear cause tear film instability independent of hyperosmolarity. Together tear hyperosmolarity and tear film instability are the core mechanisms that induce ocular surface damage in dry-eye disease. These two factors activate epithelial mitogen-activated protein kinases (MAPK) and NFκB that produce the inflammatory mediators interleukin 1 (IL-1) and tumor necrosis factor-α (TNF-α) and activate matrix metalloproteinases (MMPs). The inflammatory mediators have two major effects: (1) activation of ocular surface sensory nerves causing neurogenic inflammation and antidromic release of sensory neurotransmitters, further amplifying the production of signaling phosphoproteins and inflammatory mediators; and (2) damaging the ocular surface epithelia by inducing loss of goblet cells and glycocalyx mucins from the ocular surface epithelia and epithelial cell apoptosis. (Modified from: The definition and classification of dry eye disease: report of the Definition and Classification Subcommittee of the International Dry Eye WorkShop (2007). Ocul Surf 2007;5:75–92.)

Two important questions about the pathophysiology of the lacrimal gland in dry-eye disease remain unanswered. First, what initiates age-related and non-Sjögren dry eye? Second, which cellular mechanisms are altered in these types of dry eye to cause the decrease in lacrimal gland secretion and damage to the ocular surface?

Acknowledgment

The author thanks Robin Hodges for her contributions to the manuscript and NIH EY06177 for funding.

Key references

A complete list of chapter references is available online at www.expertconsult.com. See inside cover for registration details.

1. The definition and classification of dry eye disease: report of the Definition and Classification Subcommittee of the International Dry Eye WorkShop (2007). Ocul Surf 2007;5:75–92.

3. Mircheff AK, Wang Y, Jean M de S, et al. Mucosal immunity and self-tolerance in the ocular surface system. Ocul Surf 2005;3:182–192.

4. Research in dry eye: report of the Research Subcommittee of the International Dry Eye WorkShop (2007). Ocul Surf 2007;5:179–193.

7. Gulati A, Sullivan R, Buring JE, et al. Validation and repeatability of a short questionnaire for dry eye syndrome. Am J Ophthalmol 2006;142:125–131.

8. Gulati A, Dana M. Keratoconjunctivitis sicca: clinical aspects. In: Foster C, Azar D, Dohlman C (eds) Smolin and Thoft's The Cornea. Philadelphia: Lippincott Williams & Wilkins, 2005:603–627.

12. Schaumberg DA, Sullivan DA, Buring JE, et al. Prevalence of dry eye syndrome among US women. Am J Ophthalmol 2003;136:318–326.

15. Management and therapy of dry eye disease: report of the Management and Therapy Subcommittee of the International Dry Eye WorkShop (2007). Ocul Surf 2007;5:163–178.

21. Paulsen FP, Schaudig U, Thale AB. Drainage of tears: impact on the ocular surface and lacrimal system. Ocul Surf 2003;1:180–191.

22. McDermott AM, Perez V, Huang AJ, et al. Pathways of corneal and ocular surface inflammation: a perspective from the Cullen Symposium. Ocul Surf 2005; 3(Suppl.):S131–S138.

23. Hodges RR, Dartt DA. Regulatory pathways in lacrimal gland epithelium. Int Rev Cytol 2003;231:129–196.

25. Hodges RR, Shatos MA, Tarko RS, et al. Nitric oxide and cGMP mediate alpha1D-adrenergic receptor-stimulated protein secretion and p42/p44 MAPK activation in rat lacrimal gland. Invest Ophthalmol Vis Sci 2005;46:2781–2789.

27. Chen L, Hodges RR, Funaki C, et al. Effects of alpha1D-adrenergic receptors on shedding of biologically active EGF in freshly isolated lacrimal gland epithelial cells. Am J Physiol Cell Physiol 2006; 291:C946–C956.

29. Ubels JL, Hoffman HM, Srikanth S, et al. Gene expression in rat lacrimal gland duct cells collected using laser capture microdissection: evidence for K+ secretion by duct cells. Invest Ophthalmol Vis Sci 2006;47:1876–1885.

38. Sullivan DA. Tearful relationships? Sex, hormones, the lacrimal gland, and aqueous-deficient dry eye. Ocul Surf 2004;2:92–123.

39. Zoukhri D, Hodges RR, Byon D, et al. Role of proinflammatory cytokines in the impaired lacrimation associated with autoimmune xerophthalmia. Invest Ophthalmol Vis Sci 2002;43: 1429–1436.

CHAPTER 15

Immune mechanisms of dry-eye disease

Austin K Mircheff and Joel E Schechter

Clinical background

Key symptoms and signs

The symptoms of dry-eye disease are discussed in detail in Chapter 14. A point that bears emphasis is that patient presentation is extremely variable. Patients may experience troublesome symptoms but present none of the standard clinical signs and even have increased fluid production; may report symptoms and show ocular surface pathology but have normal fluid production; or may show decreased fluid production but deny symptoms.

Historical development

Papers describing fibrotic and atrophic changes in the lacrimal glands of aged subjects began appearing in the late nineteenth century. In 1903 Schirmer noted that fluid production varied widely among normal individuals but tended to decrease with increasing age and to decrease more severely in women. Later investigators[1] substantiated Schirmer's conclusions. In the 1930s, Sjögren introduced the terms "keratoconjunctivitis sicca" (KCS) and "sicca complex," and reported findings from patients with the sicca complex and arthritis, including documentation of inflammatory changes in glands obtained from several of the affected individuals.

The concept of autoimmune diseases emerged in the subsequent decade, along with the discovery that patients' sera frequently contained antibodies directed against certain tissues or intracellular structures. Bloch and Bunim[2] showed that the sicca complex and glandular histopathology occurred in patients with other autoimmune diseases in addition to rheumatoid arthritis. Bloch et al[3] reported that the sicca complex and autoantibody titers also occurred in patients with no sign of autoimmune disease affecting other tissues. The distinction between primary Sjögren's syndrome and secondary Sjögren's syndrome was established by the mid-1970s.

The nature of lacrimal gland atrophy and dysfunction outside the setting of Sjögren's syndrome and other inflammatory diseases has been somewhat controversial. Examining lacrimal gland and salivary gland histology in autopsy subjects, Waterhouse[4] found at least slight adenitis in the lacrimal glands of between 8% and 22% of men in different age groups, with no indication of an age-associated increase. In contrast, the frequency of adenitis, which he interpreted as an autoimmune phenomenon, increased in women, from 22% in women younger than 44 years to 65% in women 75 and older. Whaley et al[5] determined the frequency of decreased Schirmer test scores and increased rose Bengal staining in inpatients hospitalized for various indications but explicitly excluding autoimmune diseases. Because they found no correlation between the ocular surface findings and various autoantibodies, they concluded that dry-eye disease in their subjects was due to atrophic changes, rather than autoimmune phenomena. Subsequent postmortem and biopsy studies, discussed in detail in the section on pathology below, documented the frequency of age-associated fibrosis and parenchymal atrophy, and they generally also demonstrated associations with increased lymphocytic infiltration.

A development in oral pathology is of interest in this context. Daniels and Whitcher[6] described histopathological features of labial salivary glands from patients who could and could not be diagnosed as having Sjögren's syndrome on the basis of serum autoantibodies and clinical diagnoses of xerostomia and dry eye. Their conclusion might seem paradoxical to those who have been taught that the pathophysiology of Sjögren's syndrome is autoimmune-mediated destruction of the secretory parenchyma: While parenchyma was replaced by lymphocyte aggregates, Sjögren's syndrome cases were distinguished by an absence of acinar atrophy or ductal dilatation, even in parenchymal areas immediately adjacent to large aggregates.

Epidemiology

This topic is reviewed in Chapter 14.

Genetics and risk factors

There is a significant genetic influence on the incidence of Sjögren's syndrome, since having a first-degree relative with an autoimmune disease increases the risk sevenfold.[7] An association between human leukocyte antigen (HLA) DR alleles and autoantibodies is recognized,[8] but other reported genetic associations have been controversial.[9] Having delivered a baby doubles the risk for developing Sjögren's syndrome 2.1-fold.[7]

There appear to be no reports of genetic factors influencing dry-eye disease not associated with autoimmune diseases. Other risk factors are discussed in Chapter 14.

That most dry-eye patients, and the large majority of patients with Sjögren's syndrome, are women prompted studies of sex steroid actions in animal models (Box 15.1).

Androgens clearly influence immune cell activity in the lacrimal glands and the status of the ocular surface.[10-13] Rocha et al[14] proposed that androgens exert their influences by controlling expression of immunomodulatory mediators by parenchymal cells; this important concept is discussed at length in the section on pathophysiology, below. However, much remains to be learned about mechanisms underlying the androgens' influences. Gonadectomizing or hypophysectomizing experimental animals causes significant biochemical and functional changes[15,16] but does not cause acinar atrophy or fibrosis on the scale of the changes that occur in the aging human lacrimal gland or normally aging rats[17] and mice.[18]

Other hormones also influence lacrimal gland and ocular surface cytophysiology and immunophysiology. Mathers et al[19] found that lacrimal fluid production correlates positively with increasing serum testosterone only in premenopausal women. In contrast, in all groups studied, i.e., premenopausal, postmenopausal without hormone replacement therapy, and postmenopausal with hormone replacement therapy, all measures of lacrimal function correlate negatively with increasing levels of serum prolactin (PRL). Notably, all subjects in this study had PRL values within the normal range.

Findings on the actions of estrogens defy explanations based on a single hormone-regulated process. Women with premature ovarian failure present increased signs and symptoms but produce fluid at normal rates.[20] On the other hand, estrogen replacement therapy is associated with exacerbation of dry-eye symptoms in older women.[21]

Differential diagnosis, treatment, and prognosis

These topics are addressed in Chapter 14. The extent to which dry-eye disease occurs in association with local and systemic inflammatory diseases should be noted.

Pathology

Lacrimal gland

Most studies of the histopathology of the human lacrimal gland in normal aging have confirmed the earlier finding that aging is associated with increased fibrosis, ductal pathology, acinar atrophy, and infiltration of immune cells. Damato et al[22] and Pepose et al[23] described the presence of lymphoid aggregates or foci, and, occasionally secondary follicles, even in individuals without a history of autoimmune disease. Roen et al[24] and Obata[25] noted the frequent occurrence of ductal dilatation, and Obata also documented the frequency of fatty infiltration. In an analysis of postmortem lacrimal glands, Obata et al[26] found that diffuse fibrosis, diffuse acinar atrophy, and periductal fibrosis were more frequent in the orbital lobes of elderly women, and in the palpebral lobes of aging men. They also noted that the frequency of lymphoid foci increased with age and, as Wieczorek et al[27] had found, that most foci were located near intralobular or interlobular ducts, i.e., those within, but at the periphery of, a lobule.

Nasu et al[28] compared lacrimal glands from subjects with autoimmune diseases and with no history of autoimmune diseases. They concluded that the entire population shared common histopathological features and differed only by degree. Although the incidence of lymphoid foci was highest in patients with Sjögren's syndrome and other autoimmune diseases, only 36% of lacrimal glands from subjects without autoimmune diseases appeared to be free of infiltrates. In the remainder, the incidence and severity of infiltration were highest among those older than 40 years and the incidence was nearly identical in males (63.9%) and females (62.8%).

The immunohistopathology of the lacrimal glands in patients with Sjögren's syndrome presents some diversity. Pflugfelder et al[29] found that, of 6 patients, lymphocytic infiltration was diffuse in 4 and focal in 2. Tsubota et al[30] compared the histopathological features of the lacrimal glands of subjects with Mikulicz's disease and Sjögren's syndrome, which share several features, including massive infiltration by essentially identical proportions of CD4+, CD8+, and CD21+ lymphocytes. Whereas fluid production is severely impaired in patients with Sjögren's syndrome, patients with Mikulicz's disease retain exocrine function, and their ocular surfaces appear normal.

Conjunctiva and cornea

The corneal and conjunctival epithelia undergo marked morphological changes in dry-eye disease. The number of goblet cells in the conjunctival epithelia decreases; cells in the superficial conjunctival epithelial layers flatten, such that the epithelium thins even as the number of strata increases; cells in the most superficial layer lose most of their microvilli and separate from their normally close attachment to the penultimate layer; hyaline bodies, suggested to represent the residua of defunct goblet cells, appear in the epithelium; and vacuoles and other inclusions appear within the cytoplasm.[31,32] The lamina propria underlying areas of affected epithelium becomes increasingly populated by lymphocytes and leukocytes.[33] Subsequent studies have confirmed that increased numbers of lymphocytes are present within the conjunctiva of patients with dry-eye disease. Epithelial cells expressing HLA DR (human major histocompatibility complex (MHC) class II) molecules were present in conjunctival impression cytology specimens from 50% of patients[34] and in brush cytology specimens from 66% of patients[35] with idiopathic dry-eye disease.

Etiology

Explicit concepts are emerging for the mechanisms by which environmental stresses, iatrogenic factors, allergy and infection, and endocrine changes can initiate dry-eye disease. Before presenting these concepts, it is appropriate to review physiological principles and cytophysiological mechanisms that influence disease development.

Pathophysiology

Nexus between the visual system and the mucosal immune system

The normal ocular surface fluid provides a microenvironment for the living epithelial cells exposed in the interpalpebral regions of the cornea and conjunctiva. Figure 15.1 illustrates the general wiring scheme by which perception of irritation or dryness in the cornea or conjunctiva elicits production of lacrimal fluid.

The epithelia of the lacrimal glands, ocular surface, and lacrimal drainage system form a topological continuum with the mucosae of the respiratory system and the gastrointestinal system. The ocular surface system, like the respiratory and gastrointestinal systems, contains organized inductive sites for adaptive mucosal immunity, and it also performs both innate and adaptive mucosal immune effector functions. Even as the lacrimal epithelia perform the exocrine functions associated with production of the ocular surface fluid, they devote much of their cytophysiology to accomplishing mucosal immune effector functions.

Cytophysiological apparatus

Lacrimal epithelial cells employ ion pumps, symporters, exchangers, and channels that are common to essentially all nucleated cells. They generate vectorial ion fluxes by using transport vesicles to insert specific ion transporters into the basal, lateral and apical domains of their plasma membranes. Figure 15.2 illustrates the disposition of the ion transporters as an apparatus for secreting Cl^- ions and K^+ ions through the cells and Na^+ ions through the paracellular pathway. This apparatus is distinct from the apparatus that secretes proteins.

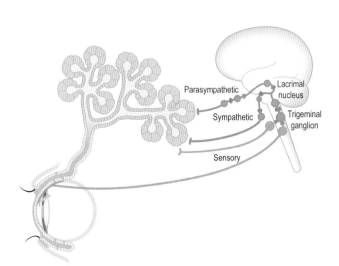

Figure 15.1 Wiring of a physiological servomechanism. A perception of irritation or dryness by sensory nerve endings in the cornea and conjunctiva elicits afferent signals, which travel through the trigeminal ganglion to reach a lacrimal center in the brainstem. (Note that sensory nerve endings are also present in the lacrimal gland.) Like sensory information from the viscera, signals from the ocular surface are processed and lead to the generation of efferent autonomic secretomotor signals, even when there is no conscious awareness that the status of the ocular surface has deviated from its homeostatic setpoint. The secretomotor signals reach the lacrimal glands by way of both sympathetic and parasympathetic nerves, which release their neurotransmitters in the general vicinity of, but do not form synapses with, parenchymal epithelial cells.

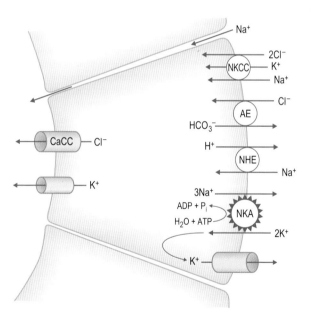

Figure 15.2 The cytophysiological apparatus for exocrine secretion of Cl^- ions, Na^+ ions, and, in ductal cells, K^+ ions. Secretion of the ions creates the osmotic driving force that causes water to move from the interstitial space to the lumen of the acinus–duct system. Recent studies indicate that the Na^+/H^+ exchanger (NHE) and the Cl^-/HCO_3^- exchanger (anion exchanger, AE) work in concert[36] and in parallel with the $Na^+K^+2Cl^-$ symporters (NKCC)[37,38] to drive Cl^- ions from the interstitial fluid to the cytosol, against an unfavorable electrochemical potential difference. Secretagogue-mediated opening of apical Cl^- channels allows Cl^- ions to flow into the lumen. Flux of Na^+ ions through the paracellular pathway dissipates the lumen-negative transepithelial voltage difference that results from the transcellular flux of Cl^- ions. Apical K^+ channels and K^+-Cl^- symporters are primarily found in ductal epithelial cells.[38] (Not illustrated is the fact that the transporters spend 90% of their time in the intracellular compartments depicted in Figure 15.3. Secretagogue stimulation recruits more Na,K-ATPase (NKA) pump units to the basal lateral plasma membrane and activates NHE exchangers in the basal lateral membrane.)

The organelles that lacrimal epithelial cells use to secrete proteins are also common to most cell types. However, by using transport vesicles to transfer products between specific organelles, they organize the organelles into apparatus to perform an exocrine function. Figure 15.3 illustrates this

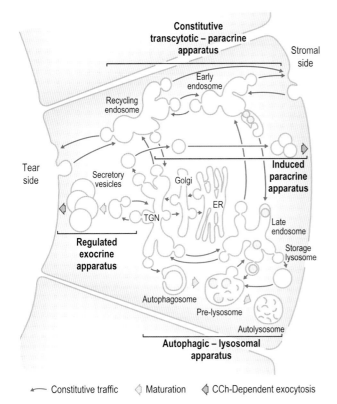

Figure 15.3 Cytophysiological apparatus for exocrine secretion of glycoproteins, transcytotic secretion of secretory component and secretory IgA, paracrine secretion of signaling mediators, and catabolism of cellular proteins, lipids, and carbohydrates. The apparatus are essentially the same in acinar cells and duct cells, but the exocrine and paracrine secretory products differ.

The glycoproteins that each epithelial cell secretes and the proteins it uses in its ion-transporting apparatus are assembled in the common biosynthetic apparatus, which consists of the endoplasmic reticulum (ER) and the Golgi complex. The products then traffic to the *trans*-Golgi network (TGN), which is the most complex of the cells' several sorting nexuses. The TGN sorts specific products into distinct microdomains, and in these microdomains the transport vesicles form that will traffic to the other organelles.

The immature secretory vesicle is the entry compartment of the classic exocrine secretory apparatus for glycoproteins. The late endosome and the isolation membrane are the entry compartments of the autophagic-lysosomal apparatus. The recycling endosome and early endosome comprise both a transcytotic secretory apparatus and, simultaneously, a paracrine secretory apparatus. Under certain circumstances, both physiological and pathophysiological, the cell is induced to express a second paracrine secretory apparatus.

Autoantigens that are present in the cytosol, as well as autoantigens that are embedded in the lipid bilayers of membrane-bound organelles, enter the luminal spaces of the membrane traffic apparatus through the process of autophagy and through the formation of multivesicular bodies. Both processes are of interest. Formation of multivesicular bodies in lacrimal gland epithelial cells has not been studied, but it is a fundamental cytophysiological process with potentially important implications for autoantigen exposure. Like proteins that are released to the fluid phase, the proteins in microvesicles that may be released from the cell can be taken up, processed, and presented by antigen-presenting cells.

dynamic apparatus. The regulated exocrine apparatus exocytoses proteins, including signaling mediators, into the nascent ocular surface fluid. The transcytotic apparatus takes dimeric IgA (dIgA) up from the stromal fluid and exocytoses secretory IgA (sIgA) at the apical membrane; it also functions as a paracrine secretory apparatus, which exocytoses extracellular matrix components and signaling mediators into the stromal space (Box 15.2). A novel paracrine apparatus, discussed below, is induced under certain physiological and pathophysiological conditions. The autophagic-lysosomal apparatus mediates the catabolic turnover of glycoproteins and phospholipids; it communicates with the transcytotic paracrine apparatus at the late endosome.

The lacrimal gland's innate mucosal immune effector function is to secrete bacteriostatic and bactericidal effector molecules. These include lactoferrin, lactoperoxidase, and lytic enzymes, such as lysozyme and other glycohydrolases, proteases, and phospholipases. Its adaptive mucosal immune function is to deliver sIgA into the ocular surface fluid.

The transcytotic paracrine apparatus that delivers IgA to the ocular surface fluid is described in detail in Box 15.3. The authors[39-41] have proposed that, because this apparatus communicates with the autophagic lysosomal apparatus at the late endosome, it also mediates the secretion of autoantigens to the underlying stromal space. Moreover, the unique strategy lacrimal epithelial cells use to regulate secretion of sIgA and secretory component acutely may give them a propensity to generate and secrete autoantigen fragments that contain otherwise cryptic epitopes.

The task of delivering of sIgA to the ocular surface fluid requires that lacrimal parenchymal cells maintain the stromal space as a niche for dIgA-secreting plasmacytes. They do so by secreting paracrine mediators that induce plasmablasts to undergo terminal differentiation and additional mediators that support the survival of mature plasmacytes. While both acinar and ductal epithelial cells secrete sIgA and

---

Box 15.2 Acute and long-term regulation of lacrimal epithelial cells

Secretagogues acutely activate:

- The ion- and water-secreting apparatus
- The exocrine apparatus for secreting proteins
- Transcytotic apparatus for secreting secretory component and secretory immunoglobulin A

Hormones, cytokines, and inflammatory mediators likely influence:

- Expression of specific components of each apparatus
- Expression of secretagogue receptors
- Expression of intracellular signaling cascades activated by secretagogue receptors

---

Box 15.3 Secretory immunoglobulin A (sIgA)

- Immobilizes microbes, preventing penetration of the epithelial barrier
- Does not fix complement
- Reduces the risk that inflammatory responses will be needed to fight infections

secretory component, they do not express the same spectra of paracrine mediators. More is known about mediators produced by duct cells, while more is known about cytophysiological mechanisms of acinar cells.

In mucosal immune effector sites transforming growth factor-β (TGF-β) conveys the signal for plasmablast differentiation. In the rabbit lacrimal gland, TGF-β expression is largely localized to interlobular duct epithelial cells. Normally, duct cells apportion TGF-β into both their exocrine secretory apparatus and their transcytotic paracrine apparatus. TGF-β is synthesized in a proform; proteolytically processed, mature TGF-β typically remains in a noncovalent complex with its latency-associated peptide. Latent TGF-β entering the stroma is thought to associate with the extracellular matrix proteoglycan, decorin, which appears to be produced by both ductal and acinar epithelial cells. Thus, decorin may create a diffusion barrier that keeps latent TGF-β concentrated in the spaces surrounding the interlobular ducts, where it would signal to plasmablasts entering the gland from venules that parallel the ducts.

TGF-β also conveys additional signals: proliferative signals to mesenchymal cells and some epithelia, and antiproliferative or proapoptotic signals to other epithelia and lymphocytes. The antiproliferative signals contribute to its immunosuppressive actions. Moreover, TGF-β can induce expression of its own mRNA in T lymphocytes and antigen-presenting cells. It appears that mucosal immune effector tissues are able to use TGF-β to induce plasmablast differentiation because they also secrete paracrine mediators that abrogate TGF-β's proapoptotic signals. In the lamina propria of the small intestine, interleukin-6 (IL-6) appears to be a major plasmacyte survival factor. In the lactating mammary gland, plasmacyte survival is supported by PRL. Schechter et al[42] demonstrated that PRL, like TGF-β, is concentrated in epithelial cells of the interlobular ducts in the rabbit lacrimal gland. Retention of TGF-β in the stromal space surrounding the interlobular ducts may minimize its deleterious actions. In contrast, PRL is thought free to diffuse from the periductal regions to the periacinar regions, where it would promote survival of plasmacytes and acinar cells.

Azzarolo and coworkers[43] found that plasmacytes in the rabbit lacrimal gland undergo apoptosis within hours after animals have been ovariectomized. Apoptosis is prevented if either dihydrotestosterone or estradiol is administered prior to ovariectomy. These findings highlight the importance of survival signals for plasmacytes, and they suggest that the sex steroids either support expression of PRL or interact with PRL to generate the survival signal.

Studies of lacrimal glands of pregnant rabbits demonstrate that the influences of epithelium-derived paracrine mediator extend beyond plasmablast differentiation and plasmacyte survival.[42,44]

As described in detail in Box 15.4, expression of both TGF-β and PRL increases during pregnancy. The increase of TGF-β appears to be driven by estradiol (E2) and progesterone (PRG), while the increase for PRL is driven, at least in part, by pituitary PRL. PRL induces expression of the novel paracrine apparatus, amplifying delivery of both mediators to the stroma and decreasing delivery of both to the ocular surface fluid. These changes are associated with significant changes in lacrimal fluid production and with a redistribution of lymphocytes and plasmacytes from periductal perive-

---

Box 15.4 Functional, cytophysiological, and immunophysiological transformations established late in pregnancy

Functional changes

- Resting fluid production decreased[44]
- Pilocarpine-induced fluid production increased[44]
- Concentration of protein in pilocarpine-induced fluid decreased[44]
- Prolactin (PRL) and transforming growth factor-β (TGF-β) contents of lacrimal gland fluid decreased[44]
- Positive rose Bengal staining occurs more frequently[44]

Cytophysiological changes

- PRL and TGF-β contents in parenchymal cells of interlobular ducts and acini increase
- PRL and TGF-β redistribute from primary localizations in apical cytoplasm to dual localizations in apical and basal cytoplasm[42]

Immunophysiological changes

- Lymphocytes and plasmacytes disperse from aggregates in stromal space surrounding interlobular ducts and become concentrated in periacinar spaces[42,44]

Current understanding of endocrine signals

- Estradiol and progesterone increase expression of TGF-β
- Elevated systemic PRL levels increase expression of PRL
- PRL induces expression of novel paracrine secretory apparatus,[45] which captures both newly synthesized PRL and PRL endocytosed from the ambient medium for secretion to the stromal space[46]

---

nular spaces to periacinar spaces. Evidence now suggests that the counterpoise between TGF-β and PRL may be a key factor determining the lacrimal gland's immunophysiological status.

Constitutive exposure of autoantigens

Experiments with several animal models have shown that activated, autoantigen-specific effector T cells can adoptively transfer disease to the lacrimal glands.[47–50] This finding indicates that potentially pathogenic autoantigen epitopes must be displayed by MHC class II on the surfaces of resident antigen-presenting cells.

Most literature on the subject posits that intracellular autoantigens become available for processing and MHC class II-mediated presentation as the result of apoptosis or necrosis. However, the authors and their colleagues have proposed that live, actively functioning lacrimal epithelial cells constantly secrete autoantigens by way of their transcytotic-paracrine apparatus. As illustrated in Figure 15.3, autoantigens that are present in the cytosol, as well as autoantigens that are embedded in the lipid bilayers of membrane-bound organelles, enter the luminal spaces of the membrane traffic apparatus through the process of autophagy and through the formation of multivesicular bodies, and they may be exocytotically secreted from the early endosome.

As detailed in Box 15.5, the traffic of transport vesicles to and from the basal-lateral plasma membrane is extensive

Box 15.5 Chronic cholinergic stimulation may lead to the appearance of otherwise cryptic autoantigen epitopes

Consequences of chronic exposure to cholinergic agonists, presumed to model chronic exposure to agonistic autoantibodies to the M3AChR:

- Decreased abundance of G_q and G_{11}, the heterotrimeric GTP-binding proteins that couple to the M3AChR, attenuates M3AChR signaling, preventing elevation of cytosolic Ca^{2+}[48]
- Activation of apparatus for exocrine protein secretion blocked
- Activation of apparatus for secreting Cl^- ions, Na^+ ions, and H_2O blocked[49]
- Traffic of vesicles recycling to and from the basal lateral plasma membrane decreases to basal rates
- Traffic of vesicles from early endosome to late endosome blocked
- Lysosomal proteases, prevented from taking normal pathway through late endosome to storage lysosome or pre-lysosome, accumulate within endomembrane compartments that remain accessible, including early endosome, recycling endosome, *trans*-Golgi network, and secretory vesicles[50]
- Traffic of identified autoantigens is also altered. Acinar cells release the autoantigens to their ambient medium, both as soluble proteins and as constituents of structures with microsomal sedimentation properties, i.e., structures that might be microvesicles

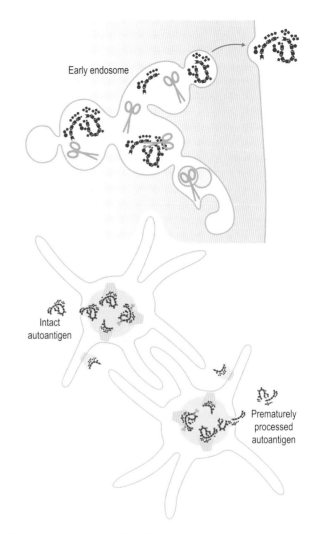

Figure 15.4 Lacrimal epithelial cells are thought to secrete autoantigens by way of transport vesicles that bud from the early endosome. When stimulation (Boxes 15.5 and 15.6) causes catalytically active lysosomal proteases to accumulate in the endosomes, they may hydrolyze peptide bonds in the exposed sequences that normally contain dominant T-cell epitopes. Subdominant, i.e., previously cryptic, epitopes may survive and associate with the peptide binding grooves on antigen-presenting cell major histocompatibility complex class II.

and dynamic, as is traffic to the late endosome. As illustrated in Figure 15.4, chronic stimulation may both increase the secretion of autoantigens to the stroma and cause the secretion of autoantigen fragments that contain previously cryptic epitopes.

Induced capacity to present autoantigen epitopes directly to T cells

The transcytotic paracrine apparatus appears also to allow acinar cells to present autoantigen epitopes directly to CD4+ T cells. Studies with thyroid epithelial cells led Bottazzo and coworkers[51] to suggest that parenchymal cells that have been induced to express MHC class II may be able to present autoantigen epitopes directly to CD4+ T cells. Epithelial cells from rat and rabbit lacrimal gland spontaneously express MHC class II when they are isolated and placed in primary culture. As noted above, conjunctival epithelial cells from patients with dry-eye disease express MHC class II. Large proportions of epithelial cells in the majority of cadaver donor lacrimal glands studied by Mircheff et al[52] expressed MHC class II. Moreover, the number of positive cells generally correlated with the number of lymphocytes present. As explained in Box 15.7, it appears that acinar cells isolated from rabbit lacrimal gland function as surrogate antigen-presenting cells and stimulate the proliferation of pathogenic CD4+ effector T cells in ex vivo models.

The focal organization of lymphocytes in Sjögren's syndrome, and the fact the B cells, CD4+ T cells, and dendritic cells are present in the foci would seem to imply that B-cell activation and autoantibody production are driven by autoantigens and immune complexes that are released into the stromal space, rather than by autoantigen epitopes displayed on the surfaces of parenchymal cells. Nevertheless, the robustness of MHC class II expression by epithelial cells in infiltrated lacrimal glands is consistent with the notion that the lymphocytic infiltration in the aging human lacrimal gland is driven, at least in part, by parenchymal cells functioning as surrogate antigen-presenting cells.

Maintaining homeostatic states

Although lacrimal epithelial cells secrete autoantigens and can be induced to secrete previously cryptic epitopes and to function as surrogate antigen-presenting cells, none of these events in isolation is likely to be the trigger for autoimmune disease.[53] Recent experiments, described in Box 15.8, suggest that the TGF-β secreted by ductal epithelial cells enforces tolerance to the lacrimal autoantigens.

Box 15.6 Transcytotic secretion of sIgA and paracrine secretion of autoantigens

A novel mechanism for acutely regulating transcytotic secretory immunoglobulin A secretion has implications for the autoantigens lacrimal epithelial cells expose. The transcytotic-paracrine apparatus is illustrated in Figure 15.3

- Upon reaching the *trans*-Golgi network (TGN), newly synthesized pIgR enter microdomains, forming transport vesicles that will be targeted to traffic to the exocrine secretory apparatus, the paracrine secretory apparatus, and perhaps also the autophagic lysosomal apparatus
- In immature secretory vesicles, secretory component (SC) portion is proteolytically severed from the membrane-spanning domain and released into the fluid phase. Immature secretory vesicles mature through return of excess membrane to the TGN. Secretagogues induce mature secretory vesicles to fuse with the apical plasma membrane, exocytosing SC along with lactoferrin, lysozyme, lactoperoxidase, and other products
- pIgR trafficking to the early endosome may return to the TGN, presumably by way of the recycling endosome; may traffic to the basal lateral plasma membrane; or enter tubular extensions that separate from the early endosome and form multivesicular bodies by invaginating small vesicles from their limiting membranes
- Multivesicular bodies traffic to prelysosomes, which fuse with storage lysosomes to gain a full complement of proteases, glycohydrolases, and phospholipases that will hydrolyze pIgR
- pIgR trafficking to the recycling endosome may recycle to the TGN; recycle to the early endosome; or undergo proteolytic processing to release SC. Transport vesicles that bud from the recycling endosome and traffic to the apical plasma membrane fuse with it to exocytose SC into the lumen of the acinus duct system
- Plasmacytes populating the stromal spaces secrete dimeric IgA. Binding of dIgA to pIgR at the basal lateral membrane is thought to direct traffic of the complex away from the late endosome and toward the recycling endosome, so that sIgA is exocytosed at the apical plasma membrane
- Acute stimulation with CCh curtails traffic to the late endosome and prelysosome, increasing pIgR traffic to the recycling endosome, and therefore increasing secretion of SC. Chronic exposure to M3AChR agonists persistently blocks traffic to the degradative compartments, but also suppresses expression of pIgR

Box 15.7 A rabbit model of autoimmune lacrimal gland disease induced by autoadoptive, ex vivo to in vivo, transfer

- Acinar cells are isolated from the inferior lobe of one lacrimal gland, obtained through a transconjunctival incision
- Isolated acinar cells express major histocompatibility complex (MHC) class II, which circulates through the network of endomembrane compartments, where it binds autoantigen epitopes, and traffic to the plasma membrane. This appears to allow isolated acinar cells to function as surrogate autoantigen-presenting cells
- Lymphocytes from peripheral blood proliferate in co-cultures with acinar cells from the same donor animal (autologous mixed-cell reaction). Proliferating cells transfer disease to the donor animal's remaining lacrimal gland, the corneas, and conjunctivae, whether injected directly into the remaining lacrimal gland or injected subcutaneously[46]

Box 15.8 An ex vivo rat model of immunoregulation

Acinar cells from rat lacrimal glands express major histocompatibility complex (MHC) class II when placed in primary culture. However, rather than becoming immunoactivating, they become immunoregulatory and immunosuppressive. They:

- Inhibit, rather than stimulate, proliferation of lymphocytes in autologous mixed-cell reactions
- Secrete soluble mediators that inhibit the proliferation of lymphocytes in mixed-cell reactions containing acinar cells and lymphocytes from rabbits
- Secrete soluble mediators that inhibit mixed-cell reactions containing ex vivo matured dendritic cells and lymphocytes from rats
- Secrete soluble mediators, including transforming growth factor-β, that control phenotypic expression of dendritic cells maturing ex vivo, permitting expression of surface MHC class II but suppressing expression of CD86[53]

Figure 15.5 summarizes the theory that TGF-β mediates the generation of regulatory antigen-presenting cells, which in turn mediate the generation of regulatory CD4+ T cells. That regulatory T cells contribute to maintaining immuno-homeostasis is indicated by observations that it is necessary to deplete regulatory T cells before adoptive transfer of activated effector T cells is able to induce disease in the models described by Niederkorn et al[48] and Jiang et al[50] and by the recent report that autoimmune disease arises spontaneously in CD25 knockout mice.[54]

Paracrine mediation of endocrine triggers

As described in detail in Box 15.4, during pregnancy increased systemic PRL, perhaps interacting with increased E2 and PRG, increases expression of PRL in lacrimal duct epithelial cells[42,44] and appears to induce both ductal and acinar cells to express the novel paracrine secretory apparatus.[45,46] In contrast, it appears that the increase of TGF-β expression in the ducts is mediated by E2, PRG, or E2 and PRG acting in concert, independently of PRL. The role PRL is thought to play maintaining plasmacyte survival by abrogating proapoptotic signals from TGF-β was discussed above. However, PRL is a proliferation factor for T lymphocytes[55]; it induces T cells to express interferon-γ (IFN-γ); and it alters the phenotypic expression of dendritic cells to favor T_H1 polarization.[56] The authors tested the hypothesis that excessive levels of PRL within the lacrimal gland abrogate regulatory signals and initiate autoimmune activation by using an adenovirus vector to transduce cDNA for rabbit PRL into the lacrimal glands of ovary-intact, nonpregnant female rabbits.[57] Transient overexpression of PRL led to an acute increase in lymphocytic infiltration, which then evolved into a chronic, low-grade infiltration. In different settings, the infiltrates were associated with a predominantly T_H1 cytokine profile; a mixed T_H1 and T_H2 profile; and a profile characterized by increases in the expression of tumor necrosis factor-α (TNF-α), TGF-β, IL-1β, and IL-6, but not the T_H1 cytokine, IFN-γ,

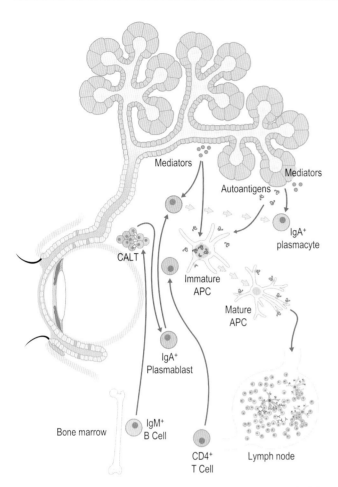

Figure 15.5 Paracrine mediators secreted by interlobular duct epithelial cells regulate plasmacytes, dendritic cells, and T cells entering the lacrimal gland. This theory posits that, as immature antigen-presenting cells (APC) enter the periductal stromal space of the lacrimal gland, they are induced by transforming growth factor-β (TGF-β) to become regulatory APC, which will constitutively express TGF-β. They take up autoantigens, then mature and traffic to the draining lymph nodes, where they will present epitopes to CD4⁺ T cells, inducing them to differentiate as regulatory cells. Induced regulatory cells that subsequently enter the lacrimal gland reinforce the TGF-β-mediated signal, inducing the next generation of immature APC to mature as regulatory APC. In the lymph nodes as well as the lacrimal glands, the induced regulatory cells compete with activated, epitope-specific effector T cells for MHC class II-mediated antigenic stimulation. CALT, conjunctiva-associated lymphoid tissue.

or the T_H2 cytokines, IL-4 and IL-10. These findings suggest that several different immunopathophysiological processes might arise in response to systemic endocrine changes or local processes that increase expression of PRL without coordinately increasing expression of TGF-β. E2 and PRG levels decline abruptly at parturition, whereas the systemic PRL level remains elevated during lactation and declines rather gradually during a nonlactating puerperium. An appealing hypothesis, which has not yet been tested, is that the interval between parturition and the return to normal PRL levels and normal cycling is a period of increased risk for autoimmune activation. The analogous hypothesis is that the loss of steroid hormone support for ductal TGF-β expression during normal aging should be investigated, but the immunopathophysiological processes of aging are likely to be considerably more complicated.

Environmental triggers

Observations that adoptively transferring activated effector T cells induces autoimmune lacrimal gland pathophysiology, cited above, suggest that activated effector T cells must be able to abrogate the immunosuppressive actions of both epithelial TGF-β and the resident population of regulatory T cells to proliferate and determine the phenotypic expression of the new generation of maturing antigen-presenting cells. Thus, the phenomenon of adoptive transfer offers a plausible explanation for the initiation of lacrimal gland disease in secondary Sjögren's syndrome and other inflammatory diseases.

Dursun et al[58] and Barabino et al[59] found that exposing mice to increased flow of dehumidified air causes dry-eye disease. Dursun and coworkers also treated the mice with scopolamine, with the goal of paralyzing lacrimal gland exocrine function and thereby exacerbating the desiccation of the ocular surface. In this model, the lacrimal glands become infiltrated with lymphocytes.[48] Adoptive transfer provides a possible link between environmental stresses, as well as allergy and infection, at the ocular surface and the initiation of autoimmune disease. The cytophysiology of conjunctival epithelial cells has not been elucidated to the same level of detail as in the lacrimal gland. However, like the lacrimal glands, the conjunctivae in humans and rabbits support resident populations of IgA⁺ plasmacytes. The apicalmost epithelial cell layers express pIgR and use a transcytotic apparatus to deliver sIgA into the ocular surface fluid. Therefore, it is reasonable to infer that, like lacrimal epithelial cells, conjunctival epithelial cells also secrete autoantigens to their stroma. As Stern and coworkers[60] proposed, factors which decrease lacrimal fluid production, such as age-related atrophy, drug side-effects, and iatrogenic sensory denervation, may lead to desiccation, causing corneal and conjunctival epithelial cells to release inflammatory mediators, and perhaps also causing sensory nerve endings to release inflammatory transmitters and neuropeptides. Mediators that increase in the mouse model of desiccating stress include IL-1, TNF-α, IL-6, IL-2, IL-12, and IFN-γ.[61] The likely scenario is that the inflammatory mediators abrogate the normal influences of TGF-β and the resident population of regulatory T cells, causing the new generation of antigen-presenting cells to mature with immunoactivating phenotypes that stimulate epitope-specific effector T cells in the lymph nodes. In such cases, dry-eye disease is not the passive consequence of failed lacrimal exocrine function, but, rather, the manifestation of pathophysiological processes that evolve in tandem in the lacrimal gland and the ocular surface tissues.

Chronic disease processes

A number of mechanisms contribute to positive-feedback loops that expand and maintain immunopathophysiological processes. Desiccation at the ocular surface generates efferent secretomotor signals to the lacrimal gland. As described above, chronic stimulation decreases lacrimal fluid production and may also cause lacrimal epithelial cells to secrete autoantigen fragments containing previously cryptic epitopes. Most patients with Sjögren's syndrome produce autoantibodies against M_3AChR. Whether these are inhibitory or agonistic, they likely decrease fluid production and exacerbate ocular surface desiccation.

Rolando et al[62] found that water evaporates from the ocular surface fluid more rapidly in patients with dry-eye disease, and Mathers[63] found that meibomian gland dysfunction is associated with increased evaporation. Thus, meibomian gland impairment, whether it is the consequence or the initial trigger of an inflammatory process,[64] contributes to a positive-feedback loop.

Zoukhri and coworkers[65] have shown that IL-1β acts on parasympathetic nerve endings in the lacrimal gland to block the release of acetylcholine and that both IL-1 and TNF-α impair acinar epithelial cells' ability to activate their exocrine secretory apparatus in response to acute stimulation with CCh. Other studies indicate that acinar cells undergo significant cytophysiological changes when they are chronically stimulated with histamine or serotonin, the receptors for which appear to couple to heterotrimeric GTP-binding proteins other than G_q and G_{11}.[66] Elevated concentrations of both decrease cells' ability to activate the Cl^- secretory apparatus in response to optimal doses of CCh.[40]

Preliminary experiments indicate that certain mediators induce ex vivo acinar cells to express inflammatory cytokines, suggesting that local feedback loops between parenchymal cells and immune cells may influence the nature of the immunopathophysiological process.

Summary

Despite the multiplicity of signaling and immune cell traffic loops that connect the ocular surface tissues and lacrimal glands, immunopathophysiological processes in the former are not always accompanied by failures of exocrine function in the latter. Two principles seem likely to account for complex clinical presentation of dry-eye disease.

First, immunopathophysiological processes in the lacrimal glands and conjunctivae are fundamentally local, maintained by interactions between parenchymal cells and immune cells, and they can be diverse, with diverse spectra of cytokines and inflammatory mediators. It may be that in some cases the ocular surface tissues are diseased but lacrimal glands are not, or that the lacrimal gland's host immunopathophysiological processes do not impair their exocrine functions. This point is illustrated by the persistence of lacrimal fluid production in patients with Mikulicz's disease, patients with premature ovarian failure, and some patients with ocular surface abnormalities that destabilize the fluid film.

Second, lacrimal epithelial cells use fundamentally different cytophysiological apparatus for secreting proteins and for producing fluid. The changes that occur during pregnancy indicate that the capacity to produce fluid can be unaffected, or even enhanced, at the same time that basal fluid production decreases and the apparatus for exocrine proteins secretion is largely replaced by a paracrine secretory apparatus. One wonders whether some of the aging lacrimal glands with atrophic acini but intact ducts might still be producing fluid.

Key references

A complete list of chapter references is available online at www.expertconsult.com. See inside cover for registration details.

3. Bloch KJ, Buchanan WW, Wohl MJ, et al. Sjögren's syndrome. A clinical, pathological, and serological study of sixty-two cases. Medicine 1965;44:187–231.

10. Sullivan DA, Hann LE. Hormonal influence on the secretory immune system of the eye: endocrine impact on the lacrimal gland accumulation and secretion of IgA and IgA. J Steroid Biochem 1989;314:253–262.

11. Sullivan DA, Edwards JA. Androgen stimulation of lacrimal function in mouse models of Sjögren's syndrome. J Steroid Biochem Mol Biol 1997;60:237–245.

19. Mathers WD, Stovall D, Lane ZA, et al. Menopause and tear function: the influence of prolactin and sex hormones on human tear production. Cornea 1998;17:353–358.

20. Schaumberg DA, Buring JE, Sullivan DA, et al. Hormone replacement therapy and dry eye. JAMA 2001;286:2114–2119.

26. Obata H, Yamamoto S, Horiuchi H, et al. Histopathologic study of human lacrimal gland. Ophthalmology 1995;102:678–686.

44. Ding C, Chang N, Fong Y-C, et al. Interacting influences of pregnancy and corneal injury on rabbit lacrimal gland immunoarchitecture and function. Invest Ophthalmol Vis Sci 2006;47:1368–1375.

45. Wang Y, Chiu CT, Nakamura T, et al. Elevated prolactin redirects secretory vesicle traffic in rabbit lacrimal acinar cells. Am J Physiol Endocrinol Metab 2007;292:E1122–E1134.

48. Niederkorn JY, Stern ME, Pflugfelder SC, et al. Desiccating stress induces T cell-mediated Sjögren's syndrome-like lacrimal keratoconjunctivitis. J Immunol 2006;176:3950–3957.

49. Thomas PB, Zhu Z, Selvam S, et al. Autoimmune dacryoadenitis and keratoconjunctivitis induced in rabbits by subcutaneous injection of autologous lymphocytes activated ex vivo against lacrimal antigens. J Autoimmun 2008; 31:116–122.

53. de Saint Jean M, Nakamura T, Wang Y, et al. Suppression of lymphocyte proliferation and regulation of dendritic cell phenotype by soluble mediators from rat lacrimal epithelial cells. Scand J Immunol 2009;70:53–62.

60. Stern ME, Beuerman RW, Fox RI, et al. The pathology of dry eye: the interaction between the ocular surface and lacrimal glands. Cornea 1998;17:584–589.

65. Zoukhri D, Macari E, Choi SH, et al. c-Jun NH2-terminal kinase mediates interleukin-1β-induced inhibition of lacrimal gland secretion. J Neurochem 2006;96:126–135.

66. McDonald ML, Wang Y, Selvam S, et al. Cytopathology and exocrine dysfunction induced in ex vivo rabbit lacrimal gland acinar cell models by chronic exposure to histamine or serotonin. Invest Ophthalmol Vis Sci 2009;50:3164–3175.

CHAPTER 16

Disruption of tear film and blink dynamics

Jianhua Wang and Anuj Chauhan

The topic of ocular tear film breakup has long been the subject of considerable attention due to its implications both in contact lens design and in the study of corneal dewetting. A better understanding of the causes of the breakup could enhance lens design and guide research toward improved dry-eye treatment options. The integrity of the pre-corneal tear film is vitally important both optically, in providing a smooth optical surface, and physiologically, in preventing corneal desiccation. The breakup time (BUT) of this film, clinically defined as the period between the last blink and the first instance of film breakup, averages 10 seconds in normal humans.[1] Because this is greater or comparable to the average interblink period of 5–10 seconds, the tear film is normally sufficiently stable.[2] Patients with dry eye, on the other hand, are characterized by a pre-corneal tear film that does not maintain integrity in the interblink period. In these patients, the breakup time may be as low as 1–2 seconds,[1] and corneal dewetting thus occurs between blinks (Box 16.1).

Structure of tear film

The ocular tear film is composed of three layers. Contacting the corneal epithelium is a hydrophilic mucous layer approximately 0.02–0.05 μm thick.[3] As the underlying cornea itself is extremely hydrophobic, this layer is believed to provide a wetting substrate for the aqueous layer above it.[3–5] Lying on this layer is a relatively thick aqueous layer that comprises the bulk of the tear film. Between this layer and the air is a 0.1–0.2-μm thick lipid layer that retards tear evaporation.[2,3]

Tear film thickness and tear volumes on the ocular surface

There has been no consensus on the thickness of human tear film for a long time due to the lack of direct visualization and measurement. Clearly, the thickness of the tear film and thinning rate hold the key to understanding the dynamics of the tear system in protecting the ocular surface. The indirect or invasive methods used to measure the layer resulted in thickness estimates from approximately 3 μm[6] to 40 μm.[7]

The early measurements of tear film thickness (TFT) used invasive methods that potentially disturbed the tear film. Both Mishima[8] and Benedetto et al[9] measured fluorescence after instilling fluorescein and reported a TFT of 4 μm; however, the tear film might have been diluted by the saline-fluorescein instillation. Using confocal microscopy, Prydal et al[7] reported thickness values of 41–46 μm. For rabbits, Mishima[8] used fine glass filaments and fluorometry to measure a TFT thickness of 7 μm. This thickness has been widely cited in the literature, although whether the rabbit tear film differs from that in humans is unknown. By applying an absorbent paper disc to the cornea,[10] human TFT was found to be approximately 8 μm, which could be an overestimate if reflex tears were generated and/or if the fluid was drawn from the tear film surrounding the disc or epithelium. Chen et al[11] used an in vivo cryofixation method to examine the tear film in rat corneas. They found that the tear film varied from 2 to 6 μm in thickness on the corneal surface. Using a modified, noninvasive optical coherence tomography (OCT) instrument, Wang et al[12] studied 80 human eyes and found the thickness of the tear film to be 3.3 μm, which is in agreement with King-Smith et al's estimate[6] of 3 μm determined by an interferometric method in vivo. In another study using a real-time anterior-segment OCT, Wang et al[13] measured TFT and found the layer to be 3.4 μm.

The total tear volume is estimated over the exposed ocular surface and tear menisci to be about 2–4 μl, including the tear fluid volume of 1 μl.[14–16] In another study using photography,[17] tear volume in the lower tear meniscus was estimated at about 0.5 μl, which appears to be too low compared to others.[18,19] The distribution is about equal in these three compartments.[16] Although there are some exchanges and renewal, the system is balanced with a fixed amount in each compartment regardless of blinking. However, the system changes when extra tears are produced or added.[20]

In the normal tear system, a small amount of tears such as 3 μl may be enough for the ocular surface to remain wet.[21] This figure of basal tear volume is slightly lower than the values reported by Mishima et al[14] using a fluorescein method. Each blink redistributes and mixes the tears[22] and the lid movement facilitates the action of the drainage system by compressing the canaliculi and lacrimal sac to expel the tears from the system.[23]

Box 16.1 Tear film and tear breakup

- Tear film is about 3–7 μm with lipid, aqueous, and mucous layers
- Small amount of tear volume is needed on the ocular surface
- Average 10 seconds of tear breakup may be sufficient for protecting ocular surface

---

Box 16.2 Mechanisms of tear breakup

- There are many mechanisms of tear breakup
- The thin tear film is stable and not likely to break, except by mechanisms that draw fluid out of the tear film such as evaporation
- The presence of a mucin-covered hydrophilic surface makes tear breakup unlikely
- The breakup time may depend strongly on the initial tear film thickness

---

Tear film breakup mechanisms
(Box 16.2)

The presence of mucins on the corneal surface renders the surface hydrophilic, i.e., the surface energy of mucin-covered cornea surface is lower if it is in contact with water compared to the surface energy if it is in contact with air. In this scenario, the thin tear film is stable and so not likely to break, except by mechanisms that draw fluid out of the tear film such as evaporation. A number of researchers have measured evaporation rates from tear films, and under normal circumstances, the measured values are significantly lower than the lacrimal secretion.[24] However damage to the lipid layer can lead to a substantial increase in evaporation rates.[24,25]

Since the presence of a mucin-covered hydrophilic surface makes tear breakup unlikely, some researchers have speculated that destruction of the mucin layer is perhaps the first step in the breakup. Holly and Lemp[5] showed that the underlying corneal epithelium is extremely hydrophobic in the absence of coating mucus, but that mucus itself is highly wettable. In a series of papers, they proposed a mechanism in which lipids from the outer film layer diffuse rapidly through the aqueous layer and deposit on the mucous layer, converting it to a hydrophobic substrate.[3,26] However, a theoretical analysis of the fluid flow in the tear film shows that this mechanism is physically inconsistent.[27] Moreover the low solubility of lipids in tears makes the process of lipid deposition on the mucus unlikely.

Proposing an alternative mechanism, Lin and Brenner[28] conducted a theoretical analysis of the film under the influence of van der Waals dispersion forces. They calculated the minimum stable film thickness for a number of retarded Hamaker constant values and reported that by this method a minimum constant of 10^{-13} erg/cm would be necessary to break a 7-μm thick film. To rupture a 4-μm thick film in 50 seconds, their method requires the Hamaker constant to be about 3×10^{-13} erg/cm.[2] This constant, however, has been estimated to have a maximum value of about 10^{-19} erg/cm,

about 6 orders of magnitude smaller than that required by Lin and Brenner.[27] This mechanism thus appears to be insufficient to produce film breakup under physiological conditions in a reasonable time span.

Sharma and Ruckenstein[2] showed that the mechanism proposed by Lin and Brenner cannot produce breakup in a clinically consistent time span with a realistic Hamaker constant. As an alternative, they propose a double-layer, double-step mechanism for breakup.[2] In their mechanism, they initially neglected the aqueous layer in order to show rapid breakup of the mucin layer. They performed a stability analysis on the mucus–cornea system and established that the mucous layer can break locally due to van der Waals interactions with the underlying corneal epithelium. They calculated that this breakup can occur within time periods consistent with clinical observation (4–50 seconds) with a Hamaker constant they believed to be reasonable for this system (10^{-14} to 10^{-13} erg for a mucous layer thickness of 200–500 Å). They then cited experimental evidence to support a near-spontaneous aqueous film rupture once the mucous layer has been broken. However, their own stability analysis shows that in order for this breakup to occur within a reasonable time span, the retarded Hamaker constant for the cornea–aqueous layer system must be about 3×10^{-13} erg/cm, about six orders of magnitude larger than the estimated value of 10^{-19} erg/cm. A further mechanism is thus still necessary to break up a micrometers-thick aqueous film over such a substrate. The BUT predicted by this mechanism depends strongly on the initial TFT. If the starting film thickness is reduced to a fraction of a micron, the breakup may occur in a reasonable time for physiological Hamaker constants.

Recently, Zhu and Chauhan[29] have shown that an increase in evaporation rate or a decrease in tear production rate leads to thinner tear films. Also, a number of reports show a clear relationship between evaporation rates and dry eyes.[30] So it may be argued that dry-eye sufferers have significantly thin tear films, which makes them susceptible to tear breakup. However, clinical studies also show that there is no significant difference between volumes of dry-eye sufferers and normal subjects.[30] Furthermore, even if the thickness of the tear film in mathematical models is reduced to a fraction of a micron, breakup still does not occur in a few seconds, unless the Hamaker constant is artificially large. It should be noted that the TFT at the intersection of the meniscus and the tear film becomes very thin immediately after a blink. This thin region is commonly referred to as a "black line," and it has been suggested that the tear film breakup is initiated in this region.[30]

However, the tear breakup on dry-eye sufferers happens in other locations also, implying that the "black line" cannot be the main contributor to tear breakup. Most studies of thin film breakup have relied upon analysis of systems in which the tear film lies upon a uniform nonwetting surface. In reality, corneal surface is expected to be patchy with both physical and chemical heterogeneities. The chemical heterogeneities drive flow from the less wettable region to the more wettable region due to gradients in surface energies in a manner analogous to the Marangoni flow.[31] The growth rates of the instabilities driven by surface energy gradients can be significantly larger than those for homogeneous surface[32] and vary inversely as the potential difference (thickness or wettabilility differences) introduced by the heterogeneities.[33] Several papers have investigated the instabilities driven by physical heterogeneities as well as a combination of physical and chemical heterogeneities.[31-38] These studies listed above and others have demonstrated that both physical and chemical variations on a surface can have a significant impact on breakup of thin films. However, even after incorporating chemical and physical gradients, the value of Hamaker constant required to drive breakup in a few seconds is larger than 10^{-17} J, which is an unreasonably large value.

A complete description of the mechanisms that can lead to tear film breakup in reasonable times with physiologically reasonable parameters is still lacking. While none of the theories are able to explain all observations related to tear breakup, each provides useful insight into the process, and it is likely that the actual breakup is caused by a combination of all the factors and mechanisms cited above.

Future directions on the mechanism

Other mechanisms that could lead to thinning of the tear film are local evaporation and fluid flow driven by Marangoni gradients created by variations in lipid concentrations. With each blink, the lipid layer is largely wiped off the aqueous layer and deposited at the terminal area of the blink. Immediately after the blink, the lipids redistribute themselves across the eye due to the action of surface tension gradients (the Marangoni effect). This redistribution will carry with it some of the aqueous layer itself, causing deformation and localized thinning and thickening of the film. After the film has thinned due to the Marangoni flow, the breakup could be caused by the mechanisms proposed above. This mechanism of thinning driven by Marangoni gradients has not been sufficiently explored in the context of tear film breakup due to lipid spreading. Some researchers have reported observing lipid aggregates in dry-eye sufferers and images of breakup suggest that the breakup is initiated around these aggregates. This observation reinforces the importance of Marangoni gradients because it is feasible that the lipid aggregates provide a continuous source of lipids to the surface immediately surrounding the aggregates. The higher concentration of the lipids will reduce the surface tension, driving fluid flow away from the aggregates and causing film thinning and potential breakup.

Another potential breakup mechanism that has not received much attention is the possibility of nonuniform mucin deposition leading to hydrophobic patches on the cornea. During the blink, the coating on the hydrophobic patches may not be as thick as on the remaining cornea. In fact it is feasible that microbubbles may become trapped on the hydrophobic patches of the cornea, leading to rapid breakup after eye opening. The hydrophobic patches may be redistributed during the blinks, leading to variations in the locations of the breakup from blink to blink.

While the detailed mechanism that leads to tear breakup is not completely understood, it is clear that the quality and quantity of tears are the most important variables that have an impact on tear film disruption and breakup. Issues related to dynamics and tear film regulation are discussed below.

Box 16.3 Regulated tear dynamic system

- The tear system is a highly regulated dynamic system with the interaction between tears and blinking
- Constant tear renewal with high-quality fresh tears is essential to maintain the ocular surface wet during the interblink period
- Tear volume and distribution on the ocular surface alter by blinking

---

Dynamic tear system with regulation

The tear system is a highly regulated dynamic system with an interaction between tears and blinking (Box 16.3). The system includes tear secretion, distribution, drainage, absorption, and evaporation, with mostly a dynamic balance in healthy eyes. The dynamic balance is maintained with a certain amount of the tears on the ocular surface in three compartments: upper and lower tear menisci and precorneal tear film. The system is also kept balanced with tear renewal between fresh tears from the secretion and tear loss due to evaporation, drainage, and absorption. The constant tear renewal with high-quality fresh tears is essential to keep the ocular surface wet during the interblink period, so that sharp vision and ocular comfort are maintained. Each blink initiates a cycle of tear secretion, spreading and drainage of tears and evaporation, which happens immediately after eye opening.[23,39,40] Any alterations in blinking might affect the tear distribution, secretion, and drainage, leading to changes in the protection of the ocular surface. McDonald and Brubaker[41] demonstrated that upper and lower menisci draw fluid from the preocular tear film and swell with time after a blink. Slit-lamp photography[42] and video meniscometry[43-46] have also been used to measure the tear meniscus around the lower eyelid and changes in the dynamics were found.

These techniques have the disadvantage of using visible light and/or introducing fluorescein dye into the eye, which may induce reflex tearing and alter the test results. Most of these studies reported the static values of various lower tear meniscus parameters some time after blinking. Using real-time OCT, Wang et al imaged the tear film and tear menisci around the upper and lower eyelids simultaneously for the first time.[13] The changes in the tears impacted by blink were clearly visualized (Figure 16.1).[16] The device is a noncontact and noninvasive modality which has been validated with good repeatability for measuring the TFT and tear meniscus.[47] Using this method, the changes of TFT impacted by blinking and eye opening can be studied (Figure 16.2).[16] The effect of blinking on tear menisci can also be tracked (Figure 16.3).[16] Tear volume was found to be altered by blinking and the tear distributions with outcomes (gain or loss) during normal blinking and delayed blinking were reported previously (Figure 16.4).The relationship between TFT and tear menisci[47] and the changes in tear dynamics impacted by the blink after the instillation of artificial tears were studied.[20] The responses of the tear system to different artificial tears were also investigated, and different dynamic responses to different artificial tears were found.[48]

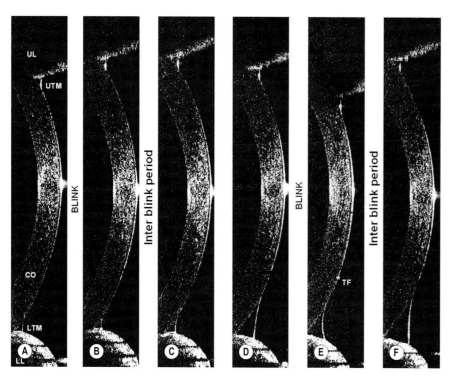

Figure 16.1 Optical coherence tomography (OCT) images obtained during normal and delayed blinks. A vertical 12-mm OCT scan was performed across the corneal apex during normal (A–C) and delayed (D–F) blinks. Images (A) and (D) were obtained immediately before blinks and images (B) and (E) were obtained immediately after blinks, at the beginning of the interblink period. Images (C) and (F) were obtained immediately before eye closure, at the end of the interblink period. Note the decrease of lower tear meniscus after blink (E compared to D), and increase at the end of eye opening (F) compared to the beginning of eye opening (E). Also note the less prominent changes in the upper tear meniscus compared to the lower tear meniscus (D–F). CO, cornea; UL, upper eyelid; LL, lower eyelid; TF, tear film (marked with an asterisk); UTM, upper tear meniscus; LTM, lower tear meniscus. (Reproduced with permission from Palakuru J, Wang J, Aquavella J. Effect of blinking on tear dynamics. Invest Ophthalmol Vis Sci 2007;48:3032–3037.)

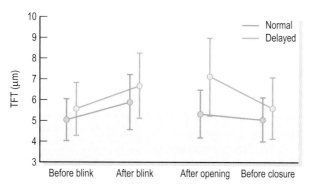

Figure 16.2 Changes in tear film thickness (TFT) during normal and delayed blinks in 21 subjects. Data were from 2 blinks and 1 interblink interval. TFT increased after blinks ($P < 0.05$) and decreased ($P < 0.05$) during the open-eye period. There were no significant differences between normal and delayed blinks ($P < 0.05$), though there was a trend of higher values during delayed blinks. Bars denote 95% confidence interval. (Redrawn with permission from Palakuru J, Wang J, Aquavella J. Effect of blinking on tear dynamics. Invest Ophthalmol Vis Sci 2007;48:3032–3037.)

> **Box 16.4 Effects of blinking on tear dynamics**
>
> - During normal blinking, the upper meniscus is smaller than the lower meniscus and neither showed significant changes with relation to blinking in healthy eyes
> - Tear film thickens after blinks and thins during open-eye periods

method and demonstrated thinning of the tear film during the open-eye period. They suggested that the rate of thinning may depend on the initial thickness of the tear film. Palakuru et al[16] found thickening of tear film after blinks and thinning during open-eye periods. The thinning rate was about 4.0 μm/min in this study.[16,50] During normal blinking, the upper meniscus is smaller than the lower meniscus and neither showed significant changes with relation to blinking.[16] This is strong evidence indicating a dynamic balance of the tear system in healthy adults.

Delayed blinking

When the blink is delayed, such as when the eye is intentionally held open for a longer time, the dynamics of the tear volume is altered due to reflex tearing and possibly decreased drainage, which was found to be dependent on blink frequency.[51] Changes in the lower tear meniscus over time occur during blinking.[17,46,52,53] Doughty et al[52] found there were no time-related changes of lower tear meniscus over 20 seconds in elderly Caucasians. However, in normal human eyes, during the delayed blink period, significant variations of the lower tear meniscus occur (Figure 16.4).[16] This difference may indicate the different dynamics between elderly and young healthy people. In elderly people, tear volume changes minimally during delayed blinking,[52] whereas young people may produce a lot of tears during the period

Effect of blinking on tear dynamics

Normal blinking

To ensure adequate wetting of the ocular surface, blinking causes a minimal change in tear volume on the ocular surface. With normal blinks, a full coverage of the ocular surface is maintained during the open-eye period, and the ocular surface is protected (Box 16.4). TFT varies over time, with thinning during interblink intervals and thickening after blinks (Figure 16.2).[16] Benedetto et al[49] used a fluorophotometric method and observed thinning of the tear film following a blink. Nichols et al[50] used an interferometric

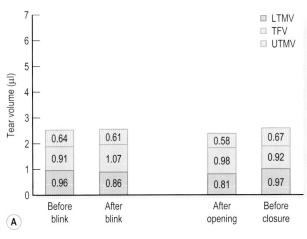
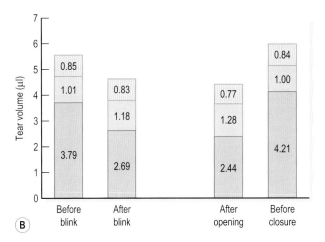

Figure 16.3 Total tear volume during normal and delayed blinks in 21 subjects. The upper tear meniscus volume (UTMV), tear film volume (TFV) and lower tear meniscus volume (LTMV) were estimated during normal (A) and delayed (B) blinking. The total tear volume was greater during delayed blinking compared to normal blinking ($P < 0.01$). Most of the change was due to increases in the LTMV (B). Both UTMV and LTMV were higher ($P < 0.001$) during delayed blinking (B) compared to normal blinking (A). The UTMV and LTMV increased significantly at the end of the open-eye period compared to the beginning during delayed blinking ($P < 0.05$). TFV, tear film volume; LTMV, lower tear meniscus volume; UTMV, upper tear meniscus volume. Note the different scales for upper (left) and lower (right) tear menisci. (Redrawn with permission from Palakuru J, Wang J, Aquavella J, Effect of blinking on tear dynamics. Invest Ophthalmol Vis Sci 2007;48:3032–3037.)

Box 16.5 Reflex tearing as an indicator of tear reserve

- Reflex tearing occurs during delayed blinking and may indicate a tear reserve
- The upper tear meniscus would not be able to hold much fluid
- The tears appear to travel from the upper tear meniscus to the lower tear meniscus through the canthi, rather than through the corneal surface

Box 16.6 Tear distribution and drainage

- The tear drainage system has a reserve capacity in removing excessive tears out of the eye
- The magnitude of the tear output due to blinking appears to be dependent on the total overloaded tear volume
- Great fluid redistribution occurs between the tear film and tear menisci when the system is overloaded

---

when the eye is held open, resulting in significant changes in the tear system (Figures 16.1–16.4).[16]

Reflex tearing may indicate a tear reserve (Box 16.5). Video recording showed the early postblink temporal changes of the lower and upper tear menisci in the 10 seconds following a blink in young adults.[53] The changes may be influenced by gravity, which moves the tears from the tear film to the lower tear meniscus, whereas few changes occur in the upper tear meniscus (Figure 16.4).[16] The results of the tearing may also be independent on the period when the eye is held open, since different observations of the changes in the tear menisci were reported.[16,53] If the eye was held open for about 10 seconds, as reported in the study of Johnson and Murphy,[53] similar changes were obtained between upper and lower tear menisci. If the eye was held open for longer, greater changes in the lower tear meniscus were evident, due to a large amount of tears added into the system and the limit of the upper tear meniscus.[16] The upper tear meniscus would not be able to hold much fluid. When the upper meniscus swells and the radius of curvature increases, the capillary pressure decreases to draw fluid towards the upper meniscus[41,42,54] and gravity exerts a significant effect to draw fluid down to the lower tear meniscus. The lower tear meniscus is capable of holding a large amount of fluid because of its structure, with the aid of the gravity. The rapid swelling of the lower tear meniscus during reflex

tearing, with small changes in the upper tear meniscus, indicates that both tear menisci are connected. The tears appear to travel from the upper tear meniscus to the lower tear meniscus through the canthi, rather than through the corneal surface. This may prevent visual blur during the eye-opening period if there is excessive tearing.

During delayed blinking, after a period of time with the eye open, tearing supplies additional volume to the ocular surface, most of which is in the lower tear meniscus (Figure 16.3).[20] However, tear film volume was found not to increase dramatically because the tears travel through the connection between the upper and lower eyelids.[16] Once the volume collected in the lower tear meniscus reaches a level, the tear film volume appears to increase after a blink.[16] This indicates that blinking is essential to spread tears from the menisci to the ocular surface.

Blinking with overloaded artificial tears

To keep a dynamic balance with a small amount of tears, the drainage system is thought to remove little fluid with each blink under normal circumstances (Box 16.6).[23] The phenomenon has been supported by the fact that there were no significant changes in tear volume in tear meniscus and tear film during normal blinking imaged with OCT.[16] While spreading during blinking and evaporation during

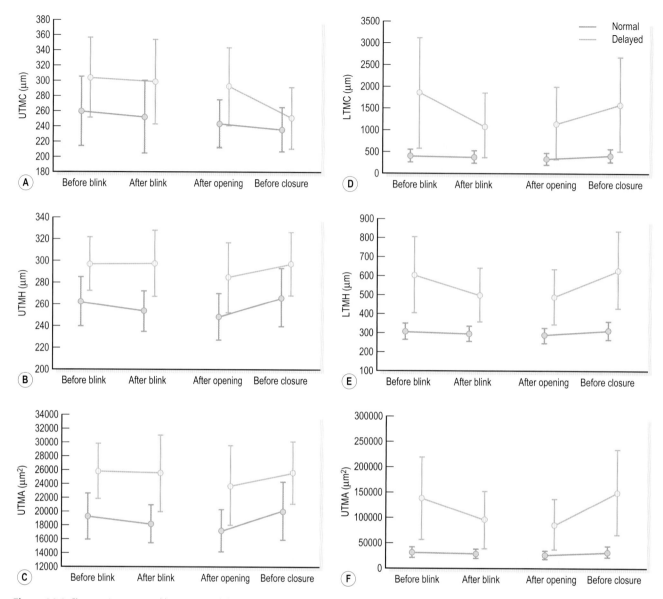

Figure 16.4 Changes in upper and lower menisci during normal and delayed blinks in 21 subjects. (A) Upper tear meniscus curvature (UTMC) before blinking was not significantly different from that after blinking during either normal or delayed blinks. Similarly, the UTMC did not change after eye opening and before the next closure for delayed or normal blinks. The upper tear meniscus height (UTMH: B) and upper tear meniscus area (UTMA: C) during delayed blinking were greater than the comparable values during normal blinking ($P < 0.005$). During the delayed blinking, the UTMH (B) and UTMA (C) increased during the open-eye period ($P < 0.005$). (D) Lower tear meniscus curvature (LTMC) before blinking was not significantly different from that after blinking during either normal or delayed blinking. Similarly, the LTMC (D) did not change significantly during the open-eye period. During delayed blinking, lower tear meniscus height (LTMH: E) was greater before blinking than that after blinking ($P < 0.05$). In contrast, during delayed blinking, LTMH (E) and lower tear meniscus area (LTMA: F) increased during the open-eye period ($P < 0.01$). Bars denote 95% confidence interval.

eye opening may cause variations in tear volumes in each compartment, it remains unknown how the surface keeps wet with such a small volume in a dynamic way. Clearly, the tear components and the ocular surface with its special structure like microvilli play a significant role. This mystery makes it complicated to restore the protection of the tears in dry-eye patients. The increase in tear volume within a short period of time may not be enough to protect the ocular surface from drying for a long time. The restoration of the tear system may be much more complex than had been thought.

The tear drainage system has a reserve capacity in removing excessive tears from the eye.[21,51,55,56] Zhu and Chauhan[55] calculated tear output and/or drainage rate due to blinking and found the rate increases by factors that ranged from 3 to 50 for overloaded tear volume. By repeated instillation of saline solution over a period of time, a blink output of 2 μl in the horizontal position and 4 μl in the upright position have been documented.[51,56] Using OCT, the blink output was found to be significantly increased during reflex tearing due to delayed blinking[21] and after instillation of drops.[20] Palakuru et al[20] found that the magnitudes of the tear output due to blinking appeared to depend on the total overloaded tear volume. More output due to blinking was found with higher tear volume.[20] Since the major tear volume was found in the lower tear meniscus, it can be hypothesized that the lower tear volume may regulate the drainage system that may be dependent on lower tear meniscus volume.

Although the tear film and the tear menisci are physically and functionally interconnected,[18,57] they appear to respond differently to blinking under different conditions, as shown in previous studies.[20,21] When limited tears were added continuously into the system, as occurs during delayed blinking, the lower tear meniscus swelled first while other compartments, including the tear film and the upper tear meniscus, remained relatively unchanged.[21] However, when a large amount of tears was added, as occurs when a drop is instilled, all compartments increased in volume, with the majority of the changes in the lower tear meniscus and tear film.[20] Under both conditions, blinking appears to play almost no role in upper tear meniscus volume since it remained almost unchanged. However, under the latter condition with excessive tears, blinking caused the increases in both upper tear meniscus and tear film volume. Under both conditions, blinking caused a decrease in lower tear volume, possibly mainly due to drainage and evaporation. Clearly, blinking induces fluid redistribution among compartments and activates the drainage system to remove excessive fluid. It is not clear about the role of evaporation during such a short period of the blink since no data are available in the literature. In addition to the loss of tears from the lower tear meniscus volume, the lower tear meniscus volume appears to supply fluid to the tear film and upper tear meniscus if excessive tears are present. A portion of the decrease in lower tear meniscus volume after a blink was found to be due to redistribution to the tear film and upper tear meniscus.[20]

With the limited tears available during delayed blinking, it appears that both upper and lower tear menisci provide fluid to the tear film.[21] This explains why tear loss from the lower tear meniscus was larger than that in total tear volume. However, the tear film volume may also depend on other sources. King-Smith et al[58] proposed that the TFT may also depend on the amount of fluid under the lid, and blinking causes deposition of the fluid. In a previous study,[19] TFT was increased when artificial tears were added into the lower tear meniscus. During the open-eye period, tear secretion, redistribution due to gravity, evaporation, and drainage occur. This period is of much greater duration than the blink itself, and most of the tear drainage may occur in the very first instant during the opening of the lid.

The tear volume during the open-eye period has been reported to be mainly influenced by tear secretion, evaporation, and absorption.[22] Redistribution of tears also affects the tear volume in different compartments.[22] The tear film begins to thin during the open-eye period.[50,58] This complex process involves mechanisms such as evaporation, dewetting, pressure gradient flow, Marangoni flow, and gravity.[50] Flow in the middle of the film has been suggested to be mediated by gravity which is proportional to the thickness of the tear film.[53] Thus the change in volume of the tear film during normal blinking could be negligible because of large flow resistances in thin films.[53] On the other hand, with thicker tear films, gravity may play a significant role in thinning.[53,59] Palakuru et al[16] found a significant reduction in TFT at the end of the open-eye period after drop instillation. The tear film was also found to be redistributed into the lower tear meniscus, most likely due to fluid flow.[20] The flow towards the lower tear meniscus appears to be aided by gravity

whereas the flow towards the upper tear meniscus goes against the force of gravity.[53] This explains the unequal changes in upper and lower tear menisci during the open-eye period. With a large amount of instilled tears, as tested in this study,[20] a greater decrease in tear film volume at the end of the open-eye period occurred compared with that during delayed blinking.[21] This indicates that great fluid redistribution occurs between the tear film and tear menisci when the system is overloaded. It appears that there is a threshold of total tear volume that is required to increase the tear film volume. Thus, TFT may not change when the total tear volume is less than approximately 5–7 μl.[20,21] Because normal tear volume is about 3 μl,[21] it may require doubling the production of tears to increase TFT, as shown during delayed blinking[21] and immediately after drop instillation.[20]

The tear film is a couple of microns thick and covers the entire ocular surface. Its integrity is maintained during eye opening between blinks and the ocular surface is protected. In healthy eyes, the long-lasting film is formed and renewed by spreading by the eyelid during blinking with supply from other compartments like tear menisci, secreted mainly from the lacrimal glands. If the breakup of the tear film occurs before the next blink, the ocular surface may be impaired, resulting in dry-eye symptoms. Many mechanisms have been proposed to resolve the puzzle of tear breakup. Clearly, the quality and quantity of the tears play roles and interaction between blinking and tears also has some impact on tear breakup. A balanced tear system needs to be maintained with a limited variation in tear volume and continuous renewal of the tear film. The tear film thins during eye opening and thickens after blinking. The thinning of the tear film may be the result of numerous factors, such as tear quality, tear volume, and blinking. Many factors can impact tear distribution on the ocular surface. The structures and locations (upper or lower) of the tear menisci determine the tear distribution during normal and delayed blinking. The upper lid may not hold much fluid and the lower lid can host a large amount of tears if excessive tears are present. Both the upper and lower tear menisci are connected through both canthi, during the open-eye period, and tears could travel through these connections without disturbing vision during eye opening. Blinking mixes and distributes the tears for a fresh and uniform tear film with no need for a large amount of tears.

In conclusion, the thin tear film on the ocular surface is essential for maintaining ocular health and sharp vision. The tear film forms and breaks during the blink cycle and blinking plays an important role. A minimal quality and quantity of tears appears to be necessary to form a long-lasting tear film. The blink dynamics and tear film breakup are intimately linked. The quality and/or quantity of tears are compromised; the tear film becomes susceptible to tear film breakup. Tear volume in both upper and lower tear menisci may regulate the TFT with the aid of blinking. When excessive tears are present, increased drainage capability takes action to remove the tears and restore the tear volume to a regular level. Reflex tearing may be an indicator of tear reserve and occurs during delayed blink. Upper and lower tear menisci are linked through both canthi to facilitate tears traveling in between without disturbing the vision. The detailed mechanism of tear breakup is not completely understood; further studies are needed to model the tear system with consideration of all impacting factors.

Key references

A complete list of chapter references is available online at www.expertconsult.com. See inside cover for registration details.

1. Dogru M, Ishida K, Matsumoto Y, et al. Strip meniscometry: a new and simple method of tear meniscus evaluation. Invest Ophthalmol Vis Sci 2006;47: 1895–1901.

2. Sharma A, Ruckenstein E. Mechanism of tear fiml rupture and formation of dry spots on cornea. J Colloid Interface Sci 1985;106:12–17.

3. Holly FJ, Lemp MA. Tear physiology and dry eyes. Surv Ophthalmol 1977;22:69–87.

4. Dohlman CH, Friend J, Kalevar V, et al. The glycoprotein (mucus)content of tears from normals and dry eye patients. Exp Eye Res 1976;22:359–365.

5. Holly F, Lemp M. Wettability and wetting of corneal epithelium. Exp Eye Res 1971;11:239–250.

6. King-Smith PE, Fink BA, Fogt N, et al. The thickness of the human precorneal tear film: evidence from reflection spectra. Invest Ophthalmol Vis Sci 2000;41:3348–3359.

12. Wang J, Fonn D, Simpson TL, et al. Precorneal and pre- and postlens tear film thickness measured indirectly with optical coherence tomography. Invest Ophthalmol Vis Sci 2003;44:2524–2528.

14. Mishima S, Gasset A, Klyce SD, et al. Determination of tear volume and tear flow. Invest Ophthalmol 1966;5:264–276.

15. Mathers WD, Lane JA, Zimmerman MB. Tear film changes associated with normal aging. Cornea 1996;15:229–234.

16. Palakuru J, Wang J, Aquavella J. Effect of blinking on tear dynamics. Invest Ophthalmol Vis Sci 2007;48:3032–3037.

22. Zhu H, Chauhan A. A mathematical model for ocular tear and solute balance. Curr Eye Res. 2005;30:841–854.

31. Konnur R, Kargupta K, Sharma A. Instability and morphology of thin liquid films on chemically heterogeneous substrates. Phys Rev Lett 2000;84:931–934.

45. Yokoi N, Bron AJ, Tiffany JM, et al. Relationship between tear volume and tear meniscus curvature. Arch Ophthalmol 2004;122:1265–1269.

50. Nichols JJ, Mitchell GL, King-Smith PE. Thinning rate of the precorneal and prelens tear films. Invest Ophthalmol Vis Sci 2005;46:2353–2361.

55. Zhu H, Chauhan A. A mathematical model for tear drainage through the canaliculi. Curr Eye Res 2005;30:621–630.

CHAPTER 17

Abnormalities of eyelid and tear film lipid

Gary N Foulks and Douglas Borchman

Clinical relevance of lipids in the tear film

Lipids play a critical role in the health of the eyelids and the tear film. Abnormalities of these lipids are common in the general population and provoke frequent disease manifested by clinical conditions of eyelid inflammation and tear film instability. Such conditions, although not life-threatening, cause considerable irritation to patients and interference with their quality of life. The most common clinical problems are meibomian gland disease (MGD) and dry-eye disease, but focal lesions of hordeola and chalazia are also often a nuisance.

Normal anatomy and production

Lipids are normally produced by the meibomian glands of the eyelid and the main and accessory lacrimal glands, as well as epithelial cells of the ocular surface. The lipids are distributed in five pools including within the eyelid, the eyelid margin, the surface of the tear film, within the aqueous layer of the tear film, and on the ocular surface.

Most of the lipid is thought to be produced by the meibomian glands of the eyelid, although contributions are also made by the main lacrimal gland, the glands of Wolfring, and the glands of Krause.[1] The meibomian glands are modified sebaceous glands, that is, tubuloacinar, holocrine glands whose acini discharge their entire contents in the process of secretion. They are distributed vertically in the substance of the tarsal plate of the eyelid with their openings on the eyelid margin just posterior to the eyelash follicles. There are about 30–40 glands in the upper eyelid and 20–30 glands in the lower eyelid.[2] Their secretion is conditioned by hormonal influences particularly of androgens with neural control by parasympathetic, sympathetic, and peptidergic innervations.[2-7]

It is estimated that there are over 30 000 molecular species of lipids in human meibum,[8] which complicates their quantification. The accuracy and precision of measurements of the lipid composition of meibum are also complicated by the large variation in composition from person to person,[9] and the paucity of sample.[10] Because of these complications, it is not surprising that the value reported for the predominant class of meibum lipid, esters, composes between 20 and 80% of the meibum.[9-11] There is also loose agreement on the composition of other meibum lipids; for instance, alkanes compose 0–36% of the meibum (Box 17.1).[9-11] In an older study using column chromatography, phospholipids constituted as much as 16% of meibomian gland secretions[10]; however, more sensitive mass spectroscopic techniques indicate that phospholipids are not present.[12] Of the total lipid hydrocarbon chains 58% are saturated. Most of the saturated hydrocarbon chains are in the form of sterol esters, which are 85% saturated.[10] The wax esters and triglycerides are the least saturated, at 22% and 38%, respectively.[10]

Chromatographic[13] and spectroscopic data[14,15] indicate major compositional differences between the lipids in tears and meibum. This is consistent with the compositional differences reported in the only comprehensive study of tear fluid lipids.[16]

Meibum normally has a melting point between 19 and 39°C.[17-20] At ambient lid temperature, the lipid is about 37% ordered, in between a solid (gel phase) and liquid (liquid crystalline phase; Box 17.2).[15] As the temperature increased from 25 to 45°C, lipid delivery to the margins was observed to increase.[21] Under similar conditions, other studies show a concomitant decrease in the refractive index,[22] hydrocarbon disorder,[15] and meibum lipid hydrocarbon motion.[14] This raises the possibility that hydrocarbon chain order and motion could contribute to the delivery of meibum lipid from the meibomian glands to the lid margins.

The function of the meibomian gland secretion is most importantly to retard evaporation of the tear film by distribution across the surface of the tear film. The secretions also function to provide a smooth optical surface for the cornea at the air–lipid interface, enhance stability of the tear film, enhance spreadability of the tear film, prevent contamination of the tear film by sebum of the cutaneous sebaceous glands, and to help seal the eyelid margin during eyelid closure (Table 17.1). Although the initial concept of the tear film as that of a three-layer structure of surface lipid layer, bulk aqueous layer, and ocular surface-wetting mucin layer has been replaced by the characterization of the tear film as a lipid-coated hydrated mucin gel with multiple interacting components of electrolyte, protein, and lipid entities, the

Box 17.1 Composition of meibum

Conflicting information[9,10]
>30 000 molecular species present[8]
Esters: 20–80%[9–11]
   Sterol esters 85% saturated[10]
   Wax esters 22% saturated[10]
   Triglycerides 38% unsaturated[10]
Alkanes: 0–36%[9–11]
Phospholipids: 0%[12]

Box 17.2 Properties of meibum

Melting point: 19–39°C[17–20]

At ambient lid temperature: 37% ordered lipid[15]

(in between gel phase and liquid crystalline phase)

As temperature increases:

- Delivery to eyelid margin increases
- Refractive index decreases
- Lipid becomes more disordered
- Lipid motion increases

Table 17.1 Functions of the meibomian gland lipid secretions

1.	Retard evaporation of the preocular tear film
2.	Maintain smooth optical surface of the eye at the air–lipid interface
3.	Enhance stability of the tear film
4.	Enhance spreadability of the tear film
5.	Prevent contamination of tear film by cutaneous sebum
6.	Seal the apposed margins of the eyelids during eyelid closure

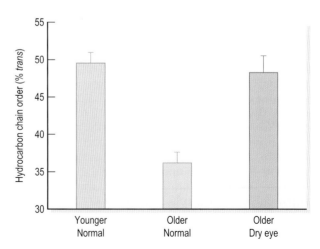

Figure 17.1 Fourier transform infrared demonstration of trans versus gauche rotamers of lipid conformation.

lipid component is still responsible for stability of the tear film and protection of the ocular surface.[23]

Changes occurring with age

The tear film is incredibly stable in infancy yet with advancing years such tear stability decreases. This progressive instability is associated with changes in the conformation of the lipids of the tear film and meibomian gland secretion. With increasing age, the ordering of the lipid changes from that of a more ordered conformation to that of a less ordered conformation as determined by Fourier transform infrared spectroscopy (FTIR) (Figures 17.1 and 17.2).[14,15] If the lipid disorder is maintained by the lipid on the tear film surface, lipid–lipid interactions would be weaker with increasing age (Box 17.3). Hence, the rate of evaporation would be expected to be greater since water escaping through the lipid layer would have to pass through lipid less tightly packed. Furthermore, if lipid–lipid interactions are weaker, one might expect that this could contribute to faster tear breakup times observed with age.

Figure 17.2 Lipid conformation changes occurring with age and meibomian gland dysfunction. as measured by Fourier transform infrared analysis.

> **Box 17.3 Changes of meibomian gland secretion with age**
>
> - More ordered conformation (trans) changes to less ordered conformation (gauche) (as measured by Fourier transform infrared (FTIR) spectroscopy (Figures 17.1 and 17.2)[14,15]
> - Decrease in ordering of lipid correlates with decreased tear film stability
> - Decrease in ordering of lipid correlates with increased tear evaporation

Lipid–protein interactions

Lipocalin, present in tears, is capable of sequestering cholesterol, fatty acids, glycolipids, and glycerophospholipids.[24] Lipid binding promotes protein conformational changes.[25] It has been proposed that lipocalin scavenges lipid from the corneal surface[26] and may enhance the transport and equilibration of lipid in the lipid surface layer. An in vitro fluorescent probe study[14] shows components in tears bind to the surface of tear film lipids. If similar interactions occur in vivo at the tear film lipid–aqueous interface, they would reduce the rate of evaporation. Mucins, lysozyme, lipocalin and other proteins present in tears could potentially bind to tear film surface lipids.

Changes occurring with disease

The most characteristic clinical change associated with lipid abnormalities of the eyelid and tear is tear film instability. Tear film instability is a hallmark feature of dry-eye disease as well as MGD.[27] Tear breakup time of less than 2–3 seconds often accompanies dry eye and MGD compared to normal tear breakup times of greater than 10–20 seconds. This functional disturbance seen in dry-eye disease can be due either to inadequate volume of secreted aqueous tear that is below that necessary to sustain the normal evaporative rate (aqueous-deficient dry eye), or to overly rapid evaporation of the tear film (evaporative dry eye). In the case of MGD, the functional disturbance of tear film instability is most likely due to increased evaporation of the tear film.[28,29]

In 18 of 20 patients with meibomian dysfunction, an infrared study showed lipid order (stiffness) increased (Figure 17.2). As discussed in the previous paragraph regarding lipid melting, stiffer meibum lipid could impede the flow of meibum, resulting in less lipid on the lid margin, creating a higher rate of tear evaporation (Box 17.4).

Specific abnormal polar lipids have been reported in meibum of patients with dry eye associated with meibomianitis by chromatography techniques, but the precise meaning of such findings is unclear, since subsequent mass spectroscopy studies have shown very little polar lipid in meibomian secretion.[12,30]

Clinical manifestation of disease: dry-eye disease and meibomian gland disease

The most common clinical manifestations of abnormality of the lipids in the eyelid and tear film are evaporative dry-eye

> **Box 17.4 Changes of meibomian gland secretion with disease**
>
> - Clinically, the most prominent change of the tear film is decreased stability
> - This decreased stability is associated with increased evaporation of tears
> - In 18 of 20 patients with meibomian dysfunction, infrared study showed lipid order (stiffness) increased in meibomian gland secretion (Figure 17.2)
> - In patients with meibomitis, breakdown of the more complex lipid structures (triglycerides) into diglycerides and increased free fatty acids proves irritative to the tissues and ocular surface[43]

> **Box 17.5 Categories of meibomian gland disease[2]**
>
> Congenital absence
> Dystichiasis
> Obstructive
>   Simple
>   Epithelial hypertrophic plugging
>   Inspissated meibomian secretion
>   Cicatricial
>   Postinflammatory
>   Medication-induced (13-*cis* retinoic acid; chlorobiphenyls)[44–48]
> Hypersecretory
>   Meibomian seborrhea
>   Rosacea

disease and MGD. Dry eye is etiopathologically categorized into aqueous production-deficient or evaporative dry eye.[27] The evaporative aspect of dry eye occurs in many dry-eye sufferers and the most common cause of evaporative dry eye is meibomian gland dysfunction.[2,27] Dry-eye disease has been documented by numerous epidemiological studies to affect 7–30% of the older (>55 years) population depending upon geographic location.[31] It is more frequent in women, particularly those who are postmenopause.[32]

Several clinical studies have identified MGD as a frequent problem in the general population, with prevalence at 39% of patients (Box 17.5). MGD occurs most frequently in older men but also affects postmenopausal women. MGD is often a major reason for discontinuing contact lens wear.[33–36]

The clinical characteristics of meibomian gland disease

MGD includes a broad spectrum of etiopathogenic events that are discussed in depth elsewhere.[2] Nonetheless a brief synopsis identifies the most common pathogenic events as obstructive, hypersecretory, infectious, inflammatory, or obliterative (Table 17.2). Obstructive disease can occur due to hypertrophy of the epithelium lining the orifice of the meibomian gland or due to inspissation of the secretion produced[2,37,38–40] (Figure 17.3). Clinical evaluation of the

Table 17.2 Classification of meibomian gland disease

Reduced number of glands: congenital absence or deficiency	
Replacement of glands: dystichiasis, metaplasia	
Meibomian gland dysfunction:	
Hyposecretory*	
Hypersecretory*	
Obstructive	
Simple	Cicatricial
Primary	
Epithelial proliferation	
Inspissated secretion	
Secondary	
Local disease	Chemical burns
Systemic disease	
Seborrheic dermatitis	
Rosacea	
Atopy	
Icthyosis	
Psoriasis	
Anhidrotic ectodermal dysplasia	
Ectrodactyly syndrome	
Turner syndrome	
Toxic	
13-*cis* retinoic acid	
Polychlorinated biphenols	
Epinephrine (rabbit)	
Other	
Internal hordeolum	
Chalazion	
Concretions	

Modified from Foulks GN, Bron AJ. Meibomian gland dysfunction: a clinical scheme for description, diagnosis, classification, and grading. Ocul Surf 2003;1:107–126.
*Conditions have not been validated clinically.

Box 17.6 Therapeutic options for meibomian gland disease[49]

Physical measures
    Heat application
    Massage of eyelids
Medicinal measures
  Antibiotics
    Tetracyclines (tetracycline, doxycycline, minocycline)
    Macrolides (azithromycin, erythromycin)
  Anti-inflammatory agents
    Corticosteroids
    Ciclosporin
    Macrolides (azithromycin)
Nutriceutical measures
    Omega-3 essential fatty acids
Hormonal measures
    Androgenic steroids

the complex lipids into more inflammation-provoking small digylcerides and free fatty acids (Figure 17.6).

Analysis of the lipid secretion during active inflammation of the eyelid (blepharitis or meibomianitis) has revealed breakdown of the more complex lipid structures (triglycerides) into diglycerides and increased free fatty acids that prove irritative to the tissues and ocular surface.[43] This breakdown can occur both due to the presence of lipase enzymes of colonizing bacteria and due to tissue lipases associated with inflammation.

Less common but very important pathophysiology that is productive of MGD is obliteration of the glandular tissue. This occurs primarily by toxicity to external agents or cicatrization of the tissue due to longstanding inflammation. The most notable toxins are 13-*cis* retinoic acid (Accutane) or exposure to chlorobiphenyl chemicals.[44–48] Loss of meibomian gland structure is visible with transillumination of the eyelid and persistent dry-eye irritation is a consequence of the toxic exposure.

Therapeutic implications

Attempts to treat clinical disease of the meibomian glands include physical, medicinal, nutritional, and hormonal measures[49] (Box 17.6). Physical treatment options include thermal and mechanical techniques designed to express inspissated secretions and thus relieve meibomian gland congestion. The simplest physical method is application of a warm compress to the eyelids followed by mechanical lid massage to express the melted secretions. The lipid secretions vary in melting temperature, but application of external heat increases the flow of the secretion from the glands and provides comfort.[50] Although effective in melting and expressing secretions when done properly in most cases, this therapy depends entirely upon patient understanding and compliance. It is helpful to reinforce the demonstration of the proper technique with a patient handout summarizing the disease concepts and the massage techniques. If self-treatment fails to relieve meibomian gland congestion and

abnormal secretions is usefully described as clear, turbid, turbid with clumps, or solid (paste-like).[2] Associated inflammatory changes include telangiectasis of the eyelid margin or more severe changes of notching, dimpling, or scarring of the eyelid margin if the disease has been chronic (Figure 17.4). Since the meibomian eyelid secretions are a rich cholesterol-containing culture medium for bacteria, stasis of the secretions can be accompanied by bacterial superinfection, most commonly by *Staphylococcus* species.[41,42] Such focal infections can produce hordeola (styes) of the eyelid with associated swelling, erythema, and pain (Figure 17.5). A more chronic inflammation due to the stasis of the lipid secretion in the meibomian glands is a lipogranulomatous reaction (chalazion) that is probably due to breakdown of

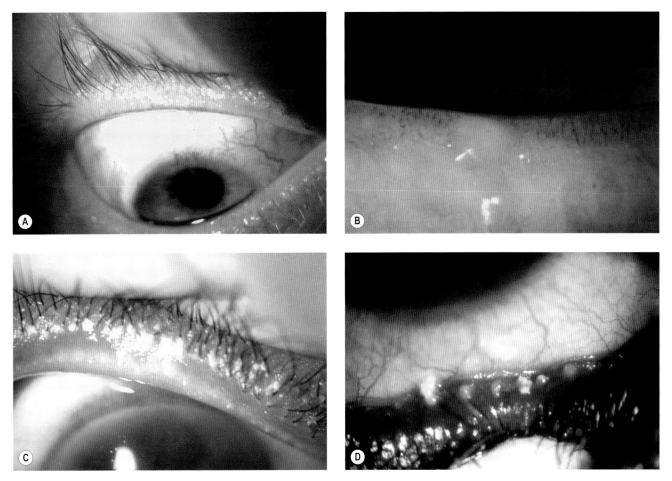

Figure 17.3 Character of stages of abnormal meibomian gland disease secretions: (A) clear; (B) turbid; (C) turbid with clumps; (D) solid (paste-like). (Reproduced with permission from Foulks GN, Bron A. Meibomian gland dysfunction: a clinical scheme for description, diagnosis, classification, and grading. Ocular Surf 2003;1:107–126.)

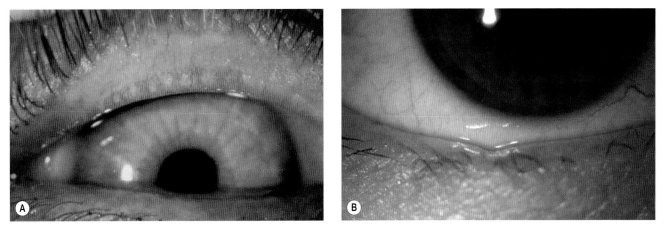

Figure 17.4 (A) Eyelid margin telangiectasia; (B) eyelid margin notching due to chronic meibomian gland disease.

plugging of the orifices persists, the ophthalmologist can express the secretions in the office by compressing the eyelid between two cotton-tipped applicators. Topical anesthetic drops should first be instilled into the conjunctival cul-de-sac for patient comfort. This in-office maneuver may open the gland orifices and facilitate the efficacy of the patient's efforts.

When physical measures alone are not effective in controlling the disease, systemic treatment with oral antibiotics is usually the next option. The tetracycline family of drugs is the most used and most effective since there is not only an antibacterial effect on any infecting organisms, but also the calcium and magnesium-chelating properties of the drug inhibit the lipolytic enzymes that break down the complex

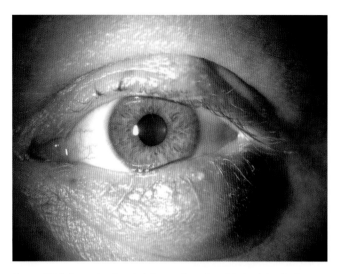

Figure 17.5 Example of acute inflammation of eyelid gland: hordeolum.

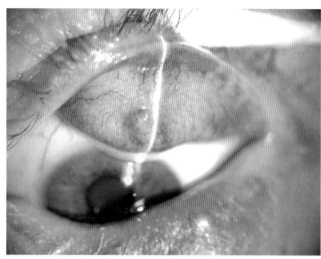

Figure 17.6 Example of chronic inflammation of meibomian gland of eyelid: chalazion.

lipids into the more inflammatory diglycerides and fatty acids. Bacterial lipolytic exoenzymes such as triglyceride lipase, and fatty wax and cholesteryl esterases can contribute to breakdown of the normal meibum's complex lipids into potentially inflammatory smaller free fatty acid fragments. Dougherty et al[51,52] demonstrated that S. aureus, coagulase-negative staphylococci, and Propionibacterium acnes all produce such enzymes, and that similar secretional lipid profile abnormalities occur in patients with blepharitis or meibomianitis in which coagulase-negative staphylococci predominate.

Attempts to use topical measures to stabilize the tear film while other treatment modalities are in progress include over-the-counter formulations that include lipid emulsions. Refresh Endura (Allergan, Irvine, CA) has been shown to prolong tear breakup time, as has a metastable emulsion, Soothe (Bausch & Lomb, Rochester, NY).[53,54] Another lipid-containing formulation, Freshkote (Focus Laboratories, North Little Rock, AR) has been reported to improve symptoms in dry-eye patients.

Systemic therapy with antibiotics such as tetracycline, doxycycline, and minocycline reduces meibomian gland inflammation and the associated symptoms of ocular irritation.[51] Tetracycline has been shown to decrease S. epidermidis lipase activity in vitro, and it is thought that its related compounds act similarly. Such treatment can return the lipid profile of the meibomian secretion to a more normal composition.[43]

Omega-3 essential fatty acid supplements have been advocated for treatment of chronic MGD.[55] Limited small studies have been completed but such supplements have been shown to improve symptoms in patients with dry eye.[56] The active components of these preparations are probably linolenic acid and its congeners. This family of essential fatty acids provides the building blocks for the prostaglandins that modulate tissue inflammation. These essential fatty acids have been shown in other tissue systems to reduce inflammation and exert beneficial effects on vascular, cardiac, and other physiologic functions.[57] Linoleic and oleic acids, unsaturated fatty acids, have been shown to inhibit keratinocyte proliferation

and are present in normal human meibomian secretions.[58] Although no controlled clinical trials have validated the efficacy of fatty acid supplements for control of meibomian gland dysfunction, a pilot study of 8 patients with refractory meibomitis who received dietary supplements of linoleic and linolenic fatty acids showed improved clinical symptoms, despite only minimal improvement in the slit-lamp appearance of the meibomian glands.[44] This symptomatic improvement could be attributed to the supplements' anti-inflammatory and antikeratinizing effects, but controlled trials are necessary to validate this hypothesis.

Control of inflammation associated with MGD can be achieved with topical corticosteroids and topical ciclosporin.[59,60] The chronic use of corticosteroids is to be avoided given the risks of cataract and glaucoma, but topical ciclosporin has been used safely for prolonged periods.

Given the evidence that decreased androgenic hormonal influence on meibomian gland secretion and inflammation may result in disease, supplementation of androgen by topical administration has been advocated.[4-7] Application of topical testosterone to the external eyelid skin has been reported to improve symptoms of dry eye and such improvement could be a sign of stimulation of meibomian gland function.[61] Controlled clinical trials will be needed to verify such a beneficial effect.

Future research and management

The 2007 Report of the International Dry Eye Workshop[62] has identified a need for additional information about the biology of ductal keratinization in MGD as well as more detailed information about the structure and function of the lipid layer in the tear film. The powerful techniques of fluorescence, FTIR, nuclear magnetic resonance, and mass spectroscopies argue in favor of a better understanding of the composition, structure, and function of meibomian gland lipids and the lipids of the tear film. Our understanding of the age-related changes and changes occurring with disease will increase our ability to manage and treat the disease.

Conclusion

Lipids play an important role in the stability of the tears and the health of the eyelid margin. Interactions of the lipids with proteins such as mucin and lipocalin in the tear film provide additional stabilization of the tear film, in addition to limitation of evaporation of the tear film. Disease of the glands of the eyelid margin is a common clinical problem associated with compositional and functional changes of the lipids produced by the glands of the eyelid margin. Our understanding of the composition, structure, and function of the lipids helps explain the behavior of the lipids and their response to changes in temperature.

The implications of the structure and function of lipid behavior to therapy of eyelid margin disease and dry eye are important both to direct clinical treatment and also to develop better medications to control those diseases.

Key references

A complete list of chapter references is available online at www.expertconsult.com. See inside cover for registration details.

2. Foulks GN, Bron AJ. Meibomian gland dysfunction: a clinical scheme for description, diagnosis, classification, and grading. Ocular Surf 2003;1:107–126.

7. Sullivan DA, Sullivan BD, Evans JE, et al. Androgen deficiency, meibomian gland dysfunction, and evaporative dry eye. Ann NY Acad Sci 2002;966:211–222.

9. Tiffany JM. Individual variations in human meibomian lipid composition. Exp Eye Res 1978;27:289–300.

10. Nicolaides N, Kaitaranta JK, Rawdah TN, et al. Meibomian gland studies: comparison of steer and human lipids. Invest Ophthalmol Vis Sci 1981;20:522–536.

12. Butovich IA, Uchiyama E, McCulley JP. Lipids of human meibum: mass-spectrometric analysis and structural elucidation. J Lipid Res 2007;48:2220–2235.

14. Borchman D, Foulks GN, Yappert MC, et al. Spectroscopic evaluation of human tear lipids. Chem Phys Lipids 2007;147:87–102.

15. Borchman D, Foulks GN, Yappert MC, et al. Temperature-induced conformational changes in human tearlipids hydrocarbon chains. Biopolymers 2007;87:124–133.

21. Nagymihalyi A, Dikstein S, Tiffany JM. The influence of eyelid temperature on the delivery of meibomian oil. Exp Eye Res 2004;78:367–370.

26. Glasgow BJ, Marshall G, Gasymov OK, et al. Tear lipocalins: potential lipid scavengers for the corneal surface. Invest Ophthalmol Vis Sci 1999;40:3100–3107.

29. Mathers WD, Lane JA. Meibomian gland lipids, evaporation, and tear film stability. Adv Exp Med Biol 1998;438:349–360.

30. Shine WE, McCulley JP. Meibomianitis: polar lipid abnormalities. Cornea 2004;23:781–783.

35. Ong BL, Larake JR. Meibomian gland dysfunction: some clinical, biochemical and physical observations. Ophthalm Physiol Opt 1990;10:144–148.

39. Jester JV, Nicolaides N, Kiss-Polvolgyi I, et al. Meibomian gland dysfunction II. The role of keratinization in a rabbit model of MGD. Invest Ophthalmol Vis Sci 1989;30:936–945.

43. McCulley JP, Shine WE. Changing concepts in the diagnosis and management of blepharitis. Cornea 2000;19:650–658.

51. Dougherty JM, McCulley JP, Silvany RE, et al. The role of tetracycline in chronic blepharitis. Inhibition of lipase production in staphylococci. Invest Ophthal Vis Sci 1991;32:2970–2975.

CHAPTER 18

Dry eye: abnormalities of tear film mucins

Ann-Christin Albertsmeyer and Ilene K Gipson

In 2007, the *Report of the International Dry Eye Workshop* (DEWS)[1] defined dry eye as "a multifactorial disease of the tears and ocular surface that results in symptoms of discomfort, visual disturbance, and tear film instability, with potential damage to the ocular surface. It is accompanied by increased osmolarity of the tear film and inflammation of the ocular surface." The comprehensive DEWS report summarizes the current knowledge of the disease, its classification, symptoms and signs, epidemiology, diagnostic methods, and management and therapy. Research into dry eye is also summarized, and a hypothesis as to the mechanisms of dry eye is put forward (Figure 18.1). As indicated in Figure 18.1, mucin loss from the tear film and the ocular surface glycocalyx is proposed to be a core mechanism of the disease. This chapter will describe current understandings of the ocular surface and tear mucins – focusing on their character, origins, and alterations in drying eye diseases – as well as therapeutics targeted toward mucin restoration.

The Ocular Surface System

The tear film is essential for vision, functioning to maintain hydration and lubrication of the surface of the eye and to provide the major refractive surface for the visual system. The tear film is composed of many products, all produced by the epithelia of the Ocular Surface System[2,3]; these include water, protective antimicrobials, cytokines, lipids, and mucins (Box 18.1).

The Ocular Surface System is responsible for producing and maintaining the all-important tear film on the surface of the cornea (Figure 18.2). The system includes the surface or glandular epithelia of the cornea, conjunctiva, lacrimal glands, accessory lacrimal glands and meibomian glands, the nasolacrimal duct, as well as the eyelashes, with their associated glands of Moll and Zeis. Also included are the extracellular matrices and their resident cells, which underlie the epithelia, the vasculature, and migrating immune system cells, which survey the tissues. All components of the system are integrated functionally by continuity of the epithelia, by innervation from the trigeminal nerves, and by the endocrine, vascular, and immune systems.[2]

The rationale for the concept of "the Ocular Surface System" is that *all* regions of the epithelia are derived from the surface ectoderm, that each region is continuous with another, and that all regions produce components of the tear film. For example, the hydrophilic mucins, responsible for holding tears on the surface of the eye, are products of the conjunctival and corneal epithelia. Water and protective proteins are secreted by the epithelia of the lacrimal and accessory lacrimal glands, and the superficial lipid layer, which prevents tear evaporation, is provided by the epithelia of the meibomian glands.[2] When one or more components of the system is defective, the normal function of the ocular surface tear film is disrupted, which can result in chronic dry-eye disease and, at end stage, loss of the tear film with keratinization of the epithelia.

The early hypothesis of tear film structure separated the several secreted components into different layers: the lipid, aqueous, and mucin layers. While it is known that the superficial lipid layer, a product of the meibomian glands, is a distinct layer at the tear surface, recent data suggest that the aqueous tears are a mixture of lacrimal fluid and soluble mucins, without a distinct mucin layer (Figure 18.3).[4] The interface between the tear film and the corneal and conjunctival epithelia is composed of the hydrophilic and heavily glycosylated glycocalyx, a major component of which is membrane- or cell surface-associated mucins (MAMs).

Mucins expressed by the ocular surface epithelium

Mucins are high-molecular-weight glycoproteins. The common features of the 20 mucin gene products known to date are: (1) the presence of tandem repeats of amino acids, in their protein backbone, that have high levels of serine, threonine, and proline – with the serines and threonines being sites for O-glycan attachment; and (2) a major portion of mass of mucin molecules being made up of O-linked carbohydrate (Box 18.2).[5] The heavy glycosylation of mucins gives molecules of this class their hydrophilic, lubricating character.

As indicated above, two types of mucins have been identified: secreted and cell-associated or membrane spanning. To date, 7 mucins have been described as secreted mucins and 10 as membrane-associated; several mucins remain uncharacterized as to type. Human mucins have been designated in

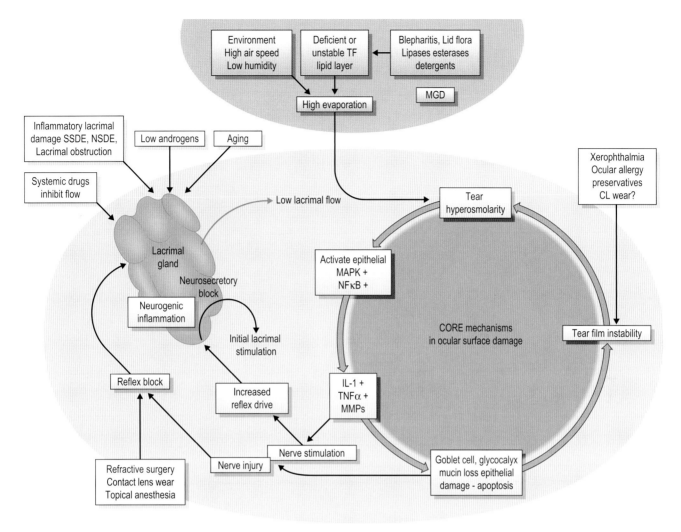

Figure 18.1 Diagram proposing multifactorial mechanisms of dry eye. The core mechanisms are those that are involved in the ocular surface epithelial damage that causes dry-eye symptoms. Central to the core mechanism is tear hyperosmolarity, caused by high evaporation or low lacrimal fluid flow. Tear hyperosmolarity causes damage, pursuant inflammatory responses and/or loss of surface mucins. Loss of mucins in turn causes tear film instability. Damage to the ocular surface epithelium can be the cause of nerve stimulation that results in a cascade of effects to the ocular surface system (see Figure 18.2). Several etiologies can cause tear hyperosmolarity through evaporation or low tear fluid. These include meibomian gland disease (MGD), environmental factors, aging, inflammation and contact lens (CL) wear. TF, tear film; SSDE, Sjögren's syndrome dry eye; NSDE, non-Sjögren's dry eye; MAPK, mitogen-activated protein kinase; IL-1, interleukin-1; TNF-α, tumor necrosis factor-α; MMPs, matrix metalloproteinases. For a complete description of the mechanisms of dry eye, see the 2007 Report of the International Dry Eye WorkShop.[3] (Modified from Research in dry eye: report of the Research Subcommittee of the International Dry Eye WorkShop. Report of the International Dry Eye WorkShop (DEWS). Ocul Surf 2007;5:75–92. © Ethis Communications (2007).)

Box 18.1 The Ocular Surface System

The Ocular Surface System is responsible for producing and maintaining the all-important tear film on the surface of the cornea. The tear film is essential for vision, functioning to maintain hydration and lubrication of the surface of the eye, and to provide the major refractive surface for the visual system. All components of the system are integrated functionally by continuity of the epithelia, by innervation from the trigeminal nerves, and by the endocrine, vascular, and immune systems

Box 18.2 Mucins expressed by the ocular surface epithelium

The high-molecular-weight glycoproteins, known as mucins, share two common features: (1) the presence of tandem repeats of amino acids in their protein backbone that have high levels of serine, threonine, and proline – with the serines and threonines being sites for O-glycan attachment; and (2) a mass primarily made up of O-linked carbohydrates. Two types of mucins have been identified: secreted, and membrane-associated or membrane-spanning. Of the 20 mucins identified to date, 7 have been described as secreted and 10 as membrane-associated; several mucins remain uncharacterized as to type. Mucins are named in order of their characterization – MUC1, MUC2, etc. The ocular surface epithelia express mucins of both types. The major mucin of the conjunctival goblet cell is the secreted mucin MUC5AC. Three major membrane mucins expressed by the ocular surface epithelia include MUCs 1, 4, and 16

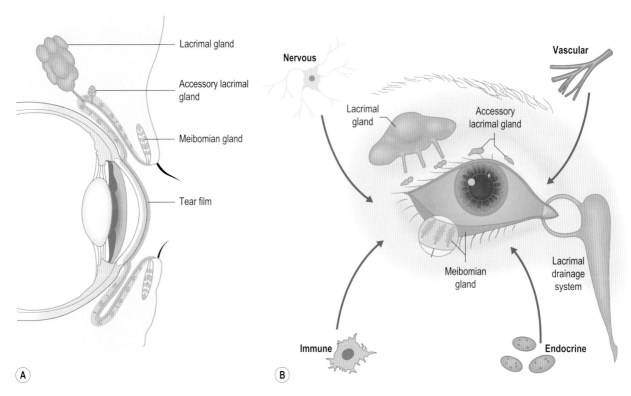

Figure 18.2 Diagrams depicting the Ocular Surface System. (A) A diagram of a sagittal section through the eye demonstrates the continuity of the ocular surface epithelium (pink). Regional specialization in the continuous epithelia includes the meibomian gland, conjunctiva, lacrimal glands, and corneal epithelia. Each region of the ocular surface epithelium contributes components to the tear film (blue). The frontal diagram of the eye (B) demonstrates the components of the ocular system. The function of the different components of the system is integrated by the nerves, the vascular system, as well as the immune and endocrine systems. (Modified from Gipson IK. The ocular surface: the challenge to enable and protect vision: the Friedenwald lecture. Invest Ophthalmol Vis Sci 2007;48:4390–4398. © The Association for Research in Vision and Ophthalmology (2007).)

order of discovery as MUC1, -2, -3, etc., with mouse homologs designated Muc1, -2, etc.

Secreted mucins

Of the secreted mucins, two types have been characterized: the so-called large, gel-forming mucins and the small, soluble mucins (one of each type is expressed by the ocular surface epithelia). The large, gel-forming mucins include MUCs 2, 5AC, 5B, 6, and 19, and the smaller, soluble mucins MUCs 7 and 9.

The five large mucins are termed gel-forming because they are responsible for the rheological properties of mucus. They share common structural motifs, including cysteine-rich, von Willebrand factor-like D domains at the amino terminal and carboxy termini that allow intermolecular associations among mucins of the same gene product. They are encoded by the largest genes known (15.7–17 kb), and their deduced proteins are at least 600 kDa. These gel-forming mucins are expressed by the goblet cells of the conjunctival, respiratory, gastrointestinal, and endocervical epithelia. However, there is a tissue- and cell-specific pattern of expression of specific mucins. The major mucin of this class expressed by the goblet cells of the conjunctiva is MUC5AC (Figure 18.4).[6] For a complete description of the structure of MUC5AC, see Gipson and Argüeso[7] and Gipson.[4]

The second category of secreted mucins, small soluble mucins, includes MUC7 and MUC9, which are present pre-dominantly as monomeric species and lack cysteine-rich D domains. MUC7 is produced by lacrimal gland epithelia,[8] but MUC7 is not present in the tear film.[9]

Membrane-associated mucins

The 10 mucins that have been categorized as cell MAMs include MUCs 1, 3A, 3B, 4, 12, 13, 15 16, 17, and 20. Mucins of this type are present on all the wet-surfaced epithelia of the body. All MAMs have a short cytoplasmic tail, and the majority have a large, extended extracellular domain, also known as the ectodomain, which is formed by heavily O-glycosylated tandem repeats of amino acids. The ectodomains may extend 200–500 nm from the cell surface and comprise a major portion of the glycocalyx. The ectodomain functions as a protective, disadhesive surface, preventing cell and pathogen adherence.[10] Ectodomains of MAMs are found in fluids at the surface of wet-surfaced, mucosal epithelia, including the tear film. The ectodomains are proteolytically cleaved or released from the apical membranes, giving rise to the soluble form, or in some instances (particularly MUC1), the soluble form may be a result of splice variants that lack the membrane-spanning domain.[4]

MUC1, MUC4, and MUC16 are MAMs that are expressed by ocular surface epithelia (Figure 18.5). MUC1 mRNA is expressed by all the epithelia of the Ocular Surface System. The protein is expressed in apical surface cells of the corneal epithelium and in apical and subapical cells of the

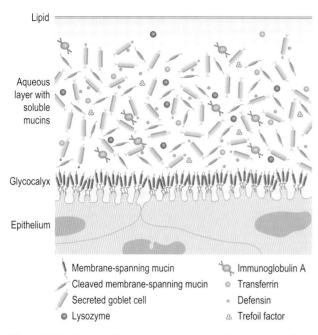

Membrane-spanning mucin
Cleaved membrane-spanning mucin
Secreted goblet cell
Lysozyme
Immunoglobulin A
Transferrin
Defensin
Trefoil factor

Figure 18.3 Diagram of the structure and composition of the tear film and the apical surface of the cornea, with emphasis on the mucin components. Goblet cell mucin MUC5AC is shown as being soluble in the tear fluid rather than as a distinct layer beneath the aqueous layer, as previously described (for review, see Gipson and Argüeso[7]). The membrane-spanning mucins form the glycocalyx at the tear–epithelial interface, where they form a hydrated, lubricating barrier that also prevents pathogen adherence. These membrane-spanning mucins are tethered to the tips of the surface membrane ridges, termed microplicae (see Figure 18.6). (Modified from Gipson IK. The ocular surface: the challenge to enable and protect vision: the Friedenwald lecture. Invest Ophthalmol Vis Sci 2007;48:4390–4398. © The Association for Research in Vision and Ophthalmology (2007).)

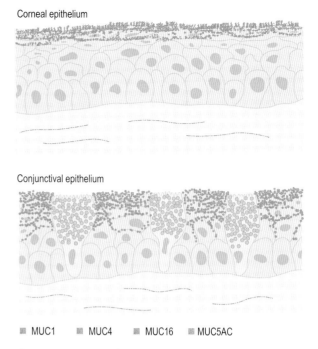

MUC1   MUC4   MUC16   MUC5AC

Figure 18.4 Diagram of sections of corneal and conjunctival epithelia demonstrating cellular localization of mucin expression. The apical cells of the stratified corneal and conjunctival epithelium express three membrane-associated mucins: MUC1, MUC4, and MUC16. These membrane-tethered mucins provide a barrier to protect the ocular surface against pathogen invasion and provide a hydrating, lubricating surface. The conjunctival epithelium also has interspersed within it goblet cells that produce the large mucin MUC5AC. MUC5AC is secreted into the tear film. The lids move the soluble mucin over the surface of the eye to trap and remove foreign debris. (Modified from Gipson IK. Distribution of mucins at the ocular surface. Exp Eye Res 2004;78:379–388. © Elsevier (2004).)

conjunctival epithelium.[4] MUC4 protein is most prevalent in conjunctival epithelium with a diminished amount in the cornea. MUC16 protein is present in apical cells of corneal epithelia and in apical and subapical cells of conjunctival epithelia.[4] The membrane mucins, MUCs 1, 4, and 16, are considered to be multifunctional molecules, with the glycosylated region of their ectodomain serving to prevent adhesion of cells/pathogens, and their juxtamembrane region and cytoplasmic tail serving additional functions. In studies of nonocular epithelia, MUC1 has signaling capabilities through its cytoplasmic tail, and MUC4 has been shown to have an epidermal growth factor (EGF)-like domain present extracellularly near its membrane-spanning domain.[4] Studies of MUC16 function in human corneal epithelial cells have shown that it provides a disadhesive, protective barrier to the epithelial membrane, since, in siRNA knockdown experiments, the binding of *Staphylococcus aureus* was significantly increased with MUC16 suppression.[11] Knockdown of MUC16 also allows penetrance of rose Bengal dye, a dye that is used in the diagnosis of dry eye.[11] MUC16 is especially prevalent on the tips of microplicae at the tear film interface, and its cytoplasmic tail is linked to the actin cytoskeleton through a class of linker molecules known as ERMs (Figure 18.6).[11]

Through their hydrophilic carbohydrates, membrane mucins hold water on the cell membrane to provide surface hydration on the eye as well as build an antiadhesive surface for the movement of secreted mucins across the ocular surface during the blink. The fact that there are several mucins of this class present at the tear film interface indicates their importance in protection and hydration of the ocular surface.

Detection of mucins in tear fluid

Tear fluid contains, in addition to the secreted goblet cell mucin MUC5AC, ectodomains of the MAMs MUCs 1, 4, and 16.[9] To measure and detect levels of MUC5AC in tears, an enzyme-linked immunosorbent assay (ELISA) was developed using antibodies specific to the N-terminal domain of MUC5AC. Pretreatment of tear proteins with neuraminidase to remove terminal sugars enhanced antibody binding.[12] Within an individual, the level of MUC5AC is consistent over several samples, but there is variation among individuals in amount of MUC5AC in tears. MUC5AC in tears can also be assayed by immunoblot analysis of tear proteins separated on agarose gels.[9] Low levels of gel-forming mucin MUC2 RNA and protein have also been detected in conjunctival RNA[13] and tears,[9] respectively, but the cellular source of the mucin is unknown. The amount of ectodomains of the MAMs in tears, MUCs 1, 4 and 16, also varies among individuals, with MUC16 being the most prevalent.

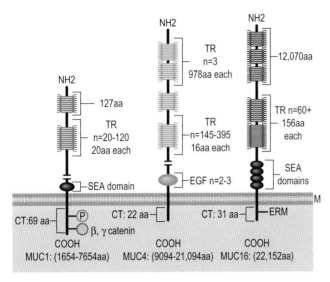

Figure 18.5 Diagram showing the structural motifs within the three membrane-associated mucins expressed by the ocular surface epithelia. A common characteristic of all mucins is the presence of a large ectodomain at the amino terminus (NH_2) that has a variable number (n) of tandem repeats (TR) of amino acids rich in serine and threonine that are highly O-glycosylated ($\curlyvee$). Each has a membrane-spanning domain (M) and a short cytoplasmic tail (CT) at the carboxy terminus (COOH). MUC1 CT has 69 amino acids, phosphorylation sites (P) and a β, γ catenin-binding site. MUC4 has several epidermal-like growth factor (EGF)-like domains in the ectodomain area near the membrane. MUC16 has several sea urchin, enterokinase, agrin (SEA) module domains in the ectodomain (MUC1 has only one) near the membrane, and its CT has an ERM-binding domain that links it to the actin cytoskeleton.

Alteration of mucins in ocular surface diseases

Dry eye

Characteristic symptoms of dry-eye syndrome are stinging, burning, or foreign-body sensation. These symptoms are ascribed to the fact that either there are not enough tears to keep the surface wet and comfortable, or that tears are not being retained at the ocular surface. The absence and alteration of mucins, which are especially responsible for retaining water/tears at the ocular surface, is considered one of the core mechanisms of dry eye (Figure 18.1; Box 18.3).[3] The current understanding of mucin character and patterns of expression at the ocular surface, and the development of assay methodologies, make it possible to measure specific mucins in patients with drying ocular surface diseases. The variation in mucins in patients with dry eye ranges from a decreased number of goblet cells in the conjunctival epithelium, with concomitant alteration in the amount of MUC5AC mucin mRNA and protein, to alteration in distribution and/or glycosylation of MAMs.

Decreased goblet cells and levels of goblet-cell-associated mucin MUC5AC

It has long been known that goblet cells are lost in the conjunctival epithelium in severe dry eye, such as that in

Box 18.3 Alteration of mucins in ocular surface epithelium

Dry-eye syndrome, perhaps the most common of the ocular surface diseases, is characterized by stinging, burning, or foreign-body sensation – symptoms ascribed to the fact that either there are not enough tears to keep the surface wet and comfortable, or that tears are not being retained at the ocular surface. Current understanding of mucin character and patterns of expression at the ocular surface, as well as the development of assay methodologies, makes it possible to measure specific variation in mucins in patients with dry eye. Studies of mucins in dry eye suggest that there is an alteration in amount of secreted mucin on the ocular surface, and either alteration in amount or glycosylation of membrane-associated mucins

Sjögren's syndrome and in cicatrizing diseases. Recent data indicate that in patients with Sjögren's syndrome, the number of RNA transcripts for MUC5AC in the conjunctival epithelium, detected by real-time polymerase chain reaction, as well as the protein levels of MUC5AC in the tear fluid, measured by ELISA, are significantly lower than in normal individuals.[12] In another study, a reduction of MUC5AC-positive conjunctival cells, as detected by flow cytometry of impression cytology samples, was found in patients with dry eye.[14] The data in these studies correlate with a decrease in the density of goblet cells in the conjunctival epithelium, thus indicating that the assay of MUC5AC mucin in tear fluid provides a noninvasive method for assessing goblet cell density. With increasing severity of the disease, the number of goblet cells decreases further and as a consequence squamous metaplasia and keratinization of the ocular surface occur.

Alteration of membrane-associated mucins

Not only is goblet cell density and, thus, MUC5AC mucin reduced in dry eye, but MAMs also appear to be altered. Assay of MUC16 distribution on the surface of the conjunctiva has been done on impression cytology samples of normal subjects and patients with non-Sjögren's dry eye, using an antibody designated H185, which recognizes a carbohydrate epitope on MUC16.[15] The typical binding pattern in apical cells of conjunctival epithelium of H185 antibody is altered in patients with non-Sjögren's dry eye.[16] The pattern of binding changes from a "cobblestone" binding pattern on the surface to one in which apical cell surface binding is increasingly reduced with severity of dry eye (Figure 18.7).[16] It is not clear whether alteration in the binding pattern in dry eye is due to decreased expression of MUC16, increased shedding of its ectodomain into the tear film, or alteration of glycosylation of the mucin, such that the carbohydrate epitope recognized by the H185 antibody is lost.

Alteration of glycosylation of mucins

The character of the O-glycans on specific mucins can vary among different epithelial types and with disease. Although there is no direct evidence of alteration of O-glycans on specific mucins in dry eye, there is evidence that the expression of the enzymes that add sugars to O-glycans is altered in ocular cicatricial pemphigoid.[17] In addition, lectin binding to conjunctival goblet cells is altered in dry-eye patients, as

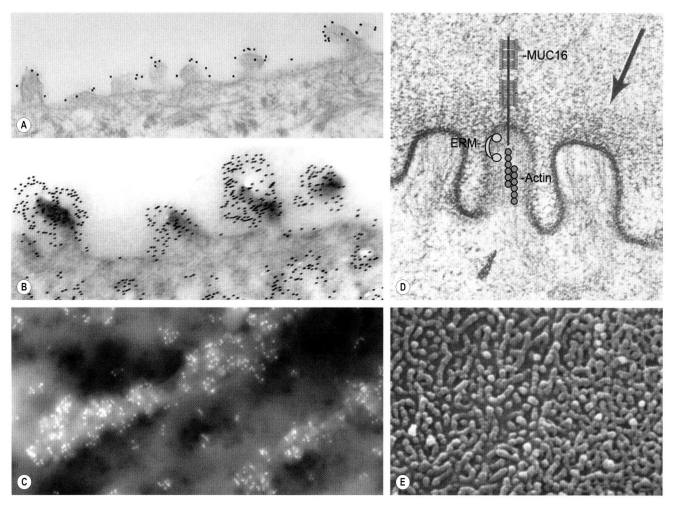

Figure 18.6 Electron micrographs demonstrating presence of the membrane-spanning mucin MUC16 on surface microplicae of corneal epithelial cells. (A) and (B) are transmission electron micrographs showing immunogold labeling of MUC16 protein and the H185 carbohydrate epitope of MUC16, respectively. (C) Field emission scanning electron micrograph of a microplica with immunogold labeling of MUC16 protein. The arrow in the electron micrograph (D) points to the electron-dense glycocalyx, where the membrane-spanning mucins are concentrated. The overlay diagram of MUC16 on the microgram demonstrates that its ectodomain (in red) extends into the glycocalyx and that its short cytoplasmic tail is linked to the actin cytoskeleton, through ERMs, the ezrin, radixin, moesin class of molecules, known to link molecules to the actin cytoskeleton. For reference, (E) is a scanning electron micrograph of corneal epithelial cell microplicae. (Reproduced with permission from Gipson IK. Distribution of mucins at the ocular surface. Exp Eye Res 2004;78:379–388. © Elsevier (2004).)

compared to normal subjects, suggesting an alteration in MUC5AC glycosylation.[18] A decrease in a sialylated Lewis A carbohydrate epitope on glycoconjugates/mucins in tears from patients with dry-eye syndrome has also been detected.[19]

Taken together, these studies of alterations of mucins in dry eye suggest that, not only is there an alteration in amount of secreted mucin on the ocular surface, but the membrane mucins are also altered, and glycosylation of both the mucin types appears to be altered.

Vitamin A deficiency (animal models)

Studies in animal models have shown that vitamin A influences the expression and production of membrane-associated and secreted mucins. Rats fed a casein-based vitamin A-deficient diet lost expression of the secretory mucin rMuc5AC and the MAM rMuc4 after 15–20 weeks;

however, the membrane-spanning mucin rMuc1 was not affected.[20] Similar results were obtained in vitro, using a human conjunctival epithelial cell line.[21] Expression of both MUC4 and MUC16 is regulated by retinoic acid, with the MUC16 regulation being mediated by secretory phospholipase A2. It is probable that the keratinization of the ocular surface in humans with vitamin A deficiency is accompanied by loss of mucin expression.

Therapeutics for dry eye targeted toward mucin production

Artificial tears have been and still are the main therapy for dry eye, but recently several drugs/agents have been developed to induce mucin expression or secretion. These drugs target both secretory and MAM types (Box 18.4).

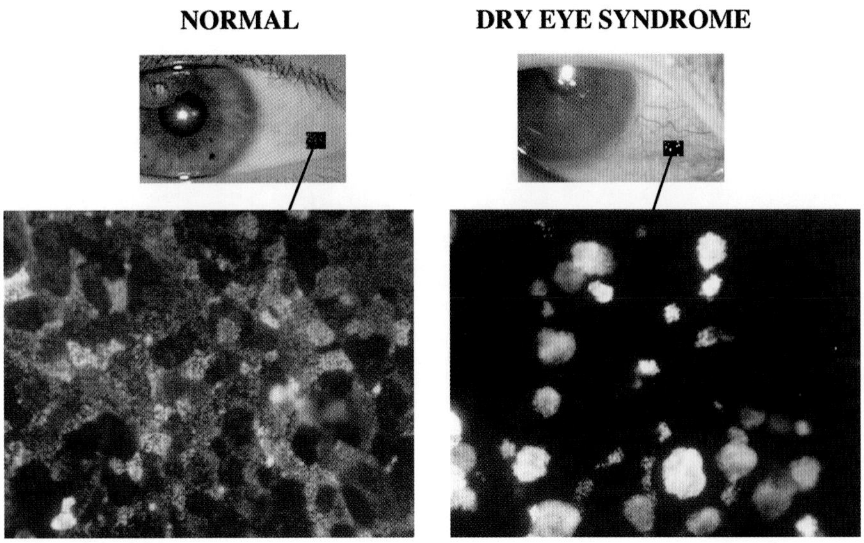

NORMAL   **DRY EYE SYNDROME**

Figure 18.7 Micrographs showing the changes in membrane-associated mucins on the conjunctival surface in patients with dry-eye syndrome. The lower micrographs were derived from impression cytology of the conjunctival epithelium from a normal subject and a patient with non-Sjögren's dry eye. MUC16 was localized using an antibody designated H185, which recognizes a carbohydrate epitope on the mucin. The apical cells from the normal subject appear in a typical cobblestone pattern. This typical pattern is lost in patients with dry-eye syndrome, where apical cells lose their binding to H185, but goblet cells have enhanced binding (for complete details, see Danjo et al[16]). (Reproduced with permission from Gipson IK. The ocular surface: the challenge to enable and protect vision: the Friedenwald lecture. Invest Ophthalmol Vis Sci 2007;48:4390–4398. © The Association for Research in Vision and Ophthalmology (2007).)

Box 18.4 Therapeutics for dry eye targeted toward mucin production

Artificial tears have been and still are the main therapy for dry eye, but recently several drugs/agents have been developed to induce mucin expression or secretion. These drugs target both secretory and membrane-associated mucin types. Current treatments used or being explored include the following: ciclosporin A (topical), P2Y2 receptor, the eicosanoid 15-(S)-HETE, gefarnate, corticosteroids, autologous serum, and vitamin A (retinoic acid)

Dry-eye syndrome is associated with inflammation and an increased expression of several inflammatory markers (human leukocyte antigen (HLA)-DR, intercellular adhesion molecule-1) by conjunctival epithelial cells.[3] Topical treatment with the immunosuppressive agent ciclosporin A, used for treating inflammatory diseases such as rheumatoid arthritis and psoriasis, has been reported to be clinically effective in patients with dry eye.[22,23] It reduces the amount of inflammatory markers,[24] and after a 6-month treatment there is an increase in the number of goblet cells in the conjunctiva.[25] Reduction of inflammation by ciclosporin A may result in an increase in goblet cell differentiation in the conjunctival epithelium. A topical emulsion ciclosporin A (Restasis: Allergan, Irvine, CA) is currently the only drug approved by the US Food and Drug Administration for dry eye.

The nucleotide P2Y2 receptor, found in many cell types,[26] is expressed by corneal and conjunctival epithelia of rabbit and monkeys.[27] Adenosine triphosphate and uridine 5′-triphosphate are P2Y2 receptor agonists that stimulate mucin secretion through a poorly understood mechanism in human conjunctiva.[28] A stable P2Y2 receptor agonist INS365 increases tear secretion in a rat dry-eye model[29]; however, it is not known if this drug influences goblet cell MUC5AC expression or whether it affects shedding of the MAM from the ocular surface. Clinical trials using INS365 for dry eye are under way.

As a metabolite of arachidonic acid, the eicosanoid 15-(S)-hydroxy-5,8,11,13-eicosatetraenoic acid (HETE) is known to be a stimulator of mucus secretion in airway epithelia.[30] Topical application of 15-(S)-HETE to the rabbit ocular surface has been reported to enhance the thickness of the mucin layer on the corneal epithelial cell surface.[31] In human conjunctiva, this agent has been reported to increase the amount of MUC1 protein, as measured by dot-blot assay,[13,32] but there was no observable effect on MUCs 2, 4, 5AC, or 7. These data suggest that 15-(S)-HETE has an effect on some of the MAMs, but not on the secreted mucins.

Gefarnate is widely used to treat patients with gastritis or gastric ulcers. Its mechanism of action is to enhance mucous secretion in the stomach (as reviewed by Nakamura et al[33]). Treatment with gefarnate (3.7-dimethyl-2.6-octadienyl-5.9.13-trimethyl-4.8.12-tetradecatrienoate) in animal models showed an increased presence of mucin-like proteins on the cornea, reduced desiccation in rabbit cornea and, after 7 days, an increased goblet cell density in the conjunctiva.[33,34] Other studies showed an induction of goblet cell secretion and differentiation, and after 4 weeks, the amount of MUC5AC in tears of monkeys had also increased.[35]

Anti-inflammatory drugs such as corticosteroids reportedly have a positive influence on dry-eye disease.[36,37] A comparison of the efficacy of corticosteroid fluoromethalone to treatment with the nonsteroidal anti-inflammatory fluribiprofen in keratoconjunctivitis sicca patients revealed that the corticosteroid was more efficacious.[37] The corticosteroid provided the greatest increase in goblet cell numbers as well as a decrease in HLA-DR-positive cells and symptom severity.

Autologous serum is a potential treatment for dry-eye diseases, since it contains a number of growth factors, vitamin A, and anti-inflammatory factors known to affect mucin gene expression. Protein and mRNA levels of MUCs 1, 4, and 16 in cultured human conjunctival epithelial cells are upregulated by serum, although studies concerning secreted mucins have not been performed.[38] Several clinical reports describe the efficacy of applying autologous serum to treat Sjögren's dry eye,[39,40] suggesting that the treatment may be related to upregulation of MAMs.

It is well known that vitamin A is essential for maintenance of a healthy, differentiated ocular surface. Vitamin A deficiency in humans leads to keratinization. As stated earlier, in animal models, a vitamin A-free diet causes a loss of expression of Muc5AC and Muc4 in ocular surface epithelia, while Muc1 levels are not altered. The retinoid is used as a treatment for severe squamous metaplasia,[41,42] and it is also reported that treatment with 100 nM retinoic acid causes higher expression of MUC4 and -16 mRNA and protein in cultured human conjunctival epithelial cells.[38]

Summary

Alteration in production of both secreted and MAMs has been reported to occur in dry eye. Loss of secreted goblet cell mucins and goblet cells leads to surface keratinization, and loss of the membrane-spanning mucins can cause damage, as indicated by rose Bengal staining. Therapies targeted toward amelioration of inflammation appear to replenish the mucin-producing goblet cells, while retinoids and autologous serum appear to upregulate mucins of the membrane-associated type.

Key references

A complete list of chapter references is available online at www.expertconsult.com. See inside cover for registration details.

1. Research in dry eye: report of the Research Subcommittee of the International Dry Eye WorkShop. Report of the International Dry Eye WorkShop (DEWS). Ocul Surf 2007;5:179–193.

2. Gipson IK. The ocular surface: the challenge to enable and protect vision: the Friedenwald lecture. Invest Ophthalmol Vis Sci 2007;48:4390–4398.

3. Report of the International Dry Eye WorkShop (DEWS). Ocul Surf 2007;5: 67–202.

8. Jumblatt MM, McKenzie RW, Steele PS, et al. MUC7 expression in the human lacrimal gland and conjunctiva. Cornea 2003;22:41–45.

10. Gipson IK, Hori Y, Argüeso P. Character of ocular surface mucins and their alteration in dry eye disease. Ocul Surf 2004;2:131–148.

13. Jumblatt JE, Cunningham LT, Li Y, et al. Characterization of human ocular mucin secretion mediated by 15(S)-HETE. Cornea 2002;21:818–824.

15. Argüeso P, Spurr-Michaud S, Russo CL, et al. MUC16 mucin is expressed by the human ocular surface epithelia and carries the H185 carbohydrate epitope. Invest Ophthalmol Vis Sci 2003;44: 2487–2495.

16. Danjo Y, Watanabe H, Tisdale AS, et al. Alteration of mucin in human conjunctival epithelia in dry eye. Invest Ophthalmol Vis Sci 1998;39:2602–2609.

17. Argüeso P, Tisdale A, Mandel U, et al. The cell-layer- and cell-type-specific distribution of GalNAc-transferases in the ocular surface epithelia is altered during keratinization. Invest Ophthalmol Vis Sci 2003;44:86–92.

18. Versura P, Maltarello MC, Cellini M, et al. Detection of mucus glycoconjugates in human conjunctiva by using the lectin-colloidal gold technique in TEM. II. A quantitative study in dry-eye patients. Acta Ophthalmol (Copenh) 1986;64:451–455.

22. Sall K, Stevenson OD, Mundorf TK, et al. Two multicenter, randomized studies of the efficacy and safety of cyclosporine ophthalmic emulsion in moderate to severe dry eye disease. CsA Phase 3 Study Group [published erratum appears in Ophthalmology 2000;107:1220]. Ophthalmology 2000;107:631–639.

25. Kunert KS, Tisdale AS, Gipson IK. Goblet cell numbers and epithelial proliferation in the conjunctiva of patients with dry eye syndrome treated with cyclosporine. Arch Ophthalmol 2002;120:330–337.

37. Avunduk AM, Avunduk MC, Varnell ED, et al. The comparison of efficacies of topical corticosteroids and nonsteroidal anti-inflammatory drops on dry eye patients: a clinical and immunocytochemical study. Am J Ophthalmol 2003;136:593–602.

40. Tsubota K, Goto E, Fujita H, et al. Treatment of dry eye by autologous serum application in Sjögren's syndrome. Br J Ophthalmol 1999;83: 390–395.

42. Soong HK, Martin NF, Wagoner MD, et al. Topical retinoid therapy for squamous metaplasia of various ocular surface disorders. A multicenter, placebo-controlled double-masked study. Ophthalmology 1988;95:1442–1446.

Steroid-induced glaucoma

Abbot F Clark, Xinyu Zhang, and Thomas Yorio

Overview

Glucocorticoids (GCs) regulate normal physiological processes such as carbohydrate, lipid, and protein metabolism. However, GCs are most often used therapeutically because of their broad anti-inflammatory and immunosuppressive activities (Table 19.1). GCs block the production of proinflammatory molecules such as prostaglandins and cytokines, inhibit/decrease edema, block inflammatory and immune cell trafficking and activation, as well as inhibit the late stages of inflammation such as myofibroblast activation and scarring (Box 19.1). There are a variety of synthetic GCs with differing potencies, metabolic profiles, and biological half-lives (Table 19.2). The widespread use of GCs for a variety of clinical conditions led to the discovery of significant side-effects associated with prolonged therapy, including metabolic effects (osteoporosis, myopathy, hyperglycemia, redistribution of body fat, and thinning of skin) and immunosuppression. Prolonged ocular administration of GCs (more commonly seen with topical ocular or intravitreal administration) can cause the development of posterior subcapsular cataracts, and the subject of this chapter, ocular hypertension and iatrogenic open-angle glaucoma in susceptible individuals.

Clinical background

Key symptoms and signs

The elevated intraocular pressure (IOP) and secondary glaucoma due to GC administration mimics the clinical presentation of primary open-angle glaucoma (POAG) in many ways. Affected individuals are unaware that they have ocular hypertension because the IOP increase is painless. The elevated IOP is due to impaired aqueous humor outflow. The IOP elevation causes very similar irreversible optic nerve head cupping and visual field loss. GC-induced ocular hypertension is different from POAG in that the damage to the aqueous outflow pathway is usually reversible upon discontinuation of GC therapy. However, there are instances of permanent IOP elevation in some patients treated with prolonged GC therapy.

A number of factors determine the ocular hypertensive effects of GC therapy. Elevated IOP generally develops weeks to months after GC administration. The degree of IOP elevation also depends on the potency and dose of GC used as well as the frequency of dosing and route of administration. For example, intravitreal injections of the potent GC triamcinolone acetonide have been increasingly used to treat conditions of retinal edema and choroidal neovascularization, resulting in the increased prevalence of GC-induced ocular hypertension. This route of administration can lead to significantly elevated IOP in 10–40% of patients, who often require treatment with glaucoma medications or even filtration surgery.[1] Although infrequent, even the use of intranasal and inhaled GCs can elevate IOP in certain individuals.

Epidemiology

There are population differences in this ocular response to GCs.[2,3] Normal individuals receiving topical ocular administration of a potent GC for 4–6 weeks could be categorized into three groups: ~5% were high responders (IOP elevation of >15 mmHg or IOP >31 mmHg), 33% were moderate responders (IOP elevation 6–15 mmHg or IOP >20 mmHg), while those remaining were considered nonresponders (no effect of IOP elevation <6 mmHg). In contrast, the majority of POAG patients are high-to-moderate responders, and interestingly, descendants of POAGs are more likely to be GC-responsive compared to the normal population. There may be a genetic predilection for the development of GC-induced ocular hypertension, and this merits additional research.

Treatment

IOP elevation resulting from GC use is treated by halting, decreasing, or removing the source of the steroid, standard ocular hypotensive agents, or, if necessary, surgery. Anecortave acetate (AA) is an IOP-lowering cortisone currently in clinical trials; it lowers IOP in GC-induced ocular hypertensive and in glaucoma patients. It is an analog of cortisol acetate, which has been modified to remove GC activity.[4] Topical ocular administration of AA lowers IOP in dexamethasone (DEX)-induced ocular hypertensive rabbits, and in an open-label, compassionate-use clinical study, topical ocular AA lowered the IOPs of patients with GC-induced ocular hypertension (Clark et al, unpublished oberservation), and in an open-label, compassionate-use clinical study, topical ocular AA lowered the IOPs of patients with

Table 19.1 Ocular diseases treated by glucocorticoids

Blepharitis

Conjunctivitis

Keratitis

Scleritis

Uveitis (anterior and posterior)

Macular edema

Choroidal neovascularization associated with age-related macular degeneration

Optic neuritis

Endophthalmitis

Table 19.2 Glucocorticoids used for ocular therapy

Prednisolone acetate (topical ocular 0.125% and 1% suspensions)

Prednisolone sodium phosphate (topical ocular 0.125% and 1% solutions)

Dexamethasone (topical ocular 0.1% suspension)

Dexamethasone (intravitreal implant 350 and 700 mg)

Dexamethasone sodium phosphate (topical ocular 0.1% solution; 0.05% ointment)

Loteprednol etabonate (topical ocular 0.2% and 0.5% suspensions)

Rimexolone (topical ocular 1% suspension)

Fluorometholone (topical ocular 0.1% and 0.25% suspensions; 0.1% ointment)

Fluorometholone acetate (topical ocular 0.1% suspension)

Medrysone (topical ocular 1% suspension)

Triamcinolone acetonide (10 mg/ml and 40 mg/ml injectable)*

Fluocinolone acetonide (intravitreal implant 0.59 mg)

*Used off-label; currently not approved for ophthalmic use.

Box 19.1 Overview of steroid glaucoma

- Glucocorticoid-induced ocular hypertension is an important side-effect of glucocorticoid therapy
- Iatrogenic form of secondary open-angle glaucoma
- Clinically similar to primary open-angle glaucoma (POAG)
- Differences in individual susceptibility:
  - Approximately 40% of the general population are steroid responders
  - Almost all POAG patients are steroid responders

GC-induced ocular hypertension.[5] Physician investigational new drug clinical studies suggest that a single anterior juxtascleral depot administration of AA lowers IOPs in patients with ocular hypertension due to intravitreal treatment with potent GCs[5] and in POAG patients.[6] Because of these positive preliminary studies, AA is currently in phase II clinical studies for both GC-induced ocular hypertension and in patients with POAG.

Box 19.2 Pathology of steroid glaucoma

- Glucocorticoid-induced ocular hypertension due to decreased aqueous humor outflow
- Associated with morphological and biochemical changes in the trabecular meshwork
- Glucocorticoid-induced ocular hypertension occurs in multiple species (human, monkey, bovine, cat, dog, rat, mouse)
- Glucocorticoid-induced ocular hypertension occurs in isolated perfusion-cultured human eyes

Pathology

The elevated IOP caused by GC administration is associated with morphological and biochemical changes in the trabecular meshwork (TM), the tissue involved in impaired aqueous humor outflow (Box 19.2).[3] There is increased deposition of extracellular material in the uveal meshwork and juxtacanalicular tissue of eyes with steroid glaucoma compared to age-matched control eyes. Some of this material has a characteristic "fingerprint" pattern.[7] There is also a decrease in intertrabecular spaces and an apparent "activation" of trabecular cells (TM cells have a more extensive Golgi apparatus and rough endoplasmic reticulum).

Humans are not the only species to develop GC-induced ocular hypertension. Topical ocular administration of potent GCs can elevate IOP in rabbits[8,9] and cats.[10] Interestingly, topical ocular administration of DEX to cynomolgus monkeys elevated IOP by >5 mmHg in 40% of the dosed animals,[11] very similar to the responder rate in normal human subjects. IOP lowered to normal levels after discontinuing steroid administration. The responder/nonresponder status remained the same when the animals were rechallenged with DEX administration. In addition, DEX-induced ocular hypertension has been shown in isolated (ex vivo) perfusion-cultured human eyes. An average 17 mmHg increase was seen in ~30% of the DEX-treated eyes compared to controls,[2] a responder rate that mimics that seen in humans. This GC-mediated ocular hypertension was associated with thickening of trabecular beams, decreased intertrabecular spaces, and increased deposition of extracellular material in the juxtacanalicular connective tissue.

Etiology

Endogenous glucocorticoids and glaucoma

In addition to the ability of GCs to induce ocular hypertension, the endogenous GC cortisol has also been implicated in the development of POAG. There have been several reports of increased levels of the cortisol in the plasma[12–14] and aqueous humor[14] of POAG patients compared to age-matched controls. However, others studies have not found this association. Diurnal and stress-induced changes in plasma cortisol levels further complicate potential disease associations. Early reports of increased lymphocyte sensitivity to GCs in POAG patients suggested an increased systemic GC sensitivity,[15] although other studies failed to support this finding. A new study showed that POAG patients were more sensitive to GC-induced cutaneous vasoconstriction compared to age-matched controls,[16] and it will be interesting to see if this initial discovery can be independently verified. In addition, there have been several reports that steroid responsiveness is a risk factor for the development of POAG.[17,18]

Both the physiologic and pharmacologic effects of GCs are mediated by the GC receptor, which is a ligand-dependent transcription factor. It is therefore not surprising that GCs alter the expression of hundreds of TM cell genes.[19–22] This altered expression includes both upregulated and downregulated genes in diverse categories and pathways, consistent with the pleotrophic effects of GCs on the TM. As previously discussed, the expression of certain genes involved in extracellular matrix (ECM) metabolism is altered by DEX treatment, including increased expression of ECM (FN1, COL8A, LUM) and proteinase inhibitor genes (SERPINA3), and decreased expression of proteinase genes (MMP1, TPA, ADAMTS5). A number of growth factor pathway genes are also altered, such as decreased expression of insulin-like growth factor (IGF1)-binding protein 2 (IGFBP2), IGF1, hepatocyte growth factor (HGF) and BMP2. Altered expression of several cytoskeletal genes (ACTA2, FLNB, NEBL) may be associated with GC-mediated reorganization of TM cell microfibrils and microtubules. In addition, DEX induced the expression of a number of stress-related genes (e.g., increased expression of SAA1, SAA2, methalothioneins, and ceruloplasmin).

Myocilin (MYOC) was first identified as a major GC-responsive gene and protein in the TM.[23,24] This gene is one of the most abundantly expressed genes in human TM tissues and is also found in the aqueous humor. In addition to induction in cultured TM cells, GCs also increase MYOC expression in the TM of perfusion-cultured human anterior segments and in monkeys treated systemically with GCs.[25] Although the MYOC promoter contains partial GC response elements (GREs), GC induction of MYOC requires additional RNA and protein synthesis, and therefore this induction is indirect.[26] Although MYOC was originally proposed to be the major mediator of GC-induced ocular hypertension, there is still no compelling evidence showing that it plays any role in this GC-mediated event. In fact, genetically overexpressing or knocking out MYOC in mice had no effect on IOP.[27,28] However, MYOC was the first glaucoma gene identified[29] and is responsible for approximately 4% of POAG.[11] Glaucomatous mutations in MYOC result in a gain-of-function phenotype, leading to nonsecretion[30] and mistargeting of MYOC,[31] which is normally a secreted glycoprotein. Expression of glaucomatous MYOC also induces the endoplasmic stress response in cultured TM cells.[32]

Pathophysiology

Effects of GCs on the trabecular meshwork (Box 19.3)

The GC-induced decrease in conventional aqueous outflow and GC-induced morphological changes in the TM point to the TM as being the target tissue involved in GC-induced

Table 19.3 Effects of glucocorticoids on the trabecular meshwork

Cellular effects	Inhibition of cell proliferation
	Inhibition of phagocytosis
	Inhibition of migration
	Increased cell and nucleus size
	Increased Golgi, endoplasmic reticulum, and vesicles
ECM metabolism	Increased ECM synthesis (FN, LM, collagen)
Decreased ECM turnover (decreased MMPs and tPA; increased PAI-1 and TIMPs)	
Cytoskeleton	Reorganization of actin cytoskeleton (CLANs)
	Increased microtubule tangles
Gene expression	Altered expression of hundreds of genes
	Increased myocilin expression

ECM, extracellular matrix; FN, fibronectin; LM, laminin; MMPs, matrix metalloproteinases; tPA, tissue plasminogen activator; PAI-1, plasminogen activator inhibitor-1; TIMPs, tissue inhibitor of matrix metalloproteinase; CLANs, cross-linked actin networks.

Box 19.3 Glucocorticoid (GC) effects on the trabecular meshwork (TM)

- TM cells have GC receptors and are targets of GC activity
- GCs alter the expression of hundreds of TM cells, genes, and proteins
- GCs alter TM cell functions (decrease proliferation and phagocytosis)
- GCs increase extracellular matrix deposition
- GC reorganize the actin cytoskeleton
- GCs alter cellular junctions

---

ocular hypertension. TM cells and TM tissues express GC receptors,[33,34] which are essential for GC responsiveness. As seen in many other tissues, GCs have a wide variety of diverse effects on TM cells and TM tissues[3] (Table 19.3). GCs alter several TM cellular functions, including proliferation, phagocytosis, and cell shape and size (Table 19.3). The potent GC DEX inhibited TM cell proliferation induced by a number of different growth factors, and at least part of this activity was mediated by DEX inhibition of growth factor receptor expression.[35] DEX also inhibited TM cell migration[36] and significantly increased TM cell and nucleus size.[37] In addition, DEX inhibited TM cell phagocytosis in a perfusion culture ex vivo system.[38] DEX also induced ultrastructural changes in cultured TM cells, including proliferation of the Golgi apparatus, stacking of the endoplasmic reticulum, and increased numbers of secretory vesicles, which provides morphological support for the increased ECM deposition seen after DEX treatment.[37,39]

One of the hallmarks of steroid-induced glaucoma is the deposition of ECM material in the TM. Aqueous humor outflow in the TM is regulated by the ECM.[40] The overall increased deposition of ECM in the TM of steroid-induced ocular hypertensive eyes could be due to increased ECM synthesis and/or decreased degradation. The synthesis of fibronectin,[37,41,42] laminin,[43] collagen,[44] and elastin[45] was increased in DEX-treated TM cells. GCs also affect ECM turnover. In addition to decreasing matrix metalloproteinase (MMP) and tissue plasminogen activator expression,[46] GCs also increase the expression of plasminogen activator inhibitor-1 (Clark, unpublished observation) and tissue inhibitors of MMPs.[47] GCs alter TM cell glycosaminoglycan (GAG) metabolism, decreasing hyaluronan and increasing chondroitin sulfate and GAGase-resistant material.[48]

The TM cytoskeleton regulates aqueous humor outflow.[49] The cytoskeleton also regulates a number of cell functions, including proliferation, migration, phagocytosis, and cell size/shape, all of which are affected in TM cells treated with GCs. GC treatment reorganizes the actin cytoskeleton to form cross-linked actin networks (CLANs) in cultured TM cells.[36,37] CLANs are geodesic dome-like structures, and GC induction of CLANs is unique to TM cells, not occurring in a variety of other ocular and nonocular cells. The dose, time, and potency dependency for GC-induced CLAN formation are very similar to GC-induced ocular hypertension, and like GC-induced ocular hypertension, CLANs in TM cells are reversible after GC withdrawal.[36] DEX-induced CLANs are also seen in perfusion-cultured eyes.[42] Interestingly, very similar cytoskeletal changes, including CLANs, are present in cultured glaucomatous TM cells[42] and in glaucomatous TM tissues.[49] In addition to reorganizing the actin cytoskeleton, DEX treatment of cultured human TM cells alters microtubules to form microtubule tangles.[50] However, we do not know whether DEX directly alters microtubules or whether this microtubule change is indirectly due to CLAN formation. These GC-induced changes in the TM cytoskeleton may make these cells more resistant to cytoskeletal disrupting agents. DEX-treated TM cells were more resistant to microtubule disrupting agent (i.e., ethacrynic acid and ethylene glycol tetraacetic acid)-induced cellular retraction.[51]

Glucocorticoid mechanism of action

The most widely accepted mechanism for transducing GC signals into cellular responses is via a cognate cellular GC receptor (GR) molecule. GR belongs to the family of intracellular ligand-inducible transcription factors termed the steroid/vitamin D/retinoic acid superfamily.[52–54] The superfamily encompasses the steroid receptor family and the thyroid/retinoid/vitamin D (or nonsteroid) receptor family. The class of steroid hormone receptors includes GR forms α and ß, progesterone receptor (PR) forms A and B, mineralocorticoid receptor (MR), androgen receptor (AR), and estrogen receptor (ER) forms α and ß. Like other members of this receptor superfamily, GR protein is composed of structurally and functionally defined domains. The amino-terminal part of the protein contains a major transactivation domain responsible for gene activation, whereas the central part includes a highly conserved cysteine-rich DNA-binding domain, composed of two highly conserved zinc fingers. The zinc fingers consist of two zinc ions coordinated with eight cysteine residues to form two peptide loops, which bind cooperatively to half-sites in specific palindromic sequences in the promoter regions, known as GC response elements (GRE), and this specific DNA association induces receptor dimerization.[52,55] The moderately conserved carboxy-terminal includes ligand-binding domain, which possesses the essential property of hormone recognition and ensures both specificity and selectivity of the physiologic response.[56–58] This region also contains sequences that are involved in nuclear translocation, receptor dimerization, heat shock protein (Hsp) 90 binding, and transactivation.[59–62]

The classic model for steroid/thyroid hormone action involves a ligand-induced conformational change in the receptor that allows the receptor–hormone complex to bind to its cognate hormone response element (HRE) in the promoter region of a target gene. The interaction of the activated receptor with the basal transcriptional apparatus alters transcription of hormone-sensitive genes.[54,63] The ligand-binding domain can be thought of as a molecular switch that, upon binding ligand, shifts the receptor to a transcriptionally active state.

Alternative GR transcripts

The full-length human GR has two isoforms, GRα and GRβ, which originate from the same gene by alternative splicing of the GR primary RNA transcript.[64–69] There is also alternative translation initiation from a downstream, in-frame ATG codon.[70] Alternative translation initiation produces two GR protein products, the longer protein (777 amino acids), initiated from the first ATG codon (Met 1), termed as GR-A, and the shorter protein (751 amino acids), termed as GR-B. A and B receptor isoforms have been consistently identified for both GRα and GRß in various tissues and cell lines.[70–73] When expressed in vitro in mammalian cells, the A and B forms are generated in approximately equivalent levels from a single cDNA. However, the GR-B form appears to be more susceptible to degradation and is more effective than GR-A in gene transactivation, but not in transrepression.[70]

GRα

GRα is the major GR transcript that has GC-binding activity.[64] Because of its predominant expression, ligand-binding activity, and transcriptional function, most of the physiological and pharmacological effects of GCs are directly mediated by GRα. GRα is expressed in most human tissues and cell lines. Unlike most members of the steroid receptor superfamily, GRα resides predominantly in the cytoplasm of cells in the absence of ligand as a multiprotein heterocomplex that contains Hsp 90, Hsp70, immunophilin, and several other proteins.[74–77] Hormone binding to GRα causes a conformation change and activation of GRα. The activated GRα can alter gene expression via GRE-dependent (classical) and GRE-independent (nonclassical) mechanisms.

GRE-dependent pathway

Activated GRα translocates to the nucleus via retrograde transport along microtubules. Once in the nucleus, GRα can bind to specific palindromic DNA sequences (GRE) as a homodimer on the promoter region of target genes, where it interacts with the basal transcription apparatus to induce transcription of the target genes.[78] In addition, GRα also functions as a negative regulator of transcription in a specific subset of GC-responsive genes, which contain a negative GRE (nGRE).[79,80]

GRE-independent pathway

There is an additional way for GRα to inhibit rather than activate gene expression. GRα can inhibit the expression of genes that do not contain nGRE. GCs are known to suppress the expression of proinflammatory cytokines, which are key regulators of the immune response. However, the majority of proinflammatory genes that are suppressed by GCs lack nGRE in their promoter regions.[81–83] Instead, GRα physically interacts with other transcription factors to prevent them from binding to their response elements of genes. The powerful GC-mediated anti-inflammatory actions and immune suppression are mediated via this GRE-independent pathway.[84–86]

GRß

In contrast, GRß was thought to be a nucleus-localized orphan receptor lacking ligand-binding activity and gene transcription regulation and, hence, it was suggested that GRß was generally of little physiological importance. However, there is increasing evidence that this view is incorrect.[87–89] GRß can act as a dominant negative regulator to antagonize the function of GRα.[66,90] Increased GRß expression has been associated with a variety of GC-insensitive conditions.[91–99] We reported that decreased expression of GRß in glaucomatous TM cells was associated with increased GC sensitivity in glaucoma.[73,100] These reports suggest a potential physiological consequence to changes in GRß expression. In addition, GRß has been reported to bind a ligand and has the ability to regulate gene expression on its own,[101] suggesting that GRß may regulate GC responsiveness beyond its ability to manipulate the function of GRα. GRß may compete with GRα for GRE binding because GRß has an intact DNA-binding domain. Alternatively, GRß may complex with activated GRα to form transcriptional impaired GRα-GRß heterodimers, as has been demonstrated in corticosteroid-insensitive cells[70,102] (Figure 19.1).

GRß role in glucocorticoid-resistant diseases

GCs are routinely used as anti-inflammatory drugs, and GC resistance poses a serious clinical problem. A number of clinical studies have reported an association between GRß expression and GC insensitivity. Increased expression of GRß appears to be responsible for unresponsiveness

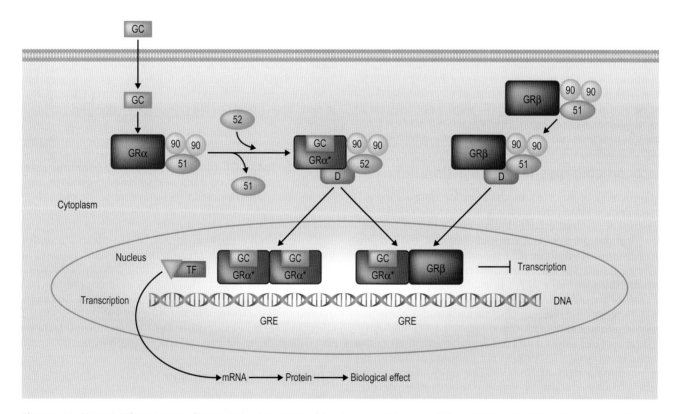

Figure 19.1 GRα and GRß mechanism of action. Both splice variants of the glucocorticoid receptor (GRα and GRß) reside in the cytoplasm as multimeric complexes, interacting with heat shock protein (Hsp) 90[66] and immunophilin FKBP51.[26] A glucocorticoid (G) freely permeates the membrane and binds to and activates GRα, causing the exchange of FKBP51 for FKBP 52.[27] This conformational change allows the activated GRα (GRα *) complex to bind dynein (D) and translocate into the nucleus via microtubules. Once inside the nucleus, activated GRα dimerizes and binds to glucocorticoid response elements (GRE) on specific genes. This complex, along with other transcription factors (TF) and RNA polymerases, generates specific mRNAs that are translated into proteins, ultimately causing the glucocorticoid-mediated biological effect.

In contrast to GRα, GRß does not bind glucocorticoids. However, GRß acts as a dominant negative regulator of GC activity. The GRß–Hsp 90–FKBP51 complex is translocated to the nucleus via dynein and microtubules. Although it is unclear exactly how GRß interferes with GRα function, one hypothesis is that GRß forms heterodimers with GRα, which are unable to turn on gene expression.

to anti-inflammatory GC therapy in diverse clinical conditions, including asthma, inflammatory bowel disease, rheumatoid arthritis, ulcerative colitis, chronic lymphocytic leukemia, and microbial antigen-induced GC-insensitivity.[91,95,96,98,99,103,104] GRß may be a key modulator of the development of these immune-related GC-resistant diseases.[105-108] In addition, increased expression of GRß is associated with disease pathogenesis. However, there is considerable controversy about the expression and physiological significance of GRß.[109-113]

GRß role in glaucoma and enhanced TM cell sensitivity to GC (Box 19.4)

There are differences in steroid sensitivity between the glaucomatous and normal populations[14]; however the molecular basis of the increase in IOP experienced by patients with glaucoma and subjects receiving GCs is not well understood. We have reported[73] that glaucomatous TM cells derived from donors with a documented history of glaucoma had a relatively lower expression of GRß, particularly lower in the nucleus, than did normal TM cells derived from normal donors. Glaucomatous TM cells were more susceptible to DEX induction of transiently expressed GRE-luciferase construct than were normal TM cells. Transfection of glaucomatous TM cells with an GRß expression vector suppressed the GC induction of the luciferase reporter gene and decreased the GC induction of MYOC and fibronectin, two glaucoma-associated genes in TM cells. A decrease in phagocytic activity has been proposed in the pathogenesis of glaucoma,[38,114] although one study did not find any difference in phagocytic activity between normal and glaucomatous eyes.[38] GCs suppress TM cell phagocytosis in perfusion-cultured eyes.[115] We have also reported[100] different phagocytic abilities between cultured normal TM and glaucomatous TM cells, with a reduced phagocytosis in glaucomatous TM cells. The glaucomatous TM cells were more responsive to DEX-induced suppression of phagocytosis compared to normal TM cells. Increased expression of GRß decreased this DEX response, and consequently these cells retained their phagocytic activity even following the DEX challenge.

Several mechanisms may be responsible for higher levels of GRß found in normal compared to glaucomatous TM cells. Expression of GRß could be regulated by alternative splicing efficiency through variations in splice sites, altered expression of splicing factors, or the presence of functional polymorphisms in splicing factors. GRß mRNA stability appears to be controlled by a 3′ untranslated region (UTR) single nucleotide polymorphism (SNP) and this SNP may vary between normal subjects and patients with glaucoma.

Box 19.4 Potential role for GRβ

- GRβ = alternative splice form of the glucocorticoid receptor
- Dominant regulator of glucocorticoid activity
- Implicated in a variety of steroid-resistant diseases
- Decreased levels in glaucomatous trabecular meshwork cells make these cells more sensitive to detrimental effects of glucorticoids

---

Genotyping studies are currently in progress to determine whether there are disease-associated polymorphisms in any of these sites in patients with glaucoma. Differences in the nuclear translocation of GRß may also explain the differential expression in normal versus glaucomatous TM cells. The expression level of GRß in TM cells can regulate the cell's ability to respond to GC, and GRß inhibit not only the DEX-induced gene expression but also DEX-suppressed phagocytic activity. The lower expression of GRß in glaucomatous TM cells could contribute to increased susceptibility of glaucoma patients to chronic endogenous cortisol exposure (years) or to exogenous pharmacological GC treatment, which may lead to the increased aqueous humor outflow resistance and elevated IOP.

Interestingly, recent reports showed that, in the absence of GC, GRα was sequestered in the cytoplasm, and nuclear GRß acted as a transcriptional repressor of cytokine genes through the recruitment of histone deacetylase complexes.[116] GRß, expressed in the absence of GRα, can regulate the expression of a number of diverse genes.[101] These studies suggest that GRß can act as an orphan receptor, representing new constitutive activator/repressor activity, along with being a repressor for ligand-activated GRα. In addition, RU-486 was able to bind to GRß and stimulate gene transcription, despite only having a partial ligand-binding domain in its carboxy terminus. We also observed that, in the presence of FK506, DEX treatment induced nuclear translocation of GRß as it does to GRα,[117] indicating that DEX might be a ligand for GRß in the presence of FK506. Our understanding of the physiological significance of GRß is expanding.

Differences in tissue/cell responses to GCs

Although almost all mammalian cells and tissues contain GRs, the biological responses to GCs are often widely divergent between different cell types. Indeed, GCs have a broad array of life-sustaining functions and are also frequently used as therapeutic compounds. Variations in tissue sensitivity and responses are essential for maintaining tissue homeostasis under both basal and stress conditions. Numerous pathologic conditions can be caused by either GC resistance or GC hypersensitivity. In human, generalized GC resistance can be due to inactivating mutations of the GR gene, but this syndrome is rare.[118] A number of factors contribute to tissue-specific GC responses, many of which involve specific steps of the GR signaling pathway, including: ligand availability, ligand-binding activity, receptor isoform expression, intracellular trafficking, promoter association, interactions with tissue-specific cofactors, and clearance of the receptor from the target genes.[119,120]

One regulatory mechanism to change cellular responses to GCs occurs via GR phosphorylation, which influences multiple functions of the GR protein, including affinity for ligand binding, intracellular trafficking, and transcriptional activity.[121-125] Several protein kinases, such as the p38 mitogen-activated protein kinase (MAPK),[126] cell cycle-dependent kinases (CDK), and other mitogen-activated kinases have been reported to phosphorylate the GR.[124,127-130] These regulatory mechanisms appear to be in tissue-specific fashions; for example, CDK5 functions specifically in the central nervous system.[120]

Selective glucocorticoid receptor agonists – future directions

GCs are used in the management of a wide range of inflammatory diseases and immunosuppressive agents, including a number of conditions affecting the eye, as noted above. Their complex actions have been attributed to a variety of cellular mechanisms, including direct effects on plasma membranes, interactions with transcription factors, genomic effects mediated by the GC response element and, more recently, a membrane-bound GC receptor.[131] The classical genomic effects can be attributed to two types of responses, transactivation or transrepression of selective genes. GC-mediated receptor transactivation may explain many of their side-effects, whereas the repression of key inflammatory transcription factors, including activator protein 1 (AP-1) and nuclear factor kappa-light-chain-enhancer of activated B cells (NF-κB), is linked to their anti-inflammatory activity.[132] Therefore, selective agents that can distinguish the gene-repressive actions from the transcriptional activation pathways will be desirable. However, separation of the desirable effects from the undesirable effects is difficult since unwanted side-effects can be seen with both types of activity. Common ocular side-effects of prolonged GC therapy include steroid-induced ocular hypertension and posterior subcapsular cataracts. Moreover, depending on the dose and duration of therapy, one can get infections, disturbed wound healing, and hypertension.[133] The search for novel formulations is still a major interest of the pharmaceutical industry, particularly those clinical uses that might separate the desired gene-repressive anti-inflammatory activity from the gene activation activity that appears to promote side-effects. Much has been learned from using a mouse model where the GC receptor was mutated in the dimerization portion of the molecule, which prevented GRE transactivation activity but allowed the receptor to bind other transcription factors and repress gene expression.[134] Treatment of these mice with a GC generated anti-inflammatory activity, as in wild-type mice. However, these mice were not without all potential side-effects because chronic treatment with a GC resulted in the induction of GC-dependent osteoporosis.[135] This suggests that some of the transactivation activity may not be the result of the dimerization of the receptor, and other mechanisms may still exist for gene activation. Therefore, this model may not be as useful to tease out the different pathways for drug development.

A number of compounds have been produced to separate potent anti-inflammatory activity from side-effects, and there appears to be a beneficial ratio of desired over undesirable actions.[136] It remains uncertain if these differences reside in the different pathways of genomic transrepression versus transactivation or the result of differences in receptor affinities or differences in receptor expressions. It will also be important to determine what pathways and cellular mechanisms are responsible for the anti-inflammatory versus each of the side-effects following GC administration. Since GCs induce the expression of a wide variety of cellular proteins, some of which may still be important for anti-inflammatory activity, it may be extremely difficult to separate out the undesirable actions totally. However, it is worth the effort to identify selective GC receptor agonists with much reduced side-effects. For the eye, the ability to retain the anti-inflammatory actions while reducing the potential for developing glaucoma or cataract will be ideal. Certainly, the search is still on for such a compound.

Key references

A complete list of chapter references is available online at www.expertconsult.com. See inside cover for registration details.

2. Clark AF. Steroids, ocular hypertension, and glaucoma. J Glaucoma 1995;4:354–369.

3. Wordinger RJ, Clark AF. Effects of glucocorticoids on the trabecular meshwork: towards a better understanding of glaucoma. Prog Retin Eye Res 1999;18:629–667.

4. Clark AF. Preclinical efficacy of anecortate acetate. Surv Ophthalmol 2007;52(Suppl. 1):S41–S48.

11. Fingert JH, Clark AF, Craig JE, et al. Evaluation of the myocilin (MYOC) glaucoma gene in monkey and human steroid-induced ocular hypertension. Invest Ophthalmol Vis Sci 2001;42:145–152.

17. Kitazawa Y, Horie T. The prognosis of corticosteroid-responsive individuals. Arch Ophthalmol 1981;99:819–823.

29. Stone EM, Fingert JH, Alward WL, et al. Identification of a gene that causes primary open angle glaucoma. Science 1997;275:668–670.

36. Clark AF, Wilson K, de Kater AW, et al. Glucocorticoid-induced formation of cross-linked actin networks in cultured human trabecular meshwork cells. Invest Ophthalmol Vis Sci 1994;35:281–294.

66. Oakley RH, Sar M, Cidlowski JA. The human glucocorticoid receptor beta isoform. expression, biochemical properties, and putative function. J Biol Chem 1996;271:9550–9559.

73. Zhang X, Clark AF, Yorio T. Regulation of glucocorticoid responsiveness in glaucomatous trabecular meshwork cells by glucocorticoid receptor-beta. Invest Ophthalmol Vis Sci 2005;46:4607–4616.

100. Zhang X, Ognibene CM, Clark AF, et al. Dexamethasone inhibition of trabecular meshwork cell phagocytosis and its modulation by glucocorticoid receptor beta. Exp Eye Res 2007;84:275–284.

103. Oakley RH, Jewell CM, Yudt MR, et al. The dominant negative activity of the human glucocorticoid receptor beta isoform. specificity and mechanisms of action. J Biol Chem 1999;274:27857–27866.

113. Webster JC, Oakley RH, Jewell CM, et al. Proinflammatory cytokines regulate human glucocorticoid receptor gene expression and lead to the accumulation of the dominant negative beta isoform: a mechanism for the generation of glucocorticoid resistance. Proc Natl Acad Sci USA 2001;98:6865–6870.

117. Zhang X, Clark AF, Yorio T. FK506-binding protein 51 regulates nuclear transport of the glucocorticoid receptor beta and glucocorticoid responsiveness. Invest Ophthalmol Vis Sci 2008;49:1037–1047.

131. Stahn C, Lownberg M, Hommes DW, et al. Molecular mechanisms of glucocorticoid action and selective glucocorticoid receptor agonists. Mol Cell Endocrinol 2007;275:71–78.

CHAPTER 20

Biomechanical changes of the optic disc

Ian A Sigal, Michael D Roberts, Michael JA Girard, Claude F Burgoyne, and J Crawford Downs

Clinical background

Lowering intraocular pressure (IOP) remains the only proven method of preventing the onset and progression of glaucoma, yet the role of IOP in the disease remains controversial. This largely arises from the wide spectrum of individual susceptibility to IOP wherein a significant number of patients with normal IOPs develop glaucoma (e.g., normotensive glaucoma), and other individuals with elevated IOP show no signs of the disease. It is therefore important to understand the relationship between IOP and glaucomatous optic neuropathy when IOP is only one of several factors that influence the disease (Box 20.1). IOP is, by definition, a mechanical entity – the force per unit area exerted by the intraocular fluids on the tissues that contain them. Glaucomatous optic neuropathy is a biologic effect – likely the result of an IOP-related cascade of cellular events that culminate in damage to the retinal ganglion cell (RGC) axons. One of the challenges of biomechanics is to understand how the mechanics are transduced into a biological response and/or tissue damage. How does this take place? Why is there such a wide range in susceptibility to IOP? Why does elevated IOP lead to that particular cascade of events and not another? What can we do to predict, detect, and stop the progression of glaucomatous damage? Unfortunately we do not have answers to these questions, but in recent years there has been considerable progress towards understanding of the role of IOP in glaucoma. In this chapter, we focus on two main themes: what is known about how IOP-related forces and deformations are distributed in the posterior pole and optic nerve head (ONH), and what is known about the response of the living system.

Pathology

From a biomechanical perspective, the ONH is a natural site of interest when studying IOP effects because it is a discontinuity in the corneoscleral shell. Such discontinuities are often weak spots in mechanically loaded systems because they give rise to significant stress concentrations.[1] In addition, it is the ONH, the lamina cribrosa (LC) in particular, that is the principal site of RGC axonal insult in glaucoma.[2] Nevertheless there is evidence both for[3] and against[4] direct,

IOP-induced damage to the retinal photoreceptors, and it is likely that there are also important pathophysiologies within the lateral geniculate and visual cortex.[5]

Etiology

We have proposed that the ONH be understood as a biomechanical structure, and that the mechanical effects of IOP on the tissues of the ONH, namely forces and deformations, are central determinants of both the physiology and pathophysiology of the ONH tissues and their blood supply at all levels of IOP (Figure 20.1). Within this framework, the susceptibility of a particular patient's ONH to IOP-related insult is a function of the biomechanical response of the constituent tissues and the resulting mechanical, ischemic, and cellular events driven by that response. Experienced over a lifetime at physiologic levels of IOP, these events underlie normal ONH aging. Hence, eyes with a particular combination of tissue geometry and stiffness may be susceptible to glaucomatous damage at normal IOP, while others may have a combination of ONH tissue geometry and stiffness that render them impervious to any deleterious effects of high IOP.

We believe that the mechanical and vascular mechanisms of glaucomatous injury are inseparably intertwined: IOP-related mechanics determines the biomechanical environment within the ONH, mediating blood flow and cellular responses through various pathways. Reciprocally, the biomechanics depend on tissue anatomy and composition, which are subject to change through cellular activities such as remodeling. The interrelationship between mechanics and physiology could be particularly strong within the LC due to its complexity. The LC is composed of a three-dimensional (3D) network of beams of connective tissue, many containing capillaries, that provides functional and structural support to the RGC axons. IOP-related forces within the LC could deform the beams containing capillaries, diminishing the blood supply to the laminar segments of the RGC axons. Conversely, primary insufficiency in the blood supply to the laminar region could introduce cell-mediated connective tissue changes that could remodel the extracellular matrix (ECM), making the laminar beams more prone to failure, and limit the diffusion of nutrients to adjacent RGC axons.

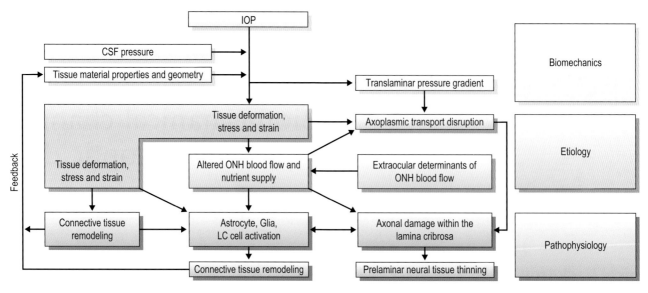

Figure 20.1 Intraocular pressure (IOP) acts mechanically on the tissues of the eye, producing deformations, strain, and stress within the tissues. These deformations depend on the particular geometry and material properties of the tissues of an individual eye. In a biomechanical paradigm, the stress and strain will alter the blood flow (primarily), and the delivery of nutrients (secondarily) through chronic alterations in connective tissue stiffness and diffusion properties. IOP-related stress and strain could also induce connective tissue damage directly (lamina cribrosa beam failure), or indirectly (cell-mediated), and eventually connective tissue remodeling that alters the geometry and tissue mechanical response to loading. This feeds back directly on to the mechanical effects of IOP, or indirectly by affecting IOP regulation.

Box 20.1 Why study optic nerve head biomechanics?

- Intraocular pressure (IOP) is the principal risk factor for the onset and progression of glaucoma
- IOP is a mechanical entity that induces glaucomatous damage through a variety of mechanisms
- Biomechanical analysis of the effects of IOP on the optic nerve head and sclera will help us understand how IOP leads to glaucoma, and why some individuals are more susceptible to IOP-induced glaucomatous damage than others

Box 20.2 Basic concepts in mechanics

- Strain is a measure of the local deformation
- Stress is a measure of the forces per unit area
- Stress and strain are related to each other through the material properties
- Ocular tissues are complex materials that are nonlinear, anisotropic, viscoelastic, and inhomogeneous
- A nonlinear material varies in stiffness as it deforms
- An anisotropic material exhibits different stiffness in different directions
- A viscoelastic material exhibits higher stiffness when loaded quickly rather than slowly

---

Before proceeding with a presentation of the mechanical effects of IOP on the eye and ONH, we review the basic concepts of mechanics relevant to this analysis.

Basic concepts in mechanics

The following are fundamental terms and concepts from mechanics that may not be familiar to clinicians (Box 20.2). The interested reader may pursue these ideas in greater depth by referring to appropriate textbooks.[1]

Stress is a measure of the forces transmitted through, or carried by, a material or tissue. Specifically, stress is the force divided by the cross-sectional area over which it acts. For example, pressure is a stress and can be expressed in pounds per square inch (psi).

Strain is a measure of the local deformation induced by an applied stress. It is computed as the change in length of a material divided by its resting length, and is often expressed as a percentage. For example, a wire that was originally 10 mm long that is stretched an additional 1 mm exhibits 10% tensile strain.

In addition to tension and compression, a material can undergo shear. Tension, compression, and shear are often referred to as the three modes of stress and strain.[6] However, these three modes are not independent, as shown in Figure 20.2.

It has been established that the biologic response of tissues and cells depends strongly on the mode of the strain stimulus (tension, compression, or shear), as well as on their magnitudes and temporal profiles.[7,8] It is therefore of interest to determine which modes of strain and stress the tissues of the ONH are exposed to as IOP is elevated. Note that strains are generally not homogeneous. When the LC deforms, some regions could be highly strained in different modes, whereas others remain largely unaffected. This is important because the biological effects on cells are likely to be strongly dependent on the local levels of strain or stress rather than on global levels.

We would also like to emphasize that mechanical stress, which represents forces, is not synonymous with notions of stress typically used in physiologic or metabolic contexts (e.g., ischemic or oxidative stress). Mechanical stress cannot be measured directly, and we believe it is strain that damages tissues. However, stress is often used to predict the sites of

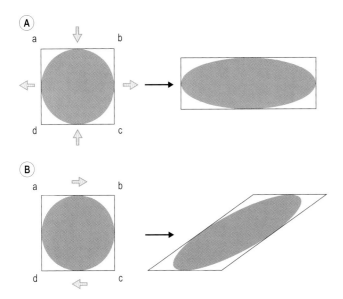

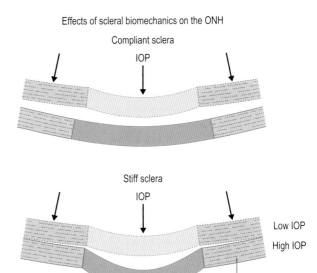

Effects of scleral biomechanics on the ONH

Figure 20.2 Schematic illustration of tissue straining in two dimensions. (A) A square tissue region *abcd* is deformed by forces that act normal to the faces of the square, represented by the black arrows. The tissue experiences tensile stretching in one direction and compression in another. Superimposed on the square tissue region is a circle that deforms with the tissue. (B) The same tissue region is deformed by shearing forces that act tangential to the faces of the square. However, as this region deforms it not only experiences shear, but also extension and compression, as can be verified by noting how the distances between *ac* and *bd* change. (Adapted from Sigal IA, Flanagan JG, Tertinegg I, et al. Predicted extension, compression and shearing of optic nerve head tissues. Exp Eye Res 2007;85:312–322.)

Figure 20.3 Influence of scleral mechanics on optic nerve head mechanics. Intraocular pressure (IOP) induces large deformations on a compliant sclera (top); these deformations are transmitted to the scleral canal, resulting in a large scleral canal expansion that pulls the lamina cribrosa (LC) taut despite the direct posterior force of IOP on the LC. Conversely, a stiff sclera deforms little under IOP (bottom), with small scleral canal expansions and little lateral stretching of the LC, thus allowing the LC to be displaced posteriorly by the direct action of IOP on its anterior surface.

and failure in engineering structures[1] and has been correlated to damage in tissues,[9] so it may be that, while strain is causing the damage, stress is a better predictor of the sites of that damage.[10]

Stress and strain (i.e., forces and deformation) in a material are related to each other through material properties, and this constitutive relationship is intrinsic to each material. For a given load, a material that exhibits large strains is thought of as compliant. Conversely, a material that exhibits small strains for the same load is termed stiff. A stiff tissue such as sclera can have high stress but low strain, while an equal volume of compliant tissue, like retina, might have high strain even at low levels of stress. The simple description above does not account for many of the complexities in material properties that occur in soft biologic tissues, such as anisotropy, nonlinearity, and viscoelasticity (Box 20.3). These complexities are likely to be fundamental to understanding ocular mechanics and will be discussed in the context of scleral biomechanics below.

Scleral biomechanics

From a mechanical perspective, the eye is a pressure vessel, on which IOP produces deformation, strain, and stress. Through computational modeling, the sclera has been shown to have a strong influence on how the LC deforms when IOP changes (Box 20.4). Therefore, understanding the mechanical behavior of the sclera is essential to understanding IOP-induced LC deformations. One of the mechanisms

---

Box 20.3 Optic nerve head (ONH) biomechanics are not trivial

- ONH biomechanics are complex, with the tissues simultaneously subject to tension, compression, and shear
- At present, it is difficult to measure the response of the lamina to changes in intraocular pressure (IOP), and therefore computational modeling is being used
- These models suggest that IOP-related stresses and strains within the connective tissues of the ONH are substantial, even at normal IOP

Box 20.4 Importance of the sclera

- The sclera is the main load-bearing tissue of the eye and deformations of the sclera are transmitted to the optic nerve head at the scleral canal wall
- As such, the mechanical properties and behavior of the sclera have a strong influence on how the optic nerve head responds to changes in intraocular pressure

---

by which scleral biomechanics can influence the response of the LC to IOP is illustrated in Figure 20.3.

Alas, describing the mechanical behavior of soft tissue such as the sclera is a formidable undertaking that demands extensive experimental and mathematical efforts. The first step in characterizing scleral material properties is the development of an experimental mechanical test to measure the deformation of the tissue subjected to loads (e.g., uniaxial, biaxial, or pressurization tests). The second step is the development of a constitutive model (i.e., relationship between stresses and strains) which describes the tissue mechanical behavior as observed in the experiment and provides a mathematical representation of the tissue's material properties.

Historically, the sclera has been described as a thin-walled, spherical pressure vessel obeying the analytical equation known as Laplace's law. Laplace's law is useful to estimate the state of stress in nonbiological pressure vessels, but it is inadequate for describing many aspects of the eye's mechanical response to variations in IOP. The sclera has been shown to exhibit several properties that violate the assumptions of Laplace's law. First, the eye is a pressure vessel of nonuniform thickness.[11-13] Second, in terms of its material properties, the sclera is nonlinear,[14-16] anisotropic,[16,17] and viscoelastic.[18-20] These concepts are fundamental to understanding scleral and ONH biomechanics, and below we present them in greater detail.

Nonlinearity is a property exhibited by most soft tissues, often as a consequence of collagen fibers within the tissue[1] (Figure 20.4). In a pressure vessel with linear material properties, the stiffness would remain constant during pressure-induced deformation, whereas a nonlinear pressure vessel would experience either softening or stiffening as it deforms. Recent experiments have shown that the sclera exhibits a considerable increase in stiffness, at least fivefold, when exposed to an acute elevation of IOP from 5 to 45 mmHg.[15] This dramatic change shows the substantial impact that collagen fibers can have on scleral stiffness and deformation.

Anisotropy, as opposed to isotropy, is the property by which materials exhibit different stiffness in different directions. For thin biological tissues, anisotropy is primarily dictated by the organization of their fibrous structure, which is confined within the plane of the tissue, as illustrated in Figure 20.4. Unlike the cornea, scleral collagen fiber orientation has not been fully characterized. However, it has been shown through computational modeling that collagen fiber orientation and distribution are major determinants of scleral deformation.[21] Further experimental work is needed to characterize better scleral anisotropy and its effects on LC biomechanics.

Viscoelastic materials, such as the sclera, exhibit higher resistance to deformation when loaded quickly rather than slowly. Downs and coworkers characterized the viscoelastic material properties of normal rabbit and monkey peripapillary sclera[18,22] and found that the material properties of peripapillary sclera are highly time-dependent (viscoelastic). This behavior protects ocular tissues from large deformations during short-term spikes in IOP, which occur during blinks, eye rubbing, or high-speed impacts.

These three aspects of the sclera's material properties – nonlinearity, anisotropy, and viscoelasticity – affect IOP-induced scleral deformations, but they are not the only important determinants of the eye's mechanical response. Material properties may be combined with thickness and shape to define another useful concept, that of structural, or effective, stiffness.

Studies of the scleral thickness of human[13,23] and monkey[11,12] eyes show that, on average, the human sclera is about twice as thick as the monkey sclera. The sclera is thinnest near the equator (as thin as 100 μm in both species) and thickest in the peripapillary region (average of 1000 μm in the human and 450 μm in the monkey). Large variations

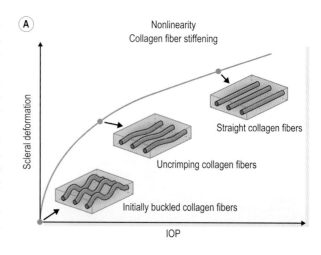

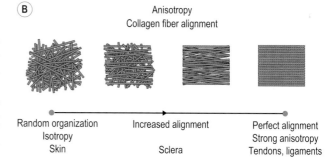

Figure 20.4 (A) Nonlinearity is a property that sclera exhibits, in which the relationship between loading and deformation is not linear. At low intraocular pressure (IOP), collagen fibers are initially crimped, which makes the sclera more compliant. As IOP increases, the scleral collagen fibers uncrimp and eventually become straight, resulting in a dramatic increase in scleral stiffness (an increase in the amount of IOP elevation necessary to produce the same deformation). (B) Schematic illustration of the various degrees of planar anisotropy present in thin soft tissues. Skin has a highly disorganized arrangement of collagen fibers and therefore resists loads similarly in many directions, a property known as isotropy. In contrast, tendons have well-organized collagen fibers running principally in the longitudinal direction, and therefore these tissues sustain loads differently along and across their length, a property known as anisotropy. The sclera is thought to have a collagen fiber alignment that is between those of skin and ligaments.

in peripapillary scleral thickness occur naturally and in pathologic conditions (e.g., myopia[24]), and have been hypothesized to be an important determinant of individual susceptibility to IOP.[25,26] Figure 20.5 illustrates how IOP-related stress is distributed in the peripapillary sclera in two situations: homogeneous thickness with a circular scleral canal, and inhomogeneous thickness with an elliptical scleral canal.

Optic nerve head and lamina cribosa biomechanics

Models of the optic nerve head

Initial experimental studies of ONH biomechanics were often designed to examine and quantify a posterior deformation of the LC in response to an acute increase in IOP. Unfortunately, it is difficult to take measurements of the LC directly because it is fragile and relatively inaccessible, and

Constant thickness

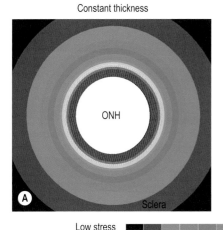

Variable thickness

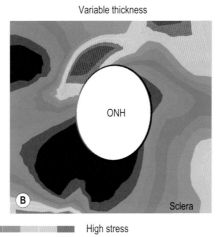

Low stress ▰▰▰▰▰▰▰▰▰▰▰▰▰▰▰ High stress

Figure 20.5 The thickness of the peripapillary sclera and the size and shape of the scleral canal influence the magnitude and distribution of intraocular pressure-related stress within the peripapillary sclera, and within the optic nerve head (ONH). Plots of stress within three-dimensional biomechanical models of the posterior sclera and ONH illustrate how stress concentrates around the scleral canal. (A) An idealized model with a circular canal and a perfectly spherical scleral shell wall of uniform thickness. (B) An elliptical scleral canal with anatomic variations in scleral shell thickness. In both cases, the stresses concentrate around the canal, but the more realistic model shows stress that varies substantially around the canal and can extend further out into the sclera. For clarity, only the scleral tissues are shown.

Box 20.5 The role of imaging

- Models have suggested that the intraocular pressure-induced displacements of the optic nerve head surface might not be a good surrogate for those of the underlying lamina
- Advances in imaging such as deep-scanning ocular coherence tomography show promise for imaging the acute deformations of the lamina

Box 20.6 Parameterized models

- Parametric computational models of the optic nerve head (ONH) identified the five most important determinants of ONH biomechanics (in rank order) as:
  1. The compliance of the sclera
  2. The size of the eye
  3. Intraocular pressure
  4. The compliance of the lamina cribrosa
  5. The thickness of the sclera

---

therefore experimental efforts used one of two approaches: histological examination of ONH tissues fixed at different IOPs[27,28] or measurement of acute deformations of the ONH surface through imaging, and using these deformations as a surrogate for the deformations of the underlying LC.[29]

Both approaches produced interesting results. For example, histology-based studies found that acutely elevating IOP produced a posterior deformation of the LC (12–79 μm in humans,[27,30] and 10–23 μm in monkeys[31]). However, these studies also highlighted the large variability in ONH geometry between individuals and the difficulties inherent in histomorphometry, which complicates distinguishing the effects of IOP from the natural differences between eyes. Imaging-based studies were subject to the assumption that IOP-induced deformations of the ONH surface are a good surrogate for deformations of the LC. Some experiments, as well as the modeling studies we describe below, have suggested that IOP-induced deformations of the ONH surface are not good predictors of LC deformations (Box 20.5).

Recently, there have been advances in direct imaging of the acute deformations of the LC itself using second harmonic imaging[32] or deep-scanning ocular coherence tomography[33] (Figure 20.6). Although promising, these technologies are still in development and have been unable to characterize the response of the ONH tissues to IOP.

In the absence of robust experimental methods for measuring the response of ONH tissues to acute IOP changes, several researchers have adopted a modeling approach to characterize the mechanical behavior of the ONH. Some of the models have been analytical,[34,35] but the majority are numerical.[36,37] While analytic approaches are attractive for their elegance, numerical models can incorporate more complex and realistic ONH geometry and material properties, such as variable sclera thickness, anisotropy, and nonlinearity.

An early example of numerical modeling is the work of Bellezza et al.[36] They used a model to study the effects of the size and eccentricity of the scleral canal on the mechanical response of the ONH, and found that IOP-related stresses within the connective tissues of the ONH could be substantial, up to two orders of magnitude larger than IOP, even at low levels of IOP. Models with larger canal diameters, more elliptical canal openings, and thinner sclera all showed increased stresses in the ONH and peripapillary sclera for a given IOP increase. The models of Bellezza et al were highly idealized with a rudimentary description of the LC, but were the first to leverage the power of numerical models for the analysis of ONH biomechanics. Sander et al developed the most advanced analytic models to date, and arrived at similar conclusions.[34]

Sigal et al developed a more comprehensive generic model to study ONH biomechanics[37] (Box 20.6 and Figure 20.7). Unlike the initial models by Bellezza et al, these models incorporated a simplified central retinal vessel and pre- and postlaminar neural tissues, which allowed them to compare the simulated IOP-induced displacements and deformations of the ONH surface with those of the LC. The central retinal vessel had only a minimal effect on ONH biomechanics and was not included in later models. More importantly, they found that the IOP-induced deformations of the ONH surface and LC, although related, are somewhat decoupled, and therefore that the displacements of the ONH surface might not be a good surrogate for those of the LC. This result was later also obtained with more complex models with eye-specific geometry of the ONH (described below), and observed in recent experiments.[33]

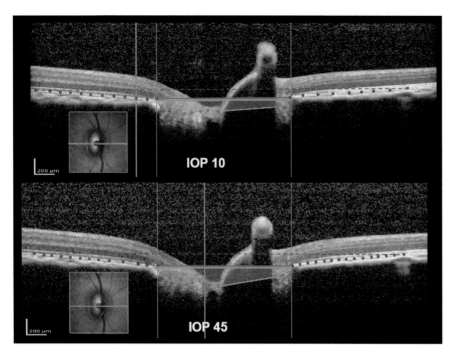

Figure 20.6 High-resolution Spectralis (Heidelberg Engineering, Heidelberg, Germany) ocular coherence tomographic (OCT) B-scans of a normal monkey eye obtained at 10 mmHg (top) and 45 mmHg (bottom) intraocular pressure (IOP). Bruch's membrane and the anterior lamina cribrosa (LC) surface have been delineated (red and green dots, respectively). The area enclosed by the anterior surface of the LC and a plane defined at Bruch's membrane (BM) opening (area shaded green) is larger in the scan at 45 mmHg. There was no detectable lateral expansion of the scleral canal (vertical green lines), suggesting that the increase in IOP produced posterior laminar deformation. Using a second reference plane parallel to BM opening (dashed red lines), it is also visible that the BM is outwardly bowed at high IOP, which suggests that there is IOP-induced posterior deformation of the peripapillary sclera. While choroidal compression may contribute to this finding, we believe that the behavior of BM is principally related to the behavior of the sclera. The parameters computed from the images are volumetric, but are shown here in cross-section for clarity.

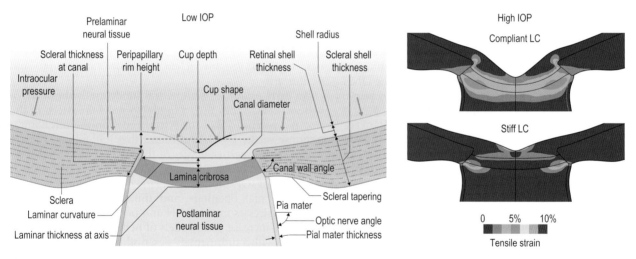

Figure 20.7 Generic models allow variation of parameters (left) to assess their independent, or combined, effects on optic nerve head biomechanics. Contour levels of tensile strain computed for an increase in intraocular pressure of 25 mmHg for two models that only differ in laminar stiffness (right). For clarity the deformation of the loaded models has been exaggerated five times, and an outline of the undeformed geometry has been overlaid. A more compliant lamina cribrosa is subject to higher strain and larger posterior deformation.

In a later study, Sigal et al[26] parameterized various geometric and material details of their model, and varied them independently to assess their impact on a host of outcome measures, including changes in the shape of the ONH tissues (such as cup-to-disc ratio), and stress and strain within the LC and neural tissues. This work identified the five most important determinants of ONH biomechanics (in rank order) as: the compliance of the sclera, the size of the eye, IOP, the compliance of the LC, and the thickness of the sclera. Their study was the first to quantify the important role of scleral properties on ONH biomechanics that we have described above. Parametric studies such as these are important because they can be used to identify the biomechanical factors that warrant more in depth study, as well as those factors that are unlikely to have a significant influence, thus providing information useful for focusing future experimental efforts.

Parametric models have also been leveraged to quantify the strength of the interactions between the factors that affect ONH biomechanics, that is, how the level of one factor influences another.[38] An example is represented by the concept of structural stiffness discussed above, where the mechanical response of the sclera depends on its thickness and on its material properties. Increasing the stiffness or thickness of the sclera independently leads to reduced deformations transmitted to the ONH. However, if the sclera is stiff, then its thickness has very little effect, or if the sclera is thick then its stiffness matters less. Identifying the strong interactions between factors is important because it facilitates interpretation of experiments that find, or fail to find, correlations between parameters and effects.

Notwithstanding their advantages over analytic models, the generic numeric models cannot, by design, make predictions of the biomechanics of a specific eye, and ultimately it is specific eyes for which we would like to predict the effects of IOP. To address this limitation eye-specific models have been developed based on 3D reconstructions of monkey[39-41] and human[6,42-44] eyes, with a long-term goal of building models based on clinical imaging of living eyes and using them in the determination of interventional target IOP.

Sigal and coworkers reconstructed eye-specific models of human eyes based on histological sections of donor tissue (Figure 20.8).[42] These models were similar to their generic models in the sense that that they incorporated load-bearing (sclera, LC, and pia mater) as well as pre- and postlaminar neural tissues into the analyses. They used these models to study the relative influences of geometry and material properties on the response of the ONH to changes in IOP.[43,44] Their results were somewhat surprising in that the differences in geometry between individual ONHs had a more limited influence on ONH biomechanics than the properties of the surrounding sclera. They also found, consistent with the results obtained using generic models, that the IOP-induced deformations of the ONH surface are likely not a good surrogate for the deformations of the LC. Eye-specific models also show that as IOP increases the scleral canal expands, tautening the LC, and that the magnitude of the compressive strains is higher than that of the tensile or shear strains.[6] Although it is now clear that the various modes of strain (tensile, compressive, and shear) are related and all occur simultaneously within the ONH, their relative magnitudes in the models could have been a consequence of the assumed material properties. The models of Sigal et al have some limitations: the reconstruction methods might not have removed all the artifacts that arise due to warping of the histological sections during preparation; and since the models are reconstructed from donor human eyes, the studies were unable to test some hypotheses in the development of glaucoma.

Models of the lamina cribrosa

A different approach for eye-specific finite element (FE) modeling has been adopted by Burgoyne and coworkers that focuses only on the collagenous load-bearing tissues of the sclera and LC.[45] Using a microtome-based technique to compile consecutive episcopic images of a surface-stained, embedded tissue block face, they are able to reconstruct the details of the laminar microarchitecture in three dimensions at high resolution. The ability to gather data from contralateral normal and glaucomatous monkey eyes makes this approach especially powerful and has provided insight into tissue-level morphometric changes that occur in response to chronic IOP elevations.[39-41]

The first use of these reconstructions in the context of FE analysis has been to define descriptions of the LC that capture the inhomogeneity of the LC connective tissue structure (Figure 20.9). In these models, the regional variations in LC connective tissue volume fraction and predominant

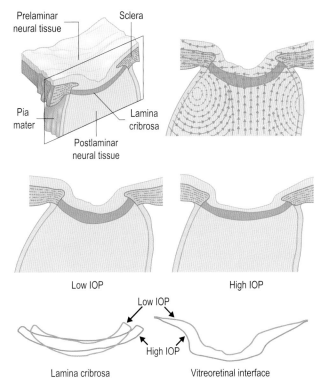

Figure 20.8 Eye-specific model reconstructed from an ostensibly healthy human donor eye simulated for an increase in intraocular pressure (IOP) from 5 to 50 mmHg. The top left image is a three-dimensional view of the model cut sagittally to show the interior. As IOP is increased the tissues deform. The displacement vectors are shown on the top right overlaid on a sagittal cross-section. The vectors were computed in three dimensions, with their two-dimensional projections shown. Vector lengths are proportional to the magnitude of the total displacement, with the scale exaggerated for clarity. The middle row shows the sagittal cross-sections of the model at low (left) and high (right) IOP. Deformations are exaggerated fivefold for clarity. Visible are effects such as the rotation of the sclera, the flattening of the cup, the thinning of the lamina cribrosa (LC) and prelaminar neural tissues and the anterior movement of the central regions of the optic nerve relative to the LC. To highlight the deformations of the LC and vitreoretinal interface these are shown in the bottom row, with low (green) and high (red) IOP outlines overlaid. The outlines show the stretching of the LC in the plane of the sclera, and the deepening of the cup. Note that these simulations were carried out assuming incompressible materials, and therefore that the thinning of the LC and the prelaminar neural region does not represent a reduction in tissue volume, only a redistribution.

laminar beam orientation are analyzed in small regions, the "elements," to define local material properties for the laminar regions of the model. Thus, regions within the LC with higher and lower porosity behave mechanically with greater and lesser compliance, respectively, and regions that exhibit strong directional orientation of laminar beams resist deformation more strongly, i.e., are stiffer, in those directions. This approach has demonstrated the importance of representing regional LC connective tissue inhomogeneity and anisotropy into models to capture the biomechanical behavior of the LC[46] (Box 20.7). These models have also suggested that the LC may become more compliant in the early stage of glaucoma development despite an apparent increase in laminar connective tissue.

The continuum-level method described above homogenizes small elemental regions of LC microarchitecture into a bulk description of their effective material properties,

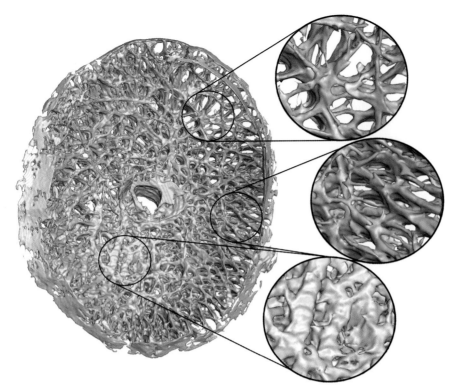

Figure 20.9 High-resolution three-dimensional reconstruction of the lamina cribrosa from a monkey eye obtained using an episcopic serial imaging technique optimized for connective tissue detection. Note the regional variation in both connective tissue density and predominant laminar beam orientation throughout the lamina cribrosa. These spatial variations in microarchitecture will affect the regional deformation and load-bearing characteristics of the lamina cribrosa both as a whole and at the level of the individual laminar beams. These data have been used to develop finite element models describing both the macro- and beam-level mechanical environment in the optic nerve head, such as those shown in Figure 20.10.

Box 20.7 The important role of laminar microstructure

- Models that incorporate the details of the microstructure of the lamina cribrosa have shown that beam-level stresses and strains are likely to be substantially higher than those computed with continuum-level models

---

precluding an analysis of the beam-level mechanical environment within the LC. To address this limitation, Downs and colleagues have developed a microscale modeling approach based on a substructuring paradigm. In this technique, continuum element-level displacement predictions from a parent model serve as inputs to corresponding element-sized micromodels so that resultant stresses and strains within laminar beams may be calculated (Figure 20.10). This technique not only reveals the complexity of IOP-related stresses and strains within the LC beams themselves, but also shows that beam-level stresses and strains are higher than those calculated using models that do not explicitly model the LC beams.[47] Furthermore, these micro-FE models predict that there are individual laminar beams with levels of IOP-related strain that are likely pathologic. While still in its early stages, this work holds the possibility of testing hypotheses about failure mechanisms and cellular responses at the level of the laminar beams.

In a complementary approach to the substructuring method described above, Kodiyalam and coworkers have developed a technique to analyze the entire LC using voxel-based FE models derived from the serial data sets described above.[48] These models are generated by directly converting image voxels into finite elements, and are analyzed using specialized algorithms optimized for the computational demands of this approach. Analysis of these voxel models is computationally intensive and requires massive storage and computer cluster resources to manage. Like the substructuring method, this approach explicitly represents the beams of the LC and therefore may be useful for characterizing the mechanical environment to which astrocytes are exposed. In its current implementation, these voxel models also account for a highly compliant neural tissue component within the porous LC space and may therefore provide insight into the effect of the translaminar pressure gradient on axoplasmic flow, and the tissues and cells of the ONH.

Pathophysiology

Other measures of acute intraocular pressure-related changes in the optic nerve head

ONH, retinal, and choroidal blood flow are also affected by acute IOP elevations. For example, studies using microspheres[49] have suggested that volume flow within the prelaminar and anterior laminar capillary beds is diminished once ocular perfusion pressure (defined as the systolic arterial blood pressure plus one-third of the difference between systolic and diastolic pressures minus IOP) falls below 30 mmHg.

While a direct link to mechanical strain has not been established, axonal transport is compromised in the LC at physiologic levels of IOP[50] and is further impaired following acute IOP elevations.[2,51] In a biomechanical context, several explanations might account for these observations. First, as the LC pores change conformation due to IOP-related mechanical strain, slight constriction of the axon bundles within these pores may occur, directly hindering axoplasmic

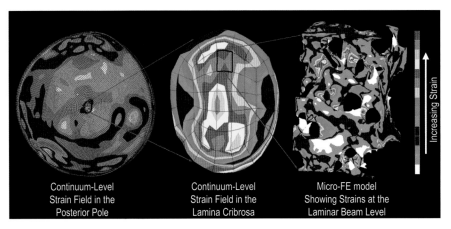

Continuum-Level
Strain Field in the
Posterior Pole

Continuum-Level
Strain Field in the
Lamina Cribrosa

Micro-FE model
Showing Strains at the
Laminar Beam Level

Increasing Strain

Figure 20.10 Multiscale modeling of the mechanical environment of the lamina cribrosa. The image on the left shows the strain distribution within a continuum-level model of the connective tissues of the posterior pole of the eye. Note that thickness variations in the sclera give rise to a nonuniform distribution of strain within the shell and that the strains are lower in the sclera than in the more compliant lamina cribrosa. The middle image shows a detail of the strain field within the continuum representation of the lamina cribrosa. While this portion of the finite element model has been assigned regional material properties related to the amount and orientation of the laminar beams (based on three-dimensional reconstruction data, such as that in Figure 20.9), the continuum description represents a bulk homogenization of the specific microarchitecture in each element. The right image shows the distribution of strains in a micromodel that captures the explicit laminar beam microarchitecture associated with a particular element of the laminar reconstruction. At this scale the strain distribution is complex.

transport. Second, it may be that the IOP-related reduction in blood flow in the laminar region impairs the mitochondrial metabolism that drives axoplasmic transport. Finally, axoplasmic transport could be sensitive to the magnitude of the translaminar pressure gradient, such that the active transport mechanisms within the bundles are required to overcome the resistance of the pressure gradient to drive axoplasmic flow.

In summary, while connective tissue dynamics should, by themselves, directly and indirectly influence astrocyte and glial metabolism and axonal transport, glaucomatous damage within the ONH may not necessarily occur at locations with the highest levels of IOP-related connective tissue strain or stress, but rather at those locations where the translaminar tissue pressure gradient is greatest and/or where the axons, blood supply, and astrocytes and glia have been made most vulnerable. Further studies are necessary to elucidate the link(s) between IOP, mechanical strain, blood flow, astrocyte and glial cell homeostasis, and axoplasmic transport in the ONH, in both the physiologic and diseased states.

Cellular mechanics

Laminar astrocytes have been shown to respond to changes in hydrostatic or barometric pressure.[52] However, the uncertain role of hypoxia and the lack of astrocyte basement membrane deformation in the barometric pressure model has led to questions concerning the true nature of the insult delivered to the cells in the hydrostatic pressure model. Instead, recent studies have concentrated on genomic and biochemical characterization of ONH astrocytes grown on membranes subjected to controlled levels of strain.[53] In vitro techniques face the difficulty of subjecting the cells to the complex, multimode, 3D strain fields that exist within the ONH. Subjecting the cells to this environment while still being able to test their response is a major challenge for both biology and engineering. We expect that, in time, strain predictions from computational FE models and data on

IOP fluctuation from telemetric IOP monitoring studies will allow these experiments to model physiologic and pathophysiologic conditions more closely in the normal and glaucomatous eye.

Restructuring and remodeling of the optic nerve head

Normal aging

As demonstrated in the previous sections, the connective tissues of the ONH experience substantial levels of IOP-related stress and strain, even at physiologic levels of IOP. We propose that exposure to these levels of stress and strain over a lifetime results in a host of gradual changes to both connective tissues and vasculature that underlie the process of normal aging in the ONH. Thus the biological processes associated with glaucomatous damage and remodeling of ONH tissues occur in tandem with the normal physiologic remodeling processes associated with aging and it is therefore important to characterize the age-related changes that occur in the ONH connective tissues.

At the cellular level, age-related changes in the ONH include increased collagen deposition in the laminar ECM and thickening of associated astrocyte basement membranes.[54,55] Mechanically, it has also been shown that the LC and sclera become more rigid with age.[54] All of these changes may act in concert with age-related decreases in volume flow within the laminar capillary network to compromise nutrient diffusion across the laminar ECM to the axonal bundles in older patients.

Alterations in connective tissue architecture, cellular activity, axoplasmic transport, and blood flow in early glaucoma

Pathophysiologic levels of stress and strain can induce aberrant changes in cell synthesis and tissue composition and microarchitecture that exceed the effects of normal aging.

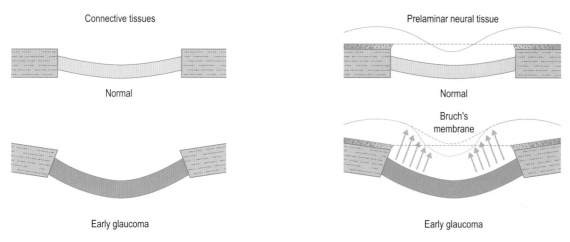

Connective tissues   Prelaminar neural tissue

Normal   Normal

Bruch's membrane

Early glaucoma   Early glaucoma

Figure 20.11 Remodeling and restructuring of the optic nerve head (ONH) in early experimental glaucoma. Sagittal-section diagrams of the ONH, showing the peripapillary sclera (hatched) and the lamina cribrosa for normal and early glaucoma eyes. Left: the early glaucoma eye has undergone permanent changes in ONH geometry, including thickening of the lamina, posterior deformation of the lamina and peripapillary sclera, and posterior scleral canal expansion. Right: recent work has also shown that, although the cup deepens relative to Bruch's membrane opening (dashed purple line), as can be detected by longitudinal confocal scanning laser tomography imaging (orange line) in early glaucoma, the prelaminar neural tissues are actually thickened rather than thinned. (Reprinted with permission from Yang H, Downs JC, Bellezza AJ, et al. 3-D histomorphometry of the normal and early glaucomatous monkey optic nerve head: prelaminar neural tissues and cupping. Invest Ophthalmol Vis Sci 2007;48:5068–5084.)

Two important pathophysiologies can follow in glaucoma: (1) mechanical yield and/or failure of load-bearing connective tissues in the ONH, and (2) progressive damage of adjacent axons by multiple mechanisms (Figure 20.1). Importantly, changes that compromise the load-bearing function and alter the stress and strain environment within the ONH connective tissues may act in a mechanical feedback manner to degrade further the biomechanical and cellular milieu.

Early glaucomatous damage has not been rigorously studied in humans because of the paucity of well-characterized cadaveric eye specimens with early damage. Analysis of early experimental glaucoma in monkeys with moderate IOP elevations has revealed several aspects of the early changes in ONH and peripapillary scleral connective tissue architecture and material properties. These changes (Figure 20.11) include: (1) thickening of prelaminar neural tissues[40]; (2) enlargement and elongation of the neural canal[39]; (3) posterior deformation and thickening of the LC with mild posterior deformation of the scleral flange and peripapillary sclera[41]; (4) hypercompliance of the LC in some animals[31]; and (5) alterations in the viscoelastic material properties of the peripapillary sclera[18,22] (Box 20.8).

The effects of early glaucoma on cellular activity, axoplasmic transport, and blood flow have not been rigorously documented in the monkey model. In the rat eye, however, genomic techniques have been used to characterize changes in the genome of ONH tissues (within which a minimal LC exists in the rat) following exposure to experimentally elevated IOP.[56] Within eyes that exhibited an early focal stage of orbital optic nerve axon loss an increase in gene expression was noted for several ECM components, including tenascin C, fibulin 2, and the matrix metalloproteinase inhibitor tissue inhibitor of metalloproteinase 1 (TIMP-1), along with increased expression of genes governing the initiation of cell division. In a rat optic nerve transection model, differences in gene expression patterns suggested that the

---

Box 20.8 Restructuring and remodeling of the optic nerve head with glaucomatous progression

- As glaucoma progresses, the optic nerve head remodels and restructures
- In the monkey model, compared to their contralateral normal control eyes, early glaucoma eyes exhibit a thicker lamina, posteriorly deformed lamina, and peripapillary sclera, posterior scleral canal expansion, and thickened prelaminar neural tissues

---

focal axon loss mentioned above was due to IOP effects rather than simply axonal loss.

Alterations in connective tissue architecture, cellular activity, axoplasmic transport, and blood flow in later stages of glaucomatous damage

The classic morphological description of glaucomatous damage – profound posterior laminar deformation, excavation of the scleral canal beneath the optic disc margin, and compression of the LC – derives largely from human and monkey eyes with moderate, severe, and end-stage glaucomatous damage.[57,58] These studies often encompass a broad range of glaucomatous damage to specimens which unfortunately have a poorly characterized IOP history. Thus, a temporal narrative of the progression of events in the IOP-insulted ONH has not emerged. Nevertheless, histologic studies have reported that several consistent phenomena occur in glaucomatous tissue, including withdrawal of astrocyte processes from laminar beams,[59] astrocyte basement membrane disruption and thickening, degradation of elastin within the laminar beams, physical disruption of the laminar beams, and remodeling of the ECM.[60,61] It is reasonable to assume that many of these effects are due to IOP-induced alterations in the synthetic activities of resident cell populations.[59,62]

Alterations in axoplasmic transport at the LC[63] level have been described in human and monkey eyes exposed to chronic IOP elevation, along with a complicated array of ONH, retinal, and choroidal blood flow alterations.[64] However, because direct observation of ONH blood flow at the level of the peripapillary sclera and the LC capillaries level is not yet technically feasible, a rigorous study of the primary effect of IOP on blood flow remains elusive. Techniques to elucidate the relationships between ONH blood flow, ONH connective tissue integrity, ONH glial cell activity, and RGC axonal transport within individual human and animal eyes are needed to unify our understanding of the multiple levels of interaction in this system.

One link between IOP-related strain in the ONH and concomitant cellular response may be found in the study of the spatial distribution of integrin types within the nerve head. Integrins are proteins that span the basement membranes of laminar astrocytes and capillary endothelial cells to bind to ligands in the ECM, providing a direct interaction between the cell cytoskeleton and the substrate to which the cell is attached. As such, integrins are ideally suited to act as critical components within a mechanosensory system that transduces IOP- and blood flow-related changes in the ONH into subsequent cellular activity. Morrison has described the location and alteration of integrin subunits in normal and glaucomatous human and monkey eyes[65] and has proposed that they are an important link between LC deformation and damage, LC connective tissue remodeling, and LC astrocyte-mediated axonal insult in glaucoma.

Future directions

Clinical implications

There are currently no science-based tools to predict the level of IOP at which an individual ONH will be damaged. As described herein, computational modeling is a tool for predicting how a biological tissue with complex geometry and material properties will behave under varying levels of load. The goal of modeling eyes from human donors and monkeys with experimental glaucoma is to learn what aspects of neural, vascular, and connective tissue architecture are most important to the ability of a given ONH to maintain structural integrity, nutritional and oxygen supply, and axoplasmic transport at physiologic and non-physiologic levels of IOP. In the future, clinical imaging of the ONH will seek to capture the architecture of these structures so as to allow clinically derived biomechanical models of individual patient risk. Eventually knowledge of the relationship between IOP, mechanical strain, systemic blood pressure, and the resultant astrocyte and axonal mitochondrial oxygen levels will drive the clinical assessment of safe target IOP. Clinical characterization of the actual IOP insult through telemetric IOP monitoring will eventually allow better-controlled studies of individual ONH susceptibility. Finally, these modeling-driven targets for clinical imaging of subsurface structures will likely allow early detection of LC deformation and thickening. Once clinically detectable, early stabilization, and perhaps reversal, of these changes will become a new endpoint for target IOP lowering in most ocular hypertensive and all progressing eyes.

Basic research directions

From an engineering standpoint, large challenges remain to achieve basic and clinical knowledge regarding: (1) the mechanisms and distributions of IOP-related yield and failure in the laminar beams and peripapillary sclera; (2) the mechanobiology of the astrocytes, glia, scleral fibroblasts, and LC cells; (3) the mechanobiology of axoplasmic flow within the LC; (4) the fluid dynamics governing the volume of blood flow within the laminar capillaries and scleral and laminar branches of the posterior ciliary arteries; and (5) nutrient diffusion to the astrocytes in young and aged eyes. We predict that knowledge gained from these studies will importantly contribute to new therapeutic interventions aimed at the ONH and peripapillary sclera of glaucomatous eyes.

Key references

A complete list of chapter references is available online at www.expertconsult.com. See inside cover for registration details.

2. Minckler DS, Bunt AH, Johanson GW. Orthograde and retrograde axoplasmic transport during acute ocular hypertension in the monkey. Invest Ophthalmol Vis Sci 1977;16:426–441.

6. Sigal IA, Flanagan JG, Tertinegg I, et al. Predicted extension, compression and shearing of optic nerve head tissues. Exp Eye Res 2007;85:312–322.

11. Downs JC, Blidner RA, Bellezza AJ, et al. Peripapillary scleral thickness in perfusion-fixed normal monkey eyes. Invest Ophthalmol Vis Sci 2002;43:2229–2235.

15. Girard MJA, Downs JC, Bottlang M, et al. Peripapillary and posterior scleral mechanics: part II: experimental and inverse finite element characterization. Exp Eye Res 2009;88:799–807. J Biomech Eng 2009;131:051012.

20. Siegwart JT Jr, Norton TT. Regulation of the mechanical properties of tree shrew sclera by the visual environment. Vision Res 1999;39:387–407.

25. Burgoyne CF, Downs JC, Bellezza AJ, et al. The optic nerve head as a biomechanical structure: a new paradigm for understanding the role of IOP-related stress and strain in the pathophysiology of glaucomatous optic nerve head damage. Prog Retin Eye Res 2005;24:39–73.

26. Sigal IA, Flanagan JG, Ethier CR. Factors influencing optic nerve head biomechanics. Invest Ophthalmol Vis Sci 2005;46:4189–4199.

40. Yang H, Downs JC, Bellezza AJ, et al. 3-D histomorphometry of the normal and early glaucomatous monkey optic nerve head: prelaminar neural tissues and cupping. Invest Ophthalmol Vis Sci 2007;48:5068–5084.

53. Kirwan RP, Fenerty CH, Crean J, et al. Influence of cyclical mechanical

strain on extracellular matrix gene expression in human lamina cribrosa cells in vitro. Mol Vis 2005;11:798–810.

58. Quigley HA, Hohman RM, Addicks EM, et al. Morphologic changes in the lamina cribrosa correlated with neural loss in open-angle glaucoma. Am J Ophthalmol 1983;95:673–691.

59. Hernandez MR. The optic nerve head in glaucoma: role of astrocytes in tissue remodeling. Prog Retin Eye Res 2000; 19:297–321.

63. Quigley HA, Addicks EM. Chronic experimental glaucoma in primates. II. Effect of extended intraocular pressure elevation on optic nerve head and axonal transport. Invest Ophthalmol Vis Sci 1980;19:137–152.

65. Morrison JC. Integrins in the optic nerve head: potential roles in glaucomatous optic neuropathy (an American Ophthalmological Society thesis). Trans Am Ophthalmol Soc 2006;104:453–477.

CHAPTER 21

Pigmentary dispersion syndrome and glaucoma

Michael G Anderson

Overview

Pigment dispersion syndrome (PDS) and its potential sequela, pigmentary glaucoma (PG), are characterized by disruption of the iris pigment epithelium (IPE) and subsequent deposition of the dispersed pigment throughout the anterior chamber. Once thought to be rare, PDS is now appreciated to be a very common condition. In most people, PDS can exist for long periods of time without contributing to further pathology. However, in some people the accumulation of pigment and debris liberated from the IPE is accompanied by elevated intraocular pressure (IOP) and increased risk of glaucoma. Current theories of the pathophysiology of PDS and PG are dominated by a hypothesis first postulated by Campbell that pigment dispersion is initiated by mechanical abrasion between the iris and anterior packets of lens zonules.[1] While this hypothesis explains several clinical features of the disease and has gained wide acceptance, several gaps in knowledge still remain. This chapter reviews the current state of knowledge and draws attention to lingering questions relevant to the basic mechanisms of PDS and PG.

Clinical background

Key symptoms and signs

The key feature of PDS and PG is shedding of melanin pigment from the IPE with subsequent accumulation on anterior-segment structures (Box 21.1). Although dispersed pigment can be widely distributed, it tends to accumulate in characteristic regions. One particularly recognizable sign of PDS is a narrow, vertical, spindle-shaped brown band of pigment deposited on the central corneal endothelium (referred to as a "Krukenberg's spindle"; Figure 21.1). Dispersed pigment is also found scattered on the surface of the iris (Figure 21.2), in the trabecular meshwork (especially inferiorly), and at the junction of the posterior lens capsule and zonules (referred to as a "Scheie's stripe"). Radial, midperipheral, slit-like iris transillumination defects are typically present (Figure 21.3). PDS is asymptomatic. The majority of PDS cases do not progress to PG and the prognosis is usually good.

However, in some PDS cases IOP becomes elevated and PG may ensue. The key signs of PG match those for PDS, but may also involve large fluctuations in IOP, optic nerve head cupping, and visual field changes. Like most forms of glaucoma, PG is asymptomatic for many people. Patients may present with symptoms related to episodic rises in IOP, such as colored halos around lights and blurred vision.

Historical perspective

Current knowledge of PDS and PG began with important contributions from Krukenberg, who in 1899 reported spindle-shaped pigment deposition on the cornea,[2] and von Hippel, who in 1901 suggested that pigment accumulations obstructing aqueous humor outflow could lead to elevated IOP.[3] By 1949, Sugar and Barbour recognized patients sharing Krukenberg's spindles, trabecular pigment accumulation, and open angles, naming the condition "pigmentary glaucoma."[4] The IPE was subsequently recognized as the source of liberated pigment, which Campbell proposed in 1979 to involve mechanical rubbing between anterior packets of lens zonules and the peripheral iris in predisposed eyes.[1] Although originally described as rare, Ritch et al have documented that PDS is in fact a very common condition[5] and have thus drawn attention to the need for a better understanding of factors determining whether or not PDS progresses to PG.

Epidemiology

The epidemiology of PDS and PG suggests a multifactorial disease process. PDS is extremely common in the general population. For example, a screen conducted by Ritch et al in New York found PDS in 2.45% of people examined.[5] In contrast, PG is less common. Studies examining the conversion rate from PDS to PG have yielded varying results, with studies of patients in glaucoma specialty practices yielding conversion rates from 35% to 50%,[6–8] whereas a community-based study found a conversion rate of only 10% at 5 years and 15% at 15 years.[9]

PG is particularly likely to affect young myopic males. PDS is most commonly observed in patients 30–50 years old.[4,6,9–11] While PDS occurs in approximately equal numbers of men and women, progression to PG is more likely to occur in men.[4,9–11] PDS and PG are both associated with

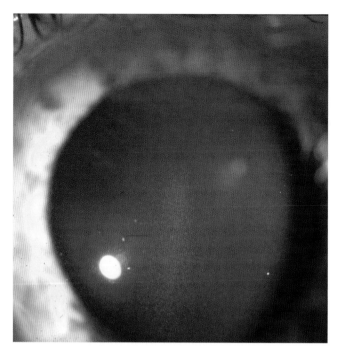

Figure 21.1 Krukenberg's spindle. Dispersed pigment often accumulates as a vertically oriented spindle-shaped brown band on the central corneal endothelium. (Courtesy of Dr. WLM Alward, Department of Ophthalmology and Visual Sciences, University of Iowa.)

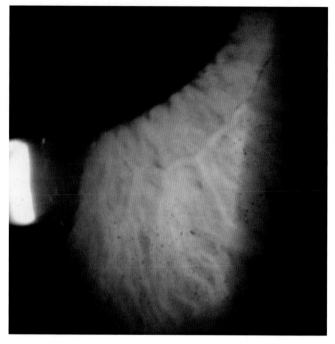

Figure 21.2 Dispersed pigment on iris. Multiple small clumps of dispersed pigment are typically visible across the surface of the iris. (Courtesy of Dr. WLM Alward, Department of Ophthalmology and Visual Sciences, University of Iowa.)

Box 21.1 Key signs

Signs of pigment dispersion syndrome

- Krukenberg's spindle
- Dispersed pigment on iris
- Darkly pigmented trabecular meshwork
- Dispersed pigment of anterior lens capsule
- Scheie's stripe

Signs of pigmentary glaucoma

- Pigment dispersion syndrome
- Fluctuations in intraocular pressure
- Optic nerve head cupping
- Visual field changes

---

myopia.[4,6,9,11] However, it is unclear whether myopia contributes to the likelihood of progression from PDS to PG, with some studies finding severe myopia predictive of progression[6] and others finding no statistically significant correlation with conversion.[9]

Genetics

PG is believed to be strongly influenced by heredity, but definitive mutations associated with the disease have not yet been identified. Several families affected by PG have been described. In some pedigrees, inheritance appears to follow an autosomal-dominant mode of inheritance.[12–14] However, some pedigrees are consistent with recessive inheritance[15] and other authors report that the majority of cases appear sporadic.[16] Positive family histories for glaucoma among PG patients vary widely, with studies reporting a positive family

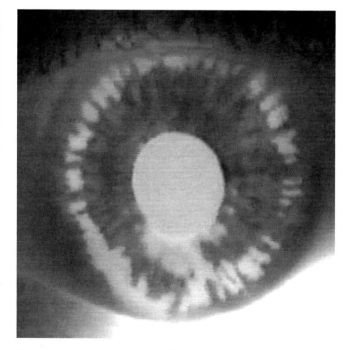

Figure 21.3 Iris transillumination defects characteristic of pigment dispersion syndrome (PDS). Single frame from infrared videography of a patient with PDS. Radial, midperipheral, slit-like iris transillumination defects correspond in number and location to anterior packets of lens zonules. (Courtesy of Dr. WLM Alward, Department of Ophthalmology and Visual Sciences, University of Iowa.)

history for glaucoma in 16–48% of cases.[9,11] These disparate observations might be explained in several ways, including incomplete penetrance of a dominant disorder, multigenic influences, and complex gene–environment interactions, to name a few. Promising findings have reported linkage to loci at chromosomal locations 7q36[12] and 18q22.[17] Mutations at these loci have not yet been identified. To date, the potential importance of these loci has neither been replicated nor refuted by other groups, leaving their potential role in most cases unclear.

Diagnostic workup

Initial diagnosis of PDS is typically based entirely on slit-lamp examination. Classical features contributing to diagnosis include: (1) presence of a Krukenberg's spindle; (2) dense trabecular pigmentation; (3) presence of Scheie's stripe; and (4) radial, slit-like, midperipheral iris transillumination defects. However, many patients will not simultaneously exhibit all four features.[9] Posterior bowing of the midperipheral iris, which likely contributes to mechanical abrasion between the iris and lens zonules, is often detectable (Figure 21.4). The extent of pigment dispersion is an important component of diagnosis as small amounts of pigment accumulation within the trabecular meshwork are also part of the normal aging process. Because PDS tends to become quiescent with advancing age, older patients with glaucoma may have only subtle features of PDS and may be misdiagnosed with primary open-angle or normal-tension glaucoma. Diagnosis of PG involves PDS, plus signs of glaucoma. Approximately 17% of PDS cases have PG at the time of initial diagnosis, suggesting that screening for glaucoma at the initial examination is warranted.[9]

Clinical signs of PDS and PG have been reported to show pronounced ethnic variability.[18,19] For example, the slit-like midperipheral iris transillumination defects identifiable by slit-lamp exam are frequently absent in African-Americans[19] and Chinese.[18] Variable iris transillumination related to iris color has previously been observed in other populations, with 25% of blue irides and 68% of brown irides lacking slit-like defects.[11] Thus, the frequent absence of iris transillumination defects in African-Americans and Chinese might partially be explained by darker iris colors. Use of sensitive infrared cameras to supplement traditional slit-lamp exams helps to detect iris transillumination defects in African-Americans with PDS, though the defects were not always the classic slit-like defects typical of PDS in Caucasians.[20] PDS and PG have previously been thought to be quite rare in African-Americans.[4,10] However, PDS might instead be underdiagnosed due to the difficulty of detecting these iris transillumination defects in African-Americans.[20]

Differential diagnosis

Differential diagnosis of PDS and PG includes exfoliation syndrome, uveitis, melanoma, iris and ciliary body cysts, trauma, postoperative conditions, and age-related changes. Exfoliation syndrome in particular involves substantial dispersion of pigment and some eyes have signs of both PDS and exfoliation syndrome.[21] The extent of iridocorneal angle pigmentation occurring in exfoliation syndrome can correlate more strongly with presenting IOP than does the amount of exfoliative material on the anterior lens capsule,[22] suggesting that the pigment dispersion occurring in exfoliation syndrome is also of pathologic relevance.

Treatment

In the absence of elevated IOP or progressive optic nerve damage, PDS typically does not require any treatment. Regular follow-up is suggested to monitor for possible progression to PG. Treatment for PG follows the same regime as open-angle glaucoma, but with some special considerations.[23] Miotics can decrease iridozonular contact and may prevent further progression of the disease, although use of this class of agents is limited because they can also worsen myopia and increase the risk of retinal detachment. Prostaglandin analogs such as latanoprost are effective in managing IOP in PG,[24] although these agents often also cause increased iridial pigmentation: in the context of PDS iris disease the long-term consequences of this pigmentation are largely unknown. When treated surgically, PG patients who have trabeculectomy are more likely to have issues with hypotony maculopathy because they tend to be young and myopic.

Pathology

A key finding in current theories of PDS and PG came from Campbell's 1979 histologic study of human eyes with PG.[1] In studying the normal anatomy of anterior zonules among

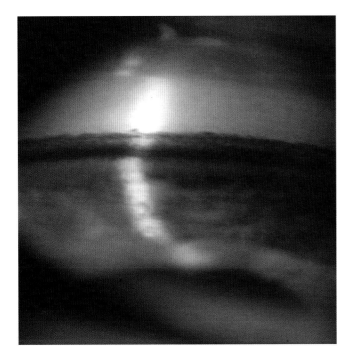

Figure 21.4 Posterior bowing of iris viewed by gonioscopy. Following the trajectory of the slit of light from the pupil toward the periphery highlights the iris concavity frequently observed in pigment dispersion syndrome. (Courtesy of Dr. WLM Alward, Department of Ophthalmology and Visual Sciences, University of Iowa.)

eyebank eyes, Campbell noted that zonules inserted on the anterior lens surface were not in single strands, but were organized into packets of zonules. The number of these packets ranged from 65 to 80, precisely the same as the number of slit-like iris transillumination defects observed in PG. This led to the hypothesis that if contact between the zonules and iris were to occur, this abrasion could account for the iris transillumination defects and dispersion of pigment observed in PDS and PG. In testing this by studying the pathology of eyes with radial slit-like iris transillumination defects, it was indeed found that wherever there was a slit-like transillumination defect, there was also a closely apposed packet of zonules. Combined with an observation that patients with PG frequently show peripheral iris concavity, this work led to the theory that mechanical rubbing between anterior packets of lens zonules and the IPE in predisposed eyes is the cause of pigment dispersion in PDS and PG.

Additional insight into the pathology of PDS and PG has come from several studies examining tissue with microscopy. Throughout the iris, there are radial defects of the IPE. Within these defects, cells are either missing or have disrupted membranes that cause extrusion of pigment.[1,25,26] The iris stroma in the area of the defects is sometimes affected and is typically infiltrated with pigment-engulfed macrophages.[1,25,26] Some studies note the presence of irregular iris melanosomes.[26,27] The trabecular meshwork is densely pigmented, with dispersed pigment found free, in macrophages, or phagocytosed by endothelial cells lining the trabecular beams.[25–28] In some eyes, it appears that pigment engulfment by trabecular endothelial cells is followed by a loss of cellularity and regional collapse of trabecular sheets.[29]

Etiology

The etiology of PDS is incompletely understood, but can be explained in part by the unique anatomical and physiological phenomenon of reverse pupillary block.[30] According to this hypothesis, irides predisposed to PDS come into close physical contact with the lens and adopt a ball-and-valve-like relationship (Figure 21.5). The close contact of the iris and lens restricts the flow of aqueous humor, except during events such as eye blinks which squeeze aqueous humor into the anterior segment. During eye blinks, aqueous humor is forced into the anterior segment, causing an increase in the volume of aqueous humor in the anterior segment and elevated IOP relative to the posterior segment. This pressure differential promotes a backward bowing of the midperipheral iris against packets of lens zonules. Patients with PDS tend to have more posterior iris insertions[31] and deeper anterior chambers,[32] which might promote reverse pupillary block. Thus, reverse pupillary block addresses why the iris often becomes bowed posteriorly in PDS to allow mechanical rubbing against the anterior packets of lens zonules.

In recent years, ultrasound biomicroscopy has allowed iris pathology in PG to be studied in new ways.[31,33–35] Recurrent findings in these studies are that iris concavity is common[33,35] and that the iris tends to have a more posterior insertion[31] in eyes of PDS patients compared to

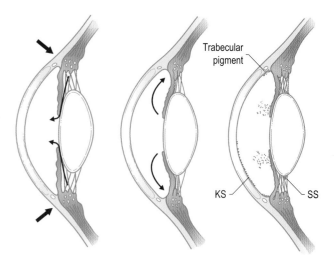

Figure 21.5 Mechanism of reverse pupillary block contributing to pigment dispersion syndrome. Left image: close physical contact between the iris and lens prevents aqueous humor flow in predisposed eye. During eye blinks, pressure from the eyelids (large arrows) squeezes aqueous humor into the anterior segment (small arrows). Middle image: a pressure differential between the anterior and posterior segment causes posterior bowing of the iris and allows mechanical abrasion between the iris pigment epithelium and anterior packets of lens zonules. Right image: mechanical rubbing causes pigment dispersion. Dispersed pigment tends to accumulate in the trabecular meshwork, on the corneal endothelium as a Krukenberg's spindle (KS), and at the junction of posterior lens capsule and zonules as a Scheie's stripe (SS). (Redrawn from the figure kindly provided by Dr. WLM Alward, Department of Ophthalmology and Visual Sciences, University of Iowa.)

controls. A similar trend holds true in ultrasound studies of patients with asymmetric PDS; the eye with worse pigment dispersion tends to have significant differences in iris concavity and have a more posterior insertion.[33] Although midperipheral iris concavity and posterior iris insertions are not observed in all patients that have been examined, these findings are consistent with the etiology suggested by Campbell[1] and Karickoff[30] that pigment dispersion often involves mechanical irideozonular abrasion in predisposed eyes.

When PDS progresses to PG, the etiology of the resulting glaucoma is related to increased IOP. One of the greatest risk factors for predicting conversion of PDS to PG is IOP at initial examination.[9] Among PG patients, elevations in IOP typically correlate to the amount of trabecular meshwork pigmentation.[1,8,11] Therefore, it appears that directly, or indirectly, pigment accumulations within the irideocorneal angle are the primary insult initiating this stage of disease.

Pathophysiology

Liberation of iris pigment

The combined work of Campbell[1] and Karickhoff[30] leads to a "mechanical rubbing hypothesis" stating that mechanical irideozonular abrasion in predisposed eyes underlies the pathophysiology of pigment dispersion. Some of the strengths often ascribed to the mechanical rubbing hypothesis are that it explains why PDS is often associated with myopia (increased iris–lenticular contact), why PDS often regresses with age (loss of accommodation with the onset of presbyopia), why some PDS patients have relatively deep anterior chambers with posteriorly located irides (anatomical variations that would promote rubbing), and why PDS is typically described as more common among males (males tend to have comparatively larger irides which may be more prone to backward bowing). Thus, the scenarios suggested by the mechanical rubbing hypothesis could logically explain many associations of PDS and PG.

However, experimental and clinical support for the mechanical rubbing hypothesis has not been universal and much remains unknown.[35-39] PDS does not develop in everyone with a relatively posterior iris insertion, concave iris configuration, or myopia. There are also other clinical features not at all accounted for in the mechanical rubbing hypothesis, including a propensity for retinal lattice degeneration.[10] Furthermore, even in the PDS cases associated with anatomical or physiological conditions likely to promote mechanical rubbing, the genetic or environmental factors leading to these circumstances are completely unknown. In sum, additional risk factors predisposing the iris toward pigment dispersion likely remain to be identified and many important questions remain to be studied.

Recent genetic studies conducted with mice have suggested new hypotheses contributing to PDS pathophysiology. Among published reports, pigment dispersion in mice has been observed in a small number of different mouse strains,[40-43] including several with mutations influencing melanosomes.[40,41] For example, DBA/2J mice exhibit pronounced accumulations of dispersed iris pigment (Figure 21.6) and progressive transillumination defects.[41,44,45] Genetic experiments have clearly defined that pigment dispersal in DBA/2J mice results from the digenic interaction of two mutations in genes encoding melanosomal proteins, *Gpnmb* and *Tyrp1*.[41] These genes appear to trigger iris disease through a mechanism involving aberrant melanosomal processes related to pigment biosynthesis.[41] This hypothesis is further supported by the recent identification of pigment dispersion in several additional strains of mice with mutations influencing melanosomes.[40] Combined, these findings identify an additional insult capable of predisposing irides to pigment dispersion. The extent to which these processes might contribute to human PDS is currently unknown.

Pigment-related insults to intraocular pressure

Once pigment is liberated from the IPE, some eyes progress toward elevated IOP, while in others, PDS can persist for extended periods of time without further incident. Despite its importance, the pathophysiology influencing these different outcomes remains only partially understood. The simplest explanation for pigment-related changes in IOP is that dispersed pigment accumulated within the trabecular meshwork physically blocks aqueous humor outflow. In support of this, in some patients vigorous exercise can briefly lead to temporary "pigment storms" and elevations in IOP.[46,47] The rapid and temporary nature of these linked events is consistent with physical obstruction to aqueous outflow caused by accumulations of pigment within the trabecular meshwork.

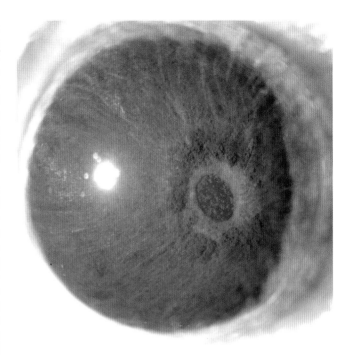

Figure 21.6 Iris disease and pigment dispersion in DBA/2J mouse. As a consequence of a pigment-dispersing iris disease, DBA/2J mice develop a form of pigmentary glaucoma. Indices of disease present in this eye of a 13-month DBA/2J mouse include dispersed pigment across the lens and iris, the presence of multiple pigment-engulfed clump cells, and iris atrophy that is particularly pronounced near the pupillary margin. This eye also has peripheral anterior synechiae that are causing the pupil to be acentric.

Contrasting this, modeling studies suggest that the amount of pigment chronically present in the juxtacanalicular tissue would likely have a negligible influence on trabecular meshwork permeability.[48] Thus, while dispersed pigment can acutely influence IOP through simple physical blockade, this does not seem likely to be the major mechanism causing progression of PDS to PG in most human eyes with chronic pigment dispersion.

Animal studies of PDS suggest that the IOP response to dispersed pigment is a multistep process. Experimental studies in living cynomolgus monkeys have found that injecting pigment into the anterior chamber will result in trabecular meshwork pigmentation, but no lasting changes in outflow facility.[49] This inducible model results in PDS, but not PG. Likewise, changes in genetic background can genetically convert the DBA/2J mouse model of PG into a model of only PDS.[50] These experiments demonstrate that progression of PDS to PG can be genetically modified. Together, these animal studies indicate that PG is not typically caused solely by physical obstruction to aqueous humor outflow. Rather, the damaging aspects of pigment dispersion appear to result from complex reactions to the dispersed pigment. In the future, identification of the mechanisms mediating these responses will likely bring important new insight into the pathophysiology of PDS.

In conclusion, many aspects of PDS pathophysiology can be explained by mechanical abrasion of the IPE against anterior packets of lens zonules. Iris concavity allowing mechanical irideozonular rubbing is likely promoted by the process of reverse pupillary block. However, additional risk factors likely also exist. The detrimental influences of dispersed pigment appear to involve a complex reaction to pigment. Defining the precise events dictating whether or not PDS progresses to PG remains a significant challenge to our understanding of these diseases. In years to come, technological advances such as high-density genome-wide arrays will bring new opportunities to study the heredity of PDS and PG in humans, while newly described mouse models will allow complementary mechanistic studies into the molecular events influencing PDS and PG.

Key references

A complete list of chapter references is available online at www.expertconsult.com. See inside cover for registration details.

1. Campbell DG. Pigmentary dispersion and glaucoma. A new theory. Arch Ophthalmol 1979;97:1667–1672.

5. Ritch R, Steinberger D, Liebmann JM. Prevalence of pigment dispersion syndrome in a population undergoing glaucoma screening. Am J Ophthalmol 1993;115:707–710.

6. Farrar SM, Shields MB, Miller KN, et al. Risk factors for the development and severity of glaucoma in the pigment dispersion syndrome. Am J Ophthalmol 1989;108:223–229.

9. Siddiqui Y, Ten Hulzen RD, Cameron JD, et al. What is the risk of developing pigmentary glaucoma from pigment dispersion syndrome? Am J Ophthalmol 2003;135:794–799.

10. Ritch R. A unification hypothesis of pigment dispersion syndrome. Trans Am Ophthalmol Soc 1996;94:381–405; discussion 409.

12. Andersen JS, Pralea AM, DelBono EA, et al. A gene responsible for the pigment dispersion syndrome maps to chromosome 7q35–q36. Arch Ophthalmol 1997;115:384–388.

22. Shuba L, Nicolela MT, Rafuse PE. Correlation of capsular pseudoexfoliation material and iridocorneal angle pigment with the severity of pseudoexfoliation glaucoma. J Glaucoma 2007;16:94–97.

25. Fine BS, Yanoff M, Scheie HG. Pigmentary "glaucoma." A histologic study. Trans Am Acad Ophthalmol Otolaryngol 1974;78:OP314–OP325.

26. Kampik A, Green WR, Quigley HA, et al. Scanning and transmission electron microscopic studies of two cases of pigment dispersion syndrome. Am J Ophthalmol 1981;91:573–587.

30. Karickhoff JR. Pigmentary dispersion syndrome and pigmentary glaucoma: a new mechanism concept, a new treatment, and a new technique. Ophthalm Surg 1992;23:269–277.

36. Balidis MO, Bunce C, Sandy CJ, et al. Iris configuration in accommodation in pigment dispersion syndrome. Eye 2002;16:694–700.

39. Krupin T, Rosenberg LF, Weinreb RN. Pigmentary glaucoma: facts versus fiction. J Glaucoma 1994;3:273–274.

40. Anderson MG, Hawes NL, Trantow CM, et al. Iris phenotypes and pigment dispersion caused by genes influencing pigmentation. Pigment Cell Melanoma Res 2008;21:565–578.

48. Murphy CG, Johnson M, Alvarado JA. Juxtacanalicular tissue in pigmentary and primary open angle glaucoma. The hydrodynamic role of pigment and other constituents. Arch Ophthalmol 1992;110:1779–1785.

49. Epstein DL, Freddo TF, Anderson PJ, et al. Experimental obstruction to aqueous outflow by pigment particles in living monkeys. Invest Ophthalmol Vis Sci 1986;27:387–395.

CHAPTER 22

Abnormal trabecular meshwork outflow

Paul A Knepper and Beatrice YJT Yue

Clinical background

Primary open-angle glaucoma (POAG) is the most common type of glaucoma, particularly in populations with European and African ancestry. This disease is the leading cause of blindness in African-Americans. The major risk factors for POAG include intraocular pressure (IOP) elevation and aging. The prevalence of POAG increases from 0.02% at ages 40–49 to 2–3% for persons over the age of 70,[1] and the incidence of ocular hypertension increases from 2% to 9% over the same time span.[2]

Pathophysiology

Anatomical and physiological background

The trabecular meshwork (TM), a specialized tissue at the chamber angle, is the major site for regulation of the normal bulk flow of the aqueous humor.[3] It functions as a self-cleaning, unidirectional, pressure-sensitive, low-flow (2 μl/min/mmHg) biologic filter for the aqueous humor, and contributes thereby to control of the IOP.[3] The TM tissue is divided into the uveal meshwork, corneoscleral meshwork, and juxtacanalicular connective tissue (JCT) regions (Figure 22.1). In the uveal and corneoscleral meshwork, sheets of trabecular beams that contain lamellae made of connective tissue or extracellular matrix (ECM) materials are lined by TM cells. In the JCT region, the cells reside relatively freely and are embedded in the ECM. In the Schlemm's canal (SC), there are endothelial cells also referred to as inner wall cells[4,5] (Figure 22.2). The aqueous humor flows through the TM and the SC into collector channels and aqueous veins, and the outflow resistance is believed to locate largely in the JCT/SC area.[4,5] In normal outflow homeostasis, a pressure gradient exists between the anterior chamber and the episcleral veins. It is likely that the pressure gradient and the resistance to aqueous outflow are altered in various types of glaucoma (Box 22.1).

Effects of disease

To facilitate comparisons and to offer mechanistic clues, biochemical changes such as up- or downregulation of genes/proteins that have been reported in POAG in the aqueous humor, TM, optic nerve, and blood are organized into three categories: (1) ECM elements and remodeling; (2) cell signaling molecules; and (3) changes related to stress and aging, and listed respectively in Tables 22.1,[6-21] 22.2,[22-31] and 22.3.[32-43]

What follows are discussions of cellular mechanisms in the TM system that may affect the aqueous humor outflow pathway. Although discussed under separate headings, the mechanisms that include the ECM composition, turnover, and modulation, cell adhesion, cytoskeletal structure, and intracellular signaling are all interconnected. The effects or influences of aqueous humor components and stress-inducing conditions are also described.

Trabecular meshwork and Schlemm's canal cell profiles

TM cells are unique and have the capacity to perform a variety of functions, including phagocytosis, migration, elaboration of metabolic, lysosomal, and matrix-degrading enzymes, and production of ECM elements.[44,45] TM cells incorporate acetylated low-density lipoprotein (LDL),[45] as do vascular endothelial cells (VEC) in culture. However, they do not stain for factor VIII antigen, a characteristic VEC marker. Neither do TM cells form an endothelium as tight as that of cultured VEC. TM cells on the other hand phagocytose more avidly than VEC.

TM cells are essential for maintenance of the normal aqueous humor outflow system.[44,45] Disturbances in the vitality and functional status by genetic predisposition, aging, or other insults may result in obstruction of the aqueous outflow, leading to IOP elevation and glaucomatous conditions. In vivo, TM cells have limited proliferative activity. A continuous loss of TM cells occurs during adulthood.[44,46] In patients with POAG, the cell loss and disruption of the endothelial covering are striking.[47] Areas in which the trabecular beams are denuded of cells are associated with a major loss of outflow channels, which represents a possible mechanism for the decreased outflow facility in POAG.

While TM cells are highly specialized, adaptive, and multifunctional cells, SC cells are pressure-sensitive endothelial cells of vascular origin. SC cells endocytose LDL and acetylated LDL and organize in the presence of Matrigel into

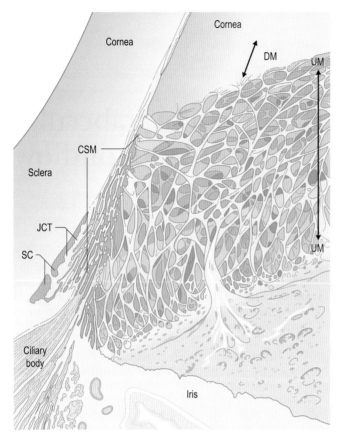

Figure 22.1 Three-dimensional drawing of the aqueous outflow pathway depicting the structural elements of the trabecular meshwork. The uveal meshwork (UM) is a loose lattice of delicate rope-like components in continuity from the base of the iris to Descemet's membrane (DM). The corneoscleral meshwork (CSM) is more tightly packed and consists of sheets of trabecular lamellae. The juxtacanicular connective tissue (JCT) forms a thin band of connective tissue adjacent to the aqueous collector channel known as Schlemm's canal (SC). (Adapted from Weddell JE. The limbus. In: Hogan MJ, Alvarado JA, Weddell JE (eds) Histology of the Human Eye. Philadelphia: WB Saunders, 1971:112–182.)

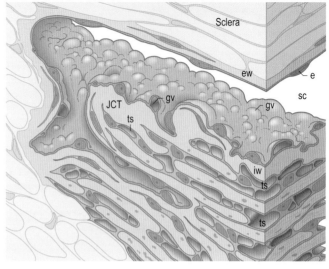

Figure 22.2 Three-dimensional drawing of the corneoscleral meshwork, the juxtacanicular connective tissue (JCT), and Schlemm's canal (SC). Note the trabecular spaces (ts), intervening endothelial processes, the inner wall (iw), the external wall (ew), and the endothelium (e) of the SC. Giant vacuoles (gv), common on the inner wall of the SC, are pressure-sensitive. The aqueous outflow pathway is complex; there are at least three layers of organization. The first layer is formed by a series of perforated trabecular lamellae. Interposed between the last trabecular lamellae and the inner wall of the SC is a thin cellular zone with an abundant extracellular matrix, the JCT, which is a highly fibrillar, cellular, and glycosaminoglycan-enriched area. (Adapted from Weddell JE. The limbus. In: Hogan MJ, Alvarado JA, Weddell JE (eds) Histology of the Human Eye. Philadelphia: WB Saunders, 1971:112–182.)

Box 22.1 Trabecular meshwork cells and glaucoma

- Essential for maintenance of the normal aqueous humor outflow system
- Disturbances by genetic predisposition, aging, or other insults may result in obstruction of the aqueous outflow, leading to intraocular pressure elevation and glaucomatous conditions
- Limited proliferative activity in vivo
- Continuous loss of trabecular meshwork cells occurs during adulthood

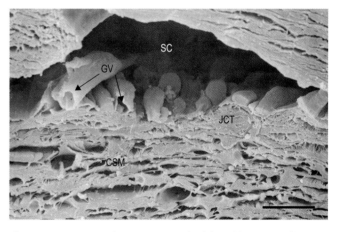

Figure 22.3 Scanning electron micrograph of the Schlemm's canal (SC) and the juxtacanicular connective tissue (JCT) of a primate eye (*Macaca fascicularis*). The endothelia of the inner wall of SC are elongated and form transient giant vacuoles (GV) that respond to intraocular pressure changes and serve as a pressure-sensitive marker of pressure between JCT and SC. Note the organization of the corneoscleral meshwork (CSM) lamellae, trabecular spaces, and relative compactness of the JCT as aqueous passes through the interstices of the aqueous pathway. Scale bar, 10 μm.

multicellular tubelike structures.[48] In situ, cells in the various regions of TM and those in SC appear to be interconnected by cell processes (Figure 22.3).[49] The SC/TM configuration is pressure-sensitive. If the IOP is exceedingly elevated, the SC/TM may be forced on to the outer wall, effectively preventing outflow of the aqueous humor.

ECM composition, turnover, and modulation

The ECM components in the TM are essential for maintenance of the normal aqueous humor outflow.[45,50–52] In the TM of POAG eyes, excessive, abnormal accumulations of certain ECM materials as well as decreases of other ECM

Table 22.1 Biochemical changes in extracellular matrix (ECM) elements and remodeling in primary open-angle glaucoma

	Aqueous humor	Trabecular meshwork	Optic nerve	Systemic (blood)
ECM elements				
CD44		↓[8]		
Cochlin		↑[9]		
Chondroitin sulfate		↑[10]		
Collagen type IV		nc[11]		
Elastin		↑[12]	↑[13]	
Fibronectin	nc[14]	nc[11]		
Hyaluronic acid	↓↓[15]	↓↓↓↓[10]	↓[16]	
GAGase-resistant material		↑↑↑↑[10]		
Tenascin			↑[17]	
Thrombospondin-1		↑[18]		
ECM remodeling enzymes and inhibitors				
MMP-1		↑[19]	↑[20]	
MMP-3	nc[21]	↑[19]	↑[20]	
MT1-MMP				↑[22]
TIMP-1	nc[21]	↑[19]		
TIMP-2	↑[23]			

The increase or decrease in the reported biochemical changes is expressed as statistically significant ↑ or ↓. Wherever possible, a twofold change is denoted by two arrows, a threefold change by three arrows, and a fourfold change by four arrows, and nc indicates no change. GAGase, glycosaminoglycan-degrading enzyme, MMP, matrix metalloproteinase, MT1-MMP, membrane type 1-MMP, TIMP, tissue inhibitor for MMP.

Table 22.2 Changes in cell signaling molecules in primary open-angle glaucoma

	Aqueous humor	Trabecular meshwork	Optic nerve	Systemic (blood)
Endothelin-1	↑[24]			↑[25]
Hepatocyte growth factor	↑[26]			
Interleukin-2				↑[27]
Phospholipase A2	↑[28]			
Soluble CD44	↑↑[29]			
Transforming growth factor-β_2	↑[30]			
Thymulin				↑↑↑[31]
Tumor necrosis factor-α			↑[20]	
Vascular endothelial growth factor	↑[32]			↑[33]

The increase or decrease in the reported changes is expressed as statistically significant ↑ or ↓. Wherever possible, a twofold change is denoted by two arrows, and a threefold change by three arrows.

materials (Table 22.1) have been documented.[6–21,45,50–52] The ECM produced by the cells is an intricate network composed of an array of multidomain macromolecules such as collagens, cell-binding glycoproteins, and proteoglycans. The macromolecules link together covalently or noncovalently to form a structurally stable composite. Recent studies have also revealed that ECM is a dynamic entity of key importance

in all biological systems, determining and controlling the behavior and biologic characteristics of the cells.

One key component of the TM is proteoglycans, which are macromolecules consisting of a core protein to which glycosaminoglycan side chains are covalently attached. This class of molecules has been implicated in the maintenance of resistance to aqueous humor outflow ever since Barany,[53]

Table 22.3 Changes related to stress and aging in primary open-angle glaucoma

	Aqueous humor	Trabecular meshwork	Optic nerve	Systemic (blood)
Acetylcholinesterase				↑[34]
αB-Crystallin		↑[35]		
3-α-Hydroxysteroid dehydrogenase				↓[36]
Ascorbic acid	↑↑↑[37]			
Cortisol				↑[38]
Fatty acid				
Eicosapentaenoic				↓[39]
Docosahexaenoic				↓[39]
Omega-3				↓[39]
Glutathione	↑↑↑[40]			↓[41]
Hypoxia-inducible factor-1α (HIF-1α)			↑[42]	
Nuclear factor-κB (NF-κB)		↑[43]		
Nitric oxide	↑[44]			
Senescence-associated β-galactosidase	↑[45]			

The increase or decrease in the reported changes is expressed as statistically significant ↑ or ↓. Wherever possible, a twofold change is denoted by two arrows, a threefold change by three arrows.

in the 1950s, demonstrated that perfusion of the anterior chamber with testicular hyaluronidase greatly reduced the outflow resistance in enucleated bovine eyes. In the TM tissue, proteoglycans form gel-like networks that may function as a gel filtration system. The major types identified include chondroitin, dermatan, and heparan sulfate proteoglycans.[45,50] These proteoglycans may represent decorin, biglycan, versican, perlecan, and syndecan.[45,50]

The relative amounts of each type of glycosaminoglycan in the TM tissue have been determined.[45,50] Hyaluronic acid and chondroitin-dermatan sulfates are the major constituents, and heparan sulfate and keratan sulfate are present in much smaller amounts. A depletion in hyaluronic acid and an accumulation of chondroitin sulfates and undigestible glycosaminoglycan material have been associated with POAG conditions.[8,45] Both chondroitin sulfate and hyaluronic acid have been shown to contribute to flow resistance and influence flow rate in vitro[54] (Figure 22.4). The flow rate was decreased when hyaluronic acid and chondroitin sulfate were used at POAG concentrations.[56] Delays to achieve steady-state level were also observed with increased pressure in in vitro studies.[54] Of note, the level of an ectodomain fragment of hyaluronic acid receptor CD44 (sCD44) was found to be elevated (Table 22.2) in the aqueous humor of POAG patients[27] and the concentration was correlated with visual field loss.[27] sCD44 is cytotoxic to TM cells, but the toxicity can be blocked by hyaluronic acid.[55] The decreased hyaluronic acid may thus result in diminished protective capacity and further deterioration in POAG conditions.

Fibronectin, laminin, and vitronectin, and matricellular proteins that include tenascin, SPARC, and thrombospondin-1 have been localized in the TM.[16,45,50] These glycoproteins are crucial in biologic processes such as cell attachment, spreading, and cell differentiation. Overexpression of fibronectin and laminin as well as collagen type IV resulted in a decrease in the TM cell monolayer permeability.[45,56] The expression of thrombospondin-1 has in addition been shown to be increased[16] in the TM of POAG eyes (Table 22.1).

Elastin is localized to the central core of sheath-derived plaques or elastic-like fibers in the TM.[45,50] Fibrillin-1, a component of microfibrils, has been found in both the core and the surrounding sheath of the elastic-like fibers. Fibrillin-1 and type VI collagen are also constituents of long-spacing collagens found in the TM.[45,51] It is believed that the collagen fibers and elastic-like fibers are organized in the TM to accommodate resilience and tensile strength, providing a mechanism for reversible deformation in response to cyclic hydrodynamic loading. In trabecular lamellae and in JCT regions, accumulation of long spacing collagens and sheath-derived plaques has been documented in POAG and aged eyes.[45,51]

The ECM is constantly modified by the surrounding cells through enzymes such as matrix metalloproteinase (MMP) family member and inhibitors such as tissue inhibitors for matrix metalloproteinase (TIMPs) found in the TM.[45,50] Ongoing ECM turnover, initiated by MMPs, appears to be essential for maintenance of the aqueous outflow homeostasis. MMP-3, and possibly also MMP-9, may be responsible for the efficacy of laser trabeculoplasty, an alternative treatment to reduce IOP in patients with glaucoma.[45,50] Addition or induction of MMP-3 in perfused human anterior-segment organ cultures increases, whereas blocking the endogenous activity of the MMPs in the TM reduces, the aqueous humor outflow facility.[45]

The ECM in the TM may also be remodeled in response to exogenous stimuli such as glucocorticoids and oxidative stress.[45] Mechanical stretch caused an increase in MMP-1 and MMP-3 activities and alteration of ECM molecules including

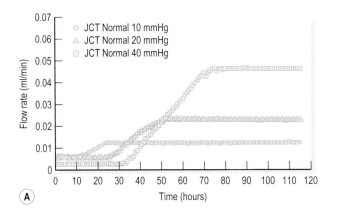

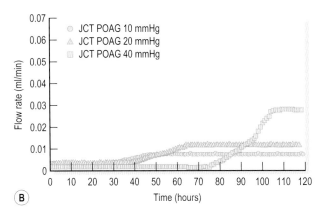

Figure 22.4 Reconstitution of hyaluronic acid and chondroitin sulfate at the normal (A) and primary open-angle glaucoma (B) juxtacanicular connective tissue (JCT) concentration and the effect of 10, 20, and 40 mmHg pressure on the flow rate. The flow rate was measured using an in vitro microtest chamber. The initial flow rate of the normal JCT at 10 mmHg was 6.7 μl/min and the lag time required to obtain the steady-state flow was 26 hours. In contrast, the initial flow rate of the primary open-angle glaucoma (POAG) JCT at 10 mmHg was 3.7 μl/min and the lag time required to obtain steady-state flow rate was 46 hours. As hydrostatic pressure was increased to 20 or 40 mmHg, the flow rate and the lag time of the POAG JCT were markedly slower than the normal JCT. (Reproduced from Knepper PA, Fadel JR, Miller AM, et al. Reconstitution of trabecular meshwork GAGs: influence of hyaluronic acid and chondroitin sulfate on flow rates. J Glaucoma 2005;14:230–238.Copyright 2005 J Glaucoma.)

proteoglycans and matricellular proteins.[45,57] The ECM is modulated by cytokines. The most studied cytokine in the TM is TGF-ß. A higher than normal level[28] of TGF-ß$_2$ was found in the aqueous humor of patients with POAG (Table 22.1). TGF-ß$_2$ upregulated ECM-related genes in TM cell cultures. In TGF-ß$_2$-perfused organ cultures, focal accumulation of fine fibrillar extracellular material was observed in TM tissues. Furthermore, TGF-ß$_2$ perfusion reduced outflow facility and elevated IOP. These results suggest that the increased TGF-ß$_2$ level in the aqueous humor may be related to the pathogenesis of glaucoma. Other cytokines such as interleukin-1α (IL-1α) and tumor necrosis factor-α (TNF-α) also modulate the ECM, probably via regulation of MMP and TIMP expressions.[45,58] The cochlin deposits in the glaucomatous TM (Table 22.1) appear to increase with age and

---

Box 22.2 Extracellular matrix components in the trabecular meshwork

- Important for normal aqueous humor outflow
- Proteoglycans help maintain resistance to aqueous humor outflow by forming a gel-like network that may function as a gel filtration system
- Glycoproteins are involved in cell attachment, spreading, and cell differentiation
- Modification via enzymes, e.g., matrix metalloproteinases and their inhibitors
- Remodeling in response to stretch, glucocorticoids and oxidative stress, and cytokines

---

are associated with proteoglycans. Such deposits have been proposed to contribute to the increase of ECM resistance to outflow and the POAG pathology (Box 22.2).[7]

Cell adhesion

Cell adhesion molecules including integrins, cadherins, and selectins mediate binding interactions at the extracellular surface and determine the specificity of cell-to-cell and cell-to-ECM recognitions. TM cells that line the trabecular beams are continually subjected to flows of the aqueous humor and IOP fluctuations. The lining integrity against stress is achieved by adhesion of cells to the matrices through cell surface receptors along with cell junctions between the cells. Disruption in these adhesions would possibly lead to cell loss, denudation of the beams, and pathology. TM cells in culture express a variety of integrins and form focal adhesions upon attachment to ECM proteins.[45]

SC cells have been shown to extend cytoplasmic processes into the JCT space (Figure 22.3), while JCT processes attach also to the trabecular lamellae processes.[4,5,49] Freeze-fracture and electron microscopy studies have described adherens junctions, gap junctions, and tight junctions in the outflow pathway.[45] Proteins that form adherens junctions such as intercellular cell adhesion molecule (ICAM)-1, N-CAM and N-cadherin are expressed in TM cells or tissues.[45,59,60] SC cells express platelet-endothelium cell adhesion molecule-1 (PECAM-1) and vascular endothelial (VE)-cadherin.[48] Gap junction protein connexin43 has also been localized in TM cells for communication with each other. Both TM and SC cells also express zonular occludens-1, an associated protein of calcium-sensitive tight junctions. Administration of glucocorticoid such as dexamethasone resulted in an increased expression of ZO-1, formation of a greater number of tight junctions, and an increase in fluid flow resistance.[45]

Selectins such as E-selectin (endothelial leukocyte adhesion molecule-1 or ELAM-1) are cell adhesion molecules that mediate interactions with complex carbohydrate moieties. Upregulation of selectins has been observed in TM tissues in POAG eyes.[42,60] The upregulation could be related to transcription factor NF-κB[42] (Table 22.3), reflecting stress response of the cells.

A number of studies have shown that the outflow facility is modified via alterations in cell-matrix and/or cell-cell adhesions.[45,52] For instance, depletion of extracellular calcium by dissociating cell-cell junctions decreases outflow resistance.[45,52] Perfusion of the Hep II domain of fibronectin[59] in human anterior-segment cultures increases outflow facility perhaps by mechanisms that involve loss of focal adhesions and/or disruption of adherens junctions in TM cells.

Cytoskeletal structure

The physiologic roles of the actin cytoskeleton of TM cells in association with outflow facility[52,61] and glaucoma have drawn considerable attention. Agents that affect the actin cytoskeleton, such as chelating reagents and cytoskeleton-active drugs including cytochalasin B and latrunculin A and B have been demonstrated to increase the aqueous outflow in relatively short-term perfusion organ culture or in vivo animal studies.[45,52,61] The increase was often associated with morphologic changes, such as separation of junctions between TM cells and breaks between SC cells. Sulfhydryl-reactive compounds, including iodoacetamide, N-ethyl maleimide, and ethacrynic acid,[61] can also influence the outflow system. A common mechanism seems to involve changes in cell shape and cell adhesion through cytoskeletal elements. Significantly, glucocorticoids alter F-actin architecture and promote cross-linked actin network (CLAN) formation in human TM cell and tissues.[62] Moreover, glaucomatous eyes, compared to normals, displayed an overall more disordered F-actin architecture in SC and JCT cells.[63] These studies collectively underscore the notion that the actin architecture is an important mediator of the aqueous outflow pathway (Box 22.3).

Intracellular signaling

Signal transduction via members of the Rho family of small guanosine triphosphatases (GTPase) has been shown to be of vital importance in the outflow system.[52,64] In the active GTP-bound state, Rho GTPases interact with and activate downstream effectors such as Rho kinase to modulate the assembly of actin structures. RhoA, for example, regulates formation of stress fibers and focal adhesions to coordinate cellular processes including adhesion, migration, and morphologic changes. In TM cells, a decrease in actin stress fibers and focal adhesions has been shown to occur with treatment of Rho kinase inhibitors Y-27632 and H-1152, and gene transfer of dominant negative RhoA and dominant negative Rho-binding domain of Rho kinase.[52,64] These cellular changes are associated with reduced myosin light-chain (MLC) phosphorylation, and/or enhanced outflow facility.[52] Conversely, molecules including sphengosine-1-phosphate and endothelin-1 that activate Rho/Rho kinase signaling pathway through G-protein-coupled receptors promote MLC phosphorylation, and in turn decrease the aqueous humor outflow facility.[52,61,64]

Box 22.3 Effects on cytoskeletal structure

- Modulating actin cytoskeleton with chelating reagents, sulfhydryl-reactive compounds, and cytoskeleton-active drugs increases aqueous outflow
- Mechanism is likely changes in cell shape and cell adhesion through cytoskeletal elements

---

Signaling molecule such as protein kinase C (PKC) also has a role in the outflow regulation.[45,64] PKC has additionally been shown to be involved in upregulation of MMP-3 and MMP-9 levels mediated by cytokines IL-1ß and TNF-α after laser trabeculoplasty. Extracellular signal-regulated kinase (ERK), mitogen-activated protein kinase (MAPK), c-Jun N-terminal kinase (JNK), and p38 MAPK pathways are also necessary in addition for the signal transduction.[65]

Aqueous humor components

The aqueous humor contains albumin as a major constituent. Other components encompass hydrogen peroxide (H_2O_2), ascorbic acid, growth factors such as TGF-ß, heptocyte growth factor and vascular endothelial growth factor, and molecules including MMPs, proteinase inhibitors, sCD44, and hyaluronic acid.[66,67] A recent study has demonstrated that addition of normal aqueous humor rather than the standard fetal bovine serum to monolayers of TM cultures decreases cell proliferation, and produces changes in cellular and molecular characteristics to mimic more closely the TM physiologic profiles in situ.[67]

Increased levels of TGF-ß$_2$, sCD44, endothelin-1, IL-2, phospholipase 2, thymulin (Table 22.2), glutathione, ascorbic acid (Table 22.3), and a decreased level of hyaluronic acid (Table 22.1) have been reported in the aqueous humor of POAG eyes. Since TM cells are in constant contact with the aqueous humor, it is expected that altered levels and/or activities of aqueous humor components would have an impact on the behavior and activities of these cells. The sCD44 found in the POAG aqueous humor is hypophosphorylated.[68] The hypophosphorylated form has high cytotoxicity and low hyaluronic acid-binding affinity and is suggested to represent a pathophysiologic feature of the disease process.[68]

Aging, oxidative stress, and other insults

TM cellularity is reduced with aging.[46] Morphologic studies have also revealed thickened basement membranes and accumulation of sheath-derived plaques and long spacing collagens in the TM of aged eyes.[51] Cultured TM cells from old donors show a decline in proteasome activity and acquisition of the senescence phenotype including reduced proliferative capacity and enlarged cell morphology.[69] A decrease of TM cellularity and an accumulation of ECM have also been documented in POAG eyes.[47,51] The number of senescent cells which stain positive for senescence-associated ß-galactosidase is increased (Table 22.3) in the TM of POAG eyes,[43] supporting further that POAG is an age-related disease.[70]

Oxidative damage has been implicated to contribute to the morphologic and physiologic alterations in the aqueous outflow pathway in aging and glaucoma.[71] The TM is known to be exposed to 20–30 µM H_2O_2 present in the aqueous humor and is subjected to chronic oxidative stress.[45] Enzymes that are involved in the protection against oxidative damage, including catalase, glutathione reductase, superoxide dismutase, and glutathione peroxidase, have been studied in the TM. The specific activity of superoxide dismutase, but not catalase, was shown to decline with age in human TM tissues.[72] TM cells also synthesized a specific set of proteins, such as aB-crystalline, that may act as molecular chaperones to prevent oxidative or heat shock damage.[33] Markers of oxidative damage,[71] abnormalities in mitochondrial DNA,[73] and diminished blood levels of oxidant scavengers glutathione[39] are found in POAG patients. It appears that oxidative stress that exceeds the capacity of TM cells for detoxification is involved in damaging the cells and alteration of the aqueous humor outflow.

Conclusions

This chapter summarizes the current knowledge regarding major cellular mechanisms in the TM that may regulate the aqueous humor outflow pathway. Not included are the roles of serum proteins, immune response, adrenergic receptors and other important intracellular or intercellular regulators such as prostaglandins.

To varying degrees the precise roles of cellular mechanisms described above and their direct links to the outflow resistance still remain to be established. Nevertheless, a theme applicable perhaps to both POAG and other neurodegenerative diseases has emerged that selective cell vulnerability occurred as a result of dysfunctional pathways, stress, aging or other insults may eventually lead to disease process. Biochemical changes listed in Tables 22.1–22.3 indicate that diverse pathways/mechanisms/molecules including proinflammatory cytokines are involved, triggering dysregulation of normal defense mechanisms, faulty signaling, and/or progressive fibrosis to increase the outflow resistance and elevate IOP. A deeper understanding of the various mechanisms is a prerequisite for the design of novel gene therapies or other treatment modalities for glaucoma.

Key references

A complete list of chapter references is available online at www.expertconsult.com. See inside cover for registration details.

2. Quigley HA. Open-angle glaucoma. N Engl J Med 1993;328:1097–1106.

3. Bill A. The drainage of aqueous humor. Invest Ophthalmol Vis Sci 1975;14:1–3.

4. Johnson M. What controls aqueous humor outflow resistance? Exp Eye Res 2006;82:545–557.

25. Yang J, Patil RV, Yu H, et al. T cell subsets and sIL-2R/IL-2 levels in patients with glaucoma. Am J Ophthalmol 2001;31:421–426.

41. Tsai DC, Hsu WM, Chou CK, et al. Significant variation of the elevated nitric oxide levels in aqueous humor from patients with different types of glaucoma. Ophthalmologica 2002;216:346–350.

42. Wang N, Chintala SK, Fini ME, et al. Activation of a tissue-specific stress response in the aqueous outflow pathway of the eye defines the glaucoma disease phenotype. Nature Med 2001;7:304–309.

43. Liton PB, Challa P, Stinnett S, et al. Cellular senescence in the glaucomatous outflow pathway. Exp Geront 2005;40:745–748.

45. Yue BYJT. Cellular mechanisms in the trabecular meshwork affecting the aqueous humor outflow pathway. In: Albert DM, Miller J (eds) Albert and Jakobiec's Principles and Practice of Ophthalmology, 3rd edn. Oxford: Elsevier, 2007:2457–2474.

47. Alvarado J, Murphy C, Juster R. Trabecular meshwork cellularity in primary open-angle glaucoma and non-glaucomatous normals. Ophthalmology 1984;91:564–579.

49. Johnstone MA. The aqueous outflow system as a mechanical pump: evidence from examination of tissue and aqueous movement in human and non-human primates. J Glaucoma 2004;13:421–438.

50. Acott TS, Writz MK. Biochemistry of aqueous outflow. In: Ritch R, Shields MB, Krupin T (eds) The Glaucomas, 2nd edn, vol. 1. St. Louis: CV Mosby, 1996: 281–305.

52. Tan JCH, Peters DM, Kaufman PL. Recent developments in understanding the pathophysiology of elevated intraocular pressure. Curr Opin Ophthalmol 2006; 17:168–174.

53. Barany EH. The effect of different kinds of hyaluronidase on the resistance to flow through the angle of the anterior chamber. Acta Ophthalmol 1956;33: 397–403.

65. Kelley MJ, Rose A, Song K, et al. p38 MAP kinase pathway and stromelysin regulation in trabecular meshwork cells. Invest Ophthalmol Vis Sci 2007;48: 3126–3137.

68. Knepper PA, Miller AM, Wertz CJ, et al. Hypophosphorylation of aqueous humor sCD44 and primary open angle glaucoma. Invest Ophthalmol Vis Sci 2005;46:2829–2837.

CHAPTER 23

Pressure-induced optic nerve damage

James C Tsai

Clinical background

Glaucoma is a disease characterized by "a progressive, chronic optic neuropathy in adults where IOP [intraocular pressure] and other unknown factors contribute to damage and which in the absence of other identifiable causes, there is characteristic acquired atrophy of the optic nerve and loss of retinal ganglion cells (RGCs)."[1] The progressive loss of RGCs and their axons produces characteristic damage of optic nerve (e.g., disc cupping and/or retinal nerve fiber layer defects) and corresponding visual field defects. Based upon its definition of a multifactorial optic neuropathy, glaucoma is diagnosed based on structural and functional criteria rather than the IOP level (Box 23.1). A recently proposed "glaucoma continuum" hypothesis characterizes patients along a path from undetectable disease to early mildly symptomatic disease to profound functional impairment.[2]

In the majority of cases, primary open-angle glaucoma (POAG) has few detectable symptoms until considerable vision loss and/or visual field loss has occurred.[3] However, in certain patients, patients may become aware of early visual defects close to central fixation. In patients with POAG, the elevated pressure may not cause the eye discomfort associated with cases of angle closure glaucoma attack. Table 23.1 outlines some ocular areas that deserve special attention during clinical slit-lamp examination of patients with POAG, including the presence of open normal-appearing anterior-chamber angles. Nevertheless, the best means to diagnose glaucoma is to have a high level of suspicion for patients with progressive optic nerve damage (Table 23.2).

It is important to note that a high percentage of glaucoma is found in patients who never manifest elevated IOPs. Historically, "glaucoma" was defined as a disease of elevated IOP above 21 mmHg (the statistical upper 95th percentile of IOP in normal subjects). Blockage of the trabecular meshwork (TM) to aqueous flow was believed to lead to chronic IOP elevation that directly caused the observed optic nerve damage and corresponding loss of peripheral vision. However, population-based studies have shown that one-third or more of persons with open-angle glaucoma (OAG) have normal levels of IOP.[1] Thus, the current definition of OAG is no longer synonymous with "elevated IOP" but that of a pressure-associated optic neuropathy. While POAG is known to occur throughout the entire spectrum of IOP,[1,4] the Collaborative Normal Tension Glaucoma Study Group designation may be clinically useful since it may denote patients in whom there may be additional non-IOP risk factors.[5]

POAG affects more than 2.5 million Americans over the age of 40 with 130 000 functionally blind (defined by central vision < 20/200 or constricted visual field less than 10°).[6] Table 23.3 demonstrates the incidence and prevalence of OAG with age and race. Glaucoma is the second leading cause of blindness worldwide, affecting an estimated 60.5 million people worldwide by 2010.[4] The percentage of undiagnosed patients in the USA ranges from 56% to 92%.[7,8] African-Americans are four to six times more likely to develop glaucoma and subsequent blindness,[9] while older Hispanic patients have a severalfold increase.[7,8]

Pathology

The visible portion of the optic nerve head (ONH) is referred to as the optic disc. The physiologic cup, a central depression in the optic disc, is a pale area partially or completely devoid of axons with exposure of the lamina cribrosa, pores in the posterior sclera that allow passage of the RGC axons and central vessels (Figure 23.1). The nerve tissue between the cup and the disc margin is defined as the neuroretinal rim, an important landmark for assessment of the integrity of the disc structure.

Glaucomatous optic neuropathy (GON) refers to excavation (depression) of the physiologic cup at the lamina cribrosa associated with chronic degeneration of the neuroretinal rim and subsequent loss of RGCs (visible as nerve fiber layer defects).[10] Amyloid precursor protein (amyloid-beta) has also been observed to be present, similar to that observed in Alzheimer's disease and other neurodegenerative diseases.[11] While initial experimental primate studies showed a selective loss of magnocellular bodies and axons, recent contrast sensitivity testing of glaucoma patients suggests nonselective impairment of the low-spatial-frequency components of both magnocellular and parvocellular pathways, presumably mediated by cells with larger receptive fields.[12]

In addition to death of RGCs, there is atrophy and loss of target neurons in the lateral geniculate nucleus of the brain.

Table 23.1 Slit-lamp evaluation

Ocular structure	Possible abnormalities
Cornea (epithelium and endothelium)	Edema, abnormal stromal thickness, Fuchs' corneal endothelial dystrophy, peripheral anterior synechiae associated with iridocorneal endothelial syndromes, pigment deposition on the corneal endothelium, keratic precipitates
Anterior chamber	Peripheral and axial anterior-chamber depth to establish normal values and to rule out a narrow chamber; axial depth to determine position of lens and possible narrowing of angle; changes in axial anterior-chamber depth that may be indicative of malignant glaucoma
Iris	Transpupillary iris transillumination to uncover peripupillary defects and pigmentary dispersion syndrome; evaluate texture of iris, and determine presence of nevi or membranes
Lens	Exfoliation on anterior surface of lens; exfoliation or pigment on the zonules; pigment deposited between posterior lens surface, zonules, and hyaloid; all other lenticular opacities

Reproduced with permission from Epstein DL. Examination of the eye. In: Epstein DL, Allingham RR, Schuman JS (eds) Chandler and Grant's Glaucoma, 4th edn. Baltimore, MD: Williams and Wilkins; 1997:33–40.

Box 23.1 Glaucoma is a complex multifactorial disease of later age onset

Glaucoma is likely caused by several or more contributing risk factors, not all of which will be present to the same degree in every patient. While our current definition of open-angle glaucoma is no longer synonymous with "elevated intraocular pressure," multiple randomized prospective clinical studies conducted across the glaucoma continuum have demonstrated the pressure-associated nature of the disease

---

Studies utilizing experimental primate models of glaucoma show reduced dendrite complexity by 47% and 41% in magnocellular layer 1 and parvocellular layer 6, respectively in experimental animals compared to controls.[13] Clinicopathology demonstrates neural degeneration in the brain involving the intracranial optic nerve, lateral geniculate nucleus, and visual cortex.[14]

Etiology

Randomized, prospective, multicenter clinical trials conducted across the glaucoma continuum (i.e., ocular hypertension to advanced OAG) demonstrate the benefits of lowered IOP. Based upon the results of multiple prospective studies, IOP has been shown to be the major risk factor for the development and progression of POAG.[5,15–17] In particular, these studies showed that normal IOP is part of the

Table 23.2 Evidence of progressive optic nerve damage

Optic disc or retinal nerve fiber layer
- Diffuse or focal narrowing or notching of disc rim (especially at the inferior or superior poles)
- Diffuse or localized abnormalities of the retinal nerve fiber layer (especially at the inferior or superior poles)
- Nerve fiber layer hemorrhage(s)
- Asymmetric appearance of the optic disc rim between fellow eyes (suggesting loss of neural tissue)

Abnormalities in visual field*
- Nasal step or scotoma
- Inferior or superior arcuate scotoma
- Paracentral scotoma
- Generalized depression
- Persistent worsening of the correct-pattern standard deviation (CPSD) on automated threshold perimetry

*In the absence of other explanations for a field defect.
Reproduced with permission from American Academy of Ophthalmology Preferred Practice Patterns Committee Glaucoma Panel. Preferred Practice Patterns. Primary Open-Angle Glaucoma. San Francisco, CA: American Academy of Ophthalmology, 2005.

Table 23.3 Summary of incidence and prevalence data for open-angle glaucoma

Study	Incidence for all ages	Prevalence
Quigley[‡]	1.1 per 100 000/year among whites	1.55% among whites over 40*
	3.9 per 100 000/year among blacks	4.6% among blacks over 40[†]
Baltimore Eye Survey[§]	Not applicable	1.29% among whites over 40
		4.3% among blacks over 40
The Beaver Dam Eye Study[¶]	Not applicable	2.9% among whites

*Median age–adjusted prevalence.
[†]Overall age-adjusted prevalence.
Data compiled from:
[‡]Quigley HA, Vitale S. Models of open-angle glaucoma prevalence and incidence in the United States. Invest Ophthalmol Vis Sci 1997;38:83–91.
[§]Tielsch JM, Sommer A, Katz J, et al. Racial variations in the prevalence of primary open-angle glaucoma. The Baltimore Eye Survey. JAMA 1991;266: 369–374.
[¶]Klein BEK, et al. Prevalence of glaucoma. The Beaver Dam Eye Study. Ophthalmology 1992;99:1499–1504.

pathogenic process of OAG and that IOP reduction favorably influences the disease course.[5,16] In the Collaborative Normal Tension Glaucoma Study, over 20% of patients continued to progress despite adequate IOP reduction of greater than 30%.[5] Approximately 50% of untreated normal-tension glaucoma patients did not progress over the 5-year period, while 5% rapidly progressed, and 45% slowly progressed.[18] Moreover, a faster rate of progression occurred in women and in patients with migraine and optic disc hemorrhages.[18]

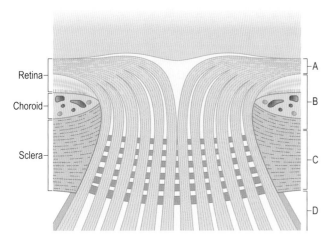

Retina

Choroid

Sclera

Figure 23.1 Optic nerve head regions. (A) Surface nerve fiber layer; (B) prelaminar region; (C) lamina cribrosa region; (D) retrolaminar region.

In eyes with early glaucoma, diurnal IOP is higher, 24-hour change of habitual IOP less, and posture-dependent IOP pattern around normal awakening time different when compared to normal eyes.[19] In the Early Manifest Glaucoma Trial (EMGT), long-term IOP variation was not found to be an independent risk factor for glaucomatous progression after accounting for mean IOP in statistical models.[20] A retrospective analysis of data from the Advanced Glaucoma Intervention Study (AGIS) showed that long-term IOP fluctuation was associated with visual field progression in patients with low mean IOP but not in patients with high mean IOP.[21] Further study is needed to explain the discrepancy among these various studies regarding the relative importance of IOP variation (independent of mean IOP) for glaucomatous progression.

Goldmann applanation tonometry is the most precise method for IOP measurement though its accuracy is affected by central corneal thickness (CCT).[22] Increased CCT alters the tonometrically measured IOP by overestimating its value, while thinner CCT may be a risk factor for OAG independent of the tonometric artifact.[22,23] Randomized clinical trials have demonstrated the importance of CCT in risk models for glaucoma in patients with ocular hypertension and for visual field progression in patients with OAG.[23,24] At present, it is unclear whether CCT might serve as an additional surrogate factor and/or be associated with ONH structural characteristics that may affect glaucoma risk and/or progression (e.g., posterior sclera thickness near the lamina cribrosa region).

Genetic risk factors

The genetic contributions to POAG are complex, resulting from interactions of multiple genetic factors and susceptibility to environmental exposures.[25] Abundant evidence supports a familial aggregation for POAG and its increased risk among first-degree relatives.[26] When juvenile OAG is detected in families, the disease generally exhibits autosomal-dominant inheritance, whereas when primary congenital glaucoma is detected in families, it generally exhibits auto-

somal-recessive inheritance.[25] Based on later onset and heterogeneous factors, POAG is not a simple genetic trait, but has a complex multifactorial pattern of inheritance from the interplay of multiple genetic and environmental factors.[27] However, specific environmental modifying features have not been clearly identified in patients with POAG.[27]

A small number of single-gene defects are associated with a small proportion of OAG overall. While at least 14 genetic loci are associated with POAG, glaucoma-predisposing genes have only been identified in three of these loci (MYOC, OPTN, WDR36).[25] Defects in myocilin (MYOC) were observed in 20% of patients with juvenile OAG and 3–5% of adult-onset POAG.[28] MYOC is one of the olfactomedin domain-containing glycoproteins involved in the extracellular matrix of the aqueous outflow pathways. Specific mutations in MYOC are linked to gain-of-function association with the peroxisomal targeting signal type 1 receptor (PTS1R).[29] Mutations in WDR36 on 5q22.1, located within the chromosomal region GLC1G, were initially reported with POAG,[30] though subsequent studies have failed to confirm this original finding.[31] Finally, mutations in optineurin (OPTN) are observed in patients with normal IOP levels,[32] though these mutations have not been seen with increased frequency in more typical high-tension POAG.[33]

Genes for OAG have been identified by candidate gene screening (e.g., MYOC) and by linkage analysis (e.g., OPTN).[27] A recent genome-wide search yielded multiple single-nucleotide polymorphisms (SNPs) in the 15q24.1 region associated with exfoliation glaucoma, a common secondary OAG characterized by abnormal fibrillar deposits on the lens and in the TM.[34] Two nonsynonymous SNPs identified in exon 1 of the gene lysyl oxidase-like 1 (LOXL1) account for more than 99% of the disease. The LOXL1 gene product catalyzes the formation of elastin fibers that are major components of the deposits in exfoliation glaucoma.[34] Exfoliation is discussed further in Chapter 24.

Vascular factors

Vascular dysregulation, leading to low perfusion pressure and/or insufficient autoregulation, may play a role in the pathogenesis of OAG.[35,36] Though previous prevalence surveys and clinical trials have failed to show an association between cardiovascular disease and the occurrence or progression of OAG, the Barbados Eye Studies and the EMGT reported positive associations.[24,37] In the African-descent participants of the Barbados Eye Studies, risk factors for long-term OAG incidence included lower systolic blood pressure, and particularly lower ocular perfusion pressures, which more than doubled risk.[37] In the EMGT, predictive factors for long-term glaucoma progression included lower systolic perfusion pressure, cardiovascular disease history in patients with higher baseline IOP, and lower systolic blood pressure in patients with lower baseline IOP.[24]

Pathophysiology of glaucoma

In the majority of cases, glaucoma is a disease of aqueous outflow resistance (Figure 23.2), leading to an elevated level of IOP that is a major risk factor for the development of

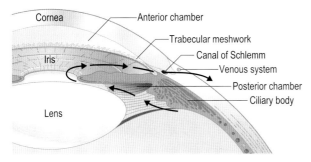

Figure 23.2 Glaucoma is a disease of aqueous outflow resistance. The increased resistance to outflow occurs at the juxtacanalicular region of the trabecular meshwork (TM) and is associated with TM cellular loss, deposition of plaque material, and morphologic and biochemical changes in the extracellular matrix. The changes likely involve transforming growth factor-β_2 (TGF-β_2), thrombospondin-1, and connective tissue growth factor.

GON. Apoptosis-mediated RGC loss in glaucoma could occur from damage to the axon or to its cell body, and there is evidence supporting both of these possibilities (Figure 23.3). Pressure-induced optic nerve damage is mediated by multiple inciting factors (Box 23.2).

Axonal damage

Axonal injury may be signaled to the cell body by injury or disruptions in axonal transport, thereby causing dysfunction of important neuronal processes. Glaucoma, like most complex diseases, results from multiple contributing factors that may not comprise the same set in all patients. The current model, based on ONH biomechanical structure,[38] incorporates multiple contributing factors including aging, connective tissue mechanics, immune cellular responses, RGC axonal transport, blood flow/vascular compromise, and nutrient delivery between laminar astrocytes. There exist substantial IOP-related stress/strain forces within the ONH even at low levels of IOP.

Mechanical factors

IOP elevation is hypothesized to affect axonal transport by compression of ONH tissues (axons, glia, or capillaries) via stress forces generated sufficiently at normal IOP (and intensified at higher levels). The resultant accumulation of retrogradely transported axonal factors includes brain-derived neurotrophic factor (BDNF), a neurotrophin important for RGC survival (its depletion initiates RGC apoptotic death).[39,40] In acute and chronic glaucoma models, interruption of BDNF retrograde transport and accumulation of the tyrosine kinase receptor B (TrkB) occurs at the ONH.[40] The dynein motor complex mediates retrograde axonal transport in RGCs and also accumulates at the ONH with experimental IOP elevation.[41]

In experimental GON, enhanced elastic synthesis is detected in laminar astrocytes.[42] ONH astrocytes also increase expression of the transcription factors c-Fos and c-Jun associated with activation of ERK-MAPK and MAPKp38.[43] Under conditions of elevated IOP, ONH astrocytes lose gap junction intercellular communication via activation of the epidermal growth factor receptor (EGFR) pathway and tyrosine

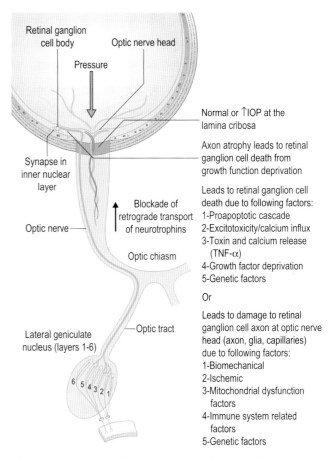

Figure 23.3 Damage to the optic nerve caused by intraocular pressure.

> ### Box 23.2 Pressure-induced optic nerve damage is mediated by multiple inciting factors, including those mediated by biomechanical, ischemic, mitochondrial, and immune system effects
>
> Since one-third or more persons afflicted with open-angle glaucoma have normal levels of intraocular pressure, multiple factors are likely contributory, including connective tissue biomechanics, immune cellular responses, retinal ganglion cell axonal transport mechanisms, volume flow of blood, and nutrient delivery between laminar glial cells. While proven therapy to date for glaucoma entails the lowering of intraocular pressure, our enhanced understanding of its pathophysiology will lead to the future development of novel therapies for the disease

phosphorylation of connexin-43 (CX43).[44] Thus, reactive astrocytes might influence progression of GON even after IOP is lowered.

Ischemia factors

In a nonhuman primate model, chronic ischemia induced by local administration of endothelin-1 (ET-1) leads to significant loss of ONH axons with varying regional susceptibility.[45] In diseased human optic nerves, increased endothelin B receptor (ETbR) expression occurs.[46] The increased ETbR immunoreactivity co-localizes with astrocytic processes, suggesting a role for the glia–endothelin system in the pathogenesis of neuronal degeneration. Tissue ischemia increases neurotrophin and high-affinity Trk receptor expression by central nervous system neurons and glial cells (e.g., astrocytes).[47]

Low cerebrospinal fluid pressure

A recent retrospective case-control study has shown that patients with POAG have low cerebrospinal fluid opening pressure on lumbar puncture compared with a group without glaucoma.[48] In glaucoma, it is hypothesized that elevated IOP blocks traffic within the lamina cribrosa, causing disruption to both anterograde and retrograde axoplasmic transport. Low cerebrospinal fluid is thought to work in concert with IOP to produce an unacceptable high translaminar pressure gradient across the lamina, further disrupting the axoplasmic transport of neurotrophins, thereby leading to RGC apoptosis. In the above study, multivariate analysis showed that larger cup-to-disc ratio was also associated with lower cerebrospinal fluid pressure.

Mitochondrial dysfunction factors

The association of polymorphisms in mitochondrial (mt) DNA in a small subgroup of patients with OAG suggests that oxidative stress and mitochondrial dysfunction are potential risk factors.[49] Increased accumulations of advanced glycation endproducts (AGEs) and their receptor (RAGE) are observed in RGCs and glial cells, primarily Müller cells.[50] The presence of these advanced glycation endproducts suggests an accelerated aging process and evidence of oxidative stress in glaucoma.

Immune system-mediated factors

Patients with POAG have an increased prevalence of monoclonal gammopathy, elevated serum titers of autoantibodies to optic nerve and retina antigens, heat shock proteins, and abnormal T-cell subsets.[51,52] Microglial cells are known to produce neurotoxic molecules, including cytokines such as tumor necrosis factor (TNF)-α, reactive oxygen species (ROS), and nitric oxide (NO), all implicated in the process of GON.[53,54] In vitro findings demonstrate that rat retina and ONH glial cells exposed to ROS upregulate major histocompatibility complex (MHC) class II molecules.[55]

RGC death

Axonal injury may lead to RGC loss by several pathways, including interruption of neurotrophic factors (e.g., BDNF) to the cell bodies, induction of injury pathways, and apoptosis/autophagy (Box 23.3). The resultant RGC death, accompanied by alterations in the supportive glial cells, occurs via a complex apoptotic mechanism triggered by multiple stimuli and interplay of diverse cellular events.[56] While the mechanisms of axonal damage and RGC death are linked, they are separate and may include different elements (see Chapter 42). For example, in DBA/2J mice deficient in the proapoptotic molecule BCL2-associated X protein (BAX), both BAX +/− and BAX−/− mice are protected from RGC death but not axonal degeneration.[57] Furthermore, BAX deficiency protects RGC cells after axon injury by optic

nerve crush, but not N-methyl-D-aspartate (NMDA)-induced excitotoxicity.

The molecular mechanism of RGC death is hypothesized to be similar to that found in Alzheimer's disease. In ocular hypertensive rat models, caspase-3 activation occurs with increased generation of caspase-3-mediated amyloid precursor cleavage product (delta C-APP).[58] Consistent with apoptosis in neurodegeneration, RGCs are terminal uridine deoxynucleotidyl transferase dUTP nick end labeling (TUNEL)-positive, with increased caspase-3 and decreased Bcl-2.[59] Elevated IOP also triggers cleavage of the autoinhibitory domain of the protein phosphatase calcineurin (CaN); the CaN-mediated mitochondrial apoptotic pathway leads to dephosphorylation of the proapoptotic Bcl-2 family member, Bad, increased cytoplasmic cytochrome c, and RGC death.[60]

The role of glutamate excitotoxicity remains in serious doubt since subsequent studies have failed to confirm the original finding of elevated glutamate levels in the vitreous humor of patients with glaucoma.[61] In this theory, neuronal cell damage is mediated by overactivation of NMDA-type glutamate receptors, leading to excessive calcium influx through the receptor-associated ion channels. NMDA-mediated RGC death is dependent on activation of matrix metalloproteinase-9 via neuronal nitric oxide synthase (nNOS).[62] Increased intracellular calcium accumulation leads to a myriad of apoptotic pathways including activation of caspase 6, m-calpain, and ubiquitin protein degradation.[63]

Experimental animal models suggest simultaneous upregulation of proapoptotic and pro-survival genes. RGC death involves activation, at different time points, of multiple proapoptotic and pro-survival pathways.[64] Gene array RNA profiles also show simultaneous upregulation of proapoptotic genes from the p-53 pathway, as well as pro-survival genes (i.e., IAP-1).[65] The simultaneous upregulation of IAP-1, an endogenous caspase inhibitor, suggests an intrinsic feedback-neuroprotective mechanism.

Secondary RGC death may also result from exposure to light, as well as growth factor deprivation and toxins released from damaged astrocytes. Visible light, in an intensity-dependent and trolox-inhibitable manner, reduces RGC viability, affects mitochondrial function, and increases the number of TUNEL-positive cells.[66] Growth factor deprivation after serum withdrawal in RGC cells induces apoptotic cell death (via mitochondrial pathways) with activation of caspase-3, -8, and -9.[67]

Box 23.3 The molecular mechanisms underlying retinal ganglion cell (RGC) loss in open-angle glaucoma involve apoptosis

Though the final common pathway of apoptotic-mediated RGC death is agreed upon, the site of initial cellular insult has not been clearly elucidated and may involve axonal injury and/or cell body damage. Axonal injury might be signaled to the ganglion cell body by disruptions in axonal transport, thereby causing dysfunction of important neuronal processes and withdrawal of neurotrophins critical for RGC survival

---

There is increasing evidence that TNF-α, a cytokine known to be released by ocular glia, is associated with RGC loss in glaucoma. In a laser irradiation-induced murine model of ocular hypertension, increased levels of TNF-α lead to microglial activation, loss of oligodendrocytes in the optic nerve, and loss of RGCs.[68] A similar sequence of biological events occurs after injection of TNF-α in mice with normal IOP. Conversely, no loss of RGCs above baseline is observed in the setting of elevated IOP when animals are treated with TNF-α inhibitors or knockout mice unable to produce TNF-α are studied.[68]

Summary and conclusions

Similar to other complex diseases of later age onset, POAG is likely caused by several or more contributing risk factors, not all of which will be present to the same degree in every patient. While our current definition of OAG is no longer synonymous with "elevated IOP," multiple randomized prospective clinical studies conducted across the glaucoma continuum (i.e., ocular hypertension to advanced OAG) have demonstrated the effectiveness of lowering IOP in preventing disease occurrence and progression. While the final common pathway involves pressure-induced optic nerve damage, multiple inciting factors are present, including those mediated by biomechanical, ischemic, mitochondrial, and immune system effects. The molecular mechanisms underlying OAG have as the final common pathway apoptotic-mediated RGC death, though the initial cellular insult may result from axonal injury and/or cell body damage. Axonal injury might be signaled to the ganglion cell body by disruptions in axonal transport, thereby causing dysfunction of important neuronal processes and withdrawal of neurotrophins critical for RGC survival. Since one-third or more persons afflicted with OAG have normal levels of IOP, multiple factors are likely contributory, including connective tissue biomechanics, immune cellular responses, RGC axonal transport mechanisms, volume flow of blood, and nutrient delivery between laminar glial cells. While proven therapy to date for glaucoma entails the lowering of IOP, our enhanced understanding of its pathophysiology will lead to the future development of novel therapies for the disease.

Acknowledgments

Support for the author's research was provided by a Challenge grant from Research to Prevent Blindness, Inc. (New York, NY) and the Eye Bank for Sight Restoration (New York, NY). The author also thanks Juliann Boccio for her assistance in illustrating Figures 23.2 and 23.3.

Key references

A complete list of chapter references is available online at www.expertconsult.com. See inside cover for registration details.

5. Collaborative Normal Tension Glaucoma Study Group. The effectiveness of intraocular pressure reduction in the treatment of normal-tension glaucoma. Am J Ophthalmol 1998;126:498–505.

13. Gupta N, Ly T, Zhang Q, et al. Chronic ocular hypertension induces dendrite pathology in the lateral geniculate nucleus of the brain. Exp Eye Res 2007;84:176–184.

15. Kass MA, Heuer DK, Higginbotham EJ, et al. The Ocular Hypertension Treatment Study: a randomized trial determines that topical ocular hypotensive medication delays or prevents the onset of primary open-angle glaucoma. Arch Ophthalmol 2002;120:701–713; discussion 829–830.

24. Leske MC, Heijl A, Human L, et al. Predictors of long-term progression in the early manifest glaucoma trial. Ophthalmology 2007;114:1965–1972.

25. Wiggs JL. Genetic etiologies of glaucoma. Arch Ophthalmol 2007;125:30–37.

34. Thorleifsson G, Magnusson K, Sulem P, et al. Common sequence variants in the LOXL1 gene confer susceptibility to exfoliation glaucoma. Science 2007;317:1397–1400.

37. Leske MC, Wu SY, Hennis A, et al. Risk factors for incident open-angle glaucoma. The Barbados Eye Studies. Ophthalmology 2008;115:85–93.

38. Burgoyne CF, Downs JC, Bellezza AJ, et al. The optic nerve head as a biomechanical structure: a new paradigm for understanding the role of IOP-related stress and strain in the pathophysiology of glaucomatous optic nerve head damage. Prog Retin Eye Res 2005;24:39–73.

39. Quigley HA, McKinnon SJ, Zack DJ, et al. Retrograde axonal transport of BDNF in retinal ganglion cells is blocked by acute IOP elevation in rats. Invest Ophthalmol Vis Sci 2000;41:3460–3466.

48. Berdahl JP, Allingham RR, Johnson DH. Cerebrospinal fluid pressure is decreased in primary open-angle glaucoma. Ophthalmology 2008;115:763–768.

50. Tezel G, Luo C, Yang X. Accelerated aging in glaucoma: immunohistochemical assessment of advanced glycation end products in the human retina and optic nerve head. Invest Ophthalmol Vis Sci 2007;48:1201–1211.

55. Tezel G, Yang X, Luo C, et al. Mechanisms of immune system activation in glaucoma: oxidative-stress-stimulated antigen presentation by the retina and optic nerve head glia. Invest Ophthalmol Vis Sci 2007;48:705–714.

56. Wax MB, Tezel G. Neurobiology of glaucomatous optic neuropathy: diverse cellular events in neurodegeneration and neuroprotection. Mol Neurobiol 2002;26:45–55.

65. Levkovitch-Verbin H, Dardik R, Vander S, et al. Experimental glaucoma and optic nerve transection induce simultaneous upregulation of proapoptotic and prosurvival genes. Invest Ophthalmol Vis Sci 2006;47:2491–2497.

68. Nakazawa T, Nakazawa C, Matsubara A, et al. Tumor necrosis factor-alpha mediates oligodendrocyte death and delayed ganglion cell loss in a mouse model of glaucoma. J Neurosci 2006;26:12633–12641.

CHAPTER 24

Exfoliation (pseudoexfoliation) syndrome

Robert Ritch and Ursula Schlötzer-Schrehardt

Introduction (Box 24.1)

Exfoliation syndrome (XFS) is an age-related disease characterized by the production and progressive accumulation of a fibrillar extracellular material in many ocular tissues. First described in 1917 by Lindberg,[1-3] it is the most common identifiable cause of open-angle glaucoma worldwide, comprising the majority of glaucoma in some countries.[4] Its incidence increases progressively with age, while its widespread distribution, frequency, and association with other diseases are still poorly understood. The discovery in 2007 of nonsynonymous single-nucleotide polymorphisms (SNPs) in the lysyl oxidase-like 1 (*LOXL1*) gene is expected to make a major impact not only in understanding XFS, but also in leading to new avenues of therapy.

Clinical background

Key symptoms and signs

All anterior-segment structures are involved in XFS. The diagnosis is made by finding typical white deposits of exfoliation material (XFM) on the anterior lens surface and/or pupillary border. The diagnosis should be suspected in the absence of XFM when ancillary pigment-related signs are present, which define patients as "exfoliation suspects."[5]

The classic pattern consists of three distinct zones that become visible when the pupil is fully dilated: a central disc, an intermediate clear zone created by the iris rubbing XFM from the lens surface during its normal excursions, and a granular peripheral zone (Figures 24.1 and 24.2). XFM is often found at the pupillary border (Figure 24.3).

Pigment loss from the pupillary ruff and iris sphincter region and its deposition on anterior-chamber structures are hallmarks of XFS (Box 24.2). As the iris scrapes XFM from the lens surface, the material on the lens causes rupture of iris pigment epithelial cells, with concomitant pigment dispersion into the anterior chamber. This leads to iris sphincter transillumination, loss of the ruff, increased trabecular pigmentation (Figure 24.4), and pigment deposition on the iris surface. Pigment dispersion in the anterior chamber is common after pupillary dilation and may be profuse. Marked intraocular pressure (IOP) rises can occur after pharmacologic dilation, and IOP should be measured routinely in all patients after dilation. XFM may be detected earliest on the ciliary processes and zonules, which are often frayed and broken (Figure 24.5). Spontaneous subluxation or dislocation of the lens can occur.

An increasing number of reported systemic associations includes transient ischemic attacks, hypertension, angina, myocardial infarction, stroke, asymptomatic myocardial dysfunction, Alzheimer's disease, and hearing loss (Box 24.3).[6-12] Some of these associations have been disputed and there is as yet no clear evidence of increased mortality in patients with XFS, which one might expect with these associations, nor has there been shown a clear-cut association of XFS with a systemic disease with conclusive evidence of a functional deficit caused by the presence of XFS.

Epidemiology

The prevalence of XFS increases steadily with age in all populations. The reported prevalence both with and without glaucoma has varied widely, reflecting true differences due to racial, ethnic, or other as yet unknown factors; the age and sex distribution of the patient cohort or population group examined; the clinical criteria used to diagnose XFS; the ability of the examiner to detect early stages and/or more subtle signs; the method and thoroughness of the examination; and the awareness of the observer.[13] It comprises as much as 50% or more of the open-angle glaucoma in some countries, including Norway, Ireland, Greece, and Saudi Arabia. Previously thought rare in Africa, recent reports indicate that it comprises 25% of open-angle glaucoma in Ethiopia[14] and in South African Zulus.[15] In the USA, it is much more common in Caucasians than in persons of African ancestry, comprising about 12% of glaucoma populations.[16-18] There are ethnic variations within countries and geographic variations even within adjacent towns in the same area.[19] In central Norway, the prevalence in two adjacent towns (20%) was twice that in a third, adjacent town. In Nepal, XFS was found in 12% of members of one ethnic

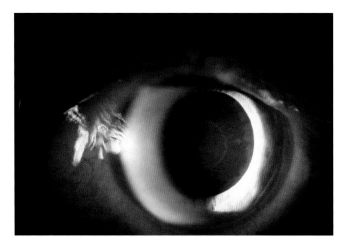

Figure 24.1 Classic appearance of exfoliation syndrome.

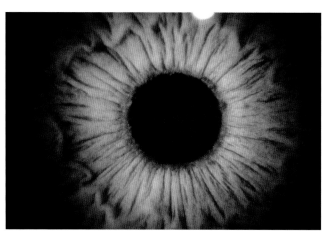

Figure 24.3 Exfoliation material at the pupillary border. The pupillary ruff has been nearly completely disintegrated.

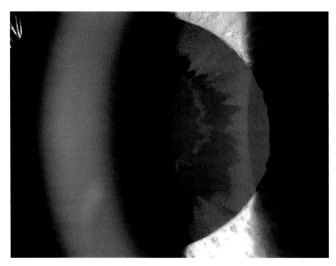

Figure 24.2 Peripheral granular zone. The edge of the central disc also shows granularity in this photograph, but this is not always present. It suggests a decreased pupillary excursion over time, so that the exfoliation material is not scraped from the edge of the central disc and gradually builds up. The same appearance is seen in the central disc after long-standing miotic treatment.

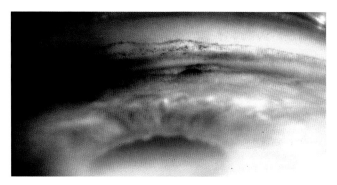

Figure 24.4 Typical angle appearance in an eye with exfoliation syndrome. The pigment on the trabecular meshwork is dark brown and smudgy. Pigment is present on Schwalbe's line and above that, on the peripheral corneal shelf (Sampaolesi line).

Box 24.2 Importance of pigment dispersion

Pigment loss from the pupillary ruff and iris sphincter region and its deposition on anterior-chamber structures lead to iris sphincter transillumination, loss of the pupillary ruff, pigment dispersion in the anterior chamber after pupillary dilation, and increased trabecular pigmentation, the degree of which has been reported to correlate with the presence and severity of glaucoma

Box 24.1 Definition

Exfoliation syndrome is an age-related disease characterized by the production and progressive accumulation of a fibrillar extracellular material in many ocular tissues and is the most common identifiable cause of open-angle glaucoma worldwide, comprising the majority of glaucoma in some countries

Box 24.3 Systemic associations

An emerging clinical spectrum of associations with cardiovascular and cerebrovascular diseases elevates exfoliation syndrome to a condition of general medical importance. Systemic associations include transient ischemic attacks, circulatory abnormalities, myocardial dysfunction, Alzheimer's disease, and hearing loss. The discovery of nonsynonymous single-nucleotide polymorphisms (SNPs) in the lysyl oxidase-like 1 (LOXL1) gene should lead to understanding of these associations and to new avenues of therapy

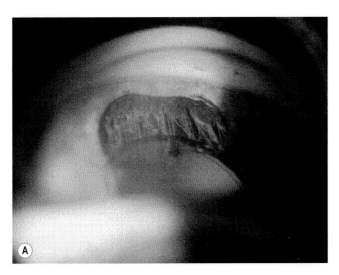

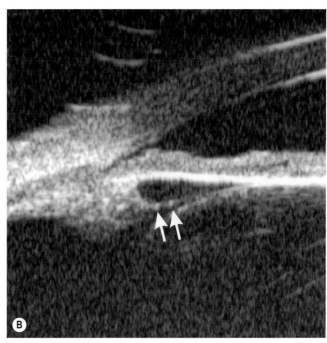

Figure 24.5 (A) The zonules are frayed, broken, and disintegrating. (B) Ultrasound biomicroscopy.

Box 24.4 Prognosis

The prognosis of exfoliative glaucoma is more severe than that of primary open-angle glaucoma at all levels of presentation and treatment

---

group, the Gurung, and only 0.24% of non-Gurung of similar ages.[20] Although common in Japan and Mongolia, it is rare in southern China.[21]

The prevalence of XFS in glaucoma patients is significantly higher than in age-matched nonglaucomatous populations. Approximately 25% of XFS patients have elevated IOP and one-third of these have glaucoma. This is approximately six times the chance of finding elevated IOP in eyes without XFS. It has been estimated (Lindberg Society) that clinically detectable XFS affects approximately 60–70 million people, so that there should be some 5–6 million persons with exfoliative glaucoma, or nearly 10% of the world's glaucoma.

Prognosis

The prognosis of exfoliative glaucoma (XFG) is more severe than that of primary open-angle glaucoma (POAG) (Box 24.4). Patients with XFS are twice as likely to convert from ocular hypertension to glaucoma and, when glaucoma is present, to progress.[22,23] The mean IOP is greater in normotensive patients with XFS than in the general population and greater in XFG patients at presentation than in POAG patients. At any specific IOP level, eyes with XFS are more likely to have glaucomatous damage than are eyes without XFS. There is greater 24-hour IOP fluctuation, greater visual field loss and optic disc damage at the time of detection, poorer response to medications, more rapid progression, greater need for surgical intervention, and greater proportion of blindness.[23]

Treatment of exfoliative glaucoma

The sole focus of therapy in XFG should not be the reduction of IOP. Understanding the mechanisms leading to elevated IOP in XFS could allow us to develop new and more logical approaches to therapy.

Most ophthalmologists approach medical treatment with topical prostaglandin analogs and aqueous suppressants. In addition to lowering IOP, prostaglandin analogs may interfere with the disease process. Latanoprost treatment had a marked effect on the aqueous concentration of transforming growth factor (TGF)-ß$_1$, matrix metalloproteinase (MMP)-2, and tissue inhibitor of matrix metalloproteinase-2 (TIMP-2) in XFG patients.[24] Aqueous suppressants do not interfere with the mechanism of pigment liberation and trabecular blockage. Cholinergic agents, on the other hand, not only lower IOP, but by increasing aqueous outflow, should enable the trabecular meshwork to clear more rapidly, and by limiting pupillary movement, should slow the progression of the disease. Aqueous suppressants result in decreased flow through the trabecular meshwork. Treatment with aqueous suppressants may lead to worsening of trabecular function.[25] Pilocarpine 2% qhs can provide sufficient limitation of pupillary mobility without causing visual side-effects. A prospective trial (International Collaborative Exfoliation Syndrome Treatment Study) comparing latanoprost and 2% pilocarpine qhs versus timolol/Cosopt for patients with XFS and ocular hypertension or glaucoma has been completed and the data are currently being analyzed (Box 24.5).

Box 24.5 Mechanism of glaucoma and directed therapy

Blockage of aqeous outflow by a combination of pigment and exfoliation material in the intertrabecular spaces and juxtacanalicular meshwork is believed to be the major cause of elevated intraocular pressure. Therapy designed to prevent this buildup (directed therapy) is a major goal for the future. At the present time, 2% pilocarpine given at bedtime suffices to produce a 3-mm nonreactive pupil throughout the day and limits release of pigment and exfoliation material

Argon laser trabeculoplasty (ALT) is particularly effective, at least early on, in eyes with XFS. Approximately 20% of patients develop sudden, late rises of IOP within 2 years of treatment.[26] Continued pigment liberation may overwhelm the restored functional capacity of the trabecular meshwork, and maintenance of miotic therapy (again 2% pilocarpine qhs) to minimize pupillary movement after ALT might counteract this. Selective laser trabeculoplasty needs further evaluation as an effective and safe alternative to ALT in the treatment of XFG.

Trabeculectomy results are comparable to those in POAG. Trabeculotomy is also successful.[27] Jacobi et al[28] described a procedure termed trabecular aspiration, designed to improve outflow facility by eliminating the trabecular blockage by pigment and XFM. Deep sclerectomy and similar procedures including a deroofing of Schlemm's canal are becoming popular choices in some centers owing to the reduced risk profile of nonpenetrating surgery. In one series, XFG patients had significantly better success than POAG patients following deep sclerectomy with an implant.[29] Moreover, phacoemulsification combined with penetrating and nonpenetrating procedures does not seem to influence success rate adversely.

Etiology

Several lines of evidence, including regional clustering, familial aggregation, and genetic linkage analyses, had previously supported a genetic predisposition to XFS.[30] Recently, a genome-wide association study detected two common SNPs in the coding region of the *LOXL1* gene on chromosome 15q24 that were specifically associated with XFS and XFG in two Scandinavian populations from Iceland and Sweden, accounting for virtually all XFS cases.[31] These disease-associated polymorphisms appeared to confer risk of glaucoma mainly through XFS. The combination of alleles formed by the two coding polymorphisms determined the risk of developing XFG, which is increased by a factor of 27 if the high-risk haplotype is present. Individuals carrying two copies of this high-risk haplotype would have a 700-times increased risk of developing XFG. Moreover, these genetic alterations also lead to decreased tissue expression of *LOXL1* dependent on the individual haplotype. These genetic findings have been confirmed in populations of European descent in Iowa,[32] New York,[33] Utah,[34] Boston,[35] and Australia.[36] One different SNP and one common SNP have been reported in a Japanese population.[37] The *LOXL1* gene

variations are not associated with POAG or primary angle closure.[38]

LOXL1 is a member of the lysyl oxidase family of enzymes, which are essential for the formation, stabilization, maintenance, and remodeling of elastic fibers and prevent age-related loss of tissue elasticity.[39] It is involved in cross-linking tropoelastin to mature elastin using elastic microfibrils as a scaffold,[40] thus serving both as a cross-linking enzyme and as a scaffolding element which ensures spatially defined elastin deposition.[41] The functional consequences of the *LOXL1* gene variants in XFS are not yet known; however, inadequate tissue levels of LOXL1 could predispose to impaired elastin homeostasis and to increased elastosis. Genetic variation in *LOXL1* may be a factor in spontaneous cervical artery dissection, a cause of stroke in younger patients.[42] Reduced LOXL1 levels are also found in patients with varicose veins and venous insufficiency.[43] Overactivity of lysyl oxidase, with localization of the enzyme in blood vessel walls and in plaque-like structures, has been found in Alzheimer's disease.[44] Mice deficient in LOXL1 develop pelvic organ prolapse secondary to a generalized connective tissue defect,[45] and women with prolapse have reduced mRNA for LOXL1.[46] Marked elastosis with elastic fiber degeneration has been observed in the skin and connective tissue of the lamina cribrosa in XFS eyes.[47] Although further studies correlating the genetic variants and tissue alterations associated with XFS are needed, these new findings already provide a basis for both genetic testing and novel treatment approaches.

Various nongenetic factors, including dietary factors, autoimmunity, infectious agents, and trauma, have also been hypothesized to be involved in the pathogenesis of XFS. Reports dealing with sunlight exposure (ultraviolet radiation) are conflicting. Eskimos are the only people reported to have no XFS, but it is common in Lapps living at the same latitude.[48] Persons living at lower latitudes develop XFS at younger ages, whereas those living at higher altitudes had a greater prevalence in two series[49,50] but not in a third.[51] In one series, XFS was detected more frequently in eyes with blue irides versus brown irides.[52] Herpes simplex virus type 1 was detected by polymerase chain reaction in 13.8% of iris and anterior capsule specimens of patients with XFS compared to 1.8% of controls.[53] Younger patients have developed XFS after penetrating keratoplasty using buttons from elderly donors.[54-57] Altogether, it appears that XFS represents a complex, multifactorial, late-onset disease, involving both genetic and nongenetic factors in its pathogenesis.

Pathogenesis of exfoliation syndrome and exfoliative glaucoma

A precise understanding of the pathogenesis of XFS remains elusive. However, the pathologic process in intra- and extraocular tissues is characterized by the progressive accumulation of an abnormal fibrillar matrix, which is the result of either an excessive production or an insufficient breakdown or both, and which is regarded as pathognomonic for the disease based on its unique light microscopic and ultrastructural criteria.

Ultrastructure and composition of exfoliation material

Exfoliation fibers are clearly distinguishable from any other known form of extracellular matrix. Light microscopy reveals XFM to be periodic acid–Schiff (PAS)-positive, eosinophilic, bush-like, nodular, or feathery aggregates on the surfaces of anterior-segment tissues. On transmission electron microscopy, the aggregates consist of randomly arranged, fuzzy fibrils, 25–50 nm in diameter, frequently with 20–25 or 45–50 nm cross-banding. These composite fibers are generally associated with 8–10 nm microfibrils, which resemble elastic microfibrils and which aggregate laterally into mature fibers. However, the microfibrillar core of the complex fibers is usually hidden by a coating of electron-dense amorphous material.

The exact chemical composition of XFM remains unknown. Indirect histochemical and immunohistochemical evidence suggests a complex glycoprotein/proteoglycan structure composed of a protein core surrounded by abundant glycoconjugates, including various glycosaminoglycans (heparin sulfate, chondroitin sulfate, hyaluronan) indicating excessive glycosylation.[58] The protein components contain epitopes of the elastic fiber system, such as elastin, tropoelastin, amyloid-P, and vitronectin.[59] Components of elastic microfibrils, such as fibrillin-1, microfibril-associated glycoprotein (MAGP-1), and the latent TGF-ß-binding proteins (LTBP-1 and LTBP-2), are associated with XFM deposits in intra- and extraocular locations and co-localize with latent TGF-ß$_1$ on exfoliation fibers.[60–63]

A recent direct analytical approach using liquid chromatography coupled with tandem mass spectrometry (LC-MS/MS) showed XFM to consist of the elastic microfibril components fibrillin-1, fibulin-2, and vitronectin, the proteoglycans syndecan and versican, the extracellular chaperone clusterin, the cross-linking enzyme lysyl oxidase, and some other proteins, confirming many of the previously reported immunohistochemical data.[63] Together, these findings support the notion that XFM represents an elastotic material arising from abnormal aggregation of elastic microfibril components interacting with multiple ligands.

Origin of exfoliation material

Ocular XFM is closely associated with the nonpigmented ciliary epithelium, pre-equatorial lens epithelium, iris pigment epithelium, trabecular and corneal endothelia, and virtually all cell types in the iris stroma and vasculature, all showing signs of active fibrillogenesis.[23,64] Passive distribution of XFM by the aqueous humor may be responsible for abnormal deposits on the central anterior lens capsule, the zonules, the anterior hyaloid surface, vitreous, and intraocular lenses. In extraocular locations, fibers are found in close proximity to connective tissue fibroblasts, vascular wall cells, smooth and striated muscle cells, and cardiomyocytes.[65,66]

Molecular pathogenesis

Differential gene expression

With gene expression analyses, XFS tissues contained a number of differentially expressed genes, which were mainly

involved in extracellular matrix metabolism and in cellular stress.[67,68] One set of genes consistently upregulated in anterior-segment tissues comprised the elastic microfibril components fibrillin-1, LTBP-1 and LTBP-2, the cross-linking enzyme transglutaminase (TGase)-2, TIMP-2, TGF-ß$_1$, several heat shock proteins (Hsp 27, Hsp 40, Hsp 60), proinflammatory cytokines, apolipoprotein D, and the adenosine receptor (AdoR)-A3. Genes reproducibly downregulated in XFS tissues included TIMP-1, the extracellular chaperone clusterin, the antioxidant defense enzymes glutathione-S-transferases (mGST-1, GST-T1), components of the ubiquitin-proteasome pathway (ubiquitin conjugating enzymes E2A and E2B), several DNA repair proteins (ERCC1, hMLH1, GADD 153), the transcription factor Id-3, and serum amyloid A1.

Together, these findings provide evidence that the underlying pathophysiology of XFS is associated with an excessive production of elastic microfibril components, enzymatic cross-linking processes, overexpression of TGF-ß$_1$, a proteolytic imbalance between MMPs and TIMPs, low-grade inflammatory processes, increased cellular and oxidative stress, and an impaired cellular stress response, as reflected by the downregulation of antioxidative enzymes, ubiquitin-conjugating enzymes, clusterin, and DNA repair proteins (Box 24.6).

Pathogenetic factors and key molecules

Factors which might stimulate the synthesis and stable deposition of XFM include growth factors, a dysbalance of MMPs and TIMPs, and increased cellular and oxidative stress conditions (Figure 24.6).

Apart from increased concentrations of various growth factors (basic fibroblast growth factor (bFGF), hepatocyte growth factor (HGF), connective tissue growth factor (CTGF), in the aqueous humor of XFS patients,[69,70] TGF-ß$_1$, a major modulator of matrix formation in many fibrotic diseases, appears to be a key mediator in the XFS process. It is significantly increased in the aqueous humor of XFS patients, in both its latent and active form, it is upregulated and actively produced by anterior-segment tissues, and it regulates most of the genes differentially expressed in XFS eyes, e.g., fibrillin-1, LTBP-1 and -2, TGase-2, and clusterin.[71,72] Binding of TGF-ß$_1$ to XFM via the TGF-ß binding proteins LTBP-1 and -2 may represent a mechanism of regulation of growth factor activity in XFS eyes. Whereas the TGF-ß$_3$ isoform was also reported to be significantly increased in aqueous humor of XFS patients,[73] levels of TGF-ß$_2$ were significantly higher in the aqueous humor of POAG patients but not that of XFS patients.

Changes in the local MMP/TIMP balance and reduced MMP activity in aqueous humor and tissues may further

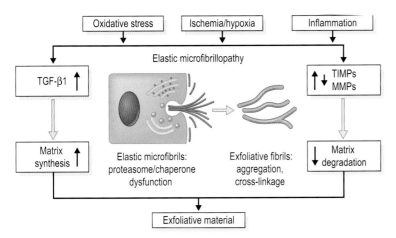

Figure 24.6 Summary of pathogenetic concept of exfoliation syndrome.

promote abnormal matrix accumulation in XFS. Significantly increased concentrations of MMP-2, MMP-3, TIMP-1, and TIMP-2 were detected in aqueous humor of XFS patients with and without glaucoma compared to controls.[74,75] However, levels of endogenously active MMP-2, the major MMP in human aqueous humor, were significantly decreased, as was the ratio of MMP-2 to TIMP-2, resulting in a molar excess of TIMP-2 over MMP-2. An imbalance of MMPs and TIMPs has been also reported in meshwork specimens from XFG patients.[76]

There is increasing evidence that cellular stress conditions (oxidative stress, ischemia/hypoxia) are involved in the pathobiology of XFS. Significantly reduced levels of antioxidants (ascorbic acid, glutathione) and increased levels of oxidative stress markers (8-isoprostaglandin-$F_2\alpha$, malondialdehyde) in aqueous humor, serum, and tissues indicate a faulty antioxidative defense system and increased oxidative stress in the anterior chamber of XFS eyes.[77-81]

Development of glaucoma

Friction between the iris and the lens surface leads to disruption of the iris pigment epithelium at the sphincter region and concomitant dispersion of pigment into the anterior chamber. Blockage of aqueous outflow by a combination of pigment and XFM deposited in the intertrabecular spaces, and XFM in the juxtacanalicular meshwork and beneath the endothelium of Schlemm's canal is believed to be the major cause of elevated IOP.

Increased outflow resistance both in the trabecular meshwork and in the uveoscleral pathways,[82] most probably from blockage of the outflow channels by XFM, leads to elevated IOP. Aggregates of XFM are found in the anterior portions of the ciliary muscle, on the inner surface of the trabecular meshwork, beneath the inner and outer wall of Schlemm's canal, and in the periphery of intrascleral aqueous collector channels and aqueous veins (Figure 24.7).[83] Accumulation of XFM in the meshwork may derive from both passive deposition from the aqueous on the surface of the uveal meshwork and local production by trabecular and Schlemm's canal endothelial cells in the juxtacanalicular tissue and canal wall. Progressive accumulation of XFM in the subendothelial space leads to a marked thickening of the juxtacanalicular tissue, the site of greatest resistance to

aqueous outflow (Figure 24.8). Concomitant disruption and breakdown of the normal elastic fiber network surrounding Schlemm's canal appear to result in a progressive destabilization and disorganization of the normal tissue architecture. Collapse of aqueous veins due to perivascular accumulation of elastotic material can also occasionally be observed.

The amount of XFM within the juxtacanalicular region correlates with the presence of glaucoma, the average thickness of the juxtacanalicular tissue, and the mean cross-sectional area of Schlemm's canal, and also with the IOP level and the axon count in the optic nerve.[83,84] These findings suggest that therapeutic efforts to improve outflow need to address the alterations in the juxtacanalicular area to obtain lasting IOP reduction.

In addition to XFM and pigment obstruction of the meshwork, increased aqueous protein concentrations and cellular dysfunction may also contribute to elevated IOP. Several members of the phospholipase A2 enzyme family, which play a major role in phospholipid metabolism and membrane homeostasis, are significantly decreased in the trabecular meshwork of exfoliative glaucoma patients compared to normal controls or POAG patients.[85] These observations may indicate abnormal physiological functions, decreased structural stability and flexibility, and reduced protection against oxidative stress in trabecular meshwork cells of XFG eyes.

Increased trabecular pigmentation is a prominent and early sign of XFS. In patients with clinically unilateral XFG, the pigment is usually denser in the involved eye. Eyes with POAG or eyes without glaucoma tend to have less pigmentation than eyes with XFG. Glaucomatous damage is usually more advanced in the eye with greater pigmentation. Pigment dispersion and deposition in the trabecular meshwork may lead to acute pressure rises after pupillary dilation.

Although XFG is characteristically a high-pressure disease with a predominant mechanical component of optic nerve damage, pressure-independent (e.g., vascular) risk factors, and structural alterations of the lamina cribrosa may further increase the individual risk for glaucomatous damage. In a prospective study of patients with clinically unilateral involvement, in whom IOP was equal throughout the follow-up period, disc changes took place only in the involved eye, suggesting that the exfoliative process itself

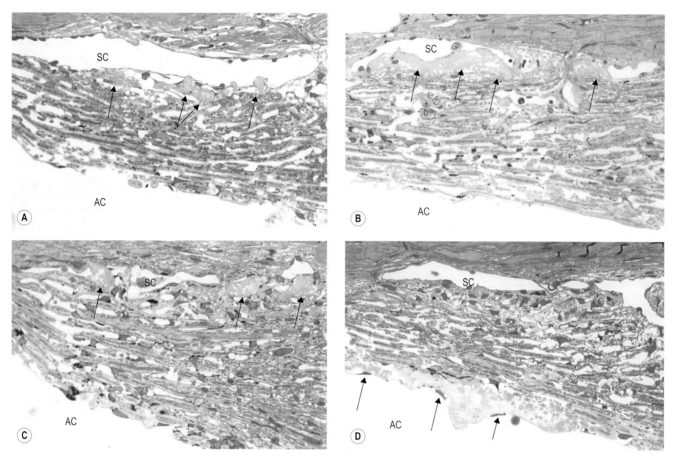

Figure 24.7 Light microscopic semithin sections showing involvement of the trabecular meshwork and Schlemm's canal in exfoliation syndrome. AC, anterior chamber; SC, Schlemm's canal (toluidine blue; magnification ×250). (A) Accumulation of small deposits of exfoliative material (arrows) in the juxtacanalicular meshwork. (B) Accumulation of large masses of exfoliative material (arrows) in the juxtacanalicular tissue. (C) Disorganization of Schlemm's canal area by exfoliative material accumulation (arrows) in the juxtacanalicular tissue. (D) Pretrabecular deposits of exfoliative material overgrown by migrating corneal endothelial cells.

may be a risk factor for optic disc changes.[86] Marked elastosis in the connective tissue sheets of the lamina cribrosa of XFS eyes may adversely affect tissue elasticity and increase the susceptibility of optic nerve fibers towards mechanical and vascular damage (Figure 24.9).[87,88] Moreover, accumulation of XFM in the walls of retrobulbar vessels increased the rigidity of their walls.[89] The recently identified sequence variants in the *LOXL1* gene and reduced tissue levels of LOXL1, a key enzyme in elastic fiber homeostasis, may predispose to these elastotic matrix processes characterizing XFS and possibly contribute to glaucoma development in XFS patients.

Angle closure is also associated with XFS. Ritch[89] found either clinically apparent XFS or XFM on conjunctival biopsy in 17 of 60 (28.3%) consecutive patients with uncomplicated primary angle closure glaucoma or occludable angles. Pupillary block may be caused by a combination of posterior synechiae, increased iris thickness or rigidity, or anterior lens movement secondary to zonular weakness or dialysis.[90]

Vacular abnormalities in XFS

An emerging clinical spectrum of associations with cardiovascular and cerebrovascular diseases elevates XFS to a condition of general medical importance. XFS is associated with ocular ischemia, particularly iris hypoperfusion and anterior-chamber hypoxia,[91] and with a reduced ocular and retrobulbar micro- and macrovascular blood flow ocurring in both patients with and without glaucoma.[92] Blood flow of the lamina cribrosa and neural rim decreases with increasing glaucomatous damage.[93] In clinically unilateral cases, ipsilateral pulsatile ocular blood flow and carotid blood flow are reduced.[94,95] Recently, pathological carotid artery function as well as altered parasympathetic vascular control was reported.[96] In a large study, XFS was reported to be an important risk factor for coronary artery disease.[97]

The vasoactive peptide endothelin-1 is significantly increased in the aqueous of XFS patients,[98] while levels of nitric oxide, a potent physiological vasodilator, were decreased in a small number of XFS patients.[99] This imbalance may play a role in the obliterative vasculopathy of the iris causing local ischemia early in the disease process. Elevated homocysteine levels in the aqueous humor of patients with XFS[100,101] may further contribute to ischemic alterations, such as endothelial dysfunction, oxidative stress, enhancement of platelet aggregation, reduction of nitric oxide bioavailability, and abnormal perivascular matrix metabolism. These findings have been summarized in a recent editorial.[102]

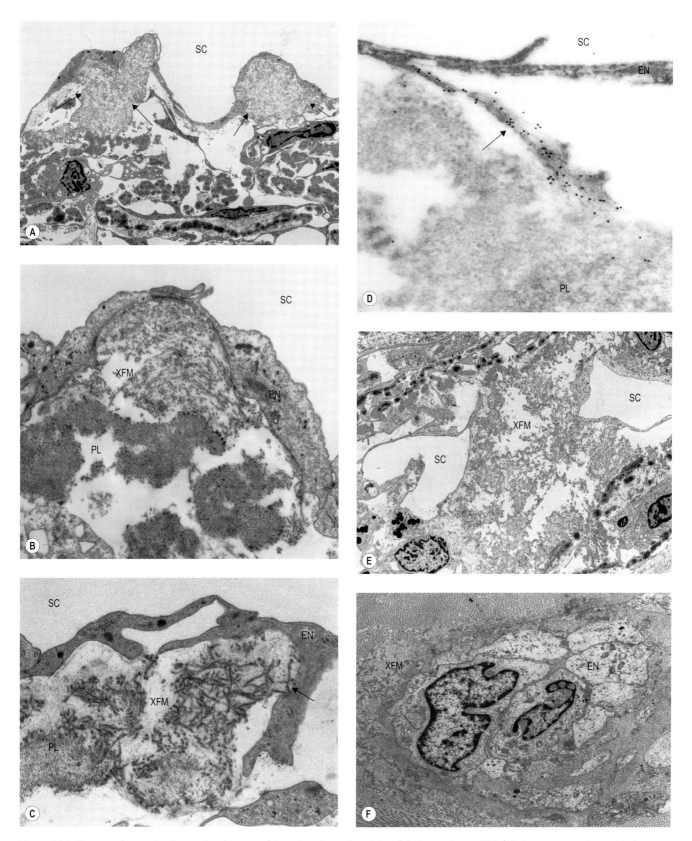

Figure 24.8 Electron micrographs showing involvement of the trabecular meshwork in exfoliation syndrome. (A) Exfoliative aggregates (arrows) in the subendothelial juxtacanalicular tissue along the inner wall of Schlemm's canal (SC). (B) Accumulation of exfoliative material (XFM) between inner-wall endothelium (EN) of Schlemm's canal (SC) and plaque material (PL). (C) Apparent production of exfoliative fibrils (XFM, arrow) by an endothelial cell (EN) lining Schlemm's canal (SC). (D) Normal fibrillin-1 immunopositive (immunogold labeling) elastic fiber bundle (arrow) connecting Schlemm's canal endothelium (EN) and juxtacanalicular plaques (PL). (E) Focal collapse and splitting of Schlemm's canal (SC) lumen by massive accumulation of XFM. (F) Collapse of aqueous vein showing accumulation of XFM in their periphery.

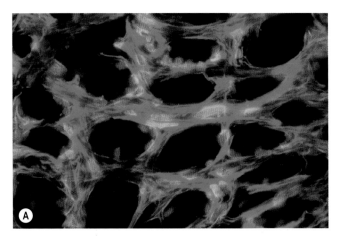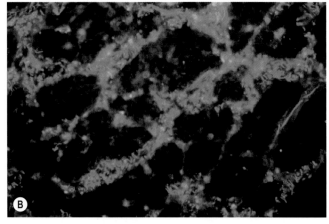

Figure 24.9 Elastosis of the lamina cribrosa in exfoliative glaucoma. (A) Elastic fibers (antielastin immunofluorescence labeling) in the connective-tissue beams of the lamina cribrosa of a normal eye. (B) Breakdown of elastic fibers in the lamina cribrosa beams of an eye with exfoliative glaucoma (magnification ×250).

Key references

A complete list of chapter references is available online at www.expertconsult.com. See inside cover for registration details.

2. Lindberg JG. Clinical investigations on depigmentation of the pupillary border and the translucency of the iris in cases of senile cataract and in normal eyes in elderly persons (1917) (reprinted). Acta Ophthalmol 1989;67(Suppl 190):1–96.

4. Ritch R. Exfoliation syndrome: the most common identifiable cause of open-angle glaucoma. J Glaucoma 1994;3: 176–178.

5. Prince AM, Streeten BW, Ritch R, et al. Preclinical diagnosis of pseudoexfoliation syndrome. Arch Ophthalmol 1987;105:1076–1082.

6. Mitchell P, Wang JJ, Smith W. Association of pseudoexfoliation with increased vascular risk. Am J Ophthalmol 1997;124:685–687.

23. Ritch R, Schlötzer-Schrehardt U. Exfoliation syndrome. Surv Ophthalmol 2001;45:265–315.

31. Thorliefsson G, Magnusson KP, Sulem P, et al. Common sequence variants in the LOXL1 gene confer susceptibility to exfoliation glaucoma. Science 2007;317: 1397–1400.

47. Netland PA, Ye H, Streeten BW, et al. Elastosis of the lamina cribrosa in pseudoexfoliation syndrome with glaucoma. Ophthalmology 1995;102: 878–886.

64. Naumann GOH, Schlötzer-Schrehardt U, Küchle M. Pseudoexfoliation syndrome for the comprehensive ophthalmologist: Intraocular and systemic manifestations. Ophthalmology 1998;105:951–968.

65. Streeten BW, Li ZY, Wallace RN, et al. Pseudoexfoliative fibrillopathy in visceral organs of a patient with pseudoexfoliation syndrome. Arch Ophthalmol 1992;110:1757–1762.

66. Schlötzer-Schrehardt U, Koca MR, Naumann GOH, et al. Pseudoexfoliation syndrome. Ocular manifestation of a systemic disorder? Arch Ophthalmol 1992;110:1752–1756.

67. Zenkel M, Poschl E, von der Mark K, et al. Differential gene expression in pseudoexfoliation syndrome. Invest Ophthalmol Vis Sci 2005;46:3742–3752.

78. Koliakos GG, Konstas AGP, Schlötzer-Schrehardt U, et al. 8-Isoprostaglandin F2a and ascorbic acid concentration in the aqueous humour of patients with exfoliation syndrome. Br J Ophthalmol 2003;87:353–356.

82. Gharagozloo NZ, Baker R, Brubaker RF. Aqueous dynamics in exfoliation syndrome. Am J Ophthalmol 1992;114: 473–478.

84. Gottanka J, Flügel-Koch C, Martus P, et al. Correlation of pseudoexfoliation material and optic nerve damage in pseudoexfoliation syndrome. Invest Ophthalmol Vis Sci 1997;38:2435–2446.

101. Vessani RM, Liebmann JM, Jofe M, et al. Plasma homocysteine is elevated in patients with exfoliation syndrome. Am J Ophthalmol 2003;136:41–46.

CHAPTER 25

Angle closure glaucoma

Shamira Perera, Nishani Amerasinghe, and Tin Aung

Overview

Primary angle closure glaucoma (PACG) is an important cause of glaucoma worldwide, especially in East Asia,[1-3] and the leading cause of bilateral glaucoma blindness in countries such as Singapore, India, and China.[2-4] Recent population-based surveys have shown that PACG is most commonly an asymptomatic disease, and the visual morbidity of the condition may be related to the finding that the asymptomatic form of the disease is visually destructive.[5]

Clinical background

Under the International Society for Geographical and Epidemiological Ophthalmology (ISGEO) classification system, there are three stages for angle closure glaucoma (ACG)[6] (Box 25.1):

1. Primary angle closure suspect (PACS) is the term for an eye in which contact between the peripheral iris and posterior trabecular meshwork is considered possible, but there are no other abnormalities in the eye.[5,7] There has been some debate recently regarding the diagnostic criteria for PACS. While 270° of iridotrabecular contact (where the posterior trabecular meshwork is not visible on gonioscopy) has been used as the minimum criterion for angle closure under the ISGEO system, this has been suggested to be too strict as eyes with lesser extent of closure may still have peripheral anterior synechiae (PAS).[8] An alternative definition is one in which 180° is the cutoff for defining angle closure. Such a definition was recently used in population-based surveys in India[9] and Singapore.[10]

2. Primary angle closure (PAC) is present when there are features in the eye indicating that trabecular meshwork obstruction by the peripheral iris has occurred. Such features include PAS, increased intraocular pressure (IOP), iris whorling, glaucomflecken (Figure 25.1), lens opacities, or excessive pigment deposition on the trabecular meshwork. Importantly, the optic disc does not have signs of glaucomatous damage during this stage.

3. PACG is PAC with evidence of glaucomatous optic neuropathy (GON) and visual field loss compatible with glaucoma.

Epidemiology

Age

The risk of angle closure increases with age.[11,12] This appears to be due to progressive shallowing of the anterior chamber as the lens grows in thickness and moves forwards.[13]

Ethnicity

The highest rates of ACG have been found in the Inuits.[14,15] High rates of angle closure have also been described in East Asian populations from Mongolia,[1] Singapore (Chinese),[11] Myanmar[16] and Hong Kong,[17] and the rate is lower amongst Indians,[4,18] Thais,[19] and Malays.[11] Several population-based studies have shown that the predominant form of ACG in Asia is asymptomatic and not acute angle closure. ACG prevalence is even lower amongst Europeans, with a prevalence of about 0.1% in people over 40 years.[20-22] The fact that angle closure is more common among Chinese, even after adjusting for axial length and anterior-chamber depth (ACD), suggests that mechanisms for angle closure may differ across racial/ethnic groups, and that factors such as thicker iris or ciliary body anatomy may have an important role in causing the disease.[23]

Clinical assessment

Gonioscopy

Gonioscopy is the main clinical method of assessing the angle. It visualizes the angle through a contact lens at the slit lamp. Various grading schemes categorize eyes on the basis of the width of the anterior-chamber angle. For example, the Spaeth classification assesses the insertion of the iris, the angular width of the angle recess, and the configuration of the peripheral iris. The Schaffer classification assesses the possibility of closure depending on which angle structures are visible (Figure 25.2).

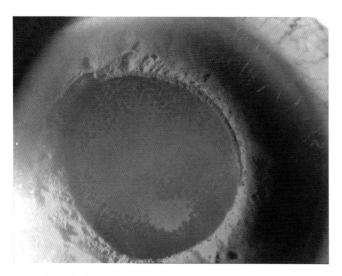

Figure 25.1 A slit-lamp photograph of an eye in acute angle closure. The pupil is mid dilated and there is glaucomflecken – ischemic anterior lens cortex fibers.

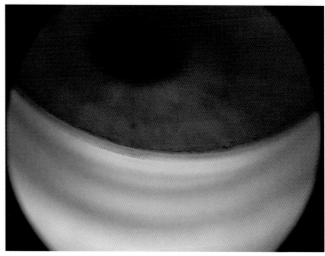

Figure 25.2 A EyeCam view of a wide-open inferior angle where the ciliary body band can be seen. This eye is extremely unlikely to proceed to primary angle closure.

Box 25.1 International Society for Geographical and Epidemiological Ophthalmology (ISGEO) classification of primary angle closure

Primary angle closure suspect (PACS)	• Contact between peripheral iris and posterior trabecular meshwork is considered possible • Eye otherwise normal
Primary angle closure (PAC)	• PACS with evidence of trabecular meshwork obstruction by peripheral iris by peripheral anterior synechiae, raised intraocular pressure, iris whorling, glaucomflecken, iris opacities, or excessive pigment deposition on the trabecular surface • No optic disc or visual field damage
Primary angle closure glaucoma (PACG)	• PAC with evidence of glaucomatous optic neuropathy

Peripheral anterior synechiae

PAS are present when the peripheral iris attaches anteriorly in the angle extending over the trabecular meshwork. PAS may be localized or extensive, pinpoint or broad. The ideal method to assess for PAS is dynamic indentation gonioscopy.

Anterior-segment optical coherence tomography (ASOCT) and ultrasound biomicroscopy (UBM)

AS-OCT and UBM are new and promising technologies for angle assessment. AS-OCT images the angle using infrared light in a noncontact fashion. Like the UBM, semi-automated image analyses can be performed. However,

unlike the UBM it cannot image the ciliary body. The UBM requires a water bath to be placed on the eye of the supine patient before scanning occurs. Research comparing UBM, AS-OCT, and gonioscopy shows that AS-OCT and UBM are good at identifying narrow angles, but AS-OCT overidentifies subjects as having closed angles compared to gonioscopy.[24,25]

Scanning peripheral anterior-chamber (SPAC) depth analyzer

The SPAC takes rapid slit measurements of the central and peripheral ACD which are compared to a normative database, and a risk assessment for angle closure is produced.[26] SPAC is sensitive, but overestimates the proportion of narrow angles relative to gonioscopy and the modified van Herick grading system for peripheral ACD assessment.[27]

Provocative testing

Provocation tests consist of placing subjects suspected as having angle closure into situations where there is a high chance of iridotrabecular contact. Examples include a dark room, prone positioning, and after pharmacologic pupil dilatation. However, provocative tests have not been shown to be consistently useful in correctly identifying those who are safe or at risk of angle closure.[28]

Acute primary angle closure

Acute primary angle closure (APAC) presents with ocular pain, nausea and vomiting, intermittent blurring of vision with haloes noted around lights, and IOP usually much greater than 21 mmHg. Typically, there is marked conjunctival injection, corneal epithelial edema, a mid dilated unreactive pupil, a shallow anterior chamber, and the presence of a closed angle on gonioscopy (Figure 25.3).

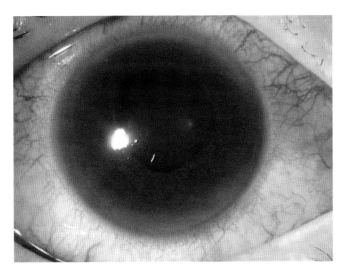

Figure 25.3 This slit-lamp photograph depicts an eye in acute primary angle closure. The cornea displays microcystic edema. The iris is mid dilated and there is conjunctival injection.

Box 25.2 Management of angle closure glaucoma

Laser

Laser peripheral iridotomy (PI)

Argon laser peripheral iridoplasty

Medical therapy

Surgery

Trabeculectomy

Lens extraction for angle closure

Combined lens extraction and trabeculectomy surgery

Treatment of angle closure glaucoma (Box 25.2)

Laser

Laser peripheral iridotomy (LPI)

The aim of an LPI is to eliminate pupil block. The iridotomy is usually placed between 11 and 1 o'clock so as to minimize visual disturbance. In thick brown irides, sequential use of argon laser to photocoagulate and pit the iris, and subsequent use of the Nd:YAG laser to create a patent hole has been described.[29] In blue irides where less power is required, Nd:YAG laser may be all that is necessary. Postlaser IOP spikes can be alleviated by brimonidine or apraclonadine perioperatively.[30]

If LPI fails or is unfeasible, surgical iridectomy may be pursued. No difference in terms of visual acuity or IOP has been observed between LPI and surgical iridectomy in a 3-year randomized controlled trial of unilateral APAC.[31]

Studies have shown that 58% of APAC subjects need further treatment of some type whilst 32% need surgery after an APAC attack treated with LPI. However, for patients with chronic PACG, 90% of patients need medications or surgery after LPI.[32]

Complications of LPI include increased IOP; laser burn to cornea, lens, or retina; development of posterior synechiae; and the development of a ghost image in the inferior field of vision. Other rare complications include progression of cataract opacity and corneal decompensation.[33]

Argon laser peripheral iridoplasty

This may be indicated if the angle remains appositionally closed with high IOP. Iridoplasty involves the placement of circumferential low-energy laser burns which pull the adjacent iris out of the angle.

For cases of APAC, iridoplasty lessens the reliance on systemic medications[34] which have side-effects, especially in elderly patients with systemic comorbidity. Medical therapy has a relatively slow onset, and 60% of APAC patients treated medically may still develop chronic PACG.[35] In a randomized controlled trial from Hong Kong, iridoplasty was found to be better in reducing the IOP in the initial 2 hours after presentation of APAC. It was also found to lead to a low percentage of cases with subsequent PAS.[35]

Medical therapy

Residual chronic PACG after iridectomy or iridotomy is common in Asian patients and is usually due to lens factors, plateau iris, or trabecular meshwork damage.[36]

Topical beta-blockers, prostaglandin analogs, carbonic anhydrase inhibitors, and alpha-2-agonists can be used in angle closure patients in the same way as for primary open-angle glaucoma (POAG) management.

Latanoprost has been shown to be more effective than timolol in lowering IOP in Asian PACG eyes,[37] even in eyes with 360° of PAS.[38] Pilocarpine constricts the pupil and pulls the iris away from the trabecular meshwork. However, long-term use can result in posterior synechiae and can make cataract surgery more difficult. Miotic agents have not been shown to prevent progression of angle closure, and should not be used in place of an iridotomy.

Follow-up evaluation of treated PACG/APAC

Patients should have regular IOP checks (to detect asymptomatic rises in IOP) and indentation gonioscopy. Those with residual open angle after laser iridotomy and raised IOP and/or GON are managed similarly to those with POAG.

Plateau iris

Plateau iris is considered when the iris root is rotated forwards and centrally in a particular configuration. The iris surface is relatively flat and the anterior chamber is usually deep. The angle is narrow. Dynamic gonioscopy reveals a double-hump sign where the peripheral iris drapes over the anteriorly rotated ciliary processes. These patients tend to be female and younger and may have a family history of ACG. There is usually some element of pupil block. Cataract extraction may not be so useful in eyes with plateau iris as iridociliary apposition still occurs,[39] whereas argon laser peripheral iridoplasty may be effective in opening up the angles.[40]

Surgery

Trabeculectomy

Trabeculectomy is indicated when there is a failure of medical or laser treatment, or poor compliance or intolerance to medical treatment leading to poorly controlled glaucoma and continuing optic disc and visual field damage.

Lens extraction for angle closure

Lens extraction deepens the anterior chamber, decreases angle crowding, and relieves pupil block.[41] Lai et al[42] showed that this leads to a decrease in IOP, and a reduced requirement for antiglaucoma medications in PACG. Cataract surgery is technically difficult in PACG eyes because of frequently coexisting shallow anterior-chamber, large bulky lens, iris atrophy secondary to ischemia, and zonular weakness. This surgical option may be particularly useful in the setting of mild optic disc damage in PACG with coexisting cataract, but there is little evidence for its effectiveness in more severe cases of PACG.

Combined lens extraction and trabeculectomy surgery

This has been shown to have similar complication rates in PACG and POAG eyes[43] and allows for an improvement in the visual acuity of PACG patients. Combined surgery may also prevent IOP spikes postoperatively and widens the angle.

Goniosynechialysis

This procedure involves stripping PAS from the angle wall, utilizing an instrument to peel PAS gently from the trabecular meshwork. However goniosynechialysis can cause IOP spikes, cataract, and hyphema. Goniosynechialysis can be combined with cataract surgery and has been found to be useful when PAS has been present for less than 1 year.[44]

Management of acute primary angle closure

The main aims of APAC treatment are to reduce the IOP, reduce inflammation, and reverse the angle closure. The patient is kept supine to allow gravity to aid in posterior movement of the lens and be reassessed regularly. Analgesics and antiemetics are used for symptomatic relief.

Medical therapy includes some of the following agents, based on the patient's overall medical status:

- Topical beta-adrenergic antagonists
- Topical alpha2-adrenergic agonists
- Topical or systemic carbonic anhydrase inhibitors
- Topical miotics
- Systemic hyperosmotic agents

Hyperosmotic agents such as mannitol 20% (or glycerol orally) can be used if the IOP remains high for too long. Hyperosmotic agents reduce vitreous volume by causing an osmotic diuresis. In one study, 44% of APAC patients required an osmotic agent to reduce IOP,[45] sometimes in multiple administrations. Topical steroids should be used to reduce the sometimes marked inflammatory response.

The fellow eye of APAC requires prophylactic treatment with an LPI, since half of these will otherwise suffer an acute attack within 5 years.[46]

Surgery for acute primary angle closure

Lens extraction for APAC

Lens removal serves to deepen the anterior chamber and open up the drainage angle. There is limited information whether primary cataract extraction as initial treatment is useful in APAC, but it is an option for refractory cases after attempting to break the pupillary block.[47] The optimum timing of lens extraction in such cases is not known; the risks and technical difficulties of surgery have to be weighed against the need to reduce IOP.[48]

Long-term prognosis after APAC

In one study, in the long term (4–10 years) following an APAC attack, 18% of eyes were blind, 48% of eyes developed serious GON, and 58% of eyes had vision worse than 20/40.[49]

Etiology (Box 25.3)

Ocular biometry

Eyes with angle closure tend to share certain biometric characteristics. These include shallow central ACD, thick lens, anterior lens position, small corneal diameter and radius of curvature, and short axial length.[13,50] Of these, a shallow ACD is regarded as the most important risk factor in most ethnic groups, and explains the high prevalence of PACG in Inuits, who have the shortest ACDs.[51] A shorter ACD is more commonly found in females and those with increasing age,[52] explaining their increased risk of angle closure in these groups. The lens is also more anteriorly placed in PACG eyes and is thicker than normal.[53] Some, but not all, studies have shown Chinese and Indian populations to have shorter axial lengths[21] and, furthermore, eyes with extremely short axial lengths are more affected by APAC than by chronic asymptomatic angle closure.[28,54,55] Other studies have shown that a more anterior lens position is responsible for a greater proportion of the differences between angle closure and normal eyes.[35]

Genetics

A more anterior position of the lens, increased lens thickness, and shallow ACD are seen out of proportion in close relatives of patients with ACG as compared to the general population.[56–59]

The inheritance of PACG is believed to be polygenic,[60–63] although both autosomal-dominant and recessive inheritance patterns have been seen in pedigrees. Sihota et al[64] found that the ACD is shallowest, lens is thickest, and axial length shortest in family members having PACG, and these

---

Box 25.3 Risk factors for angle closure

- Increasing age
- Female gender
- Ethnicity:
  - Inuit
  - East Asian
- Biometry and ocular anatomy:
  - Hyperopia
  - Shallow anterior-chamber depth
  - Shorter axial length
- Genetic factors

gradually move towards normal values in suspected and unaffected family members. Amongst Chinese twins, additive genetic effects appear to be the major factor in the variation of ACD and relative ACD (defined as ACD/axial length).[65]

No genetic associations have yet been conclusively proven for PACG. Two studies have reported that PACG subjects may carry a mutation in the myocilin gene (MYOC)[66,67]; however other analysis has not supported this in Chinese patients with chronic PACG.[68] Linkage with a locus at 10q for PACG has been reported,[69] as has an association between a single-nucleotide polymorphism in the matrix metalloproteinase 9 (MMP-9) gene and APAC.[70]

Pathophysiology

Primary angle closure

Ritch and Lowe described the four main mechanisms of angle closure resulting in iris blocking aqueous outflow through the trabecular meshwork. Treatment for each level of the block is necessary[71] and each level of the block may have a component of the preceding level (Box 25.4a).

Level I: iris and pupil

Pupil block is the most common mechanism of angle closure.[72] There is resistance to aqueous flow through the pupil in the area of iridolenticular contact. This causes a limitation of aqueous flow from the posterior chamber to the anterior chamber, and creates an increased pressure gradient between the anterior and posterior chambers with resultant anterior bowing of the iris (bombé), narrowing of the angle, and iridotrabecular contact. Laser iridotomy or surgical iridectomy relieves the pressure difference between the anterior and posterior chambers caused by pupil block. Consequently, the iris becomes flatter and the iridocorneal angle widens.

Level II: ciliary body

An abnormal ciliary body position leads to anteriorly positioned or rotated ciliary processes, pushing the peripheral iris into the angle. This condition is also known as plateau iris. Gonioscopy will show the iris root angulated forward and centrally, giving the appearance of a "double hump." Plateau iris syndrome occurs when angle closure with raised IOP develops in an eye with plateau iris configuration despite a patent iridotomy. As laser iridotomy only relieves pupil block, laser iridoplasty has been suggested as the treatment of choice for plateau iris.[73] Iridociliary cysts, tumors, or edema may mimic plateau iris configuration.[74]

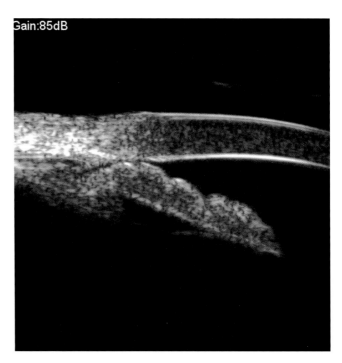

Gain:85dB

Figure 25.4 Ultrasound biomicroscopy image of plateau iris causing angle closure.

A study in Singapore using standardized UBM criteria found plateau iris (Figure 25.4) in about a third of PACS eyes after LPI,[75] confirming that non pupil block mechanisms are important in angle closure in Asians. However, this may not be pertinent to other populations.[76]

Level III: lens-induced glaucoma

A large intumescent lens or an anteriorly subluxed lens[51] may push the iris and ciliary body forward, triggering acute or chronic ACG (phacomorphic glaucoma) (Figure 25.5). Treatment involves removing the lens.

Level IV: malignant glaucoma/retrolenticular

In this condition, a pressure difference is created between the vitreous and aqueous compartments due to aqueous misdirection into the vitreous. Anterior rotation of the ciliary body with forward rotation of the lens–iris diaphragm causes anterior lens displacement and angle closure by pushing the iris against the trabecular meshwork. A shallow supraciliary detachment may be present and it is this effusion that is thought to cause the anterior rotation of the ciliary body.[51]

Medical treatment with cycloplegics, hyperosmotic and ocular hypotensive agents helps reverse the abnormal anatomy. Vitrectomy is indicated if Nd:YAG laser anterior hyaloidotomy or posterior capsulotomy (in pseudophakic patients) fails.

Choroidal effusion

Quigley et al[77] proposed several contributing risk factors for PACG/APAC: small eye size, choroidal expansion, and poor vitreous conductivity. Choroidal expansion causing anterior rotation of the ciliary body and iridolenticular forward movement is thought to be the mechanism by which scleri-

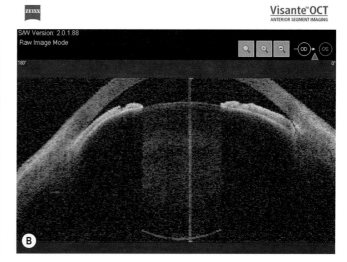

Figure 25.5 (A) UBM image of a subluxed lens, pupil block and a closed angle. (B) ASOCT image of the same eye showing a very large intumescent lens. The angles are closed asymmetrically.

tis, sulfa drugs, and panretinal photocoagulation cause secondary angle closure. Uveal effusion has been found in untreated PACG/APAC eyes prior to LPI by UBM,[78,79] but it is not known if this is a cause or effect of PACG/APAC.[80] Alternatively, the accumulation of suprachoroidal fluid could be secondary to rapid changes in IOP, exudation from uveal vessels, a congestion of the choroidal circulation due to high IOP, or the effect of topical pilocarpine and oral acetazolamide.

Causes of secondary angle closure (Box 25.4b)

Secondary angle closure glaucoma with an anterior pulling mechanism without pupil block

This occurs when the trabecular meshwork is obstructed by iris tissue or a membrane. Examples are neovascular glaucoma, where a fibrovascular membrane occludes the trabecular meshwork. Iridocorneal endothelial syndrome (ICE) occurs when a progressive endothelial membrane formation

> **Box 25.4b Causes of secondary angle closure**
>
> * With an anterior pulling mechanism without pupil block
> * With a posterior pushing mechanism without pupil block

occludes the trabecular meshwork. Epithelial ingrowth after intraocular surgery or the formation of inflammatory membranes may also cause this secondary angle closure. Rarer causes are aniridia and endothelial posterior polymorphous dystrophy.

Secondary angle closure with a posterior pushing mechanism without pupil block

Causes are iris and ciliary body cysts, silicone oil, or expansile gas injected in the vitreous cavity, uveal effusions due to inflammation, scleral buckling (by the resultant increased choroidal venous) pressure and retinopathy of prematurity.[51]

Key references

A complete list of chapter references is available online at www.expertconsult.com. See inside cover for registration details.

6. Foster PJ, Buhrmann R, Quigley HA, et al. The definition and classification of glaucoma in prevalence surveys. Br J Ophthalmol 2002;86:238–242.

8. Foster PJ, Aung T, Nolan WP, et al. Defining "occludable" angles in population surveys: drainage angle width, peripheral anterior synechiae, and glaucomatous optic neuropathy in east Asian people. Br J Ophthalmol 2004;88: 486–490.

25. Radhakrishnan S, Goldsmith J, Huang D, et al. Comparison of optical coherence tomography and ultrasound biomicroscopy for detection of narrow anterior chamber angles. Arch Ophthalmol 2005;123:1053–1059.

36. Ritch R, Lowe RF. Angle-closure glaucoma: therapeutic overview. In: Ritch R, Shields MB, Krupin T (eds) The Glaucomas, 2nd edn. St. Louis: Mosby, 1996:1521–1531.

40. Ritch R, Tham CC, Lam DS. Long-term success of argon laser peripheral iridoplasty in the management of plateau iris syndrome. Ophthalmology 2004;111: 104–108.

42. Lai JS, Tham CC, Chan JC. The clinical outcomes of cataract extraction by phacoemulsification in eyes with primary angle-closure glaucoma (PACG) and co-existing cataract: a prospective case series. J Glaucoma 2006;15:47–52.

43. Aung T. In: Weinreb RN, Friedman DS, editors. Angle Closure and Angle Closure Glaucoma. Consensus Series 3. The Hague, Netherlands: Kugler Publications, 2006:27–35.

45. Choong YF, Irfan S, Manage MJ. Acute angle closure glaucoma: an evaluation of a protocol for acute treatment. Eye 1999;13:613–616.

65. He M, Wang D, Zheng Y, et al. Heritability of anterior chamber depth as an intermediate phenotype of angle-

closure in Chinese: the Guangzhou Twin Eye Study. Invest Ophthalmol Vis Sci 2008;49:81–86.

71. Ritch R, Lowe RF. Classifications and mechanisms of the glaucomas. In: Ritch R, Shields MB, Krupin T (eds) The Glaucomas, 2nd edn. St. Louis: Mosby, 1996:752.

72. Nolan WP, Foster PJ, Devereux JG, et al. YAG laser iridotomy treatment for primary angle closure in East Asian eyes. Br J Ophthalmol 2000;84:1255–1259.

74. Foster P, He M, Liebmann J. In: Weinreb RN, Friedman DS (eds) Angle Closure and Angle Closure Glaucoma. Consensus Series 3. The Hague, Netherlands: Kugler Publications; 2006:20.

75. Kumar RS, Baskaran M, Chew PTK, et al. Prevalence of plateau iris in primary angle closure suspects an ultrasound biomicroscopy study. Ophthalmology 2008;115:430–434.

76. He M, Foster PJ, Johnson GJ, et al. Angle-closure glaucoma in East Asian and European people. Different diseases? Eye 2006;20:3–12.

79. Sakai H, Morine-Shinjyo S, Shinzato M, et al. Uveal effusion in primary angle-closure glaucoma. Ophthalmology 2005;112:413–419.

CHAPTER 26

Central nervous system changes in glaucoma

Yeni H Yücel and Neeru Gupta

Clinical background

Glaucoma is the leading cause of irreversible blindness and is estimated to affect approximately 67 million people worldwide.[1] The pathological correlate of disease is the loss of retinal ganglion cells (RGCs)[2,3] and their optic nerve axons. Glaucoma is a silent, slowly progressive disease that causes irreversible vision loss. Elevated intraocular pressure (IOP) is a major risk factor. Other risk factors include family history of glaucoma, black race, increasing age, myopia, and abnormal blood pressure.

Key components of the clinical assessment for glaucoma include measurement of IOP, and examination of the optic nerve head. The diagnosis is made based on visualizing characteristic patterns of damage to the optic nerve head. Features of glaucomatous optic neuropathy include evidence of retinal nerve fiber layer loss, excavation and cupping of the nerve head, focal or diffuse loss of the neuroretinal rim, and disc hemorrhage (Box 26.1). These findings correlate with visual field deficits in a retinotopic fashion when vision loss is present. A complete eye assessment that includes the anterior-chamber angle helps to determine whether these changes are secondary to specific etiologies such as angle closure glaucoma, or whether the entity is primary open-angle glaucoma in which no abnormality is detected other than optic nerve head pathology and possibly elevated IOP.

All treatments for glaucoma are based on lowering IOP by pharmacological agents in the form of eye drops or surgical methods. Glaucoma may also occur in patients without evidence of elevated IOP, so-called low-tension glaucoma, where the IOP lies within the range observed in the general population. Large randomized prospective clinical trials have demonstrated that reducing IOP helps protect vision loss compared to untreated patients, including those without obvious elevated IOP.[4-7] Many patients, however, continue to lose sight in spite of adequate IOP-lowering treatment.[4-7] In this context, factors other than IOP that are implicated in RGC injury and death in glaucoma are under active investigation. Understanding how and why glaucoma progresses will propel the development of novel adjunctive treatments to prevent blindness.

Retinal pathology in glaucoma

The pathologic basis for vision loss in glaucoma appears to be RGC injury and death.[2] The RGC injury in glaucoma is typically slow, partial, and progressive, accounting for specific patterns of vision loss that deepen and expand over time. Some evidence suggests that RGC death is apoptotic in nature,[2] and primary mechanisms leading to programmed cell death have been reviewed elsewhere.[3] Experimental work performed in glaucoma models with elevated IOP has been optimized over the years to study the sequence of pathological events triggered by IOP elevation.[8-11]

As RGCs die, histological examination of the optic nerve head reveals progressive optic nerve head excavation, with progressive tissue atrophy and gliosis. In the retina, there is reduced density of surviving RGCs and thinning of the inner nerve fiber layer. These changes are likely due to atrophy and/or loss of the RGC cell body.[12,13] Previous morphological studies demonstrated increased susceptibility of larger optic nerve fibers to IOP and this was interpreted as selective injury to magnocellular neurons.[14,15] However, it is now accepted that cell atrophy may have accounted for some of these observations, and recent studies show that at least 10 RGC types in nonhuman primates are larger than magnocellular RGCs.[16]

In addition to inner retinal pathology, photoreceptor pathology in glaucoma has been reported[17,18] but remains controversial.[19] Horizontal cell abnormality was reported previously in two glaucoma eyes with elevated IOP requiring enucleation.[20] A recent report demonstrated abnormal phosphorylation of tau protein involving the horizontal cells of human glaucoma surgical enucleation specimens (Box 26.2).[21]

Pathological events associated with RGC death include glial cell alteration at the optic nerve head,[22,23] disruption of axonal transport mechanisms leading to growth factor deprivation,[24] oxidative stress,[25] glutamate excitotoxicity,[26] immune alterations,[27] and vascular pathology[23,28] (Figure 26.1).

Etiology

The cause of open-angle glaucoma is not clearly established. The major risk factor, elevated IOP, can be considered as the

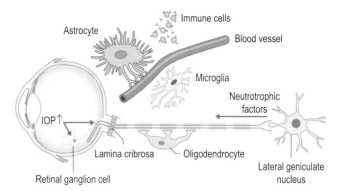

Figure 26.1 Multiple cell types and mechanisms implicated in neural degeneration in visual pathways in glaucoma. IOP, intraocular pressure.

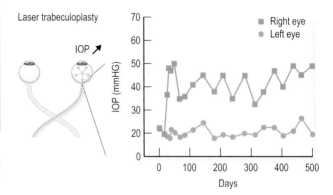

Figure 26.2 Laser-induced injury to the right eye induces elevated intraocular pressure (IOP). IOP is monitored in the experimental right and fellow nonglaucoma eyes over time.

cause of the glaucomatous injury in many cases. Support for this comes from nonhuman primate studies in which damage from elevated IOP closely mimics human glaucoma. In this model, IOP elevation is caused by laser-induced scarring of trabecular meshwork in the eye.[9,29] The IOP elevation is typically induced in one eye, and eye pressure is chronically monitored during experiment (Figure 26.2). The experimental primate model of glaucoma is highly relevant to human disease due to similar anatomy and physiology of central visual pathways,[30] characteristic glaucomatous optic nerve changes as observed in human glaucoma,[9,31,32] and visual deficits similar to those observed in glaucoma patients.[33] In addition to IOP, optic disc changes[34,35] and visual electrophysiological changes[36-38] can be monitored in vivo. After chronic exposure to elevated IOP there is blocked anterograde transport to the lateral geniculate nucleus (LGN)[39] and retrograde transport at the level of the lamina cribrosa,[40-43] RGC death,[2] and atrophy of surviving cell bodies and dendrites.[12,44,45]

Anatomy and pathophysiology

The unmyelinated RGC axon inside the eye becomes myelinated as it leaves the eye beyond the lamina cribrosa. The RGC axon is long and forms the intraorbital, intracanalicular, and intracranial components of the optic nerve, optic chiasm, and optic tract (Figure 26.3 and Box 26.3). In primates most RGC axons are retinogeniculate, and target the LGN directly,[46] while a remaining 10% target other subcortical structures including the superior colliculus, pretectal nuclei, accessory optic system, and suprachiasmatic nucleus.[47]

The LGN conveys visual information received from the retina to the primary visual cortex in humans and nonhu-

man primates. This structure is composed of neuronal cell bodies arranged into six anatomically segregated layers that carry signals from the three major magno-, parvo-, and koniocellular vision pathways. Each LGN layer receives input from one eye only: layers 2, 3, and 5 receive input from the ipsilateral eye, and layers 1, 4, and 6 from the contralateral eye. In the two most ventral layers, magnocellular neurons convey motion information, and in the four remaining dorsal LGN layers, parvocellular neurons convey red–green color information. Koniocellular neurons are found intercalated between principal layers and convey blue–yellow color information.[48] Eighty percent of neurons in the LGN are relay neurons that comprise the axons of the optic radiations to the primary visual cortex. Approximately 20% of LGN neurons stay within the LGN: these are GABAergic interneurons.[49] Of the total input to the LGN, less than 10% derive from RGCs, with the remaining 90% coming from GABAergic interneurons, cortical, and subcortical synaptic inputs.[50]

Transsynaptic degeneration of the lateral geniculate nucleus in glaucoma

Transsynaptic degeneration is a phenomenon in which injured neurons spread injury to previously uninjured neurons connected by a synapse. Within the central nervous system, injury typically spreads from a population of neurons to other anatomically and functionally connected neurons.[51–53] This pathological process accounts for the progressive cognitive decline in diseases such as Alzheimer's disease.[53] Transsynaptic degeneration likely plays a role in

Box 26.3 Anatomy and pathophysiology

- Most of the retinal ganglion cell axon lies outside the eye, forming intraorbital, intracanalicular, and intracranial components of the optic nerve, optic chiasm, and optic tract
- Most retinal ganglion cells terminate in the lateral geniculate nucleus
- In the lateral geniculate nucleus, there is anatomic segregation of functionally distinct visual channels, namely the magno-, parvo-, and koniocellular pathways

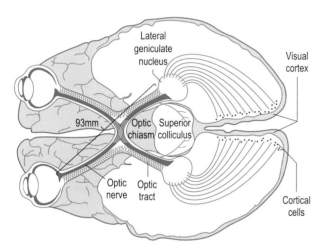

Figure 26.3 Retinal ganglion cell axons forming intraorbital, intracanalicular, and intracranial portions of the optic nerve, optic chiasm, and optic tract measure approximately 93 mm in total.

the progressive loss of vision in glaucoma. Evidence from independent laboratories confirms that RGC damage leads to injury to target neurons of the LGN. Experimental work in models with elevated IOP has helped us to understand the sequence of pathological events triggered by IOP elevation.[8–11,54] Attention to pathology within the length of the RGC axon and also its LGN target has shed new light on the progressive nature of central visual changes in glaucoma.

Evidence of transsynaptic degeneration in glaucoma comes mainly from the monkey model of glaucoma. Elevated IOP causes varying degrees of injury to myelinated optic nerve fibers behind the globe, most of which are destined for the LGN. Using established histomorphometric techniques (Figure 26.4), the degree of damage ranges from no loss of optic nerve fibers to total replacement of axons by glial scar in this model.[32]

Examination of the LGN following elevated IOP reveals metabolic changes detected by altered cytochrome oxidase enzyme activity in LGN layers connected to the experimental eye.[55,56] Size measurement of LGN neurons connected to the glaucoma eye in this model shows significant atrophy of neurons,[57] and relay neurons[58] in magno- and parvocellular layers. Furthermore, quantitative assessment by three-dimensional morphometric techniques revealed significant loss of neurons in both magno- and parvocellular layers (Figure 26.5).[57,59] A linear relationship between LGN neuron loss and mean IOP was observed.[60] Surviving neurons also showed increasing atrophy with mean IOP more pronounced in parvocellular layers.[58]

In the koniocellular pathway, a selective marker for these neurons, called alpha subunit of type II calmodulin-dependent protein kinase (CaMK-II alpha), showed reduced immunoreactivity in the LGN.[60] In ocular hypertensive monkeys without evidence of optic nerve fiber loss, decreased LGN immunoreactivity of this major postsynaptic density protein[60] suggests early neurochemical alterations in the blue–yellow pathway in response to elevated IOP. In this group of ocular hypertensive monkeys, marked alterations

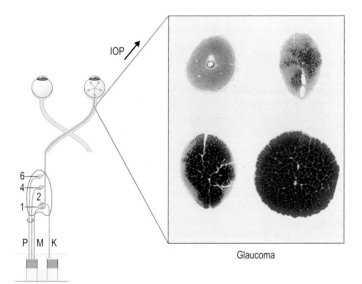
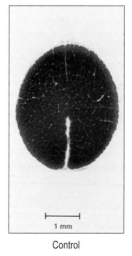

Figure 26.4 Following intraocular pressure elevation, glaucomatous optic nerves show overall atrophy and varying degree of optic nerve fiber loss compared to the normal optic nerve on the right (myelin stain in black). The bar indicates 1 mm. IOP, intraocular pressure. (Reproduced with permission from Yücel YH, Kalichman MK, Mizisin AP, et al. Histomorphometric analysis of optic nerve changes in experimental glaucoma. J Glaucoma 1999;8:38–45.)

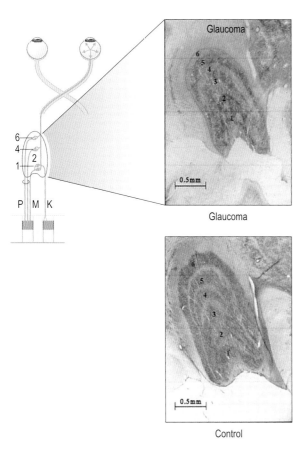

Figure 26.5 Cross-sections of the right lateral geniculate nucleus in control (lower panel) and glaucomatous monkeys (top panel) show the laminar arrangement of the neuronal cell bodies. Compared to the control, in glaucoma, overall atrophy is observed. Parvalbumin-positive relay neurons in layers 1, 4, and 6 are decreased in number. (Reproduced with permission from Yücel YH, Zhang Q, Gupta N, et al. Loss of neurons in magno and parvocellular layers of the lateral geniculate nucleus in glaucoma. Arch Ophthalmol 2000;118:378–384.)

> ### Box 26.4 Transsynaptic degeneration of the lateral geniculate nucleus in glaucoma
>
> - The spread of disease from injured neurons to connected neurons, known as transsynaptic degeneration, is a feature of neurodegenerative diseases and glaucoma
> - In glaucoma, degenerative neuron changes appear diffuse, affecting all major vision pathways
> - Early neurochemical changes have been observed in blue–yellow koniocellular neurons of the lateral geniculate nucleus (LGN) in glaucoma
> - Major changes in metabolic activity in addition to neurochemical changes have been observed in ocular dominance columns driven by the glaucomatous eye in the primate glaucoma model
> - Some mechanisms of injury common to neurodegenerative diseases also appear relevant to glaucomatous injury

Visual cortex changes in glaucoma

Relay neurons of the LGN project to the primary visual cortex. Here, neurons are arranged into six layers subdivided into sublayers. The M, P, and K geniculate axons terminate in sublayers of layer 4 and superficial layers in eye-specific columns called ocular dominance columns.[66] In monkeys with unilateral glaucoma, a relative decrease in metabolic activity has been detected with cytochrome oxidase activity in ocular dominance columns driven by the glaucomatous eye, compared to those driven by the fellow nonglaucoma eye[55,56,60,67] (Figure 26.6). Neurochemical changes in the visual cortex involving growth cone-associated protein-43 (GAP-43) and inhibitory neurotransmitter receptor γ-aminobutyric acid (GABA) A receptor subtype are additional evidence of neuroplasticity in the primate visual system.[68] Apart from these neurochemical changes, direct evidence of neuron loss in the primary visual cortex in primate glaucoma is lacking. However, relative differences in metabolic activity of ocular dominance columns between the glaucoma and nonglaucoma eye appeared more pronounced with increasing optic nerve fiber loss.[60]

---

were noted in the dendrites, with measurable reduced dendrite complexity and field area in the magno- and parvocellular layers of the LGN.[61] These findings suggest that not all LGN changes are attributable to deafferentation within the visual system. Transsynaptic degeneration of the LGN in primate glaucoma appears to affect the three major vision channels, namely the magno, parvo- and koniocellular pathways (Box 26.4).[60] While changes to relay neurons in experimental glaucoma are described above, it is not known whether GABAergic interneurons in the LGN are also altered in glaucoma, as has been observed following enucleation and monocular deprivation.[62]

Glial cells including astrocytes and NG-2 cells appeared altered in experimental glaucoma in the optic tract and LGN.[54,63] Other studies show the involvement of other cell types such as microglia[64] and vascular[65] cells in the LGN in glaucoma. Mechanisms related to transsynaptic degeneration in glaucoma may be relevant to strategies aimed at preventing the spread of disease to visual centers in the brain and presumably disease progression.

Central visual system changes in human glaucoma

Decreased LGN neuron density was reported in humans, with more pronounced effect in magnocellular layers,[69] a subject of considerable controversy.[70,71] Recent findings in human glaucoma support observations of central visual pathway neural degeneration in experimental primate glaucoma.[72] In an index human glaucoma case, postmortem analysis of the visual system revealed neuropathology in the prechiasmal intracranial optic nerve, LGN, and visual cortex and correlated with visual field defects in a retinotopic fashion.[72] Thus, in this case with superior bilateral visual field defects, marked inferior optic nerve atrophy and decreased phosphorylated neurofilament, neuron atrophy in the lateroposterior LGN and marked thinning of the inferior bank of the primary visual cortex was noted. In a study of human primary open-angle glaucoma patients with vision loss, atrophy of the LGN by magnetic resonance imaging has been reported.[73] Functional neuroimaging (fMRI) showed

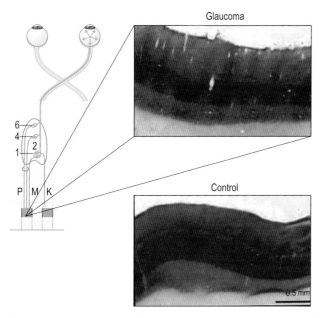

Glaucoma

Control

0.5 mm

Figure 26.6 Normal primate visual cortex section stained with a metabolic activity marker, cytochrome oxidase shows continuous and homogeneous dark staining. In contrast, glaucomatous visual cortex shows alternating light and dark bands corresponding to ocular dominance columns driven by the glaucoma and nonglaucomatous fellow eyes, respectively. (Reproduced with permission from Yücel YH, Zhang Q, Weinreb RN, et al. Effects of retinal ganglion cell loss on magno-, parvo-, koniocellular pathways in the lateral geniculate nucleus and visual cortex in glaucoma. Prog Retin Eye Res 2003;22:465–481.)

Box 26.5 Central visual system changes in human glaucoma

- In postmortem human glaucoma, degenerative changes have been noted in the lateral geniculate nucleus (LGN) and the visual cortex
- In patients with glaucoma, atrophy of the LGN by MRI has been detected
- In vivo studies of the visual cortex by functional MRI have detected functional changes in glaucoma

---

decreased blood oxygen level-dependent (BOLD) signal in human primary visual cortex in patients with primary open-angle glaucoma (Box 26.5).[74] Thus, pathology in central vision centers is present in at least some glaucoma patients.

Mechanisms of transsynaptic degeneration in glaucoma

Common mechanisms implicated in neurodegenerative diseases such as Alzheimer's disease may also play a role in transsynaptic degeneration in experimental primate glaucoma. There is evidence that oxidative injury[65] and glutamate excitotoxicity[75] are implicated in transsynaptic degeneration in experimental primate glaucoma.

In oxidative injury, reactive oxygen species accumulate, altering cellular and molecular pathways to induce cell death.[76] Oxygen species can react with nitric oxide to form

---

Box 26.6 Mechanisms of transsynaptic degeneration in glaucoma

- There is evidence that excessive glutamatergic stimulation is implicated in transsynaptic degeneration in glaucoma
- Reduced trophic factor support from the degenerating lateral geniculate nucleus in glaucoma may promote retinal ganglion cell susceptibility

---

peroxynitrite, and this mediates protein nitration to produce nitrotyrosine.[77] In neurodegenerative diseases, the finding of nitrotyrosine is considered a footprint of oxidative injury.[78] Nitrotyrosine found in LGN neural parenchyma and blood vessels in layers connected to the glaucomatous eye implicates oxidative injury in transsynaptic degeneration in primate glaucoma.[65] The additional finding that oxidative injury was also observed in LGN layers connected to the nonglaucomatous eye may relate to blood vessel changes that do not respect layer specific organization (Box 26.6).[65]

Glutamate is the major neurotransmitter of the central nervous system, and the glutamatergic system is responsible for excitatory neurotransmission in the brain. Excessive stimulation by glutamate may lead to neuron toxicity called "excitotoxicity," characterized by intracellular calcium overload and neuron death.[79] Glutamate excitotoxicity is implicated in a number of neurodegenerative diseases,[79] and also in glaucomatous neural degeneration in the retina and optic nerve.[26] Memantine, an open channel blocker of the N-methyl-D-aspartic acid (NMDA) subtype, is a pharmacological agent capable of blocking overstimulation of the glutamatergic system. Memantine may block NMDA receptors in the LGN,[80] retina,[81] and visual cortex[82] because it crosses the blood–brain barrier in monkey glaucoma. Surviving LGN relay neurons in monkeys with glaucoma given daily doses of memantine showed attenuated atrophy, compared to vehicle-treated glaucoma monkeys.[75] Statistically significant differences in absolute neuron numbers compared to vehicle-treated glaucoma animals were not observed, suggesting that blocking excitotoxicity by memantine (4 mg/kg) had no significant effect on neuronal death in LGN in experimental glaucoma.

The altered LGN and visual cortex damage in glaucoma may reduce trophic support to surviving RGCs, increasing their susceptibility to injury, with worsening of disease. The exact role of trophic factors in transsynaptic degeneration is not known; however, ocular delivery of BDNF has been shown to have a protective effect on RGCs.[83] BDNF may serve as an anterograde trophic factor for survival of target neurons, as seen during development.[84] Neurotrophic factors may have multiple neural targets, such as LGN,[85] intracortical circuitry, and subcortical afferents.[86]

Clinical implications

The clinical finding of optic nerve head damage indicates injury at a point closest to the RGC cell body in the eye; however, depending on the severity of the disease, it may extend anywhere from the retina to the visual cortex in the brain.

Box 26.7 Clinical implications

- Glaucoma is a neurodegenerative disease affecting visual neurons in the eye and brain
- Early intervention to lower intraocular pressure in glaucoma and prevent the spread of damage to target neurons is an important therapeutic strategy
- Progressive damage in glaucoma despite adequate intraocular pressure control may be explained by ongoing central neural degeneration
- There is a strong need for neuroprotective agents to target neural degeneration in glaucoma
- Functional deficits in glaucoma may be unveiled by a multidisciplinary approach to retinogeniculocortical pathway involvement
- In human primary open glaucoma there is evidence of structural atrophy of the lateral geniculate nucleus and functional change in the visual cortex

Box 26.8 Conclusions

- Visual field loss in moderate to advanced glaucoma is a reflection of damage throughout the visual pathway
- A better understanding of brain changes in glaucoma may contribute to novel strategies to diagnose, manage, and follow disease
- Intraocular pressure (IOP)-lowering strategies combined with therapies to protect retina and central visual system neurons offer new opportunities to prevent blindness from glaucoma
- In glaucoma, features of progressive loss of visual neurons, transsynaptic degeneration in the visual system, and abnormal protein accumulation make it the most common neurodegenerative disease

In patients with inadequate IOP control and progressive loss of RGCs, degeneration in the visual system might be expected. Thus, treatment to lower IOP prior to significant RGC loss would help to prevent the spread of injury from RGCs to their target neurons in the brain. Furthermore, in patients with well-controlled IOP and progressive glaucomatous damage, transsynaptic central degeneration triggered by RGC injury helps to explain the progressive nature of the disease. Future more comprehensive treatment strategies to treat glaucoma may need to protect neurons in the retina and central visual system (Box 26.7).[87] Clinical trials in glaucoma with memantine, an NMDA open channel blocker, have recently failed to show significant effect as detected by primary outcomes. At this time, there is no neuroprotective agent that has proven to help preserve vision in glaucoma patients.

The retinogeniculocortical involvement in glaucoma might be exploited to uncover specific functional neural deficits in patients, including cortical binocular functions such as stereovision[88–90] or other pathway-specific functions. Nongeniculocortical pathways involved in eye movements and reflexes and circadian rhythms may also be worth exploring in glaucoma. Multifocal and evoked electrophysiological measurements may be relevant to the detection of dysfunction along visual pathways.[91]

The loss of visual field in moderate to advanced disease is likely a representation of damage to central visual pathways in glaucoma. Increased susceptibility of RGCs to ongoing glaucomatous injury has been described as a determinant in progression of the disease.[92] We suggest that degeneration with neuronal loss and atrophy of target neurons in the LGN may alter the normal function of surviving RGCs in glaucoma. In fact, degenerative changes in RGCs are observed following the loss of target cells in the LGN[93–95] and lesions of the striate cortex.[96,97] Changes in the visual

stations may deplete growth factor sources to be transported back to the retina, contributing to the susceptibility of surviving RGCs to ongoing glaucomatous injury and progression, and studies are needed to test this hypothesis.

Conclusion

While RGC death is central to the pathology in glaucoma, depending on the severity of disease, injury may extend anywhere from the retina to the visual cortex in the brain. It is likely that by the time visual field deficits are detected, central nervous system pathology is present. Lowering IOP is an important strategy to prevent RGC death in the eye, and may reduce the risk of central nervous system degeneration in glaucoma. In patients with progressive vision loss despite adequate IOP control, secondary pathological changes in the brain are likely. Thus, IOP-lowering strategies combined with therapies to protect retina and central visual system neurons offer new opportunities to prevent blindness from glaucoma (Box 26.8).

Numerous similarities exist between glaucoma and neurodegenerative diseases[98]: the selective loss of neuron populations; transsynaptic degeneration in which elevated IOP and injury to RGCs can trigger injury in distant connected neurons; common mechanisms of cell injury and death, including abnormal protein accumulation. There is a need to understand factors other than IOP involved in disease progression in patients. Approaching glaucoma as a neurodegenerative disease that considers eye and central visual pathway damage may help to identify future strategies to prevent progressive blindness from glaucoma.

Acknowledgment

This work was supported in part by the Glaucoma Research Society of Canada, Canadian Institutes of Health Research, and The Nicky and Thor Eaton Fund and Dorothy Pitts Fund.

Key references

A complete list of chapter references is available online at www.expertconsult.com. See inside cover for registration details.

21. Gupta N, Fong J, Ang LC, et al. Retinal tau pathology in human glaucomas. Can J Ophthalmol 2008;43:53–60.

55. Vickers JC, Hof PR, Schumer RA, et al. Magnocellular and parvocellular visual pathways are both affected in a macaque monkey model of glaucoma. Aust NZ J Ophthalmol 1997;25:239–243.

56. Crawford ML, Harwerth RS, Smith EL 3rd, et al. Glaucoma in primates: cytochrome oxidase reactivity in parvo- and magnocellular pathways. Invest Ophthalmol Vis Sci 2000;41:1791–1802.

57. Weber AJ, Chen H, Hubbard WC, et al. Experimental glaucoma and cell size, density, and number in the primate lateral geniculate nucleus. Invest Ophthalmol Vis Sci 2000;41:1370–1379.

58. Yücel YH, Zhang Q, Weinreb RN, et al. Atrophy of relay neurons in magno- and parvocellular layers in the lateral geniculate nucleus in experimental glaucoma. Invest Ophthalmol Vis Sci 2001;42:3216–3222.

59. Yücel YH, Zhang Q, Gupta N, et al. Loss of neurons in magnocellular and parvocellular layers of the lateral geniculate nucleus in glaucoma. Arch Ophthalmol 2000;118:378–384.

60. Yücel YH, Zhang Q, Weinreb RN, et al. Effects of retinal ganglion cell loss on magno-, parvo-, koniocellular pathways in the lateral geniculate nucleus and visual cortex in glaucoma. Prog Retin Eye Res 2003;22:465–481.

61. Gupta N, Ly T, Zhang Q, et al. Chronic ocular hypertension induces dendrite pathology in the lateral geniculate nucleus of the brain. Exp Eye Res 2007;84:176–184.

65. Luthra A, Gupta N, Kaufman PL, et al. Oxidative injury by peroxynitrite in neural and vascular tissue of the lateral geniculate nucleus in experimental glaucoma. Exp Eye Res 2005;80:43–49.

67. Crawford ML, Harwerth RS, Smith EL 3rd, et al. Experimental glaucoma in primates: changes in cytochrome oxidase blobs in V1 cortex. Invest Ophthalmol Vis Sci 2001;42:358–364.

68. Lam DY, Kaufman PL, Gabelt BT, et al. Neurochemical correlates of cortical plasticity after unilateral elevated intraocular pressure in a primate model of glaucoma. Invest Ophthalmol Vis Sci 2003;44:2573–2581.

72. Gupta N, Ang LC, Noel de Tilly L, et al. Human glaucoma and neural degeneration in intracranial optic nerve, lateral geniculate nucleus, and visual cortex. Br J Ophthalmol 2006;90:674–678.

73. Gupta N, Greenberg G, de Tilly LN, et al. Atrophy of the lateral geniculate nucleus in human glaucoma detected by magnetic resonance imaging. Br J Ophthalmol 2009;93:56–60.

74. Duncan RO, Sample PA, Weinreb RN, et al. Retinotopic organization of primary visual cortex in glaucoma: Comparing fMRI measurements of cortical function with visual field loss. Prog Retin Eye Res 2007;26:38–56.

98. Gupta N, Yücel YH. Glaucoma as a neurodegenerative disease. Curr Opin Ophthalmol 2007;18:110–114.

CHAPTER 27

Retinal ganglion cell death in glaucoma

Heather R Pelzel and Robert W Nickells

Clinical background

Glaucoma is a collection of optic neuropathies that exhibit similar clinical phenotypes of thinning of the nerve fiber layer and excavation or cupping of the optic nerve head. Collectively, the glaucomas are a relatively common, but serious, blinding disease that is anticipated to affect nearly 80 million individuals worldwide by the year 2020.[1] The most prevalent form of this disease is known as primary open-angle glaucoma (POAG). It is often associated with elevated intraocular pressure (IOP) and has no distinguishing pathology in the angle of the eye, which is defined as the junction between the iris and cornea, and is the location of the aqueous outflow channels that are critical to IOP homeostasis. In addition to POAG, there are several other varieties of this disease. These include normal-tension glaucoma (NTG), which is associated with IOPs at or below the population average, angle closure glaucoma (ACG), and secondary glaucomas resulting from pigment dispersion or pseudoexfoliation, which are associated with the accumulation of debris in the angle leading to obstruction of the outflow pathways and the elevation of IOP. Clearly, there are a variety of factors at play that affect an individual's susceptibility to the effects of IOP. Not surprisingly, family history of glaucoma is a major risk factor and glaucoma is often considered a complex genetic chronic neurodegenerative disease of the central nervous system (CNS).[2]

Pathology

The common feature of all forms of glaucoma is the progressive degeneration of the optic nerve and retinal ganglion cells (RGC) in the retina. This loss of RGCs occurs through an apoptotic-like pathway.[3,4] In this chapter, we will discuss the current knowledge of ganglion cell death in the context of elevated IOP and damage to the optic nerve. The relationship between IOP and initiation of the disease is not well understood. Although increased IOP is the most important risk factor, the majority of individuals with ocular hypertension will never develop the disease. Alternatively, lowering IOP, which is the only current treatment for glaucoma, is an effective therapy for most forms of the disease, even for people with NTG. Recent findings may suggest new ways to help early diagnosis of the disease and provide therapeutic options in addition to lowering IOP.

Etiology

RGCs are CNS neurons that transmit visual signals processed in the retina to the visual centers of the brain. Although the mechanism of insult that initiates apoptosis in the RGCs of a glaucomatous eye is not well understood, there are two predominant theories – mechanical damage of RGC axons in the region of the optic nerve head and vascular disturbances in the optic nerve head leading to ischemia in the retina that directly affects RGCs. In humans, it is thought that mechanical damage occurs at the lamina cribrosa where the axons pass through the laminar plates. Pressure on this series of collagenous plates may cause conformational changes in the pores through which bundles of axons pass, thus leading to compression of the axons. The compression could compromise the transport of small molecules, such as neurotrophins, through the axonal process. The loss of neurotrophic support to neuronal soma likely plays a role in the response of the cell body to axonal damage. A similar pattern of damage is seen in mouse models of glaucoma, but the mouse laminar region does not contain collagenous plates. Instead, bundles of murine axons in the optic nerve are surrounded by sheaths of glial cells.[5] Focal damage to these discrete bundles leads to wedge-shaped sectors of RGC loss in the retina (Figure 27.1).

Both mechanical damage and ischemia could lead to activation of the supporting glial cells in the optic nerve. It is well established that glia in the CNS become activated in response to damaging stimuli, and several studies have shown that this is also the case in glaucoma.[6–8] For example, Hernandez et al have shown that at least 150 genes are upregulated in astrocytes from a glaucomatous optic nerve head.[6] More recently, Johnson et al have shown that glial changes in the early glaucomatous optic nerve head include the upregulation of genes involved in cell proliferation, suggesting that this behavior of glia is one of the earliest events associated with optic nerve head pathology.[9] Although it is possible that glial cells are exerting a protective effect on adjacent axons, several studies have suggested that they are triggering the damage to these axons. There are several theories as to how this is accomplished, ranging from direct transmission of neurotoxic compounds, such as nitric oxide,[8,10] to a passive role, such as reducing energy available to the axons due to decreased glycogen breakdown or stimulating vasoconstriction of capillaries surrounding axons in the lamina. The stimulation of vasoconstriction by the glia could be a link between mechanical damage and ischemic damage during glaucoma.

Pathophysiology

Compartmentalized self-destruct pathways and degeneration

Whitmore and colleagues have proposed the idea of addressing glaucoma as a neurodegenerative disease in which destruction of the neuron occurs compartmentally. Specifically, compartmental degeneration of the axon, synapse, and dendrites can occur independently of somal loss (Box 27.1).[11] Autonomous axonal degeneration has already been shown to occur in a mouse model of progressive motorneu-

ronopathy.[12] In a murine model of inherited glaucoma, Libby et al have shown that axonal loss occurs independently of somal loss, not just spatially but also via a distinct molecular pathway.[13] In this latter model, which will be discussed in more detail below, the loss of the proapoptotic protein BAX prevents somal loss following increased IOP, but does not prevent axonal degeneration. In addition, experiments using a primate model of experimental glaucoma have shown that damage to the dendritic arbor sometimes precedes damage to ganglion cell bodies.[14] Currently, no studies have shown definitively that synaptic degeneration plays a role in glaucoma pathophysiology, but this cannot be ruled out as a possibility.

Wallerian degeneration versus die-back

Damaged axons usually degenerate in one of two basic patterns: wallerian degeneration or "die-back." Each pattern of degeneration appears to be dependent on the severity of damage to the axons.[15] Wallerian degeneration generally occurs in severely damaged axons and is characterized by a rapid loss of axonal structure throughout the length of the axon. Die-back occurs in axons with more moderate injury and is characterized by a slower retrograde degeneration that proceeds from the synapse to the soma. Although it is not known how axons in a glaucomatous human eye degenerate, clues to this process have come from recent studies in DBA/2J mice. These mice develop an iris atrophy, which leads to an accumulation of pigment in the trabecular meshwork causing an increase in IOP and an optic neuropathy that is similar to human pigmentary glaucoma. It appears that damage to the axon is relatively mild in this chronic model of ganglion cell loss, as the observed axonal degeneration exhibits a pattern similar to die-back[16] (Figure 27.1). In contrast, a more severe insult to the optic nerve, such as axotomy, causes the axons to degenerate in a wallerian pattern.[15] If ganglion cells in a glaucomatous retina undergo this same type of slow axonal degeneration as in the DBA/2J mice, it may provide an explanation for the presence of visual field defects in individuals with no detectable loss of ganglion cells.[17] That is, the axon has already begun to degenerate, so there is no connection to the visual centers of the brain, even though there appear to be unaffected ganglion cell bodies in the retina.

Box 27.1 Degeneration pathology

- Retinal ganglion cell (RGC) degeneration occurs compartmentally, with the different regions of the nerve responding to the initiating insult in a semi-independent manner
- As demonstrated in *Bax* knockout mice, axonal degeneration and somal degeneration are autonomous processes. The destruction of one compartment of the neuron does not guarantee degradation of another
- Damage to the axon precedes damage to the cell soma in models of experimental glaucoma
- The pattern of damage in DBA/2J mice, which shows wedge-shaped regions of ganglion cell loss, suggests that the initial site of damage is at the optic nerve head where axons for these cells are bundled. This is consistent with early speculation that the lamina cribrosa is the initial site of damage in glaucoma
- Selective loss of small- versus large-body RGCs is controversial

---

Figure 27.1 Patterns of ganglion cell somal and axonal loss in DBA/2J mice. (A–D) Correlation between patterned cell and axon loss in the DBA/2J mouse model of glaucoma. The retinas were stained for ganglion cell-specific βGEO enzyme activity and the optic nerves were silver-stained after being cross-sectioned immediately posterior to the laminar region. (A, B) Uniform staining throughout the retina is matched by even staining of the axonal bundles in an unaffected eye. (C, D) Two wedge-shaped regions of soma loss (* in C) correlate with two regions of axonal loss in the optic nerve head (* in D).

(E) Dieback degeneration of optic nerves in a mouse model of glaucoma. Optic nerves were labeled postmortem with crystals of 1,1'-dioctadecyl-3,3,3',3'-tetramethylindocarbocyanine perchlorate (DiI) placed at the optic nerve head. These are whole-mount preparations of the left optic nerve from five individual mice. The orientation of each nerve is arranged so that the chiasm is at the top of the panel and the globe is at the bottom. In this analysis, optic nerve (ON) integrity is scored from 1 (most normal) to 5 (complete degeneration). Progressive retrograde degeneration is evident as a loss of DiI labeling as the nerve deteriorates.

(F) Longitudinal, silver-stained section of an optic nerve of a young DBA/2J mouse. Note, the retina has been removed from this preparation. Region A begins at the ON head. Regions B and C contain the laminar region of the ON and clearly show discrete bundling of the axons. Region D represents the postlaminar, myelinated section of the ON. Axons are no longer organized in bundles at this point. Sections shown in (B) and (D) of this figure were cut through region C of the ON. Wedge-shaped loss of somas in the retina is indicative that discrete bundles of axons are being damaged in the glaucomatous DBA/2J mouse. Since discrete axon bundles only occur in the laminar region of this ON, it suggests that this is the initial site of damage in glaucoma in this animal model.

In (B) and (D), the central retinal artery (A) and vein (V) are indicated. In E, bar = 0.5 mm (A–E: modified from Schlamp CL, Li Y, Dietz JA, et al. 2006. Progressive ganglion cell loss and optic nerve degeneration in DBA/2J mice is variable and asymmetric. BMC Neurosci 2006;7:66.)

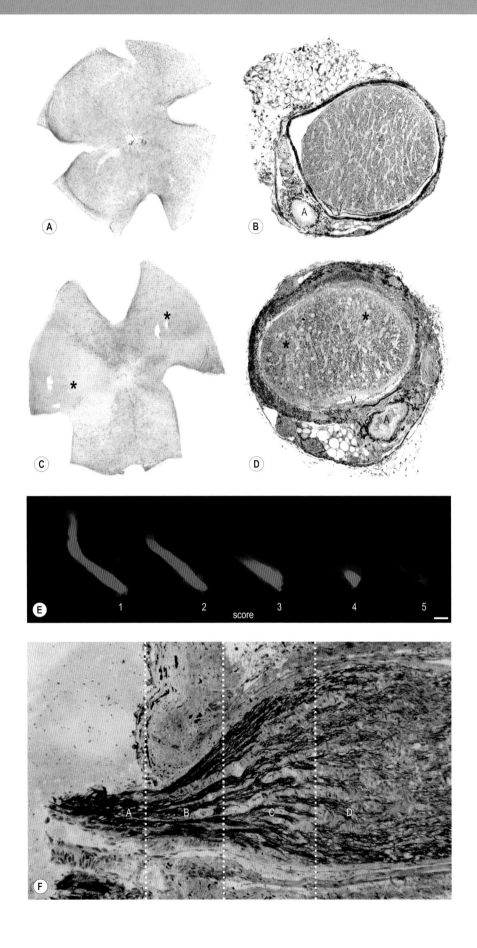

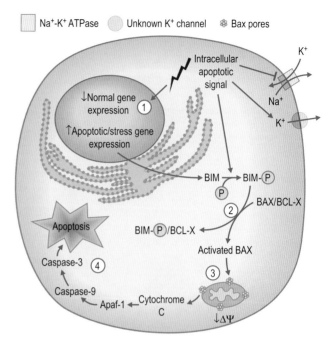

> **Box 27.2 Rules of apoptosis**
>
> - Changes in gene expression are an important early event in apoptosis. These changes, which are marked by the downregulation of normal ganglion cell gene expression, take place before the committed stage of apoptosis
> - Loss of retinal ganglion cells in mouse models of glaucoma occurs via the intrinsic apoptotic pathway, which must proceed through a stage of mitochondrial dysfunction
> - BH3-only proteins mediate the activation of the proapoptotic protein BAX. BAX plays a critical role in mitochondrial dysfunction during apoptosis
> - Activation of the caspase cascade enables the cell to autodigest itself and complete the apoptotic process

Figure 27.2 The intrinsic pathway of apoptosis. The apoptotic pathway begins with an unknown intracellular apoptotic signal that triggers several events in the cell. The first is the inhibition of the Na$^+$-K$^+$ ATPase and the activation of an unknown K$^+$ channel. The combination of these two events leads to a decrease in intracellular potassium levels due to the efflux of K$^+$. The other main event that is triggered is a change in normal gene expression. This is the first of four stages in the apoptotic pathway. The second stage involves the activation of downstream effectors. The diagram represents the indirect model of activation of BAX. BAX activation leads to the third stage of mitochondrial dysfunction, which includes a decrease in mitochondrial membrane potential and an increase in mitochondrial membrane permeability. Several molecules, including cytochrome c, are released due to the increase in permeability. Cytosolic cytochrome c allows the formation of the apoptosome with Apaf-1, procaspase-9, and adenosine triphosphate (ATP), which is the beginning of stage 4. Stage 4 continues with the activation of the caspase cascade, leading to activation of other digestive enzymes. All of these activated enzymes act to autodigest the cell and prepare it for phagocytosis.

Selectivity of ganglion cell loss

Some controversy exists over whether or not some ganglion cells are more susceptible to apoptosis in glaucomatous conditions (Box 27.2). Early studies indicated that large ganglion cell and nerve fibers were selectively lost in experimental glaucoma of nonhuman primates and human glaucoma.[18–21] In support of these observations, another study showed a selective loss of anterograde axonal transport to the magnocellular layer of the dorsal lateral geniculate nucleus, which is the target area for the largest RGCs.[22] A caveat of these early studies is that the conclusions were based only on size comparisons between average cell diameters in unaffected and glaucomatous eyes. A potential confounder of this phenomenon is that damaged RGCs atrophy prior to succumbing to apoptosis. Two different studies compared midget and parasol cell soma size and dendritic features to determine if the larger parasol cells were selectively destroyed.[14,23] These studies found that both RGC populations underwent shrinkage and loss in approximately the same proportions. In addition to this, a study by Jakobs et al[24] used several labeling methods to identify different subtypes of RGCs in the DBA/2J mouse retina and found that the loss of RGCs was not limited to any particular subtype. A more complete discussion of the process of cell shrinkage is made in a following section.

Intrinsic versus extrinsic apoptosis

Apoptosis occurs via one of two major pathways. The first pathway occurs when the cell senses intracellular stress, hence the name intrinsic apoptosis. The intrinsic pathway relies on control by the members of the *Bcl2* gene family and involves deregulation of mitochondrial function leading to activation of a cascade of proteases called caspases, initially triggered by caspase-9. In contrast, the extrinsic pathway is initiated by cell surface signaling following the binding of an extracellular ligand to a "death receptor." This signal leads directly to the caspase cascade via activation of caspase-8, without involvement from the mitochondria. Although the two pathways can operate independently, there is some crossover. For example, caspase-8 can process the *Bcl2* family member, Bid, into its active form, tBid, causing amplification of the cell death process by activation of the intrinsic pathway. Like the majority of neurons, it is believed that RGCs die using the intrinsic pathway of apoptosis (Figure

27.2). The main evidence for this comes from *Bax* knockout mice. The prevalent theory of *Bax* function in an apoptotic cell is the creation of a pore in the mitochondrial outer membrane by oligomerized BAX proteins. This pore allows the release of small molecules, such as cytochrome c, that are critical for downstream events in the apoptotic pathway. The absence of *Bax* function prevents the loss of RGCs in both acute and chronic models of optic nerve damage.[13,25]

The intrinsic pathway follows a basic temporal order of four stages.[26] The first stage involves changes in gene expression, including both the downregulation of normal gene expression and the upregulation of stress response and proapoptotic genes. The second stage is characterized by the activation of downstream effector molecules. These activated molecules lead to the mitochondrial involvement that is indicative of stage 3. The fourth and final stage involves activation of caspases and endonucleases and is triggered by the release of molecules from the mitochondria. Each of these stages of the intrinsic pathway will be discussed in more detail below.

Stage 1: changes in gene expression

As stated above, the first stage in the intrinsic pathway is characterized by changes in gene expression. In all cases of RGC death due to induced or spontaneous glaucomatous conditions, a common response has been a decrease in normal gene expression and an increase in stress and pro-apoptotic genes. Some of the normal genes whose expression is known to decrease include *Thy1, NF-L, BclX$_L$, Fem1c, Brn3b*, and *TrkB receptor*.[27–32] Napankangas et al[33] have shown that expression of the proapoptotic factors, *Bim* and possibly *Bax*, increase after injury. An increase in the expression of a variety of stress response genes has also been shown, including *Hsp72*,[34] alpha and beta crystallins,[35] and several iron-regulating genes.[36,37] The clinical importance of the downregulation of normal gene expression during this stage in the apoptotic pathway is not clear. As more therapies become available for blocking cell loss, however, a greater understanding of how to reactivate silenced genes is likely to become more relevant. Glimpses of this have been observed in the effects of glaucoma in *Bax* knockout mice; the RGCs in these mice undergo some changes in gene expression even though there is no somal loss.[27] The fact that rescued ganglion cells in *Bax* knockout mice are affected by early apoptotic events suggests that researchers need to address the difference between mere survival of ganglion cells and the retention of normal function.

Stage 2: downstream effectors

The second stage of the intrinsic pathway involves the activation of downstream effectors, several of which are members of the *Bcl2* family. The *Bcl2* family is divided into three sub-families. The pro-survival family, including BCL-2 and BCL-X, and the proapoptotic family, including BAX and BAK, share three conserved BCL homology (BH) domains, termed BH1, BH2, and BH3. The third family, the BH3-only proteins, are also proapoptotic, but are structurally unlike the other two families, except for the conserved BH3 domain.[38] The BH3 domain plays the important role of allowing *Bcl2* family members to interact with each other via the presence of an amphipathic alpha helix that can bind to a hydrophobic groove formed by the BH1, BH2, and BH3 domains.[38] There are two proposed models for how down-stream activation occurs.[37] In the direct model, BH3-only proteins, termed "sensitizers," bind BCL-X and displace "activator" molecules. These "activator" molecules, which are also BH3-only proteins, then bind directly to the proapoptotic proteins BAX and BAK. In the indirect model, the BH3-only proteins function only to bind the antiapoptotic proteins and prevent them from contacting and desensitizing the proapoptotic proteins. Most of the current experimental literature points to the indirect model of BAX/BAK activation.[39]

Stage 3: mitochondrial involvement

Mitochondrial dysfunction is a distinct feature of RGC death in glaucoma. The evidence for this is a loss of the electrochemical gradient across the mitochondrial inner membrane, the generation of reactive oxygen species, and the release of cytochrome c. Many of the changes in mitochondria, particularly the release of cytochrome c, are mediated by the proapoptotic protein, BAX. Although it had been shown that BAX played an important role in the apoptotic loss of RGCs,[13,25] it had not been definitively demonstrated that mitochondria were involved until a study done by Mittag et al in a rat model of glaucoma.[40] In this work, the mitochondrial membrane potential was determined in rats with chronically elevated IOP and compared between cells in the late stages of apoptosis and cells from unaffected fellow eyes. This study showed that the mitochondrial membrane potential was decreased by approximately 17.5% in cells in the RGC layer of the experimental eye. In a follow-up study, Tatton et al suggest that this decrease in mitochondrial membrane potential implied an increase in mitochondrial permeability, possibly due to the affects of BAX on the permeability transition pore complex.[41] However, the predominant theory on mitochondrial permeability during apoptosis is the formation of pores in the outer mitochondrial membrane by BAX oligomerization. An increase in the permeability of the outer mitochondrial membrane is permissive for the release of several factors important to the apoptotic pathway, including cytochrome c and apoptosis initiation factor.[41]

Stage 4: caspase activation

In the intrinsic pathway, caspase activation requires the formation of an activating complex called an apoptosome. This complex is made up of four components, including cytochrome c, apoptosis-activating factor 1 (Apaf-1), adenosine triphosphate (ATP), and procaspase-9.[42] Once all of the components are in place, Apaf-1 provides a scaffold that repositions procaspase-9, allowing it to cleave itself autoproteolytically into the active form (caspase-9). In turn, caspase-9 cleaves caspase-3, which activates endonucleases and other caspases. Each caspase has reportedly specific targets, while the active endonucleases digest DNA within the intact nucleus.[43] This latter event is one of the hallmarks of apoptosis, which results in the classic pyknotic nucleus referred to by pathologists, and the ability of researchers to label dying cells with terminal nucleotidyl transferase using the terminal uridine deoxynucleotidyl transferase dUTP nick end labeling (TUNEL) method. Overall, the activation of the caspase cascade results in the autodigestion of the cell itself.

Cell shrinkage

Cell shrinkage, including chromatin condensation and membrane blebbing, occurs late during the cell death pathway, typically as a result of caspase-mediated degradation events (Box 27.3). Several of these morphological changes are considered classic descriptors of this process of cell death. Recent studies, however, have demonstrated that overall cell shrinkage can occur very early and may actually be an intracellular apoptotic trigger.[44] RGC shrinkage occurs prior to the appearance of other apoptotic hallmarks in various mouse and primate models of experimental glaucoma, including *Bax*-deficient RGCs that cannot fully execute the apoptotic program[14,23,24] (Figure 27.3). Cell shrinkage appears to have a temporal order with changes in the dendritic arbor and soma occurring concurrently followed by changes in prelaminar (intraretinal) axon diameter.[14] Although there are few theories for why this apoptotic cell shrinkage occurs, it could be linked to an efflux of intracellular potassium,[44] associated with trophic factor depriva-

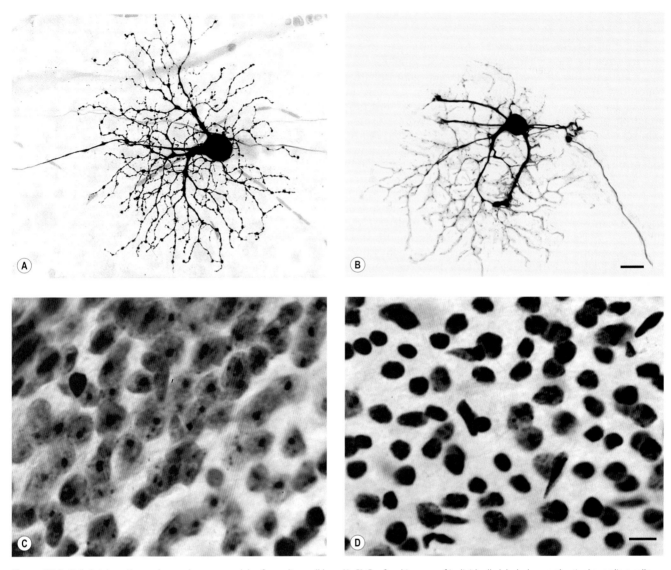

Figure 27.3 Cell shrinkage in monkey and mouse models of ganglion cell loss. (A, B) Confocal images of individually labeled parasol retinal ganglion cells from the midperipheral region of the superotemporal retinas of a rhesus monkey. The retinal ganglion cell (RGC) in (A) is from a control eye with an intraocular pressure (IOP) of < 21 mmHg and a cup:disc ratio (C:D) of ~0.3. The RGC in (B) is from an eye with experimental glaucoma. This eye had an average IOP of 46 mmHg for 2.5 weeks and a C:D of 0.9. In the cell from the glaucomatous eye, there was shrinkage of the cell body, dendritic tree, and proximal axon. On average, eyes with a C:D ratio > 0.8 exhibit a 43.2% reduction in soma size and a 42.4% reduction in the area of the dentritic field. (C, D) Nissl-stained retinal wholemounts from *Bax* knockout mice 2 weeks after optic nerve crush. This is a representative view of the ganglion cell layer in a control retina (C), and an experimental retina (D). The average nuclear area in the contol retinas is 44.50 μm^2. After crush in the *Bax* knockout animals, there is no loss of RGCs, but there is a decrease in average nuclear area to 26.55 μm^2. This emphasizes the fact that shrinkage is occurring early in the cell death pathway and not at the end since the apoptotic pathway in these cells is blocked prior to mitochondrial involvement.

The scale bar for (A, B) is 12 μm and is shown in (B). The scale bar for (C, D) is 10 μm and is shown in (D). (A and B are reproduced with permission from Weber AJ, Kaufman PL, Hubbard WC. Morphology of single retinal ganglion cells in the glaucomatous primate retina. Invest Ophthalmol Vis Sci 1998;39:2304–2320.)

tion.[11] In fact, it is possible that these two events may be linked, with glial activation as the common stimulus. The fact that somal changes appear to occur prior to any damage to the axonal transport system indicates that damage to RGCs may be detectable before any perimetric loss of vision occurs, and possibly before the cell death pathway is activated. If this is the case, a small window of time exists for the treatment of glaucoma prior to irreversible damage to these neurons. The problem, of course, is detecting these minute changes in ganglion cell appearance in time to treat the damaged cells effectively.

Future therapies/clinical management

Although it is not currently possible to visualize changes in ganglion cell morphology in the living eye, new retinal imaging technology is closer to turning this feat into reality. Two prospective scenarios for the early detection of glaucoma are emerging from new research. The first involves the use of adaptive optics technology with ophthalmoscopy. Scientists using this method have been able to visualize individual photoreceptors at a high enough resolution to

Box 27.3 Cell shrinkage and apoptosis

- Cell shrinkage is a phenomenon that occurs very early in the apoptotic pathway, and can still occur if the process is blocked in BAX-deficient ganglion cells
- Cell shrinkage appears to be mediated by rapid changes in ion concentration across the ganglion cell plasma membrane, mediated by changes in voltage-gated K^+ channels
- The role of the cell shrinkage phenomenon in the apoptotic program is not well understood, but blocking it has been shown to prevent apoptosis[43]
- Cell shrinkage may provide early gross morphological changes in the ganglion cells that could be detected using new imaging technologies like adaptive optics
- Blocking cell shrinkage could become an important pharmacologic target for the treatment of glaucoma

identify the spatial arrangement of the different types of cones, as well as measuring capillaries as small as 6 μm in diameter.[45] Although researchers have not yet been able to produce images of individual ganglion cells, this goal is a main focus of improving this technology. Recently, adaptive optics was used to visualize the nerve fiber layer as an individual three-dimensional entity.[46] The second emerging technique also involves the use of a confocal scanning laser ophthalmoscope with the apoptotic specific fluorophores bound to dying cells.[47] Using this technology, researchers were able to watch the progression of apoptosis in RGCs following optic nerve transection.

As this new retinal imaging technology becomes available, it may be possible to screen individuals for glaucoma before they experience loss of vision or, at the very least, to detect damage to the RGCs prior to soma loss, which could have substantial benefits. The early detection of RGC damage, for example as these cells undergo preapoptotic shrinkage, could be followed up with therapies to block cell death. One promising possibility for blocking cell death is inhibiting BAX, which has been shown to prevent RGC loss in murine glaucoma models.[13,25]

Although much about the complex pathway of RGC death in glaucoma remains a mystery, the progress in knowledge that has been made in the last 15 years provides the promise that the intricacies of the pathway will some day be elucidated.

Key references

A complete list of chapter references is available online at www.expertconsult.com. See inside cover for registration details.

2. Wiggs JL. Genetic etiologies of glaucoma. Arch Ophthalmol 2007;125:30–37.
4. Quigley HA, Nickells RW, Kerrigan LA, et al. Retinal ganglion cell death in experimental glaucoma and after axotomy occurs by apoptosis. Invest Ophthalmol Vis Sci 1995;36:774–786.
11. Whitmore AV, Libby RT, John SW. Glaucoma: thinking in new ways – a role for autonomous axonal self-destruction and other compartmentalised processes? Prog Retin Eye Res 2005;24:639–662.

13. Libby RT, Li Y, Savinova OV, et al. Susceptibility to neurodegeneration in a glaucoma is modified by Bax gene dosage. PLoS Genet 2005;1:17–26.
14. Weber AJ, Kaufman PL, Hubbard WC. Morphology of single retinal ganglion cells in the glaucomatous primate retina. IOVS 1998;39:2304–2320.
16. Schlamp CL, Li Y, Dietz JA, et al. Progressive ganglion cell loss and optic nerve degeneration in DBA/2J mice is variable and asymmetric. BMC Neurosci 2006;7:66.

38. Adams JM, Cory S. The Bcl-2 apoptotic switch in cancer development and therapy. Oncogene 2007;26:1324–1337.
44. Bortner CD, Cidlowski JA. Cell shrinkage and monovalent cation fluxes: role in apoptosis. Arch Biochem Biophys 2007;462:176–188.

CHAPTER 28

Wound-healing responses to glaucoma surgery

Stelios Georgoulas, Annegret Dahlmann-Noor,
Stephen Brocchini, and Peng Tee Khaw

Clinical background

Scarring constitutes the major threat to long-term success after most forms of glaucoma filtration surgery (GFS). Successful modulation of scarring increases the percentage of patients achieving final intraocular pressures (IOPs) that are associated with virtually no glaucoma progression. Antifibrotic agents for inhibition of scarring of trabeculectomy blebs are widely used worldwide, and their use is now well established, although they are linked to severe complications such as leakage, infection, hypotony, and endophthalmitis. These complications may lead to irreversible blindness. In addition, as surgery still fails in some individuals, despite maximal doses of current antifibrotics, more effective and selective therapeutic agents are sought.

Pathology

Hemostasis, inflammation, cell proliferation, and remodeling are the main phenomena observed in wound healing. After injury, formation of fibrin clots takes place with activation of the clotting cascade. This mechanism reduces blood loss. At the same time, neutrophils, macrophages, and lymphocytes are attracted to the region (inflammatory phase). Following these phenomena, the proliferative phase occurs: this comprises re-epithelialization and formation of granulation tissue and involves migration of fibroblasts, keratinocytes, and vascular endothelial cells to the wound region from neighboring tissues. Finally, in the remodeling phase, remodeling of the tissue takes place and involves the formation of scar tissue (Figure 28.1). Many different cell types participate in the healing process, including fibroblasts, keratinocytes, endothelial cells, neutrophils, macrophages, lymphocytes, and mast cells.

Pathogenesis

Inflammation

The grading system used in our long-term Medical Research Council trial showed a good correlation between inflamma-

tion and long-term outcome (www.blebs.net) (Figure 28.2). This finding agrees with many studies that have reported that inflammatory cells and mediators released during and after surgery stimulate the scarring cascade. Topical steroids applied as part of the routine postoperative management are effective in reducing inflammation.[1] Additionally, IOP reduction has been achieved with intrableb triamcinolone acetonide injection at the conclusion of GFS, and this constitutes a relatively safe method for steroid administration.[2] Topical nonsteroidal anti-inflammatory drugs may be effective,[1] but their use is still controversial.

The use of other agents, including ciclosporin and cyclooxygenase-2 inhibitors, against inflammation has been suggested (Box 28.1).[3] For the inhibition of inflammatory cytokines, a novel approach has been attempted with the development of dendrimers: hyperbranched nanomolecules that can be chemically synthesized to have precise structural characteristics. In our in vivo model of GFS, water-soluble conjugates of D(+)-glucosamine and D(+)-glucosamine 6-sulfate with immunomodulatory and antiangiogenic properties applied together enhanced the long-term success of GFS from 30% to 80%.[4] This experimental result is far more effective than that seen with conventional steroids (Figure 28.3).

Fibrin and hemostasis

Fibrin constitutes an important part of wound healing. Fibrinolytic agents are effective in lysing blood clots after surgery,[5] and, in the short term, these agents may lower IOP. The main side-effects that may deter the use of these agents are an increased risk of prolonged bleeding as well as the fact that fibrin breakdown molecules may have a longer-term stimulatory effect on the induction of scarring (Box 28.2).[6]

Cytokines, chemokines, and growth factors

Large numbers of growth factors or cytokines are contained in the tissues in a wound and this is the case in GFS and in the aqueous flowing through the bleb (Box 28.3).[7] Transforming growth factor-β (TGF-ß) in wound healing has been shown to be more stimulatory than other growth factors and cytokines found in the aqueous.[8] TGF-ß may even reverse the effect of mitomycin C (MMC) in vivo.[8] Recent finding

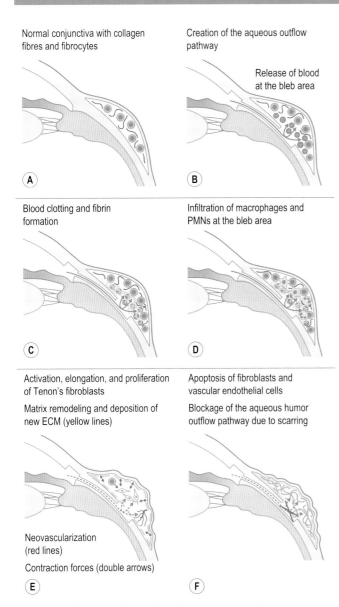

Figure 28.1 Sequence of wound-healing phenomena after glaucoma filtration surgery.

Normal conjunctiva with collagen fibres and fibrocytes

Creation of the aqueous outflow pathway

Release of blood at the bleb area

Blood clotting and fibrin formation

Infiltration of macrophages and PMNs at the bleb area

Activation, elongation, and proliferation of Tenon's fibroblasts

Matrix remodeling and deposition of new ECM (yellow lines)

Neovascularization (red lines)

Contraction forces (double arrows)

Apoptosis of fibroblasts and vascular endothelial cells

Blockage of the aqueous humor outflow pathway due to scarring

---

Box 28.1 Modulation of inflammation

• Steroids (intrableb triamcinolone acetonate injection)	Present mainly intracellular activity by alteration of gene expression. Clinically beneficial for intraocular pressure reduction[2]
• Synthetic derivatives of glucocorticoids	1. Inhibit macrophage function and reduce the recruitment of leukocytes and neutrophils in wounds 2. Decrease vascular permeability, leakage of plasma, and clotting factors 3. Inhibit the arachidonic acid pathway and subsequently the production of prostaglandins and leukotrienes
• Nonsteroidal anti-inflammatory drugs	1. Inhibition of cyclooxygenase, leading to reduction of prostaglandins, prostacyclin, and thromboxane A 2. Inhibition of platelet aggregation and function
• D(+)-glucosamine and D(+)-glucosamine 6-sulfate dendrimers	D(+)-glucosamine and D(+)-glucosamine 6-sulfate dendrimers have immunomodulatory and antiangiogenic properties, respectively[4]
• Ciclosporin A	Inhibition of lymphocyte-mediated immune responses
• Amniotic membrane	Potent anti-inflammatory properties, maintenance of oxygenation and moisture, and mechanical protection of covered tissues

---

Box 28.2 Fibrin and hemostasis

• Heparin[79]	Anticoagulant. Inhibits soluble thrombin, not fibrin-bound thrombin
• Recombinant Hirudin	Naturally occuring anticoagulant from the leech *Hirudo medicinalis*. Direct irreversible thrombin inhibitor
• Tissue-type plasminogen activator	Lyses blood clots after surgery and may lower intraocular pressure
• Urokinase or single-chain urokinase-type plasminogen activator	Thrombolytic (fibrinolytic) agent

Side-effects of anticoagulants and thrombolytic agents

Risk of further bleeding

Fibrin breakdown molecules may induce scarring

---

of enhanced expression of TGF-ß-RII receptors in failed blebs indicates the importance of TGF-ß in scarring after GFS.[9] Modulation of the activity of growth factors may be a useful therapeutic strategy for the inhibition of fibrosis.

Because TGF-ß in the eye seems to be involved in many pathways that are vital for the scarring process,[8] we performed several studies using a variety of biological mechanisms to block TGF-ß activity, including antisense oligonucleotides[10] and a human monoclonal antibody against the active form of human TGF-ß₂, the predominant isoform in the aqueous (Lerdelimumab, TrabioR, Cambridge Antibody Technology, Cambridge, UK). The theoretical advantage of antibodies includes a self-regulating concept, only working when levels of the target protein are high (Figure 28.4). In an in vivo model of conjunctival scarring, the administration of this antibody significantly improved GFS outcome[11] and appeared much less destructive to local tissue than MMC. A pilot clinical study of this antibody in

GFS demonstrated the absence of significant side-effects, inflammatory reaction, and cystic bleb formation. However, two larger randomized controlled trials have not shown a significant effect on the outcome of GFS.[12] Based on the data obtained from an earlier study,[11] we believe that the dose used was not sufficient. Further studies from our lab have shown a significantly enhanced effect with a prolonged dosing regimen,[13] and the data also suggested an enhanced effect in the GFS outcome when the antibody is combined with intraoperative 5-fluorouracil (5-FU).

Small interfering RNA against TGF-ß receptor II mRNA reduced the production of TGF-ß receptor II, the expression

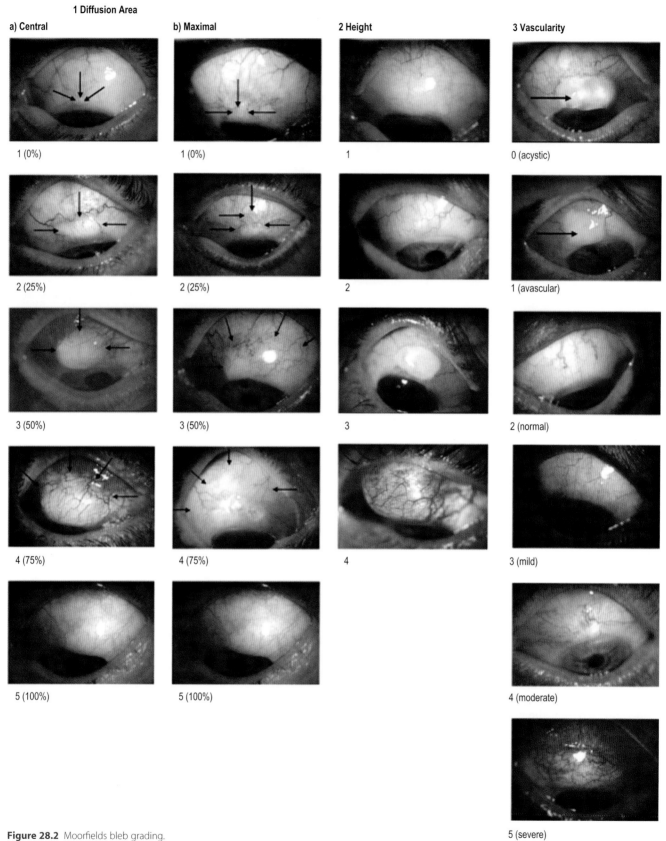

Figure 28.2 Moorfields bleb grading.

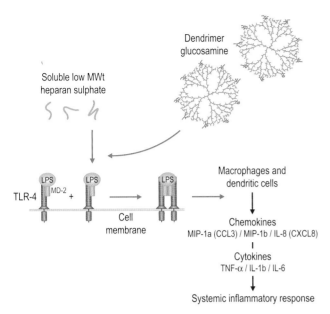

Figure 28.3 Branched dendrimers carrying drugs to enhance binding and efficacy.

and deposition of fibronectin, the migration of human corneal fibroblasts, inflammation and deposition of extracellular matrix (ECM) in an in vivo model of subconjunctival scarring after GFS.[14]

Transglutaminases are calcium-dependent enzymes which cross-link proteins using ε-(γ-glutamyl)-lysine bonds. Transglutaminase (tTgase) and its end product ε-(γ-glutamyl)-lysine were detected in scarred tissue of failed trabeculectomy blebs.[15] Since vertebrates lack enzymes capable of hydrolyzing these bonds, the protein cross-linking created by transglutaminases seems to be unbreakable. tTgase cross-links fibronectin and collagen-3; these proteins are produced by human Tenon's fibroblasts (HTFs) in vitro and have been detected in the scar tissue deposited in the bleb area after GFS. In the same study, TGF-ß$_2$ was shown to stimulate the expression of tTgase and, subsequently, the cross-linking of fibronectin in vitro,[15] leading to the conclusion that inhibition of TGF-ß$_2$ activity could extend the success of the surgery as this pathway might lead to enhanced cross-linking of the newly formed scar tissue in vivo.

The main intracellular TGF-ß signaling pathway runs through proteins that activate transcription of the genes that encode the Smad proteins. Of particular relevance is Smad-3, which is essential for TGF-ß-induced production of ECM proteins.[16,17] Targeting intracellular signaling downstream of the TGF-ß receptor could be another effective strategy. Inhibiting Smad3 in immediate postoperative applications might prove beneficial.[18] Smad-7, acting differently from Smad-3, is another potential therapeutic target. As TGF-ß can suppress its action through the induction of Smad-7 (negative-feedback loop), gene transfer of the Smad-7 gene has been shown in animal models to have a protective effect against the development of lung, liver, and renal fibrosis.[19]

P38 MAP kinase (MAPK) is believed to trigger the transcription of Smad-2/3, facilitate the phosphorylation and activation of Smad-3 and, subsequently, the formation of Smad-3/4 complex, which is important for the development of the fibrotic reaction. The Smad-3 signaling pathway is important in retinal fibrosis. Inhibition of Smad-3 is associated with a reduction of a cellular fibrotic reaction.[20] Adenoviral transfer by intravitreal application of a dominant negative p38MAPK gene demonstrated reduced fibrotic reaction of retinal pigment epithelium cells after retinal detachment.[21] In later studies, adenoviral gene transfer of the same gene was applied to in vitro cultured HTFs[22] and in an in vivo conjunctival scarring model in mice.[23] Reduction of the differentiation of fibroblasts to myofibroblasts and decline of the connective tissue growth factor (CTGF) and of the monocyte chemoattractant protein (MCP-1) expression were the main in vitro findings. Inhibition of conjunctival scarring was observed in vivo. As MCP-1 is a chemoattractant for macrophages, one of the main sources of TGF-ß, the reduction in levels of MCP-1 through inhibition of p38MAPK, seems to reduce the levels of TGF-ß; hence, it plays a favorable role in conjunctival scarring.[24–26] Furthermore, the recent finding that the antiglaucoma drug latanoprost, a prostaglandin F$_{2\alpha}$ analog, induces formation of stress fibers in HTFs in vitro as well as contraction of collagen I gels mediated by HTFs in vitro is indicative of the important role of MAPKs in subconjunctival scarring. The contraction of collagen I gels by latanoprost was blocked by inhibitors of MAPKs, Rho-activated kinase, myosin light chain (MLC).[27] Moreover, the findings of this in vitro study point out potential induction of scarring by latanoprost in vivo. This conclusion agrees with previous findings that long-term antiglaucoma treatment represents a risk factor in scarring after GFS[28] and that eyes treated with latanoprost after surgery were observed to have smaller decrease of IOP compared to the ones that did not receive latanoprost.[29]

CTGF influences ECM production and subsequent fibrosis. TGF-ß$_1$ triggers the expression of CTGF, which is also necessary for TGF-ß stimulation of myofibroblast differentiation and collagen contraction.[30] Inhibition of this factor could be a possible future therapeutic target.[31] Lovastatin, a member of the drug class of statins, was shown to inhibit the TGF-ß-induced CTGF transcription, α-smooth-muscle actin (SMA) expression and, subsequently, the HTF differentiation to myofibroblasts as well as collagen contraction in vitro.[32]

Rho is a small GTPase that has been implicated in the formation of stress fibers and focal adhesions, actin cytoskeleton remodeling, and cell contractility. TGF-ß increases cell tension in HTF cultures and contraction in HTF collagen I gels by triggering the activation of Rho. Rho activates the serine-threonine Rho-associated kinase (ROCK), which enhances cytoskeletal tension and results in actomyosin-mediated contraction. ROCK inhibitors reduce cell tension and inhibit the TGF-ß-mediated p-38 activation, α-SMA expression, and HTF development of enhanced contractile abilities characteristic of the so-called myofibroblast phenotype."[22] ROCK inhibitor Y-27632 inhibited contraction of HTF-seeded collagen I gels and α-SMA expression by HTFs in vitro. In vivo, application of Y-27632 after GFS significantly increased the survival of the blebs compared to controls. Furthermore, reduction of collagen I deposition and scarring in the treated blebs compared to controls was observed in histological analysis.[33] ROCK inhibitors may block TGF-ß-induced scarring by downregulating pathways that are generating mechanical tension and thereby improve the success of GFS.

Box 28.3 Cytokines, chemokines, and growth

• Recombinant human monoclonal antibody against active transforming growth factor (TGF-ß₂)	Inhibition of TGF-ß₂ activity[13]
• Small interfering RNA (SiRNA) against TGF-β mRNA	Inhibition of transcription of the mRNA with subsequent inhibition of synthesis of the protein TGF-ß[10]
• SiRNA against TGF-β II receptor mRNA	Reduction of inflammation and extracellular matrix deposition in vivo.[13] Increased presence of TGF-β II receptors in the failed blebs
• Tranilast ((N-(3′,4′-dimethoxycinnamoyl) anthranilic acid)	Inhibition of TGF-ß activity[82]
• Genistein: isoflavone from soy products	Inhibition of TGF-ß activity, tyrosine kinases, matrix metalloproteinases, and angiogenesis[83]
• Suramin: polycyclic trypan dye derivative	Inhibition of TGF-ß activity and reduction of fibrosis after experimental glaucoma filtration surgery[83]
• Conversion of angiotensin I to II	Angiotensin II regulates TGF-ß₁ expression via angiotensin receptor ligand binding, which contributes to myofibroblast conversion
• Chymase inhibitors: chymase is an enzyme released by mast cells	Chymase activates angiotensin I to angiotensin[84]
• Smad-7 gene transfer	Suppression of TGF-β action and protection against the development of lung, liver, and renal fibrosis[19]
• Rho-associated kinase (ROCK) inhibitors (mainly Y-27632)	Control of GTPase Rho activation, which is triggered by TGF-β. Inhibition of human Tenon's fibroblasts collagen I contraction in vitro and increase of bleb survival in vivo[33]
• Decorin	Small proteoglycan, natural inhibitor of TGF-β. Delay of intraocular pressure increase and decrease of fibrosis after glaucoma filtration surgery
• Ribozymes: RNA molecules which can cleave specific bonds in other RNA molecules	Cleavage of TGF-ß-mRNA with subsequent inhibition of synthesis of the protein TGF-ß
• Aptamers ARC126 and ARC127	Platelet-derived growth factor (PDGF) activates ocular fibroblasts. ARC126 and ARC127 bind and block PDGF-B[36] and may improve the success of glaucoma filtration surgery
• Adenoviral transfer of a dominant negative p38MAPK gene	Inhibition of Smad3 activation. Reduction of the differentiation of fibroblasts to myofibroblasts in vitro and reduction of conjunctival scarring in vivo[21]
• Simvastatin, Inhibitor of the enzyme, HMG-CoA reductase	Inhibition of the connective tissue growth factor gene and protein expression, a downstream mediator of TGF-ß[85]
• Lovastatin	Inhibition of TGF-β-induced connective tissue growth factor transcription, α-smooth-muscle actin (α-SMA) transcription and human Tenon's fibroblasts differentiation to myofibroblasts[86]
• Follistatin	Inhibitor of activin A. Reduction of liver and lung fibrosis[41] Potential application in GFS

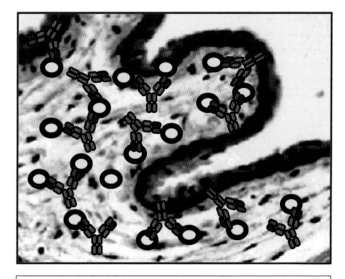

High TGF-β2 levels

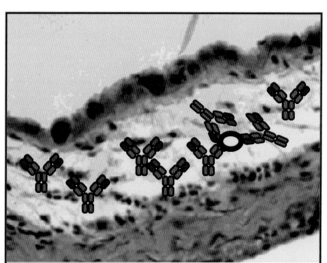

Low TGF-β2 levels

Figure 28.4 Antibody only working in the presence of high concentrations of antigen.

Myofibroblasts express a platelet-activating factor (PAF) nuclear receptor and tumor necrosis factor-ß (TNF-ß) receptors; PAF and TNF-ß cause time-dependent myofibroblast apoptosis. Future therapeutic approaches may take advantage of the expression of these receptors.[34]

Platelet-derived growth factor (PDGF) has been found to activate certain ocular fibroblasts. Some ocular fibroblasts express high levels of PDGF receptor beta. When stimulated, these fibroblasts proliferate, migrate, produce ECM molecules and cause contraction, fibrosis, and the development of fibrotic membranes such as those observed in proliferative vitreoretinopathy (PVR).[35] Aptamers, nucleic acid-based macromolecules with similar functions as monoclonal antibodies (high affinity and specificity for target proteins), are capable of recognizing, binding, and blocking PDGF-B. Two aptamers, ARC126 and ARC127, have been tested in animal models of PVR,[36] and may also be useful in GFS.

Bone morphogenic proteins (BMPs) are growth factors that are vital for cell proliferation, differentiation, apoptosis, angiogenesis, and other biological functions.[37] Activins are dimeric proteins that participate in cell differentiation and proliferation, apoptosis, inflammation, and neurogenesis.[38] Investigation of the expression of many members of BMPs and activins in normal and scarred conjunctival tissue revealed enhanced mRNA and protein levels of BMP-6 and activin A in scarred compared to normal conjunctiva.[39] The use of follistatin, an inhibitor of activin bioactivity, was shown to be effective in decreasing liver and lung fibrosis.[40,41] Based on the above findings, the inhibition of BMP-6 and activin A could be a future therapeutic option for the control of scarring after GFS.[39]

Fibroblast proliferation and vascularization

The antimetabolites 5-FU and MMC are the main agents currently used to inhibit scarring and subsequent IOP increase and blindness after trabeculectomy. Lately, mechanisms of prolonged release of 5-FU and MMC are sought (Box 28.4). We have achieved the formulation of tablets that release 5-FU for more than 8 hours in our lab model, which mimics the bleb. Prolonged release of 5-FU may enhance the success of trabeculectomies.[42] Slow-release MMC-loaded hydrogels were shown to inhibit cell proliferation in an in vitro model. In the future, these gels, placed in the bleb, could find an application in GFS in humans.[43] It was recently reported that repeated exposure of HTFs in vitro to MMC increases the expression of P-glycoprotein, a protein that creates multidrug resistance by lowering intracellular concentration of various drugs. This finding may explain failure of repeated trabeculectomies despite the application of MMC. 5-FU seems to be a better option for repeated trabeculectomies as it does not increase the expression of P-glycoprotein.[44]

Paclitaxel, an antineoplasmatic agent that prevents mitosis by blocking the depolymerization of intracellular microtubules, inhibits HTF proliferation and prolongs the success of GFS. But as paclitaxel is hydrophobic, its administration in the subconjunctival area is not easy. Polyanhydride disks[45] and carbopol 980 hydrogel[46] containing paclitaxel have been tested, with encouraging results comparable to the antiscarring effects of MMC, although the development of severe inflammation, especially in the case of polyanhydride disks, has been reported.[45]

Box 28.4 Fibroblast proliferation and neovascularization

• Mitomycin C-loaded hydrogels	Inhibit cell proliferation in vitro
• Slow-release 5-fluorouracil tablets	May enhance the success of trabeculectomy[42]
• Photodynamic therapy	BCECF-AM: fluorescent probe. When applied locally in its inactive form diffuses into adjacent cells and is cleaved and rendered fluorescent by intracellular esterases. After illumination (activation) with blue light, it exerts a photo-oxidative effect; only cell destructive within the targeted cells[53]
• Paclitaxel (Taxol): first isolated from the bark of the Pacific yew tree, *Taxus breviofolia*, Taxaceae	Inhibits depolymerization of intracellular microtubules and subsequently prevents mitosis[45,87]
• Bleomycin: group of related glycopeptide antibiotics isolated from *Streptomyces verticillus*	Inhibits cell replication and survival through DNA binding. Creates free radicals, which cause single- and double-strand breaks which lead to inhibition of DNA synthesis[40,88]
• Thiotepa: synthetic antimitotic agent similar to nitrogen mustards used in chemical warfare	Polyfunctional alkylating agent
• Retinoic acid and its derivative, vitamin A	Retinoic acid regulates gene expression by binding to nuclear transcription factors
• Interferon-α (IFN-α): recombinant protein mimicking the effects of natural IFN-α	IFN-α regulates cell proliferation and differentiation by affecting several cellular communication and signal transduction pathways[89]
• Lectins (phytoagglutinins): proteins that agglutinate erythrocytes and other cells	The mushroom lectin from *Agaricus bisporus* binds to galactosyl-ß-1,3-N-acetyl-galactosamine-alpha (Gal-Gal-NAc) and has a strong antiproliferative effect. The exact mechanism of action is unknown[90]
• Saporin: derived from the plant *Saponaria officinalis*	Ribosome inactivating protein → cell proliferation inhibitor
• Antiproliferative gene p21(WAF-1/Cip-1)	p21(WAF-1/Cip-1) is a transcription factor that mediates cell cycle arrest in response to cellular stress. Transfection using an adenoviral system resulted in inhibition of scarring[55]
• Bevacizumab (Avastin) intrableb or intravitreal injection(s)	Inhibition of vascularization and reduction of intraocular pressure[58,60,62]
• Ranibizumab needling in failed blebs	Intraocular pressure and vascularity reduction[59]

Beta-irradiation, by inhibiting the proliferation of fibroblasts,[47] significantly improved the success of GFS in a large African trial using a dose based on our laboratory studies.[48,49] It may also be useful in pediatric GFS.[37]

Photodynamic therapy with a diffuse blue light coupled with a photosensitizing agent has been used in order to kill fibroblasts.[50] Many studies have demonstrated that photodynamic therapy reduces neovascularization and maturation of scar tissue after GFS. Intraoperative photodynamic therapy using preoperative subconjunctival application of ethyl etiopurin[51] and BCECF-AM as photosensitizers[52] have proven to be safe and effective against scarring after GFS in vivo. Pilot clinical trials of intraoperative photodynamic therapy with locally administered BCECF-AM have shown promising results.[53] Furthermore, postoperative photodynamic therapy has been reported to be effective against neovascularization and scarring. Intravenous administration of the photosensitizer verteporfin in the early postoperative period to occlude the newly formed capillaries in the bleb area had favorable results in the modulation of wound healing in rabbits after GFS.[54]

Additionally, future interesting experimental strategies to modulate proliferation include overexpressing genes that inhibit fibroblast proliferation, such as p21 WAF-1/CIP-1 introduced via an adenovirus system,[55] antagonizing integrins and their receptors,[56] or altering intracellular gene transcription.[57]

It has recently been demonstrated that bevacizumab (Avastin), a humanized monoclonal antibody that is used in the eye for the treatment of proliferative (neovascular) diseases, could potentially inhibit scarring after GFS. Subconjunctival injections of Avastin administered in failed blebs of patients with primary open-angle glaucoma, normal-tension glaucoma, or exfoliation syndrome revealed significant decrease of IOP and of vascularity 1 month postinjection.[58] Similar findings regarding IOP and vascularity reduction were observed after bleb needling with antivascular endothelial growth factor treatment (ranibizumab) in patients with failed blebs.[59] Furthermore, application of bevacizumab injections combined or not with 5-FU application during trabeculectomy extended the survival of the bleb in an in vivo GFS model.[60] Moreover, it has been suggested that intravitreal administration of bevacizumab at the same time as trabeculectomy augmented with MMC in patients with neovascular glaucoma may be effective in inhibition of neovascularization and in modulation of scarring.[61] It is likely that bevacizumab may control scarring by inhibiting fibroblast proliferation and their contractile ability as well as by inducing fibroblast death, as has been observed after administration of bevacizumab in HTF cultures.[62]

Matrix and cell-mediated contraction

Tissue contraction constitutes a critical component of GFS failure, as revealed by bleb analysis using carefully graded masked digital photographs. We have developed a more detailed understanding of the processes that occur during tissue contraction and have recently been able to image cells and matrix simultaneously during the process of contraction (Figure 28.5). The matrix metalloproteinases (MMPs) are the main enzymes responsible for the ECM degradation among all the proteinases that participate in ECM turnover

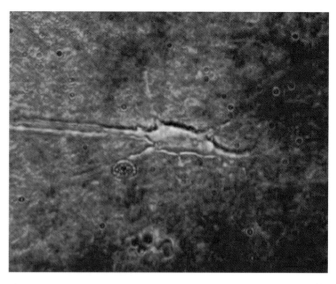

Figure 28.5 Fibroblast and matrix imaged simultaneously.

Box 28.5 Modulation of matrix deposition and cell-mediated contraction

• Colchicine: plant alkaloid of *Colchicum autumnale* L., Liliaceae	Depolymerization of microtubules, results in the inhibition of cellular migration, proliferation, and contraction[87]
• Etoposide: anticancer agent	Stabilizes a normally transient DNA–topoisomerase II complex, thereby increasing double-stranded DNA breaks[67]
• D-penicillamine: degradation product of penicillin	Prevents collagen cross-linking and makes collagen more susceptible to cleavage[91]
• ß-aminoproprionitrile (BAPN)	Inhibits the enzyme lysyl oxidase, which catalyzes the initial step in collagen cross-linking[91]
• Fibrostatin-c: produced by *Streptomyces catenulae* subsp. *Griseospor*	Inhibits prolyl-4-hydroxylase[92]
• Matrix metalloproteinase inhibitors	Enzymes with zinc-containing catalytic site expressed during embryogenesis, tissue remodeling, and repair. Inhibition of enzymes prevents collagen contraction and prevents scarring in a model of glaucoma surgery[63–66]
• Minoxidil: pyrimidine derivative	Inhibits the enzyme lysyl oxidase, which catalyzes the initial step in collagen cross-linking

---

(Box 28.5). Cell-mediated collagen contraction can be reduced using MMP inhibitors.[63] In an experimental model of GFS, the repeated administration of MMP inhibitor injections led to a dramatic reduction of scarring with retention of normal tissue morphology. This action is equivalent to MMC, but without the deleterious side-effects.[64,65] MMP inhibition also results in a reduction of collagen synthesis in vitro,[63] which may help to explain the dramatic reduction in scar tissue formation in vivo.[64] Recently, our group has formulated a novel prolonged-release MMP inhibitor tablet that was placed at the subconjunctival space after GFS in our in vivo model. It was surprisingly shown that the prolonged release of MMP inhibitor resulted in significantly extended survival of the bleb and lower IOP compared to both the negative (water sponge) and the positive control (MMC 0.2 mg/ml group). Histology revealed decreased collagen deposition and number of fibroblasts at the blebs treated with the MMP inhibitor tablet compared to the positive and negative control blebs.[66]

Other agents such us Taxol and etoposide (microtubule-stabilizing agents) have been used in models of GFS and they prolong bleb survival.[67] ß-aminopropionitrile and D-penicillamine interfere with molecular cross-linking of collagen, and there is experimental and clinical evidence that they may work in GFS.[67]

Using surgical and anatomical principles to modify therapy

Minimizing tissue damage during surgery is of obvious relevance to the outcome of GFS, and we have shown that simple changes in surgical and antimetabolite application technique can radically reduce side-effects even when the same concentrations of antimetabolites are used[68] (Figure 28.6). Amniotic membrane, used as a physical spacer, may increase the success of GFS, as it appears to have antiangiogenic, anti-inflammatory, and antifibrotic characteristics. Amniotic membrane has been tested in both animal models of GFS[69] and in humans,[70,71] with encouraging results. Lately, two pieces of amniotic membrane soaked in MMC were sutured, one under the scleral flap and one into the subconjunctival space, in a study performed in trabeculectomies of high-risk patients (who had had two or more trabeculectomies with MMC). After 6–18 months, IOP was found to be significantly reduced.[72] A bioequivalent gel may, in future, perform the function of amniotic membranes. Gas, such as perfluoropropane or sodium hyaluronate 2,3%, may improve subconjunctival drainage spaces with resultant creation of more diffuse blebs (Figure 28.7).[73,74] Creation of a subscleral aqueous outflow channel with femtosecond laser in an in vivo study was shown to decrease IOP significantly.[75] Devices made of relatively inert materials already used in other spaces, such as the suprachoroidal space, may also facilitate aqueous outflow by keeping the surgical field free of scar tissue (Box 28.6). However, in many cases the continuous inflammatory reaction due to the presence of the biomaterial leads to excessive scarring and poor postoperative results.

Conclusions and future directions

New treatments and refining existing treatments to prevent scarring after disease, trauma, or surgical intervention represent the aim of many scientific groups worldwide. More effective drug delivery methods are sought for post-GFS management because it is clearly vital for the prevention of blindness. The long-term requirement of treatment and the narrow therapeutic window of drugs in current use still limit the control of scarring. Sustained-release delivery systems,

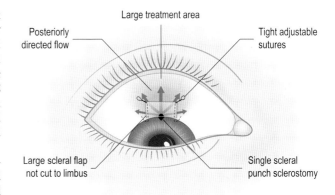

Figure 28.6 Changes in surgical technique leading to better outcomes.

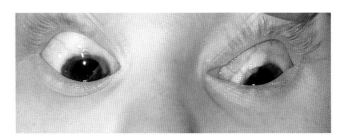

Figure 28.7 Dramatic change in bleb appearance with change in MMC treatment area.

including liposome encapsulation,[76] microspheres,[77] scleral plugs,[78] and biodegradable implant polymers, may have a significant future role. With our ability to combine agents will come better efficacy. An example is the combination of 5-FU and heparin to prevent PVR.[79]

The ability to control fibrotic processes fully in the eye offers the tantalizing prospect of 100% success of glaucoma surgery with pressure around 10 mmHg associated with minimal progression over a decade. For that reason, in addition to traditional chemical drugs, the development of new technologies such as dendrimers, antibodies, aptamers, ribozymes, gene therapy with viral vectors, and RNA interference is necessary and opens the door to achieve this aim. Finally, most exciting is the prospect that neutralizing the fibrotic response to disease and injury will allow us to revert to the "fetal" mode when regeneration is the "normal" process, such as shown in a recent report which demonstrated that induction of bcl-2 gene expression together with downregulation of gliosis results in axonal regeneration in mice.[80] Modifying matrix and cell conditions allows intrinsic stem cells to differentiate into different cells of the retina like lower species, which can regenerate a severely damaged complex retina and possibly the optic nerve.[81]

Acknowledgments

The authors acknowledge the support of the Medical Research Council, Moorfields Trustees, the Haymans Trust, Ron and

Box 28.6 Glaucoma filtration surgery

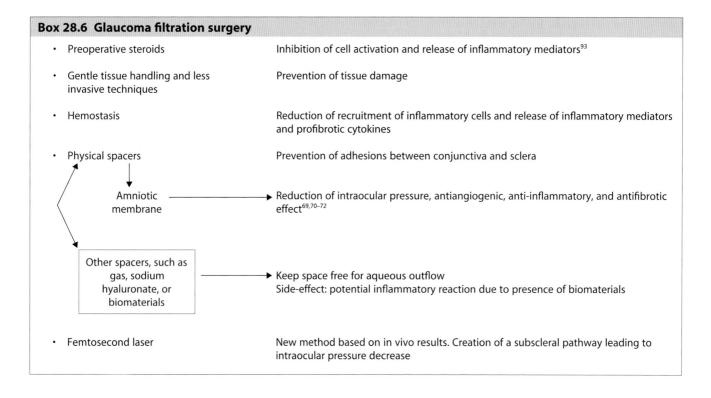

• Preoperative steroids	Inhibition of cell activation and release of inflammatory mediators[93]
• Gentle tissue handling and less invasive techniques	Prevention of tissue damage
• Hemostasis	Reduction of recruitment of inflammatory cells and release of inflammatory mediators and profibrotic cytokines
• Physical spacers	Prevention of adhesions between conjunctiva and sclera
Amniotic membrane	Reduction of intraocular pressure, antiangiogenic, anti-inflammatory, and antifibrotic effect[69,70–72]
Other spacers, such as gas, sodium hyaluronate, or biomaterials	Keep space free for aqueous outflow Side-effect: potential inflammatory reaction due to presence of biomaterials
• Femtosecond laser	New method based on in vivo results. Creation of a subscleral pathway leading to intraocular pressure decrease

Liora Moskovitz Foundation, the Michael and Ilse Katz Foundation, the Helen Hamlyn Trust in memory of Paul Hamlyn, Fight for Sight (UK), School of Pharmacy University of London, and the AG Levendis Foundation. This research has received a proportion of its funding from the Department of Health's National Institute for Health Research Biomedical Research Centre at Moorfields Eye Hospital and the UCL Institute of Ophthalmology. The views expressed in this publication are those of the authors and not necessarily those of the Department of Health.

Key references

A complete list of chapter references is available online at www.expertconsult.com. See inside cover for registration details.

4. Shaunak S, Thomas S, Gianasi E, et al. Polyvalent dendrimer glucosamine conjugates prevent scar tissue formation. Nat Biotechnol 2004;22:977–984.

7. Chang L, Crowston JG, Cordeiro MF, et al. The role of the immune system in conjunctival wound healing after glaucoma surgery. Surv Ophthalmol 2000;45(1):49–68.

12. Khaw PT, Grehn F, Hollo G, et al. A phase III study of sub-conjunctival human anti-transforming growth factor beta(2) monoclonal antibody (CAT-152) to prevent scarring after first-time trabeculectomy. Ophthalmology 2007;114(10):1822–1830.

13. Mead AL, Wong TTL, Cordeiro MF, et al. Anti-Transforming growth factor–β2 antibody: a new post operative anti-scarring agent in glaucoma surgery. Invest Ophthalmol Vis Sci 2003;44: 3394–3401.

14. Nakamura H, Siddiqui SS, Shen X, et al. RNA interference targeting transforming growth factor-beta type II receptor suppresses ocular inflammation and fibrosis. Mol Vis 2004;4:703–711.

17. Massague J. Wounding Smad. Nat Cell Biol 1999;1:E117–E119.

28. Broadway DC, Grierson I, O'Brien C, et al. Adverse effects of topical antiglaucoma medication. II. The outcome of filtration surgery. Arch Ophthalmol 1994;112:1446–1454.

49. Kirwan JF, Constable PH, Murdoch IE, et al. Beta irradiation: new uses for an old treatment: a review. Eye 2003;17: 207–215.

55. Perkins TW, Faha B, Ni M, et al. Adenovirus-mediated gene therapy using human p21WAF-1/Cip-1 to prevent wound healing in a rabbit model of glaucoma filtration surgery. Arch Ophthalmol 2002;120:941–949.

63. Daniels JT, Cambrey AD, Occleston NL, et al. Matrix metalloproteinase inhibition modulates fibroblast-mediated matrix contraction and collagen production in vitro. Invest Ophthalmol Vis Sci 2003; 44:1104–1110.

64. Wong TT, Mead AL, Khaw PT. Matrix metalloproteinase inhibition modulates postoperative scarring after experimental glaucoma filtration surgery. Invest Ophthalmol Vis Sci 2003;44:1097–1103.

65. Wong TT, Mead AL, Khaw PT. Prolonged antiscarring effects of ilomastat and MMC after experimental glaucoma filtration surgery. Invest Ophthalmol Vis Sci 2005;46:2018–2022.

68. Wells AP, Bunce C, Khaw PT. Flap and suture manipulation after trabeculectomy with adjustable sutures: titration of flow and intraocular pressure in guarded filtration surgery. J Glaucoma 2004;13: 400–406.

79. Asaria RH, Kon CH, Bunce C, et al. Adjuvant 5-fluorouracil and heparin prevents proliferative vitreoretinopathy: results from a randomized, double-blind, controlled clinical trial. Ophthalmology 2001;108:1179–1183.

81. Lawrence JM, Singhal S, Bhatia B, et al. MIO-M1 cells and similar muller glial cell lines derived from adult human retina exhibit neural stem cell characteristics. Stem Cells 2007;25(8):2033–2043.

CHAPTER 29

Blood flow changes in glaucoma

Leopold Schmetterer and Mark Lesk

Clinical background

The idea that factors other than elevated intraocular pressure (IOP) contribute to the pathophysiological processes underlying glaucoma was formulated more than 150 years ago. Von Graefe was the first to recognize that glaucoma can occur despite normal IOP.[1] Only 1 year later Jaeger proposed the vascular concept as cause for normal-tension glaucoma (NTG).[2] The prevalence of NTG as estimated from different studies differs significantly. On average it is now assumed that 30–40% of all primary open-angle glaucoma (POAG) patients have normal IOP,[3] a proportion that rises to 90% in Japan.[4]

The fact that optic nerve head damage and loss of visual field are not related only to elevated IOP is also seen from other arguments. On the one hand a large number of subjects have elevated IOP without showing signs of glaucoma, a condition known as ocular hypertension. The rate of conversion from ocular hypertension to glaucoma is small. Therefore, a large proportion of ocular hypertensive patients never develop glaucoma. On the other hand several multicenter trials have shown that a large proportion of patients with glaucoma progress despite IOP-lowering therapy.[5,6]

In this chapter the evidence that reduced blood flow plays a role in the glaucomatous process will be summarized. Unfortunately, measurement of ocular blood flow is difficult and currently available techniques are not suitable for clinical practice. This makes it difficult to discern whether a specific patient shows signs of vascular dysregulation (Box 29.1) in the optic nerve head or retina. Hence, the diagnosis of vascular dysregulation in glaucoma patients largely relies on indirect evidence and a thorough evaluation of medical history plays a key role. Patients with vascular dysregulation often suffer from a history of cold hands. Migraine, a risk factor for the progression of NTG, can also be found in some glaucoma patients with vascular dysregulation. Obviously, measurement of systemic blood pressure is required in patients with potential vascular involvement. Ideally, a 24-hour ambulatory blood pressure profile is recorded together with a 24-hour IOP profile. This allows for identification of periods of nocturnal hypotension and low ocular perfusion pressure (OPP), which are likely associated with ischemic conditions at the level of the eye.

When discussing the potential therapeutic implications of ocular blood flow disturbances in glaucoma one first has to consider that lowering IOP, the hallmark of glaucoma therapy, has a vascular consequence in itself. Any reduction in IOP, whether achieved pharmacologically or surgically, induces an increase in OPP. In addition, a number of drug classes that may induce direct vasodilatation at the posterior pole of the eye have been identified. The best evidence is available for carbonic anhydrase inhibitors and calcium channel blockers. Given that reduced perfusion and vascular dysregulation are risk factors for glaucoma there is a clear rationale behind such treatment. On the other hand, results of large-scale clinical trials showing that improving ocular blood flow is associated with beneficial effects on visual fields are lacking. Is it conceivable to assume that vasodilator treatment is beneficial for glaucoma? At least some studies show that short-term improvements of visual fields in glaucoma are closely related to vasodilatation, particularly in vasospastic subjects. However, vasodilator therapy could also induce negative effects, including disturbance of autoregulatory mechanisms, increase of capillary hydrostatic pressure, or shunting of blood to other vascular beds. Hence, large-scale clinical trials are urgently required. At the moment any attempted vasodilator treatment in glaucoma patients needs to be done under careful monitoring of visual fields and drug-related adverse events, but may be tried in patients who progress despite optimal IOP reduction. It may currently be more fruitful to evaluate patients for nocturnal hypotension and to treat this, if present, in collaboration with other physicians.

Pathology

The specific tissue changes characteristic for glaucoma are covered in other chapters of this book. Clinical findings suggesting that vascular phenomena are important in glaucoma include the common finding of flame hemorrhages of the optic nerve head neuroretinal rim in open-angle glaucoma patients (Figure 29.1).[7] A flame hemorrhage is commonly followed by the appearance of a new nerve fiber layer defect and subsequent progressive visual field loss, suggesting that a vascular phenomenon is contributing to disease progression. These hemorrhages are interpreted as a sign of vascular

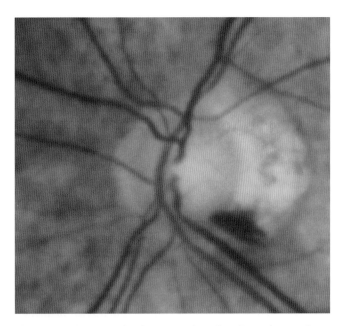

Figure 29.1 Optic nerve head neuroretinal rim flame hemorrhage and beta-peripapillary atrophy.

Box 29.1 Clinical findings in systemic vasospasm (vascular dysregulation)

- Cold hands and feet, more frequently than the average person
- Raynaud's syndrome
- Low blood pressure, especially at night
- Local vasoconstriction of conjunctival blood vessels
- Migraine
- Variant angina
- Vasospasm induced by cold, mechanical stress, or by emotional stress
- Reduced feeling of thirst
- Low body mass index

Box 29.2 Clinical vascular findings in primary open-angle glaucoma/normal-tension glaucoma

Ocular

- Neuroretinal rim flame hemorrhages
- Local constriction of peripapillary retinal arteries
- Peripapillary chorioretinal atrophy
- Low ocular perfusion pressure
- Reduced perfusion of the ocular vasculature

Systemic

- Low blood pressure
- Nocturnal hypotension
- Cold hands and feet
- Migraine
- Cardiovascular disease

Box 29.3 Clinical characteristics of four glaucoma disk types (data from Broadway et al[10])

Focal ischemic

Focal notch or acquired pit of the optic nerve head, some peripapillary atrophy

- Vasospasm
- Cold hands and feet
- Migraine
- Rim flame hemorrhages
- Two-thirds are female

Senile sclerotic

Shallow saucerized cupping, peripapillary atrophy around most of the disk

- Older age
- Systemic cardiovascular disease
- Hypertension
- Reduced blood flow in the ophthalmic artery
- Slower rate of progression

Myopic disk

Tilted disk with a crescent of peripapillary atrophy

- Younger age
- Some vasospasm
- Myopia
- Two-thirds are male

Concentric cupping

Round, concentric cup without localized rim thinning

- Younger age
- Markedly elevated intraocular pressure
- Low prevalence of vascular risk factors

strain in the optic nerve head, but their cause and mechanism are unknown. Arterial narrowing may also be seen overlying the disk in glaucoma.[8] Beta-peripapillary atrophy is associated with glaucomatous optic nerve changes and is linked to glaucoma progression[9] (Figure 29.1). This atrophy is hypothesized to be vascular in origin, because it is characterized histologically as a loss of choriocapillaris (Box 29.2).

Attempts have been made to characterize specific phenotypes in optic disk appearance associated with the presence of vascular risk factors[10] (Box 29.3). According to this work glaucomatous optic nerve head appearance has been divided into four subtypes: (1) focal glaucomatous optic disk; (2) myopic glaucomatous optic disk; (3) senile sclerotic optic disk; and (4) generalized enlargement of the optic disk cup. The vast majority of glaucomatous disks, however, appear to have features of two or more of these disk types. However, some risk factors were associated with a higher prevalence of a specific disk appearance. Ischemic heart disease was more prevalent among patients with senile sclerotic glau-

coma in comparison with the other groups. A suggestion of a greater prevalence of systemic hypertension in the senile sclerotic group and of migraine and vasospasticity in the focal glaucomatous group was also observed. Larger studies are required to characterize in more detail which risk factors

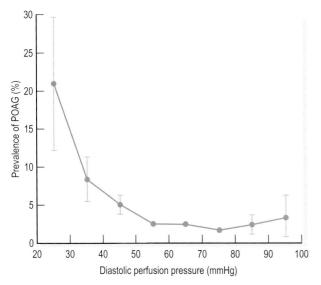

Figure 29.2 Systemic vascular findings in glaucoma. There is a sixfold risk of glaucoma for subjects with the lowest ocular perfusion pressure. POAG, primary open-angle glaucoma. (Baltimore Eye Survey: reproduced with permission from Tielsch JM, Katz J, Sommer A, et al. Hypertension, perfusion pressure, and primary open-angle glaucoma. A population-based assessment. Arch Ophthalmol 1995;113:216–221.)

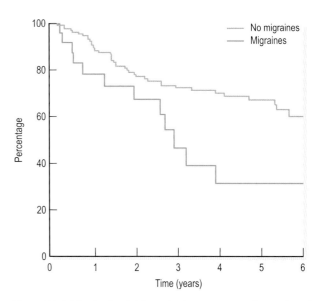

Figure 29.3 Migraine is a risk factor for the progression of normal-tension glaucoma. (Collaborative Normal Tension Glaucoma Study: reproduced with permission from Drance S, Anderson DR, Schulzer M, et al. Risk factors for progression of visual field abnormalities in normal-tension glaucoma. Am J Ophthalmol 2001;131:699–708.)

are associated with specific optic disk appearance and patterns of visual field loss.

Etiology

A number of vascular risk factors for the prevalence, incidence, and progression of POAG have been identified.

Low systemic blood pressure

Systemic blood pressure has been closely linked to prevalence of open-angle glaucoma. Epidemiologic studies indicate a markedly increased prevalence of glaucoma in people with lower diastolic OPP. In the Baltimore Eye Study, there was a sixfold increased risk of OAG in subjects having the lowest diastolic OPPs[11] (Figure 29.2). These findings were confirmed in different populations in the Egna-Neumarkt Eye Study[12] and the Rotterdam Eye Study.[13] The Barbados Study of Eye Disease subsequently observed an elevated incidence of OAG in subjects with low OPP and low blood pressure.[14] The Early Manifest Glaucoma Trial demonstrated an increased risk of glaucoma progression in patients with low OPP.[15] Low OPP appears to be the most important vascular risk factor for POAG.

High blood pressure

While in general lower blood pressures and OPPs are associated with glaucoma, epidemiological evidence suggests that systemic hypertension may play a role as well,[11,12] particularly in older patients. This association is hypothesized to result from a breakdown of vascular autoregulation in long-standing hypertension. One needs, however, to consider that there is a correlation, albeit weak, between IOP and systemic blood pressure.[12]

> **Box 29.4 Evidence for vascular etiology of glaucoma from the Collaborative Normal Tension Glaucoma Study (data from Drance et al[17] and Anderson DR and Drance SM, 2003)**
>
> Greater rate of progression in:
> - Migraineurs
> - Patients with disk hemorrhages
> - Women (vascular mechanism?)
>
> Lesser response to intraocular pressure therapy if:
> - History of disk hemorrhage
> - Family history of stroke
> - Personal history of cardiovascular disease

Vasospasticity and migraine

Vasospasticity or vascular dysregulation is associated with POAG.[16] In the Collaborative Normal Tension Glaucoma Study, there was a 2.5-fold risk of visual field progression in patients reporting a history of migraine[17] (Figure 29.3 and Box 29.4). Schulzer et al[18] defined two populations of glaucoma patients: those with predominantly atherosclerotic workups and those with peripheral vasospasm (Figure 29.4). While there was no correlation between the maximum known IOP and the degree of visual field damage in the atherosclerotic group, there was a strong positive correlation in the vasospastic group. The authors interpreted their findings to suggest that, while in atherosclerotic patients optic nerve damage might be IOP-independent, in vasospastic patients the IOP damage was IOP-dependent. Hafez et al[19] subsequently demonstrated that, in OAG, there exists a correlation between the degree of vasospasticity and the amount

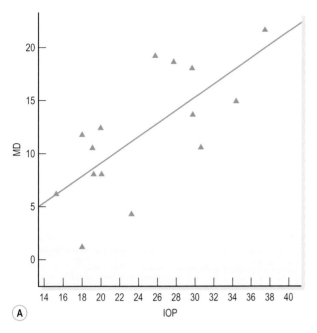
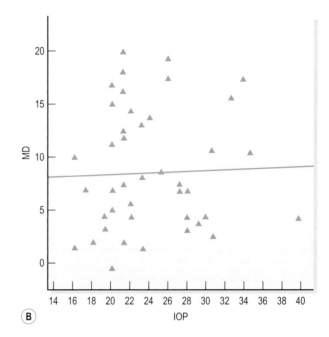

Figure 29.4 (A, B) Evidence for two populations of glaucoma patients: vasospastic patients with pressure-dependent glaucoma and atherosclerotic patients with pressure-independent glaucoma. (Reproduced with permission from Schulzer M, Drance SM, Carter CJ, et al. Biostatistical evidence for two distinct chronic open angle glaucoma populations. Br J Ophthalmol 1990;74:196–200.)

of change of neuroretinal rim blood flow upon IOP reduction. In other words, neuroretinal rim blood flow may be more sensitive to changes in IOP in vasospastic patients than in nonvasospastic patients.

Anticardiolipin antibodies

Anticardiolipin antibodies (ACA) are present in acquired prothrombotic syndromes and are linked to ischemic stroke, myocardial infarction, and systemic lupus erythematosus, but it is not known if they are causal or merely a sign of ongoing vascular inflammatory disease. A recent prospective clinical trial found a strong association between positive ACA and progression of open-angle glaucoma, although the prevalence of positive ACA was low in the study population.[20] This suggests that vascular inflammatory factors may be linked to OAG, although at this time it is impossible to know whether they are causal or secondary to neurovascular damage.

Ocular blood flow and visual field progression

In order to prove definitively that abnormal ocular blood flow contributes to the pathophysiology of glaucoma a prospective large-scale clinical trial is required. Such a trial would test the hypothesis that reduced blood flow is an independent risk factor for glaucoma. There are some small-scale studies that examined this. In a prospective study of 44 newly diagnosed OAG patients, a lower diastolic velocity and higher resistivity index in the ophthalmic artery were associated with markedly greater risk of visual field progression over a 7-year follow-up.[21] This is in good agreement with other data showing that reduced diastolic velocity in the central retinal artery is associated with progression of the disease.[22] Martinez and Sánchez also studied OAG patients

> **Box 29.5 Vascular phenomena associated with visual field progression in glaucoma**
>
> - Migraine
> - Low ocular perfusion pressure
> - Low blood pressure
> - Nocturnal hypotension
> - Anticardiolipin antibodies
> - Neuroretinal rim flame hemorrhages
> - Reduced blood flow in the ophthalmic artery
> - Reduced blood flow in the central retinal artery

prospectively and found that patients with subsequent visual field progression had significantly greater resistance indexes in the ophthalmic artery at baseline.[23] Another small-scale study suggested that patients with the smallest improvements in optic nerve head blood flow in response to initial IOP reduction had the greatest risk of visual field progression over 4.5 years[24] (Box 29.5).

Pathophysiology

Although there is a large body of evidence that glaucoma is associated with reduced blood flow to the posterior pole of the eye in general and the optic nerve head specifically, it is currently assumed that the disease process is more closely linked to vascular dysregulation. Vascular dysregulation refers to an abnormal vasoconstrictor or vasodilator response to stimulations such as changes in perfusion pressure, increase in neural activity, or changes in neural input. The reason for this vascular dysregulation in glaucoma is not entirely known, but may in some patients be related to a phenomenon called primary vasospastic syndrome.[25] There is a longstanding discussion whether reduced blood flow in glaucoma is a primary phenomenon playing a causal role in the disease process or secondary due to optic nerve atrophy and loss of retinal ganglion cells. Since it has widespread systemic manifestations, vascular dysregulation is, however, unlikely to be a direct consequence of the ocular morphological changes associated with the disease.

Pressure autoregulation

A variety of experiments indicate that pressure autoregulation is to some extent altered in patients with POAG. A study performing 24-hour ambulatory blood pressure monitoring and diurnal measurement of the IOP revealed significant blood pressure drops during the night, which were more pronounced in patients with NTG than in patients with anterior optic neuropathy.[26] In patients with arterial hypertension receiving oral hypotensive therapy a significant association between progressive visual field loss and nocturnal hypotension was seen. This observation played a key role in the formulation of the hypothesis that nocturnal systemic hypotension may be associated with episodes of nocturnal ischemia at the level of the optic nerve head contributing to glaucomatous damage (Figure 29.5).[27]

Only recently this concept was expanded by introducing the idea that increased fluctuations of OPP may generally represent a risk factor for glaucoma. A study by Plange and coworkers[28] confirmed increased blood pressure dipping during the night in NTG, but also showed a generally increased variability of blood pressure over 24 hours. This was confirmed and extended in larger study populations,[29,30] where fluctuations in OPP were consistently associated with parameters of visual field damage and optic nerve head remodeling.

Using single-point laser Doppler flowmetry it was observed that glaucoma patients with systemic hypertension have higher blood flow values than glaucoma patients without systemic hypertension.[31] Although such data must be interpreted with caution, because laser Doppler flowmetry does not provide absolute blood flow measurements, they indicate an abnormal association between blood pressure and blood flow, suggesting a breakdown of autoregulation in glaucoma. In addition, it has been argued that systemic antihypertensive treatment may even further decrease optic nerve head blood flow in glaucoma, thereby increasing the risk of progression.[31] These data were confirmed in a much larger study population using scanning laser Doppler flowmetry (Figure 29.6).[32] This abnormal relation between ocular hemodynamic parameters and systemic blood pressure appears to be directly related to the disease process. In a study using color Doppler imaging a negative association between resistance index in the ophthalmic artery and central retinal artery was only observed in patients with progressive

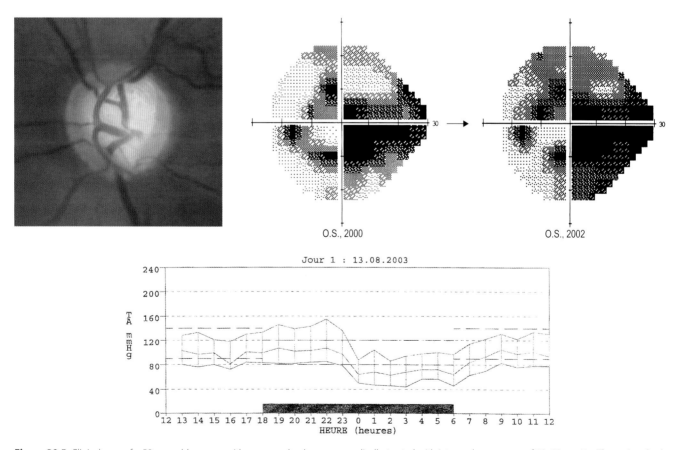

O.S., 2000   O.S., 2002

Figure 29.5 Clinical case of a 59-year-old woman with open-angle glaucoma, medically treated with intraocular pressures of 11–12 mmHg. The patient had visual field progression associated with nocturnal hypotension.

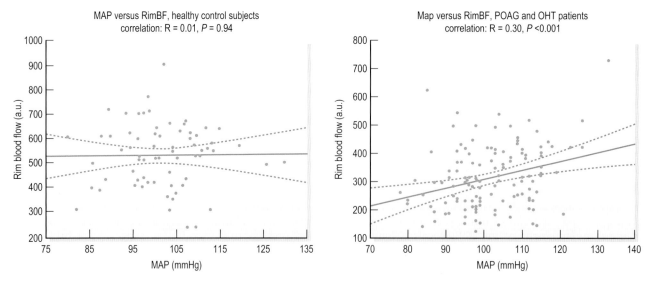

Figure 29.6 (A, B) Abnormal association between optic nerve head blood flow and systemic blood pressure in patients with primary open-angle glaucoma (POAG) or ocular hypertension (OHT) as compared to healthy control subjects indicating vascular dysregulation. MAP, mean arterial pressure. (Reproduced with permission from Fuchsjäger-Mayrl G, Wally B, Georgopoulos M, et al. Ocular blood flow and systemic blood pressure in patients with primary open-angle glaucoma and ocular hypertension. Invest Ophthalmol Vis Sci 2004;45:834–839.)

visual field damage, but not in patients with stable visual fields.[33]

Finally, a number of studies investigated the response of ocular blood flow parameters in response to experimentally induced changes in perfusion pressure. Both an increase and a decrease in blood pressure have been induced, leading to vasoconstriction or vasodilatation as part of the autoregulatory response, respectively. The first study indicating impaired retinal blood flow autoregulation in glaucoma used the blue-field entoptic technique during an experimental increase in IOP.[34] The maximum increase in IOP at which retinal white blood cell flux remained constant was higher in healthy controls than in glaucoma patients. Evidence for reduced retinal autoregulation in glaucoma was also seen in a study employing the retinal vessel analyzer.[35] During a step increase in IOP the reaction of retinal vessel diameters was less pronounced in glaucoma patients than in healthy controls.

A variety of studies used changes in posture to induce changes in OPP, because they can easily be implemented with minimal discomfort for the participating subjects. In a color Doppler imaging study an abnormal velocity response to posture was observed in the central retinal artery, but not in the ophthalmic artery.[36] An abnormal response to changes in posture was also seen in patients with OAG using combined measurements of retinal blood velocities and retinal vessel diameters.[37] Only a few studies tried to investigate optic nerve head blood flow in glaucoma patients during artificial changes in perfusion pressure. Indication of abnormal autoregulation at the level of the optic nerve head was observed in a study using scanning laser Doppler flowmetry after a therapeutic IOP reduction.[19,38]

Endothelial dysfunction

The mechanism behind abnormal autoregulation in patients with glaucoma is largely unknown. In recent years, however,

it has been hypothesized that it may be related to endothelial dysfunction. This concept has recently been reviewed in some detail.[39] Endothelial dysfunction refers to a number of complex biochemical alterations resulting in the inability of endothelial cells to perform their normal physiological function. These alterations are initiated by increased oxidative stress leading to pathological alterations in the cellular balance of mediators produced by endothelial cells. Diseases of chronic endothelial dysfunction such as atherosclerosis, systemic hypertension, or diabetes are characterized by a decrease in the biosynthesis and/or bioavailability of nitric oxide (NO), and increased superoxide and endothelin production.

In the eye the vascular endothelium plays a key role in the regulation of blood flow both under physiological conditions and in response to changes in perfusion pressure and agonists.[40] In glaucoma endothelial dysfunction can involve various tissues and is not limited to vascular functions. It has for instance been shown that endothelial leukocyte adhesion molecule-1 (ELAM-1), the earliest marker for the atherosclerotic plaque in the vasculature, is consistently present on trabecular meshwork cells in the outflow pathways of eyes with glaucoma, providing an interesting link between increased IOP and vascular diseases.[41] In the present chapter, however, the focus will be directed towards the vascular aspects of endothelial dysfunction in glaucoma. A variety of studies indicate alterations of the l-arginine/NO system in glaucoma. In POAG patients, decreased aqueous humor total nitrite levels were found to be indicative of reduced NO production.[42] An in vitro study, however, reported increased levels of the three isoforms of NO synthase in the optic nerve head of patients with glaucoma.[43] One needs, however, to consider that in this experiment the most pronounced changes were reported for NO synthase-1 (neuronal NO synthase) and NO synthase-2 (inducible NO synthase).

In vivo studies also revealed that glaucoma patients show signs of an abnormal l-arginine/NO system, mainly based

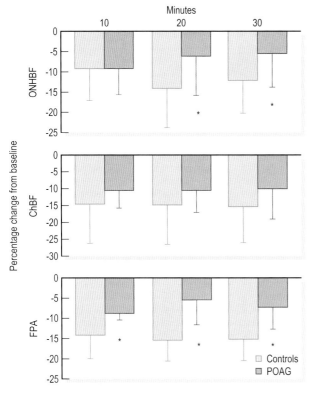

Figure 29.7 Abnormal response of ocular blood flow parameters to systemic nitric oxide synthase inhibition in patients with primary open-angle glaucoma (POAG) as compared to healthy control subjects indicating endothelial dysfunction. (Reproduced with permission from Polak K, Luksch A, Berisha F, et al. Altered nitric oxide system in patients with open-angle glaucoma. Arch Ophthalmol 2007;125:494–498.)

Box 29.6 Native molecules that alter ocular blood flow

- Nitric oxide*
- Endothelin-1*
- Estrogens*
- CO_2*
- O_2
- Adenosine
- Angiotensin II
- Thromboxane
- Dopamine
- Serotonin
- Histamine

*Evidence exists that this molecule may be involved in the pathogenesis of glaucoma.

NO synthase-3 alleles was significantly different in subjects who had glaucoma with migraine when compared with control subjects without glaucoma.

Endothelin-1 has been hypothesized to act as a contributor to glaucoma pathophysiology.[49] The possible involvement of the endothelin system is not limited to the vascular effects of the peptides, but may also comprise interaction with neurotrophic support, astrocyte activation, tissue remodeling, and cell death. A complete discussion of this topic is, however, beyond the scope of the present chapter. Hence, the focus is directed towards the vascular aspects of the endothelins. Early studies revealed that patients with NTG show elevated basal plasma ET-1 concentrations.[50,51] Increased plasma ET-1 levels were also found in progressive POAG patients, but not in stable patients.[52] Increased plasma levels of ET-1 are, however, found in a variety of cardiovascular and neurological diseases and are far from being specific for glaucoma. Hence, increased ET-1 plasma levels in glaucoma more likely reflect sites of locally increased ET-1 production rather than directly contributing to the disease process. This is compatible with ET-1 primarily being a paracrine factor and the observation that glaucoma patients show increased ET-1 aqueous humor levels.[53,54]

More importantly there is evidence for altered regulation of the endothelin system and abnormal vascular responses to the peptide. In healthy subjects a change from the supine to the upright position is associated with an increase in ET-1 plasma levels, which is absent in patients with NTG.[55] In response to cooling POAG patients showed an increase in ET-1 plasma levels, which was absent in healthy control subjects.[56] In addition, POAG patients with acral vasospasm showed more visual field deterioration after cooling than patients without acral vasospasm. Altered vasoreactivity to endothelins or their receptor antagonists was reported in different studies. In vitro, arteries dissected from gluteal fat biopsies of patients with NTG showed an enhanced reactivity to ET-1.[57] In vivo reduced vasodilator responses to a specific ETA receptor antagonist were observed in the forearm of NTG patients, whereas the response to ETB receptor antagonists was preserved.[58] In addition, glaucoma patients with lower systemic blood pressures were more sensitive to the vasoconstrictor effects of ET-1 in the forearm than patients

on an abnormal vascular response to either agonists that induce NO-dependent vasodilatation or NO synthase inhibitors. In patients with NTG a number of studies indicate generalized endothelial dysfunction as evidenced from experiments assessing forearm blood flow. Reduced vasodilator responses in the forearm of patients with NTG were observed after intra-arterial administration of acetylcholine[44] and after hyperemia.[45] In patients with POAG an altered response of ocular blood flow to a systemically administered NO synthase inhibitor was shown (Figure 29.7).[46] Whereas in this study the systemic hypertensive response to NO synthase inhibition was comparable between POAG patients and age-matched healthy controls, the glaucomatous group showed reduced response in terms of ocular hemodynamic parameters. This is well compatible with the hypothesis of reduced endothelial NO production in the ocular vasculature.

The hypothesis that the L-arginine/NO system is involved in the pathogenesis of glaucoma has been supported by a number of genetic case-control studies. In an early study sequence analysis demonstrated a C/T substitution at the 5′ sequence position nucleotide -690 from the transcription start site, which lies between the cAMP regulatory element and an activator protein-1 binding domain in the NO synthase-3 gene.[47] This polymorphism was significantly associated with POAG. Logan et al[48] found that the distribution of

with higher blood pressures.[59] Such an association between systemic blood pressure and ET-1 reactivity was absent in the healthy control group.

Additional evidence for the involvement of the endothelin system in glaucoma pathophysiology arises from genetic studies. In patients with NTG the GG genotype of the ETA receptor (c+70G) was associated with more pronounced visual field loss, indicating that it is related to progression of the disease.[60] In another South-east Asian population another polymorphism (c+1222T) of the ETA receptor gene was significantly associated with NTG.[61] Other studies, however, failed to detect an association between genetic variants in the ET-1 gene and glaucoma[47,48] (Box 29.6).

Conclusion

Numerous studies now indicate vascular dysregulation in glaucoma, which is unlikely to be a consequence of the disease process. A direct link between vascular dysregulation and progression of the disease has not been provided, but a number of indirect observations point in this direction. Investigating ocular blood flow regulation in clinical practice in glaucoma patients is not easy, because it is dependent on significant instrumental requirements, but it has rewarded us with numerous insights into the mechanisms underlying the disease.

Key references

A complete list of chapter references is available online at www.expertconsult.com. See inside cover for registration details.

9. Jonas JB. Clinical implications of peripapillary atrophy in glaucoma. Curr Opin Ophthalmol 2005;16:84–88.

10. Broadway DC, Nicolela MT, Drance SM. Optic disk appearances in primary open-angle glaucoma. Surv Ophthalmol 1999;43(Suppl. 1):S223–S243.

11. Tielsch JM, Katz J, Sommer A, et al. Hypertension, perfusion pressure, and primary open-angle glaucoma. A population-based assessment. Arch Ophthalmol 1995;113:216–221.

15. Leske MC, Heijl A, Hyman L, et al. Predictors of long-term progression in the early manifest glaucoma trial. Ophthalmology 2007;114:1965–1972.

16. Flammer J, Pache M, Resink T. Vasospasm, its role in the pathogenesis of diseases with particular reference to the eye. Prog Retin Eye Res 2001;20:319–349.

17. Drance S, Anderson DR, Schulzer M, et al. Risk factors for progression of visual field abnormalities in normal-tension glaucoma. Am J Ophthalmol 2001;131:699–708.

21. Galassi F, Sodi A, Ucci F, et al. Ocular hemodynamics and glaucoma prognosis: a color Doppler imaging study. Arch Ophthalmol 2003;121:1711–1715.

27. Graham SL, Drance SM. Nocturnal hypotension: role in glaucoma progression. Surv Ophthalmol 1999;43(Suppl. 1):S10–S16.

30. Choi J, Kim KH, Jeong J, et al. Circadian fluctuation of mean ocular perfusion pressure is a consistent risk factor for normal-tension glaucoma. Invest Ophthalmol Vis Sci 2007;48:104–111.

32. Fuchsjäger-Mayrl G, Wally B, Georgopoulos M, et al. Ocular blood flow and systemic blood pressure in patients with primary open-angle glaucoma and ocular hypertension. Invest Ophthalmol Vis Sci 2004;45:834–839.

38. Hafez AS, Bizzarro RL, Rivard M, et al. Changes in optic nerve head blood flow after therapeutic intraocular pressure reduction in glaucoma patients and ocular hypertensives. Ophthalmology 2003;110:201–210.

39. Resch H, Garhofer G, Fuchsjäger-Mayrl G, et al. Endothelial dysfunction in glaucoma. Acta Ophthalmol 2009;87:4–12.

44. Henry E, Newby DE, Webb DJ, et al. Peripheral endothelial dysfunction in normal pressure glaucoma. Invest Ophthalmol Vis Sci 1999;40:1710–1714.

46. Polak K, Luksch A, Berisha F, et al. Altered nitric oxide system in patients with open-angle glaucoma. Arch Ophthalmol 2007;125:494–498.

49. Yorio T, Krishnamoorthy R, Prasanna G. Endothelin: is it a contributor to glaucoma pathophysiology? J Glaucoma 2002;11:259–270.

Biochemical mechanisms of age-related cataract

David C Beebe, Ying-Bo Shui, and Nancy M Holekamp

Clinical background

A cataract is any opacification of the lens. Visually significant cataracts may be present at birth or may occur at any time thereafter, but incidence increases exponentially after 50 years of age.[1] Age-related cataracts are responsible for nearly half of all blindness worldwide.[2,3] As longevity increases, the impact of cataracts on society is expected to increase. At present, surgical removal of the lens opacity with implantation of an intraocular lens (IOL) is the standard of care throughout most of the world where cataract surgery is available. Although this is usually a safe and effective treatment, intraocular surgery is an expensive and technically challenging solution for such a widespread problem. Rare but serious surgical complications include intraocular infection and inflammation and swelling of the retina (cystoid macular edema). Secondary opacification of the lens tissue remaining after surgery may occur (secondary cataract or posterior capsular opacification), the frequency of which depends on the age of the patient, the experience of the surgeon, and the type of IOL. Secondary cataract is treated by laser-mediated disruption of the posterior capsule of the lens, a procedure that requires expensive equipment and may incite further complications. There is no recognized medical treatment for age-related cataracts. For these reasons, identifying interventions to prevent or delay lens opacities represents an exceptional opportunity to reduce morbidity, increase productivity, and reduce health care costs.

The lens comprises an anterior layer of epithelial cells covering a mass of elongated fiber cells (Figure 30.1). Fiber cells are responsible for the transparency and refractive properties of the lens. The entire lens is surrounded by a thick, acellular capsule that provides structural support to the lens cells and a site of attachment for the zonular fibers that anchor the lens to the ciliary body. The lens grows linearly throughout life by the proliferation of epithelial cells near the equator and the differentiation of their progeny into fiber cells.[4,5] Fiber cells are laid down in concentric shells over pre-existing layers of fiber cells (Figure 30.1). As part of their differentiation, fiber cells degrade their nuclei, mitochondria, and other membrane-bound organelles, preventing the synthesis of new proteins.[6] Enzyme systems in mature fiber cells soon become nonfunctional. To maintain homeostasis (and transparency), most fiber cells depend on the metabolic activities of the epithelium and a thin layer of metabolically competent superficial fiber cells.

This chapter outlines the major risk factors for age-related cataract, identifies areas where more knowledge is needed, and highlights promising opportunities for prevention. The information provided is not meant as a complete review of the biochemical mechanisms that may contribute to cataract formation, which would be a much larger undertaking. Instead, it explores the results of epidemiologic studies, biochemical and biophysical analyses of human lenses, and selected animal studies, to suggest the likely causes and potential treatment of clinically significant cataracts in humans.

Pathology

"Age-related cataract" encompasses at least three distinct diseases (Box 30.1). Although each involves opacification of lens fiber cells, these opacities occur in different regions of the lens, have different risk factors, and involve different pathologic mechanisms. Interventions to delay or prevent age-related cataracts must take into account these different pathologies. The three types are nuclear, cortical, and posterior subcapsular cataracts.

In most western populations, nuclear cataracts are the commonest reason for cataract surgery. Opacities occur in the central region of the lens, the lens nucleus, in fiber cells that were produced before birth (Figure 30.2). Opacification of the nucleus is associated with increased light scattering, caused by the aggregation or condensation of lens proteins, and increased coloration. Nuclear cataracts are associated with relatively minor effects on cell structure.[7,8] In some populations, nuclear color may be responsible for most of the opacity, resulting in "brunescent" nuclear cataracts.

Cortical cataracts are the commonest reason for cataract surgery in many Asian populations and are frequently seen in western countries. They begin in the outer third of the lens, in cells that were generated postnatally. Cortical opacities are associated with gross disruption of the structure of fiber cells, local proteolysis, and protein precipitation.[9-11] Opacities usually begin in small foci near the lens equator, then spread along the length of the fiber cells toward the optic axis and circumferentially to adjacent fiber cells (Figures 30.1 and 30.2). Cortical cataracts may progress for years

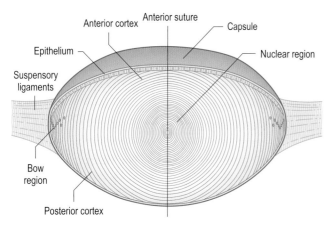

Figure 30.1 Diagram showing the major structural features of the human lens. The diagram is not to scale; the epithelium and superficial, nucleated fiber cells comprise a smaller proportion of the adult lens than in the illustration.

Box 30.1 Age-related cataract is at least three diseases

The three types of age-related cataract (cortical, nuclear, posterior subcapsular) occur in different regions of the lens, cause opacity by different mechanisms, and have different environmental, societal, and genetic risk factors. Studies that consider "cataract" as a single entity are likely to miss important relationships

---

before they impinge on the optic axis and become visually significant.

Posterior subcapsular cataracts typically account for less than 10% of age-related cataracts. They arise from epithelial cells that fail to differentiate properly into fiber cells.[12,13] These cells migrate or are carried by their neighbors to the posterior pole of the lens, where they swell and form a plaque that scatters light (Figure 30.2). Because these plaques are in the optic axis, they significantly degrade vision, even when quite small.

Etiology

Other than age, lower socioeconomic status and poorer nutrition are often associated with increased risk of all types of age-related cataract.[3] However, the specific components of these societal risks have been difficult to identify. Attempts to prevent or slow the progression of age-related cataracts by dietary supplementation have had modest success, at best.[14–19]

Many studies have shown that women are at greater risk of age-related cataracts, although this has not been a universal finding. Protective effects of hormone replacement therapy have been small or inconclusive.[20–22] Given the natural, long-term exposure of women to estrogenic steroids, it is difficult to argue that these hormones offer significant protection against age-related cataract. It seems more likely that, if there is a role of female sex steroids in cataract, the decline in estrogen levels at menopause may increase risk.

The possibility that male sex hormones protect against cataract seems plausible, but has been little explored.[23]

Beyond these more general risks, each type of age-related cataract is associated with a distinct spectrum of environmental risk factors. The most consistent positive association with lifestyle and nuclear cataracts is smoking. Since smoking is preventable, it represent an important, though challenging, opportunity for intervention. Nuclear cataracts are more prevalent in warmer climates.[24] Whether this is due to ambient temperature or to other nutritional or societal risks has not been established. Cortical cataracts are associated with greater sunlight exposure and diabetes. Although a contribution of sunlight exposure to cortical cataracts is well established, greater sunlight exposure accounts for only a small increase in the risk of cortical cataracts in a typical population.[25–28] Numerous studies have shown that even the highest level of sunlight exposure represents no detectable increased risk for the development of nuclear or posterior subcapsular opacities.[29] Posterior subcapsular cataracts are most often associated with diabetes and therapeutic treatment with steroids or ionizing radiation. When diabetes is reasonably well controlled, it presents only a modest increase in the risk of age-related cataracts.[30] Most of the increase in cataract surgery in diabetics is due to posterior subcapsular opacities. Steroid-induced posterior subcapsular cataracts have typically been associated with long-term systemic administration, but are becoming more prevalent due to the increasing popularity of high-dose intraocular steroids to treat retinal inflammation and neovascularization.[31,32] Because the biology of these cataracts is less well understood than other types, studying cataracts induced by steroids during retina therapy or in animal models[33] may offer an opportunity for understanding better the pathobiology of this disease.

Environmental risk factors provide clues to the etiology of age-related cataracts (Box 30.2). Unfortunately, we know little about the biochemical mechanisms by which smoking contributes to nuclear cataracts or sunlight promotes cortical cataracts. Therefore, these risk factors have, so far, told us little about the pathogenic mechanisms underlying these diseases. Equally important, environmental factors that do not increase the risk of cataracts tend to rule out certain pathways in the cause of that type of cataracts. For example, the biochemical effects of sunlight exposure do not contribute significantly to the risk of nuclear or posterior subcapsular opacities. Therefore, it is reasonable to conclude that light-generated free radicals, for example, are not central to the etiology of these diseases.

As important as they may eventually be for understanding cataract etiology, environmental factors appear to account for a relatively small percentage of age-related cataracts. Other variables, many of which are less easily modified, are more significant contributors to the burden of disease. Among the most significant is genetic variation (Box 30.3).

Studies that measured the incidence of specific types of cataract in families, or between monozygotic (identical) and dizygotic (fraternal) twins, showed that approximately half of the risk of cortical and at least one-third of the risk of nuclear cataracts can be attributed to heredity.[34–38] Increased risk of nuclear or cortical cataract was genetically separable in these populations, underscoring the distinct nature of these diseases. Although the subject of ongoing

Scheimpflug

Retro-illumination

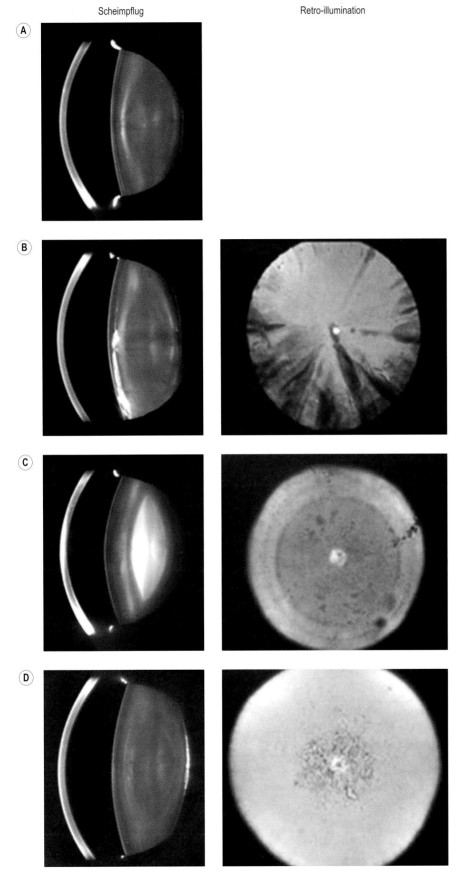

Figure 30.2 Clinical images showing a normal, older human lens (A) and lenses with cortical cataract (B i and ii), nuclear cataract (C i and ii), or posterior subcapsular cataract (D). Scheimpflug images show cross-sections of the lens through the optic axis. In these images, increased brightness is due to increased light scattering. Retroillumination images show the light reflected back through the lens from the retina. In these images, decreased brightness is due to the absorption or scattering of light by the lens. (Courtesy of Dr. Yasuo Sakamoto, Kanazawa Medical University, Japan.)

Box 30.2 The contributions of environmental and societal risk factors

Epidemiologic studies in populations around the world have identified recurring risk factors for the different types of age-related cataracts. Nuclear cataracts are often associated with smoking, poorer nutrition, and living in a warmer climate. Common risk factors for cortical cataracts include higher sunlight exposure and diabetes. Posterior subcapsular cataracts are associated with diabetes, use of immunosuppressive and intraocular steroids, and therapeutic radiation to the head. Anatomic factors, like lens thickness and the stability of the vitreous gel, also seem to contribute to the risk of nuclear and cortical cataracts. Surprisingly, the biochemical links that connect these risk factors to age-related cataracts are generally not known

Box 30.3 The potential importance of genetics

Studies of the prevalence of age-related cataracts in families and cohorts of twins demonstrated the importance of hereditary factors. Identifying the underlying genes may be valuable for preventing all types of age-related cataracts. Gene products usually function in metabolic pathways. Knowing these pathways may permit the suppression or augmentation of the biochemical reactions that make the lens more susceptible to or protect it from cataracts, respectively

studies, the genes associated with the increased risk of age-related cataracts have not been identified in published studies.

Genetic risk factors may seem to present intractable barriers to treatment, especially for a common disease. However, understanding the genetics of age-related cataract may hold significant promise for therapeutic intervention or prevention. It is not always necessary to correct a genetic alteration at the DNA level to treat a gene-based disease. It may be sufficient to understand the pathway in which the defective gene acts, then design therapies that compensate for that defect to restore the function of the pathway. Genetic studies can also identify genes and pathways that protect against age-related cataracts. Enhancing the function of the pathways that, when impaired, increase the risk of cataracts, or augmenting pathways that normally protect against cataract could provide effective means to delay cataract formation in all individuals. For these reasons, identifying the genes responsible for promoting cataract or protecting the lens from cataract represents one of the most promising areas for future advances.

Epidemiologic studies have also identified anatomic risks for cataract. In a cross-sectional analysis of participants in the Beaver Dam Eye Study, individuals with thinner lenses were at much increased risk of cortical cataract, while those with thicker lenses had significantly more nuclear cataracts.[39] Five-year follow-up of this population showed that individuals were more likely to develop cortical cataracts if their lenses were initially smaller.[40] Those with larger lenses were more likely to develop nuclear cataracts. Similar associations between lens size and cataract have been identified in cross-

sectional and prospective studies in Japan and Singapore[41] (K Nagai, K Sasaki, H Sasaki, personal communication). The reasons underlying the association between smaller (or thinner) lenses and cortical cataract have not been explored. Possible connections between larger lens size and nuclear cataract may involve the lens "diffusion barrier," discussed below in the section on the natural history of nuclear opacification.

Like lens fiber cells and the proteins within them, the vitreous gel that lies between the lens and the retina is made early in life and is never regenerated or replenished. Gradual collapse (also called syneresis) of the vitreous body occurs to a greater extent in older individuals, presenting increased risk of retinal detachment, macular hole, and other retinal complications.[42,43] The extent of vitreous liquefaction varies greatly in older individuals.[42,44] Those with a more liquefied vitreous are at increased risk of nuclear cataracts.[44,45] The increase in the length of the eye that occurs in high myopia (severe near-sightedness) is associated with early degeneration of the vitreous body and increased risk of nuclear cataract.[41,46-48] The possible physiologic relationship between the structure of the vitreous body and nuclear cataract is discussed below in the section on oxygen and cataracts.

Pathophysiology of age-related cataract

Oxidative damage

All cataracts involve damage of lens cells and/or lens proteins, leading to increased light scattering and opacification. Much of this damage can be traced, directly or indirectly, to oxidative or free radical-mediated effects. However, it has been difficult to show that oxidative damage initiates human cataract formation, rather than being the final "executioner" of transparency. In fact, the lens appears to be remarkably well protected from oxidative stress. It is essential to discover how these protective mechanisms are broken down or overcome to understand cataract etiology. We discuss some of the likely causes for different types of age-related cataracts, linking them to oxidative or free radical damage when appropriate.

Sunlight, aging, and cortical cataracts

Although exposure to higher levels of sunlight over a lifetime is one of the best-validated environmental risks of cortical cataract, the mechanism by which light exposure contributes to cortical opacities in humans is not understood. We do not know if sunlight has its effect by damaging DNA, inhibiting enzyme activity, decreasing protein stability, increasing lipid oxidation, or some combination of these. We do not even know whether it is the direct interaction of light with the lens or another component of the anterior segment, the iris for instance, that increases cataract risk. Unlike the skin, which shows clear evidence of light-induced DNA damage in sun-exposed areas,[49,50] no similar "signature" of light damage has been identified in cortical cataracts. Paradoxically, the equatorial region of the lens, where cortical cataracts originate, is better protected from light exposure than regions that show no apparent susceptibility to sunlight-induced cataract, like the nucleus. Dark iris color, which might be expected to protect the lens from light exposure, has been identified as a risk factor for cortical cataracts in some studies,[26,51] although not in others.[52,53] Lack of understanding of the causal chain between sunlight exposure and cortical cataract formation in humans makes it difficult to speculate whether there are biochemical similarities between the cause of sunlight-induced cortical cataracts and the cortical cataracts that are associated with smaller lens size, diabetes, or genetic variation. Each of these disparate risk factors may contribute separately to cortical cataract or may be connected through an, as yet, unidentified mechanism.

An alternative view of cortical cataract formation is based on the frequent occurrence of these cataracts at the onset of presbyopia. Shearing force between the soft cortex and stiffer nucleus, generated during attempted accommodation in the increasingly presbyopic eye, could cause local rupture of cortical fiber cells.[54–57] This initially focal damage then spreads along damaged fiber cells and to nearby fiber cells, leading to the spoke-like pattern of damage that is often seen in cortical opacities. If this view is correct, it can be related to the epidemiologic risk factors for cortical cataracts. The increased glycation of lens proteins seen in diabetics might further stiffen nuclear fiber cells or weaken cortical fiber cells. Smaller lens size might be associated with higher strain on the lens during disaccommodation, as the zonules of smaller lenses could be more taut. High sunlight exposure could exacerbate the hardening of the lens nucleus, thereby indirectly contributing to cortical cataracts without exposing the cortical cells to light. Further tests of this view of cortical cataract formation seem warranted.

Diabetes and cataract

Diabetes is one of the most widely recognized risk factors for age-related cataracts, although other diabetic complications are more clinically significant.[30,58–60] Rapid-onset, uniformly distributed cortical opacities are seen in patients or experimental animals with acute hyperglycemia. While this type of opacity is important because it may alert patients to the need for treatment, it is not the typical presentation for diabetic patients with reasonably well-controlled blood glucose.[30] In general, diabetics have earlier-onset opacities than nondiabetics. These are usually cortical or posterior subcapsular cataracts. Although nuclear cataracts can occur in diabetics, epidemiologic studies suggest that diabetes may provide modest protection against nuclear opacification.[61] Because they impair vision at an earlier stage, posterior subcapsular cataracts often account for a disproportionate percentage of cataract surgery in diabetics.[60,62]

The natural history of nuclear opacification

With increasing age, the lens nucleus gradually increases in opacity and hardness in all individuals.[63–65] When nuclear opacities become visually significant they are often called nuclear sclerotic cataracts. Thus, nuclear cataract formation can be thought of as an acceleration or exacerbation of changes that occur during aging. This is not the case for cortical and posterior subcapsular cataracts. Although more cortical and posterior subcapsular cataracts occur in older individuals, most older patients will never have even a trace of either type.[44] In this way, nuclear cataracts are fundamentally different from cortical or posterior subcapsular cataracts.

Increasing nuclear opacification correlates with a decline in reduced glutathione and an increase in the oxidized form of this important intracellular antioxidant in the lens nucleus.[66,67] Experimental depletion of glutathione causes rapid opacification of the lens.[68] Glutathione is synthesized and converted to its protective, reduced form in the metabolically active cells near the lens surface. It then diffuses through abundant gap junctions in the fiber cell membranes to the center of the lens, where it can protect lens crystallins and membrane proteins from oxidation. Once glutathione is oxidized, it diffuses down its concentration gradient to the lens surface, where it can again be reduced (Figure 30.3). This glutathione cycle slows with age, due to a decrease in the apparent viscosity of the lens cytoplasm, appearing as a diffusion barrier between cells at the lens surface and the nucleus[69,70] The resulting decrease in access of reduced glutathione to the nucleus places the proteins there at greater risk of oxidative damage. It is likely that this decline in antioxidant capacity contributes to the age-related increase in opacification and hardening of the nucleus, seen in virtually all lenses. Other antioxidant systems may decline with aging,[71,72] possibly contributing to increased risk of nuclear cataract.

Oxygen, the vitreous body and nuclear cataracts

During hyperbaric oxygen (HBO) therapy, patients breathe pure oxygen at two or more times atmospheric pressure. This is likely to cause oxygen levels around the lens to increase dramatically, since intraocular oxygen levels increase greatly when patients breathe 100% oxygen at normal pressure.[73] If HBO treatment is protracted, the refractive power of the lens increases, causing a "myopic shift."[74–76] This effect may reverse after therapy is discontinued.[74,77] If therapy persists for over a year, the lens develops increased nuclear opacity or frank nuclear cataract.[74] In these cases, it appears that exposure to elevated oxygen causes rapid hardening of the lens, the presumed cause of the myopic shift[76] and progression to nuclear cataracts (Box 30.4). Both are typical properties of age-related nuclear cataracts. However, these pathological changes occur more rapidly after HBO treatment than during aging.

The lens normally exists in a hypoxic environment.[73,78–80] Given the demonstrated toxicity of oxygen to the lens, it is worth considering how the low level of oxygen around the lens is maintained. Recent measurements in patients undergoing cataract or glaucoma surgery revealed that oxygen levels in the posterior chamber, the space between the ciliary epithelium, iris, and lens, and in the anterior chamber, at the anterior surface of the lens, are also usually less than 1% (Siegfried et al, unpublished results). In rabbits and

235

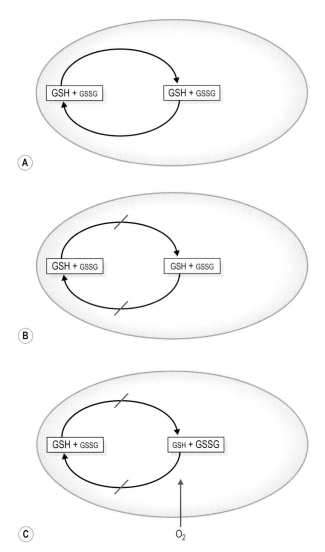

Box 30.4 The vitreous body, oxygen, and nuclear cataracts

The lens is normally in a severely hypoxic environment, which is likely to protect its constituents from oxidative damage. Exposure to excess oxygen causes nuclear opacification. Degeneration or destruction of the vitreous gel, as occurs with aging or after vitrectomy, exposes the lens to more oxygen and increases the risk of nuclear cataracts. Preservation or replacement of the vitreous gel or interventions that preserve the hypoxic environment around the lens are likely to reduce the prevalence or progression of nuclear cataracts

Figure 30.3 Diagrams representing the distribution of reduced (GSH) glutathione, and its oxidized form (GSSG) in young and older lenses and the hypothetical role of oxygen in altering the ratio of these metabolites in the lens nucleus. (A) The distribution of GSH and GSSG in young lenses. (B) The distribution of GSH and GSSG in older lenses. (C) The distribution of GSH and GSSG in older lenses exposed to increased oxygen. Oxygen or its metabolites diffuse from the vitreous body to the center of the lens, reducing GSH and increasing GSSG, which is postulated to lead to nuclear opacification. The red bars in (B) and (C) represent the barrier to diffusion resulting from the increased viscosity of the lens cytoplasm that occurs with age.

humans, oxygen levels in the vitreous body at the posterior of the lens are normally very low, ~1% or less.[78] These measurements suggest that oxygen levels are already low in freshly secreted aqueous humor, placing the entire anterior of the lens in a hypoxic environment. They also suggest that the vitreous body protects the lens from exposure to the higher levels of oxygen found near the surface of the retinal vessels.[81,82]

Diverse studies suggest that the gel structure and biochemical activities of the vitreous body protect the human lens from oxygen and the formation of nuclear cataracts. As indicated above, severe myopia is associated with early degeneration of the vitreous body and increased risk of nuclear cataract.[41,48,83] Examination of eyes postmortem

showed that the level of vitreous degeneration varied greatly in older individuals.[42,44] Increased liquefaction of the vitreous body was associated with increased nuclear opacification, but not with other types of cataract.[44] Many studies have shown that removal of the vitreous body during retinal surgery (vitrectomy) leads to the formation of nuclear cataracts within 2 years in 60–98% of older individuals.[84–88] However, if retinal surgery is performed without damaging the structure of the vitreous body, there is no detectable increase in nuclear opacification.[89] Oxygen levels near the lens increase dramatically during vitrectomy and remain significantly elevated for years after destruction of the vitreous gel.[73] Recent studies showed that the vitreous body metabolizes oxygen in a reaction that is dependent on the high level of ascorbate (vitamin C) that is normally present there. Vitrectomy and the slower degeneration of the vitreous gel seen during aging are associated with decreased levels of ascorbate, decreased ability of the vitreous to consume oxygen and increased risk of nuclear cataract.[90] Therefore, the gel structure of the vitreous body appears to maintain low oxygen levels at the posterior of the lens and protects the lens against nuclear cataract. A model that provides a possible explanation for the protective effect of the vitreous gel is shown in Figure 30.4.

Recent studies showed that elevating the level of oxygen around the rodent lens markedly increases its rate of growth, especially in older individuals.[91] If a similar relationship between oxygen and lens growth exists in humans, the increased oxygen levels that accompany the degeneration of the vitreous body could lead to larger lenses. Summarizing from the data mentioned above, larger lens size is associated with increased risk of nuclear cataract. Oxygen exposure causes a myopic shift, similar to that which occurs early in the formation of a nuclear cataract. In these cases, the myopic shift is probably due to hardening of the lens, thereby increasing its refractive power. Hardening of the lens decreases the rate of diffusion from the lens surface to the nucleus. Larger lens size and decreased diffusion through lens cytoplasm should reduce the level of reduced glutathione in the lens nucleus, thereby hastening nuclear opacification (Figure 30.3). It seems possible that exposing the lens to increased oxygen accelerates nuclear cataract formation by directly causing oxidative damage and/or by making the lens more susceptible to oxidative damage.

If the vitreous gel protects the lens against nuclear cataract formation, it follows that factors that promote the stability of the vitreous body could decrease the risk of nuclear cata-

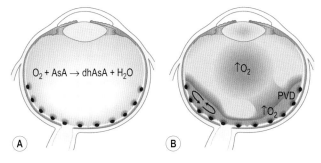

Figure 30.4 Diagram illustrating the proposed effect of vitreous degeneration on the distribution of oxygen in the eye. (A) The vitreous gel is intact, there are standing gradients of oxygen near the retinal vessels, and some of the oxygen that diffuses into the vitreous gel is consumed by reacting with ascorbate (AsA). The ultimate products of this reaction are dehydroascorbate (dhAsA) and its eventual degradation products and water. After extensive vitreous liquefaction (B) due to syneresis of the vitreous gel, the vitreous separates from the retina (posterior vitreous detachment; PVD), allowing fluid to circulate in the fluid-filled spaces at the surface of the retina and within the liquid parts of the vitreous body. This overwhelms the ability of ascorbate to maintain low oxygen, increases the Po_2 near the lens, and results in nuclear cataract formation.

ract. This makes it important to understand why the vitreous body degenerates at an early age in some individuals and remains intact in others. Some of the hereditary risk of nuclear cataracts might result from genetic variations that promote the early degeneration of the vitreous gel. Smoking might increase the risk of nuclear cataracts by promoting vitreous degeneration, although this possibility has not been examined. In summary, interventions that preserve or restore the mechanical and biochemical properties of the vitreous body should protect against age-related nuclear cataract.

Summary and conclusions

Age-related cataract is at least three different diseases. Each occurs in different locations in the lens, involves a distinct pathogenic mechanism, and is associated with different risk factors. Although several common environmental risk factors have been identified, each appears to contribute to a relatively small fraction of the total cataract burden. Heredity plays a major role in the risk of age-related cataract. Identifying the genes involved may lead to treatments that augment or suppress the pathways in which these genes function. Much research has centered on the potential role of oxidative stress and sunlight in cataract etiology. Greater sunlight exposure accounts for only a small percentage of cortical cataracts and constitutes little or no risk for the other types. Little evidence has been offered for increased oxidative stress as an inciting factor in cortical or posterior subcapsular cataract. Anatomic changes with aging, particularly hardening of the lens nucleus and degeneration of the vitreous body, provide insight to the etiology of nuclear cataracts and suggest interventions for their prevention. Closer collaboration between basic scientists, clinicians, epidemiologists, and geneticists could help clarify the etiology of age-related cataracts and provide the first steps toward delaying or preventing them.

Acknowledgments

Support for the authors' research was provided by Research to Prevent Blindness, the Department of Ophthalmology and Visual Sciences, the Barnes Retina Institute Research Fund, and NIH grants EY015863, EY04853, and core grant EY02687.

Key references

A complete list of chapter references is available online at www.expertconsult.com. See inside cover for registration details.

17. AREDS. A randomized, placebo-controlled, clinical trial of high-dose supplementation with vitamins C and E and beta carotene for age-related cataract and vision loss: AREDS report no. 9. Arch Ophthalmol 2001;119:1439–1452.

26. AREDS. Risk factors associated with age-related nuclear and cortical cataract: a case-control study in the Age-Related Eye Disease Study, AREDS report no. 5. Ophthalmology 2001;108:1400–1408.

27. West SK, Duncan DD, Munoz B, et al. Sunlight exposure and risk of lens opacities in a population-based study: the Salisbury Eye Evaluation project. JAMA 1998;280:714–718.

30. Bron AJ, Sparrow J, Brown NA, et al. The lens in diabetes. Eye 1993;7:260–275.

34. Hammond CJ, Duncan DD, Snieder H, et al. The heritability of age-related cortical cataract: the Twin Eye Study. Invest Ophthalmol Vis Sci 2001;42:601–605.

35. Hammond CJ, Snieder H, Spector TD, et al. Genetic and environmental factors in age-related nuclear cataracts in monozygotic and dizygotic twins. N Engl J Med 2000;342:1786–1790.

40. Klein BE, Klein R, Moss SE. Lens thickness and five-year cumulative incidence of cataracts: The Beaver Dam Eye Study. Ophthalm Epidemiol 2000;7:243–248.

44. Harocopos GJ, Shui Y-B, McKinnon M, et al. Importance of vitreous liquefaction in age-related cataract. Invest Ophthalmol Vis Sci 2004;45:77–85.

55. Michael R, Barraquer RI, Willekens B, et al. Morphology of age-related cuneiform cortical cataracts: the case for mechanical stress. Vision Res 2008;48:626–634.

64. Heys KR, Cram SL, Truscott RJ. Massive increase in the stiffness of the human lens nucleus with age: the basis for presbyopia? Mol Vis 2004;10:956–963.

67. Truscott RJW. Age-related nuclear cataract – oxidation is the key. Exp Eye Res 2004;80:709–725.

73. Holekamp NM, Shui YB, Beebe DC. Vitrectomy surgery increases oxygen exposure to the lens: a possible mechanism for nuclear cataract formation. Am J Ophthalmol 2005;139: 302–310.

74. Palmquist BM, Philipson B, Barr PO. Nuclear cataract and myopia during hyperbaric oxygen therapy. Br J Ophthalmol 1984;68:113–117.

89. Sawa M, Ohji M, Kusaka S, et al. Nonvitrectomizing vitreous surgery for epiretinal membrane: long-term follow-up. Ophthalmology 2005;112: 1402–1408.

90. Shui et al. Arch Ophthalmol (in press)

CHAPTER 31

Posterior capsule opacification

Judith West-Mays and Heather Sheardown

Clinical background

Cataract, a pathology of the ocular lens, is the leading cause of blindness worldwide despite the availability of effective surgery in developed countries.[1,2] According to the World Health Organization,[1,2] up to 40 million people are blind worldwide, and of these, 47% of them are blind due to cataract. A total of 82% of the blind are more than 50 years of age. Thus, the number of blind people worldwide, and likely those with cataracts, is expected to increase further as the population ages. Cataract surgery provides quick restoration of vision and is the most frequently performed surgical procedure in the developed world.[3] However, it is not without its problems and can lead to a number of complications, the most common of which is secondary cataract, also known as posterior capsular opacification (PCO).[4-7]

Modern cataract surgery, also known as extracapsular cataract extraction (ECCE), involves removing a circular anterior portion of the lens capsule, breaking up and removing the fiber mass it contains, and placing a synthetic lens implant (intraocular lens: IOL) into the remaining capsular bag (Figure 31.1). This newer procedure replaced intracapsular cataractous lens extraction (ICCE), in which the whole lens and capsule were removed and often resulted in a number of significant complications, including retinal detachment and macular edema.[8,9] ECCE avoids such complications, yet frequently leaves behind lens epithelial cells (LECs) on the remaining portion of the anterior capsule; these cells can proliferate, transdifferentiate, and migrate on to the otherwise cell-free zone of the posterior capsule surface (Figure 31.1; Box 31.1). Here the cells deposit aberrant matrix and also cause capsular wrinkling, two important features of PCO.[7] Both of these events obstruct or alter the path of light entering the eye by decreasing the amount of available light, decreasing contrast and color intensity, and increasing light scatter, culminating in a reduction in visual acuity[10] (Figure 31.1). The time between surgery and PCO development varies considerably, ranging from a few months to 4 years.[8] Interestingly, the visual symptoms do not always correlate with the degree of PCO observed, and some patients with significant PCO as determined by slit-lamp examination are less symptomatic as compared to others who have only mild haze observed.[8]

PCO was diagnosed following the beginnings of ECCE surgery and was fairly common in these early days (late 1970s and early 1980s) with incidence in up to 50% of patients.[11] Advances in IOL design and surgical technique over the last 20 years have resulted in a dramatic reduction in reported PCO rates, to occurrence in 14–18% of patients.[6,7] However, PCO remains a major medical problem with profound consequences for the patient's well-being and is a significant financial burden due to the costs of follow-up treatment. The most common postoperative treatment for PCO is neodymium-doped yttrium aluminum garnet (Nd-YAG) posterior capsulotomy.[8] This treatment involves using the Nd-YAG laser to cut an opening in the posterior capsule to clear the visual axis and restore vision. Complications, although rare, include IOL damage and pitting, postoperative IOP elevation, cystoid macular edema, retinal detachment, and IOL subluxation. Access to this procedure is also not widely available in developing countries.[8]

Pathology

The intact lens is composed of an anterior monolayer of epithelial cells (referred to earlier as LECs) and an underlying fiber cell population, making it a relatively simple tissue (Figure 31.2). The lens continues to grow throughout life, albeit at a much slower rate in the adult. This continued growth is attributed primarily to the proliferation of the LECs in the germinative zone of the lens, a region just anterior to the lens equator.[12] In PCO, LECs from the anterior and equatorial regions left behind after surgery have the capacity to survive, proliferate, and transdifferentiate. Cells derived from the anterior lens epithelium, referred to as "A cells," are those thought to transdifferentiate into spindle-shaped myofibroblasts, through a process known as epithelial-to-mesenchymal transformation (EMT) (Figure 31.2). These myofibroblasts express contractile elements such as alpha-smooth-muscle actin (α-SMA), and are therefore thought to contribute to the capsular wrinkling detected in PCO.[13,14] Unlike epithelial cells, myofibroblasts also stop producing type IV collagen and the highly organized crystallin proteins and begin to secrete abnormal amounts of extracellular matrix (ECM) proteins, including type I and type III collagen. The abnormal ECM deposition contributes to the capsular fibrosis observed in PCO.

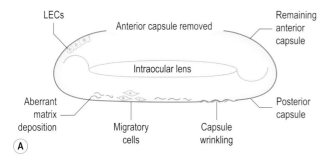

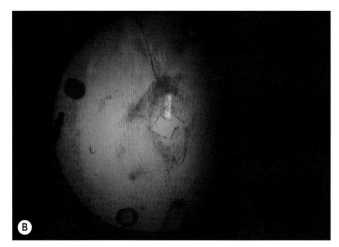

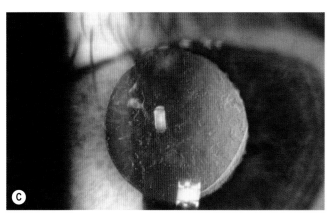

Figure 31.1 (A) Schematic diagram of the capsular bag with an implanted intraocular lens (IOL) following surgery. Remaining lens epithelial cells (LECs) on the anterior lens capsule can proliferate, transition, and then migrate to the posterior capsule where they multilayer and deposit aberrant matrix. (Modified from Wormstone IM. Posterior capsule opacification: a cell biological perspective. Exp Eye Res 2002;74:337–347.) (B) The clinical appearance of a posterior capsular opacity as viewed through the slit-lamp biomicroscope. (Courtesy of Mike Feifarek, MD.) (C) Appearance of posterior capsular opacification with retroillumination. (Courtesy of Rakesh Ahuja, MD.)

In PCO, the "E cells" are those derived from the pre-equatorial region of the lens. Although fibrosis may also occur in these cells, they have a stronger tendency to form "epithelial pearls" (also called Elschnig pearls) in which the cells transform into swollen and opacified cells known as "bladder cells" or "Wedl cells" that do not express α-SMA and are considered to be LECs attempting to form fiber cells.[8,13] Thus, clinically, two morphological types of PCO have been documented, including wrinkling and fibrosis of

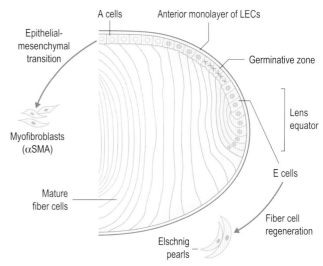

Figure 31.2 Schematic diagram of the adult mammalian lens. The germinative zone, just anterior to the lens equator, is where the majority of the active proliferation takes place in the adult lens. Following cataract surgery, cells from the anterior monolayer, referred to as "A cells," are those thought to undergo epithelial to mesenchymal transition into myofibroblasts, expressing alpha-smooth-muscle actin (αSMA). The "E cells" are derived from the pre-equatorial region of the lens and tend to transition into fiber-like cells, referred to as Elschnig pearls. LECs, lens epithelial cells.

Box 31.1 Clinical background

- The most common complication of primary cataract surgery is secondary cataract, also known as, posterior capsular opacification (PCO)
- PCO results from lens epithelial cells remaining on the anterior capsule following cataract surgery; these cells migrate on to the posterior capsule, deposit aberrant matrix, and cause capsular wrinkling

---

the capsule, from the transformed A cells, and epithelial pearls from improper proliferation and differentiation of E cells. The former phenomenon is often referred to as fibrotic PCO, whereas the latter is called regeneratory PCO.

Etiology

As discussed above, considerable evidence has shown that the LECs remaining after cataract surgery are the cells that contribute to the development of PCO. The histology surrounding these cells has been relatively well documented. However, knowledge regarding the mechanisms that lead to their survival and fibrotic phenotype is more limited. What is clear is that age plays an important role in the incidence of PCO, with patients over the age of 40 having a significantly lower incidence than those under 40 (Box 31.2).[8,15,16] Furthermore, in pediatric patients PCO occurrence is nearly universal if the posterior capsule is left intact, as is the case in ECCE surgery. This difference may be related to the role of inflammation in PCO, since children and younger patients typically have a more marked inflammatory response after cataract surgery. Another contributing factor may be that the LECs in younger patients produce more autocrine growth factors that stimulate their survival and fibrotic phenotype.[7] The potential consequences of these factors are discussed in greater detail in the next section on pathophysiology.

Changes in surgical technique and design and placement of IOLs have been important in minimizing PCO. Surgical improvements include the implementation of hydrodissection-enhanced cortical cleanup, a technique allowing for more efficient removal of the cortex and LECs, and placement of the IOL in the capsular bag such that direct contact is made with the posterior capsule.[17] A surgical approach, referred to as continuous curvilinear capsulorrhexis (CCC), has aided with the IOL placement. In this case, a continuous circular tear is made in the anterior capsule of the cataractous lens to allow for phacoemulsification (surgical breakup) and removal of the lens material, while maintaining the integrity of the posterior capsule. The diameter of the CCC incision is slightly smaller than that of the IOL inserted such that a tight fit is made, sequestering the IOL in the bag from the surrounding aqueous humor.[3,8] This type of placement of the IOL is thought to act as a barrier, preventing the edge of the anterior capsule from adhering and fusing to the posterior capsule. It is also thought to prevent the posterior capsule from being exposed to any inflammatory or fibrotic mediators in the aqueous humor. The development of newer surgical techniques is also being considered, such as primary posterior capsulorrhexis, which would prophylactically eliminate the possibility of PCO.

Considerations for the IOL design have also been important for minimizing PCO. Numerous studies have examined the role of IOL materials, both the optic and the haptic, on the development of PCO. Foldable IOL materials can be broadly categorized into three areas: silicone materials, hydrogel materials, and nonhydrogel acrylic materials. A range of materials exists in each of the categories. Regardless of the material type, however, all are susceptible to PCO to some extent and as a result a number of clinical studies have examined the role of IOL material in PCO development. While material specific effects have been shown in some cases, there are a number of contradictions in the literature and it is far from clear whether one material is superior to the others with respect to PCO prevention. Much of the contradiction has occurred due to the lack of appropriate controls, and that factors such as lens design were not kept constant in these studies. The work of Nishi et al[18,19] suggests that the effects of materials are much less significant than design effects. However, there are some limited data suggesting that silicone IOLs may have lower PCO rates than acrylic.[20]

The majority of recent studies have focused on IOL design effects. The observation that the incorporation of a square edge in an acrylic IOL[21] results in a significantly lower incidence of PCO has led to significant changes in lens design.

Implantation of sharp-edged IOLs causes postoperative capsular bag closure, fusion, and wrapping of the bag around the optic periphery, resulting in the tight apposition of the posterior capsule along the posterior optic rim. This barricades lens epithelial cell migration, effectively inhibiting PCO caused by migration and proliferation of residual lens cells into the area between the lens capsule and the IOL.

The effect of incorporating a square edge has been shown for various materials, including silicones[20] and polymethyl methacrylate (PMMA).[22] Results also suggest that an edge effect is present in acrylic lens materials,[23,24] although the effect is less clear with these materials.[25] The work of Hayashi and Hayashi[26] suggests that an anterior round edge and a posterior square edge are particularly advantageous. There is some controversy, however, as to whether the square-edged IOLs lead to an increased incidence of anterior capsular contraction (ACC), which can hinder postoperative procedures such as fundoscopy, retinal photocoagulation, and vitreal surgery.[27,28] The area of anterior capsule opening (ACO), related to ACC, has in fact been shown to be independent of the incidence and severity of PCO.[26]

Surface modification of IOL materials is used to improve lens properties for various reasons, including to allow for ease of insertion and to reduce tackiness (Box 31.3). Modification of the IOL materials has also been used as a method of reducing PCO. Modification with cell-resistant polymers, such as polyethylene oxide[29] and poly methacryoyloxyethyl phosphorylcholine (MPC),[30] provided in vitro results suggesting that adhesion of lens cells is inhibited. However, others have demonstrated that polyethylene glycol (PEG) coatings, even at high density, are not sufficient to inhibit completely protein adsorption or cell adhesion.[31,32] Various patents have examined the modification of IOL materials with materials which can lead to interactions with the lens capsule. These include tackiness coatings,[33] functional end groups which react with the components of the capsule,[34] and biological glues to stimulate adhesion to the lens capsule.

Pathophysiology

Primary cataract surgery often results in a breach of the blood–aqueous barrier and a subsequent influx of inflammatory cells, erythrocytes, and other cell types into the aqueous humor. A consequence of this is a reported increase in the protein levels in the aqueous humor. In fact, some proteins are only detected in the aqueous humor following such trauma to the eye.[7] The implanted IOL can also elicit an inflammatory response as a foreign body and thereby further contribute to the increased cellularity and protein content in the aqueous humor following surgery.[7,13] The production of these proteins/peptides, namely growth factors and cytokines, has been the focus of much of the research related to PCO. Numerous studies using multiple models have therefore been aimed at determining which factors control the pathophysiological features of PCO, namely LEC proliferation, migration, and EMT.

Transforming growth factor-ß (TGF-ß), specifically isoforms 1 and 2, is detected in the aqueous humor under normal circumstances, mainly in their latent forms, whereas the active forms have been detected in the ocular media from patients following cataract surgery.[35,36] TGF-ß 1 and 2 can affect multiple cellular processes, including cell adhesion, proliferation, apoptosis, migration, and fibrosis.[37,38] In particular, it is the strong association of TGF-ß with fibrosis that has caused increased attention regarding the role that it may play in promoting PCO. Multiple models have been developed to investigate this, many of which involve the seeding of LECs on to structures such as Plexiglas, plastic, or bovine capsules with or without IOLs to determine their effects on proliferation and migration.[39,40] A capsular bag model similar to that produced in vivo following cataract surgery has also been developed to monitor LEC migration as it occurs during PCO from the anterior equatorial margin on to the posterior capsule.[41–43] Other derivations of this capsular bag model have been undertaken by Wormstone et al[44] and Saxby et al.[45] Importantly, utilizing their capsular bag model, Wormstone et al[14] were able to demonstrate that addition of TGF-ß accelerated LEC transformation and capsule wrinkling, both of which are thought to induce light scattering. Furthermore, co-culturing with an anti-TGF-ß antibody (CAT-152) suppressed TGF-ß-induced development of PCO, implicating TGF-ß in its etiology.[14]

Additional support for the involvement of TGF-ß in PCO includes the fact that connective tissue growth factor (CTGF), a factor closely associated with TGF-ß, has been detected in human postmortem capsular bags.[46] TGF-β has been shown to induce CTGF and CTGF on its own has been shown to induce EMT, reminiscent of that induced by TGF-β (Box 31.4). Thus, CTGF may serve as mediator of TGF-β's effects on LECs and may play a prominent role in PCO; however this has yet to be confirmed.

Basic fibroblast growth factor (FGF-2) and acidic FGF (FGF-1) are additional growth factors detected in the ocular media bathing the lens and are known to regulate normal lens structure and function. FGF-2 has been shown to stimulate LEC proliferation, migration, and differentiation in vitro.[47] These three different cellular responses to FGF occur in a sequential fashion as the concentration of FGF is increased. For example, when LEC explants from the rat lens are cultured with a lower concentration of FGF, LEC proliferation is induced whereas a higher concentration of FGF stimulates differentiation of LECs into lens fiber cells.[47] Interestingly, an FGF concentration gradient is evident in

Box 31.4 Pathophysiology

- Primary cataract surgery often results in an influx of inflammatory cells, erythrocytes, and other cell types into the aqueous humor and an accompanying increase in the production of autocrine and paracrine growth factors and cytokines, including transforming growth factor-β (TGF-β, fibroblast growth factor (FGF), epidermal growth factor (EGF), hepatocyte growth factor (HGF) and connective tissue growth factor)
- TGF-β accelerates lens epithelial cell (LEC) transformation and causes capsule wrinkling
- FGF has been shown to exacerbate the ability of TGF-β to induce posterior capsular opacification (PCO) by promoting LEC survival
- Like FGF, HGF and EGF have been shown to regulate LEC proliferation and likely act together with FGF to promote LEC proliferation during PCO

Box 31.5 Matrix metalloproteinases (MMPs) and posterior capsular opacification (PCO)

- MMPs are a family of zinc-dependent matrix-degrading enzymes, involved in multiple fibrotic diseases, with emerging roles in a variety of cataract phenotypes, including PCO
- Broad-spectrum and specific MMP inhibitors (MMPIs) have been shown to suppress the development of PCO effectively in an vitro animal model setting

vivo with lower levels in the aqueous humor and higher levels in the vitreous humor.[47] Thus, the concentration of FGF in the aqueous is thought to stimulate LEC proliferation. Indeed, FGF has been shown to exacerbate the ability of TGF-ß to induce PCO in vitro, and this is thought to occur due to the fact that FGF promotes LEC survival by counteracting the apoptotic effects of TGFß.[48,49]

Hepatocyte growth factor (HGF) and its receptor, c-met, have been found to be expressed in human postmortem capsular bags and LECs remaining on the anterior and posterior capsules showed elevated levels following surgical trauma.[7] Like FGF, HGF has also been shown to regulate LEC proliferation and likely acts together with FGF to promote LEC proliferation during PCO. Similarly, the application of epidermal growth factor (EGF) to LECs has been shown to induce proliferation. In some cases, EGF was also found to induce LECs to differentiate into lens fiber-like lentoid bodies in vitro, which could have relevance to the appearance of regenerated lens fiber cells observed in the capsular bag in some cases of PCO.

The matrix metalloproteinases (MMPs) are a family of zinc-dependent matrix-degrading enzymes, involved in multiple diseases, including fibrosis, and emerging roles in a variety of cataract phenotypes, including PCO (Box 31.5).[50] In particular, the gelatinases, MMP-2 and MMP-9, have been shown to be induced by TGF-ß in capsular bags.[14,51] Studies that directly test whether MMPs promote PCO include that in which the broad-spectrum MMP inhibitor, GM6001, was shown to inhibit LEC migration significantly on human donor lens capsules.[51] A significant reduction in capsular contraction was also observed in the GM6001-treated capsular bags. The ability of MMPIs to prevent another related, fibrotic cataract, anterior subcapsular cataract (ASC), has also been shown. Like PCO, ASC involves a transformation and proliferation of LECs and an aberrant deposition of matrix beneath the anterior lens capsule. A common model of ASC, employing excised rat lenses cultured with active TGF-β, was used to provide further evidence for a causative role(s) for MMPs in the development of ASC: Dwivedi and colleagues[52] showed that co-treatment of excised rat lenses with TGF-β and either of two commercially available MMP inhibitors (MMPIs), GM6001, a broad MMPI, or a MMP2/9-specific inhibitor, significantly suppressed formation of the cataractous plaques typically observed in ASC.

As outlined above, the cellular changes that occur in PCO are likely regulated in a paracrine manner by factors in the ocular media. Interestingly, while the levels of these factors peak shortly after cataract surgery, and typically return to basal levels within a few weeks or months, PCO can develop years after.[53] This suggests that the events contributing to PCO persist after the initial exposure to paracrine factors. Thus, it is proposed that autocrine signals from the LECs themselves also contribute to PCO. Indeed, it has been shown using a human capsular bag model that LECs cultured in serum-free media, and devoid of any proteins/peptides, proliferate well on the capsule.[44] Candidate autocrine signaling systems in the capsular bag include those normally expressed in the native lens epithelium, including EGF and its receptor EGFR, FGF and the FGF receptor 1, and also HGF and the c-met receptor.[7]

In summary, significant progress has been made in identifying the factors that contribute to the development of PCO. While surgical and IOL improvements have significantly minimized the incidence of PCO, it still remains an important problem. A number of pharmacological antagonists have thus been explored, including agents that affect cell growth, such as ethylenediaminetetraacetic acid (EDTA), and thapsigargin, as well as those that inhibit multiple aspects of PCO, including LEC proliferation, migration, EMT, and capsular contraction, such as the MMPIs, and the proteosome inhibitor, MG132.[51,54–56] However, to date, agents that inhibit PCO have not gone beyond phase I clinical trials (Box 31.6). Delivery of these agents is likely to be a key factor in their success in the clinic. Potential delivery mechanisms include injection into the anterior chamber or incorporation of the agent into the irrigation solution used during surgery, or modification of the IOL. The most promising of these appears to be delivery from an IOL, which offers the advantage of controlled release of the modulating agent and perhaps reduced toxicity to surrounding ocular tissues. Of course an important requirement for this type of delivery system would be that, following incorporation of the agent in the IOL, the optic of the IOL would need to retain its transparency.

Box 31.6 Treatment

- A number of pharmacological antagonists to posterior capsular opacification have been explored but none has gone beyond phase I clinical trials
- Delivery of these agents is likely to be a key factor in their success in the clinic
- The most promising is delivery from an intraocular lens, which offers the advantage of controlled release of the modulating agent and perhaps reduced toxicity to surrounding ocular tissues

---

Key references

A complete list of chapter references is available online at www.expertconsult.com. See inside cover for registration details.

5. Kappelhof JP, Vrensen GF. The pathology of after-cataract. A minireview. Acta Ophthalmol 1992;(Suppl.):13–24.

7. Wormstone IM. Posterior capsule opacification: a cell biological perspective. Exp Eye Res 2002;74:337–347.

8. Pandey SK, Apple DJ, Werner L, et al. Posterior capsule opacification: a review of the aetiopathogenesis, experimental and clinical studies and factors for prevention. Ind J Ophthalmol 2004;52:99–112.

11. Apple DJ, Solomon KD, Tetz MR, et al. Posterior capsule opacification. Surv Ophthalmol 1992;37:73–116.

13. Saika S. Relationship between posterior capsule opacification and intraocular lens biocompatibility. Prog Retin Eye Res 2004;23:283–305.

14. Wormstone IM, Tamiya S, Anderson I, et al. TGF-beta2-induced matrix modification and cell transdifferentiation in the human lens capsular bag. Invest Ophthalmol Vis Sci 2002;43:2301–2308.

19. Nishi O, Nishi K, Menapace R, et al. Capsular bending ring to prevent posterior capsule opacification: 2 year follow-up. J Cataract Refract Surg 2001;27:1359–1365.

31. Chen H, Brook MA, Chen Y, et al. Surface properties of PEO-silicone composites: reducing protein adsorption. J Biomater Sci Polym Ed 2005;16:531–548.

35. Wallentin N, Wickstrom K, Lundberg C. Effect of cataract surgery on aqueous TGF-beta and lens epithelial cell proliferation. Invest Ophthalmol Vis Sci 1998;39:1410–1418.

44. Wormstone IM, Liu CS, Rakic JM, et al. Human lens epithelial cell proliferation in a protein-free medium. Invest Ophthalmol Vis Sci 1997;38:396–404.

51. Wong TT, Daniels JT, Crowston JG, et al. MMP inhibition prevents human lens epithelial cell migration and contraction of the lens capsule. Br J Ophthalmol 2004;88:868–872.

52. Dwivedi DJ, Pino G, Banh A, et al. Matrix metalloproteinase inhibitors suppress transforming growth factor-beta-induced subcapsular cataract formation. Am J Pathol 2006;168:69–79.

55. Duncan G, Wormstone IM, Liu CS, et al. Thapsigargin-coated intraocular lenses inhibit human lens cell growth. Nat Med 1997;3:1026–1028.

CHAPTER 32

Diabetes-associated cataracts

Peter F Kador

Clinical background

Diabetes mellitus (DM) is an expanding major health problem. By the year 2030, it is anticipated that the worldwide incidence of DM will roughly double to 366 million, with 75% of all diabetics residing in developing countries.[1] Diabetic adults 18 years of age and older have a 21% increased prevalence of visual impairment while those 50 years or older have a higher prevalence of vision loss from retinopathy, cataracts, and glaucoma.[2] Cataracts develop earlier and more rapidly in diabetics. According to the Wisconsin Beaver Dam Study, the Australian Blue Mountains Eye Study, the Barbados Eye Study, the French Pathologies Oculaires Liées à l'Age (POLA) Study, and the West African Countries (Ghana and Nigeria) Study, diabetics have up to a fivefold increase in the prevalence of cataracts with cortical and/or posterior subcapsular opacities, with women developing cataracts slightly more than men.[3-5]

It is anticipated that the worldwide increase in DM will lead to an upsurge of cataracts and need for cataract surgery. While cataract surgery generally results in a favorable visual outcome, the visual potential in diabetics is often less and the surgical management more complex because of pre-existent retinopathy, macular edema, or prior laser surgery.[6] Hyperglycemia along with the duration of DM are important risk factors for cataract development (Box 32.1). The risk for cataracts is reduced fivefold when children and adolescents with type 1 DM are treated with intensive insulin therapy while tight control of hyperglycemia in adults with type 2 DM lowers the need for cataract extraction.[7,8]

Pathology

Precataractous changes

Clear lenses in diabetics are often larger in size with a widened subcapsular clear zone (Box 32.2). The cortex and nucleus of these lenses are also more fluorescent due to protein glycation that is proportional to glycemic control. This fluorescence is reduced with tight control.[9] Transient refractive changes are also linked to glycemic control, with hyperglycemia primarily associated with myopia and hyperopia associated with a reduction in hyperglycemia. These changes may be linked to the lenticular accumulation of sorbitol, a sugar alcohol metabolite of glucose.[10] Sorbitol plays an osmoregulatory role in the kidney by helping cells adjust to intraluminal hyperosmolality during urinary concentration. In the lens, sorbitol may similarly diminish the dehydrational effects of increased aqueous osmolarity due to hyperglycemia.[11] Sorbitol, however, is not rapidly removed from lens cells. As a result, an osmotic gradient favoring lens hydration is formed when hyperglycemia is reduced. The osmotic differences between the lens and aqueous are accentuated by rapid decreases in blood and aqueous glucose levels and this can lead to an additional accumulation of water and hyperopia. If severe enough, these changes can result in lens opacification.

Appearance of diabetic cataracts

While hyperglycemia is the common factor in cataract development in both type 1 and 2 diabetics, the appearance of cataracts in these patients differs depending on the individual's age and the severity of the hyperglycemia (Figure 32.1). Experimental studies indicate that the appearance of diabetic cataracts is also affected by species differences, as discussed below (Figure 32.2). Clinically, the most common diabetic cataracts contain cortical and/or posterior subcapsular opacities. In children and adolescents with type 1 DM, the lenses contain numerous flaky white cortical deposits which give the appearance of a snowstorm. Alternatively, posterior subcapsular opacities with radial striae extending from the equatorial zone are present. As the opacities progress to the more advanced stages, the lens fibers become distinct with the formation of vacuoles and clefts.[12] These opacities are often referred to as "true" diabetic cataracts because they rapidly evolve bilaterally over a period of days or weeks and are osmotic in nature.[10] Cataract development in type 1 diabetics appears primarily dependent on the severity and prolonged poor control of the hyperglycemia rather than on the duration of DM.[13]

In adults, cataracts from diabetics are often difficult to differentiate from those from nondiabetics. In addition to cortical and/or posterior subcapsular opacities, adult-onset diabetic cataracts often contain nuclear sclerosis which closely resembles the typical senile cataracts of nondiabetics.[13] Comparison of posterior cortical subcapsular cataracts from elderly individuals with type 2 DM and nondiabetics shows similar morphological changes.[14] Moreover, the cataractous regions in both the diabetic and nondiabetic lenses contain similar spherical globules, which are estimated to account for most light scatter, with the remainder from fiber degeneration. Similar morphological changes have also been observed in comparisons of the inner nuclear fiber cells from diabetic and nondiabetic lenses with nuclear sclerosis. However, the epithelial cell densities are lower in cataractous lenses from diabetics compared to nondiabetics.[15]

Pathophysiology

The specific mechanism(s) of how hyperglycemia initiates human cataracts has not been established (Box 32.3). To date, sorbitol pathway hyperactivity, oxidative stress and the generation of reactive oxygen species (ROS), and nonenzymatic glycation/glycooxidation have been implicated in diabetic cataract development. These pathways are summarized in Figure 32.3.

Box 32.1 Clinical background

- Diabetics have a fivefold increase in the prevalence of cataracts with cortical and/or posterior subcapsular opacities
- The anticipated worldwide doubling of patients with diabetes by 2030 will lead to an upsurge of cataracts and need for cataract surgery
- Hyperglycemia is the primary risk factor for diabetic cataracts and its tight control reduces the risks of cataract development and progression
- Transient refractive changes can occur with hyperglycemia, primarily associated with myopia, and a reduction of hyperglycemia associated with hyperopia
- Sorbitol may serve as an osmolyte in protecting lens epithelia against dehydrational effects of hyperglycemia-increased aqueous osmolarity

---

Box 32.2 Appearance of cataracts

- Appearance of diabetic cataracts depends on age, hyperglycemia, and species
- Children and adolescents with type 1 diabetes demonstrate "snowstorm" cortical opacities or "true" osmotic cataracts where posterior subcapsular opacities with radial striae and eventually vacuoles and clefts develop
- Adults with type 2 diabetes demonstrate cortical and/or posterior subcapsular opacities, often with nuclear sclerosis, that are similar to typical senile cataracts of nondiabetics. Although morphologically similar, epithelial cell densities in cataractous lenses from diabetics are lower than those from nondiabetics

---

Box 32.3 Pathophysiology of diabetic cataracts

- The specific mechanism(s) of how hyperglycemia initiates human cataracts has not been established
- Animal studies demonstrate that sorbitol formation associated with aldose reductase (AR) activity occurs in the epithelium and superficial cortical fibers. This can initiate localized osmotic changes that trigger biochemical cascades, leading to cataract formation. Sorbitol is also produced in human epithelial cells and biochemical similarities and clinical observations have linked both AR activity and sorbitol formation with the development of diabetic cataracts
- Oxidative stress and the generation of reactive oxygen species can result from hyperglycemia-associated mitochondrial dysfunction and sorbitol accumulation-initiated endoplasmic reticular stress, both of which are localized to the lens epithelium and bow region where the endothelial cells are differentiating into lens fibers
- Protein glycation and the formation of advanced glycation end products occur in both human and animal lenses and are directly linked to the levels of hyperglycemia present. However, animal studies with aldose reductase inhibitors and the observed absence of cataracts in some diabetic animals, such as hyperglycemic mice or diabetic cats, fail to support a central role for glycation in cataract development

---

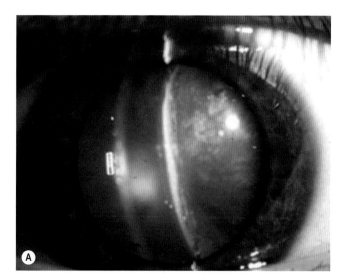 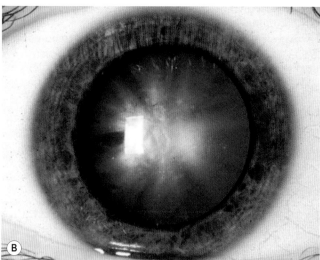

Figure 32.1 Appearance of diabetic cataracts from patients with type 1 and type 2 diabetes mellitus (DM). (A) Appearance of cataract in a 15-year-old female with type 1 DM with a fasting glucose level of 450 mg/dl. Slit-lamp examination shows markedly swollen lens with dense cortical opacities consisting of water clefts, vacuoles, and liquefied lens fibers. (Courtesy of Dr. M Datiles.) (B) Appearance of cataract in a 45-year-old female with type 2 DM showing typical radiating opacities in the cortices anteriorly and posteriorly. (Courtesy of David Cogan.)

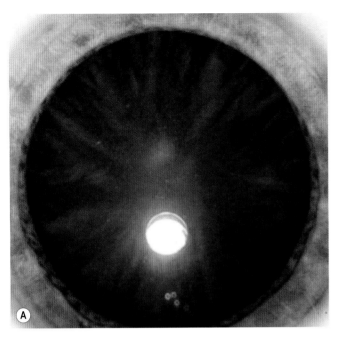

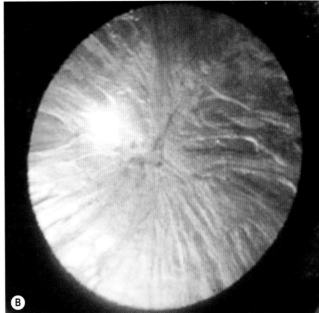

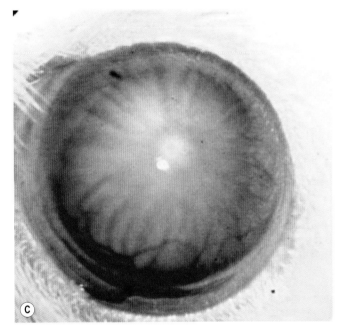

Figure 32.2 Appearance of sugar cataracts differs among different species. Shown are: (A) mature cataracts from a type 1 human with diabetes mellitus; (B) a dog fed 30% galactose diet for 38 months; and (C) a rat fed 50% galactose diet for 3 weeks.

Aldose reductase and sorbitol pathway activity

The sorbitol pathway converts glucose to fructose. In the first step, aldose reductase (AR) utilizes NADPH to reduce glucose to sorbitol. Then sorbitol dehydrogenase (SDH) using NAD^+ oxidizes sorbitol to fructose. In the lens glucose is rapidly phosphorylated by hexokinase and undergoes glycolysis. Hyperglycemia results in rapidly increased lens glucose levels because glucose uptake is insulin-independent. As a result, hexokinase becomes saturated while AR is activated through gene expression by hypertonicity changes associated with excess glucose; however, SDH is not activated. Since glucose is reduced faster than sorbitol is oxidized, the net effect is the intracellular accumulation of the osmolyte sorbi-

tol. Excess formation of sorbitol has been directly linked to the onset and progression of diabetic complications, and the clinical development of select diabetic complications has been linked to the presence of AR alleles that are associated with increased enzyme activity.[16]

The importance of AR in initiating diabetic complications such as cataracts has been experimentally established by taking advantage of the broad substrate specificity of this enzyme. In addition to glucose, AR reduces galactose to its sugar alcohol galactitol. Galactose-induced tissue changes occur faster and are more severe than glucose-induced changes.[5] This is because AR reduces galactose more rapidly than glucose and because higher intracellular levels of this osmolyte are achieved because galactitol is not further metabolized by SDH. Combining observations that similar

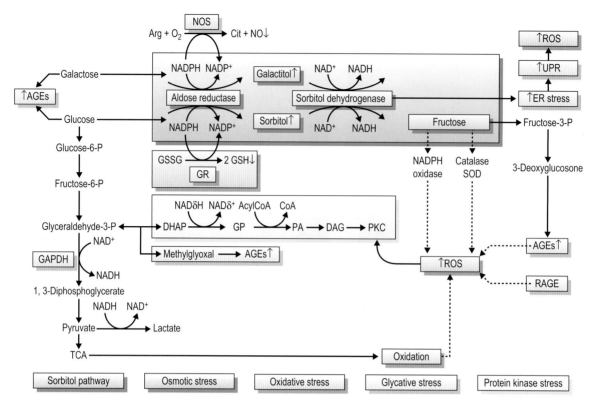

Figure 32.3 Relationship between hyperglycemia, glycolysis, polyol pathway, AGE formation, protein kinase activation and ROS generation. AGEs, advanced glycation end products; Arg, arginine; Cit, citrulline; DAG, diacylglycerol; ER Stress, endoplasmic reticulum stress; LDH, lactate dehydrogenase; DHAP, dihydroxyacetone phosphate; GP, glycerol-3-phosphate; GR, glutathione reductase; GSH, reduced glutathione; GSSG, oxidized glutathione; NO, nitric oxide O$_2$; oxygen; PA, phosphatidic acid; PKC, phosphokinase C; RAGE, receptors for advanced glycation end products; ROS, reactive oxygen species; SOD, superoxide dismutase; TCA, tricarboxylic acid cycle or citric acid cycle; UPR, unfolded protein response.

cataracts develop in diabetic and galactosemic rats and that AR is present in the lens, Kinoshita et al established that these "sugar" cataracts are initiated by the intracellular accumulation of sorbitol or galactitol.[17,18] Moreover, these authors demonstrated that the accumulation of sorbitol or galactitol results in localized lens swelling, membrane permeation, vacuole and cleft formation, intracellular biochemical changes, protein aggregation/modification, and light scatter. This is known as the osmotic hypothesis, aldose reductase hypothesis, or sorbitol hypothesis.

This hypothesis is supported by extensive studies utilizing AR inhibitors (ARIs), animal models, and in vitro lens culture studies.[18,19] Prevention studies utilizing a broad range of structurally diverse ARIs demonstrate that sugar cataracts can be dose-dependently delayed or inhibited. Animal studies show that the onset and severity of sugar cataract formation are directly linked to the levels of lens AR activity, which decreases with age.[5,20] Cataracts develop faster and are more severe in young animals and they develop faster and under milder hyperglycemic conditions in animals possessing high lens AR levels. In contrast, cataracts do not clinically appear in hyperglycemic mice where AR levels are low. However, when AR is introduced into the lenses of transgenic mice, sugar cataracts rapidly form under both diabetic and galactosemic conditions.[20,21] In vitro lens culture studies indicate that lens opacification is not only prevented by reducing lens polyol formation with ARIs, but also by preventing the formation of osmotic gradients between the lens and medium in iso-osmotic experiments.[17,19] This suggests

that lens opacification does not directly result from AR activity.

The specific mechanism(s) of how sorbitol (or galactitol) formation and increased AR activity initiate cataract formation remains unclear. While sorbitol or galactitol as osmolytes can initiate localized osmotic stress, increased flux through AR, SDH or both have also been proposed to initiate oxidative stress and generate ROS.[22] Reduced NADPH levels are associated with reduced levels of the antioxidant glutathione, the synthesis of nitric oxide (NO), and the activation of protein kinases. Since SDH only metabolizes sorbitol and not galactitol, it has also been suggested that alternate mechanisms of sugar cataract formation may occur with galactosemia linked to osmotic stress and diabetes linked to oxidative stress-associated ROS. This premise is not supported by animal studies, which show that sorbitol pathway activity is not altered by the administration of antioxidants and potent superoxide scavengers.

It has been proposed that sorbitol is formed through a free radical auto-oxidation of glucose rather than through the enzymatic reduction of glucose by AR; however, glucose auto-oxidation does not occur in the lens at physiological pH and sorbitol (or galactitol) is only enzymatically formed by AR.[13,23] Sorbitol and galactitol formation has also been linked to oxidative stress[24] and oxidative damage attributed to free radical scavenger formation has been observed in sugar cataracts . Both osmotic and oxidative stress in the lens is reduced by ARIs. Recent studies indicate that ROS is not directly generated by glucose metabolism but by the induction of endoplasmic reticular stress (ER stress) resulting from osmotic stress associated with sorbitol or galactitol formation.[25] By reducing osmotic stress, ARIs also reduce ER stress and the subsequent formation of ROS. Findings that compounds suppressing the induction of ER stress also delay sugar cataract formation support this premise.[26]

Aldose reductase and human cataracts

It is argued that sorbitol formation in the human lens is biochemically insignificant.[13] AR levels and SDH activity in the adult human lens are lower than in the adult rat lens; however, similarities between the human lens and animal models combined with recent clinical observations suggest that a role for AR cannot be ruled out. The sorbitol pathway is functional in human lens and sorbitol and galactitol accumulate in in vitro cultured human lenses and are inhibited by the addition of ARIs.[19] Sorbitol and fructose levels in lenses extracted from diabetics are also proportional to blood glucose levels at the time of extraction.[27] Moreover, cataractous lenses extracted from patients with DM accumulate higher amounts of sorbitol than cataractous lenses from nondiabetics when incubated in vitro. This suggests that AR is activated in diabetic lenses. Immunohistochemical staining for AR is also increased in lenses from diabetic versus nondiabetic patients, suggesting that AR protein levels are increased.[28] Similar increases in both immunohistochemical staining and AR activity have been observed in lenses from diabetic and galactosemic animals.[5]

The prevalence of posterior subcapsular cataracts in patients under 60 years of age with a duration of DM of 10 years has also been correlated with erythrocyte AR levels.[29] Erythrocyte AR levels have also been correlated with decreased lens epithelial cell densities in diabetics with hemoglobin A1c levels above 6.5% or with diabetic retinopathy.[30] The AR gene along with age has been reported to be an important determinant for cataract formation in type 2 diabetics.[31] Similar correlations between erythrocyte AR levels and diabetic retinopathy in type 2 diabetics[32] and

diabetic retinopathy development and increased AR activity associated with polymorphisms in the promoter region of the AR gene have been reported.[16]

Are localized osmotic changes possible in human lens?

Classical osmotic cataracts commonly develop in infants with uncontrolled galactosemia and they have been documented in cases of acute hyperglycemia in adolescent and adult diabetics. However, in older human lens sorbitol accumulation is not adequate for initiating osmotic stress over the entire lens; nevertheless, the possibility of localized osmotic stress should not be ignored. AR is localized in the epithelial cell layer and superficial fiber cells in the human, dog, and rat (Figure 32.4).[5] Specific activity of AR in the rat lens is 14-fold higher than in the dog or human lens, which are similar. In vitro cultured dog lenses primarily accumulate sorbitol in the epithelial cells and superficial cortical fibers.[33] Raman spectroscopy of diabetic rat lenses indicates that hydration is localized in primarily the lens epithelium and the bow and superficial cortical regions, but not in the nucleus.[34] Similar localized osmotic changes in the rat lens have been observed by histology. Localized osmotic changes have also been demonstrated by magnetic transfer contrast magnetic resonance imaging (MTC-MRI) in galactose-fed dog lenses.[5]

Both cultured human and dog lens epithelial cells accumulate sorbitol and when cultured in high sugar media undergo apoptosis which is inhibited by ARIs.[25,35] Lens capsules from humans and rats indicate the epithelial cell density decreases with DM and increased terminal uridine deoxynucleotidyl transferase dUTP nick end labeling (TUNEL) staining suggests that this decrease results from apoptosis. ARIs also prevented this decrease in diabetic rats.[36] In cultured human lens epithelial cells, sugar alcohol accumulation results in osmotic stress that, in turn, initiates ER stress that ultimately produces oxidative stress and ROS.[25]

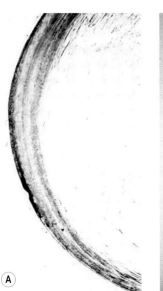

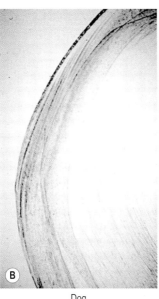

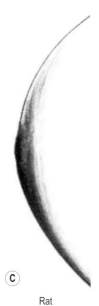

Human   Dog   Rat

Figure 32.4 Immunostaining of aldose reductase (AR) in the bow region of the human, dog, and rat lens illustrating that there is a similar distribution of the enzyme in all three lenses. AR staining was observed primarily in the epithelium and the superficial cortical fibers. Frozen sections of human lenses were treated with antibodies raised against purified human placental AR; dog with antibodies raised against purified dog lens AR; rat with antibodies raised against purified rat lens AR. The antibodies were visualized with the 3,3′-diaminobenzidine and hydrogen peroxide method (DAB-PAP). Total lens specific activity of AR with dl-glyceraldehyde as substrate was measured as human 0.39 nmol/NADPH/min/mg protein, dog 0.39 nmol/NADPH/min/mg protein, rat 5.5 nmol/NADPH/min/mg protein.

Sorbitol dehydrogenase activity

It has been suggested that SDH inhibition can ameliorate oxidative stress that leads to pseudohypoxia in diabetic tissues. In the lens, SDH inhibition actually enhances diabetic cataract formation, thus confirming the importance of sorbitol accumulation in cataract formation.[5,37]

Oxidation

ROS formation is associated with the lenticular presence of sorbitol or galactitol. Lenticular antioxidant defenses are also decreased in patients with DM. Cu, Zn-superoxide dismutase and catalase activity are significantly lower in cataractous lenses from diabetics and malondialdehyde levels, a marker of lipid peroxidation, are significantly higher. Diabetes is also associated with increased lens levels of copper and iron which can potentiate oxidative stress by participating in Fenton reactions where highly reactive hydroxyl radicals are generated from hydrogen peroxide.

Hyperglycemic-associated cellular damage may also be linked to superoxide overproduction.[38] The principal source of cellular ROS is the mitochondria and hyperglycemia-associated mitochondrial dysfunction. An alternate source of ROS, as discussed above, is the stress activation of ER. In the lens, mitochondria and ER are only found in epithelial cells and these are lost as epithelial cells differentiate into fiber cells. Therefore, ROS resulting from both hyperglycemia-induced mitochondrial dysfunction and osmotic-induced ER stress is localized to the lens epithelium and bow region where the endothelial cells are differentiating into lens fibers. Since these are the most metabolically active areas of the lens, damage to these cells is anticipated to lead to lens opacification. The observed effect of ARIs in preventing the generation of ROS under hyperglycemic conditions strongly suggests that ER stress rather than hyperglycemia-induced mitochondrial dysfunction is the primary source of ROS in the diabetic lens. Since there is no evidence that ARIs directly affect mitochondrial function, the lack of ROS generated in the presence of ARIs suggests that mitochondrial ROS production in the lens is minor.

Nonenzymatic glycation, AGE, and RAGE

Reducing sugars such as glucose can nonenzymatically react with protein amino groups to form reversible Schiff bases which rearrange to form irreversible Amadori products. The above reactions result in glycosylated hemoglobin (hemoglobin A1c) which is used as a clinical indicator of long-term hyperglycemia. Amadori products can undergo further reactions to form irreversibly cross-linked, heterogeneous fluorescent derivatives termed advanced glycation end products (AGEs). This process is accompanied by the formation of free radicals and ROS. Lens protein glycation and AGE formation are proposed to play an important role in protein modifications that result in cataract formation.[10] In addition, it has been suggested that lens cells may be disrupted by osmotic stress that is linked to glycation of lens ion pumps. Recent evidence suggests that AGEs also interact with specific soluble receptors (sRAGE). While these receptors are present in lenses, they do not appear to increase or correlate with diabetic cataract formation.[39] To date, no direct evidence demonstrating that lens glycation or AGEs directly initiates sugar cataract formation has been published. The observation that ARIs prevent sugar cataracts without reducing hyperglycemia or glycation, along with the absence of cataracts in some chronic diabetic animals such as hyperglycemic mice or diabetic cats, fails to support a central role for glycation in cataract development.[5]

Anticataract agents

Surgery is currently the only treatment for diabetic cataracts (Box 32.4). A number of pharmaceutical agents addressing the potential mechanisms of diabetic cataract formation described above have been experimentally evaluated. The results are summarized below and extensively reviewed elsewhere.[37] A number of antioxidants and aspirin are being used to treat diabetic cataracts since they are readily available over the counter or as health food supplements. Clinical observations, to date, suggest that any effect on cataract development is small and of no clinical significance.

Aldose reductase inhibitors

While animal studies demonstrate that ARIs not only delay, but actually inhibit, the development and progression of sugar cataracts in a dose-dependent manner, clinical trials evaluating ARIs on cataract development have not been conducted. It is doubtful that such a clinical trial will be conducted in the near future because the clinical time frame for diabetic cataract development has not been established. Only one ARI, epalrestat, is in clinical use. Available in Japan for the treatment of diabetic neuropathy, the potential clinical effects of ARIs on cataract may be assessed as the rate of cataract surgery is evaluated in patients administered epalrestat and future, more potent ARIs, over an extended period of years. In contrast to human cataract development, cataract formation in diabetic dogs is rapid and predictable. Currently, the topical ARI formulation Kinostat, which has been shown to reverse early sugar cataract formation,[40] is undergoing a preliminary phase I trial in diabetic dogs for the prevention of cataracts.

Antioxidants

Protection from oxidative damage and/or delayed progression of cataracts has been experimentally observed when diabetic rats were treated with antioxidant supplements that include α-lipoic acid,[41] vitamin E (α-tocopherol), its esters, vitamin E combined with vitamin C (ascorbic acid) and

---

> **Box 32.4 Treatment of cataracts**
>
> - Surgery is currently the only treatment for diabetic cataracts
> - Aldose reductase inhibitors dose-dependently inhibit the onset and progression of cataracts in animals; however, no specific clinical trials have been conducted in humans
> - A number of antioxidants have been observed to delay the progression of cataracts in diabetic animals; however, clinical observations to date suggest that any effect on cataract development is small and of no clinical significance

ß-carotene,[42] or taurine (2-aminoethanesulfonic acid), which serves as both an osmoregulator and antioxidant.[43] Carnosine (ß-alanyl-L-hystidine), and its topical prodrug formulation N-acetylcarnosine (NAC), is advertised (especially on the internet) to treat a range of ophthalmic disorders associated with oxidative stress, including age-related and diabetic cataracts.[44] No convincing animal studies or masked clinical trials have been reported. Pyruvate, a key biochemical intermediate in the glycolysis of glucose in the lens, has been reported to delay cataract formation by reducing both sorbitol levels and lipid peroxidation in diabetic rats.[45]

Glycation inhibitors

Aminoguanidine (Pimagedine) is a hydrazine derivative that reduces glycation. Aminoguanidine has been reported to delay cataract formation in mild but not severely diabetic rats or rats fed a 50% galactose-fed diet. Clinically, aminoguanidine (Pimagedine) has been evaluated on the progression of renal disease; however, two clinical trials were stopped due to lack of efficacy in diabetic kidney disease and the development of potential toxic lesions.[46] No ocular effects have been clinically reported.

Aspirin is believed to reduce glycation in lens proteins by acetylating reactive glycation sites containing ε-amino groups so that they cannot react with sugars. High concentrations of aspirin have a hypoglycemic effect and reduce AR activity. The ability of high doses of aspirin to delay cataracts in diabetic rats has been attributed to both its ability to inhibit AR and glycation. Clinical findings of aspirin on diabetic cataract are controversial. Retrospective studies suggest that cataract progression is decelerated in diabetics receiving high aspirin dosages over a number of years.[47] Several case-control studies also suggest that long-term use of aspirin-like analgesics reduces the risk of cataract in both nondiabetics and diabetics.[48] Although the Barbados Eye Study reported that aspirin reduced lens opacities in a small number of diabetic patients,[49] the largest study to date, the Early Treatment Diabetic Retinopathy Study (ETDRS) reports that aspirin did not reduce the risk of developing visually significant lens opacities.[50]

Conclusion

Cataracts that develop in humans and animals with DM differ significantly in appearance, despite the fact that their development is linked to hyperglycemia. Current hypotheses link the formation of sugar cataracts to sorbitol pathway hyperactivity, oxidative stress, and the generation of ROS and nonenzymatic glycation/glycooxidation. Experimental animal studies support a central role for AR and the generation of oxidative stress and ROS in the development of sugar cataracts. No in vivo animal data specifically link glycation or AGEs to the initiation of cataracts. The generation of ROS, polyol pathway activity, and sorbitol formation all occur in the metabolically active epithelial cell monolayer and the differentiating fiber cells at the bow and superficial cortical fiber layers. The observation linking osmotic changes to activation of ER stress and the subsequent generation of ROS provides an attractive mechanism linking AR with oxidative damage. Studies to date in the human lens have assumed that AR activity is insignificant; however, re-examination of the experimental data indicates that a localized role for AR in the human lens cannot be ruled out. More studies are needed.

There is currently no treatment for diabetic cataracts, but tight control of hyperglycemia reduces the progression of cataract development. Select antioxidants have been reported to delay the onset and progression of cataracts in animals with DM, but not in humans. Animal studies also demonstrate that ARIs not only delay, but actually inhibit, the development and progression of sugar cataracts in a dose-dependent manner. Insight into the potential of ARIs in humans may come from future studies examining the incidence of cataract surgery in patients after long-term (>5 years) use of the ARI epalrestat in Japan.

Key references

A complete list of chapter references is available online at www.expertconsult.com. See inside cover for registration details.

5. Kador PF. Ocular pathology of diabetes mellitus. In: Tasman W, Jaeger E (eds) Duane's Ophthalmology, vol. 3. Philadelphia: Wolters Kluwer/Lippicott Williams and Wilkins, 2007:1–84.

13. Bron AJ, Brown NA, Harding JJ, et al. The lens and cataract in diabetes. Int Ophthalmol Clin 1998;38:37–67.

15. Struck HG, Heider C, Lautenschlager C. [Changes in the lens epithelium of diabetic and non-diabetic patients with various forms of opacities in senile cataract.] Klin Monatsbl Augenheilkd 2000;216:204–209.

17. Kinoshita JH, Kador P, Catiles M. Aldose reductase in diabetic cataracts. JAMA 1981;246:257–261.

18. Kinoshita JH. Mechanisms initiating cataract formation. Proctor lecture. Invest Ophthalmol 1974;13:713–724.

19. Kador PF. Biochemistry of the Lens: Intermediary Metabolism and Sugar Cataract Formation. Basic Sciences. Philadelphia: WB Saunders, 1994.

20. Lee AY, Chung SK, Chung SS. Demonstration that polyol accumulation is responsible for diabetic cataract by the use of transgenic mice expressing the aldose reductase gene in the lens. Proc Natl Acad Sci USA 1995;92:2780–2784.

22. Lee AY, Chung SS. Contributions of polyol pathway to oxidative stress in diabetic cataract. Faseb J 1999;13:23–30.

25. Mulhern ML, Madson CJ, Danford A, et al. The unfolded protein response in lens epithelial cells from galactosemic rat lenses. Invest Ophthalmol Vis Sci 2006;47:3951–3959.

30. Kumamoto Y, Takamura Y, Kubo E, et al. Epithelial cell density in cataractous lenses of patients with diabetes: association with erythrocyte aldose reductase. Exp Eye Res 2007;85:393–399.

37. Kador PF, Zigler JS, Clark J, et al. Medical treatment of cataract. In: Tasman W, Jaeger EA (eds) Duane's Ophthalmology, 2nd edn. Philadelphia: Lippincott Williams and Wilkins, 2009.

CHAPTER 33

Steroid-induced cataract

Abbas Samadi

Clinical background

Since the successful use of steroids in 1948 in the suppression of clinical manifestations of rheumatoid arthritis, numerous compounds with glucocorticoid activity have been synthesized. Today, they represent standard therapy for the reduction of immune activation in asthma and inflammation associated with allergies, rheumatoid arthritis, inflammatory bowel syndromes, and other systemic diseases, plus they are used in ocular infections and allotransplantation.[1] The therapeutic usage of glucocorticoids has risen continuously in recent years. Each year 10 million new prescriptions are written just for oral corticosteroids in the USA. Overall, the total market size is considered to reach about 10 billion US dollars per year. Glucocorticoids are used in almost all medical specialties for systemic as well as topical therapies.[2]

Despite its therapeutic efficacy, glucocorticoid therapy is associated with metabolic and toxic effects. The side-effects (summarized in Table 33.1) occur with different prevalence, in different organs, and after different durations of therapy. Ocular complications of glucocorticoid therapy include cataract, glaucoma, infection, and corneal epithelial healing (Table 33.2).[3–5]

Cataracts: background

Cataracts are a clouding of the ocular lens of the eye which is most often associated with age-related oxidation and insolubilization of lens proteins. Cataracts are a major public health problem, affecting almost 50% of adults aged >65 years, and cataract extraction is the most common surgical procedure carried out in the USA.[6] Furthermore, it has been estimated that, by delaying the development of cataract formation by 10 years, 45% of these extractions would be avoided.[7] The development of cataract and its subsequent progression are influenced by multiple factors, including age, gender, diabetes, ultraviolet light exposure, smoking, a diet low in antioxidants, and steroid use.[8]

Epidemiology of the steroid cataracts

The incident of cataracts has considerably increased in recent years with widespread use of steroid therapy. Steroids typically induce cataract formation in the cortex of the posterior region of the lens, called posterior subcapsular cataract (PSC). In 1966, the incident of cataracts was 0.2% and 0.6% in young adults and those in their fifth and sixth decades, respectively.[9] In recent years, chronic use of steroids had become one of the risk factors for development of cataracts, surpassed only by diabetes, myopia, and glaucoma.[10,11] The incidence of steroid-mediated development of cataracts is expected to accelerate due to aging of the population and the associated increase of conditions that require steroid treatment. Therefore, better understanding of the mechanism of action of steroid-mediated cataracts may lead to their prevention, which would have an impact on the quality of life in the elderly.

Characteristics of steroid-induced cataract

The link between steroid use and the development of PSC was first reported in 1960 by Black and colleagues.[12] They examined 72 patients suffering from rheumatoid arthritis. In this study, 42% of the patients developed PSC whereas none of the individuals in the control group developed PSC. All cataracts were bilateral. Two subsequent papers by the same group provided a more detailed picture of glucocorticoid-mediated PSC.[13,14] The cataract which developed in these patients was characterized by "black spots or thread-like opacities" seen against the red fundus and located in the lens cortex immediately adjacent to the posterior lens capsule in the center of the field of vision. Other investigators reported "small yellow-white, highly refractile" cataracts with "small, scattered punctate vacuoles" that form a granular conglomerate.[15] Since then, numerous other studies have described an association between the use of steroids such as dexamethasone, beclomethasone, prednisone, and triamcinolone and development of cataract regardless of their route of administration.[16–18]

Steroid cataracts which present with superficial cortical vacuoles in posterior subcapsular region are referred to as "vacuolated PSC." However other conditions, such as age-related PSC, diabetes PSC, and retinitis pigmentosa associated PSC, are classified as vacuolated PSC.[19] With the exception of diabetes PSC, these other forms of vacuolated PSC appear to be clinically different in the early stage of their development. It is not clear why diabetes PSC and steroid-induced PSC share common features. The mechanism of steroid-induced cataracts has been actively investigated (Box 33.1).

Table 33.1 Glucocorticoid side-effects

Skin

Atrophy, delayed wound healing

Erythema, teleangiectasia, hypertrichosis

Skeleton and muscle

Muscle atrophy

Osteoprosis, bone necrosis

Central nervous system

Mood, behavior, memory, and cognitive disturbances

Cerebral atrophy

Eye

Electrolyte, metabolism, endocrine system

Increased Na^+ retention and K^+ secretion

Diabetes mellitus

Cushing's syndrome

Growth retardation

Adrenal atrophy

Hypogonadism, delayed puberty

Cardiovascular system

Hypertension

Thrombosis

Vasculitis

Gastrointestinal

Bleeding, peptic ulcer

Pancreatitis

Immune system

Infection

Table 33.2 Ocular effects of glucocorticoid use

Cataract

Raised intraocular pressure and glaucoma

Hypertensive retinopathy

Rebound inflammation

Delayed corneal healing

Refractive changes

Exophthalmos

Ocular muscle palsy

Pseudotumor cerebri

In early studies Black et al found that the incidence of steroid-induced cataract increased in proportion to the steroid dose. However, the dose-dependent nature of steroid-induced cataracts formation is controversial. Some investigators confirm the observation of Black et al[12] whereas others have observed no direct relationship between steroid dose and PSC severity.[20–22] It is possible that, while steroid dose is important, other factors such as age, susceptibility of the individual, genetic effects, co-medication, and duration of treatment may influence the development of PSC.

Box 33.1 Steroid-induced cataract

- Steroid cataracts which present with superficial cortical vacuoles in posterior subcapsular region are referred to as "vacuolated posterior subcapsular cataract (PSC)"
- Other conditions, such as age-related PSC, diabetes PSC, and retinitis pigmentosa-associated PSC, are also classified as vacuolated PSC
- With the exception of diabetes PSC, these other forms of vacuolated PSC appear to be clinically different in the early stage of their development

Epidemiology of route of steroid therapy and development of cataract

Systemic administration of glucocorticoids is associated with PSC development.[23–25] However, topical application[26–29] and intravitreal injection[30–32] of glucocorticoids can also induce cataract. Intravitreal glucocorticoid therapy is used for the treatment of many allergic and inflammatory disorders of the eye, such as uveitis, choroiditis, optic neuritis, and allergic conjunctivitis.

Inhaled steroids taken by asthma patients have also been related to the development of PSC.[33–35] Most recent data show that inhaled corticosteroid therapy increased significantly the risk of cataract even at low doses of beclomethasone (<500 µg/day) and reached a maximum level of 44% at doses of 1500–2000 µg/day among elderly patients.[36] The risk of cataract increased with increased dose of inhaled and nasal corticosteroid treatment. Therefore, these results have important implications for the treatment of asthma and chronic obstructive pulmonary disease in the elderly. For asthma, significant effort should be devoted to reducing the dose of inhaled corticosteroid as much as possible, perhaps by using inhaled corticosteroid in combination with long-acting bronchodilators or antileukotrienes.[37] Steroid therapy of children should be monitored more closely since PSC development occurs at a faster rate and at lower doses.[38–40] Shiono et al[41] reported that 33 (26.2%) of 126 children receiving long-term corticosteroid therapy developed PSC. Some of these patients manifest lens changes in under 6 months.[42] In the majority of cases, adverse effects of steroids were irreversible. Complete reversal of lens opacification is highly unlikely once vision is affected.

Mechanism of action of glucocorticoid-induced cataract

Steroids

Steroids are derived from cholesterol (Figure 33.1). They comprise five groups: progestagens, androgens, estrogens, mineralocorticoids, and glucocorticoids (Figure 33.2). They are produced in different tissues and have different functions. Progestagens are produced by corpus luteum, whereas androgens and estrogens are produced by testis and ovaries, respectively. Mineralocorticoids and glucocorticoids are produced by the adrenal cortex. Steroid effects on normal cell function are complex and not fully understood. Steroid

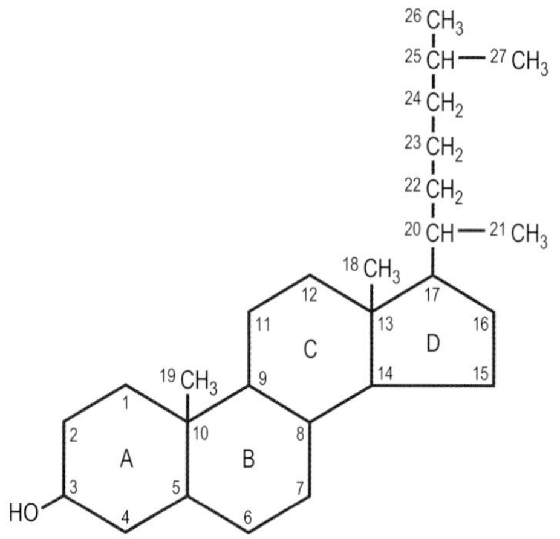

Figure 33.1 The structure of cholesterol. Letters A–D show ring designations and numbers show carbon atoms.

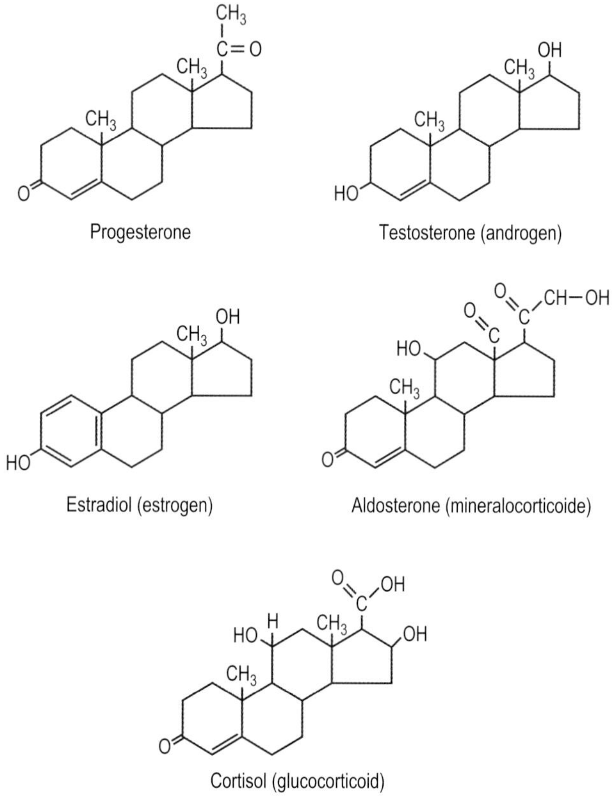

Figure 33.2 Structure of different classes of steroids.

actions may be plasma membrane-initiated, intracellular receptor-mediated (genomic), and/or posttranscriptional.

Nongenomic rapid glucocorticoid signaling

From early studies on the mechanism of actions of steroids, it became apparent that all classes of steroid hormones can induce effects that occur in a very short time frame, within minutes or even seconds of their application. These changes have been well documented in vitro on intracellular signaling pathways, and in vivo, in a wide array of human and animal models used to study biological functions such as oogenesis, vasoregulation, response to stress, and neurobehavioral changes (Box 33.2).[43,44] These rapid events do not fit the classical "genomic" model for steroid action. Nongenomic effect of glucocorticoids may contribute to insulin resistance. Reduced kinase activities of the insulin receptor (INSR) and several downstream INSR signaling intermediates (i.e., p70S6K, adenosine monophosphate-activated protein kinase, glycogen synthase kinase-3, and Fyn) were detected in adipocytes and T lymphocytes due to short-term treatment with dexamethasone.[45] Several membrane-associated proteins are involved with rapid nongenomic action of glucocorticoids. Glucocorticoid-dependent phosphorylation of caveolin and protein kinase B/Akt was reported to inhibit lung epithelial cell growth.[46] Disruption of caveolae led to dissociation of glucocorticoid action, with impaired induction of Akt activation. Glucocorticoids rapidly inhibit high-voltage-activated calcium currents in several different cell types in a G protein-dependent manner.[47,48]

Box 33.2 Nongenomic action of steroid hormones

- From early studies of the mechanism of action of steroids, it became apparent that all classes of steroid hormones can induce effects that occur in a very short time frame, within minutes or even seconds of their application
- These changes have been well documented in vitro on intracellular signaling pathways, and in vivo, in a wide array of human and animal models used to study biological functions such as oogenesis, vasoregulation, response to stress, and neurobehavioral changes

The classical corticosteroid receptor, a cytosolic protein, has also been found localized to the plasma membrane, suggesting the possibility that rapid effects of glucocorticoids may be mediated by the classical intracellular receptors associated with the cell membrane.[49] In addition, glucocorticoid signaling to the nucleus may be mediated via the membrane glucocorticoid receptor. Glucocorticoids cause rapid activation of several mitogen-activated protein kinases (MAPK), including p38, c-Jun NH_2-terminal kinase (JNK), and ERK1/2 in cultured hippocampal neurons and PC12 cells.[50,51] Activation of ERK by glucocorticoids occurs in a 1–3 hour time frame, which is not consistent with the nongenomic action of steroids.[52] Regardless, the activation and nuclear translocation of MAPK by either, or both, transcriptional and nontranscription mechanisms provide the potential for epigenetic regulation of gene expression, because MAPK can cause histone phosphorylation that can lead to modification of chromatin structure.[53] Transcriptional and nontranscriptional signaling by MAPK in human lens is not defined. It will be interesting in the future to show how these potentially distinct mechanisms of accessing the genome might interact, either positively or negatively, to formulate the resulting net regulation of gene expression by glucocorticoids in human lens.

Receptor-mediated glucocorticoid action

Classical genomic action of steroids is mediated through their receptors, ligand-regulated transcription factors that belong to the superfamily of nuclear receptors. Glucocorticoid initiates a process culminating in dimerization of glucocorticoid receptor and translocation of the ligand–receptor complex to the nucleus via the microtubule network[54]

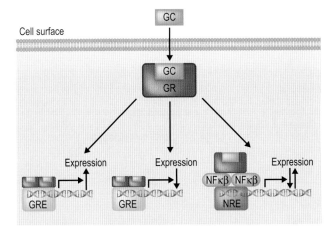

Figure 33.3 Classical mode of action of glucocorticoid hormone (GC). GC binds to its receptor, glucocorticoid receptor (GR), in the cell. GC–GR complex enters the nucleus and binds to glucocorticoid response element (GRE) in a dimer form to increase or decrease the expression of respective gene or may interact with nuclear factor kappa B (NF-κB) on the nuclear response element (NRE) to modulate cognate gene expression.

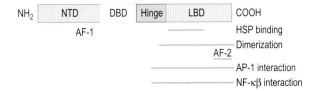

Figure 33.4 Functional domains of glucocorticoid receptor. NTD, amino terminal domain; DBD, DNA binding domain; LBD, ligand binding domain; AF-1, activation factor-1; HSP, heat shock protein.

Box 33.3 Genomic action of steroids

- Classical genomic action of steroids is mediated by nuclear receptors
- Glucocorticoid initiates dimerization of glucocorticoid receptor and translocation of the ligand–receptor complex to the nucleus
- Once in the nucleus, the activated glucocorticoid receptor associates with unique DNA sequences termed glucocorticoid response elements (GRE) in the promoter or enhancer of target genes
- Glucocorticoid receptor can be recruited to target genes either through direct DNA binding or with other DNA-bound transcription factors
- Ligand–glucocorticoid receptor promotes formation of macromolecular complex formation on DNA molecule
- The macromolecular complex includes coactivator proteins, chromatin remodeling factors, and other factors that directly or indirectly engage the transcriptional machinery

---

Box 33.4 Transactivation and transrepression of glucocorticoids

- Once bound to glucocorticoid response elements as a homodimer, glucocorticoid receptor serves as scaffold for the assembly of distinct macromolecular complexes that activates transcription of target gene (transactivation)
- The genes mainly controlled by glucocorticoid receptor transactivation are involved in metabolic regulation; for example, increasing blood glucose levels, gluconeogenesis, and mobilization of amino acids and fatty acids
- The reduction of transcription (transrepression) by glucocorticoid receptor occurs by different mechanisms. One mechanism resembles transactivation, but the receptors bind to DNA sequences distinct from positive glucocorticoid response elements

---

(Figure 33.3). Once in the nucleus, the activated glucocorticoid receptor associates with unique DNA sequences termed glucocorticoid response elements (GRE) in the promoter or enhancer region of target genes. The ligand–glucocorticoid receptor may modulate the expression of the target genes (Box 33.3).[55] The glucocorticoid receptor can be recruited to target genes either through direct DNA binding or with other DNA-bound transcription factors. Once bound to GREs as a homodimer, glucocorticoid receptor serves as scaffold for the assembly of distinct macromolecular complexes that activates transcription of target gene (transactivation). The macromolecular complex includes coactivator proteins, chromatin remodeling factors and other factors that directly or indirectly engage the transcriptional machinery.[56] The genes mainly controlled by glucocorticoid receptor transactivation are involved in metabolic regulation; for example, increasing blood glucose levels, gluconeogenesis, and mobilization of amino acids and fatty acids.[57] The reduction of transcription (transrepression) by glucocorticoid receptor

occurs by different mechanisms. One mechanism resembles transactivation, but the receptors bind to DNA sequences distinct from positive GREs (i.e., negative GRE sites or nGREs).[58]

Glucocorticoid receptor also triggers transcriptional repression through a mechanism that does not involve its direct DNA binding but rather a tethering to other DNA-bound transcription factors such as AP-1 and NF-κB.[59] Anti-inflammatory actions of glucocorticoid receptors are through modulation of AP-1 and NF-κB transcriptional activity (Box 33.4).[60]

Glucocorticoid receptors share common structural organization with other steroid receptors consisting of several modulatory domains with two highly conserved, zinc-finger DNA binding domains (DBD), a less-conserved carboxy terminal ligand binding domain (LBD), and a divergent amino terminal domain (NTD)[60] (Figure 33.4). A region rich in acidic amino acids in the NTD domain known as activation factor-1 (AF-1) is a transcriptional regulator that can be ligand-independent. Disruption of the AF-1 region reduces gene expression. A second region in the LBD domain, known as AF-2, undergoes conformational changes modulating transcriptional activator or repressor activity of glucocorticoid receptor. LBD promotes receptor dimerization and contains the sequence for heat shock protein 90 (HSP90) interaction. Maturation of proper folding of glucocorticoid receptor is provided by HSP90 interaction (Figure 33.5). In the absence of ligand, inactive glucocorticoid receptor in the cytoplasm interacts with HSP90. In addition to HSP90, other heat shock proteins (HSP70, HSP40) and co-chaperones p23, immunophilins FKBP52 and Cyp40 play key roles in the proper folding and function of glucocorticoid receptor.[61,62] For example, functional disruption of p23 gene produces a phenotype that is distinctly similar to that of mouse

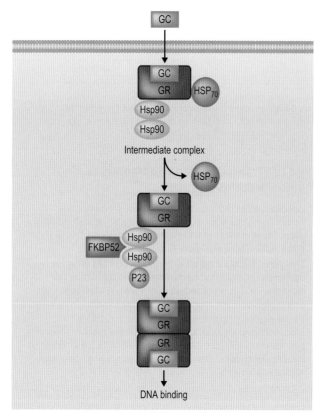

Figure 33.5 Heat shock protein contribution of glucocorticoid receptor (GR). Glucocorticoid (GC) upon entering the cell binds to its receptor. GR is a client protein for heat shock protein 90 (HSP90). HSP90 binds to this newly synthesized GR to form the intermediate complex. Upon GC–GR maturation, which involves co-chaperones FKBP52 and p53, HSP90 and FKBP52 are involved in GR movement from the cytoplasm to the nucleus.

glucocorticoid receptor knockout.[63] Since glucocorticoid receptor is well characterized in the lens, understanding the role of chaperones, co-chaperones, and immunophilins may provide key information on the mechanism of corticosteroid-induced PSC.

Posttranscriptional gene regulation is increasingly recognized as a critical component of the regulation of several genes, including inflammatory genes. For example, glucocorticoids regulate mRNA stability of cytokines (interleukins IL-1, IL-4Rα, IL-6, IL-8), cyclooxygenase-2 (COX-2), interferon-β (IFN-β), inducible nitrous oxide synthase (iNOS), and vascular endothelial growth factor (VEGF).[64]

Mechanism of glucocorticoid-induced cataract

Nongenomic effects of glucocorticoid lens epithelial cells

Recent reports indicate that lens epithelial cells express a 28-kDa membrane steroid-binding protein (MSBP).[65,66] The deduced amino acid sequence of the lens protein was extremely similar to those of other species and tissues, being 95–98% homologous with that of members. Others have reported a similar 28-kDa membrane protein in other

Box 33.5 Membrane steroid-binding protein

- Lens epithelial cells express a 28-kDa membrane steroid-binding protein
- The deduced amino acid sequence of the lens protein was extremely similar to those of other species and tissues, being 95–98% homologous with that of members
- A similar 28-kDa membrane protein has been found to be present in other tissues
- Progesterone and corticosterone bind with great affinity ($K_d = 75$ nM) to the lens epithelial microsomal membrane preparation

tissues.[67–69] Progesterone and corticosterone bind with great affinity ($K_d = 75$ nM) to the lens epithelial microsomal membrane preparation (Box 33.5).[70] The functional role of the lens epithelial cell MSBP awaits further characterization. However multiple functions of this protein have been described in other cell systems.[71,72]

Rapid nongenomic action of steroids is also reported in lens epithelial cells. Progesterone and 17 β-estradiol transiently increased intracellular calcium concentration in lens epithelial cells and this event required the presence of an inwardly directed electrochemical gradient promoting Ca^{2+} influx.[73] In addition a synthetic estradiol receptor agonist, diethylstilbestrol (DES), induced relatively rapid increases in intracellular calcium that occurred over an interval of 10–50 seconds and that persisted for several minutes. The DES-mediated increase in the intracellular calcium concentration was due to inhibition of smooth endoplasmic reticulum Ca^{2+} ATPase (SERCA).[74] These results show that progesterone and estradiol transiently increase calcium levels in the lens epithelial cells and these events are incompatible with transcriptional actions of steroid receptor.

Glucocorticoid receptor-mediated signaling in lens epithelial cells

Glucocorticoid receptor has been reported in lens epithelial cells.[75–77] A broad range of genes are up- and downregulated by glucocorticoid treatment of lens epithelial cells.[78,79] Corticosteroid-mediated upregulation of glucocorticoid-induced leucine zipper protein (GILZ), serum glucocorticoid kinase (SGK), MAK phosphatase-1 (MKP-1), and plasminogen activator inhibitor-1 (PAI-1) was confirmed by reverse transcriptase polymerase chain reaction in lens epithelial cells (Box 33.6).[78,79] Further research is required to define glucocorticoid-mediated effects of SGK and PAI-1 in lens epithelial cells. GILZ, as a transcription factor, is associated with regulation of transmembrane sodium transport, suppression of apoptosis, modification of NF-κB and AP-1 activity, and inhibition of differentiation.[80–82]

Ligand–glucocorticoid receptor regulates MKP-1 protein expression in the lens epithelial cells.[83] Phosphorylation of MAPK components, ERK, JNK, and p38 regulates activation of the MAPK pathway. MPK-1 is a phosphatase enzyme, which by removing phosphate groups reduces activation of the MAPK pathway. Glucocorticoid-dependent dephosphorylation of RAF-1, ERK1/2 was reported after 4 and 16 hours of glucocorticoid treatment.[83] No changes in basal levels of total RAF-1 and total ERK1/2 and phospho- and total JNK were observed. Similarly, glucocorticoid receptor reduces

Box 33.6 Glucocorticoid receptor in lens epithelial cell

- Glucocorticoid receptor is present in lens epithelial cells. A broad range of genes are up- and downregulated by glucocorticoid-treated lens epithelial cells
- Corticosteroids induce upregulation of glucocorticoid-induced leucine zipper (GILZ) protein, serum glucocorticoid kinase (SGK), MAK phosphatases-1 (MKP-1), and plasminogen activator inhibitor-1 (PAI-1) in lens epithelial cells

Box 33.7 Glucocorticoid reduces glutathione (GSH) in lens

- Glucocorticoid reduces GSH levels in both lens and the aqueous humor
- Pretreatment of the lenses with the glucocorticoid receptor antagonist RU486 prevents reduction of GSH concentration by glucocorticoids, leading to the conclusion that glucocorticoid-mediated cellular GSH depletion may be a glucocorticoid receptor-related event

activation of the phosphoinositide-3 kinase (PI3K)/protein kinase-B (PKB/Akt) signal transduction pathway without change in Akt protein level. The MAPK pathway is involved in cell proliferation, differentiation, motility, survival, and apoptosis. PI3K/AKT is associated with cell survival, proliferation, growth, and transformation.[84] These results indicate that glucocorticoid receptor-mediated events are associated with a decrease in activation of the MAPK and PI3K/Akt pathways. The functional significance of these changes in human lens is not known. In addition, nongenomic, rapid modulation of these survival factors in lens epithelial cells requires further investigation.

Genomic receptor-mediated oxidation stress

A general mechanism in age-related cataract is oxidation of proteins. A high concentration of the reduced form of glutathione (GH) is maintained in the lens, and it is essential for cellular antioxidant machinery. H_2O_2 is a strong oxidizing agent in the lens. It is converted to water by glutathione peroxidase enzyme utilizing GSH as a proton donor, generating oxidized glutathione (GSSG). Reduced levels of GSH lead to the oxidation of lens proteins. Steroids having glucocorticoid activity reduce the GSH levels in both lens and the aqueous humor.[85,86] Pretreatment of the lenses with glucocorticoid receptor antagonist RU486 prevents reduction of GSH concentration by glucocorticoids, leading to the conclusion that glucocorticoid-mediated cellular GSH depletion may be a glucocorticoid receptor-related event. Reduction of lens GSH may be due to receptor transrepression of glutathione peroxidase/glutathione reductase system or enzymes responsible for GSH synthesis (Box 33.7). The rate-limiting enzyme γ-glutamylcysteine synthase (γ-GCS) and glutathione synthetase (GS) are responsible for GSH synthesis starting with cysteine substrate. The γ-GCS is a heterodimer enzyme having a 73-kDa heavy (γ-GCS-HS) and a 28-kDa light subunit (γ-GCS-LS)[87]; the catalytic site is located on the γ-GCS-HS subunit. The promoter region of the γ-GCS-HS contains an AP-1 binding site and its expression is mediated by AP-1 transcription factor.[88] Therefore, glucocorticoid modulates γ-GCS-HS expression through AP-1. Whereas reduced levels of γ-GCS and GS are reported in PSC, however, no significant modulation of γ-GCS-HS expression is reported in glucocorticoid-treated lens epithelial cells. Therefore, it is unlikely that glucocorticoids reduce GSH synthesis. At this point it is not clear how glucocorticoid receptor transcriptional activity leads to a reduction in lens GSH. That it directs nongenomic binding of glucocorticoids to and modulation of enzymes related to reactive oxygen species homeostasis is an attractive hypothesis which needs to be examined.

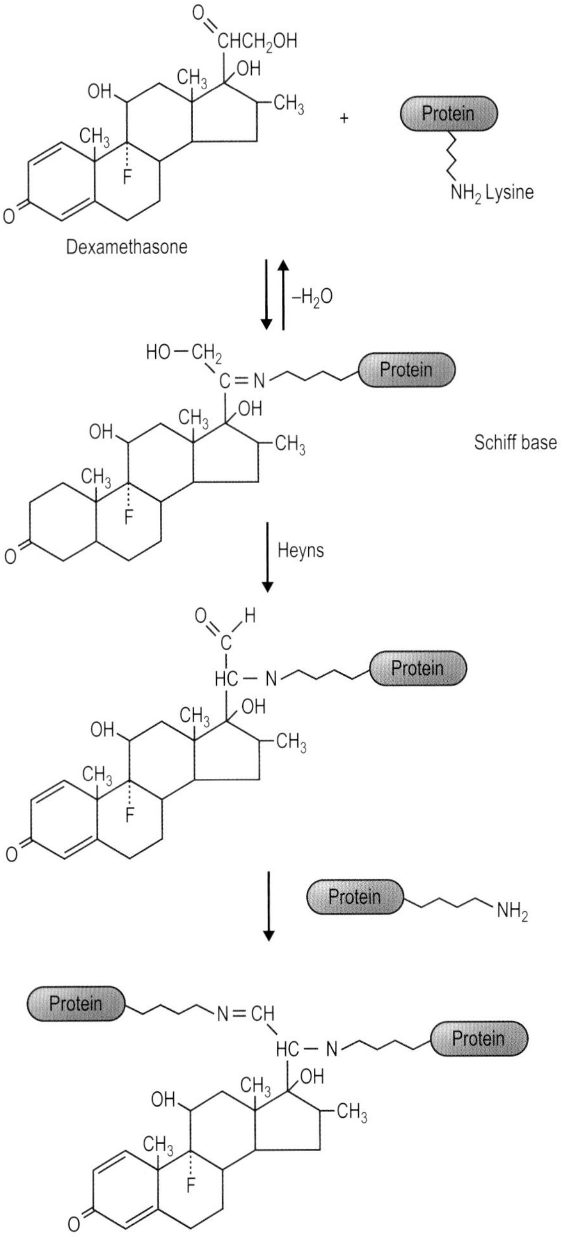

Figure 33.6 Glucocorticoid–protein adduct formation.

Glucocorticoid-mediated alteration in lens hydration

The presence of intercellular clefts, vacuoles, and swollen cells in glucocorticoid cataracts has led to the suggestion that glucocorticoid-induced alteration in the levels of expression of cell membrane channels, which are important in regulating intracellular ion and water, may change lens hydration. Glucocorticoid may alter lens hydration by modulation of expression and/or activity of cell membrane ion channels. For example, glucocorticoids increase the expression of both alpha1 and beta1 Na/K-ATPase in lens epithelial cells.[78] However, glucocorticoid may also modulate lens Na/K ATPase activity.[89] Glucocorticoids are also reported to modulate high-voltage-activated calcium currents,[90] Na/K ATPase in beta insulin-producing cells,[91] and calcium-activated potassium channels[92] in other cell systems. Further research on the effect of glucocorticoids on lens ion channels (genomic and nongenomic) is required.

Glucocorticoid–protein adduct formation

The nonenzymatic addition of small molecules can alter the conformation or function of proteins and this can contribute to the development of disease. Steroids with both a C-20 and a C-21 hydroxyl group have been shown to react with proteins to form stable adducts.[93] These reactions involved the formation of a Schiff base between a lysine residue ε-amino group of lens crystallin and the C-20 carbonyl group bond of the steroid, followed by Heyns rearrangement involving the C-21 hydroxyl group to form a stable ketoamine product (Figure 33.6). The crystallin protein undergoes a conformational change, facilitating SH cross-linking and subsequent oxidation. However, the steroid–protein adducts isolated from steroid-induced PSC human lens are small, and adducts do not appear to influence lens crystallin conformation.[94]

Conclusion

Although the development of PSC is well documented in patients receiving glucocorticoid therapy, the mechanisms of cataract formation remain to be determined. The presence of glucocorticoid receptor is documented in the lens. However, the effect of glucocorticoids on membrane-associated glucocorticoid receptor and other membrane-associated proteins remains to be determined. The nongenomic and rapid-action glucocorticoids may be directed through MSBP. Cytoplasmic glucocorticoid receptor activation is associated with changes in the gene expression that lead to: (1) cell proliferation, differentiation, and apoptosis; (2) modulation of glucose metabolism; (3) modulation of membrane channels; and (4) direct and indirect modulation of signal transduction. Although microarray studies on short lens epithelial cell exposure to glucocorticoids have provided valuable information, however, extension of these to human PSC samples may provide a better understanding of the glucocorticoid mechanism of action. The association of glucocorticoid with G-protein receptor proteins, protein tyrosine kinase receptors, lipid raft-associated proteins, transcription factors (AP-1 and NF-κB), heat shock proteins (HSP90, HSP70), and co-chaperones in the lens needs to be characterized. The etiology of steroid cataract may be due to transactivation and transrepression of genes as well as modulation of the activity of proteins and enzymes (Figure 33.7). Further elucidation of the function of MSBP may provide information on the role of nongenomic actions of glucocorticoids in lens epithelial cells.

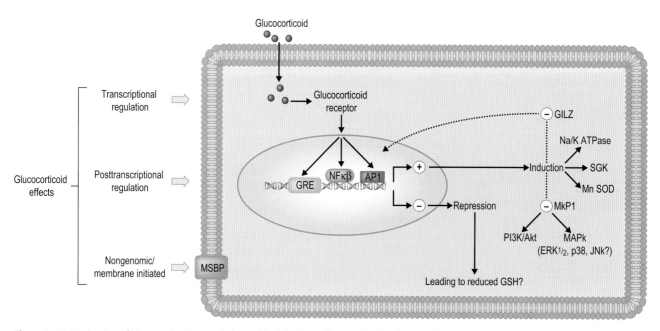

Figure 33.7 Mechanism of glucocorticoid action in lens epithelial cells, as discussed in this chapter. Glucocorticoids exert their action through multiple mechanisms mediating coordinate changes in the expression of targets genes. Upon binding to ligand, glucocorticoid receptor (GR) dimerizes and translocates to the nucleus. Hormone–GR complex binds either to the glucocorticoid response element (GRE) site or to transcription factors, such as nuclear factor kappa B (NF-κB) or activating protein 1 (AP-1), or cofactors, producing either transcriptional repression (–) or induction (+) of genes. Glucocorticoid-induced genes can also carry an inhibitory function by acting as transcriptional inhibitors (for example on glucocorticoid-induced leucine zipper (GILZ) protein), or by mediating inhibitory glucocorticoid effects downstream of transcription. Among these, induced MAP kinase phosphatase-1 mediates dephosphorylation of members of the MAP kinase family (ERKYz, p38). Finally, glucocorticoids bind to membrane steroid-binding protein (MSBP), which may mediate rapid, nongenomic membrane-initiated events. SGK, serum glucocorticoid kinase; Mn SOD, manganese superoxide dismutase.

Key references

A complete list of chapter references is available online at www.expertconsult.com. See inside cover for registration details.

1. Fauci AS, Dale DC, Balow JE. Glucocorticoid therapy: mechanism of action and clinical considerations. Ann Intern Med 1976;84:304–315.

4. Carnahan MC, Goldstein DA. Ocular complications of topical, peri-ocular, and systemic corticosteroids. Curr Opin Ophthalmol 2000;11:478–483.

5. Renfro L, Snow JS. Occular effects of topical and systemic steroids. Dermatol Clin 1992;10:505–512.

28. Costagliola C, Cati-Giovannelli B, Piccirillo A, et al. Cataracts associated with long-term topical steroids. Br J Dermatol 1989;120:472–473.

52. Revest JM, Di Blasi F, Kitchener P, et al. The MAPK pathway and Erg-1 mediate stress-related behavioral effects of glucocorticoids. Nat Neurosci 2005;8:664–672.

62. Grad I, Picard D. The glucocorticoid responses are shaped by molecular chaperones. Mol Cell Endocrinol 2007;275:2–12.

65. Cenedella RJ, Sexton PS, Zhu XL. Lens epithelia contain a high-affinity, membrane steroid hormone-binding protein. Invest Ophthalmol Vis Sci 1999;40:1452–1459.

66. Zhu Xl, Sexton PS, Cenedella RJ. Characterization of membrane steroid binding protein mRNA and protein in lens epithelial cells. Exp Eye Res 2001;73:213–219.

67. Falkenstein E, Schmieding K, Lange A, et al. Localization of a putative progesterone membrane binding protein in porcine hepatocytes. Cell Mol Biol 1998;44:571–578.

73. Samadi A, Carlson CG, Gueorguiev A, et al. Rapid, non-genomic actions of progesterone and estradiol on steady-state calcium and resting calcium influx in lens epithelial cells. Pflugers Arch 2002;444:700–709.

74. Samadi A, Cenedella RJ, Carlson CG. Diethylstilbestrol increases intracellular calcium in lens epithelial cells. Pflugers Arch Eur J Physiol 2005;450:145–154.

75. James ER, Robertson L, Ehlert E, et al. Presence of transcriptionally active glucocorticoid receptor alpha in lens epithelial cells. Invest Ophthalmol Vis Sci 2003;44:5269–5276.

79. Gupta V, Galante A, Soteropoulos P, et al. Global gene profiling reveals novel glucocorticoid induced changes in gene expression of human lens epithelial cells. Mol Vis 2005;11:1018–1040.

91. Ulrich S, Zhang Y, Avram D, et al. Dexamethasone increases Na^+/K^+ ATPase activity in insulin secreting cells through SGK1. Biochem Biophys Res Commun 2007;352:662–667.

CHAPTER 34

Presbyopia

Jane F Koretz

Overview

Presbyopia (from the Greek *presbys*, elder or old, and, *-ops*, eye) is a progressive condition where the ability to focus on nearby objects is gradually lost as part of the natural aging process. Although the development of presbyopia appears to begin in the second decade of life, it does not become a significant problem for most people until they reach their 40s, when it becomes increasingly difficult to read, sew, or use a computer without visual assistance. It is sometimes confused with far-sightedness because far vision remains relatively unaffected. However, although the eye's far point of focus is not significantly altered, the near point (the closest comfortable focus) is gradually receding toward the far point, reducing the range over which clear focus can be attained. Although presbyopia is not life- or vision-threatening, it nevertheless "represents a significant economic cost to society," as reported by the National Eye Institute (http://www.nei.nih.gov/resources/strategicplans/neiplan/frm_cross.asp). It also reduces quality of life and is a universal harbinger of middle age.

Clinical background

Key symptoms and signs

The range over which one can focus – one's accommodative amplitude – declines throughout life. A small child has an accommodative range of 15–20 D (from infinity to about 5 cm, or the tip of one's nose), while a young adult's range is about 10 D (infinity to about 10 cm), reducing to less than 1 D (infinity to about 1 meter) by about 60. Thus diminution of the ability to focus on near objects is the hallmark of presbyopia. This loss becomes particularly apparent to individuals, generally in their 40s, in the process of performing familiar tasks. It may become more difficult to focus on print at normal reading distances, particularly at low light levels, or it may take a perceptible amount of time to shift focus from one distance to another, or prolonged close work might lead to eyestrain or headache (Box 34.1). When people complain that the print is suddenly too small or their arms are too short, they are likely becoming presbyopic.

Historical development

Why does presbyopia occur? It could be argued that the impact of presbyopia was moot for prehistoric hominids, since it is unlikely that their life span in general reached into their 40s, let alone their 50s. However, as will be discussed in more detail later, the changes in the anterior segment associated with visual aging lead specifically to the preservation of far focus at the expense of near. In terms of evolutionary pressure, it is possible that maintenance of distance vision was a survival advantage in spotting and avoiding predators, as well as in locating prey. Indeed, even in modern times, average human refraction around the world is roughly 1 D hyperopic.

Epidemiology

Because presbyopia is an integral part of the human aging process, its impact is theoretically universal once middle age has been reached. There appears to be no significant difference in the progression of the condition between males and females or among different human ethnic groups. What will differ is the apparent age of onset. Some of this difference arises simply from a natural Gaussian distribution of traits across the human population, and some from an individual's lifestyle (e.g., web page designer versus national park ranger). For an emmetropic (20/20 or 6/6 visual acuity) eye, apparent onset is generally in one's 40s and progresses until total loss of objective visual range by about 60. A subjective range of about 1 D, due largely to the pinhole effect (a constricted pupil providing an increased depth of focus), remains, but will clearly be dependent on the illumination intensity of ambient light. The impact of presbyopia will be different from emmetropes for those with refractive errors, with far-sighted (hyperopic) individuals more severely affected and near-sighted (myopic) individuals less so. For hyperopes, the location of their far point is further away than for emmetropes, and their most comfortable near point will also be further away for a given age. As a result, their ability to focus on nearby objects will be diminished at an earlier age, and the apparent onset of presbyopia may be in their late 30s or even earlier. In contrast, myopes have a far point that tends to be nearby, so their receding near point does not lead to the functional visual loss experienced by their emmetropic and hyperopic friends. As a consequence, many

Box 34.1 Symptoms of presbyopia

- Age
- Decrease in ability to focus nearby
- Increase in comfortable reading distance
- Eyestrain
- Headaches after prolonged focus
- Trouble focusing when tired or stressed
- Slow response to change in focus distance
- Need for increased illumination

presbyopic myopes find themselves needing additional optical assistance only for distance viewing (e.g., driving); this "myopic advantage" is lost when invasive procedures like laser in situ keratomileusis (LASIK) and photorefractive keratectomy (PRK) have previously been used for refractive correction.

Diagnostic workup

Diagnosing presbyopia is straightforward, especially since many patients diagnose themselves. A person's age is of course a major consideration, since it is the primary risk factor. Symptoms will include the gradual onset of several of the following: decreased ability to focus on nearby objects; increase in comfortable reading distance ("arms too short"); eyestrain; headaches after prolonged visual tasks; trouble focusing when tired or stressed; slow visual response to a change in focus distance; and need for increased illumination. Further assessment can be incorporated into a standard eye exam, which may identify additional potential contributory factors. A simple reading test using well-illuminated text of graded sizes at a standard distance (e.g., 35 cm or 14 inches) can be helpful both in characterizing the degree of near-vision loss and in determining the appropriate refractive correction.

Differential diagnosis

Although presbyopia is generally an easily identified condition, there are nevertheless other potential factors affecting changes in visual range that must be considered and eliminated. These factors can include nuclear cataract development, untreated diabetes, central nervous system disorders, macular degeneration, and migraines. In general, a thorough refractive history combined with a standard ophthalmic examination that includes slit-lamp biomicroscopy and inspection of the retina should serve to eliminate most of these possibilities. Presbyopia can also be confused with hyperopia when a subject's refractive history is unknown; however, hyperopia in an adult over 35 would be indistinguishable from presbyopia, and would be treated as such.

Treatment

Because of the universality of presbyopia in older individuals, there are many different options available for mitigating its effects. Historically, the very first contribution to the treatment of presbyopia was developed in 1784, when Benjamin Franklin combined two pairs of glasses – one for distance

vision and one for close work – into the first set of bifocals (bifocles). Reading glasses, bifocals, progressives, and even trifocals, remain the most common methods for providing one or more different comfortable refractive distances for eyes that can no longer focus on near objects, and are the most versatile option for a visual system that continues to change from the onset of presbyopia into the 60s. It is possible for presbyopes to test out and buy their own reading glasses from a pharmacy or supermarket; if both eyes have similar or identical refractions, this is a reasonable if limited strategy for the long term. However, if there are significant differences between the two eyes due to refractive or other differences, or if there are special visual requirements (e.g., sustained focus on a computer monitor) it becomes important to have glasses or other optical prostheses professionally prescribed.

A second set of options involves contact lenses. There are a growing number of different designs of contact lenses available for presbyopes, either bifocal (one refractive range within the circumference of a second) or multifocal (simultaneous images at two or more different refractive powers), which have received a mixed response from users. An additional alternative is monovision contact lenses, where the refractive correction for one eye is set for focus at a distance and the other for focus nearby; although the image received by each eye is clear, the concomitant loss of depth perception has a vertiginous effect which some people cannot overcome. A general drawback to the use of contact lenses for presbyopia is the decrease in tear production with increasing age in the target population, but, like glasses, an advantage is that a change in prescription is easy to do.

A third set of alternatives involves direct alteration of the visual system. These currently include monovision through LASIK, conductive keratoplasty, or other procedures altering corneal shape (and thus refractive power), and scleral relaxation and scleral expansion surgeries. The same problem as experienced in contact lens-mediated monovision – loss of depth perception – is a consequence of surgical monovision, so it is important to ensure that this can be tolerated before the procedure is performed. Modifying scleral shape has not been very successful up to this point in treating presbyopia, although it continues to have its fervent advocates and detractors. In development are methods for altering lens properties in situ using laser techniques or replacement of the natural lens with an intraocular lens implant that restores accommodation. These and other novel approaches for the treatment of presbyopia and restoration of accommodative range continue to be designed, developed, and tested, and it is likely that effective new options for treatment will be available within the next decade (Chapter 35).

Physiology and pathophysiology

Introduction

Image formation by the human eye involves refractive contributions from both the cornea and the crystalline lens, with the cornea a passive component and the lens and associated structures an active contributor. In order to understand presbyopia, which is a natural consequence of the aging process, it is first necessary to understand accommodation, the mech-

Box 34.2 Accommodative process

- When unaccommodated, the lens is at its thinnest and flattest, while the ciliary muscle is relaxed
- Closer focus couples ciliary muscle contraction with lens elastic recovery, or "rounding up"
- The lens becomes thicker and more sharply curved
- Anterior-segment length remains almost the same, so lens center of mass is moved forward and anterior-chamber depth decreases
- Internal lens curvatures are directly related to surface curvatures, and these relationships are maintained during accommodation

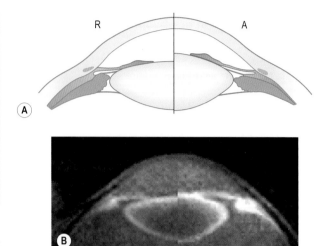

Figure 34.1 (A) Helmholtz drawing demonstrating his theory of accommodation. The left half of the image shows relaxed accommodation. The right half shows the increase in lens thickness and decrease in equatorial diameter after ciliary muscle contraction. (B) A composite of two magnetic resonance imaging (MRI) images. The left half is an image acquired with relaxed accommodation, while the subject, a young adult, views a far target. The right half is an image acquired during accommodation, while the subject views a near target. It shows an increase in lens thickness and a decrease in equatorial diameter upon ciliary muscle contraction. (Reproduced with permission from Strenk SA, Strenk LM, Koretz JF. The mechanism of presbyopia. Prog Retin Eye Res 2005;24:379–393.)

anism by which this focusing is effected, and the age-related changes in this mechanism that are associated with loss of accommodative amplitude.

Accommodation

The human focusing mechanism is the subject of qualitative, if not quantitative, agreement.[1] Focus on points closer than infinity (for the human eye, about 6 meters or 20 feet) involves an increase in the sharpness of curvature of the crystalline lens surfaces, an increased thickening of the lens along the optical axis, a shallowing of the anterior chamber, and essentially no change in the distance from the cornea to the posterior lens surface along the axis (Box 34.2). This process was, in essence, first described in the 19th century by Helmholtz (Figure 34.1) in his *Treatise on Physiological Optics*, although Helmholtz was certainly not the first to develop hypotheses about the mechanism. It is the causative factors through which these alterations in lens shape, thickness, and position relative to the cornea occur that are the subject of intense debate,[2–12] and that lead to presbyopia.

The crystalline lens is located in the anterior segment of the eye behind the iris, suspended in place by the zonules of Zinn (Figure 34.2), which connect the lens to the ciliary muscle through insertions into the collagenous lens capsule surrounding the lens fiber cells.[13] Light enters the eye through the cornea, which provides the major refractive component of the system, due in part to its small radius of curvature and to the comparatively large increase in refractive index in going from air to the cornea. The light emerging from the posterior surface of the cornea, after passing through the circular slit of the iris, arrives at the lens, which provides a variable refractive contribution to the system (Figure 34.3). When focused at infinity, the lens is at its flattest and thinnest along the optical axis, while the ciliary muscle is relaxed; closer focus involves a carefully controlled relaxation of the forces acting upon the lens, coupled to ciliary muscle contraction, and allows the lens to "round up" and increase its refractive contribution (Figure 34.4).

Modern versions of the helmholtzian model of accommodation directly couple ciliary muscle contraction, and its shift of net muscle mass anteriorly and inward, with lens elastic recovery and net anterior movement of lens mass.[12,14] In contrast, modern versions of the classic hydraulic theory, such as that proposed by D Jackson Coleman,[3,15,16] suggest that ciliary muscle contraction exerts a force on the choroid, which in turn generates an increased pressure through the

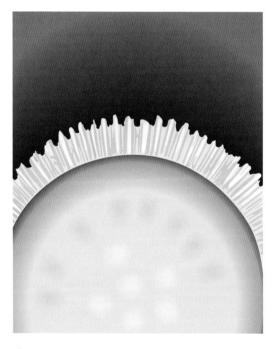

Figure 34.2 Retroilluminated image/schematic representation of the crystalline lens in the anterior segment, viewed perpendicular to its axis of symmetry. The lens is suspended within the circle of the ciliary muscle by fibers of the zonular apparatus, which serves to connect the lens capsule and muscle. (Modified from Koretz JF, Handelman GH. How the human eye focuses. Sci Am 1988;256:92–99.)

vitreous that alters lens shape by deforming the anterior hyaloid membrane; the latter acts something like a diaphragm, separating anterior and posterior segments, cradling the posterior of the lens, and being forced in an anterior direction when the vitreous-chamber pressure is

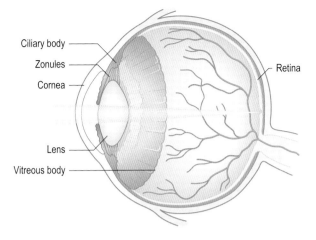

Figure 34.3 Schematic of image formation by the human eye. Light at the air–cornea interface is refracted inward, passing through the biological aperture of the iris before being further refracted through the crystalline lens to focus on the fovea. (Modified from Koretz JF, Handelman GH. How the human eye focuses. Sci Am 1988;256:92–99.)

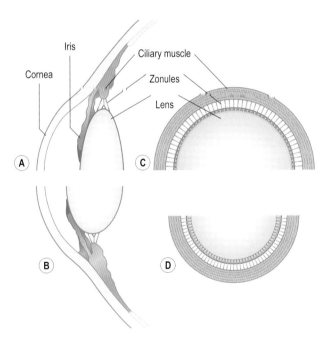

Figure 34.4 When a change of focus from far to near occurs, the lens exhibits very specific changes in shape. Its thickness increases, its equatorial diameter decreases, and its surface curvature, particularly on the anterior, becomes sharper. These changes are due to the contraction of the ciliary muscle ringing the lens equator; reduction of the diameter of the ciliary ring relaxes the zonular force acting on the lens, resulting in it "rounding up" and leading to a decrease in anterior-chamber depth. Change of focus from near to far reverses these changes, as ciliary muscle relaxation leads to increased force acting on the lens. (Modified from Koretz JF, Handelman GH. How the human eye focuses. Sci Am 1988;256:92–99.)

increased. Aside from this force application in the hydraulic theory, the other role that the ciliary muscle would play is to maintain lens position within the anterior segment. While a preponderance of data appears to support a helmholtzian representation of accommodation, it has also become evident that the support of the vitreous is a critical factor.[17] A third model of accommodation[18–20] suggests that ciliary

muscle contraction is coupled with increased equatorial zonular tension on the lens, and that presbyopia is the result of loss of the capacity to alter this tension. This model serves as the basis for the scleral expansion and scleral relaxation procedures mentioned earlier, but remains controversial because there is little or no independent verification for it.

The crystalline lens

The lens itself is not the ideally deformable material molded by changes in capsular shape, as originally suggested by Helmholtz and successors. In fact, the human lens is an intricate and highly organized structure (Figure 34.5) that grows throughout life.[21–26] New lens fiber cells differentiate from the single layer of epithelial cells found on the anterior lens surface, gradually elongating to as much as 2 mm and becoming integrated with other lens fiber cells into a flattened hexagonal packing with interconnections between each fiber cell and its six nearest neighbors. These fiber cells gradually lose their nucleus, organelles, and other inclusions while maintaining cellular protein concentrations in excess of 300 mg/ml. Such high concentrations are required of any protein solution exhibiting a significant increase in refractive index over water. Proteins that are soluble in such high concentrations and exhibit transparency in the visible spectrum under these conditions and maintain these characteristics for decades are extremely rare. An additional property of these highly concentrated solutions is that they are quite viscous. Combining the tight packing of the lens fiber cells with their viscous contents and inability to slide past each other, it is no surprise that any model of accommodation at the cellular level must involve a redistribution of material within each cell, leading to an alteration in lens fiber curvature.

Recent work by Kuszak and colleagues[27,28] has illustrated this process directly (Figure 34.6). They were able to show that the lens fiber cells are S-shaped in situ, and that they become "straighter" with accommodation, like a spring being released; this also results in the interleaved ends of the fiber cells separating from each other. This dynamic change in shape provides the ultrastructural basis for a rational explanation of lens elastic recovery, with potential energy stored in the nonaccommodated, flattened coils and released as the lens rounds up during accommodation. Thus, the lens fiber cells, individually and in combination, provide the conceptual link between the molecular (viscoelastic and optical) properties of the lens cytoplasm and its biomechanical and optical response at the whole-lens level to an accommodation stimulus.

Over the course of time, the lens undergoes specific changes which affect both its refractive capabilities and its viscoelastic (material) capacity for undergoing a change in overall shape (Figure 34.7). At the organ level, these changes have been most clearly delineated for the adult years (18–70 years). During this time the central region of the lens becomes more deeply embedded within the steadily growing lens, and the lens increases in volume and thickness with age.[29–32] This increase in thickness is uneven between the anterior and posterior, due to differences in the shape of the lens fiber cells in each region, but linear with time. Because the lens equatorial diameter remains essentially constant during this period and the distance from the cornea to the

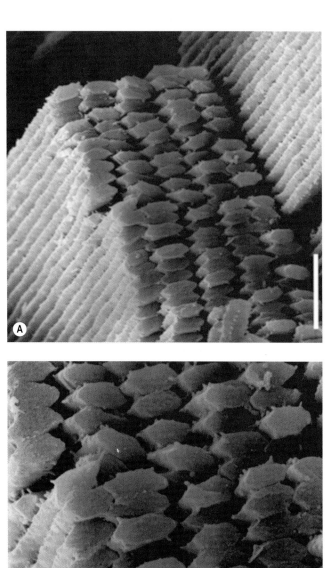

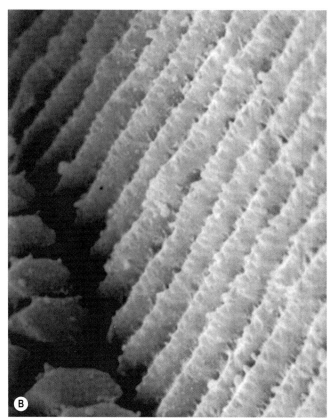

Figure 34.5 The lens is a highly organized structure, with growth taking place through the addition of differentiating lens fiber cells to the lens surface. The fiber cells (A) are arranged in a space-filling, flattened hexagonal pattern with (B) interconnections (tongue in groove and ball in socket) between fibers stabilizing geometric organization and preventing the fibers from sliding past each other (C). (Reproduced with permission from Koretz JF. Models of the lens and aging. In: Hung GK, Ciuffreda KJ (eds) Models of the Visual System. New York: Kluwer, 2002:57–103.)

lens posterior remains constant, the additional lens mass appears along the sagittal axis and leads to a steady diminution of anterior-chamber depth.[33,34]

At the subcellular and supramolecular levels, there are equivalent age-dependent processes occurring, some of which have been characterized. The highly concentrated solutions of lens proteins, primarily the lens crystallins, functionally contribute to the lens's heightened refractive index gradient. These proteins undergo a series of posttranslational modifications over time which may be associated with their longevity.[35,36] In the aging of the prepresbyopic eye, there is a slow, linear reduction in lens transparency[31]

due to lens discoloration and other chemical changes, and, more significantly, lens crystallin superaggregate formation; the latter process also contributes to an increased degree of glare, increasing night blindness, and decreasing contrast sensitivity. The rate at which these processes occur is very low, but they nevertheless affect the ability of the lens to act as a light refractor.

The increasing graininess of the lens fiber cell cytoplasm, combined with an increasing amount of superaggregated soluble and insoluble material, leads to a decreased refractive index related to the rate at which these processes occur.[37–40] At the same time, the lens surfaces are becoming

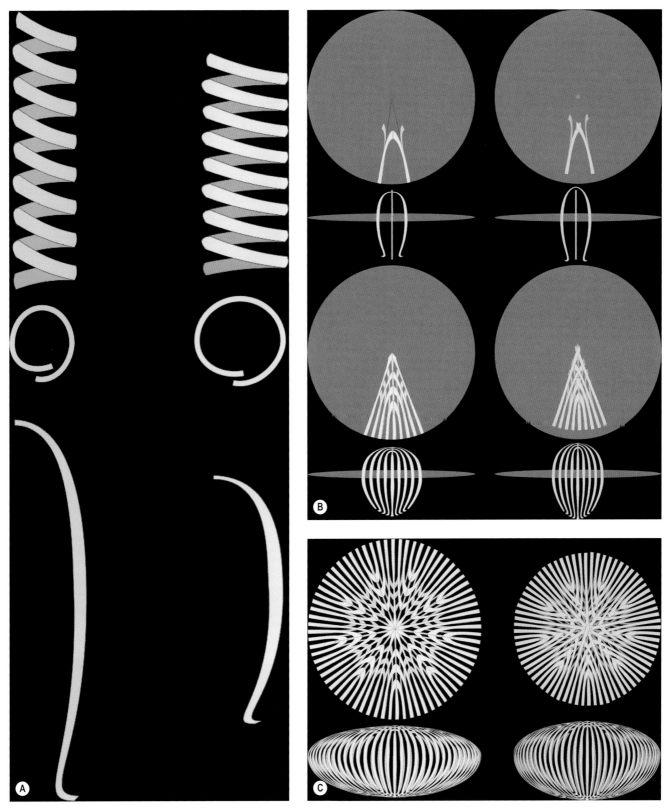

Figure 34.6 Accommodation at the lens fiber cell level. (A) The differentiated lens fiber cells are shaped like a single turn of a compressed coil, appearing as an S-shape in two dimensions. Relaxation of this coil would involve it straightening out without change in length, analogous to the redistribution of toothpaste in a tube when squeezed. (B) The ends of the fiber cells organize into sutures where they are precisely apposed. A relaxation of applied force, as in an accommodation, would allow the S-shaped cells to straighten out. Since, however, they cannot slide past each other, changes in the fibers are "accommodated" at the lens sutures, where the fiber cell tips begin to overlap. As a result (C), the lens becomes thicker and more sharply curved, while its equatorial diameter decreases. (Reproduced with permission from Tasman W, Jaeger E A (eds) Duane's Ophthalmology, 2006 edition (CD-ROM). Philadelphia: Lippincott Williams & Wilkins, 2005.)

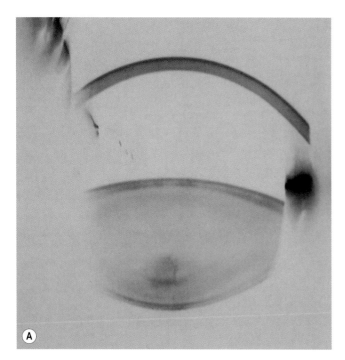

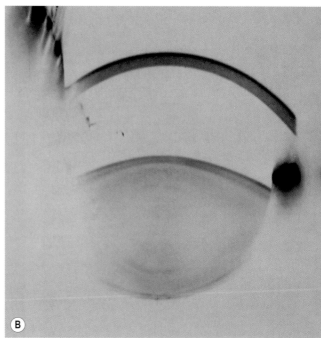

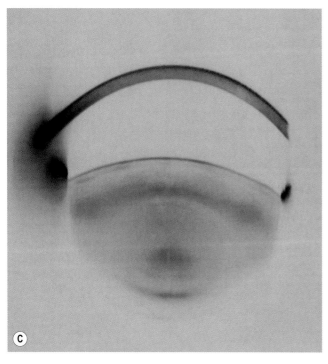

Figure 34.7 Changes in the lens and anterior segment with accommodation and age illustrated by Scheimpflug photographs from subjects aged 18 and 67 years. Accommodation by the young human lens (A: focus on infinity; B: focus at about 10 cm) involves an increase in lens sharpness of curvature, particularly on the anterior lens surface, and a shallowing of the anterior chamber. Internal lens regions also become more sharply curved, as would be expected from lens ultrastructural connections. (C) The 67-year-old subject's lens appears to have roughly the same anterior curvature as the young accommodated lens and to be at about the same distance from the cornea. However internal regions are significantly different, due in part to increased lens mass, and refractive power is equivalent to that of the young lens shown in (A). Additionally, the posterior lens surface is not fully resolved because the older anterior lens scatters so much light. (Reproduced with permission from Koretz JF. Models of the lens and aging. In: Hung GK, Ciuffreda KJ (eds) Models of the Visual System. New York: Kluwer, 2002:57–103.)

more sharply curved due to the continuing addition of new lens fiber cells.[32,41,42] Normally, one would expect that, with more sharply curved surfaces, the refractive power of the lens would increase, which would suggest that the ability to see far objects should be reduced with age, and not nearby ones. Indeed, the preservation of far vision at the expense of near despite the shape of the mature lens is the basis of Brown's "lens paradox."[43] This paradox is resolved by the fact that the gradual reduction in lens refractive power due to molecular aging processes seems almost exactly to balance the increase in the sharpness of lens curvature. In reality the balance between these two opposing trends is slightly uneven,[44,45] leading to a slight hyperopic increase of about 1 D, an additional aspect of the "myopic advantage."

In the postpresbyopic lens, these degenerative processes at the molecular level show an increase in rate. This change has been modeled either as bimodal or exponentially increasing, but whichever is used to fit the data, the critical change in slope occurs in the same decade that presbyopia becomes a significant factor in visual function. It has been suggested that the increase in the rate of these processes is due to the inability of the lens to be reshaped through the

Table 34.1 Testing the correlation between elements of the visual system and the development of presbyopia

The basic envelope – the globe and its divisions – remains essentially unchanged with age, but the geometry of the anterior segment and the properties of its components are altered

Age-independent factors
- Globe length
- Vitreous-chamber depth
- Anterior-segment length
- Corneal refractive power
- Lens equatorial diameter

Age-dependent factors

- Accommodative amplitude
- Anterior-chamber depth
- Lens thickness
- Lens refractive index gradient
- Lens shape
- Lens center of mass
- Lens transparency
- Lens elastic response
- Ciliary body/uveal tract geometry in anterior segment
- [Zonule and/or capsule material properties?]

accommodative mechanism, leading to a reduction in the efficiency of cytoplasmic "mixing" and the reliance solely on diffusion to establish and maintain chemical equilibrium throughout the lens. It is also likely that the increasing amounts of large soluble and large insoluble particles in the lens cytoplasm will affect the viscoelastic properties of the lens,[46–48] making it harder for cytoplasm to flow within the lens fiber cells and thus for lens reshaping to occur; even if it is possible for flow to occur, however, the presence of larger particles will increase both the resistance to flow and the time-dependent response to an applied stress. Thus, events at the molecular and subcellular levels, along with the overall tissue changes that occur with age,[49,50] can affect both the range of the accommodative process and the rate at which it takes place (Box 34.3).

The development of presbyopia

In order to understand the basis of presbyopia, a number of biometric studies looking for correlations between accommodative range and changes in the anterior of the eye with age have been performed. Table 34.1 provides two lists: factors that are independent of age and those that are age-dependent. Many variables associated with the lens, such as thickness, anterior and posterior central radii of curvature, and center of mass, change significantly as a function of age. Other variables showing age dependence are less explicitly associated with the lens, such as the placement of the ciliary muscle and zonular apparatus within the anterior of the eye, but will nevertheless affect the overall geometry of the system. Of course, correlation does not prove causation, but combining many of these trends together leads to models that lay the blame for presbyopia primarily on the lens. One such is the geometric model of presbyopia, formulated by Koretz and Handelman[1,12,51] on the basis of these and other biometric results combined with biomechanical modeling studies. Accommodation, according to this model, is helmholtzian, and is the result of changes in the magnitude and direction of forces applied by the ciliary muscle to the lens through the zonular fibers attached to the capsule enclosing the lens. Changes in lens shape are due to its inherent ultrastructure, since the discrete forces applied by the zonules to the capsule are evenly redistributed by its elastic properties into largely normal (perpendicular to the surface) forces. With increasing age, lens mass and thickness increase, but

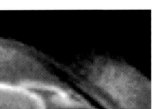

Figure 34.8 Changes in the anterior segment with age illustrated with high-resolution in vivo magnetic resonance imaging of two nonaccommodated lenses from subjects aged 26 (left) and 49 (right). Lens thickness, mass, and overall shape will change considerably, and the anterior chamber becomes shallower. Note that the ciliary muscle location relative to the cornea and lens is shifted with age as well, providing additional support for the geometric theory. (Reproduced with permission from Strenk SA, Strenk LM, Koretz JF. The mechanism of presbyopia. Prog Retin Eye Res 2005;24:379–393.)

the posterior lens surface along the optical axis remains about the same distance away from the cornea (vitreous-chamber depth is constant), resulting in a net anterior movement of lens mass. At the same time, the zonular insertions into the capsule remain in the same location relative to the

Box 34.4 Aging of accommodation

- Increasing sharpness of curvature of all lens boundaries
- Changes in lens anterior, including thickness and curvature, greater than posterior
- Decreasing overall lens power
- Loss of accommodative range, as near point approaches far point
- Reduction in steepness of lens gradient refractive index compensating for increased lens sharpness of curvature nearly exactly (solution to "Brown's lens paradox")
- Change in lens geometry relative to ciliary body, uveal tract
- Changes in ciliary body geometry

optical axis, so that the geometric relationship between the muscle, the lens, and the zonules gradually changes, and the effective mechanical advantage of the system is gradually lost (Figure 34.8). That a change in the ciliary muscle location within the anterior segment also occurs may well be due to lens growth and the concomitant application of a distorting force on the muscle to relieve extra stress; interestingly, when the lens is removed, as in cataract surgery, the ciliary muscle bounces back to its original, youthful location. This model does not explicitly require increased lens stiffness to explain presbyopia, but it is clear that such a process would be consistent (Box 34.4). Other recent models of human accommodation and presbyopia are also primarily lens-based,[12,52-54] which strongly implies that age-dependent changes in the lens and lens-associated structures directly affect loss of accommodative amplitude.

Key references

A complete list of chapter references is available online at www.expertconsult.com. See inside cover for registration details.

1. Koretz JF, Handelman GH. How the human eye focuses. Sci Am 1988;259:92–99.
2. Koretz JF, Handelman GH. Model of the accommodative mechanism in the human eye. Vision Res 1982;22:917–927.
3. Coleman DJ. Unified model for accommodative mechanism. Am J Ophthalmol 1970;69:1063–1079.
4. Koretz JF, Handelman GH. A model for accommodation in the young human eye: the effects of lens elastic anisotropy on the mechanism. Vision Res 1983;23:1679–1686.
12. Strenk SA, Strenk LM, Koretz JF. The mechanism of presbyopia. Prog Retin Eye Res 2005;24:379–393.
14. Fisher RF. The mechanics of accommodation in relation to presbyopia. Eye 1988;2:646–649.
25. Kuszak JR, Zoltoski RK. The mechanism of accommodation at the lens fiber level.

In: Ioseliani OR (ed.) Focus on Eye Research. Hauppage, NY: NovaScience, 2006:117–133.
29. Brown N. The change in lens curvature with age. Exp Eye Res 1974;19:175–183.
32. Koretz JF, Cook CA, Kaufman PL. Aging of the human lens: changes in lens shape at zero-diopter accommodation. J Opt Soc Am A Opt Image Sci Vis 2001;18:265–272.
33. Strenk SA, Semmlow JL, Strenk LM, et al. Age-related changes in human ciliary muscle and lens: a magnetic resonance imaging study. Invest Ophthalmol Vis Sci 1999;40:1162–1169.
34. Strenk SA, Strenk LM, Guo S. Magnetic resonance imaging of aging, accommodating, phakic, and pseudophakic ciliary muscle diameters. J Cataract Refract Surg 2006;32:1792–1798.

38. Moffat BA, Atchison DA, Pope JM. Age-related changes in refractive index distribution and power of the human lens as measured by magnetic resonance micro-imaging in vitro. Vision Res 2002;42:1683–1693.
43. Koretz J, Handelman GH. The lens paradox and image formation in accommodating human eyes. In: Duncan G (ed.) The Lens: Transparency and Cataract. Rijswijk: EURAGE, 1986:57–64.
45. Koretz JF, Cook CA. Aging of the optics of the human eye: lens refraction models and principal plane locations. Optom Vis Sci 2001;78:396–404.
53. Gerometta R, Zamudio AC, Escobar DP, et al. Volume change of the ocular lens during accommodation. Am J Physiol Cell Physiol 2007;293:C797–C804.

CHAPTER 35

Restoration of accommodation

Stephen D McLeod and Michelle Trager Cabrera

Clinical background

Accommodation refers to a process whereby a change in position as well as increased curvature of the crystalline lens increases the conjugation power of the eye, i.e., its ability to converge an image to focus on the retina. This process allows for the focus of a near object of regard on the retina. The first well-recognized and now widely accepted theory of accommodation was proposed by Hermann von Helmholtz in 1856. Helmholtz's theory posits that accommodation occurs through a relative rounding of the lens due to relaxation of the zonules, the fibrous elements that suspend the lens in place. The ciliary muscle attaching to the fibrous zonules contracts during accommodation, leading to relaxation of the zonules and therefore rounding of the crystalline lens. The change in shape of the lens leads to increased conjugation power of the eye, and therefore enhanced focus at near (Figure 35.1).

As humans age, a well-established age-correlated decrease in accommodation occurs starting at just over the age of 40. This process is known as presbyopia. The causes of presbyopia are varied and include changes in the lens shape, size and compliance, as well as changes in the ciliary body and zonular structure.

Based on the various etiologies of presbyopia, multiple surgical approaches have been introduced for restoring accommodation in the presbyopic or pseudophakic population with variable effectiveness. These procedures can be broadly categorized into two groups: procedures intended to enhance the change in crystalline lens shape during accommodation that is attenuated in presbyopia, and procedures whereby the rigid and enlarged crystalline lens is removed and replaced by a multifocal or accommodative intraocular lens (IOL).

Pathology

Lens changes in presbyopia

The lens increases in thickness with age, with a 60-year-old lens having on average one-third greater volume than a 30-year-old lens (Box 35.1). This is demonstrated by exten-sive cadaveric analysis, ultrasound, and scheimpflug biomicroscopy.[1,2] In theory, a larger lens is more difficult to deform than a smaller lens. Mimicking zonular forces, Glasser and Campbell[3] demonstrated that older lenses exhibit less change in focal length when stretched radially, both with and without the lens capsule. Fisher[4] has studied in great detail changes in the elasticity and water content of the lens substance, and has demonstrated constant water content with increased stiffening of the lens substance with age. By Fisher's mathematical modeling,[4] these lens changes contribute 55% of presbyopia.

Ciliary body changes in presbyopia

An age-dependent decline in ciliary body movement, amplitude, and velocity was demonstrated by Croft et al[5] through dynamic real-time videography in monkeys. This finding suggests that decreased functioning of the ciliary body itself may contribute to presbyopia. Poyer et al,[6] however, found no evidence of variable muscle function with age by observing in vitro ciliary muscle contractility induced by cholinergic agents. Examination of rhesus monkey eyes by biomicroscopy and electron microscopy revealed that posterior tendons of ciliary muscle in older monkeys exhibited increased fibrillar material compared to those of younger monkeys. Increased mechanical stiffness of the posterior insertion of the muscle with age with preserved muscle contractility may therefore contribute to presbyopia.[7]

Lens capsular changes in presbyopia

Fisher[4] postulated that, if the lens capsule is truly elastic, it can transmit radial forces from zonules to the lens and alter the lens shape during accommodation without requiring an anteroposterior force, such as vitreous pressure. Fisher[4] demonstrated that the lens capsule does have elasticity sufficient to deform the shape of the lens anteroposteriorly, as shown by centrifuging lenses to create a radial force mimicking zonules. Fisher's work demonstrated that this elasticity appears to decrease precipitously with age, a process thought to contribute at least 40% of presbyopia. The lens capsule's ability to mould the lens necessitates compliance of the lens matrix as well as sufficient force generated from the capsule. Both of these factors appear to decline with age.[2,4]

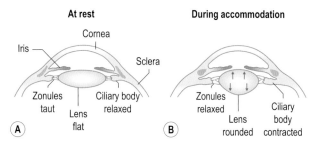

Figure 35.1 Diagram of the Helmholtz theory of accommodation. (A) A cross-section of the anterior segment during relaxation of accommodation. (B) Accommodation leads to contraction of the ciliary body muscle leading to relaxation of the zonules and rounding of the lens. The increased anteroposterior thickness of the lens increases the converging power of the eye.

Box 35.1 Anatomical changes in the eye with age

- Thickness of the crystalline lens increases
- The ciliary body muscular insertion becomes stiffer with age but the muscle itself retains contractility. Overall ciliary body muscle function decreases
- The lens capsule decreases in elasticity
- Zonular attachments migrate anteriorly

Box 35.2 Schachar's theory

- Zonular tension increases during accommodation. Increased lenticular size with age decreases zonular tension, leading to presbyopia

---

Zonular changes in presbyopia

With age, the zonular attachments to the lens migrate anteriorly, likely due to the expansion of the lens size. With a greater tangential orientation of the zonules to the lens, zonules are less able to generate force, contributing to presbyopia.[2]

Alternative theories of presbyopia

In 1994, Schachar[8] proposed a theory of accommodation that rebukes the widely accepted Helmholtz theory (Box 35.2). According to Schachar's theory, zonular tension primarily increases during accommodation. As the anterior and posterior surfaces of the lens round during accommodation, the anterior and posterior zonules, those that are visualized by biomicroscopy in vivo, relax. Meanwhile, the more important equatorial zonules increase in tension during accommodation with contraction of the ciliary body. This leads to relative flattening of the peripheral lens, but steepening of the central lens. Following this theory, increased lenticular size with age decreases equatorial zonular tension, leading to presbyopia. Scleral expansion surgery may counteract presbyopia by reinstating equatorial zonular tension.

By Schachar's theory, increased equatorial zonular tension during accommodation should pull the lens equator toward the sclera. Glasser and Kaufman's work[9] contradicts Schachar's theory by demonstrating in vivo that the lens

---

Box 35.3 Coleman's catenary theory

- Differential pressures in the anterior and posterior chambers are created during ciliary body contraction, creating a reproducible shape of the anterior lens surface important for accommodation

---

Box 35.4 Etiologies for loss of accommodation

- Normal aging process
- Pseudophakia
- Aphakia
- Changes in ciliary body functioning (spasm, paralysis, or atony)
- Cranial nerve 3 palsy

---

equator moves away from the sclera during accommodation in monkeys induced by Edinger–Westphal stimulation as well as local pharmacologic agents. Their work also revealed a downward sag of the lens with gravity during accommodation, which further challenges Schachar's theory.

Coleman proposed a theory in 1970[10] supporting a role for vitreous pressure in the processes of accommodation and presbyopia (Box 35.3). His catenary theory states that the lens, zonules, and vitreous act as a diaphragm controlling differential pressures in the anterior and vitreous chambers. Ciliary body contraction during accommodation initiates movement of the diaphragm, creating a differential pressure gradient in the eye between the anterior chamber and the vitreous cavity. Coleman asserts that this pressure gradient is crucial in establishing a reproducible "catenary" shape of the anterior lens surface during accommodation. Coleman's theory is supported by a mechanical model and demonstration of differential pressures in the two chambers during accommodation. By Coleman's model, the development of more flexible IOLs may provide some degree of accommodation.[11,12]

Mathematical modeling suggests that posterior pressure by the vitreous may be important in the process of accommodation, supporting Coleman's theory.[13] However, recent modeling with a two-dimensional axisymmetric model did not reveal an increase in refractive power with posterior lenticular pressure.[14]

Etiology

Loss of accommodation most commonly occurs by three primary mechanisms: presbyopia as a normal process of aging, pseudophakia (lens extraction followed by implantation of an artificial lens without the ability to accommodate), and aphakia (lens extraction without replacement). Less commonly, premature loss of accommodation can occur secondary to paralysis, spasm, or atony of the ciliary muscle. For example, cycloplegia with a pharmacologic agent such as atropine will paralyze the ciliary muscle and inhibit accommodation. A cranial nerve 3 palsy also paralyzes accommodation via loss of neurologic innervation of the ciliary muscle (Box 35.4).

Box 35.5 Helmholtz theory

- The equatorial zonules relax during accommodation, leading to rounding of the central lens curvature, increasing the converging power of the eye

---

Box 35.6 Extraocular changes that occur with accommodation

- Pupil size decreases
- Convergence

Box 35.7 Stimuli for accommodation

- Retinal disparity between the two eyes
- Change in angular size of an object
- Image blur

Pathophysiology

The lens

According to the Helmholtz theory of accommodation, the equatorial zonules maintain tension on the lens at rest, allowing for a relative flattening of the central curvature of the lens and an enlarged diameter. An effort to focus at near induces ciliary body contraction which paradoxically relaxes the zonules due to a centripetal movement of the muscle (Figure 35.1). In turn, the zonules release tension on the equator of the lens, allowing the lens to round up at the anterior and posterior surfaces, increasing in thickness and therefore the converging power of the eye (Box 35.5).[15]

In the modern era, through ultrasound biomicroscopy and goniovideography, Glasser and Kaufman[9] have been able to substantiate the Helmholtz theory and further characterize the accommodative process in monkeys. These investigators have documented that not only does the lens equator move away from the sclera radially during accommodation, but it also moves anteriorly due to a forward migration of the ciliary body during contraction. The contracting ciliary body, anchored to the scleral spur, trabecular meshwork, and peripheral cornea, acts as a sling to bring the lens forward during accommodation. Conversely, the elastic choroid and posterior zonules pull the lens posteriorly during relaxation of accommodation.

In addition to intraocular changes altering the lens, a number of other intraocular and extraocular changes are known to occur during accommodation to assist with viewing objects at changing distances. These factors are not considered true components of accommodation by its strict definition.

Pupil size

The pupil becomes smaller with accommodation effort by way of parasympathetic innervation of the iris sphincter from the Edinger–Westphal nucleus via the third cranial nerve.[16,17] Such a process is known to enhance depth of focus that assists with near viewing.[18] Recent work has demonstrated that the dynamic pupil near response does not change appreciably with age, and therefore likely does not contribute to or counteract presbyopia.[19] Static pupil size tends to decrease with age.[17]

Convergence

Changes in stimulation of the rectus muscles bilaterally allow for convergence of the eyes to focus on objects binocularly at varying distances. Stimuli for accommodation, both binocular and monocular, initiate convergence (Box 35.6). Therefore, accommodation within the eye and ocular convergence occur in parallel.[20]

Neural pathways in accommodation

Accommodation is initiated by voluntary effort to focus on near objects. Multiple stimuli for accommodation have been identified, but not all are well understood. It is likely that the most powerful stimulus for accommodation is retinal disparity between the two eyes as they focus on an object at varying distances. Monocular accommodation is driven by other cues for distance. For example, a change in angular size of an object has also been shown to induce accommodation even in the absence of actual distance change if all else is kept constant.[21] Image blur also induces accommodation. Placing minus lenses in front of the eye, with angular size maintained constant, appears to induce accommodation by way of blur. This effect is diminished when blur cues are blunted, such as with decreased illumination or increased depth of focus with a pinhole.[22] The mechanism by which the brain appears to recognize the appropriate direction of accommodation with blurring is unknown. Simply blurring an object without changing the refractive status of the eye or the object distance does not induce accommodation (Box 35.7).[21]

Neuronal pathways in the brain controlling accommodation are not fully understood but appear to involve primarily the Edinger–Westphal complex in the midbrain. The Edinger–Westphal complex receives inputs from the ventral and rostral midbrain, the likely location for receipt of accommodative cues such as retinal image disparity. From the Edinger–Westphal complex, the parasympathetics and third-nerve fascicles leave and synapse at the ciliary ganglion. Postsynaptic fibers continue to join the posterior ciliary nerves reaching the iris sphincter for control of pupil size as well as the ciliary body for control of accommodation[17] (Figure 35.2).

Tonic accommodation occurs at all times without any neural stimulus. Presumably baseline innervation from the midbrain is constantly firing. In a completely darkened room and without cognitive near cues, young adults are found on average to accommodate approximately 1.00 D.[20]

Restoration of accommodation

Scleral expansion surgery

Scleral expansion surgery is based on Schachar's theory[8] of accommodation that postulates that equatorial zonules increase in tension during accommodation. By this theory,

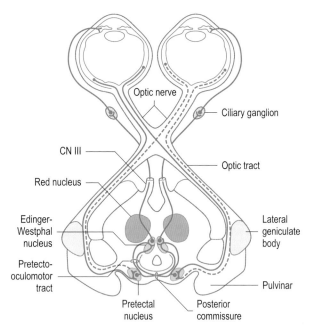

Figure 35.2 Diagram of the neural path of accommodation. CN III, third cranial nerve. (Modified from Walsh FB, Hoyt WF. Clinical Neuro-ophthalmology, 3rd edn, vol. 1. Philadelphia: Williams & Wilkins, 1969.)

Box 35.8 Scleral expansion surgery

- Relies on Schachar's theory that equatorial zonules increase in tension during accommodation
- Band implants pull sclera surrounding the zonules outward to increase zonular tension
- Encircling band implants have multiple side-effects
- More recent segmental implants (PresVIEW) may have fewer side-effects
- Further studies are needed to determine efficacy

---

as the lens enlarges with age, zonular tension decreases, leading to presbyopia (Box 35.8). Scleral expansion techniques were developed to increase the circumference of the sclera around the lens equator and ciliary body, thus increasing equatorial zonular tension, changing lens contour, and reversing presbyopia.

Scleral expansion began with simple radial incisions to the sclera. A modest accommodative effect has been reported (1.5 D of accommodation) which was lost as the sclera healed.[23] Silicone implants sewn into the incisions have been proposed to prolong the effect (over the 18 months of the study) but the measured accommodative effect has been limited (1.5 D). Subsequent encircling scleral expansion band implants have been associated with significant complications, including elevated intraocular pressure, implant extrusion, myopic shift, and anterior-segment ischemia.[23,24] Furthermore, the effectiveness of the implants has not been well established, with trials demonstrating little or no change in accommodative amplitude and a low level of patient satisfaction.[25,26]

More recently, the PresVIEW (Refocus Group, Dallas, TX) scleral implant has been developed to avoid the complications of its predecessors. The PresVIEW implant includes

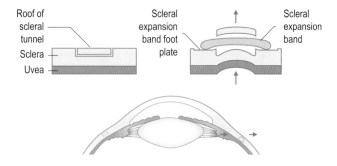

Figure 35.3 Illustration of mechanism of scleral expansion by the PresVIEW implant. First, a scleral tunnel is performed at various locations at the level of the ciliary body. Then, the scleral expansion band is inserted within the tunnel, allowing the foot plates to pull the adjacent scleral inward such that the floor of the scleral tunnel bows outward. This outward movement of sclera theoretically pulls zonules outward and increases zonular tension.

Box 35.9 Laser reduction of lens stiffness

- Photophako reduction (PPR): laser reduction of lens volume
- Photophako modulation (PPM): laser microperforations to soften the lens and increase flexibility
- Cadaver and animal studies show promise for safety and efficacy
- Concern persists for risk of cataract formation
- Further human studies necessary to determine safety and efficacy

---

four polymethyl methacrylate segments which are placed at the four oblique quadrants in partial-thickness scleral belt loops, avoiding the ciliary arteries, theoretically decreasing risk of anterior-segment ischemia. The implants are placed over scleral incisions to grasp the edge of the incisions and allow for the sclera centrally to bow outward (Figure 35.3). Phase II clinical trials show 70% of subjects with the implants having a best distance corrected near visual acuity of J3 or better compared to 4% in the control group ($P = 0.0001$).[23] Larger studies are needed to evaluate further the efficacy of this surgery. In addition, with the existence of various cadaveric and biometric evidence against Schachar's theory of accommodation,[9] the mechanism of any increased near-vision function in these subjects will need clarification.

Laser reduction of lens stiffness

In 1998, Myers and Krueger[27] proposed laser modification of the crystalline lens to treat presbyopia. By one method, called photophako reduction (PPR), accommodation is restored by laser reduction of lens volume with attention to the lens periphery. The second method, photophako modulation (PPM), seeks to soften the lens to increase flexibility, focusing on creating microperforations within the hard lens nucleus (Box 35.9). Human cadaver lenses treated with YAG laser photodisruption demonstrated significantly increased flexibility on centrifugation testing previously developed by Fisher, suggesting a potential therapeutic effect for presbyopia.[28] Although there is some promise for efficacy based on this study, there is considerable concern for iatrogenic cataract development with this treatment. In favor of the treatment, however, use of the femtosecond laser on live rabbit lenses resulted in intralenticular bubble formation that resolved without cataract formation after 3 months.[29] Further studies in humans are necessary to understand both the safety and efficacy of this treatment approach.

Intraocular lens surgery

Replacement of the lens substance by capsule-filling gel

Given that loss of lens matrix compliance appears to be in large part responsible for presbyopia, replacing the lens with pliable material has been explored extensively as a strategy to combat presbyopia. Two methods have been devised to refill the lens. By one method, a viscous material is injected into the capsule after removing the lens from a small opening in the capsule.[30,31] A second method involves insertion of a balloon filled with the viscous material into the empty capsule. Kessler first devised a method in 1964 by which the empty lens capsule is injected with a polymer mimicking the youthful crystalline lens.[32] Since then, multiple attempts have been made to achieve results for capsular refilling in animal models. Haefliger and Parel[33] have investigated direct capsule bag refilling in a primate model, and reported change in anterior-chamber depth representing accommodation under pilocarpine stimulation. Their method of evaluating accommodation has been refuted more recently because change in anterior-chamber depth may actually represent pilocarpine's effect on the position of the lens–iris diaphragm rather than definitive evidence of accommodation.[34] Nishi et al[35,36] were able to demonstrate refractive changes suggesting a small amount of accommodation by automated refractometry with pilocarpine after capsular refilling with injectable silicone in both rabbits and monkeys. Nishi's method utilized a silicone plug to prevent leakage of the injected silicone.

To avoid the technical challenges of removing a cataract from a small capsular opening and to prevent leakage of liquid from the capsular bag, a fluid-filled balloon was devised to contain the liquid artificial lens material. In rabbits, this technique failed to improve accommodation substantially and also resulted in capsular opacification.[37] Monkeys demonstrated only a modest improvement in accommodation that decreased with time with fibrosis of the lens capsule.[38]

Hettlich et al[31] devised a method of injecting a monomeric material that can be polymerized inside the capsular bag by short light exposure to avoid risk of fluid leaking out of the lens after the surgery. Containment of the artificial lens material with a balloon is no longer necessary by this method. However, beyond initial safety studies in animals, no further developments have been made using this technique.

Lens refilling by either liquid polymer injection or balloon insertion has several important drawbacks (Box 35.10). It is difficult to achieve a specific lens power with liquid polymer injection. The range of accommodation in animal models is most often minimal and frequently unpredictable. The accommodative effect appears to be unstable and short-lived due to capsular fibrotic changes. More importantly, posterior

---

> **Box 35.10 Lens refilling with a gel**
>
> - Methods include liquid polymer injection and liquid-filled balloon insertion
> - Use of balloons or silicone plugs helps counteract risk of postoperative leakage
> - Animal studies show only modest refractive results in restoring accommodation with significant capsular lens opacification postoperatively
> - Refractive results are unpredictable

> **Box 35.11 Multifocal intraocular lenses**
>
> - Utilize concentric rings of differential power to allow for far, near, and intermediate vision
> - Well-established improvement in near vision with implantation of these lenses
> - Decrease in contrast sensitivity is a significant side-effect that limits use

and anterior capsular opacification is an almost universal complication in both monkeys and rabbits in lens refilling by 3 months following surgery. Performing YAG capsulotomy may result in herniation of the lens material, negating the refractive benefits of the initial surgery.[39]

Multifocal intraocular lenses

While not actually restoring accommodation by its strict definition, multifocal IOLs have been utilized extensively to enhance near vision while maintaining distance acuity. These lenses employ concentric rings of differential refractive or diffractive power in the optic to allow for far, near, and in some cases intermediate vision (Box 35.11). Some lens designs exploit pupil size changes that naturally occur with changing distance of focus effort by assigning the lens center to near focus. While demonstrated to be effective in improving near vision and pseudoaccommodation by defocus curve analysis and subjective near vision testing, the almost universal prominent decrease in contrast sensitivity has encouraged the development of alternative modalities for restoration of accommodation.[40]

Accommodative intraocular lenses

As an alternative to capsular bag filling, Hara and colleagues proposed the implantation of a rigid optic lens implant that moves with accommodation to change the refractive status of the eye.[41] These investigators devised an implant known as the "spring IOL" with two optics connected by a polypropylene coil spring. The two optics are compressed by the capsular bag and then separated with ciliary body constriction as tension on the capsular bag is released. A modification of the original design consisted of two optics separated by four peripheral polyvinylidene fluoride haptics. The posterior optic is plano while the anterior optic contains the appropriate power for the lens complex. The haptics transmit the movement of the capsular bag due to changes in zonular tension during near activity.[41] Initial rabbit studies failed to demonstrate accommodation with these devices, likely due to species-specific limitations.[42]

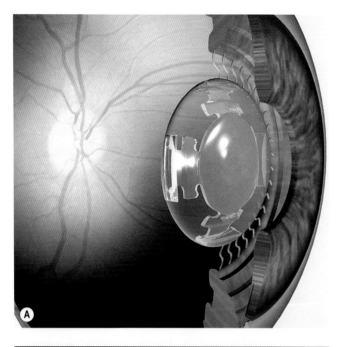

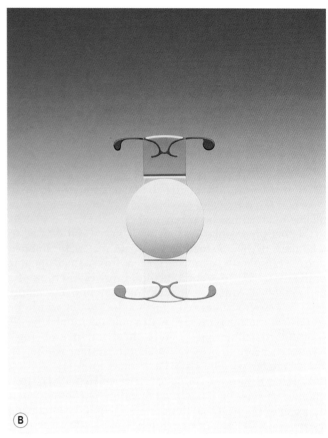

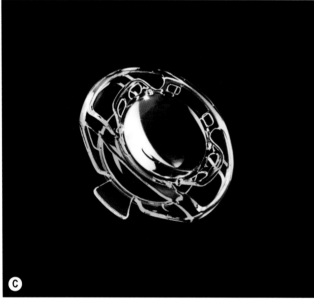

Figure 35.4 Accommodating intraocular lenses currently available or in development. (A) The 1CU implant (HumanOptics, Erlangen, Germany; image courtesy of HumanOptics). (B) The AT-45 Crystalens (Eyeonics, Aliso Viejo, CA; image courtesy of Eyeonics). (C) The Synchrony lens (Visiogen, Irvine, CA; image courtesy of Visiogen).

Subsequent developments of accommodating IOLs have relied on similar principles to the "spring IOL," utilizing a pair of hinged optics that harness the force of ciliary body contriction for axial movement and refractive change in the eye during near work. Changes in posterior vitreous pressure, as described by Coleman,[12] may also play a role in accommodating IOL movement. Clinical trials with these devices have demonstrated a modest degree of accommodation in humans. Some of these devices are still in the early stages of clinical evaluation and show promise for clinical efficacy, while others have received Food and Drug Administration approval and have entered clinical practice. See Figure 35.4 for various accommodating IOL schematics and photographs and Box 35.12.

In a recent meta-analysis of accommodating IOLs,[43] five randomized controlled trials and 15 nonrandomized con-

trolled trials were identified assessing the clinical success of the HumanOptics (Erlangen, Germany) 1CU implant (Figure 35.4A). Three of the five randomized controlled trials found a statistically significant improvement in distance corrected near visual acuity compared to control subjects with monofocal implants. Nonetheless, the mean distance corrected near visual acuity from all 20 studies is only J7. Several of these studies demonstrated axial movement of the IOL with instillation of pilocarpine, supporting the principles of design. Unfortunately, neither a mean axial movement of 1 mm or less nor a mean distance corrected near visual acuity of J7 in these studies would accomplish the goal of freedom from reading glasses.[43]

Seven nonrandomized studies of another accommodating IOL, the AT-45 Crystalens (Eyeonics, , Aliso Viejo, CA), found highly variable results in clinically demonstrated

Box 35.12 Accommodative intraocular lenses

- HumanOptics (Erlangen, Germany) 1CU implant: randomized controlled trials in humans show significant improvement in near vision and appropriate movement of lens with pilocarpine; however, most patients still require reading glasses
- AT-45 Crystalens (Eyeonics, Aliso Viejo, CA): nonrandomized controlled trials in humans show improvement in near vision to J3 in over 90% of subjects; however, variable movement of lens with pilocarpine
- Synchrony lens (Visiogen, Irvine, CA): has a high-powered plus anterior optic coupled with a compensatory minus posterior optic. Early pilot study controlled trials show 96% of subjects with J3 or better near vision; however further studies are needed
- BioComFold IOL 43E (Morcher, Stuttgart, Germany): has a peripheral bulging ring that pushes the intraocular lens forward with ciliary body constriction. Significant appropriate movement of the lens seen with pilocarpine; however no significant difference in accommodation

accommodation.[43] (Figure 35.4B). The largest study of 246 subjects found 90.1% of subjects with this lens showing a best distance corrected near visual acuity of J3 or better.[44] Biometric studies of IOL movement with pilocarpine 2% revealed conflicting results, however, with one study showing a backward movement of the IOL.[43] Although promising, randomized clinical trials with appropriate control groups are necessary to assess the AT-45 Crystalens definitively.

Utilizing a dual-optic single-piece silicone IOL design, the Synchrony lens (Visiogen, Irvine, CA) has a high powered plus anterior optic coupled with a compensatory minus posterior optic (Figure 35.4C). By ray tracing analysis, this design enhances the accommodative power of the eye without requiring an increased axial movement of the IOL.[45,46] In the pilot clinical study of 24 subjects with the Synchrony lens implant, 96% of subjects had a best distance

corrected near visual acuity of J3 or better. Subjects with the Synchrony lens implant had significantly greater accommodation measured by defocus curves compared to a control group with monofocal implants (3.22 D, range 1.00–8.00 D, compared to 1.65 D, range 1.00–2.50 D). While these results are promising, biomicroscopy to demonstrate IOL movement as well as larger clinical trials are needed to establish the efficacy of this accommodating IOL.

The BioComFold IOL 43E (Stuttgart, Germany) has a peripheral bulging ring that pushes the IOL forward with ciliary body constriction (no picture shown). Among 15 subjects implanted with the BioComFold IOL, the lens was shown to shift anteriorly to a greater degree than monofocal lenses with instillation of pilocarpine (0.72 ± 0.58 mm compared to 0.28 ± 0.38 mm); however no significant difference in accommodation measured by defocus curves was seen between the two groups.[47]

Conclusions

Restoration of accommodation is an exciting and dynamic field today. Various approaches to the reversal of presbyopia are currently in development. More sophisticated techniques accompanied by future human safety and efficacy trials are needed to elucidate the utility of modification of the crystalline lens as a technique for presbyopia reversal. Scleral expansion surgery continues to be a controversial technique and has an uncertain future. Multifocal lenses, while somewhat effective, are limited by quality of vision issues and loss of contrast sensitivity. While lens refilling techniques have largely been abandoned due to poor results in animal trials, advances in material and control of lens epithelial cell proliferation may improve performance. Multiple accommodating IOL designs are now entering the market with promising results in human clinical trials. Larger randomized controlled trials are needed to establish that these lenses provide adequate visual function to allow patients to forgo spectacle correction for the broad range of daily tasks.

Key references

A complete list of chapter references is available online at www.expertconsult.com. See inside cover for registration details.

3. Glasser A, Campbell MC. Presbyopia and the optical changes in the human crystalline lens with age. Vision Res 1998;38:209–229.
4. Fisher RF. The elastic constants of the human lens. J Physiol 1971;212:147–180.
8. Schachar RA. Zonular function: a new hypothesis with clinical implications. Ann Ophthalmol 1994;26:36–38.
9. Glasser A, Kaufman PL. The mechanism of accommodation in primates. Ophthalmology 1999;106:863–872.
10. Coleman DJ. Unified model for accommodative mechanism. Am J Ophthalmol 1970;69:1063–1079.
15. Helmholtz Hv. Treatise on Physiological Optics. New York: Dover Publications, 1962.
23. Kleinmann G, Kim HJ, Yee RW. Scleral expansion procedure for the correction of presbyopia. Int Ophthalmol Clin 2006;46:1–12.
26. Mathews S. Scleral expansion surgery does not restore accommodation in human presbyopia. Ophthalmology 1999;106:873–877.
27. Myers RI, Krueger RR. Novel approaches to correction of presbyopia with laser modification of the crystalline lens. J Refract Surg 1998;14:136–139.
32. Kessler J. Experiments in refilling the lens. Arch Ophthalmol 1964;71:412–417.
33. Haefliger E, Parel JM. Accommodation of an endocapsular silicone lens (Phaco-Ersatz) in the aging rhesus monkey. J Refract Corneal Surg 1994;10:550–555.
40. Leyland M, Pringle E. Multifocal versus monofocal intraocular lenses after cataract extraction. Cochrane Database Syst Rev 2006;CD003169.
43. Findl O, Leydolt C. Meta-analysis of accommodating intraocular lenses. J Cataract Refract Surg 2007;33:522–527.
44. Cumming JS, Colvard DM, Dell SJ, et al. Clinical evaluation of the Crystalens AT-45 accommodating intraocular lens: results of the U.S. Food and Drug Administration clinical trial. J Cataract Refract Surg 2006;32:812–825.
46. McLeod SD. Optical principles, biomechanics, and initial clinical performance of a dual-optic accommodating intraocular lens (an American Ophthalmological Society thesis). Trans Am Ophthalmol Soc 2006;104:437–452.

CHAPTER 36

Intraoperative floppy iris syndrome

Amy Lin and Roger F Steinert

Overview

Intraoperative floppy iris syndrome (IFIS) was first characterized by Chang and Campbell in 2005.[1] It is associated with the use of systemic α-receptor blockers, such as tamsulosin (Flomax), used in the medical management of benign prostatic hyperplasia (BPH). The features of IFIS are seen during cataract surgery despite proper wound construction and compose of a triad of: (1) a flaccid iris that billows in response to normal intraoperative fluid currents; (2) a strong propensity for the iris to prolapse through any or all properly constructed incisions; and (3) progressive intraoperative pupillary constriction.[1] This behavior of the iris creates a difficult situation for the surgeon and can potentially increase the complication rate. About 2% of the general cataract surgery population has some degree of IFIS.[1] Since the syndrome was first described, surgeons have devised a variety of techniques to minimize the characteristics of IFIS.

Pharmacology

The iris is a complex structure mediated by the iris dilator smooth muscle and the sphincter muscle. When the α-receptors are stimulated, the dilator smooth muscle contracts to cause pupillary dilation, and conversely, when the α-receptors are blocked, the dilator smooth muscle relaxes, causing pupillary miosis.[2] There are nine subtypes of α-receptors: α_{1a}, α_{1b}, α_{1d}, α_{2a}, α_{2b}, α_{2c}, ß_1, ß_2, and ß_3.[2] Like most tissues, multiple subtypes of adrenergic receptors exist in the iris smooth muscle. However, iris contraction is 100-fold more sensitive to α_1-antagonists than α_2-antagonists, which suggests that α_1-receptors predominate in mediating dilation.[2] Molecular, protein, and functional assays have found that the α_{1a}-receptor subtype mediates iris dilator smooth-muscle contraction in animal species.[2] It is presumed that humans have a similar α_{1a}-receptor profile in the iris dilator muscle.

Like the iris, the prostate smooth muscle is also mediated by a balance of sympathetic, parasympathetic, and other receptor systems (Box 36.1). BPH is associated with lower urinary tract symptoms such as nocturia, dysuria, and incomplete bladder emptying.[3] The main α_1-receptor subtype found in the smooth muscle of the prostate, urethra, and bladder neck is the α_{1a}-receptor.[2] Blockage of the α_{1a}-receptor relaxes the prostatic smooth muscle to relieve outflow obstruction, and enhances urine flow. Older α_1-receptor blockers such as alfuzosin (Uroxatral), doxazosin (Cardura), and terazosin (Hytrin) bind all α_1 subtypes equally.[2] Tamsulosin (Flomax) is more uroselective,[3] as it selectively binds α_{1a} and α_{1d}-receptors.[2] However, because tamsulosin is a systemic drug, it is also selective for the iris dilator smooth muscle.

It is presumed that the lack of tone in the dilator muscle of the iris due to the highly selective α_{1a}-receptor blockade is responsible for the signs of IFIS.[4] However, several studies have found that only a portion of patients on tamsulosin develop the manifestations of IFIS, and that there is a continuum of the degree of manifestation.[5-7] Of patients taking tamsulosin, the percentage of eyes of patients with no IFIS features has been found to range from 10% to 43%.[5-7] The percentage of eyes with all three characteristics of IFIS, or severe IFIS, has been reported as 30–43%.[6,7] Manivikar and Allen[8] found that 31% of eyes were well dilated and remained so throughout the surgery, 22% were well dilated but constricted during the surgery, 38% were mid dilated and remained the same or constricted further during the surgery, and 9% were poorly dilated at the outset.[8] IFIS can present in varying degrees even between the two eyes of the same patient. Complete IFIS has been reported to occur in the eye of one patient, when surgery in the fellow eye 1 week prior did not reveal any IFIS.[9]

While IFIS is clearly associated with tamsulosin, it is unclear whether or not other medications or systemic conditions can manifest an IFIS-like picture. Because the nonselective α-blockers have some affinity for the α_{1a}-receptor, one can presume that these medications may cause a minor degree of IFIS; however, multiple studies have not found an association between the nonselective α-blockers and IFIS.[1,5] It is possible that other medications may cause IFIS. Zuclopenthixol, an antipsychotic with dopaminergic, as well as α-adrenergic blockade, may be associated with IFIS.[10] However, this was found in just one patient, and thus warrants further study. Patients with diabetes and pseudoexfoliation syndrome can have poor dilation; however, these disease processes have not been implicated in IFIS.[5] Similarly, pilocarpine, a muscarinic receptor antagonist, which causes miosis, has not been associated with IFIS.[5] Furthermore, it has been reported that patients may develop IFIS

Box 36.1 Basic IFIS mechanism

- Tamsulosin (Flomax) is a highly selective α_{1a}-receptor blocker
- α_1-receptor blockade relaxes the iris dilator smooth muscle, causing miosis
- There is a broad continuum in the manifestation of the features of intraoperative floppy iris syndrome, with variation even between the eyes of the same patient

Box 36.2 Long-lasting effects of tamsulosin

- Stopping tamsulosin preoperatively does not affect the severity of intraoperative floppy iris syndrome
- Previous use of tamsulosin even years before surgery does not eliminate the manifestation of intraoperative floppy iris syndrome

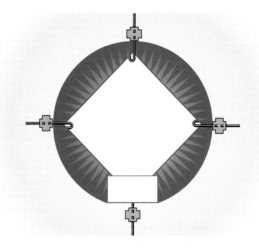

Figure 36.1 Oetting's diamond configuration of iris retractors. (Redrawn with permission from Oetting TA, Omphroy LC. Modified technique using flexible iris retractors in clear corneal surgery. J Cataract Refract Surg 2002;28:596–598.)

without any known reason.[5] There may be other issues at play in IFIS besides a simple α_{1a}-blockade of the iris dilator muscle.

Preoperative intervention

Many solutions have been proposed to minimize the effects of IFIS. The first seemingly obvious solution was to remove the offending medication. The half-life of tamsulosin is 48–72 hours.[1] Stopping tamsulosin use prior to cataract surgery may have a slight effect on improving preoperative dilation, but does not affect IFIS severity.[6] Patients have been reported to have varying degrees of IFIS even if they had not taken tamsulosin for 1–10 years.[1,7,9] It is thought that a relatively constant α_{1a}-receptor blockade while patients are on tamsulosin therapy can lead to disuse atrophy of the iris smooth muscle.[1] A lack of iris rigidity would explain the billowing of the iris to the point of prolapse through all wounds. The progressive miosis may be the natural response of the iris to its own billowing in the midst of normal irrigation currents. It is not known how long patients have to be taking tamsulosin before exhibiting the features of IFIS. It has been reported to occur after 3 months of use,[7] but there have been anecdotal reports of occurrence after less than 1 month of therapy. Currently, most surgeons do not advocate discontinuing the drug before cataract surgery because of lack of evidence of any benefit (Box 36.2).

Intraoperative measures

Prior to the description of IFIS, there were various techniques for enlarging a poorly dilated pupil. These methods included pupil stretching, sphincterotomies, and pupillary restraints such as iris hooks and pupil expansion rings (Box 36.3). As reported in Chang and Campbell's original article,[1] pupil stretching and sphincterotomies did not prevent iris prolapse or progressive pupil constriction. This phenomenon was thought to occur because the IFIS pupillary margin remained elastic, and snapped back to its original size. The authors recommended iris hooks or expansion rings for maintenance of a sufficiently large pupil. It was further rec-

Box 36.3 Interventions that may minimize the manifestations of intraoperative floppy iris syndrome

- Pupil expansion rings or iris hooks with subincisional placement
- Healon 5 to dilate pupil and tamponade iris anteriorly
- Topical atropine prior to surgery
- Intracameral phenylephrine or epinephrine

ommended that the iris hooks be oriented in the diamond configuration described by Oetting and Omphroy,[11] which has an iris retractor placed subincisionally (Figure 36.1). This technique minimizes further iris prolapse and damage to the iris by the phacoemulsification needle, as well as increasing the space accessible by the phacoemulsification needle.

Since the original IFIS article, surgeons have proposed a multitude of additional ways to maximize pupil size and prevent iris billowing and prolapse. A super-cohesive viscoelastic, such as sodium hyaluronate 2.3% (Healon 5, Advanced Medical Optics, Santa Ana, CA) has been used to augment pupil dilation intraoperatively, as well as tamponade the peripheral iris to block iris prolapse. At low flow and vacuum rates, Healon 5 resists aspiration and can stay within the eye.[4] Aspiration of the Healon 5 can be further prevented by keeping the phacoemulsification needle at, or posterior to, the level of the pupil. If aspiration does occur, the anterior chamber can be reinjected with more Healon 5, or a dispersive viscoelastic such as sodium hyaluronate 3%–chondroitin sulfate 4% (Viscoat) can be injected centrally following the initial peripheral Healon 5 injection, helping to resist aspiration and keep the original Healon 5 over the peripheral iris.[4]

If Healon 5 alone is used prior to the capsulorrhexis, capsule tearing can be more difficult because of the increased resistance within this viscoelastic environment. Arshinoff had already devised a method, termed the ultimate soft-shell technique, to simplify this step.[12] Healon 5 is injected in the anterior chamber to about 60–80% full. Then the rest of the anterior chamber is slowly filled with balanced salt solution (BSS) by aiming the injection cannula at the surface of the lens capsule, near the center. This keeps the anterior lens capsule well tamponaded during the capsulorrhexis, yet with minimal resistance to tearing.[12]

Additional pharmacologic measures to prevent IFIS manifestations have been reported. Preoperative use of topical atropine 1% twice a day for 10 days before surgery has been described to improve preoperative dilation over the standard drops of cyclopentolate and phenylephrine on the day of surgery. The dilation was maintained intraoperatively in most patients, with 19% (3/16) of patients requiring additional modifications of surgical technique.[13]

Intracameral pharmaceutical interventions for dilation have been explored. These methods may maximally stimulate the atrophic iris dilator smooth muscle. Manivikar and Allen[8] employed standard topical dilating and nonsteroidal drops on the day of surgery, but also used intracameral preservative-free phenylephrine if the pupil was small or mid dilated at the start of surgery, or if there was significant pupil constriction or iris prolapse during the surgery.[8] When intracameral phenylephrine was used at the start of surgery, there was a variable response, with some pupils staying the same size, and others dilating further. However, when intracameral phenylephrine was used when iris difficulties arose during surgery, it stopped the iris from prolapsing and dilated the pupil back to its preoperative size. This response took about 30–35 seconds for maximal effect.[8]

Because of the high acidity of dilating agents, there has been concern over toxicity. Manivikar and Allen[8] were careful to use preservative-free phenylephrine diluted to a pH of 6.4. In a letter, Shugar[14] described success in using intracameral epinephrine in the eyes of patients taking tamsulosin, with the thought that flooding the iris directly with epinephrine could overcome the α_{1a}-receptor blockade. He evaluated the pH and performed rabbit studies to investigate any potential toxicity of his solution of 1:1000 bisulfite-free epinephrine mixed in a 1:3 dilution into his intracameral anesthetic mixture of BSS plus and preservative-free lidocaine ("Shugarcaine": 3 parts BSS plus mixed with 1 part nonpreserved 4% lidocaine).[14] The pH of his solution was 6.899, well within physiologic range. He injected the solution into the anterior chambers of rabbits, and found significantly less corneal edema than compared to bisulfite-containing solutions.

Masket and Belani[15] reported success in using intracameral epinephrine diluted to 1:2500 in combination with topical use of atropine 1% for 2 days preoperatively. In 19 of 20 eyes, sufficient pupil dilation was achieved, without intraoperative constriction or billowing of the iris. One eye required iris hooks because no further dilation was achieved with intracameral epinephrine. Sodium hyaluronate 3%–chondroitin sulfate 4% (DisCoVisc), a mixed cohe-sive as well as dispersive viscoelastic was used in all cases. The pharmacologic combination of atropine and epinephrine was postulated to have worked well because of the synergistic effect of blockage of the muscarinic receptors of the iris sphincter muscle, coupled with direct stimulation of the weakened iris dilator muscle with concentrated epinephrine. Use of DisCoVisc may have been of value as well, as it mechanically dilated the pupil further and also held the iris in a favorable position during surgery.

Bimanual microincisional cataract surgery may offer some benefit in IFIS cases, as it creates a small and maximally watertight seal to prevent iris prolapse, and has a separate irrigation port which can be kept anterior to the iris to prevent billowing. Chang and Campbell[1] used this technique on four eyes, but it only helped in two of the cases. At the time of writing, there had not been any published studies regarding bimanual phacoemulsification and its role in IFIS.

Conclusions

There has been much interest in IFIS since it was first described. New techniques for preventing its manifestations continue to evolve. There are still questions surrounding the pathophysiology and variability of its clinical presentation, with ongoing studies in this area. Because of the potential increase in risk of complications during surgery, it is vital that all patients be screened for any past history of taking tamsulosin. Although tamsulosin is indicated for the treatment of BPH, it is also being used off-label in women for treatment of lower urinary tract symptoms. Knowledge of tamsulosin use is the first step in anticipating possible IFIS. A surgeon should be comfortable with various methods of dealing with IFIS to decrease the rate of complications.

Summary

IFIS has been associated with tamsulosin (Flomax), a highly selective α_1-receptor drug for BPH. Because antagonism of the α_1-receptors causes relaxation of the iris dilator muscle, it is thought that lack of iris tone causes the features of IFIS: a billowing iris, iris prolapse, and progression intraoperative miosis. There is a great variability of IFIS presentation, ranging from no manifestations to a severe degree of presentation. A patient with any present or previous history of taking tamsulosin is considered at risk for exhibiting IFIS. There are a variety of intraoperative maneuvers to help the surgeon achieve control over the abnormal iris, and thus prevent complications during cataract surgery. Anticipation of possible IFIS is the first step to a successful surgery in the setting of IFIS.

Key references

1. Chang DF, Campbell JR. Intraoperative floppy iris syndrome associated with tamsulosin. J Cataract Refract Surg 2005;31:664–673.
2. Schwinn DA, Afshari NA. α_1-Adrenergic receptor antagonists and the iris: new mechanistic insights into floppy iris syndrome. Surv Ophthalmol 2006;51: 501–512.
3. Thiyagarajan M. α-Adrenoreceptor antagonists in the treatment of benign prostate hyperplasia.

Pharmacology 2002;65:119–128.
4. Mamalis N. Intraoperative floppy iris syndrome [editorial]. J Cataract Refract Surg 2006;32:1589–1590.

5. Chadha V, Borooah S, Tey A, et al. Floppy iris behaviour during cataract surgery: associations and variations. Br J Ophthalmol 2007;91:40–42.

6. Chang DF, Osher RH, Wang L, et al. Prospective multicenter evaluation of cataract surgery in patients taking tamsulosin (flomax). Ophthalmology 2007;114:957–964.

7. Cheung CMG, Awan MAR, Sandramouli S. Prevalence and clinical findings of tamsulosin-associated intraoperative floppy-iris syndrome. J Cataract Refract Surg 2006;32:1336–1339.

8. Manivikar S, Allen D. Cataract surgery management in patients taking tamsulosin: staged approach. J Cataract Refract Surg 2006;32:1611–1614.

9. Takmaz T, Can I. Intraoperative floppy-iris syndrome: do we know everything about it? J Cataract Refract Surg 2007;33:1110–1112.

10. Pringle E, Packard R. Antipsychotic agent as an etiologic agent for IFIS. J Cataract Refract Surg 2005;31:2240–2241.

11. Oetting TA, Omphroy LC. Modified technique using flexible iris retractors in clear corneal surgery. J Cataract Refract Surg 2002;28:596–598.

12. Arshinoff SA. Using BSS with viscoadaptives in the ultimate soft-shell technique. J Cataract Refract Surg 2002;28:1509–1514.

13. Bendel RE, Phillips MB. Preoperative use of atropine to prevent intraoperative floppy-iris syndrome in patients taking tamsulosin. J Cataract Refract Surg 2006;32:1603–1605.

14. Shugar JK. Use of epinephrine for IFIS prophylaxis. J Cataract Refract Surg 2006;32:1074–1075.

15. Masket S, Belani S. Combined preoperative atropine sulfate 1% and intracameral nonpreserved epinephrine hydrochloride 1:2500 for management of intraoperative floppy-iris syndrome. J Cataract Refract Surg 2007;33:580–582.

Optic neuritis

John R Guy and Xiaoping Qi

Clinical background

Optic neuritis is an inflammatory disorder of autoimmune optic nerve demyelination. It is often the first clinical sign of multiple sclerosis (MS).[1,2] Optic neuritis is second only to glaucoma as the most common optic neuropathy in the USA. There are approximately 25 000 cases diagnosed per year. Optic neuritis patients are young, typically more than 10 years of age but less than 50 years of age. The clinical symptomatology is characterized by sudden painful visual loss in one eye, although occasionally both eyes can be simultaneously involved. The pain is usually exacerbated by eye movement. Optic neuritis associated with transverse myelitis may be due to Devics disease.

Clinical examination of patients with acute optic neuritis usually reveals a relative afferent pupillary defect (unilateral cases or bilateral cases with asymmetric involvement), visual field deficits, loss of visual acuity, contrast sensitivity, color vision, and stereopsis. The intraocular segment of optic nerve known as the optic nerve head that is visible by clinical examination with an ophthalmoscope is normal in three-quarters of cases. When swelling of the optic nerve head is present, leakage of lipid from the vasculature of the swollen disc into the neurosensory retina sometimes results in a macular star pattern. Although this is coined neuroretinitis, retinal inflammation is typically absent.

In a landmark study of almost 500 optic neuritis patients, the Optic Neuritis Treatment Trial (ONTT), visual field defects were nonspecific in approximately half the patients.[1] In those patients with defects considered specific for an optic neuropathy, one-third were altitudinal defects previously associated with another disorder, ischemic optic neuropathy, caused by infarction of the optic nerve head that also has swelling of the optic nerve head. Occasionally the visual field defects of optic neuritis may be a bitemporal hemianopsia or junctional scotoma mimicking a pituitary adenoma or other suprasellar mass such as an aneurysm compressing the optic chiasm. Such cases may be resolved by neuroimaging with magnetic resonance imaging (MRI) or computed tomography (CT), as done for two patients inadvertently entered into the ONTT who turned out to have a pituitary adenoma or aneurysm as the cause of their optic neuropathy. MRI is the imaging modality of choice, as it typically reveals contrast enhancement of the optic nerve characteristic of disruption of the blood–optic nerve barrier in most cases of acute optic neuritis.[2] For visualization of contrast enhancement of the intraorbital optic nerve, a fat suppression pulse sequence is necessary. MRI also reveals asymptomatic lesions of the intracranial white matter associated with the MS and excludes compressive lesions.

Etiology

While optic neuritis may occur in isolation or in association with MS, systemic diseases such as sarcoidosis,[3,4] collagen vascular disease,[5] or the remote effects of cancer[6] and infections including cat scratch,[7,8] human immunodeficiency virus (HIV),[9,10] syphilis,[11] retinal necrosis,[12,13] Whipple's disease,[14] or West Nile encephalitis[15] may be masqueraders of optic neuritis. They can be elucidated by atypical features such as persistence of pain, progression of visual loss beyond 2 weeks, or lack of visual recovery after 4 weeks.

Genetics

Traditionally, optic neuritis and MS have not been considered to be genetic disorders, apart from association with certain human leukocyte antigen (HLA) haplotypes. Recently, single nucleotide polymorphisms have been detected in the mitochondrial genome of some optic neuritis patients[16] and in the gene encoding the interleukin-7 receptor alpha chain (IL7R) in MS patients (Box 37.1).[17,18]

Prognosis

The prognosis of visual loss in optic neuritis is typically good.[19] Visual loss stops worsening 2 weeks after it begins and by 4 weeks most patients show signs of recovery.[20] Recovery of vision occurs in almost all patients after their initial bout of optic neuritis.[21] Still, 6% are left with 20/50 or worse, and 3% are devastated by 20/200 or worse, i.e., legal blindness. Even though visual acuity recovers to 20/20 in 70% of patients and even more (87%) recover to 20/25, most of these patients show signs of residual deficits in their contrast sensitivity, visual fields, and stereopsis 10 years later, thereby suggesting these troubling deficits are permanent. A single recurrence of optic neuritis is common (60%

Box 37.1

- Optic neuritis is an inflammatory disorder of autoimmune optic nerve demyelination that is often the first clinical sign of multiple sclerosis
- Optic neuritis is second only to glaucoma as the commonest optic neuropathy in the USA
- Traditionally, optic neuritis and multiple sclerosis have not been considered to be genetic disorders. Recently, single nucleotide polymorphisms have been detected in the mitochondrial genome of some optic neuritis patients and in the gene encoding the interleukin-7 receptor alpha chain (IL7R) in multiple sclerosis patients

Box 37.3

- The experimental autoimmune encephalomyelitis (EAE) animal model has impacted the design and direction of both basic and clinical research to understand the pathogenesis and treatment of multiple sclerosis
- The magnetic resonance imaging and reactive oxygen species histopathologic similarities of the EAE animal model to human optic neuritis suggest that EAE is the ideal model system to investigate and target the underlying mechanisms by which retinal ganglion cells and their axons are lost in optic neuritis and multiple sclerosis

Box 37.2

- The traditional view of optic neuritis and multiple sclerosis has emphasized demyelination as the primary event in the disease process
- The targeted cells appear to be the oligodendrocytes that are responsible for producing the axon's myelin. In fact, apoptosis of oligodendrocytes has been described as the earliest event in the early lesions of multiple sclerosis
- Recently this focus has changed. Axonal and neuronal loss are increasingly recognized as the primary factors contributing to persistent deficits and disability in multiple sclerosis and optic neuritis

Animal model

The experimental autoimmune encephalomyelitis (EAE) animal model has impacted the design and direction of both basic and clinical research to understand the pathogenesis and treatment of MS.[40,41] Immunomodulatory cyclophosphamide, ciclosporin A, copolymer 1, antibodies to specific lymphocyte subsets, and immunization with T-cell receptor peptides initially evaluated in EAE have been or are being applied to MS.[42] The EAE model has an additional important advantage over other animal models. The alterations in the permeability of the blood–brain barrier (BBB) play a major role in the pathogenesis of EAE-induced demyelination.[43] Comparable disruption of this barrier occurs in immune-mediated disorders such as optic neuritis and MS. In fact, optic neuritis and MS are believed to be disorders of the BBB through which ICs and humoral factors producing demyelination gain access to the central nervous system (CNS). Histopathology of inactive EAE lesions shows foci of gliosis without active inflammation that are also seen in MS. Active optic nerve lesions in EAE reveal demyelination, mononuclear cell infiltration, and phagocytosis of axons and myelin by effector macrophages.[44] These findings are also seen in MS. In EAE there is also an immunogenetically restricted recognition system that involves the major histocompatibility antigens. Helper CD4 lymphocytes first adhere to endothelial cells, and then they infiltrate the CNS. The inflammatory response is amplified by recruitment of ICs and release of mediators, such as cytokines, antibodies, and reactive oxygen species (ROS). It is presumed that similar mechanisms may contribute to the pathogenesis of MS, but this is not known because in most patients the disease is already well established at clinical presentation.[45]

Histopathologic findings of a patient with optic neuritis exhibited inflammation and demyelination that is also seen in the EAE optic nerve.[46] Since human pathologic material is generally unavailable, MRI has provided an important link of EAE to optic neuritis and MS. MRIs of the optic nerve showing contrast enhancement and demyelination are similar in EAE and human disease.[47,48] The MRI, histopathologic, and ROS similarities of the EAE animal model to human optic neuritis suggest that EAE is the ideal model system to investigate and target the underlying mechanisms by which retinal ganglion cells and their axons are lost in optic neuritis and MS (Box 37.3).

within 10 years), as are multiple recurrences. Repeated attacks can lead to more severe visual loss, and in some patients legal blindness.[22-30]

Pathophysiology

The traditional view of optic neuritis and MS emphasizes demyelination as the primary event in the disease process. The targeted cells appear to be the oligodendrocytes that are responsible for producing the axon's myelin (Box 37.2). In fact, apoptosis of oligodendrocytes has been described as the earliest event in the early lesions of MS.[31] Recently this focus has changed. Axonal and neuronal loss are increasingly recognized as the primary factors contributing to persistent deficits and disability in MS and optic neuritis,[22,32,33] as also revealed by optical coherence tomography (OCT).[24,25] Permanent disability is believed to develop when a threshold of neuronal and axonal loss is reached and compensatory responses are exhausted. There is relatively little known about the underlying molecular mechanisms involved in the neurodegeneration process and as a consequence there is no treatment for this phase of the disease. A leading hypothesis is that axons are transected by inflammatory cells (ICs).[34,35] However, this does not explain the degeneration of neurons seen well before the IC infiltration or the progressive loss of function after the inflammatory phase has subsided.[36] Mitochondria play a key role in the pathogenesis of many neurological diseases,[37] but the role of the organelle has only recently been recognized in optic neuritis and MS.[38,39]

Neurodegeneration in EAE

Axonal loss is seen in acute EAE.[49] Loss of retinal ganglion cells (RGCs) is also common to chronic EAE[50,51] as well as to relapsing/remitting EAE.[52] The incidence of optic neuritis is very high in both model systems with one significant difference. In chronic EAE, RGC loss occurs prior to the infiltration of ICs,[36] but not in relapsing and remitting EAE[52] or in myelin oligodendrocyte glycoprotein (MOG)-specific T-cell receptor transgenic mice that develop isolated optic neuritis, usually without any other characteristic lesions of EAE in the brain or in the spinal cord.[53] Mitochondrial dysfunction may play an important role in the neurodegeneration of EAE and MS and this process begins much sooner than currently believed.[54,55] Mitochondria are the primary source of cellular adenosine triphosphate (ATP), energizing neurons and axons in the CNS. Current evidence implicating mitochondria is a loss of ATPase activity in MS lesions,[39] but how? In addition, mitochondria are the primary source of cellular ROS. Increased ROS activity is linked to many neurodegenerative diseases that have as a major feature axonal and neuronal loss.[38] Still, while ROS have been recognized among the mediators of CNS injury in EAE and MS,[56-64] the contribution of mitochondria to ROS activity and cell death has received little attention. The rest of this chapter reviews the role of mitochondrial respiration, oxidative stress, and the potential effects of modulating antioxidant gene expression in the visual system of mice induced with EAE, with a focus on long-term suppression of neurodegeneration.

Mitochondrial injury in EAE starts early

ICs that cause the classical demyelination of EAE and MS are believed to be the primary source of oxidative stress.[22] IC infiltration typically begins within 1–2 weeks of antigenic sensitization for EAE. Qi and coworkers[54] focused on the role of the mitochondrion as a potential source of ROS and target of oxidative injury before this initial phase of disease. Mitochondria were isolated from the retina, optic nerve, brain, and spinal cord of animals 3 and 6 days after sensitization for EAE, then probed for ROS. At this early stage none of the animals exhibited any clinical signs of EAE. As an initial gauge of ROS activity they used the peroxynitrite-mediated nitration of tyrosine residues that was detected with an antibody directed against nitrotyrosine. Peroxynitrite formed by the reaction of two other ROS, superoxide and nitric oxide, has been implicated in the pathogenesis of EAE, optic neuritis, and MS.[65-67] They found nitration of mitochondrial proteins in the EAE nervous system began as early as 3 days after sensitization for EAE (Figure 37.1).[54] Control specimens of unsensitized animals did exhibit some mitochondrial protein nitration indicative of the basal ROS activity that occurs under normal physiologic conditions. Peroxynitrite can inactivate proteins,[68-72] but which ones?

Respiratory chain, glycolytic, and chaperone proteins are altered

Using a proteonomics approach, Qi and coworkers[54] identified the nitrated mitochondrial proteins. In situ trypsin

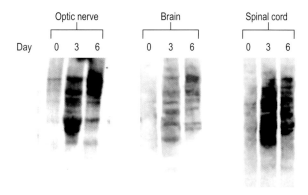

Figure 37.1 Immunoblots of mitochondria isolated from the optic nerve, brain, and spinal cord revealed peroxynitrite-mediated nitration of tyrosine residues at day 3 and day 6 after sensitization for experimental autoimmune encephalomyelitis, but not in the control specimens (day 0). (Reproduced with permission from Qi X, Lewin AS, Sun L, et al. Mitochondrial protein nitration primes neurodegeneration in experimental autoimmune encephalomyelitis. J Biol Chem 2006;20:31950–31962.)

digests of the excised protein bands were submitted for mass spectroscopy.[73] When the peptide fingerprints obtained were submitted for protein database sequence analysis the highest match was for mitochondrial heat shock protein 70 (mtHsp70) (Figure 37.2A). This chaperone is critical not only to the import of nuclear-encoded mitochondrial proteins from the cytosol, but also protein folding and assembly into the mitochondrial matrix. In vitro, loss of mtHsp70 function results in aggregation of mitochondria and profoundly alters the morphology of the organelle.[74] Qi and coworkers[54] showed these very same ultrastructural changes in the mitochondria of EAE axons.

Protein database sequence analysis of the other peptide fingerprints obtained (Figure 37.2B) included two respiratory chain complexes. They were identified as the NADPH-ubiquinone oxidoreductase B14 subunit (NDUFA6) of complex I and cytochrome c oxidase subunit IV. Loss of activity of complexes I and IV induced by ROS here potentially contributes to loss of cellular energy.[75,76] NDUFA6 is critical to the assembly of the holo complex I. Protein database sequence analysis of other peptide fingerprints obtained included the calcium-transporting ATPase and the glycolytic enzyme glyceraldehyde 3-phosphate dehydrogenase (GAPDH). Alterations in calcium sequestration, another important function of mitochondria, contribute to loss of mitochondrial membrane potential that can lead to cell death.[77,78] In addition to its role in glycolysis, translocation of nitrosylated GAPDH to the nucleus is linked to apoptotic cell death, or necrosis with ATP depletion.[79] Both mechanisms may induce loss of retinal ganglion cells in EAE.

ROS suppress oxidative phosphorylation

Exposure of RGCs to peroxynitrite for 24 hours suppressed the rate of ATP synthesis by 94%, relative to RGCs grown in normal culture media (Figure 37.3). This degree of impairment in oxidative phosphorylation is much greater than that seen in fatal neurodegenerative diseases caused by mutated mitochondrial DNA such as maternally inherited Leigh's syndrome and neuropathy ataxia retinitis pigmentosa or the blinding disease Leber hereditary optic neuropathy that

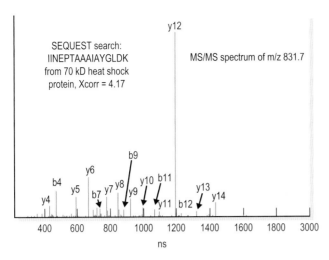

Figure 37.2 Multiple sclerosis (MS) peptide fingerprint of excised nitrated 70-kDa band (A) was identified as mtHsp70. Amino acids identified by protein database sequence analysis of mitochondrial heat shock protein 70 (mtHSP70), NADPH-ubiquinone oxidoreductase B14 subunit (NDUFA6) of complex I, cytochrome c oxidase subunit IV, and glyceraldehyde 3-phosphate dehydrogenase (GAPDH) are capitalized and underlined (B). (Reproduced with permission from Qi X, Lewin AS, Sun L, et al. Mitochondrial protein nitration primes neurodegeneration in experimental autoimmune encephalomyelitis. J Biol Chem 2006;20:31950–31962.)

primarily results in loss of RGCs.[80,81] Thus, loss of ATP synthesis induced by ROS can potentially have a severe impact on optic nerve function and cell survival in EAE and perhaps MS.

Antioxidant gene therapy suppresses loss of OXPHOS in vitro

Cellular defenses against ROS are present to some degree in all tissues and organs. They include the antioxidant enzymes superoxide dismutase (SOD), catalase, and glutathione peroxidase. Unfortunately, there are no endogenous defenses per se against peroxynitrite. However, defense against a key reactant, superoxide, leading to peroxynitrite formation does exist in all cells. SOD dismutes superoxide to hydrogen peroxide (H_2O_2) that can be further metabolized by the actions of catalase and glutathione peroxidase to water and molecular oxygen. Several isoforms of SOD exist. The manganese SOD (MnSOD), encoded by the *SOD2* gene, is exclusively mitochondrial. The copper/zinc (Cu/Zn) SOD, encoded by the *SOD1* gene, is primarily cytoplasmic, but it is also found in the mitochondrial and nuclear compartments.[82,83]

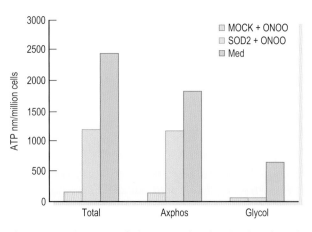

Figure 37.3 A histogram of adenosine triphosphate (ATP) synthesis shows that, relative to retinal ganglion cells (RGC-5) grown in normal culture medium (striped bar), RGC-5 cells incubated with 250 µM of peroxynitrite added to the medium and transfected with AAV-*GFP* (white bar) had depressed mitochondrial ATP synthesis. RGC-5 cells transfected with AAV-*SOD2* had partial rescue of ATP synthesis (black bar).

ROS localization in EAE

In the EAE optic nerve the distribution of inflammation and peroxynitrite-mediated protein nitration is remarkably similar to findings in a human optic neuritis specimen.[67] ROS have been linked to loss of mitochondrial membrane potential.[54] This can initiate a cascade of events leading to death of retinal ganglion cells, whose axons comprise the optic nerve.[84] Qi and coworkers[85] looked at mitochondrial membrane potential (Figure 37.4A) in the optic nerve 6 days after antigenic sensitization for EAE. Hydrogen peroxide labeled green by dichorofluordiacetate (Figure 37.4B) had a heavy presence at perineural and perivascular foci with the mitochondrial membrane potential sensing dye MitoTracker red. However, at several perivascular foci where hydrogen peroxide was highly expressed, mitochondrial membrane potential was diminished or even completely lost (Figure 37.4C). It was also found that loss of mitochondrial membrane potential detected by MitoTracker green was associated with superoxide labeled red by dihydroethidium. Thus, in vivo mitochondrial function is altered by ROS activity.

Modulation of anti-ROS genes alters acute optic neuritis

Qi and coworkers[85] examined the effect of antioxidant gene therapy in experimental optic neuritis. They found that, relative to the normal optic nerve (Figure 37.5A), a month after sensitization for EAE, filling of the optic cup and displacement of the peripapillary retina are seen in EAE (Figure 37.5B). This is illustrative of the histologic features of optic disc edema, also visible by ophthalmoscopy of optic neuritis patients. This finding was due predominantly to hydropic degeneration of axons. Relative to the normal retina (Figure 37.5E), loss of RGCs was not yet apparent (Figure 37.5F). Indicative of mitochondrial ROS activity, electron-dense cerium perhydroxide reaction product was found formed by the reaction of perfused cerium chloride and endogenous hydrogen peroxide within mitochondria (Figure 37.6), some

swollen with dissolution of cristae. These mitochondrial findings were not limited to fibers with loss of the myelin sheath, considered the hallmark of MS and EAE.[86,87] They were more widespread. Myelinated axons also contained swollen mitochondria that exhibited disorganization and dissolution of cristae, some to the point that only a double membranous bag identified the organelle.

To determine the pathogenicity of mitochondrial ROS activity in EAE, Qi and coworkers[85] suppressed antioxidant defenses in the organelle by using a ribozyme designed to target the *SOD2* mRNA for destruction. This ribozyme, delivered by the adenoassociate virus (AAV) vector, substantially reduced mitochondrial SOD activity, exacerbating mitochondrial and axonal edema and resulting in massive optic nerve head swelling (Figure 37.5C), RGC loss (Figure 37.5G), and myelin fiber loss. These findings, seen a month after EAE sensitization and intraocular injection of the AAV constructs, illustrate the detrimental role that increased mitochondrial ROS activity may play in acute EAE.

To protect the optic nerves against EAE, Qi and coworkers[85] augmented anti-ROS defenses. They found that AAV-*SOD2*-inoculated nerves exhibited less mitochondrial and axonal and disc swelling (Figure 37.5D), with 46% more myelin fiber preservation than the contralateral nerves inoculated with AAV-*GFP*. RGCs were also preserved (Figure 37.5H). The suppression of mitochondrial injury by *SOD2* was not limited to demyelinated axons. It was seen in myelinated axons, with less hydropic degeneration, disorganization, and dissolution of cristae.

Comparisons to the normal optic nerve further emphasized the importance of these findings. Relative to the normal optic nerve, acute EAE eyes lost two-thirds of their optic nerve myelin fiber area. Treatment with AAV-*SOD2* mitigated this by half, to a 50% loss relative to normal optic nerves. Thus, the protective effect achieved here approached the threshold beyond which visual loss is believed to be clinically symptomatic.[88] Therefore, *SOD2* treatment may potentially prevent irreversible visual loss, by reducing the threshold of myelin fiber injury in the optic nerve. Still, proof of a long-term protective effect is necessary for *SOD2*, a lesson learned from the opposing effects of nitric oxide in suppressing acute EAE, but aggravating remissions during chronic stages of the disease.[39]

Long-term antioxidant gene therapy suppresses optic neuritis

Optic nerve degeneration associated with optic neuritis and MS may develop after just a single attack.[89] Typically, irreversible visual loss develops after several recurrences.[90] MRI is increasingly being relied on as the tool to test the effectiveness of treatments designed to suppress MS. Qi and coworkers[85] used volume measurements of the optic nerve obtained by serial three-dimensional MRIs to follow the changes associated with EAE (Figure 37.7). MRIs of these animals were performed at 2 weeks, then 1, 3, 4, 6, 7, and 12 months following sensitization for EAE. The right eyes received intraocular injections of AAV-*SOD2*. The left eyes were injected with AAV-*GFP*. Since ocular injections may be associated with the release of growth factors that can sometimes offer a protective effect, another group of animals that received no ocular

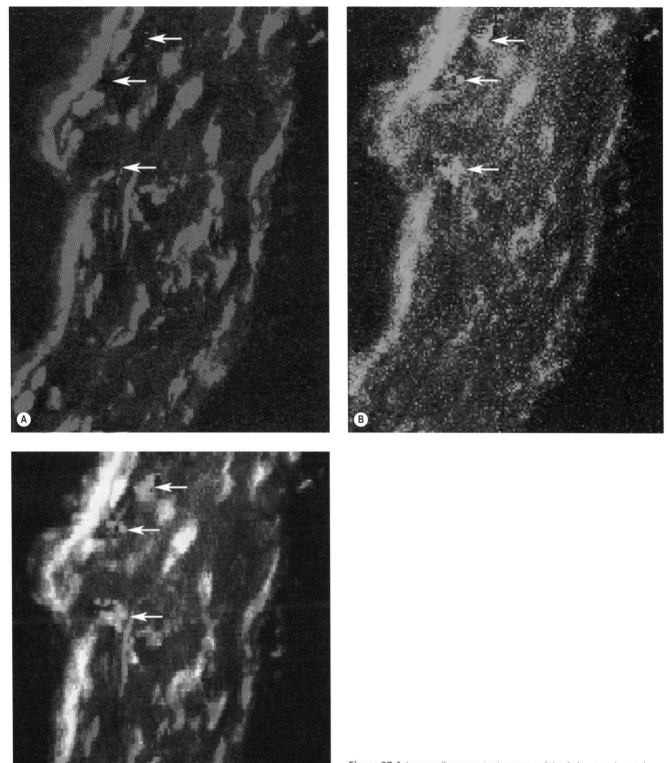

Figure 37.4 Immunofluorescent microscopy of the 6-day experimental autoimmune encephalomyelitis optic nerve shows mitochondria labeled by MitoTracker red (A); hydrogen peroxide labeled green by dichorofluordiacetate (B); often localized (C). At several perivascular foci where hydrogen peroxide was highly expressed, mitochondrial membrane potential was diminished or even completely lost (arrows). (Reproduced with permission from Qi X, Lewin AS, Sun L, et al. Suppression of mitochondrial oxidative stress provides long-term neuroprotection in experimental optic neuritis. Invest Ophthalmol Vis Sci 2007;48:681–691.)

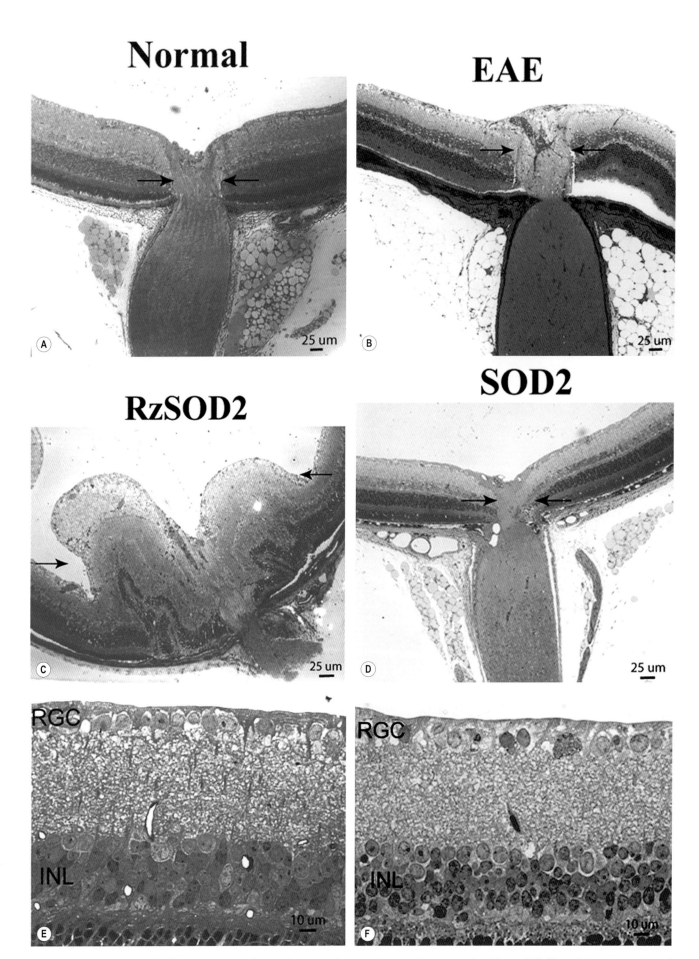

Figure 37.5 Light micrographs of the optic nerve and retina show that, relative to the normal optic nerve head (arrows) (A) filling of the optic cup (arrows) and displacement of the peripapillary retina are seen in acute experimental autoimmune encephalomyelitis (EAE) (arrows) (B). A ribozyme suppressing *SOD2* expression markedly increased optic nerve head swelling in EAE-sensitized mice (arrows) (C) while *SOD2* overexpression suppresses it (arrows) (D).

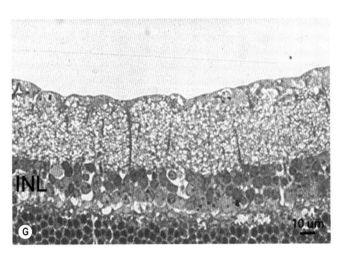

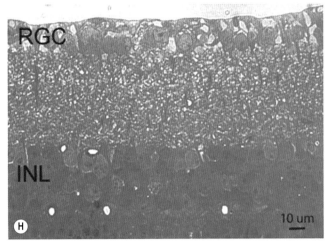

Figure 37.5, cont'd The retina of a normal animal (E) and 1-month EAE animal (F) contrast with the severe loss of the retinal ganglion cell layer in a 1-month EAE animal inoculated with the *SOD2* ribozyme (G) and with *SOD2* treatment (H). (Reproduced with permission from Qi X, Lewin AS, Sun L, et al. Suppression of mitochondrial oxidative stress provides long-term neuroprotection in experimental optic neuritis. Invest Ophthalmol Vis Sci 2007;48:681–691.)

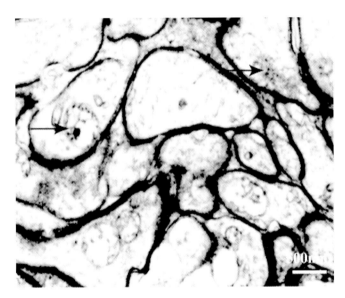

Figure 37.6 Transmission electron microscopy shows that cerium perhydroxide reaction product (arrows), formed by the reaction of endogenous hydrogen peroxide with perfused cerium chloride, is evident within mitochondria, some swollen with dissolution of cristae in the 1-month experimental autoimmune encephalomyelitis optic nerve. (Reproduced with permission from Qi X, Lewin AS, Sun L, et al. Suppression of mitochondrial oxidative stress provides long-term neuroprotection in experimental optic neuritis. Invest Ophthalmol Vis Sci 2007;48:681–691.)

initial decrease in swelling with *SOD2* treatment. Later, by the third month and beyond, Qi and coworkers[85] detected a loss of optic nerve volume. This optic nerve degeneration was suppressed by *SOD2* gene inoculation as long as 1 year after sensitization for EAE, the longest interval studied. Postmortem examinations confirmed the long-term protective effect of *SOD2*. Excised optic nerves clearly show that, relative to *GFP* inoculation, the characteristic optic atrophy was suppressed by *SOD2* gene inoculation. The effects of EAE were evident in the optic nerve, where myelin fiber area was reduced by 49% relative to normal animals, after 1 year. With *SOD2*, myelin fiber area diminished, but only by 23%. Thus, treatment offered a twofold protective effect when compared to the normal optic nerve. Relative to the EAE optic nerve, *SOD2* nerves had 51% more myelin fiber preservation, somewhat less when measured against the *GFP*-inoculated eyes (31%). Excavation of the optic nerve head, atrophy of the retrobulbar nerve (Figure 37.8A and 37.8C), and myelin fiber loss (Figure 37.9A) were suppressed with *SOD2* (Figures 37.8B and 37.8D). Degenerating axons, some with aggregation of mitochondria, hydropic degeneration, and loss of cristae, evidenced the ongoing neurodegeneration not only at 3 months, but also at 1 year after sensitization for EAE.

Antioxidant gene therapy suppresses neuronal degeneration

The protective effect of *SOD2* seen in the optic nerve was mirrored in the retina, where the RGC soma is located. Unlike their findings in acute EAE, where degeneration of the nerve fiber layer and loss of retinal ganglion cells was mainly evident in anti-*SOD2* ribozyme-inoculated eyes,[84] RGC loss predominated in the chronic stages of EAE. *SOD2* treatment preserved the nerve fiber layer and RGCs. Quantitative analysis revealed a 32% loss of retinal ganglion cells a year after sensitization for EAE, relative to normal animals (Figure 37.9B). Qi and coworkers[85] found that *SOD2* sup-

viral inoculation were sensitized for EAE. Optic nerve volumes between the right and left eyes of this group were the same throughout the course of EAE studied. Though disease activity is often variable between animals with EAE, as is often the case with MS patients, the severity of disease did not substantially vary between eyes of the same animal.

During the acute stages, 2 and 4 weeks after EAE sensitization, optic nerve volumes for the *GFP*-inoculated nerves increased relative to *SOD2* treatment, thus reflecting an

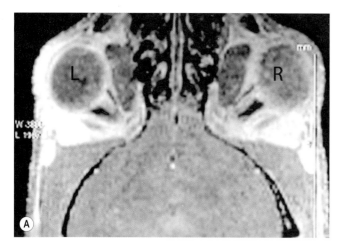

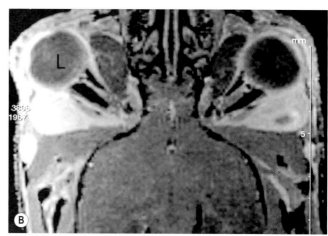

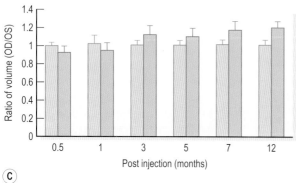

Figure 37.7 Magnetic resonance imaging (MRI) revealed slightly less swelling of the right optic nerve with *SOD2* treatment relative to the control, AAV-*GFP*-inoculated left eye, 2 weeks after experimental autoimmune encephalomyelitis (EAE) sensitization and intraocular gene injections (A). One year after sensitization for EAE, optic nerve atrophy seen on the left was suppressed by *SOD2* gene inoculation on the right (B). Histogram of MRI optic nerve volume measurements (C) of the right nerve (OD) relative to the left nerve (OS) revealed no differences in EAE animals that received no ocular injections. However, optic nerve swelling characteristic of acute EAE was suppressed by ocular gene injection of *SOD2* at 2 weeks ($P < 0.05$), but not at 4 weeks ($P > 0.05$) after sensitization for EAE. Later, optic nerve degeneration was suppressed by *SOD2* at 3 months ($P < 0.02$), 4 months ($P < 0.05$), 7 months ($P < 0.02$), and 12 months ($P < 0.002$) after sensitization for EAE. (Reproduced with permission from Qi X, Lewin AS, Sun L, et al. Suppression of mitochondrial oxidative stress provides long-term neuroprotection in experimental optic neuritis. Invest Ophthalmol Vis Sci 2007;48:681–691.)

pressed ganglion cell loss fourfold, limiting it to just 7% in EAE. Even at 1 year, retinal ganglion cells of unprotected and *GFP*-inoculated EAE animals were still undergoing apoptosis. This suggested that the neurodegenerative process was ongoing and still active even this late in the disease course, and emphasized the potential value of *SOD2* gene therapy to suppress it in EAE and perhaps patients with optic neuritis and MS.

Additional approaches to suppress axonal loss

Using a different approach for neuroprotection, Shindler and coworkers[91] found that intravitreal injections of the SIRT1 activator, resveratrol, suppressed RGC loss in SJL/J mice sensitized for EAE. Targeting mitochondria, Forte and coworkers[78] showed that transgenic mice with knockout of the gene encoding cyclophilin D that were sensitized for EAE had suppression of axonal loss in the spinal cord. Cyclophi-

> **Box 37.4 Strategies for neuroprotection tested in experimental autoimmune encephalomyelitis (EAE)**
>
> - Mitochondrial antioxidant gene therapy with *SOD2* suppressed retinal ganglion cell loss fourfold, limiting it to just 7% even 1 year after induction of EAE
> - SIRT1 activator, resveratrol, suppressed RGC loss 1 month after sensitization for EAE
> - Knockout of the gene encoding cyclophilin D that regulates the mitochondrial permeability transition pore and calcium sequestration suppressed axonal loss in the spinal cord

lin D regulates the mitochondrial permeability transition pore and calcium sequestration. Although they did not focus their studies on the retina or optic nerve, neurons isolated from transgenic knockout mice were resistant to oxidative stress and mitochondria lacking cyclophilin D had increased levels of sequestered calcium (Box 37.4).

CONTROL 3 Months

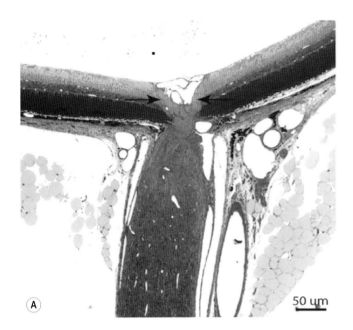

SOD2 3 Months

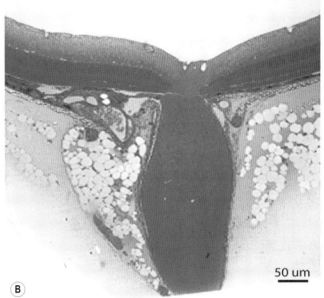

CONTROL 1 Year

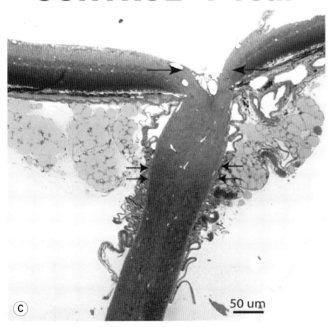

SOD2 1 Year

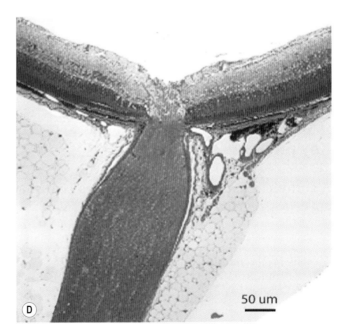

Figure 37.8 Light microscopy of the optic nerves revealed cupping (arrows) and atrophy of the AAV-*GFP*-inoculated control nerve 3 months after sensitization for experimental autoimmune encephalomyelitis (EAE) (A). Neuroprotection with *SOD2* ameliorated the optic atrophy associated with EAE (B). In control eyes injected with AAV-*GFP*, 1 year after sensitization for EAE, cupping (arrows) and atrophy of the retrobulbar nerve (double arrows) were advanced (C). Protection with *SOD2* ameliorated cupping of the optic nerve head and atrophy of the retrobulbar nerve 1 year after EAE sensitization and intraocular AAV-*SOD2* injection (D). (Reproduced with permission from Qi X, Lewin AS, Sun L, et al. Suppression of mitochondrial oxidative stress provides long-term neuroprotection in experimental optic neuritis. Invest Ophthalmol Vis Sci 2007;48:681–691.)

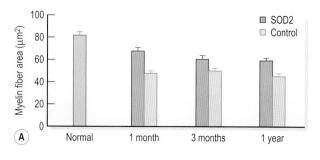

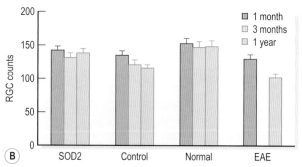

Figure 37.9 A histogram of myelin fiber area illustrates the protective effect of *SOD2* relative to control gene inoculation with AAV-*GFP* ($P < 0.001$), the uninoculated experimental autoimmune encephalomyelitis (EAE) nerve ($P < 0.005$), and the normal optic nerve ($P < 0.05$). Myelin fiber loss in EAE relative to normal is also shown ($P < 0.05$) (A). A histogram of retinal ganglion cell (RGC) counts shows the neuroprotective effect of *SOD2* relative to control treatment with AAV-*GFP* ($P < 0.005$) and uninoculated EAE ($P < 0.0001$). No significant differences were detected between *SOD2*-treated and normal optic nerve ($P > 0.05$). A one-third loss of RGCs was seen in uninoculated EAE relative to the normal optic nerve ($P < 0.0005$). Treatment with AAV-*GFP* had a mild protective effect relative to EAE eyes that received no ocular injection ($P < 0.05$) (B). (Reproduced with permission from Qi X, Lewin AS, Sun L, et al. Suppression of mitochondrial oxidative stress provides long-term neuroprotection in experimental optic neuritis. Invest Ophthalmol Vis Sci 2007;48:681–691.)

Whether neuroprotective treatments tested in the EAE animal model will suppress RGC and axonal injury that leads to permanent visual disability in optic neuritis and MS patients remains to be proven.

Conclusion

Axonal and neuronal degeneration rather than demyelination is now increasingly recognized as the primary cause of permanent visual and neurological disability in optic neuritis and MS. Currently, there is no effective treatment to suppress or repair this damage. Moreover, the mechanisms leading to neurodegeneration in optic neuritis and MS are poorly understood. Evidence demonstrates that peroxynitrite mediates nitration of key mitochondrial proteins. This commences during the earliest phase of the EAE animal model of MS, well before infiltration of ICs. Mitochondrial oxidative injury impaired mitochondrial bioenergetics and resulted in apoptosis of ganglion cells of the retina and oligodendrocytes in the optic nerve of animals with EAE. These novel findings implicate mitochondrial oxidative stress as a key event in the initiation of optic nerve degeneration and demyelination in EAE. Mitochondria play a key role in the pathogenesis of many neurological diseases, but the role of the organelle has only recently been recognized in MS. More importantly, modulation of mitochondrial gene expression effectively suppressed neurodegeneration in EAE, suggesting that antioxidant gene therapy targeted to mitochondria may be useful in patients with optic neuritis and MS.

Key references

A complete list of chapter references is available online at www.expertconsult.com. See inside cover for registration details.

1. Optic Neuritis Study Group. The clinical profile of optic neuritis. Experience of the Optic Neuritis Treatment Trial [see comments]. Arch Ophthalmol 1991;109: 1673–1678.

2. Guy J, Mao J, Bidgood WD Jr. et al. Enhancement and demyelination of the intraorbital optic nerve. Fat suppression magnetic resonance imaging. Ophthalmology 1992;99:713–719.

3. DeBroff BM, Donahue SP. Bilateral optic neuropathy as the initial manifestation of systemic sarcoidosis. Am J Ophthalmol 1993;116:108–111.

4. Galetta S, Schatz NJ, Glaser JS. Acute sarcoid optic neuropathy with spontaneous recovery. J Clin Neuroophthalmol 1989;9:27–32.

5. Dutton JJ, Burde RM, Klingele TG. Autoimmune retrobulbar optic neuritis. Am J Ophthalmol 1982;94:11–17.

6. Cross SA, Salomao DR, Parisi JE, et al. Paraneoplastic autoimmune optic neuritis with retinitis defined by CRMP-5-IgG. Ann Neurol 2003;54:38–50.

7. Bar S, Segal M, Shapira R, et al. Neuroretinitis associated with cat scratch disease. Am J Ophthalmol 1990;110: 703–705.

8. Bhatti MT, Asif R, Bhatti LB. Macular star in neuroretinitis. Arch Neurol 2001;58: 1008–1009.

9. Burton BJ, Leff AP, Plant GT. Steroid-responsive HIV optic neuropathy. J Neuroophthalmol 1998;18:25–29.

10. Larsen M, Toft PB, Bernhard P, et al. Bilateral optic neuritis in acute human immunodeficiency virus infection. Acta Ophthalmol Scand 1998;76:737–738.

11. Rush JA, Ryan EJ. Syphilitic optic perineuritis. Am J Ophthalmol 1981;91: 404–406.

12. Benz MS, Glaser JS, Davis JL. Progressive outer retinal necrosis in immunocompetent patients treated initially for optic neuropathy with systemic corticosteroids. Am J Ophthalmol 2003;135:551–553.

13. Francis PJ, Jackson H, Stanford MR, et al. Inflammatory optic neuropathy as the presenting feature of herpes simplex acute retinal necrosis. Br J Ophthalmol 2003;87:512–514.

14. Vital DD, Gerard A, Rousset H. [Neurological manifestations of Whipple disease.] Rev Neurol (Paris) 2002;158: 988–992.

15. Anninger WV, Lomeo MD, Dingle J, et al. West Nile virus-associated optic neuritis and chorioretinitis. Am J Ophthalmol 2003;136:1183–1185.

CHAPTER 38

Abnormal ocular motor control

James A Sharpe and Arun N Sundaram

Clinical background

Five eye movement systems are utilized to achieve clear vision: (1) saccadic; (2) smooth pursuit; (3) optokinetic; (4) vestibulo-ocular; and (5) vergence. Four systems generate conjugate movements, called version, but vergence achieves binocular vision by generating disjunctive eye movements that align the two foveas on an object as it approaches the head. Saccades are fast eye movements that bring the fovea to a target, while pursuit, vestibular, optokinetic, and vergence smooth eye movements prevent slippage of retinal images.[1,2] Gaze refers here to binocular movements achieved by saccades, smooth pursuit, or optokinetic tracking, and the vesitibulo-ocular reflex (VOR). This chapter reviews the pathophysiology of selected disorders of these movements caused by central nervous system lesions.

Key symptoms and signs

Central disorders of gaze impair vision by causing retinal image slip, or inability to attain foveation. The cardinal sign of disordered gaze is limitation of version. Even with a normal range of version, the quality of version can be impaired for specific ocular motor systems, for example, by slow saccades or saccadic pursuit.

Epidemiology

The epidemiology is that of the many diseases that cause gaze disorders.

Genetics

Genetic predisposition is common among neurological disorders and direct inheritance is responsible for some. Gaze palsy may be a sign of lipid storage diseases. Vertical gaze paresis with foam cells or sea-blue histiocytes in the bone marrow is a neurovisceral storage disease with profiles of lipid analysis similar to Niemann–Pick disease type C (NPC).[3] Paresis of horizontal saccades is a feature of Gaucher's disease (GD).[4] Saccade initiation failure is often the earliest neurological sign in GD type 3.

Familial paralysis of horizontal gaze is an autosomal-recessive disorder.[5,6] Aplasia of the abducens nuclei or non-decussation of motor pathways may explain the gaze palsy. Congenital ocular motor apraxia can be inherited as an autosomal-dominant trait.[7]

Spinocerebellar ataxia types 1 or 2 (SCA1, SCA2) are autosomal dominant and associated with slow saccades.[8] Progressive supranuclear palsy (PSP) with characteristic defective vertical gaze and extrapyramidal signs is associated with a mutation (S305S) in the tau gene on chromosome 17 that results in an increase in the splicing of exon 10, and the presence of tau containing four microtubule-binding repeats.[9,10] Autosomal-dominant frontotemporal dementia and parkinsonism linked to chromosome 17, and its subset of families with pallido-ponto-nigral degeneration, are a group of four repeat tauopathies that often have vertical gaze palsy identical to that in PSP.[11,12]

Diagnostic workup

Gaze deviations are manifestations of acute and often massive brain damage. Less severe disorders of gaze are apparent with subacute or chronic lesions and often signify discrete involvement of eye movement pathways. Systematic examination of saccades and smooth eye movements and brain imaging are often adequate for diagnosis. An operational classification of the direction of horizontal gaze paresis caused by lesions at different levels of the neuraxis is provided in Table 38.1.

Differential diagnosis

Gaze palsies carry the differential diagnosis of the myriad of disease processes that cause them.

Treatment

Therapy is first directed at the responsible neurological disease. Specific treatment of visual neglect resulting from nondominant parietal lobe damage and visual restoration therapy for homonymous hemianopia remain to be established by clinical trials and readers are referred to other sources.[13]

Table 38.1 Direction of horizontal gaze paresis

System involved	Frontal lobe	Parietotemporal lobes	Rostral midbrain	Pons	Cerebellum
Saccades	Contraversive	Contraversive	Contraversive	Ipsiversive	Contraversive, (acute)
Smooth pursuit	Ipsiversive or bidirectional*	Ipsiversive*	Ipsiversive or bidirectional	Ipsiversive	Ipsiversive or bidirectional
Vestibulo-ocular reflex	Spared	Spared	Usually spared	Ipsiversive	Spared

*See Table 38.2 for additional types of pursuit paresis.

Prognosis and complications

The outcomes are determined by the disease causing the gaze disorder; readers may refer to reviews of those conditions.

Etiology

Infarction, hemorrhage, demyelination, neoplasia, and neurodegenerative diseases are common brain disorders affecting gaze.

Pathophysiology

Brainstem control of horizontal saccades

The innervational change in motoneurons during all types of eye movements consists of a phasic discharge (an eye velocity command) and a tonic discharge (an eye position command). During saccades, the phasic discharge consists of a high-frequency pulse of innervation that moves the eyes rapidly against orbital viscous forces. When a new eye position is attained, a position command, called a step change in innervation, is required to sustain position against elastic restoring forces of the eye muscles.[1,2]

Saccades are generated by excitatory burst neurons in the paramedian pontine reticular formation (PPRF) that project to the ipsilateral abducens nucleus.[14] During fixation, the burst neurons are kept silent by omnipause neurons located in the midline of the caudal pons (Figure 38.1).[15] Inhibitory burst neurons, located laterally in the rostral medulla, serve to turn antagonist motoneurons off, while the excitatory burst neurons drive the agonist motoneurons.[16] Signals from the cerebral cortex and superior colliculus (SC) inhibit the pause neurons, thereby releasing the burst neurons to create the pulse. The step discharge (a position command) is generated from the pulse (a velocity command) by a neural integrator that "integrates" (in the mathematical sense) the pulse. The velocity-to-position neural integrator for horizontal saccades, smooth pursuit, and the VOR is located in the medial vestibular nucleus (MVN) and the nucleus prepositus hypoglossi, which lies just medial to it.[17]

The abducens nucleus contains both motoneurons to the lateral rectus muscle, and internuclear neurons that project in the contralateral medial longitudinal fasciculus to medial rectus motoneurons (Figure 38.1). These internuclear neurons transmit saccadic, pursuit, and vestibular signals to the medial rectus.

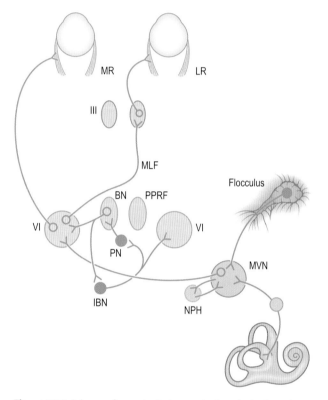

Figure 38.1 Schema of some brainstem projections for horizontal gaze. Saccades are dispatched when a trigger signal turns off pause neurons, which inhibit burst neurons. Reciprocal inhibition of antagonist muscles is achieved by excitation of inhibitory burst neurons. MR, medial rectus; LR, lateral rectus; III, oculomotor nucleus; MLF, medial longitudinal fasciculus; PPRF, paramedian pontine reticular formation; PN, pause neurons; BN, excitatory burst neurons; IBN, inhibitory burst neurons; NPH, nucleus prepositus hypoglossi; MVN, medial vestibular nucleus; VI, abducens nucleus. (Modified from Sharpe JA, Morrow MJ, Newman NJ, et al. Neuro-ophthalmology: Continuum, American Academy of Neurology. Baltimore: Williams and Wilkins, 1995.)

Brainstem paralysis of horizontal saccades

Unilateral acute lesions of the caudal pontine tegmentum cause contraversive deviation of the eyes. Because the PPRF is damaged, ipsiversive saccades are paralyzed (Table 38.1). Disruption of projections from the vestibular nuclei to the abducens nucleus, or of the abducens nucleus itself, also paralyzes ipsiversive pursuit and the VOR. The eyes cannot be brought beyond the midline toward the side of damage. Contraversive jerk nystagmus is sometimes evident.[18,19]

Box 38.1 Pontine Horizontal Gaze Paresis

- Unilateral pontine tegmental lesions paralyze conjugate ipsiversive saccades
- Medial longitudinal fasciculus lesions cause pareses of adducting saccades (internuclear ophthalmoplegia) and reduce vertical vestibulo-ocular reflex speed
- Abducens nucleus lesions paralyze ipsiversive saccades, smooth pursuit and vestibular eye motion
- Combined paramedian pontine reticular formation (or abducens nucleus) and medial longitudinal fasciculus damage on one side causes the one-and-a-half syndrome
- The one-and-a-half syndrome consists of paralyzed adduction and abduction of the eye on the lesion side, and paralyzed adduction of the contralateral eye, which is exotropic in the acute stage

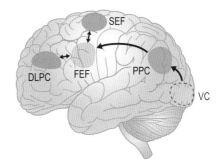

Figure 38.2 Cortical areas involved in generating voluntary and reflexive saccades to visual targets. The parietal eye field in posterior parietal cortex (PPC) governs the accuracy and latency of visually guided saccades. The frontal eye field (FEF), supplementary eye field (SEF; located in the mesial frontal cortex), and dorsolateral prefrontal cortex (DLPC) regulate voluntary and visually guided and memory-guided saccades (see text for description). VC, striate visual cortex (area V1).

Internuclear ophthalmoplegia (INO) consists of impaired adduction on the side of the lesion in the MLF and abducting jerk nystagmus of the opposite eye.[20] In total INO, adduction is paralyzed to saccadic, pursuit, and vestibular stimulation (Box 38.1). A hypertropia on the side of MLF damage, a form of skew deviation, is often present. (Skew deviation is discussed elsewhere.) Slow adducting saccades are the only manifestation of incomplete or chronic MLF lesions.[21] Convergence may be lost or spared. Lesions of the MLF disrupt the commands that ascend from the vestibular nuclei (Figure 38.1), resulting in slowed vertical pursuit and vertical VOR movements. Vertical saccades are normal. Gaze-evoked nystagmus occurs during upward, and sometimes downward, fixation.[22]

Damage to the PPRF or abducens nucleus and the MLF on one side causes paralysis of horizontal movements of the ipsilateral eye in both directions and paralysis of adduction in the opposite eye, a combination called the one-and-a-half syndrome.[23] In the acute phase the opposite eye is exotropic (Box 38.1). This "paralytic pontine exotropia" is distinguished from other types of exotropia by slowed adducting saccades in the laterally deviated eye and the horizontal immobility of the eye on the side of pontine damage.[24]

Unilateral lesions of the midbrain reticular formation cause paresis of contraversive saccades and of ipsiversive or bidirectional smooth pursuit. Such lesions are usually associated with involvement of the ipsilateral oculomotor nucleus, or vertical gaze palsy.[25]

Cerebral cortical control of saccades

The cerebral hemispheres generate contraversive saccades. The frontal eye field (FEF) is reciprocally connected with the parietal eye field (PEF) in the posterior parietal cortex and the superior temporal sulcus. The FEF projects directly to the ipsilateral SC and the midbrain tegmentum, and the contralateral pontine tegmentum.[26] The supplementary eye field (SEF) of the supplementary motor area plays a predominant role in directing voluntary sequences of saccades (Figure 38.2). The dorsolateral prefrontal cortex contributes to the advanced planning of environmental scanning using memory of target location (Box 38.2). Whereas the FEF is mainly involved in intentional saccade generation to visual targets, the PEF is more involved in reflexive visual explora-

Box 38.2 Cerebral Saccade Control

- The cerebral hemispheres generate predominantly contraversive saccades
- Parietal eye field controls reflexive saccades to visual targets and other visually guided saccades
- Supplementary eye field governs voluntary sequences of saccades
- Dorsolateral prefrontal cortex contributes to programming saccades using memory of target location
- Acute frontal or parietal lobe lesions cause transient ipsiversive gaze deviation and paresis of contraversive saccades
- Normal horizontal vestibulo-ocular reflex motion to oculocephalic maneuvers is spared with cerebral lesions but often lost toward the side of pontine tegmental lesions

tion.[27] The FEF, SEF, and SC dispatch contraversive saccades by delivering signals to the PPRF. In monkeys ablation of either the SC or the FEF produces only transient ipsiversive deviation of the eyes and reduced frequency of contraversive saccades. Bilateral ablation of the FEF and the SC produces enduring paralysis of saccades,[28] indicating that redundant, parallel pathways subserve the generation of voluntary and visually guided saccades.

Cerebral gaze paralysis

Massive acute cerebral lesions of the frontal or parieto-occipital regions cause transient ipsiversive deviation of the eyes and inability to trigger contraversive voluntary or visually guided saccades (Table 38.1 and Box 38.2). Soon after, saccades can be initiated up to the midline of craniotopic space, but not beyond. Within hours or days, a full range of saccades recovers. Sparing of horizontal VOR motion to oculocephalic stimulation distinguishes this acute hemispheric gaze palsy from that caused by unilateral damage to caudal pontine tegmentum.[18,29] Rehabilitation of contraversive saccades is nearly complete, but they are hypometric. Occasionally, thalamic hemorrhage causes transient contraversive, or "wrong-side," deviation of the eyes.[30]

Basal ganglia

The basal ganglia participate in saccadic eye movements. The pars reticulata of the substantia nigra (SNr) and globus pallidus are major outflow pathways of the basal ganglia. In monkeys, neurons of the SNr decrease their tonic discharge rate before saccades to visual, auditory, or remembered targets. The FEF projects to the caudate nucleus which in turn projects to the SNr. The SNr projects to the SC and inhibits it. Saccades are triggered when SNr inhibition of the SC is removed by suppression of the tonic activity of SNr neurons.[31]

Cerebellum

Cerebellar vermis lobules VI and VII, comprising the ocular motor vermis, and the caudal part of the fastigial nucleus and its outflow pathways control saccade accuracy. Saccadic dysmetria usually indicates a lesion of the ocular motor vermis or deep nuclei.[32,33] Overshoot dysmetria (hypermetria) is apparent when the patient makes refixation saccades between two targets. Multiple-step hypometric saccades (discussed below) occur toward the side of lesions involving the cerebellar hemisphere.

Saccadic paresis

Paresis of saccades may be evident as delay in initiating them, undershooting the target (hypometria), or slowness of their trajectories (Box 38.3).

Saccadic delay

Saccades are dispatched with latency about 200 ms after a visual stimulus. Saccadic delay in all directions can be an enduring sign of cerebral cortical and basal ganglia involvement, as in Alzheimer's disease and Parkinson's disease.[34–36] Reflexive saccades to visual targets are delayed mainly con-

tralateral to parietal lobe lesions.[37] Prolonged saccadic latency is an obvious and fundamental defect in congenital ocular motor apraxia,[38] and head motion is required to dispatch coincident saccades. Acquired ocular motor apraxia after frontal and parietal lobe damage consists of delayed and hypometric voluntary saccades with relative preservation of reflexive saccades to visual targets and intact nystagmus quick phases.[39,40]

Hypometric saccades

Saccadic refixations normally consist of one or two steps. Refixations of three or more dysmetric steps to a target are called multiple-step hypometric saccades. They occur in some normal subjects after fatigue or in advanced age.[41,42] They are conclusively abnormal if they predominate in one direction. Hypometric saccades occur contralateral to cerebral hemispheric damage and ipsilateral to cerebellar cortical lesions.[29,32,43] Omnidirectional hypometric saccades accompany bilateral cerebral, basal ganglia, or cerebellar disease.[34,35,44]

Lateropulsion of saccades is a form of dysmetria that occurs after lateral medullary infarcts, a phenomenon called ipsipulsion, in order to specify the direction of saccadic dysmetria relative to the side of the lesion.[43,45,46] It consists of a triad of: (1) overshoot of ipsiversive saccades; (2) undershoot of contraversive saccades; and (3) ipsiversive deviation of vertical saccades (Box 38.3). Lesions of the superior cerebellar peduncle and uncinate fasciculus cause contrapulsion, which is the triad of overshoot of contraversive saccades, undershoot of ipsiversive saccades, and contraversive deviation of vertical saccades.[43]

Slow saccades

Damage to excitatory burst neurons in the PPRF or to inhibitory burst neurons or to omnipause neurons (Figure 38.1) causes slow saccades.[18,47] Lesions in the pontine tegmentum such as infarcts, tumors, degenerations such as PSP, Huntington's disease,[48] and variants of spinocerebellar degenerations,[8] multiple sclerosis, lipid storage diseases, and infections (e.g., acquired immunodeficiency syndrome (AIDS), Whipple disease) cause slowing of voluntary and reflex saccades and of the fast phases of vestibular and optokinetic nystagmus.

Slow saccades are also caused by peripheral neuromuscular disease (ocular myopathy and nerve palsies).[49] Involvement of cerebral projections to the brainstem by strokes, and degenerations such as Parkinson's disease and Alzheimer's disease, causes mild, but clinically imperceptible slowing.[34,35] Mental fatigue, reduced vigilance, and ingestion of sedative drugs cause slight slowing of saccades.

Box 38.3 Saccadic Paresis

- Saccade paresis consists of delayed or hypometric or slow saccades
- Saccade delay is usually a manifestation of cerebral cortical or basal ganglia disease
- Apraxia of saccades consists of severe delay of voluntary saccades with preservation of visual triggered reflexive saccades and nystagmus quick phases. Head saccades may be required to start eye saccades
- Dysmetric saccades may be hypermetric or hypometric. Hypometria is a sign of cerebral cortical, basal ganglia, or cerebellar damage. Hypermetria is a sign of cerebellar cortical or deep nuclear involvement
- Pulsion of saccades consists of unidirectional hypermetria of horizontal saccades, with hypometria in the opposite direction, and deviation of vertical saccades toward the side of hypermetria
- Pulsion toward the side of lateral medulla and inferior cerebellar peduncle damage is called ipsipulsion. Pulsion away from superior cerebellar peduncle damage is contrapulsion
- Slow saccades signify damage to paramedian pontine reticular formation burst neurons or omnipause neurons

---

Cerebral, cerebellar, and brainstem smooth pursuit circuits

Middle temporal (MT) visual area and middle superior temporal (MST) visual area of the superior temporal sulcus and inferior parietal lobe (IPL) or area 7a contain neurons that respond to image motion and generate smooth pursuit in monkeys.[50] In humans the angular gyrus and prestriate cortical Brodmann areas 19, 37, and 39 at the temporal-occipital-parietal junction[51,52] are the homologs of

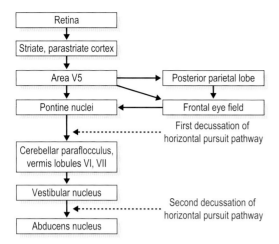

Figure 38.3 Schematic flow of visual motion and motor signals that generate smooth pursuit. Dashed lines indicate a double decussation of pathway for horizontal pursuit. (Adapted from Morrow MJ, Sharpe JA. Smooth pursuit eye movements. In: Sharpe JA, Barber HO (eds) The Vestibulo-ocular Reflex and Vertigo. New York: Raven Press, 1993:141–162.)

Table 38.2 Four classes of cerebral hemispheric pursuit paresis

Unidirectional	Saccadic pursuit toward the side of lesions to the posterior parietal and temporal lobe junction, involving V5 or ventral parietal cortex
	Contraversive smooth pursuit velocities may be normal, high, or low (but above the speed of ipsiversive smooth eye movement)
Omnidirectional	Saccadic pursuit in all directions, with bilateral focal or diffuse cerebral disease
Retinotopic	Saccadic pursuit in both horizontal directions in the contralateral visual hemifield, with unilateral lesions of striate cortex, optic radiation, or area V5
Craniotopic	Loss of pursuit contralateral to the craniotopic midline after acute hemisphere lesions

areas MT and MST (visual area V5) in the monkey brain. Area V5 and IPL project to the FEF and to pontine nuclei (Figure 38.3).

Lesions of area MT cause retinotopic pursuit defects that are related to target position on the retina. Pursuit eye movements have subnormal speed when the target falls upon the region of the visual field represented by the damaged area.[50] Retinotopic pursuit defects can be identified in the laboratory after parieto-temporo-occipital junction lesions in humans, but not by clinical examination (Table 38.2 and Box 38.4).[52] In contrast, lesions of area MST cause directional pursuit defects. Ipsiversive pursuit speed is reduced, regardless of target location on the retina.[50]

Pursuit commands are transmitted from the cerebral hemispheres to the ipsilateral dorsolateral pontine nucleus (DLPN) and nucleus reticularis tegmenti pontis (NRTP).[53] then relayed through the contralateral middle cerebellar peduncle to the flocculus and paraflocculus, vermis lobules VI, VII, and lobule IX (the uvula),[54,55] and finally to the caudal part of the fastigial nucleus and to the vestibular

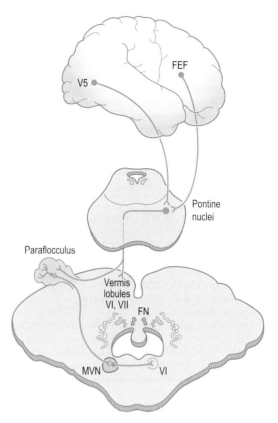

Figure 38.4 Putative pursuit pathway showing double decussation. The first decussation is from pontine nuclei (dorsolateral pontine nucleus (DLPN) and nucleus reticularis tegmenti pontis (NRTP)), the ocular motor vermis (lobules VI and VII) and to the cerebellar paraflocculus, which inhibits neurons in the medial vestibular nucleus (MVN). Excitatory projections from the MVN, the contralateral abducens nucleus (VI), constitute a second decussation. The caudal part of the fastigial nucleus (FN) processes pursuit signals from the vermis. (Modified from Sharpe JA. Neuroanatomy and neurophsiology of smooth pursuit: lesion studies. Brain Cognition 2008;68:241–254.)

nuclei (Figure 38.4). Direct connections from the vestibular nuclei to ocular motor nuclei complete the principal pursuit circuit in the brainstem. The vestibular nucleus activates the lateral rectus motoneurons and internuclear neurons in the contralateral abducens nucleus (and inhibits them in the ipsilateral abducens nucleus). The pontocerebellar projections, through the contralateral middle cerebellar peduncle, form a first decussation of the pursuit pathway, and the effect of MVN neurons on the contralateral abducens nucleus is a second decussation (Figure 38.3). The double decussation renders the pursuit pathway from the cerebral hemisphere to the abducens nucleus effectively ipsilateral.[55]

Smooth pursuit paresis

When smooth eye movements fail to match the speed of a slowly moving target, catch-up saccades compensate for the low velocity of smooth tracking, called saccadic pursuit. It is the sign of smooth pursuit paresis (Box 38.4).[55]

Unidirectional pursuit paresis

Saccadic pursuit occurs toward the side of posterior parietal and parietotemporal lobe lesions (Table 38.2), particularly

Box 38.4 Smooth Pursuit Paresis

- Saccadic tracking of a slowly moving object is the clinical sign of impaired, or paretic, smooth pursuit
- Ipsiversive pursuit defects consist of lowered smooth pursuit speed toward the side of unilateral cerebral lesions of area V5 or the frontal eye field, or their projections to the brainstem
- Ipsiversive pursuit defects are identified in response to a target moving anywhere in the visual field, either ipsilateral or contralateral to the side of the hemispheric lesion
- Retinotopic pursuit defects consist of lower smooth pursuit speed and inaccurate saccades in the area of the contralateral visual field subserved by damaged striate cortex, optic radiation, or area V5
- Craniotopic pursuit defects consist of reduced smooth pursuit speed and lowered saccade amplitudes in the hemirange of movement contralateral to unilateral acute frontal or parietal lobe lesions. They are identified in response to a pursuit target presented on the opposite side of the orbital midline
- Omnidirectional pursuit defects consist of low smooth pursuit speed in both horizontal and both vertical directions. They signify extensive unilateral or bilateral focal cerebral lesions, or diffuse cerebral cortical, basal ganglia, cerebellar, or brainstem disease

involving the angular gyrus and prestriate cortical Brodmann areas 19, 37, and 39 (area V5).[51,52] Ipsiversive saccadic pursuit is usually associated with contralateral hemianopia but the smooth eye movement disorder is independent of the visual field defect. It does not accompany hemianopia from pregeniculate or striate cortical damage.[56] Cerebral hemispheric control of smooth pursuit is not entirely ipsiversive, since unilateral lesions can cause some bidirectional impairment of horizontal smooth pursuit.[51,52,55]

Frontal lobe lesions may also cause ipsiversive pursuit paresis,[57] attributed to FEF involvement.[58] But saccadic pursuit after unilateral frontal lobe damage often appears to be bidirectional on clinical examination. Area V5 and dorsolateral frontal lobe provide two parallel routes through which cortical pursuit commands are conveyed to the brainstem. Impairment of ipsiversive pursuit accompanies posterior thalamic hemorrhage and may be explained by involvement of the posterior limb of the internal capsule which transmits pursuit commands.[51]

Optokinetic nystagmus asymmetry

Small hand-held striped tapes or drums, that are used in the clinic to test optokinetic nystagmus (OKN), activate both smooth pursuit and optokinetic smooth eye movements, but the slow phases of OKN stimulated by small targets are generated largely by the pursuit system. The pursuit system is concerned with foveal tracking of small objects, while the optokinetic system is responsible for parietinal tracking of large objects. Nonetheless small OKN stimuli are useful in the clinical setting since paretic pursuit typically accompanies impaired OKN, and asymmetry of OKN is more readily observed than is asymmetry of pursuit. Like smooth pursuit, OKN is defective when stimuli move toward the side of cerebral lesions.[59] The amplitude and frequency of the nys-

tagmus response are reduced, but the primary deficit is reduction in the slow phase velocity. By convention nystagmus direction is named by the quick phase direction; therefore, defective slow phases of OKN (and smooth pursuit) toward the side of a posterior parietotemporal lobe lesion are identified at the bedside as defective OKN beating away from the side of the lesion.

Some patients with acute unilateral parietal or frontal lobe damage do not track targets past the orbital midline into the contralateral craniotopic field of gaze. This is a craniotopic paresis of pursuit.[60] Cerebral hemispheric pursuit defects can be grouped into four categories[55,61] (Table 38.2).

Ipsiversive saccadic pursuit also occurs toward the side of lesions that involve the cerebellar flocculus/paraflocculus (Figure 38.2). Unilateral tegmental damage in the caudal pons and rostral medulla can impair contraversive smooth pursuit.[18,62] Greater paresis of contraversive pursuit after pontomedullary damage may signify disruption of excitatory projections from the vestibular nucleus to the contralateral abducens nucleus, or damage to connections with the cerebellum.

Omnidirectional pursuit paresis

Saccadic pursuit in all directions (Table 38.2) results from diffuse cerebral, cerebellar, or brainstem disease (Box 38.4); for example, multiple sclerosis,[63] Parkinson's disease,[35] Alzheimer's disease,[64] and cerebellar degenerations,[44] lower smooth pursuit speed. Similarly, advanced age, sedative drugs, fatigue, and inattention also cause saccadic tracking.[65,66] When qualified by these influences, horizontal and vertical saccadic pursuit is the most sensitive ocular motor sign of brain dysfunction.

Vestibulo-ocular reflex disorders

Head rotation elicits the angular VOR. The ratio of the output of the angular VOR (smooth eye movement speed in one direction) to the input of the reflex (head speed in the opposite direction) is its gain. VOR gain must approximate 1.0 in order to prevent slippage of retinal images and maintain clear vision. The eyes and head must also be 180° out of phase; this normal phase difference is called zero, by convention. Abnormal gain or phase of the reflex causes visual blur and oscillopsia. Nystagmus quick phases correct for failures of smooth eye movement motion to match head speeds. Imbalance of the VOR is caused by damage to the vestibular labyrinthine or nerve on one side or by asymmetric damage to its central brainstem connections to the ocular motor nuclei. This imbalance creates jerk nystagmus beating toward the side of defective vestibular smooth eye motion (Box 38.5).

Low gain of the VOR signifies bilateral peripheral vestibular or brainstem disease. Acute unilateral labyrinthine or vestibular nerve damage lowers gain acutely but compensation occurs within days or weeks so that a gain asymmetry of the reflex persists only during high frequency (>~2 Hz) head motion. High gain of the VOR (>1.0) is uncommon and is a feature of cerebellar disease.[67]

Oculocephalic reflex

The oculocephalic reflex (OCR) elicited by passive head on body rotation (doll's head reflex) tests the range of the VOR.

Box 38.5 VOR disorders

- The vestibulo-ocular reflex (VOR) achieves clear vision during head motion by moving the eye in the opposite direction at the same speed
- Abnormal VOR gain (ratio of eye velocity/head velocity) causes oscillopsia or blurring of vision
- Low VOR gain (head velocity > eye velocity) is a feature of peripheral vestibular or brainstem damage
- High VOR gain (eye velocity > head velocity) is an uncommon effect of cerebellar disease
- Abnormal gain can be detected by reduction in visual acuity during high-frequency head shaking
- Marked asymmetry of the VOR creates jerk nystagmus beating toward the direction of lowered smooth eye movement speed
- Asymmetry of the VOR can also be detected by the head impulse test and by the presence of nystagmus after head shaking

Box 38.6 Vertical Saccades Palsy

- Vertical gaze paresis indicates a bilateral or paramedian lesion, usually in the rostral midbrain tegmentum
- Upward saccadic palsy signifies damage to the posterior commissure or its adjacent fibers of passage
- Downward saccadic palsy signifies damage to neurons of the rostral intestinal nucleus of the medial longitudinal fasciculus (riMLF) and their projections to the interstitial nucleus of Cajal (INC)
- Combined upward and downward saccadic palsy indicates more extensive damage to the ventral midbrain tegmentum involving the riMLFs or their projections

Limited range of the VOR indicates disruption of brainstem VOR pathways or damage to ocular motor nerves, nuclei, or muscles. Conversely, normal range of the OCR, in the presence of limited range of saccades or smooth pursuit, indicates that a lesion responsible for the gaze paresis is supranuclear. However the OCR does not assess the VOR alone. Passive movement of the head at low frequencies activates visual following responses, both smooth pursuit and optokinetic, as well as the VOR. If the VOR is absent, visual following reflexes can move the eyes at the same velocity as the head if the motion is below 1 Hz. Only in comatose patients do low-frequency passive OCR movements test the VOR alone.

Visual acuity during head shaking

When patients are instructed to shake their head from side to side at 2–3 Hz through an amplitude of about 20°, Snellen visual acuity should remain about the same as with the head immobile. If acuity falls by two or three lines the VOR gain is low or high, or its phase is abnormal (Box 38.5). If the VOR is hyperactive (gain > 1.0), the patient perceives movement of the image in the same direction as head movement. If the VOR is hypoactive (gain < 1.0), images appear to move opposite to the direction of head motion. One can also examine the eyes for nystagmus. If the VOR is normal while the patient fixates an object during high-frequency head oscillation, the eyes should remain stable in space. Vestibular nystagmus indicates abnormal VOR gain or phase.

Ophthalmoscopy during head shaking

Another technique for detecting VOR abnormalities is examination of one fundus while the patient shakes the head from side to side at 2–3 Hz.[68] If the VOR is normal the optic disc (or other fundus landmark) remains stable. If the VOR is overactive (gain > 1.0) the disc moves in the same direction as the head whereas if the VOR is hypoactive (gain < 1.0) the disc moves opposite to the direction of head movement. Care must be taken that the head does not sway from side to side, since head translation causes the disc to move, even when the VOR is normal. This test can be difficult to perform and interpret. Patients must wear their regular glasses during the test, since the gain of the VOR is adapted according to the magnifying power of their lenses. Magnification can be predicted by the formula: magnification power $= 40/(40 - D)$, where D is the lens power in diopters. For example, a -5 D myopic patient would have a VOR gain of 0.89 in darkness, instead of 1.0.

Head-shaking nystagmus

Patients with unilateral peripheral vestibular lesions have nystagmus directed away from the affected side after vigorous head shaking.[69] The patient is instructed to shake the head through 40° of range at about 2 Hz for 20 seconds. Then, when the head is stopped, the observer examines the patient's eyes under Frenzel glasses (plus 20 lenses which magnify the eyes and blur the patient's fixation). Slow phases of head-shaking nystagmus (HSN) are directed toward the impaired ear. It lasts less than 20 seconds, and is sometimes followed by a low-amplitude reversed HSN with slow phases away from the impaired ear. After central vestibular lesions HSN may be directed in planes different from the direction of head shake or with slow phases away from the side of brainstem damage.[70]

Head impulse test

While the patient fixates a distant target the head is briskly moved to one side. The eyes should stay on target and the examiner should see only a smooth compensatory eye movement. Patients with unilateral vestibular loss make one or more saccades to bring the eyes on target when the head is moved toward the side of the impaired ear. As noted by Gauthier and Robinson, saccades in the same direction as the VOR signify inability of vestibular smooth eye movements to match head velocity.[71] Thus a patient with right vestibular neuritis will make leftward saccades during rightward head movements. Compensatory, refixation saccades during rapid horizontal head rotations indicate a horizontal semicircular canal or vestibular nerve lesion on the side toward which the head is being rotated.[72] The head must be moved at high velocity, because the VOR eventually becomes rebalanced for low-velocity head movements after unilateral peripheral vestibular damage.

Vertical gaze

As a general principle, vertical gaze is mediated by bilateral circuits and vertical gaze palsies signify bilateral or paramedian lesions (Box 38.6). Commands for vertical saccades descend from the cerebral hemispheres, and ascend from the caudal PPRF, to the rostral interstitial nucleus of the MLF (riMLF), located rostral to the third nerve nucleus, and within the MLF. Excitatory short lead burst neurons for vertical and torsional saccades reside in the riMLF.[73] Excitatory burst neurons with upward on-direction project bilaterally to oculomotor nucleus neurons (Figure 38.2), whereas neurons with downward on-directions project ipsilaterally to motoneurons of the oculomotor and trochlear nuclei[74]; this makes isolated lesions of the riMLF more likely to impair downward saccades selectively.[75]

Either a unilateral or bilateral pretectal lesion near the posterior commissure may destroy projections from both riMLF and the interstitial nucleus of Cajal (INC), selectively abolishing upward saccades. The nucleus of the posterior commissure (nPC) also contains upward short lead burst neurons that project across the commissure.[76] The nPC projects to the contralateral nPC, riMLF, and INC and intralaminar nucleus of the thalamus. Lesions of the posterior commissure paralyze upward saccades in monkeys and humans[73,77] as part of the pretectal syndrome.

The riMLF projects to the INC, which in concert with the vestibular nucleus and the paramedian tracts serves as the eye velocity-to-position integrator for vertical eye motion.[78,79] The INC is located within the MLF just caudal to the riMLF in the rostral midbrain. The INC participates in vertical gaze holding, generation of the vertical and torsional VOR, and vertical smooth pursuit.[80]

Vertical smooth pursuit channels ascend from the vestibular nuclei to the midbrain. They group of the vestibular nucleus, located at the junction of the brainstem and cerebellum, the MLF, and the superior cerebellar peduncle in monkeys carry signals for vertical pursuit. Pathways outside the MLF appear to carry much of the vertical smooth pursuit commands in humans.[22] Lesions in the pretectum that affect the posterior commissure degrade upward pursuit.[29,81] Both upward and downward smooth pursuit are limited by damage in the ventral tegmentum of the midbrain.[82,83]

Upward gaze palsy in the pretectal syndrome

The pretectal syndrome consists of paralysis of upward saccades, light-near dissociation of the pupils, retraction, and convergent oscillations of the eyes which are evoked by attempted upward saccades, and retraction of the upper

Table 38.3 Pretectal syndrome

Paralysis of upward saccades
Paralysis of upward saccades and pursuit
Paralysis of upward gaze and the vestibulo-ocular reflex
Retraction and convergence oscillations
Eyelid retraction
Light-near dissociated enlarged pupils

eyelids (Table 38.3).[84,85] Destruction of the posterior commissure is sufficient to cause the pretectal syndrome, but bilateral, or unilateral, extracommissural pretectal lesions that interrupt its fibers have the same effect. Limitation of upward gaze is also an effect of normal senescence.[42] The pretectal syndrome has the eponyms sylvian aqueduct and dorsal midbrain syndromes.

Downward gaze palsy and ventral midbrain lesions

Lesions in the rostral midbrain tegmentum, ventral to the aqueduct of Sylvius, cause selective paralysis of downward saccades by disrupting projections from the riMLF to the INC and the oculomotor and trochlear nuclei. The responsible lesions are usually bilateral infarcts, but unilateral paramedian lesions can also paralyze downward gaze or both upward and downward gaze[73,82]; the pupils are usually of medium size and poorly reactive to light and during accommodation. We term these distinct ocular motor defects the ventral midbrain syndrome.

In both the dorsal and ventral syndromes, the vertical VOR and smooth pursuit often appear to be spared. However, reduced gain, limited amplitude, and abnormal phase lead of the vertical VOR, and slow, limited pursuit, occur with ventral infarcts involving the INC and riMLF.[82,86]

Acknowledgment

This work was supported by Canadian Institutes of Health Research (CIHR) grants MT 15362, ME 5504, and MOP 57853.

Key references

A complete list of chapter references is available online at www.expertconsult.com. See inside cover for registration details.

1. Sharpe JA, Wong AM. Anatomy and physiology of ocular motor systems. In: Miller NR, Newman NJ (eds) Walsh and Hoyt's Clinical Neuro-ophthalmology. Baltimore: Lippincott, Williams and Wilkins, 2005:809–885.

2. Leigh RJ, Zee DS. The Neurology of Eye Movements, 4th edn. New York: Oxford University Press, 2006.

13. Sharpe JA. Gaze disorders. In: Noseworthy JH (ed.) Neurological

Therapeutics: Principles and Practice. London: Martin Dunitz, Taylor Francis, 2006:2028–2047.

14. Barton EJ, Nelson JS, Gandhi NJ, et al. Effects of partial lidocaine inactivation of the paramedian pontine reticular formation on saccades of macaques. J Neurophysiol 2003;90:372–386.

17. Cannon SC, Robinson DA. Loss of the neural integrator of the oculomotor system from brainstem lesions in

monkeys. J Neurophysiol 1987;57:1383–1409.

20. Baloh RW, Yee RD, Honrubia V. Internuclear ophthalmoplegia. Arch Neurol 1978;35:484–493.

22. Ranalli PJ, Sharpe JA. Vertical vestibulo-ocular reflex, smooth pursuit and eye-head tracking dysfunction in internuclear ophthalmoplegia. Brain 1988;111: 1277–1295.

52. Morrow MJ, Sharpe JA. Retinotopic and directional deficits of smooth pursuit initiation after posterior cerebral hemispheric lesions. Neurology 1993;43: 595–603.

55. Sharpe JA. Neuroanatomy and neurophsiology of smooth pursuit: lesion studies. Brain Cognition 2008;68:241–254.

69. Hain TC, Spindler J. Head-shaking nystagmus. In: Sharpe JA, Barber HO (eds) The Vestibulo-Ocular Reflex and Vertigo. New York: Raven, 1993:217–228.

73. Buttner-Ennever JA, Buttner U, Cohen B. Vertical gaze paralysis and the rostral interstitial nucleus of the medial longitudinal fasciculus. Brain 1982;105: 125–149.

CHAPTER 39

Idiopathic intracranial hypertension (idiopathic pseudotumor cerebri)

Deborah M Grzybowski and Martin Lubow

Clinical background

Key symptoms and signs

The signs and symptoms of increased intracranial pressure (ICP) are headache, subjective pulse-synchronous bruit, and papilledema (Box 39.1). Papilledema can cause fleeting visual obscurations in one or both eyes. Occasional diplopia is attributed to presumed sixth-nerve compression. Visual field loss and decreased acuity are unusual early in the course of disease, but may become devastating over time.

Historical development

Helmholtz's 1851 invention of the ophthalmoscope allowed visualization of the optic nerves, and of their dramatic engorgement with the swelling of papilledema that accompanied the increased ICP of brain tumors. The development of the first effective neurosurgical procedures by Harvey Cushing around 1910, which allowed life-saving treatment by urgent removal or decompression of such tumors, made recognition of papilledema and its connection to brain tumors critically important.[1] It was an association, which when recognized and acted upon, might save a patient's life. For that reason it became a high-priority sign in the routine medical examination, so that papilledema, or any optic disc edema, needed to be quickly categorized as "brain tumor" or "otherwise." The "otherwise" became known as pseudotumor cerebri (PTC), a brain tumor-mimicking form of papilledema. The most common cause before 1950 was bacterial meningitis, a nonsurgical cause of increased ICP, as shown by the early work of Paton and Holmes.[2] A frequent cause of meningitis, with an associated element of adjacent venous thrombosis, in that preantibiotic era, was mastoiditis. An infection of the mastoid air spaces in the petrous bone, it might start as a routine nasopharyngitis, extend to the eustachian tube and inner ear, then a petrous bone infection with mastoiditis. The sequential adjacent meningitis and lateral sinus thrombosis became recognized as "otitic hydrocephalus".[3]

All of this changed after World War II with the availability of penicillin. Bacterial meningitis and otitic hydrocephalus became unusual, but the appearance of a patient with papilledema still required a determination of brain tumor versus pseudotumor as the first diagnostic step. Despite the availability of cerebral angiography and ventriculography, many patients had exploratory craniotomies as the last step in ruling out a brain tumor and in establishing their diagnoses as pseudotumor. It was not until the evolution of neuroimaging to modern computed tomography and magnetic resonance techniques that this became unnecessary. Until then all increased ICP, meaning all papilledema, was regarded, and needed to be so regarded, as due to brain tumor.

Nomenclature for PTC syndromes is varied. "Benign intracranial hypertension" is flawed, in that the disorder is anything but benign. We prefer "idiopathic pseudotumor cerebri" or iPTC for cases where the etiology is unclear, although in deference to common use, we will use the term "idiopathic intracranial hypertension" (IIH) in this chapter. "Secondary PTC" is used when there is a detectable etiology, e.g., cerebral venous thrombosis or use of tetracycline, doxycycline, minocycline, or retinoids (Box 39.2).

Epidemiology

IIH is a disease that most frequently affects obese women of child-bearing age.[4–7] The incidence of IIH in the general population is 1 : 100 000; however, the incidence rises to 19.3 : 100 000 in women aged 20–44 who are at least 20% over ideal body weight.[8,9] The incidence of IIH appears to be rising dramatically, and the Centers for Disease Control recently released statistics indicating that the rate of obesity in the USA has doubled in the past decade.[10]

Genetics

Rare, but verified, examples of a mother with known IIH, and her son with the same diagnosis,[11] a father with a daughter,[12] and dizygotic twin brothers,[13] are consistent with a genetic link. Twins have been reported, both heterozygous

> **Box 39.1 Key symptoms and signs of increased intracranial pressure in idiopathic pseudotumor cerebri**
>
> - Increased intracranial pressure (over 250 mm H_2O)
> - Headache
> - Papilledema
> - Pulsatile bruit (noise)
> - Transient visual obscurations
> - Obesity
> - Child-bearing age
> - Female
> - Diplopia (uncommon)
> - Visual field loss (uncommon)

> **Box 39.2 Secondary causes of pseudotumor cerebri**
>
> - Head trauma (including posttraumatic brain injury)
> - Underlying disease: liver or kidney failure
> - Sleep apnea
> - Venous thrombosis (cerebral blood clots)
> - Stroke (subarachnoid hemorrhage)
> - Cystinosis
>
> **Drugs**
>
> - Accutane (isotretinoin)
> - Tetracycline
> - Growth hormone
> - Corticosteroids
> - Tetracyclines
> - ATRA (acute promyelocytic leukemia)
> - Vitamin A (hypervitaminosis A; retinoids)
> - Amiodarone
> - Nitrofurantoin
> - Nalidixic acid
> - Sulfa antibacterials
> - Leuprorelin (luteinizing hormone-releasing hormone analog)
> - Lithium
> - Levonorgestrel (Norplant)
> - Steroid withdrawal
>
> **Underlying infectious diseases**
>
> - Meningitis (bacterial or viral)
> - Lyme disease
> - Human immunodeficiency virus (HIV)
> - Poliomyelitis
> - Coxsackie B viral encephalitis
> - Guillain–Barré syndrome
> - Infectious mononucleosis
> - Syphilis
> - Malaria

and homozygous, e.g., homozygous twin sisters with similar onset of symptoms in both.[14,15]

Diagnostic workup

IIH is diagnosed when the following are all true:

1. Symptoms and signs all attributable to increased ICP or papilledema
2. No medications known to elevate ICP (see Box 39.2)
3. Normal neurological examination except for papilledema and possibly evidence of sixth-nerve dysfunction
4. Normal magnetic resonance imaging and magnetic resonance venography
5. Elevated ICP recorded during lumbar puncture in the standard lateral decubitus position (cerebrospinal fluid (CSF) opening pressure greater than 250 mm H_2O; pressures of 200–250 mm H_2O should remain suspect)
6. Normal CSF composition.

Treatment

Normalizing and maintaining the CSF pressure can be challenging. Fluid removal is often temporary, and shunting to another location is invasive and often impermanent. Medical treatment can decrease fluid formation, but does so incompletely and with side-effects that can be unpleasant and sometimes dangerous.

Most patients are managed with medical treatment to lower the CSF pressure. The typical treatment progression for IIH is shown in Box 39.3. Carbonic anhydrase inhibitors (CAIs), usually acetazolamide, are used to impair CSF formation and can improve symptoms of headache and visual obscurations in most patients. Despite unpleasant sensory disturbances (tingling fingers and toes, and taste distortions), malaise, diuresis, and even the risks of abreaction (sulfa allergies and aplastic anemia), the CAIs are the most common form of medical treatment. The effect of CAIs on CSF outflow is unknown; however, receptors for CAIs have been identified in the arachnoid membrane, suggesting a role in modulating CSF outflow.

More effective agents than CAIs are not known. Furosemide has been tried and adds little beyond the risk of potas-

> **Box 39.3 Typical treatment progression for idiopathic pseudotumor cerebri**
>
> 1. Carbonic anhydrase inhibitors (CAIs)
> 2. Other pharmaceuticals
>   a. Lasix (furosemide)
>   b. Beta-blockers (propranolol)
>   c. Octreotide (somatostatin)
> 3. Surgery
>   a. Optic nerve sheath fenestration
>   b. Neurosurgical shunts
>   i. Lumboperitoneal (LP) shunt
>   ii. Ventriculoperitoneal (VP) shunt
>   iii. Cisterna magnum shunt
>   c. Cortical venous stents

sium imbalance. Somatostatin analogs may be encouraging, demonstrated by our clinical experience with octreotide (not published),[16] but remain at the research level.

Shunting procedures include lumbar peritoneal shunts, ventriculoperiotoneal shunts, and optic nerve sheath fenestration. These procedures have significant limitations. They each need a patent opening to allow persistent drainage of CSF from the subarachnoid or intraventricular space into the peritoneal cavity or orbit. A critical limitation in both is failure to work consistently and predictably over the years.

A controversial alternative to surgery of the intracranial or orbital subarachnoid space for lowering ICP is cortical venous sinus stenting.[17-21]

Prognosis and complications

Patients with IIH are carefully followed with perimetry and fundoscopy in order to detect visual field deterioration (which may be asymptomatic until late) and worsening papilledema. Retinal nerve fiber layer analysis by optical coherence tomography is a promising complement to the clinical examination.

Pathophysiology

Normal CSF homeostasis relies on a careful balance between CSF production and absorption. Alterations in the rate of CSF formation, absorption, or outflow resistance can lead to a buildup of ICP, causing multiple neurological deficits.

While the mechanisms explaining secondary PTCs remain obscure, their clarification is a worthwhile objective. Neurophysiologists and neuroscience-oriented physicians are quick to presume that such agents somehow impair CSF outflow by damage to outflow channels. Likely that is true, but except for seeing red blood cells in the subarachnoid space and in the arachnoid villi after intracranial hemorrhage, we don't know what happens, or how it happens, at the molecular level of the CSF outflow pathways.

Isolating the "distilled" group of patients labeled as IIH now permits us to focus on their common findings and characterize them in a way that should help our clinical perspective, while recognizing that later information will regroup them more accurately. The following factors should be considered in any discussion of pathogenesis:

1. Genetics
2. Obesity
3. Retinoids
4. Hydrocephalus
5. Models.

A simplified model circuit shows the movement of CSF in Figure 39.1.[22-24] Basic fluid mechanics shows that the driving force for fluid movement is a pressure difference.[25] This implies that a pressure gradient must occur prior to any movement of CSF. Any of the fluid reservoirs shown in Figure 39.1 may be affected by changes in pressure gradients and the resultant fluid redistribution. The subarachnoid space (SAS) acts like a variable fluid capacitor, taking up excess CSF when needed or giving it up if necessary. The ability of the SAS to do so is affected by age and other factors that stiffen the arachnoid trabeculae. The vasculature responds to changes by dilation or constriction (autoregulation), with a redistribution of fluid, and a rebalance of pressure gradients, which leads us to mechanistic theories.

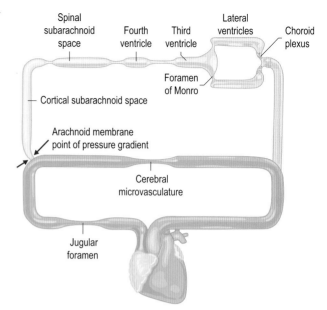

Figure 39.1 Model circuit of fluid movement between cerebrospinal fluid and vasculature.

Mechanistic theories

CSF homeostasis and raised ICP in IIH have long puzzled investigators.[24,26] CSF formation rates range from approximately 0.3 to 0.4 ml/min.[27-29] Based on this, the entire CSF volume turns over 3–4 times daily.

In a seemingly healthy patient, with all other variables unchanged, CSF pressure rise must be due to either increased CSF production or decreased CSF outflow. Increased CSF production is possible, but much less likely than decreased outflow. Several studies have shown that the rate of CSF production is either normal or slightly decreased, therefore hypersecretion of CSF as a mechanism is unlikely.[30,31] Further evidence against excessive CSF production as the mechanism of IIH lies in clinical experience, such as with choriod plexus papilloma, a condition with excessive CSF production, which does not clinically produce anything similar to IIH.[32]

Theories explaining decreased outflow relate to slowed egress through the membrane system that includes the arachnoid membrane and arachnoid granulations (AGs),[24,33-36] or increased backpressure in the cortical venous system, similar to that seen in secondary PTC due to venous thrombosis.

Vitamin A connection

Because of clinical experience with vitamin A toxicity, recent attention has focused on retinoid metabolism and transport with interesting, but still inconclusive, results. The association between secondary PTC and vitamin A has been recognized in cases of excessive dietary intake of vitamin A (hypervitaminosis A), the most prominent example of which is the well-documented vitamin A toxicity resulting from the ingestion of polar bear liver by arctic explorers and Eskimos.[37] It has since been demonstrated that bear and seal livers contain extremely high concentrations of vitamin A and can produce rapid vitamin A toxicity when consumed even in moderate doses.[38] Secondary PTC has also been reported in association with natural and synthetic retinoid-based medications, often used in dermatology in the treatment of acne (for review, see Friedman[39]). The secondary association between vitamin A and PTC in these cases is so strong that it has recently led to the investigation of serum and CSF levels of retinol and serum retinol-binding protein (RBP) levels in IIH patients without excessive vitamin A intake or supplementation.[40–42]

Several studies have examined the levels of retinol in the serum and CSF of patients with and without PTC and found conflicting results, most likely due to differences in study design and/or sample handling. Jacobson et al[40] examined only the serum levels of retinol and retinyl ester in patients with and without PTC. Selhorst et al[43] compared both serum retinol and serum RBP levels in patients with and without PTC. More recently studies have focused on CSF retinol levels. Tabassi et al[41] measured both serum and CSF retinol in 20 patients with PTC and 20 age- and body mass index-matched control patients. These studies have led to the hypothesis that perhaps patients with IIH are predisposed to vitamin A intoxication, even at normal intake levels.

Warner et al have recently reported on CSF retinol and RBP levels in several patient groups, including those with IIH.[42] In this study, the authors found that patients with IIH had significantly elevated CSF retinol levels in addition to significantly reduced CSF RBP levels compared to control patients. This led to a significantly increased CSF retinol : RBP ratio in patients with IIH. The results of this study led the authors to hypothesize that these decreased levels of CSF RBP coupled with increased CSF retinol might lead to elevated circulating levels of free, unbound retinol that could potentially be toxic to the arachnoid villi and granulations.

Important too is the 2005 review article by Helen Everts et al[44] in which they demonstrate (in rats) immunolocalization of RA biosynthesis systems to the selected tissue sites where their effects are required. The focal paracrine nature of these retinoid functions obviates the need for endocrine-type systemic circulation of retinoids or their transporters beyond the initial retinol stage. In IIH patients the tissues will be normal, but the signal transduction pathway will be abnormal and cause overproduction of RA, measurable in their CSF but probably not in their serum.[45]

No one has been able to develop an adequate demonstration of a consistent abnormality, nor to offer an adequate hypothesis to explain the role of retinoids and increased CSF pressure. This is especially troublesome in view of known examples of vitamin A toxicity, and in view of long-standing animal work in other species showing that hypervitaminosis A causes decreased CSF pressure.[46]

Vitamin A and adipocytes

Two proteins for vitamin A transport in blood and brain are transthyretin (TTR) and RBP. TTR is a critical transport protein for thyroxine and retinol. It is also an important metabolic modulator and has been linked to obesity. It is expressed in liver, and synthesized and secreted by the choroid plexus into CSF.

Studies in rats show that adipocytes synthesize RBP and store RBP and retinoids.[47] Cellular RBP (CRBP) gene expression is regulated dynamically in adipocytes by retinol uptake,

intracellular transport, and metabolism. Another rat study showed that adipocytes are dynamically involved in retinoid storage and metabolism, and synthesis and secretion of RBP.[48] This may be significant for those IIH patients who characteristically have a body mass index greater than 30. Increased numbers of adipocytes, which regulate vitamin A metabolism by altering gene expression, are critical in IIH. A Medical Research Council study was conducted in 1942 to determine time of vitamin A depletion in human volunteers. They found it very difficult to deplete vitamin A; in some cases it took over 2 years, the length of their study.[49]

The increased levels of adipocytes in obese IIH patients can dynamically regulate vitamin A metabolism by altering gene expression, and must be considered as a possible mechanism for IIH. Retinoic acids (RAs) have the ability to alter gene transcription via their receptors, which have been identified in arachnoid tissues in our unpublished data. Increases in the plasma concentration of RA isomers have been shown to upregulate expression of their receptors, suggesting that the metabolism of vitamin A can be altered or self-regulated in humans.[50] Elevated RA levels may also act directly via dynamic vitamin A-related transcriptional changes to alter CSF pressure. These transcriptional changes lead to decreased cellular viability, proliferation, cellular remodeling, adhesiveness, and a resultant decrease in membrane permeability which also contributes to elevated CSF pressure.

Vitamin A animal models

Studies on hypo- and hypervitaminosis A in animal models, including rodents, cattle, and goats, have investigated the effects of vitamin A on CSF formation and clearance rates as well as on biochemical composition of the dura mater and arachnoid villi. Several groups have investigated the association between altered vitamin A status and morphological changes in the AGs associated with changes in ICP.

Hypovitaminosis A

Increased ICP has been found in hypovitaminotic A calves[46] and in rat.[51] The effects of vitamin A deficiency on the formation and absorption of CSF by adult goats were reported by Frier et al.[52] Unlike the results previously reported for developing calves, deficient adult goats exhibited no change in CSF formation rate or ICP; however CSF outflow resistance was elevated compared to control animals. The authors conclude that adult ruminates may require a deficiency of a longer duration to produce similar effects as in younger, developing animals.

Hayes et al[53] reported the first detailed analysis of arachnoid morphology in hypovitaminotic calves and rats. They used histology with electron microscopy to examine the AGs of deficient animals. The authors of this study report that the AGs of deficient animals were larger and more readily visible, and in some cases so large that portions of the brain had herniated through the dura mater and into the dural sinus lumen. Ultrastructural analysis of the AGs revealed an overall thickening of the dura mater and subarachnoid trabeculae. The fibrous capsule and interstitial arachnoid cells appeared fibrotic, with increased collagen fibrils, tonofilaments, and glycogen granules. The general thickening of these tissues led these authors to speculate that ICP increases might be due to an overall decrease in the subarachnoid CSF space and an increased resistance to CSF outflow.

Hypervitaminosis A

Similar studies by Hurt et al on the rates of CSF formation and absorption have been performed in calves with vitamin A toxicity. They reported on the rates of CSF formation and absorption in hypervitaminosis A and found the calves had significantly decreased ICP and a decreased rate of CSF production.[54]

Frier et al[55] noted that the hypervitaminosis A toxicity reported by Hurt et al[54] was quite severe and that several animals died from the toxicity. They repeated the test in calves using mild vitamin A toxicity, and found decreased ICP. Increased CSF formation rate and increased bulk absorption of CSF were attributed to decreased resistance to CSF outflow.

Frier et al[55] studied the effects of vitamin A toxicity in adult goats. They compared the effects of vitamin A toxicity in the developing calf and found decreased ICP and increased CSF formation rate.

Finally, Gorgacz et al[56] provided a morphologic assessment of the AGs in calves with hypervitaminosis A, similar to the analysis of Hayes[57] for vitamin A deficiency. This study reported that the AGs in bovine vitamin A toxicity were significantly reduced in size with overall thinning of the cellular membranes, including a thinner fibrous capsule surrounding the granulations. In addition, the height of choroid plexus epithelial cells in hypervitaminotic calves was reduced.

Taken together, these studies on the effects of vitamin A status on CSF homeostasis in animal models initially seem to agree. They indicate that vitamin A deficiency is associated with increased ICP and is likely due to decreased absorption of CSF from increased resistance to CSF outflow. In these animal models, hypervitaminosis A is associated with a significantly reduced ICP and a decreased resistance to CSF absorption. On the other hand, production rates of CSF vary with age and species.

Vitamin A animal model conclusions

The results of animal studies are in direct contrast with human vitamin A status, where vitamin A toxicity is closely associated with increased ICP and a secondary PTC condition. It is not clear if these differences relate to fundamental differences in the transport and metabolism of vitamin A between humans and animals, variation in the degree of toxicity/deficiency, or distinctions between developing and fully mature subjects. The important points to remember from this critical analysis of animal models are:

1. There is a link between vitamin A levels and ICP
2. Vitamin A levels effect structural and morphological changes in the arachnoid tissues, as shown in animals
3. Animal models are not adequate to study human IIH.

Other mechanisms

Recent work with calcium-regulating target genes has shown that alpha-klotho, with its link to fibroblast growth factor-2, is critical to membrane regulation of calcium homeostasis and thereby CSF formation in the choroid plexus and in

membranes generally.[58,59] Interestingly there is also a link to retinoids via nuclear receptors and particularly peroxisome proliferator-activated receptor-γ.[60]

We have recently published a pathogenetic hypothesis for IIH[45] which is based on: (1) the recognition of multigenerational familial disease patterns, which confirm the hereditary nature of IIH; and (2) the demonstration of retinaldehyde, an intermediate metabolite in the retinoid pathway, as an important regulator of adipogenesis, fat storage, and insulin resistance. We hypothesize that IIH is a familial disease. It is caused by a highly conserved, tightly controlled genetic variant of the enzyme systems controlling the regulation of the retinoid intermediate metabolite retinaldehyde, and its major oxidation product, RA. We point specifically to a deficit of retinaldehyde due to inefficient enzymatic regulation, and a resultant increase in available RA in the central nervous system (CNS) due to the same inefficient enzymatic regulation and inefficient RA degradation (Figure 39.2). The decrease in retinaldehyde is known to cause obesity and insulin resistance. The increase in RA is the cause of impaired CSF outflow and thereby idiopathic increased intracranial pressure (IICP) via impaired transport of CSF through the arachnoid membrane outflow channels. Of special interest is the necessary role of estrogen in the induction of RA expression, as demonstrated, and more recently reviewed, by Li et al.[61] It suggests an explanation for the sex and the age preference of the IIH syndrome, with its onset in teenage girls, and it offers the possibility of medical treatment based on manipulation of estrogen hormone suppression and even ovarian cycle alteration to diminish the excess RA production which we hypothesize to be the cause of the IICP in these patients. These combined elements are the hallmarks of the syndrome we recognize as IIH. Localizing the metabolic defect and the enzyme variant offers the possibility of treatment and even possibly the cure of this familial syndrome. Initial treatment of IIH by diet modifications to bypass defective pathways, such as reduced retinoid intake and increased Raldh inhibitors such as citral, may be effective.[45]

CSF outflow models

Structure and function

The AGs, described by Pacchioni in 1705 as "peculiar wart-like excrescences" were functionally investigated by Key and Retzius in 1876.[56,57,62,63] They injected Berlin blue-stained gelatin into the spinal subarachnoid space (SAS) of human cadavers "at fairly low pressures (60 mmHg)" and saw the blue pass through the AGs ("die Arachnoidenzotten") into the cerebral sinus, but also into the lymphatic vessels of the frontal sinus and the nasal mucous membrane (Figure 39.3). Theirs was the first modern indication of a dual CSF drainage system in humans, demonstrating both AG and basal lymphatic outflow pathways.

Weed, working with Cushing at the beginnings of neurosurgery, used what he considered to be more informative markers, Prussian blue and ferrocyanide solutions, and again verified the AG pathway into the venous sinus.[64,65] He dismissed the basal lymphatic outflow as insignificant, and emphasized that CSF was absorbed across the arachnoid villi and into the venous system.

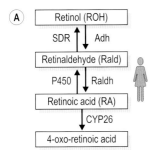 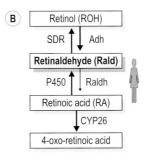 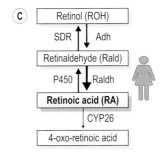

Figure 39.2 (A) Summary of retinol metabolism in a "normal" person with "normal" survival value under stress by famine. Balanced levels of retinaldehyde (Rald) and retinoic acid (RA) are present. These result in normal levels of body fat, normal insulin resistance, and normal intracranial pressures. (B) Summary of retinol metabolism in a "lean" person variant, with poor survival value for times of stress by famine. High concentrations of Rald controlled by "lean mix" on the genetic control of enzyme and cellular regulators for hydrolysis of Rald from retinol (ROH), and its subsequent metabolism to RA. Normal regulation of RA metabolism by cytochrome p450 (CYP26) enzymes also present. These result in very low levels of body fat, low insulin resistance, and normal intracranial pressure. (C) Summary of retinol metabolism in an idiopathic intracranial hypertension (IIH) patient, with excellent survival value for times of stress by famine, but at high risk for diseases attributable to the metabolic syndrome (diabetes, hypertension, atherosclerotic vascular disease) in times of plenty. Low concentrations of Rald controlled (most likely) via increased hydrolysis by a familial genetic variant of a Raldh (one of the common dehydrogenase variants), increasing RA formation and lowering Rald concentrations to produce the phenotypical IIH patient. Possible dysregulation of RA metabolism by CYP26 enzymes would also increase RA concentration. These result in metabolic syndrome and IIH with high levels of body fat, insulin resistance, and increased intracranial pressure.

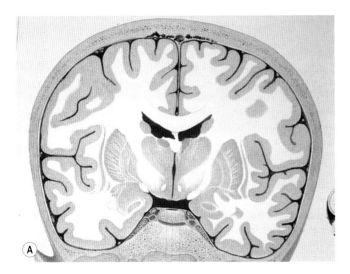

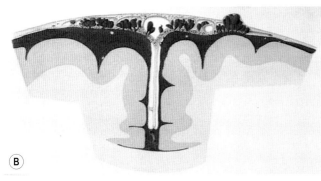

Figure 39.3 (A) Cerebrospinal fluid outflow pathway marked with Berlin blue-stained gelatin by Key and Retzius in 1875. (B) Close-up of filled subarachnoid space, arachnoid membrane, and granulations, and the superior sagittal sinus. (Courtesy of the Johns Hopkins Rare Book Collection.)

Most studies thereafter dealt with the issue of open versus closed (valved) channel mechanisms of CSF outflow through the arachnoid membrane. The open-channel theory was first proposed by Davson et al in 1973[66] and followed by others[67,68] until the electron microscope became commercially available around 1965, when numerous studies hypothesized a mechanism which utilizes valve-like structures, or closed channels.[69-73] Tripathi also detailed the analogy between outflow of aqueous humor and CSF.[72]

Ultrastructural perspectives have also shown that human AGs are different from those of other species.[74] Human AGs demonstrate a cap cell layer contacting or extending through the dura in places to provide a direct contact with the venous lumen. This combination of special anatomy, cap cells, and their location further suggests a special function in their role for CSF outflow in humans.[75-81]

More recently, research attention has returned to the basal lymphatic pathway shown earlier by Key and Retzius in 1875.[82-84] A major component via olfactory fibers through the cribriform plate has been suggested, but the microanatomy remains to be clarified. It is likely that it will turn out to be a variant of the arachnoid sleeve structure shown along the spinal nerves, where an arachnoid sheath surrounds the exiting nerve with an adjacent lymphatic channel available for passage of exiting CSF (Figure 39.4).[85-91]

The optic nerve remains a special physiological entity due to its location, its origin (white-matter tract of the CNS surrounded by CSF along its length), and the opposing pressures induced by the CSF from the subarachnoid space and intraocular pressures. Animal work has suggested that the optic nerve offers a similar pathway to adjacent lymphatics, but clinical experience demonstrates that this is not true in humans. Indeed, the cul-de-sac nature of the dural-arachnoid sleeve on the optic nerve terminating as it does at the globe is the very reason for chronic increased ICP in PTC causing nerve compression blindness. Some have claimed otherwise, but have not explained common clinical experience.[92,93]

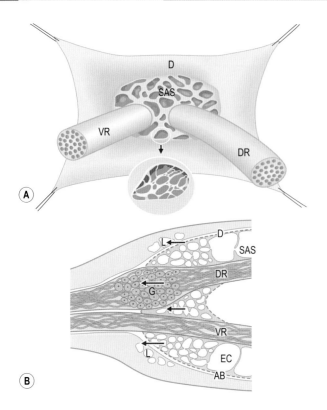

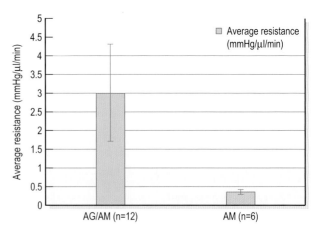

Figure 39.5 Comparison of average cerebrospinal fluid outflow resistance in physiologically perfused human arachnoid granulations in arachnoid membrane (AG/AM) and arachnoid membrane with no visible granulations (AM). Perfusion pressure was 5 mmHg (physiologic). The values are within the range of previously reported human arachnoid membrane resistance values.

Figure 39.4 (A) Schematic drawing of the spinal cerebrospinal fluid outflow pathway (arrows) along the ventral and dorsal root (VR, DR) seen from the subarachnoid space. The dura (D) is held by tenting sutures to visualize the outflow area, which, due to bulges and trabeculae of the external arachnoid layers, has a reticular appearance (magnified inset). (B) Schematic drawing of the horizontal cutting plane of (A). The median outflow area toward the endoneurium between dorsal root (DR) and ventral root (VR) can be differentiated from two lateral outflow areas of the subarachnoid space (SAS). In these areas the outer arachnoid layer forms several bulges and excavations (EC). The external arachnoid layer (AB) builds the border to the dura mater (D, white area), which becomes thinner in the distal area. Lymph vessels (L) can be found in the connective tissue around the dura mater, predominantly near spinal ganglia (G). (Modified from Voelz K, et al. A ferritin tracer study of compensatory spinal CSF outflow pathways in kaolin-induced hydrocephalus. Acta Neuropathol 2007;113:569–575.)

Studies have shown that arachnoid villi are present in the optic nerve sheaths of both humans and primates.[94,95] This is an area of controversy because it disputes clinical findings. Optic nerve surgery for PTC seems to demonstrate that the optic nerve sheaths retain CSF under increased pressure. Though villi are present, perhaps they are unable to drain at increased pressure. These seemingly confounding ideas will be explored further in the discussion of human models.

Development of arachnoid villi

Controversies over the time of appearance of arachnoid villi seem misplaced, in that their function is the issue of interest and need not depend on their enlargement or visibility as AGs later in life. Nevertheless, Le Gros Clark[96] concluded his 1920 studies with the opinion that the villi were present at birth and at times in the fetus. Visible granulations appeared variably from 4 to 18 months, when the fontanels closed. Since then Turner[97] showed arachnoid villi in developing human embryos at 12 weeks' gestation, and in term fetuses,

and in 92 other human subjects. These data suggest the potential for CSF outflow function through these structures before birth.

Human CSF outflow model

Models for human CSF outflow in vitro and ex vivo have been developed and used to verify arachnoid membrane functional characteristics.[98–101] They have shown unidirectionality of flow across the arachnoid membrane, and fluid transport via transcellular (vacuoles) and paracellular (vesicles) pathways,[97,98] both mimicking physiologic CSF passage. These findings are in agreement with earlier electron microscopic ultrastructural studies.[72,81,102]

Of special interest is our demonstration that our ex vivo perfusion model of the human arachnoid membrane alone, without visible granulations, has the capability of permitting the passage of five times the volume of outflow than the AG perfusion model (Figure 39.5; unpublished data).

Our ex vivo model shows that resistance to outflow at 15 mmHg is greater than at 5 mmHg. This might explain the disparity that is suggested with increased pressure and failure of the outflow mechanism in the optic nerve. Figure 39.6 (unpublished data) shows the increase in resistance by human arachnoid membrane with increasing pressure. We must keep in mind that the arachnoid membrane in the ex vivo model is not an exact model of in vivo functionality.

When verified by others, this CSF outflow resistance data would suggest the need to reconsider the relative distribution between the venous and the lymphatic contributions in selected age groups. The developmental status of the membrane surface used, as manifested by age and by morphology, will be important for the study of infantile hydrocephalus where, despite increase in the CSF pressure gradient (versus systemic venous and lymphatic pressures), the CSF outflow mechanism has failed.

Increased cerebral venous sinus pressure

Others have speculated that CSF absorption is decreased by increased cerebral venous pressure which decreases the

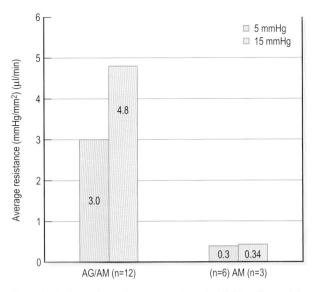

Figure 39.6 Comparison of average cerebrospinal fluid outflow resistance in physiologically perfused human arachnoid granulations in arachnoid membrane (AG/AM) and arachnoid membrane with no visible granulations (AM) at physiologic pressure (5 mmHg) and increased intracranial pressure (15 mmHg).

driving force for CSF outflow.[17,18,103] Numerous studies have reported controversial results for use of stents in PTC patients.[18,104] Conflicting results may be attributed to uncontrolled variables and differences in patient selection criteria.

King et al showed by manometry that removal of CSF in PTC patients produced a drop in proximal transverse sinus pressure. This indicates that venous outflow obstruction is reversible by reducing ICP, from which it follows that the stenosis is the effect and not the cause.[105] Three case reports by Rohr et al also indicate that the venous sinus obstruction is secondary to increased ICP.[106]

It has always been presumed, and more recently recognized, that increased ICP greater than cerebral venous pressure would collapse the low-pressure cerebral venous sinuses, and that a drop in that elevated ICP should allow those low-pressure veins to reopen, and to drain properly. This drop in pressure also affects the arachnoid membrane resistance to outflow, thereby allowing normal CSF outflow to resume through normalized arachnoid membrane. Removal of CSF can, at times, relieve IIH in a similar manner.

Key references

A complete list of chapter references is available online at www.expertconsult.com. See inside cover for registration details.

2. Paton L, Holmes G. The pathology of papilloedema: a histological study of 60 eyes. Brain 1911;33:389–432.

4. Ireland B, Corbett JJ, Wallace RB. The search for causes of idiopathic intracranial hypertension. A preliminary case-control study. Arch Neurol 1990; 47:315–320.

29. Rubin RC, Henderson ES, Ommaya AK, et al. The production of cerebrospinal fluid in man and its modification by acetazolamide. J Neurosurg 1966;25: 430–436.

38. Rodahl K, Moore T. The vitamin A content and toxicity of bear and seal liver. Biochem J 1943;37:166–168.

42. Warner JE, Larson AJ, Bhosale P, et al. Retinol-binding protein and retinol analysis in cerebrospinal fluid and serum of patients with and without idiopathic intracranial hypertension. J Neuroophthalmol 2007;27:258–262.

45. Grzybowksi, Lubow in press

46. Calhoun MC, Hurt HD, Eaton HD, et al. Rates of formation and absorption of cerebrospinal fluid in bovine hypovitaminosis A. J Dairy Sci 1967;50: 1489–1494.

53. Hayes KC, McCombs HL, Faherty TP. The fine structure of vitamin A deficiency. II. Arachnoid granulations

and CSF pressure. Brain 1971;94:213–224.

62. Key G, Retzius A. Studien in der Anatomie des Nervensystems und des Bindesgewebe. Stockholm: Samson and Wallin, 1876.

65. Weed LH. The absorption of the cerebrospinal fluid into the venous system. Am J Anat 1923;31:191–221.

71. Shabo AL, Maxwell DS. The subarachnoid space following the introduction of a foreign protein: an electron microscopic study with peroxidase. J Neuropathol Exp Neurol 1971;30:506–524.

72. Tripathi RC. The functional morphology of the outflow systems of ocular and cerebrospinal fluids. Exp Eye Res 1977;25(Suppl.):65–116.

77. Kida S, Yamashima T, Kubota T, et al. A light and electron microscopic and immunohistochemical study of human arachnoid villi. J Neurosurg 1988;69: 429–435.

78. Upton ML, Weller RO. The morphology of cerebrospinal fluid drainage pathways in human arachnoid granulations. J Neurosurg 1985;63:867–875.

81. Yamashima T. Functional ultrastructure of cerebrospinal fluid drainage channels

in human arachnoid villi. Neurosurgery 1988;22:633–641.

84. Johnston M, Zakharov A, Papaiconomou C, et al. Evidence of connections between cerebrospinal fluid and nasal lymphatic vessels in humans, non-human primates and other mammalian species. Cerebrospinal Fluid Res 2004;1:2.

91. Weller RO. Microscopic morphology and histology of the human meninges. Morphologie 2005;89:22–34.

94. Hayreh SS. Pathogenesis of oedema of the optic disc. Doc Ophthalmol 1968; 24:289–411.

98. Glimcher SA, Holman DW, Lubow M, et al. Ex vivo model of cerebrospinal fluid outflow across human arachnoid granulations. Invest Ophthalmol Vis Sci 2008;49:4721–4728.

99. Grzybowski DM, Holman DW, Katz SE, et al. In vitro model of cerebrospinal fluid outflow through human arachnoid granulations. Invest Ophthalmol Vis Sci 2006;47:3664–3672.

101. Holman DW, Grzybowski DM, Mehta BC, et al. Characterization of cytoskeletal and junctional proteins expressed by cells cultured from human arachnoid granulation tissue. Cerebrospinal Fluid Res 2005;2:9.

CHAPTER 40

Giant cell arteritis

Lynn K Gordon

Clinical background

Giant cell arteritis (GCA) is a serious and relatively common systemic vasculitis that occurs in adults older than 50 years. The key symptoms and signs of GCA include both systemic and neuro-ophthalmic manifestations (Table 40.1).[1-3] Systemic manifestations may involve a long prodromal period of multiple symptoms including weight loss, fatigue, fever, and malaise. Generalized muscle pain, claudication of the jaw or tongue, or localized scalp or temporal pain, swelling, and tenderness are also commonly observed in this disease. Ischemic manifestations from vascular compromise include blindness, stroke, aortitis with aneurysm, myocardial ischemia, and bowel infarction.[4] Neuro-ophthalmic manifestations include arteritic anterior ischemic optic neuropathy, posterior optic neuropathy, choroidal ischemia, diplopia, retinal arterial occlusions, and ocular ischemic syndromes, occuring in up to 70% of patients.[5-8] It is estimated that 15–20% of patients with GCA suffer permanent and potentially bilateral visual loss from ischemic infarction of the optic nerve.

Although the original descriptions of GCA are attributed to Hutchinison in 1890, initial references to this disease were first noted in ancient Egypt.[9,10] The hallmark granulomatous inflammation with giant cells was described in 1932 by Horton. Use of the terms temporal or cranial arteritis is commonly found in the literature but may preclude the understanding that GCA is a systemic, not localized, disease.

Epidemiology of GCA depends on geography; it is a rare disease in Japan, and the incidence in Europe increases in association with higher latitudes. Recent literature suggests that prior reports of a lower prevalence among Hispanic and Black individuals was underestimated, perhaps because of ascertainment bias.[11-13] In western countries the frequency is commonly defined at about 20 per 100 000 individuals older than age 50. However, for reasons that remain obscure, this increases over time, reaching a peak at between 70 and 80 years of age and women are twice as likely to be affected as compared to men. The cyclical increase in incidence of GCA every 7 years in the large epidemiologic Minnesota study, as well as other associations between onset of GCA and epidemics of specific bacterial or viral infections, suggests an environmental or infectious impact on disease prevalence.[14-16] Genetically there is an association between GCA

and HLA-DRB1*04.[17-19] Other associations have been reported between genetic polymorphisms in multiple genes and susceptibility to GCA or its complications. These genes include matrix metalloproteinase 9 (MMP 9),[20] platelet glycoprotein receptor IIIA,[21] interferon-γ (IFN-γ),[22] and the interleukin (IL)-10 and IL-6 promoters.[23-25]

Diagnostic evaluation of patients with suspected GCA is challenging as there are no specific laboratory examinations. On physical examination, a palpable, tender, enlarged temporal artery may be identified and the abnormal portion should be biopsied for histopathologic analysis (Figure 40.1). Histology, when positive, can be diagnostic but the characteristic giant cells identified at the junction of the intima and media are only observed in about half of the cases; the remaining positive biopsy specimens demonstrate a nonspecific mixed inflammatory response and may show disruption of the internal elastic lamina (Figure 40.2).[26-28] One potential challenge is that the lesions are not continuous and may only involve a portion of the artery, therefore a long segment of artery (greater than 15 mm) must be carefully evaluated in its entirety, and sometimes multiple biopsies increase the diagnostic yield.[28]

Some patients with suspected GCA do not have a positive biopsy and then the diagnosis is based on the clinical history, physical examination, and nonspecific laboratory diagnostic indicators of inflammation. Laboratory findings include elevations in the erythrocyte sedimentation rate (ESR), C-reactive protein (CRP), and platelet counts.[29,30] Although these are not specific for GCA, the sensitivity of an elevated ESR and CRP in a patient suspected of having GCA is greater than 99%, and the positive likelihood value of thrombocytosis alone is high in patients with other signs and symptoms referable to GCA.[31] However, it is also important to note that a normal ESR does not exclude GCA as a diagnosis and may occur in more than 15% of affected individuals. Recent improvements in imaging techniques have been applied to the diagnosis of GCA with varying results. Color duplex ultrasonography, high-resolution magnetic resonance imaging, and positron emission tomography imaging have all been reported as helpful in the diagnosis, yet the accuracy remains controversial and thus these are not routinely performed for GCA diagnosis.[32-34]

The differential diagnosis of GCA is dependent on the presenting symptoms and signs. If one considers only the ophthalmologic presentations, then there are three main

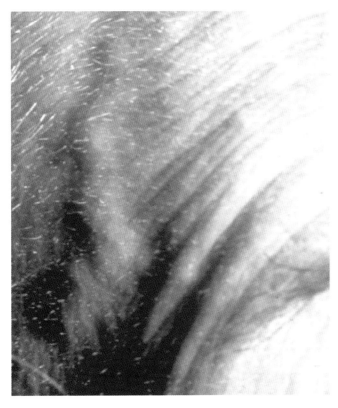

Figure 40.1 External appearance of involved artery. The photo demonstrates the characteristic irregularly enlarged and ropey appearance of a giant cell arteritis-involved artery. This would typically be tender to the touch and the pulse may be decreased or absent.

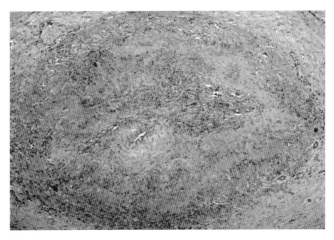

Figure 40.2 Histologic section of involved artery. In this example the lumen of the artery is nearly occluded and there is evidence for inflammatory infiltrate and giant cells.

Table 40.1 Characteristic symptoms and neuro-ophthalmic manifestations of giant cell arteritis

Symptoms	Neuro-ophthalmic manifestations
Constitutional	Anterior ischemic optic neuropathy:
Weight loss	arteritic
Fatigue	Posterior ischemic optic neuropathy
Malaise	Choroidal ischemia
Fever	Retinal artery occlusion
Jaw/tongue claudication	Strabismus
Neck pain	Acquired onset
Muscle pain	May appear as cranial nerve palsy
Scalp/temple pain	
Double vision	
Transient decreased vision	
Loss of vision	
Partial or total	
One or both eyes	

categories of subjective complaints: (1) transient visual disturbance; (2) double vision; and (3) loss of all or part of the vision in one or both eyes. The differential diagnosis for transient visual obscurations lasting several minutes includes emboli; or that lasting seconds includes swelling of the optic disc. New-onset double vision in the elderly is a common occurrence in association with medical ischemic etiologies of cranial mononeuropathies, such as hypertension or dia-

betes. However GCA is a potential diagnosis even in the presence of these common systemic diseases and must be carefully considered in each individual patient. Permanent vision loss from GCA is most frequently associated with an arteritic form of anterior ischemic optic neuropathy (AAION) characterized by swelling of the optic disc; however, it may also be secondary to posterior ischemia of the retrobulbar optic nerve or from central retinal or cilioretinal artery occlusions (Figure 40.3).[35] AAION must be differentiated from nonarteritic anterior ischemic optic neuropthy (NAION) through clinical evaluation and suspicion, an accompanying cilioretinal artery occlusion which is diagnostic of a vasculitic etiology, or through fluorescein angiography which, in the case of AAION, may demonstrate a marked delay in disc or choroidal perfusion. Formal visual field testing and analysis should be performed on any patient with suspected GCA but the defects observed may vary widely depending on the involvement of the optic nerve. Progressive loss of visual field is ominous and may be observed as evidence for worsening clinical status (Figure 40.4).

Glucocorticoids remain the primary treatment for GCA; however, the high doses and long duration that are required for effective control of disease are also associated with significant morbidity (Box 40.1). In particular, the risk of bone fractures is significant and prophylactic therapy to decrease osteoporosis should be used concomitantly with the steroid treatment. Differing opinions about the optimum initial steroid dose or route of administration remain, although there is some evidence in support for high-dose intravenous induction therapy in producing sustained remissions and decreasing the total steroid requirement.[36] Steroid-sparing agents have been attempted and clinical trials report varying conclusions regarding the utility of methotrexate, although a recent meta-analysis of the published trials supports an adjunctive role for methotrexate in GCA therapy in conjunction with steroids.[37] Recent interest in use of biologic agents in the treatment of immune-mediated disease prompted trials of agents that target tumor necrosis factor-α (TNF-α).[38,39] There have been discordant results from the clinical trials with TNF-α blockade and there have been two case reports of individuals who developed GCA while on one of

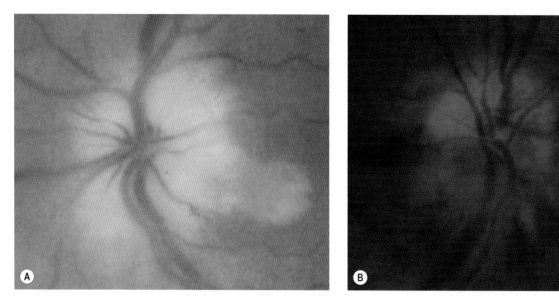

Figure 40.3 Optic disc appearance in anterior ischemic optic neuropathy (AION). (A) The optic disc is pale, swollen, and accompanied by a small vascular occlusion to the right of the disc. This is a typical appearance of an arteritic form of AION. (B) The optic disc exhibits a segmental swelling of the inferior half with peripapillary hemorrhages, typical, although not diagnostic, of the nonarteritic form of AION.

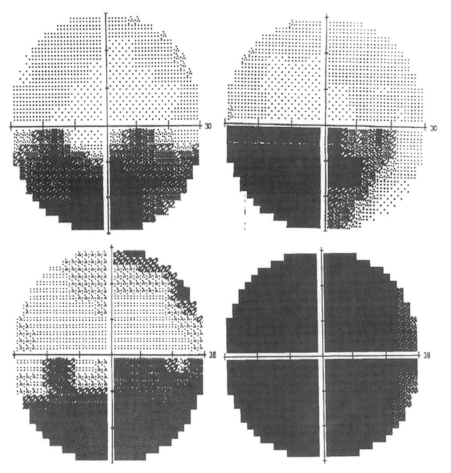

Figure 40.4 Progressive visual field changes in untreated giant cell arteritis. The figure shows the gray scale of the visual field for the right and left eyes of a patient with giant cell arteritis. On the day of presentation (day 1) the patient complained of decreased vision in both eyes and there is an altitudinal-style loss of the inferior half of the visual field in each eye. The underlying diagnosis of GCA was not made and within 2 weeks the patient lost the remaining vision in the right eye (day 13). Prompt high-dose steroid treatment was initiated and the remaining vision was spared.

the TNF-α blockers, supporting controversies in the utility of this therapy for control of GCA. A monoclonal antibody that targets the B-cell-associated CD20 was used in two patients to deplete B lymphocytes; respiratory complications were observed in one individual.[40] In addition to steroid therapy, the use of aspirin has been suggested as adjunctive therapy. Retrospective studies demonstrate that low-dose aspirin may reduce risks of ischemic complications of GCA.[41] Prospective controlled clinical trials will be required to assess the utility of aspirin in GCA.

Therapy is generally effective in reducing systemic symptoms of GCA such as fatigue, fever, headache, and jaw claudication and this therapeutic response is typically dramatic, occurring within hours to days of starting steroids. However, it is unusual for visual functions to recover following the onset of therapy; thus permanent vision loss remains a major complication of disease. In addition, progressive loss of vision may occur despite onset of steroid therapy, but will generally present within the first week.[5] If untreated or treated with insufficient immunosuppressive therapy, then the risk for loss of vision in the fellow eye within 2 weeks following AAION in the first eye is significant.[42] Long-term complications of GCA include thoracic aortic aneurysms and ischemia.

Pathology

The pathological hallmark of GCA is a granulomatous inflammatory infiltrate involving all layers of the vessel wall, in particular in the intima or media with concomitant damage or destruction of the inner elastic lamina (Box 40.2).[27] The presence of giant cells is not required in order to make the diagnosis. Skip lesions, areas without apparent evidence for inflammation, can occur in 8.5–28.3% of involved specimens. Typically the inflammatory infiltrate consists of a mixture of lymphocytes, predominantly CD4+ T cells, mononuclear cells, and occasional neutrophils and eosinophils. Some pathologic findings are preserved in biopsies of individuals who have already been on prolonged steroid therapy and may be best detected using special immunohistochemical or histologic stains. Following steroid therapy, findings common to involved arteries include loss of the internal elastic lamina and infiltration of lymphocytes, mononuclear cells, and epithelioid histiocytes in a band at the junction of the outer layer of muscle and adventitia.[26]

Etiology

The etiology of GCA is unknown but the pathophysiology of disease is mediated by an immune mechanism. What agents could initiate or modify the disease process? Several pathogens have been implicated as potential initiating agents either because of a temporal association between onset of GCA and known epidemics or because of the presence of genetic fingerprints of microbial agents in association with lesions.[14] Epidemiologic studies of large populations demonstrate a temporal correlation between the onset of GCA and various acute systemic microbial diseases, including *Mycoplasma pneumoniae*, parvovirus B19, and *Chlamydia pneumoniae*, suggesting a direct or indirect effect of infection on the clinical manifestation of GCA.[16,43,44] A number of candidate microorganisms have been entertained as specific inducing agents in GCA lesions. Genetic analysis of affected arteries yielded conflicting evidence for parvovirus DNA, herpesvirus zoster DNA, *C. pneumoniae* DNA, and yet unidentified sequences of microbial origin.[44-49] The significance of the relationship of these or other microorganisms to GCA pathogenesis requires additional future investigation.

Pathophysiology

Genetic associations

Significant evidence indicates that GCA disease susceptibility is in part mediated by expression of specific major histocompatibility complex (MHC) class 1 alleles. Immunogenetic susceptibility to GCA is suggested by association with HLA-DRB1*04 and conservation of an antigen-binding domain of the DR4 molecule.[17] Recently, independent associations of MICA A5, HLA-B*15, and HLA-DRB1*04 alleles with GCA and a synergistic increase when the MICA A5 is in combination with either the HLA-B*15 or HLA-DRB*04 alleles was observed, strengthening the associations between HLA and GCA (Box 40.3).[50]

Polymorphisms in genes that code for agents that either modify the immune response or are involved in local tissue damage have been a subject of recent interest as potential disease modifiers in GCA. Myeloperoxidase (MPO) is a molecule of interest in many inflammatory diseases; the -463 G/A MPO promoter polymorphism, G allele homozygosity is more commonly observed in individuals with GCA than in controls.[51] Multiple gelatinases, including MMP 2, 9, and 14, are observed in the inflamed GCA tissues and are also suspected of playing a role in disease pathogenesis.[52] In a limited sample from one institution, a polymorphism in a coding SNP of MMP-9 (rs2250889, G allele) is overrepresented in patients with GCA.[20] Intercellular adhesion molecule 1 (ICAM-1) is also highly expressed in GCA lesions and there is controversy as to whether a polymorphism in exon 4 is associated with either polymyalgia rheumatica (PMR), a related systemic illness without vasculitis, or GCA susceptibility.[53,54] IL-10 may act to suppress the proinflammatory cytokine IFN-γ. Two studies recently reported an increase in different polymorphisms in IL-10 in GCA patients, as compared to controls.[23,25] When a polymorphism in the first intron of the IFN-γ gene was studied, there were no associations with disease susceptibility, although there was evidence for a relationship between specific alleles and disease severity supporting a potential role for disease modification by IFN-γ.[22] Immune regulation is also achieved through the Fc-γ receptor and the FCGR2A-FCGR3A 131R-158F haplotype was associated with GCA susceptibility.[55] In combination with HLA-DRB1*04 positivity, the presence of FCGR2A-131R was associated with a multiplicative increase in GCA susceptibility. The relevance of these observations requires additional study.

Alterations in inflammatory responses

Significant progress has been achieved on the immunophenotypic features of vascular lesions and circulating mononuclear populations of patients with GCA. This characterization provides potentially important insights about the immunopathogenesis of GCA vasculitis, and points to the unresolved issue of the antigenic target in the vascular lesions.

Distinctive patterns of cytokine production and specific, topographic localization of CD4+ T cells and CD68+ macrophages indicate an immunologically active state in GCA.[56–63] Furthermore, analysis of T-cell receptors (TCR) in peripheral blood lymphocytes of GCA patients demonstrates expansion of T cells with specific TCR V domains and CD4 T-cell expansions with restricted use of Jβ genes, suggesting an antigen-specific local response.[58]

Examination of the cellular inflammatory infiltrate within GCA lesions primarily reveals macrophages and CD4+ T cells.[62] Immunohistochemistry demonstrates the diffuse presence of IL-6- or IL-1β-expressing CD68+ macrophages.[62] CD68+ cells expressing 72 kDa type IV collagenase and the inducible nitric oxide synthase (iNOS) are found in the intima and intima-media of the artery, implicating these cells in the vascular-destructive response. A chimera mouse model, in which arterial segments of human specimens were implanted into a severe combined immunodeficiency (SCID) mouse, provides information about the activity state of the resident immune cells. Adventitial dendritic cells of either PMR or GCA specimens, in contrast to normal samples, were noted to be functionally mature in their ability to stimulate T cells; suggesting that activation of these cells plays a significant role in local T-cell activation.[57]

In contrast to the common T-cell presence in affected arteries, B cells are infrequent in GCA lesions. However, identification of lesional B cells demonstrates the presence of these cells in the adventitia, both scattered and located in perivascular clusters, the same tissue microenvironment as the antigenically activated T cell. These lines of evidence strongly implicate the role of a CD4-mediated immune response in the formation of GCA vascular lesions.

Identification of the inciting antigen(s)

What is the antigenic target of this response? Evidence for a specific antigenic response in GCA comes from studies of lesional T cells.[63] Clonal expansion of CD4+ T cells bearing identical specificities has been observed in independent inflammatory foci from the same individual. Proliferation studies using T-cell lines derived from GCA-involved arteries provide additional evidence for local antigen expression and validate a microbial pathogenesis hypothesis. A proliferative response of these T-cell clones is observed in response to stimulation by exposure to autologous antigen-presenting cells and tissue extracts from autologous or nonautologous GCA or PMR-derived arteries.[64] Tissue extracts from control arteries did not produce T-cell stimulation of these clones. This important study provides strong evidence of local antigen expression in the arteries of both GCA and PMR. The observed stimulation is unlikely to be secondary to local, arterial cytokine production because inflammatory cytokines have been observed in arterial biopsies from patients with PMR as well as from patients with GCA. Furthermore, the antigen is not ubiquitously expressed, since stimulation is not observed with arterial extracts from normal individuals.

These findings suggest that vascular lesions are distinguished, compared to uninvolved sites, by the presence of antigenic targets for the disease-related immune response. It is conceivable that the vascular target is a self-antigen(s), somehow locally modified in the PMR and GCA arteries for immunogenicity. Such modifications might include structural changes to somatic proteins, and/or enhanced antigen-presenting capabilities of local resident or infiltrating cells of these vascular segments.[29] However, the GCA-associated antigen(s) has resisted efforts towards its biochemical identification, and its restriction to inflammatory lesions would be an unusual feature for self-antigens. Accordingly, there are uncertainties regarding the existence of a GCA autoantigen, and formidable technical and experimental difficulties have precluded identification of candidates. An alternative and equally compelling hypothesis, in particular in concert with the genetic evidence for microbial sequences in GCA lesions, is that vascular microbial infection and local expression of an antigen of noneukaryotic origin drive the stimulation of lesional T-cell clones.

Role for cytokines and chemokines in disease activity

Many proinflammatory cytokines and chemokines are described in tissues and serum of patients with GCA. Some evidence points to a predictive value of the levels of these agents in defining either disease severity or response to therapy. In one study, the levels of monocyte chemoattractant protein-1 (MCP-1) mRNA, as measured by quantitative reverse transcriptase polymerase chain reaction (RT-PCR), were noted to be significantly higher in individuals with GCA who experienced two relapses over the course of 1 year as compared to those in remission.[65] Systemic manifestations of GCA and PMR indicate an inflammatory response characterized by activated circulating monocytes with attendant production of IL-1 and IL-6; elevations of tissue-associated IL-1β and IL-6 mRNA correlate with increased systemic inflammation. Increased lesional TNF-α mRNA is associated with a longer duration of systemic corticosteroid requirement.[66]

It is believed that there may be a common trigger to both GCA and PMR but that the disease phenotype is controlled by additional immunologic or regulatory factors. Studies of specific GCA lesions for cytokine profiles provide additional clues about the pathogenesis of this disease. The production of IL-6 is found in both the tissue and circulation in GCA but is restricted to the circulation in PMR. Focal immunologic activation is observed in a high percentage of GCA specimens in which IL-1β, IL-6, and T-cell-derived cytokines IL-2 and IFN-γ are observed.[15,65] Although GCA lesional IFN-γ-producing cells are less than 4% of the tissue-infiltrating cells, the IFN-γ+ cells are generally CD4+ T cells (greater than 90%); these are often associated with immune-mediated diseases.[63] The IFN-γ+, CD4+ T cells are mature and show evidence of recent encounters with antigen, as demonstrated by expression of CD45RO and production of IL-2 receptor (IL-2R). Recently the role of IL-23, IL-17, and the Th17 subset of T cells has gained significant interest in immune pathogenesis of many inflammatory diseases. To date there are no reports for the role of these cells or cytokines in GCA pathogenesis.

Pathophysiology

Pathophysiology of GCA is likely controlled by multiple factors, including exposure to an initiating antigen, recruitment and activation of inflammatory cells, differentiation of macrophages and T lymphocytes into specific effector cells, proliferation of myoblasts with secondary luminal stenosis, and ischemia (Figure 40.5 and Box 40.4). Genetic factors initially support the ability of the affected individual to respond to the inciting agent and help direct the immune response towards a proinflammatory function. Disease activity or response results from a combination of activation of the immune system and modulation of local responses. Local modulation likely occurs through genetic polymorphisms in genes that control responsiveness to immune activation, cytokine production, and locally expressed proteins for tissue degradation or repair. Major advances in the field require a comprehensive understanding of disease triggers combined with advances in targeted control of inflammation.

Conclusion

GCA, a systemic vasculitis of older individuals, continues to be a disease that presents many diagnostic and therapeutic challenges. In the absence of the "gold standard"

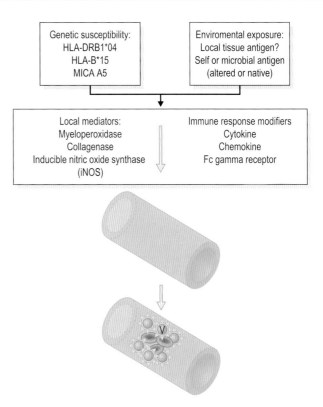

Figure 40.5 Giant cell arteritis pathogenesis. Giant cell arteritis likely results from a multifactorial insult including genetic predisposition, exposure to specific tissue-associated antigen, local tissue factors, and immune response elements that create the inflammatory arterial milieu leading to ischemia and disease manifestations.

Box 40.4 Pathophysiology of giant cell arteritis

- Genetic susceptibility
- Environmental exposure
- Possible pathogen or local tissue antigen involvement
- Immune responsiveness
- Effector tissue damage leading to ischemia

---

histopathologic arterial involvement, the diagnosis is circumstantial and based on clinical presentation in combination with nonspecific indicators of inflammatory disease such as the ESR or CRP. At the present time pharmacologic therapy continues to be based on nonspecific immunosuppression, which is often associated with high morbidity in the elderly patient population, which is at greatest risk for the disease. Many clues about pathogenesis exist; however, the specific disease pathophysiology remains elusive. Advances in the scientific understanding of disease pathophysiology are required in order to improve diagnostic confidence and therapeutic options for this serious disease.

Key references

A complete list of chapter references is available online at www.expertconsult.com. See inside cover for registration details.

2. Gordon LK, Levin LA. Visual loss in giant cell arteritis. JAMA 1998;280:385–386.

3. Hayreh SS, Podhajsky PA, Zimmerman B. Ocular manifestations of giant cell arteritis. Am J Ophthalmol 1998;125:509–520.

4. Gonzalez-Gay MA, Barros S, Lopez-Diaz MJ, et al. Giant cell arteritis: disease patterns of clinical presentation in a series of 240 patients. Medicine (Baltimore) 2005;84:269–276.

16. Petursdottir V, Johansson H, Nordborg E, et al. The epidemiology of biopsy-positive giant cell arteritis: special reference to cyclic fluctuations. Rheumatology (Oxf) 1999;38:1208–1212.

26. Font RL, Prabhakaran VC. Histological parameters helpful in recognising steroid-treated temporal arteritis: an analysis of 35 cases. Br J Ophthalmol 2007;91:204–209.

29. Gonzalez-Gay MA, Lopez-Diaz MJ, Barros S, et al. Giant cell arteritis: laboratory tests at the time of diagnosis in a series of 240 patients. Medicine (Baltimore) 2005;84:277–290.

36. Mazlumzadeh M, Hunder GG, Easley KA, et al. Treatment of giant cell arteritis using induction therapy with high-dose glucocorticoids: a double-blind, placebo-controlled, randomized prospective clinical trial. Arthritis Rheum 2006;54:3310–3318.

39. Pipitone N, Salvarani C. Improving therapeutic options for patients with giant cell arteritis. Curr Opin Rheumatol 2008;20:17–22.

50. Gonzalez-Gay MA, Rueda B, Vilchez JR, et al. Contribution of MHC class I region to genetic susceptibility for giant cell arteritis. Rheumatology (Oxf) 2007;46:431–434.

57. Ma-Krupa W, Jeon MS, Spoerl S, et al. Activation of arterial wall dendritic cells and breakdown of self-tolerance in giant cell arteritis. J Exp Med 2004;199:173–183.

59. Weyand CM, Ma-Krupa W, Goronzy JJ. Immunopathways in giant cell arteritis and polymyalgia rheumatica. Autoimmun Rev 2004;3:46–53.

64. Weyand CM, Schonberger J, Oppitz U, et al. Distinct vascular lesions in giant cell arteritis share identical T cell clonotypes. J Exp Med 1994;179:951–960.

CHAPTER 41

Ischemic optic neuropathy

Helen Danesh-Meyer

Introduction

Ischemic optic neuropathy refers to a group of conditions in which damage to the optic nerve is presumed to be secondary to ischemia of the optic nerve head (anterior ischemic optic neuropathy; AION) or retrobulbar optic nerve (posterior ischemic optic neuropathy; PION). It is clinically characterized by sudden painless loss of vision. By definition, AION presents with optic disc edema and PION without optic disc edema. AION is further subclassified as nonarteritic AION (NAION) and arteritic AION (AAION) based on the presumed underlying etiology of the latter being an inflammatory process most commonly caused by giant cell arteritis (GCA). NAION is considered to encompass diabetic papillopathy.

Nonarteritic ischemic optic neuropathy

NAION typically occurs in patients older than 50 years, with most being between 60 and 70 years.[1] The incidence in Caucasian populations is about 2.3–10.3 patients per 100 000 over the age of 50 years.[2,3] NAION is uncommon in patients under 50 but does occur.[4] It occurs predominantly in Caucasians. The clinical features of NAION are summarized in Box 41.1.

Clinical course

Progressive NAION occurs in approximately 22–27% of patients and is defined as either stepwise, episodic decrements or steady decline of vision over weeks prior to eventual stabilization. Further decline in visual acuity after 1–2 months from initial onset is rare.[5,6] The Ischemic Optic Neuropathy Decompression Trial (IONDT) reported up to 40% of patients showing an improvement of several lines of visual acuity.[7] However, this apparent visual recovery may be an adaptation to the visual field defect or eccentric fixation.[1] Younger patients with NAION (less than 50 years of age) have been reported to have better visual acuity outcomes.[5,8]

Second eye involvement occurs in approximately 15–24% of patients within 5 years of the first eye being affected.[1,7,9]

There is thought to be an increased incidence in second eye involvement in patients with poor visual acuity in the first eye and diabetes. However, the IONDT did not report age, sex, smoking history, or aspirin use to alter the incidence of second eye involvement. It has been suggested that younger patients may have a higher risk of fellow eye involvement than older patients, with rates of up to 35% fellow eye involvement within a median of 7 months being reported. Other investigators have suggested that higher rates of both anemia and type 1 diabetes mellitus are significantly associated with decreased time to second eye involvement in younger patients.[5] The recurrence rate of NAION in the same eye is approximately 3–8% with a median follow-up of 3 years from first onset.[10-12]

A classic finding on the unaffected side is a small-diameter optic disc with small or absent optic cup: this is known as "disc at risk."[13] The optic disc swelling subsides between 6 and 12 weeks, with a median time of 8 weeks, after acute disc swelling, leaving a pale atrophic-appearing optic nerve head. The time to resolution of the disc edema has been shown to be longer in diabetics, but also longer in those who have milder visual loss. It seems that corticosteroid treatment may hasten the time to resolution of the disc swelling.[14] Despite the retinal nerve fiber layer (RNFL) loss that occurs after NAION, excavation of the optic cup is rarely detected, as opposed to eyes with AAION, in which it is the most common end-stage appearance.[15]

Investigations

The diagnosis of NAION is based on clinical history and examination and there are no specific tests to confirm the diagnosis. The differential diagnosis includes an extensive list of causes of unilateral optic disc swelling (rarely, bilateral). The three most important differential diagnoses to consider are AAION secondary to GCA, and optic neuritis (Box 41.2). Figure 41.1 demonstrates the different appearance between the optic nerve head appearance in NAION and AAION.

Neuroimaging

There are a few magnetic resonance imaging (MRI) studies evaluating small series of patients with NAION.[16,17] Unlike patients with optic neuritis who had abnormal MRI in 97% of cases, patients with NAION only had an abnormal scan in 17%.[18] There are more white-matter abnormalities in patients with NAION, suggesting that it is more likely in the setting of diffuse cerebrovascular small-vessel disease.[19] Eyes with NAION have more white-matter hyperintensities, lower optic nerve volume, and magnetization transfer ratio of the chiasm than controls, likely reflecting axonal loss and demyelination.[20]

Electrophysiology

Both arteritic and nonarteritic ION have been shown to result in amplitude reduction in pattern visual evoked potential (VEP) and flash VEP.[19,21,22] This contrasts with demyelination in which there is delayed latency as well as reduced amplitude in the involved eye, and the uninvolved eye is commonly abnormal. The N95 component of the pattern electroretinogram (PERG) may be reduced in ischemic optic neuropathy,[23] while the P50 component of the PERG is more frequently affected in NAION than demyelination.[24]

Quantitative ocular imaging modalities

Quantitative techniques that measure the peripapillary RNFL thickness and/or optic disc morphology, such as optical coherence tomography (OCT, StratusOCT), scanning laser polarimetry (SLP), and confocal scanning laser ophthalmoscopy (Heidelberg Engineering retinal tomography; HRT) have been used to evaluate the optic disc and RNFL in NAION. Presently, these techniques do not assist in diagnosis or management but they may offer a quantitative measurement of ganglion cell loss in the pale optic disc and may be useful in the evaluation of patients with NAION after swelling of the optic disc has resolved.

Several studies have evaluated the correlation between RNFL thickness and visual field sensitivities using these modalities. It has been demonstrated that both SLP and OCT show strong correlations between RNFL thickness, and visual sensitivities.[25–27] OCT has also demonstrated that some patients develop subretinal fluid following NAION. The resolution of the subretinal fluid may explain some of the visual recovery that has been documented to occur.[28] The HRT has also been used to evaluate the morphology of the optic nerve head cup and disc and has shown that eyes that have had an episode of AAION show greater excavation than eyes with NAION.[29] A possible explanation is that in AAION the ischemic insult is more severe compared to NAION and consequently leads to more tissue damage. Alternatively, it may be that excavation in eyes with NAION is more difficult to detect because of the previously small or absent physiologic cup and the development of optic disc pallor (Figures 41.2–41.5).

Box 41.1 Clinical features of nonarteritic anterior ischemic optic neuropathy

	Frequency
Symptoms	
Painless loss of vision	Common
Pain on eye movement	10% of patients
Simultaneous bilateral involvement	Uncommon
Positive visual phenomenon	Very rare
Signs	
Loss of visual acuity	Two-thirds have better than 20/200 visual acuity
Dyschromatopsia	Usually in proportion to visual acuity loss
Relative afferent pupillary defect	If unilateral involvement
Visual field defect	Inferior altitudinal most common
Hyperemic disc swelling	Sectorial or diffuse
Retinal exudates	Only reported in 7%

Box 41.2 Comparison of nonarteritic anterior ischemic optic neuropathy (NAION)/arteritic anterior ischemic optic neuropathy (AAION) and optic neuritis

	NAION	AAION	Optic neuritis
Age	Most commonly over 50 years	Most commonly over 60 years	20–45 years
Disc appearance	Hyperemic Disc swelling	Pallid disc Swelling	± Swelling
Other symptoms	None	Systemic symptoms Signs of giant cell arteritis	Pain on eye movement
Laterality	Simultaneous rare, but sequential common	Simultaneous or within days of first eye involvement is not uncommon	Simultaneous uncommon
Associated features	Small disc with small cup:disc ratio in contralateral eye	Giant cell arteritis	Multiple sclerosis
Visual acuity	Majority better than 20/64 at presentation	Majority worse than 20/200 at presentation	Variable

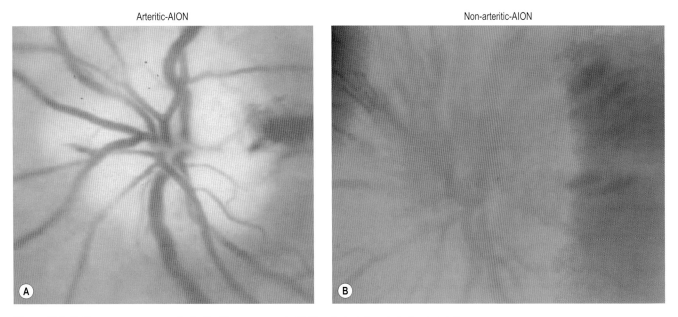

Figure 41.1 Optic nerve appearance of arteritic (A) versus nonarteritic(B) anterior ischemic optic neuropathy.

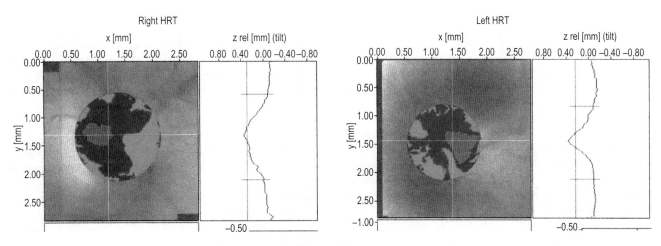

Figure 41.2 Heidelberg retinal tomograph (HRT) of patient 6 months following left nonarteritic anterior ischemic optic neuropathy. The HRT demonstrates no significant difference between the cup size in the uninvolved right optic nerve and the involved left optic nerve.

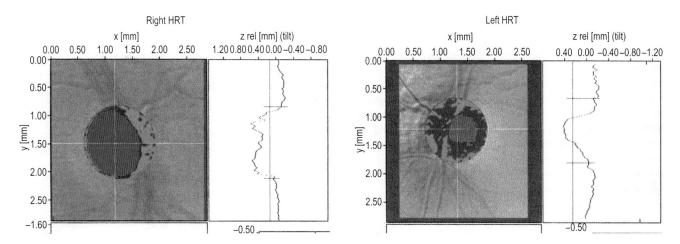

Figure 41.3 Heidelberg retinal tomograph (HRT) of patient 3 months following right arteritic anterior ischemic optic neuropathy. The HRT demonstrates a significant difference between the cup size in the involved right optic nerve and the uninvolved left optic nerve.

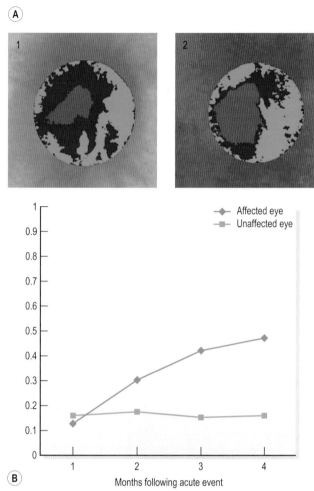
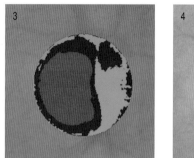
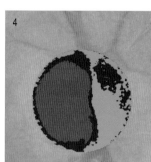

Figure 41.4 (A) Serial enlargement of the cup:disc ratio in a patient who had an episode of right arteritic anterior ischemic optic neuropathy as measured by the Heidelberg retina tomograph. The first image (1) was taken at 1 month and each serial image was taken monthly. (B) Change in the cup:disc ratio of the involved compared to the contralateral uninvolved eye.

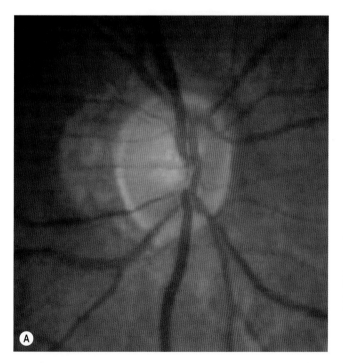
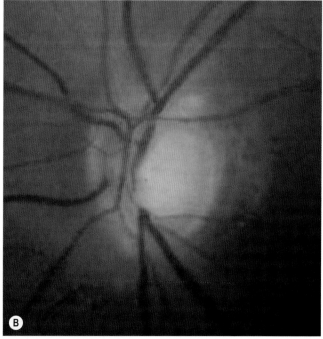

Figure 41.5 Patient who had left arteritic anterior ischemic optic neuropathy demonstrates enlargement and excavation of the optic nerve cup 4 months following the acute event. The right eye was uninvolved.

Pathology

Histology

The histopathology from cases of NAION does not provide conclusive evidence of the underlying pathophysiology with no definite histopathologic documentation of the vasculopathy that produces NAION. The largest series of eyes with histological evidence of ischemic optic neuropathy is by Knox et al[30] who collected 193 eyes over 47 years, although those cases of typical NAION were not analyzed separately. In these eyes, infarction was primarily located in the retrolaminar region of the optic nerve head with occasional extension to the laminar and prelaminar layers.

Of the few cases of clinically diagnosed NAION that have been studied histopathologically the majority have been atypical cases, including internal carotid occlusion, multiple embolic lesions, and severe blood loss. The short posterior ciliary arteries (SPCAs) were described in only one case, which was an atypical NAION associated with internal carotid artery occlusion and which demonstrated emboli within the vessels, central retinal artery (CRA), and pial vessels.[31–33]

Histopathological data from NAION patients and experimentally induced anterior optic nerve ischemia demonstrate apoptosis of the retinal ganglion cells and oligodendrocytes, associated with axonal demyelination and wallerian degeneration.[34]

In contrast, histopathological studies of AAION have demonstrated greatest signs of infarction of the optic nerve at or just posterior to the lamina cribrosa. A comparison of studies in which optic nerve tissue was obtained at various time points from the onset of loss of vision reveals progressive stages of retrolaminar liquefaction at 4 and 8 weeks and fibrosis at 4 months.[35] These optic nerve findings are associated with loss of the retinal ganglion cell layer with preservation of the other retinal layers. It has been suggested that this absence of transsynaptic degeneration in the retina may be due to the fact that the longest histological specimen was 4 months following the AAION episode and such degeneration is estimated to take 2–3 years to develop.[36] Anterograde degeneration with loss of axons and myelin in the chiasm was demonstrated to be present by 4 months. In AAION, the SPCAs have been shown to be infiltrated by chronic inflammatory cells producing segmental occlusion of multiple vessels.

Pathophysiology

Fluoroscein angiography and indocyanine green

Fluoroscein angiography provides evidence suggesting that pathophysiology of NAION involves a primary circulatory abnormality of the optic nerve head. Delayed onset of filling not seen in controls or cases of disc swelling due to causes other than NAION was demonstrated in the majority of patients (76%) with NAION during the acute phase.[37] This suggests that the delay in filling is not related to mechanical obstruction potentially caused by disc swelling.[38] Furthermore, these studies have shown that there is no consistent delayed filling in the choroidal vasculature in NAION (unlike AAION), suggesting that the vasculopathy lies within the distribution of the paraoptic branches of the SPCA after their

branching from the choroidal branches rather than in the short ciliary arteries themselves.[39]

The concept of the "watershed zone" in the pathophysiology of NAION is that the prominent dilation of the overlying optic disc vasculature that comes from the retinal circulation is analogous to the "luxury perfusion" that is seen at the junction of perfused and nonperfused areas of cerebral infarctions. However, the overlying vasculature of the optic disc that comes from the retinal circulation shows variable filling patterns ranging from impaired filling to prominent dilation. Furthermore, delayed filling of the watershed zone has been identified to occur equally frequently in normal eyes as in NAION eyes with no correlation between optic disc and choroidal filling.[42] Indocyanine green angiography angiographic studies have also shown optic disc blood flow impairment in a pattern, suggesting SPCA occlusion but no abnormality in the choroidal circulation in NAION (unlike AAION).[40]

Flow studies

With current technology, evidence for impaired vascular flow in NAION remains unsubstantiated. Several flow study instruments and techniques have been employed but all are limited in their ability to measure the blood volume in the branches' posterior ciliary arteries that supply the optic nerve. Both stationary (laser Doppler flowmetry) and scanning (Heidelberg retinal flowmeter) laser imaging methods have been used to measure surface blood flow derived from the retinal arterial circulation, but have not been able to measure the deeper layers from the SPCA which supply the optic disc. Scanning laser Doppler flowmetry technique measures only the blood flow on the surface of the optic nerve in the nerve fiber layer which is supplied by the CRA.[41] Carotid duplex studies are limited because they measure velocity rather than volume, and are not able to measure flow in the paraoptic branches which supply the optic disc.

Single-point flowmetry instruments or similar systems may allow sampling of volume in the laminar layer of the optic nerve. Using such a system in rhesus monkey eyes after manipulation of ciliary and retinal circulations, it was found that flow measurements were decreased with occlusion of the CRA, but not the posterior cerebral artery.[42] Other studies have considered flow velocity as a surrogate for volume and demonstrated changes in flow velocity in SPCA and the ophthalmic artery in NAION.[43]

Experimental ischemia of the optic nerve

Over the past years various models of optic nerve injury have been developed to investigate axonal injury to optic nerves. These include complete optic nerve transection, partial transection, optic nerve crush, and partial crush. Ischemic optic neuropathy has been modeled by infusion of endothelin-1 (ET-1) around the optic nerve head, although this produces more chronic ischemia.[44] An ischemic optic nerve model to produce rodent AION (rAION) injury may be produced by intravenous injection of rose Bengal dye followed by argon green laser application to the retinal arteries overlying the optic nerve. The laser causes the rose Bengal to release superoxide free radicals that can then cause vascular occlusion.[45]

Ischemic optic nerve injury can also be modelled in experimental animals by occluding the posterior ciliary arteries[46] or infusing vasoconstrictor ET-1 into the perineural space.[47] Since ET-1 has been reported to cause reduced blood flow in the optic nerve head and apoptotic death of retinal ganglion cells it is considered a valid model for optic nerve ischemia. Recent studies have indicated that ET-1 causes reactive astrocytosis and interferes with the anterograde axonal transport.[48] These various animal models have been widely used in studies which aimed to find out which neuroprotective agents increase retinal ganglion cell survival.

Etiology

The etiology of NAION is believed to be multifactorial, although the mechanism of neural damage is generally considered to be ischemic.

Crowded disc

The presence of a "disc at risk" is the most conclusive association with NAION. Small optic disc with a small cup-to-disc (C/D) ratio or absence of the cup is a well-recognized risk factor for NAION, with approximately 97% of eyes demonstrating small optic discs with small or absent optic cups.[49–54] It is thought that this anatomical variant causes structural crowding of the axons at the level of the cribriform plate and places the optic nerve at risk for a compartment syndrome-like phenomenon.

Diseases associated with atherosclerosis

Significant controversy exists between the association of NAION and athereosclerotic risk factors and the relationship remains uncertain. Some studies have demonstrated an association between NAION and other cardiovascular diseases such as stroke and ischemic heart disease using general population studies as controls, although this finding has been inconsistent.[55,56]

Hypertension

Systemic hypertension has been reported in 34–47% of patients, although in most studies this was compared to population-matched data. Hence, systemic hypertension as a risk factor for NAION remains unsubstantiated.[5,8,11,57,58]

Diabetes

Diabetes has been shown to be associated with NAION at all ages, with a prevalence of 24% in the IONDT study.[59]

Cerebrovascular or cardiovascular events

Studies have reported mixed findings on the prevalence of ischemic heart disease or cerebrovascular accident amongst patients with NAION.[1,58]

Hypercholesterolemia

Various studies have attempted to investigate whether elevated cholesterol and lipids are associated with NAION but have had conflicting reports.[60,61] NAION occurring at a younger age has also been reported in patients with hyperlipidemia.[62]

Hypercoagulable states

Many prothrombotic states have been reported in patients with NAION, including hyperhomocysteinemia, and prothrombotic risk factors, such as lupus anticoagulant, anticardiolipin antibodies, prothrombotic polymorphisms, and deficiencies of protein C, S, and antithrombin III, heterozygous factor V Leiden mutation, and *MTHFR* mutations in case series but not larger studies.[63–65] The presence of elevated homocysteine levels in NAION has been shown to be present in some studies,[58,59,66] but not others.[67]

Sleep apnea

Several studies have reported links between NAION and obstructive sleep apnea syndrome (SAS).[65] The risk ratio for a NAION patient to have sleep apnea has been determined to be between 2.6 and 4.9 compared to the general population. Furthermore, sleep apnea was 1.5–2-fold more frequent than the rate of the other identified risk factors typically associated with NAION (hypertension, diabetes).[68,69] However, the mechanism of this association is unclear. It is postulated that vascular changes such as acute surges in blood pressure, increased intracranial pressure, or nocturnal hypoxemia from repetitive apneic spells may contribute to local ischemia or hypoxia at the optic disc level.[70] It has been suggested that continuous positive airway pressure may prevent NAION[71] but it has been documented to occur in patients receiving such therapy.[72]

Smoking

Smoking as a risk factor for NAION also remains unsubstantiated.[73]

Medications

Phosphodiesterase inhibitor 5 (PDE5)

Several cases of NAION have been reported since 2005 in users of these agents.[74] Following a series of case reports, the World Health Organization and Food and Drug Administration have labeled the association between use of PDE5 inhibitors and risk of NAION as "possibly" causal. Evidence is primarily in the form of case reports, including a rechallenge case report[75] and a large managed-care database study.[71] It has been hypothesized that PDE5 inhibitors may accentuate the physiological nocturnal hypotension enough to decrease the perfusion pressure in the posterior ciliary arteries, resulting in ischemia to an optic nerve head and setting off the cascade of a compartment syndrome, which is thought to occur in a small, crowded optic nerve. Alternatively, activation of the nitric oxide–cyclic guanosine monophosphate (GMP) pathway may reduce optic nerve head perfusion or disrupt autoregulation.

Interferon-α

Interferon-α has been associated with the development of bilateral, sequential NAION which has been shown not only to have a temporal association, but also to recur following rechallenge. There is variable improvement on cessation of the medication. Although the mechanism is unknown, the deposition of immune complexes within the optic disc circulation has been suggested.[76,77]

Amiodarone

Amiodarone produces bilateral insidious visual loss with optic disc swelling that may persist for months despite withdrawal of the drug. The exact cause of the optic neuropathy is not known. Lipid inclusions characteristic of amiodarone

Box 41.3 Amiodarone versus nonarteritic anterior ischemic optic neuropathy (NAION)

	Amiodarone	NAION
Onset of symptoms	Insidious	Acute
Laterality	Bilateral simultaneous	Unilateral, or bilateral sequential
Resolution of edema	Months	6–8 weeks

have been found in one optic nerve studied histopathologically. Decreased vision is insidious in onset and is slowly progressive as long as the drug is taken. Optic disc swelling is bilateral and the decreased visual acuity is not usually worse than 20/200. The ingestion of the drug in the presence of bilateral optic disc edema is grounds for suspecting this diagnosis (Box 41.3).

Cataract surgery

Two types of NAION have been suggested to occur following cataract surgery. The first is an immediate type that has been variably defined to occur within 24 hours or a few days of cataract extraction. The second is a delayed NAION, although the window of suspected postoperative susceptibility has not been clearly defined.[78] The risk of the second eye experiencing NAION if the first eye experienced an episode following cataract extraction is reported to be as high as 50%.[79,80]

Blood loss

Numerous accounts in the medical literature report NAION in conditions of extreme circulatory irregularities, usually involving a combination of hypovolemia, hemodilution through aggressive volume substitution, systemic hypotension, anemia, face-down positioning, and pre-existing cardiovascular disease. The incidence of ischemic optic neuropathy (either anterior or posterior) following surgery has been approximated to 0.03–0.1%.[81,82] Protracted surgery and amount of blood loss are considered risk factors for the development of postoperative visual loss.[83,84] The underlying mechanism by which hypotension and hemodilution may lead to NAION remains unclear. Increased venous pressure due to increased interstitial fluid accumulation may "trap" the optic nerve, producing a compartment syndrome. Others have emphasized focusing on loss replacement and maintenance of normovolemia, rather than the volume of loss itself, and the duration of factors that might influence inadequate perfusion of the ophthalmic vasculature, rather than the duration of the surgery, suggesting that the duration of surgery is a surrogate for hypovolemia/hypoperfusion. Aside from correction of acute anemia, hypotension, or hypovolemia in the case of postoperative NAION, no known treatment has been proven to reverse its course.

Genetics

A genetic contribution to NAION has been increasingly explored, although presently there are no clear associations between genetic factors and NAION that have been consistently replicated. Case reports and series have identified the occurrence of NAION in more than one member of a family.[80,85–87] An association between a polymorphism in platelet glycoprotein Ibα and NAION has been identified.[88] An increased prevalence of T(-786)C polymorphisms of the endothelial nitric oxide synthase (eNOS) gene in NAION in Japanese people has also been shown.[89] The role of mitochondrial genes in NAION has also been investigated, with candidate gene-screening studies suggesting that mitochondrial genetic factors carried on the mitochondrial genome malfunction may be a risk factor for NAION, although there is likely to be interaction with other risk factors.[90,91] In a Sardinian population it has been demonstrated that the frequency of glucose-6-phosphate dehydrogenase (G6PD) deficiency in patients with NAION was significantly lower than expected, suggesting that G6PD-deficient patients may have a significantly decreased risk of having NAION.[92] Evidence indicates that G6PD-deficient patients are protected against ischemic heart and cerebrovascular disease and retinal vein occlusion. However, the reason why G6PD-deficiency may offer protection against NAION and retinal vein occlusion as a total deficiency is unclear.

Optic disc drusen

NAION seems to occur at a younger age in patients with optic disc drusen, which may be due to exaggerated crowding of the optic disc caused by the drusen.

Pathogenesis

Various theories have been proposed to explain the pathogenesis of NAION, although none does so completely. NAION is presumed to result from circulatory abnormalities within the territory of the SPCAs but the specific mechanism and location of the vasculopathy remain poorly understood.

The presence of small optic discs with small or no cup is also fundamental to explaining the pathophysiology of NAION. It may be that the structural crowding produces mechanical effects, leading to a compartment syndrome that predisposes the optic nerve to microcirculatory compromise in the laminar region.

By whatever mechanism the ischemia is produced, the result is an alteration of retinal cell metabolism, including changes in extracellular ion concentrations, depletion of growth factors, altered release of neurotransmitters, and increases in free radicals. These processes lead to axonal degeneration and progressive neuronal cell loss via apoptosis, which ultimately results in significant and permanent vision.[55]

Vasculopathic occlusion

A popular theory relates to the concept of vasculopathic occlusion in the SPCAs causing infarction of the retrolaminar region of the optic nerve head. It is suggested that atherosclerosis may predispose to decreased optic nerve head perfusion via microvascular occlusion. However, there are no histological data to confirm this hypothesis.

Nocturnal hypotension

It has been proposed that nocturnal systemic hypotension plays a role in the pathogenesis of NAION. It is recognized that sleep is associated with a "dip" in systemic blood pressure and that some people are known to have exaggerated hypotensive blood pressure dips at night. It has been hypothesized that, in such circumstances, the optic nerve circulation may be compromised. Patients at risk of showing such dips include those with systemic hypertension where the autoregulatory mechanisms of the optic disc may be impaired.[93] Aggressive antihypertensive treatment with evening dose may exaggerate such nocturnal dips. However, the evidence to support this theory is contradictory.[94,95]

Impaired autoregulation

Another theory purports that impairment of the normal autoregulatory mechanisms of the optic nerve head is responsible for NAION.[91] It has been suggested that such derangement results in release of vasoactive substances such as the endogenous serotonin which is produced during platelet aggregation within atherosclerotic plaques. This may be mediated by endothelial-derived vasoactive agents such as endothelins. Evidence to support this theory is indirect. Fundus photographs of cases of NAION show vasoconstriction in the peripapillary retinal arterioles, suggesting that some humoral factor may play a role.[96] Furthermore, it has been postulated that endothelial defects in the ocular circulation could impair the efficacy of endothelial-derived relaxation factors such as nitric oxide.[97]

Experimental animal studies provide indirect connection between autoregulation and optic nerve ischemia. Intravenous and intravitreal infusion of ET-1 in rabbits produced a decrease in blood flow measurements of the optic nerve head which was shown to be reversed by nifedipine, a calcium channel blocker.[98] It has been reported that serotonin-induced vasoconstriction occurs in CRA and posterior cerebral artery in atherosclerotic monkeys and that this is reversed by discontinuing an atherogeneic diet.[99]

Venous insufficiency

A further hypothesis put forward to explain NAION is that of venous insufficiency resulting from closure of tributary venules that receive blood from optic nerve capillaries and drain into the central retinal vein.[100] Hence, it may be that NAION is precipitated by venous insufficiency, with venous congestion causing initial disc edema. The creation of a compartment syndrome leads subsequently to cytotoxic and vasogenic (interstitial) edema, causing the infarction and tissue loss. Evidence that may support this includes the clinical characteristics of NAION, compared to AAION which is well recognized to be occlusion of the posterior ciliary arteries. In the majority of cases of NAION, the optic nerve head appearance differs from what is seen in arterial disease of the optic nerve. AAION causes a swollen disc which is pale, whereas NAION typically causes swelling with normal color or hyperemia. AAION usually causes severe visual loss, similar to the severe neuronal damage from arterial cerebral infarcts. In contrast, NAION causes less severe visual loss, akin to the moderate neuronal damage associated with cerebral venous disease. Pathophysiological evidence also provides suggestions that the etiology may be venous in origin. The vascular bed of the occlusion in AAION often includes the choroidal circulation as a result of posterior ciliary artery vasculitis. In contrast, the infarct in NAION does not fit the vascular bed of any known artery,[101] and fluorescein angiography in NAION demonstrates normal choroidal filling and mild delayed arterial filling of the anterior (prelaminar) disc alone. Finally, arterial risk factors, e.g., atherosclerotic disease, are not independent risk factors for NAION. However, further research is required to validate this theory.

Treatment

Presently, there is no treatment for NAION, although both surgical and medical interventions have been attempted. Box 41.4 outlines the various treatments trialed for NAION.

Box 41.4 Treatments investigated for nonarteritic anterior ischemic optic neuropathy

Treatment	Study design	Author	Result
Optic nerve decompression	Randomized clinical trial	Ischemic Optic Neuropathy Decompression Trial*	No benefit; may be harmful
Transvitreal optic neurotomy	Small case series	Soheilian et al[†]	Improved outcome
	Small randomized clinical trial	Soheilian et al[‡]	No benefit
Triamcinolone	Small case series	Jonas et al[§]	No benefit
Aspirin	Retrospective	Kupersmith et al[¶]	Protective effect for second eye involvement (17.5% in treated versus 53.5 untreated)
	Retrospective		No benefit

*Ischemic Optic Neuropathy Decompression Trial Research Group. Optic nerve decompression surgery for nonarteritic anterior ischemic optic neuropathy (NAION) is not effective and may be harmful. JAMA 1995;273:625–632.
[†]Soheilian M, Koochek S, Yazdani S, et al. Transvitreal optic neurotomy for nonarteritic anterior ischemic neuropathy. Retina 2003;23:692–97.
[‡]Soheilian M, Yazdani S. Alizadeh-Ghavidel L, et al. Surgery for optic neuropathy. Ophthalmology 2008;115:1099.
[§]Jonas JB, Spandau UH, Harder B, et al. Intravitreal triamcinolone acetonide for treatment of acute nonarteritic anteirior ischemic optic neuropathy. Graefes Arch Clin Exp Ophthalmol 2007;45:749–750.
[¶]Kupersmith MJ, Frohman, Sanderson M, et al. Aspirin reduces the incidence of second eye NAION: a retrospective study. J Neuroophthalmol 1997;17:250–253.

Neuroprotection

A few potential neuroprotective agents have been evaluated, but none has been shown to demonstrate therapeutic efficacy in humans.

Brimonidine

One study evaluated the effect of briminodine tartrate on the survival of retinal ganglion cell axons. The study demonstrated that the application of brimonidine eye drops for 1 week prior to an ischemic injury resulted in a statistically significant increase in survival of optic axons within the injured optic nerves. Brimonidine treatment of the eye after the ischemic injury did not result in axon rescue.[95] Another investigator found that briminodine did have a beneficial effect within 24–48 hours of injury in a rat crush model.[102]

There is a published prospective clinical trial of neuroprotection in NAION in humans using brimonidine topically.[103] This trial was halted because of difficulty in recruitment, with no significant difference between treatment and control groups. Another study compared NAION treated acutely with controls and found a trend to worse visual outcome.[104]

Estrogren

The investigation of estrogen as a neuroprotective treatment following rodent AION did not reveal any effective reduction in neuronal loss.[105]

Citicoline

Citicoline (cytidine-5′-diphosphocholine) is a candidate neuroprotective drug used in brain trauma, Parkinson's and Alzheimer's disease and was investigated in a small crossover clinical trial for the treatment of NAION. The study demonstrated changes in the PERGs, VEPs, and visual acuity parameters in the treatment group compared to pretreatment values. It is hypothesized that the drug efficacy seems to be related to its ability to stimulate some brain neurotransmitter systems, including the dopaminergic one, known to be largely expressed in both retina and postretinal visual pathways.[106]

Posterior ischemic optic neuropathy

PION is an ischemic infarct to the retrobulbar of the optic nerve which has a blood supply intraorbitally from the pial plexus and intracranially by branches of the internal carotid, anterior cerebral, and anterior communicating arteries. Clinically it is characterized by acute loss of vision with the absence of optic disc edema. Some have reported a small amount of disc edema a week or so after the acute event, presumably from propagation of damage and swelling forward from the site of the original infarct. The most important cause of PION to diagnose is GCA because it is treatable, although it can occur in the setting of surgery or spontaneously, similar to NAION. PION secondary to GCA or following surgery is usually associated with profound visual loss and minimal recovery. However, nonarteritic PION tends to be less severe and shows some improvement in 34%.[99]

Conclusion

To date, the pathogenesis of NAION remains poorly elucidated and there are no effective surgical or pharmacological therapies. Hence, understanding the pathophysiology of NAION is critical in order to identify novel therapeutic strategies.

Key references

A complete list of chapter references is available online at www.expertconsult.com. See inside cover for registration details.

1. Repka M, Savino P, Schatz N, et al. Clinical profile and long-term implications of anterior ischemic optic neuropathy. Am J Ophthalmol 1983;96: 478–483.

6. Arnold AC, Hepler RS. Natural history of nonarteritic anterior ischemic optic neuropathy. J Neuro-ophthalmol 1994; 14:66–69.

9. Newman NJ, Scherer R, Langenberg P, et al. The fellow eye in NAION: report from the ischemic optic neuropathy decompression trial follow-up study. Am J Ophthalmol 2002;134:317–328.

13. Beck R, Savino P, Repka M, et al. Optic disc structure in anterior ischemic optic neuropathy. Ophthalmology 1984;91: 1334–1337.

15. Danesh-Meyer HV, Savino PJ, Sergott RC. The prevalence of cupping in arteritic and non-arteritic anterior ischemic optic neuropathy. Ophthalmology 2001;108:593–598.

25. Danesh-Meyer HV, Carroll SC, Ku JY, et al. Correlation of retinal nerve fiber layer as measured with scanning laser polarimetry to visual fields in ischemic optic neuropathy. Arch Ophthalmol 2006;124:1720–1726.

29. Danesh-Meyer HV, Spaeth GL, Savino PJ, et al. Comparison of arteritis and nonarteritic anterior ischemic optic neuropathies with the Heidelberg retina tomograph. Ophthalmology 2005;112: 1104–1112.

49. Beck RW, Servais GE, Hayreh SS. Anterior ischemic optic neuropathy: IX. Cup-to-disc ratio and its role in pathogenesis. Ophthalmology 1987;94: 1503–1508.

50. Arnold AC. Pathogenesis of nonarteritic anterior ischemic optic neuropathy. J Neuroophthalmol 2003;23:157–163.

57. IONDT Research Group. Characteristics of patients with nonarteritic anterior ischemic optic neuropathy eligible for the Ischemic Optic Neuropathy Decompression Trial. Arch Ophthalmol 1996;114:1366–1374.

71. Margo CE, Dustin DF. Ischemic optic neuropathy in male veterans prescribed phosphodiesterase-5 inhibitors. Am J Ophthalmol 2007;143:538–539.

74. Danesh-Meyer HV, Levin LA. Erectile dysfunction drugs and risk of anterior ischaemic optic neuropathy: casual or causal association? Br J Ophthalmol 2007;91:1551–1555.

75. Bollinger K, Lee MS. Recurrent visual field defect and ischemic optic neuropathy associated with tadalafil rechallenge. Arch Ophthalmol 2005; 123:400–401.

100. Levin LA, Danesh-Meyer HV. Hypothesis: a venous etiology for non-arteritic ischaemic optic neuropathy. Arch Ophthalmol 2008;126:1586–1592.

101. Tesser RA, Niendorf ER, Levin LA. The morphology of an infarct in nonarteritic anterior ischemic optic neuropathy. Ophthalmology 2003;110: 2031–2035.

CHAPTER 42

Optic nerve axonal injury

Daniela Toffoli and Leonard A Levin

Overview

Unlike the peripheral nervous system (PNS), in which axonal injury leads to regeneration, injury to axons of central nervous system (CNS) neurons is irreversible, and usually leads to death of the cell body. The optic neuropathies, which are the main focus of this chapter, almost always involve injury to the retinal ganglion cell (RGC) axon. Etiologies include glaucoma, ischemia, compression, inflammation and demyelination, transection, infiltration, and papilledema (Box 42.1). Each of these involves axonal injury that ultimately leads to varying degrees of ganglion cell death.

Glaucoma (Chapters 19–29) is the most common of all of the optic neuropathies, ischemic optic neuropathy (Chapters 41 and 43) is the most common acute optic neuropathy in older persons, and optic neuritis (Chapter 37) is most common in the young. Compressive etiologies include neoplasms, aneurysms, and enlargement of extraocular muscles in thyroid-associated orbitopathy. Transection of the optic nerve may be partial or complete, and can occur with trauma such as bullet or knife wounds, or iatrogenically, e.g., during resection of a tumor. Infiltration of the optic nerve may involve neoplasm (e.g., gliomas or metastases) or inflammation (e.g., sarcoidosis) and usually results in a combination of compressive, inflammatory, and ischemic damage to the optic nerve. Papilledema is caused by increased intracranial pressure and the pathological mechanism of disease involves disrupted axonal transport.[1–5]

Clinical background

Historical development

The quest to understanding the mechanisms behind axonal degeneration began in the mid-1800s with the works of Augustus Waller. In 1850, he demonstrated that axons could undergo a compartmentalized degenerative process. By transecting frog hypoglossal and glossopharyngeal nerves, he noted that the distal axonal fragments (those separated from the cell soma) underwent a "curdling" and disorganization, and in 1856 noted a similar observation following transection of the rabbit optic nerve.[6] This type of axonal degeneration has been termed "wallerian degeneration." Since this time, more and more evidence has shown that axons undergo a compartmentalized degenerative process, using mechanisms distinct from those causing the degeneration and death of the cell soma.[7] Clinically, this has arisen parallel to the perception that certain CNS diseases may be considered "axogenic" diseases, or arising primarily from injury to the neuronal axon, whereas others may be considered "somagenic" diseases, which, in contrast, arise primarily from injury to the cell soma.[8]

In neuro-ophthalmic disease, the RGC body and its axon are the main targets of pathology, and just as in the rest of the CNS, the concept of somagenic versus axogenic disease applies. Diseases primarily affecting the RGC layer (somagenic diseases) are usually retinopathies, and result from injuries including ischemia, excitotoxicity, autoimmune processes, thermal and photic injury, storage diseases, neoplastic processes, nutritional deprivation, and toxins.[1] Axogenic diseases of the optic nerve and the mechanisms underlying their pathophysiology are the subject of this chapter.

Key symptoms and signs

Diseases characterized by optic nerve axonal injury are associated with abnormal visual acuity, color vision, visual field, and optic nerve head color and morphology. Ischemic, traumatic, compressive, infiltrative, inflammatory, infectious, toxic, and nutritional optic neuropathies are often associated with decreased visual acuity early in the course of disease because of significant involvement of RGCs sending axons via the papillomacular bundle. Open-angle glaucoma, papilledema, and optic disk drusen affect the papillomacular bundle much later on, thereby not initially causing reduction in visual acuity. Similarly, color vision is variably affected. Color vision loss, which usually affects the red–green axis, occurs late in glaucomatous optic neuropathy.

Optic nerve excavation and pallor, which reflect the effect of chronic loss of RGC axons, are elements that can help distinguish the various optic neuropathies. Histologically, excavation represents loss of all tissue and thus leads to the creation of an empty space, or cup, surrounded by axon-containing tissue, called the rim. Pallor is caused by axonal loss, but occurs in the presence of remaining viable glial tissue. This glial tissue takes the place of the space that would

Box 42.1 Clinical features of common axonal diseases of the retinal ganglion cell

Disease	Clinical features	Genetics	Epidemiology	Treatment	Prognosis
Glaucoma	Progressive visual field defects, starting peripherally and eventually involving fixation (and, consequently, visual acuity). Normal color vision. Characteristic disk cupping without significant rim pallor. Elevated intraocular pressure (IOP) frequently present	Family history important, and several known genes, e.g., myocilin (MYOC) for primary open-angle glaucoma; optineurin (OPTN) for primary open-angle glaucoma; CYP1B1 for congenital glaucoma	Second leading cause of blindness in the world[2]. Risk factors: Age, Race, Family history, Elevated IOP, Myopia	Lowering of IOP	Many patients progress despite lowering of IOP
Optic neuritis	Decreased visual acuity and color vision acutely. Pain on eye movements. Visual field loss, often central. Optic disk swollen in 30% of patients. Disk pallor begins weeks after attack	Similar to those of multiple sclerosis (MS), e.g., HLA complex (HLA-DR2 haplotype)	15–20% of patients with MS present with optic neuritis initially. Occurs in 50% of MS patients. Risk factors: Young adults, Female > male, MS	Intravenous methylprednisone. Disease-modifying drugs for MS	Usually complete or almost complete recovery of vision (20/40 or better). May have residual color vision or visual field deficits
Papilledema	Bilateral optic disk swelling from increased intracranial pressure. Transient visual obscurations. Relatively preserved visual acuity, color vision and field acutely. Late visual field changes: nasal depression, arcuate scotomas, concentric constriction of field	Dependent on disease causing elevated intracranial pressure	Idiopathic intracranial hypertension (obesity). Intracranial tumor. Cerebral venous thrombosis	Removal of tumor. Weight loss, acetazolamide, topiramate, lumbar peritoneal or ventriculoperitoneal shunting, optic nerve sheath fenestration	Prognosis dependent on severity and duration of intracranial hypertension. Optic atrophy and arterial narrowing are late signs
Arteritic anterior ischemic optic neuropathy	Acute loss of vision. Unilateral initially and, if untreated, bilateral in days to weeks. Headache, jaw claudication, weight loss, neck and shoulder pain. Scalp pain, myalgias, fever. Optic disk edema	Sporadic	20 cases/100 000 persons over age of 50 annually. Risk factors: Women > men, Mostly Caucasians, Age 65 or older[113]	Intravenous followed by oral corticosteroids. Temporal artery biopsy to confirm diagnosis	Profound visual loss: counting fingers to no light perception. Rarely improvement in vision. Corticosteroids prevent vision loss in second eye in most patients
Nonarteritic anterior ischemic optic neuropathy	Usually acutely decreased visual acuity. Color vision relatively preserved. Visual field defects, which are usually altitudinal. Optic disk edema	Sporadic	2.3–10.2 cases/100 000/year over 50 years of age. Mostly Caucasians[113]. Risk factors: Small cup-to-disk ratio, Diabetes, hypertension. ? Nocturnal hypotension[113,115]	No proven treatment	Visual acuity from 20/20 to light perception. 42% of patients improve by 3 lines or more. Rarely recurs in same eye. Increased risk of second eye involvement (up to 15% at 5 years)[115,116]
Compressive optic neuropathy	Slowly progressive painless decrease in visual acuity. Decreased color vision. Disk edema and/or atrophy. Central or cecocentral field defects. Also proptosis, strabismus, optociliary shunt vessels (meningiomas and gliomas)	Dependent on cause of disease	Risk factors: Middle-aged female > male for meningiomas. Neurofibromatosis 1 for gliomas. Thyroid orbitopathy	Removal or reduction of compressive mass by surgery, radiotherapy, or chemotherapy	Usually slowly progressive decrease in vision unless treatment undertaken. Gliomas may remain stable
Traumatic optic neuropathy	Acurely decreased visual acuity and color vision. Optic nerve pallor develops after a few weeks	None	Up to 5% of indirect head injuries may have a traumatic optic neuropathy[114]	No treatment shown to be superior to observation alone	Spontaneous improvement may occur, but prognosis often poor, especially if no light perception at onset
Infiltrative optic neuropathy	Subacute, chronic decrease in visual acuity and color vision. May present with headache. Other cranial nerves may be affected. Optic disk either normal or edematous	Dependent on cause of disease	Risk factors: Granulomatous disease (e.g., sarcoidosis), neoplasms (leukemia, lymphomas, metastases), optic nerve glioma	Treatment of underlying disease	Dependent on disease process

Table 42.1 Disorders with disk excavation

Glaucoma
Compressive optic neuropathies (sometimes)
Methanol optic neuropathy
Arteritic anterior ischemic optic neuropathy
Shock optic neuropathy
Dominant optic neuropathy
Leber's hereditary optic neuropathy
Periventricular leukomalacia

otherwise increase the size of the excavation, producing instead a pale area. In glaucoma, the morphology of the excavation is almost pathognomonic, although other optic neuropathies may have significant excavation (Table 42.1). Pallor of the neuroretinal rim is eventually seen in most nonglaucomatous optic neuropathies. On the other hand, cupping in the absence of pallor is typical of glaucomatous optic neuropathy. This rule is not without exception, however, as end-stage glaucoma may be associated with a pale rim (see Chapter 44).

Visual field abnormalities help to differentiate the optic neuropathies. Optic neuropathies that are caused by more anterior or optic nerve head damage usually give rise to defects that follow the RGC axon distribution pattern in the retina, or nerve fiber bundle defects. Glaucoma is the best known of these, and typically causes arcuate scotomas, nasal steps, and temporal wedges. Other neuropathies which may cause similar types of visual field changes include papilledema and optic disk drusen. In the beginning stages, papilledema may give rise to an enlarged blind spot that is refractive (due to elevation of the peripapillary retina). This is followed by nasal steps, arcuate visual field defects, and concentric constriction of the visual field. Nonarteritic anterior ischemic optic neuropathy typically gives rise to altitudinal field defects, mostly inferiorly, which may also cross the horizontal meridian and involve fixation and are therefore not strictly nerve fiber bundle defects. Optic neuropathies due to axonal injury posterior to the optic nerve head, yet anterior to the chiasm, frequently produce central scotomas or diffuse visual field loss. Included in this category are optic neuritis, compressive, infiltrative, toxic and nutritional optic neuropathies, as well as Leber's hereditary optic neuropathy and autosomal-dominant optic neuropathy.[4]

Epidemiology

See Box 42.1.

Genetics

See Box 42.1.

Diagnostic workup

The diagnosis of many axonal injuries of the optic nerve can be made on the basis of neuro-ophthalmic history and examination. Neuroimaging is typically the first step when the diagnosis is not otherwise apparent, especially when there is optic nerve edema, pallor of the neuroretinal rim, central visual field loss, or visual field loss that respects the vertical meridian. Examination of the blood or cerebrospinal fluid and other imaging techniques are determined based on the specific clinical syndrome.

Differential diagnosis

See Box 42.1.

Treatment and prognosis

Treatment and prognosis depend on specifics of the optic neuropathies. There are no proven treatments for nonarteritic anterior ischemic optic neuropathy, congenital and hereditary optic neuropathies, most traumatic optic neuropathies, and compressive optic neuropathy other than decompression of the instigating mass. Lowering the intraocular pressure has been proven to decrease the rate of progression of glaucomatous optic neuropathy. Patients with optic neuritis will recover vision more quickly when treated with intravenous corticosteroids, but the final visual outcome is the same as with placebo. Intravenous and oral corticosteroids may stop progression or save the unaffected eye in arteritic anterior ischemic optic neuropathy.

Pathology

The mechanisms responsible for optic neuropathies reflect different types of axonal injury. Major underlying causes include ischemia, demyelination, inflammation, compression, transection, glaucoma, infiltration, and papilledema. Two or more of these factors may be involved in one optic nerve disease. For example, both demyelination and inflammation are implicated in the pathogenesis of optic neuritis or other active lesions in multiple sclerosis. In multiple sclerosis, demyelination is thought to lead to loss of axonal trophic support, whereas inflammatory mechanisms may lead to either direct (immunologic attack) or indirect (through cytokines and proteolytic enzymes) axonal injury.[9] In glaucoma, increased intraocular pressure is thought to lead to mechanical deformations of axons, disrupted axonal transport, and microvacular ischemia.[10]

On a microscopic level, mitochondrial dysfunction, disruption of axonal conduction, disruption of axonal transport, and axonal transection can each result from the different types of axonal injury and contribute to the pathogenesis of the various optic neuropathies (Box 42.2). Ultrastructurally, the first sign of axotomy-induced axonal degeneration includes a rounding and swelling of the axolemma, occurring in the first 12–24 hours following injury in rats and up to 7 days for humans.[11] This is followed by calcium entry into the cell, the subsequent activation of calcium-dependent proteases (calpains), and activation of the ubiquitin proteosome system. These processes ultimately lead to the degradation of microtubules and neurofilaments, contributing to axonal disassembly. Wallerian degeneration demonstrates multiple dense bodies, neuroaxonal spheroids, and retraction balls at the sites of axonal transection.[12] Blockage of extracellular calcium channels or inhibition of the ubiquitin-proteasome system is enough to delay the

Box 42.2 Pathogenesis of common axonal diseases of retinal ganglion cells

Optic neuropathy	Pathogenesis
Glaucoma	Mechanical, ischemic, or inflammatory injury of axons at the optic disk Interruption of axonal transport Oxidative free radical generation[1]
Optic neuritis	Demyelination of optic nerve (loss of trophic factors) Immune-mediated axonal damage Axonal conduction block Mitochondrial dysfunction and energy crisis Axonal transection and loss[1,9]
Papilledema	Intra-axonal edema causing abnormalities in axonal transport[1]
Arteritic anterior ischemic optic neuropathy	Occlusion of posterior ciliary arteries and infarction of optic nerve head [4]
Nonarteritic anterior ischemic optic neuropathy	Decreased perfusion
Compressive optic neuropathies	Conduction block, ischemia, demyelination, and axonal transection
Traumatic optic neuropathies	Transection, avulsion, hemorrhage (direct injury) or stretch, compression (indirect injury)
Infiltrative optic neuropathies	Infiltration, compression of optic nerve

processes of axonal degeneration.[13,14] The importance of calcium in mediating axonal degeneration cannot be overemphasized; increasing extracellular calcium concentrations alone (in the absence of axotomy) is sufficient to cause axonal degeneration in mouse dorsal root ganglia cultures.[13]

The pathological end-stage of axonal optic neuropathy is optic atrophy, and this is discussed in Chapter 44, as well as in the pathophysiology section, below.

Etiology

A variety of risk factors have been associated with optic nerve axonal injuries, including age, sex, race, family history, ocular morphology, systemic disease, nutritional factors, exposure to toxins, and possibly other environmental factors (see Box 42.2 and individual chapters for specifics). For example, optic neuritis and Leber's hereditary optic neuropathy are more common in the young, whereas glaucoma and ischemic optic neuropathy are more prevalent in older individuals. Optic neuritis and arteritic anterior ischemic optic neuropathy are more common in women and Leber's hereditary optic neuropathy is more common in men. Examples of ocular morphology risk factors include a greater incidence of glaucoma in myopic individuals and of nonarteritic anterior ischemic optic neuropathy in those with small, crowded

optic nerve heads. Systemic disease risk factors include neurofibromatosis (optic gliomas), thyroid disease (compressive optic neuropathy), and many more. Genetic risk factors are profound in hereditary optic neuropathies, e.g., Leber's hereditary optic neuropathy and dominant optic atrophy, but play an important role in glaucoma, optic neuritis, and disk drusen. Some studies have demonstrated that genetics may also play a role in the ischemic optic neuropathies.

Pathophysiology

As discussed above, the optic neuropathies generally arise from some form of injury to retinal ganglion axons. In some cases, the site of injury is obvious, e.g., traumatic optic neuropathies. In other cases, e.g., glaucoma, there is less direct evidence that the initial sites of injury are the RGC axons within the optic nerve head. Several studies have demonstrated that early injury occurs at the lamina cribrosa in glaucoma.[15–18] Additional findings, including focal notching of the disk[19] and splinter hemorrhages,[20,21] have also helped to pinpoint the optic disk as the initial site of injury. More recent evidence from the DBA/2J mouse model of glaucoma confirms the axonal locus of injury.[22,23]

The effects of the axonal injury are numerous, not only on the optic nerve and RGCs, but also on other cells. The concept of axonal degeneration has recently been reviewed[24] (Figure 42.1). This section discusses some of the major consequences of axonal injury, focusing on the following: (1) effects on the RGC body; (2) wallerian degeneration of the axon distal to the injury site; (3) retrograde degeneration proximal to the injury site; (4) effects on other neurons; and (5) effects on nonneuronal cells. There are numerous other effects, e.g., excitability, axonal conduction, and particularly changes in the dendritic arborization,[25–27] which are areas of active study.

Effects on the retinal ganglion cell body

Axonal injury is the first step to occur in most of the optic neuropathies, and leads to RGC death.[28] Depending on the animal species affected, the distance of injury from the RGC, and the cell body size, up to 70% of ganglion cells may survive following axonal injury.[1] Studies of the time course of RGC death in rodents after optic nerve injury demonstrate a partial (20–40%) loss within the first 3–7 days, the remainder (50–90%) taking weeks to sometimes months.[29–34] Nonhuman primate RGCs die approximately 4–6 weeks after axotomy.[28,35] In humans there is sparing of some ipsilateral temporal ganglion cells 35 days after transection of the optic tract,[36] and even in absolute glaucoma some RGCs seem to survive.[37] In lower animals, e.g., goldfish and frogs, ganglion cells do not die, but hypertrophy and regenerate axons within 1–2 months.[38–40] The fact that ganglion cell death is not a necessary consequence of axotomy suggests that there are regulatory mechanisms underlying RGC survival after axonal injury.

Axonal injury following axotomy, elevated eye pressure, ocular ischemia, optic nerve crush injury, and occurring subsequent to the destruction of postsynaptic target cells has been shown to lead to RGC death through apoptosis.[41–43] As with apoptosis in other tissues, there is chromatin condensa-

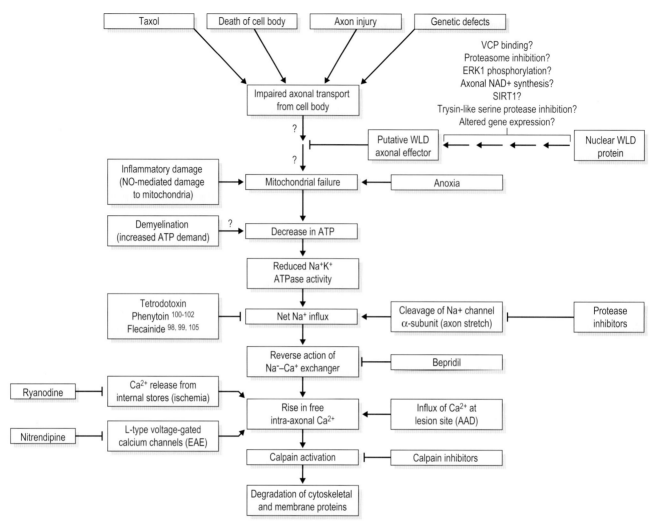

Figure 42.1 Example of some of the multiple pathways activated by axonal injury. (Redrawn from Coleman M. Axon degeneration mechanisms: commonality amid diversity. Nat Rev Neurosci 2005;6:889–898.)

tion, shrinkage, and phagocytosis by surrounding cells, and it appears to be predominantly mediated by the bcl-2 family of proteins, containing proapoptotic members Bax, Bid, and Bad and antiaptoptotic members Bcl-2 and Bcl-X, and the cysteine protease family of caspases.[44] Though the exact signaling process leading from nerve fiber layer injury to RGC apoptosis has not been elucidated, many molecular mechanisms are involved. For example, deprivation of neurotrophic factors from the target or other tissues, excitotoxicity from physiological or pathological levels of glutamate, free radical formation, increases in intra-axonal Ca^{2+}, induction of neuronal endopeptidases, accumulation of excess retrogradely transported macromolecules, and induction of p38 MAP kinase and other signaling molecules may stimulate the apoptotic pathway.[29,45–54]

Of these, the most well-studied mechanism to date involves loss of neurotrophin support from target cells. It has long been known that neurotrophic factors are essential elements in neuronal development. During development, neurons are present in excess numbers. According to the neurotrophic factor hypothesis, developing neurons compete for a limited number of target-derived neurotrophic factors that are required for survival and differentiaion. Lack of

appropriate target cell contacts leads to neurotrophin deprivation in the developing neuron, with subsequent axonal pruning and death of the cell soma by apoptosis.[55,56] Target cell integrity and neurotrophin support are also essential elements in maintaining the survival of adult RGCs.[57–59] Following nerve fiber layer injury, disruption of orthograde and retrograde axonal transport of neurotrophins can occur and this may ultimately lead to RGC neurotrophin deprivation and subsequent apoptosis. This has mostly been demonstrated with intraocular pressure elevation in primate and rat models.[60–65] Support for the role of neurotrophin dependence particularly comes from experiments using identified neurotrophic factors to rescue axotomized neurons. Purified neonatal RGCs (which are axotomized during dissociation) can be kept alive for significant periods with a cocktail of factors, including brain-derived neurotrophic factor (BDNF), ciliary neurotrophic factor, forskolin, and insulin.[66] Intraocular administration of certain neurotrophins (e.g., BDNF) delays RGC death after axotomy in adult rats[33,49] and cats,[67] and in an experimental model of glaucoma.[68] Gene delivery of BDNF to the retina or to the RGC itself also increases survival in experimental glaucoma,[69,70] as it does inhibition of apoptosis.[71]

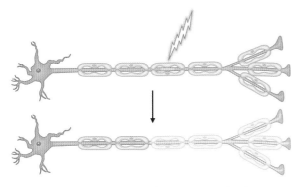

Figure 42.2 Optic nerve injury induces intra-axonal and extra-axonal pathophysiology. An early event is wallerian degeneration, in which the distal axon degenerates. (Redrawn from Di Polo A. Mechansms of neural injury in glaucoma. In: Levin LA, Weinreb RN, Di Polo A (eds) Neuroprotection for Glaucoma: A Pocket Guide. New York: Ethis, 2007.)

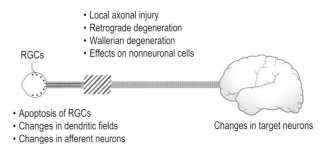

Figure 42.3 Axonal injury affects the retinal ganglion cell's axon, dendrites, and soma, other neurons, and nonneuronal cells in the optic nerve and retina.

There are likely other signals for RGC death besides neurotrophin deprivation. RGCs maintain viability for long periods of time when there is decreased axonal transport from compressive optic neuropathy or papilledema. Retrograde axonal transport is rapid, and the subacute time course by which RGCs die after axonal injury does not reflect the time course of interrupted retrograde axonal transport. RGC axotomy induces changes in responsiveness to neurotrophins independent of neurotrophin deprivation.[72] Finally, removal of the RGC axonal target, and therefore, target-derived factors, causes very slow RGC death.[57,73] These findings suggest that axotomy can signal changes at the cell body independent of neurotrophin deprivation. For example, an elevation in intracellular levels of the reactive oxygen species superoxide can occur independent of neurotrophin deprivation, and is necessary and sufficient for RGC death after axotomy.[74]

Wallerian (anterograde) and retrograde degeneration

Wallerian degeneration

Axonal injury in the CNS and PNS arising from traumatic, metabolic, toxic, inflammatory, and hereditary causes often results in a form of secondary axon pathology termed wallerian degeneration[6] (see section on historical development, above). Focal injury to the axon leads to an orderly disassembly of the distal axonal stump in the hours to days following injury (Figure 42.2). At the cellular level, there is initial disassembly of the myelin sheath, followed by swelling of the axolemma, disorganization of neurofilaments and microtubules, and mitochondrial swelling. The remaining axonal fragments then undergo phagocytosis by glial cells and macrophages, followed by apoptosis of surrounding oligodendrocytes in the CNS.[11]

The directionality of wallerian degeneration was explored by Beirowski et al,[75] who showed that, in mouse peripheral nerves, wallerian degeneration proceeds asynchronously (at different rates between different axons) and either anterogradely or retrogradely depending on whether it was a transection or crush injury that was incurred, respectively.[75] Studies performed on dorsal root ganglion nerves had shown

similar results, demonstrating that CNS transection injury causes anterograde degeneration. Wallerian degeneration may occur in a variety of diseases, including demyelinating diseases such as multiple sclerosis and Guillain–Barré, as well as following neurovascular insults, and neurodegenerative and infectious processes.[12] As would be expected, wallerian degeneration is seen in optic nerve diseases.[22,76–82]

Dying-back degeneration

Another well-characterized type of axonal degeneration occurs by a process called dying back. As opposed to wallerian degeneration, which is thought to occur due to localized injury, dying-back degeneration occurs following a chronic and more generalized form of injury to the axon. It is a slow process, occurring over weeks to months, and involves degeneration of the axon from the synaptic end towards the cell soma in a retrograde fashion. It is known to occur in peripheral neuropathies, but in recent years evidence has accrued that it also is important for the pathophysiology of CNS degenerations (e.g., Alzheimer's disease and Parkinson's disease).[7] Presumably a chronic optic nerve injury from a toxin, mitochondrial dysfunction, or nutritional deficiency could cause a parallel pathology to RGC axons.

Acute axonal degeneration

Though wallerian degeneration is the main form of axonal degeneration following axotomy, another degenerative process may occur in the acute stages of transection injury (beginning 20 minutes postinjury and lasting 5 minutes). Using in vivo time lapse imaging studies, Kerschensteiner and colleagues[82] demonstrated that a process which they referred to as acute axonal degeneration (AAD) may occur prior to wallerian degeneration following dorsal root transection in mice. AAD is thought to occur in the minutes following axotomy, causing axonal fragmentation in a bidirectional fashion in both the proximal and distal axonal stumps. This is thought to lead to retraction of the proximal axonal stump and subsequent wallerian degeneration of the distal end.[82,83]

Axonal degeneration is independent of soma degeneration

The mechanisms responsible for axonal degeneration are distinct from those causing apoptosis (Figure 42.3). Axonal degeneration often involves the calpains and/or the ubiquitin-proteosome system, unlike caspases in apoptosis.

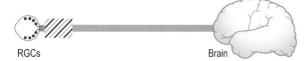

Figure 42.4 Axonal injury when apoptosis is blocked with bax knockout. The soma and proximal axon are spared (green), but the distal axon undergoes wallerian degeneration (red).

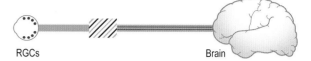

Figure 42.5 Axonal injury when wallerian degeneration is blocked in the Wld^S mutant. The distal axon is spared (green), but the proximal axon dies back and the soma undergoes apoptosis (red).

In recent years the distinction between apoptosis and axonal death has become clearer. It is now evident that, even though axonal death usually occurs following apoptosis (and vice versa), apoptosis is not a necessary requirement for axonal death. Axonal degeneration does not appear to occur due to a process of "starvation" from the cell soma, but rather seems capable of undergoing its own autonomous death process.

Blocking apoptosis

The DBA/2J Bax knockout mouse is just one of the experimental models which have helped to demonstrate this. DBA/2J mice develop elevated intraocular pressure and glaucoma as they age. DBA/2J mice crossed with mice with knockout alleles for Bax undergo axonal degeneration, but are protected from cell body apoptosis[84] (Figure 42.4). These results demonstrate that axonal degeneration is distinct from apoptosis in glaucoma and that axonal death can occur in the absence of death of the cell soma.

Other clues have emerged from bcl-2 transgenic mice. Axotomy of nerves from mice containing the human bcl-2 transgene undergo axonal degeneration at a rate comparable to wild-type mice, but are protected from apoptosis of the cell soma. This demonstrates the importance of bcl-2 in preventing cell body death but its failure to protect from axonal degeneration.[85] The pmn mouse, a mouse model of a motor neuropathy, is another example of the concept that axonal degeneration and death of the cell soma are distinct compartmentalized processes. Overexpression of the bcl-2 gene or inactivation of the bax gene in pmn mice prevents the death of the motor neuron cell bodies, but does nothing to prevent axonal degeneration.[86] These mice continue to develop weakness and eventually die at a normal rate, despite protection from neuronal apoptosis.

Wallerian degeneration slow (Wld^S) mutants

Perhaps the most impressive evidence that axonal degeneration may occur independently from death of the cell soma was demonstrated using the wallerian degeneration slow (Wld^S) strain of mice. Wld^S mice have an autosomal-dominant 85-kb tandem triplication mutation on chromosome 4 which confers delayed wallerian degeneration in both the PNS and CNS. In this strain of mice, axonal degeneration following injury or neurotrophin deprivation is delayed severalfold compared to wild-type mice, taking place several weeks after injury compared to only hours or days after. Remarkably, though axonal degeneration is delayed in these mice, death of the cell soma proceeds at a rate comparable to that of wild-type mice. That is, following injury, the process of apoptosis is not slowed or delayed in Wld^S mice.[87,88] Axonal loss is slowed in glaucoma models in mice[22] and rats[89] when on a Wld^S background (Figure 42.5).

These results provide distinct and parallel evidence that axonal degeneration and apoptosis likely occur by very different and autonomous molecular mechanisms.

The genetic mutation responsible for the delayed Wallerian degeneration phenotype is an in-frame fusion of the N-terminal 70 amino acids of the E4 ubiquitin ligase Ube4b, an 18-amino-acid linker, and the full-length nicotinamide mononucleotide adenylyl transferase 1 (Nmnat1), involved with NAD^+ synthesis.[90,91] All parts are necessary for in vivo protection of axons from wallerian degeneration, and it is likely that direction of the fusion protein to a specific subcellular compartment is necessary for full effects.[92–94] How this fusion protein blocks wallerian degeneration is an area of active research.[93,95,96]

Effects of axonal injury on other neurons

Axonal injury may also lead to the secondary degeneration of surrounding axons (which were uninjured by the primary insult). Partial optic nerve crush and transection injury models have demonstrated initial rapid injury of directly damaged axons, followed weeks or months later by degeneration of axons in adjacent areas.[97–99] This was first demonstrated following traumatic injury to the CNS[100] and is proposed to be a possible cause of continued RGC loss in optic neuropathies, particularly glaucoma, despite intraocular pressure control. Regardless of the type of injury, this secondary degeneration is believed to occur through a variety of mechanisms, including excitatory neurotransmitter (glutamate) or oxygen free release by primarily injured axons, or by changes in extracellular ion concentrations, particularly potassium levels.[51,97,101] Support for glutamate involvement stems from experiments using MK-801 (an N-methyl-d-aspartate (NMDA) receptor antagonist) following optic nerve crush injury, which has been shown to attenuate secondary degeneration.[102]

Finally, the impact of axonal degeneration is not only visible in close proximity to the initial lesion, but may also extend to target cells, located much further away. For example, the vast majority of RGCs establish terminal synapses in the lateral geniculate nucleus (LGN), and in several models of glaucoma, it has been shown that atrophy of cells in the LGN correlates with severity of RGC axon loss and of intraocular pressure (see Chapter 26).

Effects of axonal injury on nonneural cells

Though most work has focused on axonal injury and the subsequent effects on RGC death and/or survival, axonal disruption may also have consequences on surrounding retinal cells. Following optic nerve crush or spinal cord injury, for example, oligodendrocytes undergo apoptosis.

The loss of axonal contact and the decrease in neurotrophic factors are believed to lead to the initiation of the apoptotic program or of an atrophy-like resting state in oligodendrocytes following wallerian degeneration.[103-106] Members of the tumor necrosis factor cytokine receptor superfamily and other molecules are involved in nonneuronal cell death after axonal injury.[107,108]

Other cells which are affected by axonal injury in the CNS include the resident microglia. These phagocytic cells increase in size and number and undergo activation in response to wallerian degeneration, occurring several days later than the macrophage response in the PNS.[11,109] Though they undergo activation following axonal injury,[110] their phagocytic response nevertheless is limited and they incompletely clear myelin debris in the CNS.[111] This is in contrast to PNS injury, where macrophages are actively recruited from the circulation and phagocytose myelin debris in an opsonin-dependent manner.[112] Unlike in the PNS, there is a less profound influx of macrophages from the circulation during CNS injury.[11]

Key references

A complete list of chapter references is available online at www.expertconsult.com. See inside cover for registration details.

1. Levin L, Gordon L. Retinal ganglion cell disorders: types and treatments. Prog Retin Eye Res Sep 2002;21:465–484.

6. Waller AV. Experiments on the section of glossopharyngeal and hypoglossal nerves of the frog, and observations on the alterations produced thereby in the structure of their of their primitive fibers. Philos Trans R Soc Lond B Biol Sci 1850;140:423–429.

7. Raff MC, Whitmore AV, Finn JT. Axonal self-destruction and neurodegeneration. Science 2002;296:868–871.

8. Schwartz M, Yoles E, Levin LA. 'Axogenic' and 'somagenic' neurodegenerative diseases: definitions and therapeutic implications. Mol Med Today 1999;5:470–473.

11. Vargas ME, Barres BA. Why is Wallerian degeneration in the CNS so slow? Annu Rev Neurosci 2007;30:153–179.

12. Whitmore AV, Libby RT, John SW. Glaucoma: thinking in new ways–a role for autonomous axonal self-destruction and other compartmentalised processes? Prog Retin Eye Res 2005;24:639–662.

24. Coleman M. Axon degeneration mechanisms: commonality amid diversity. Nat Rev Neurosci 2005;6: 889–898.

41. Quigley HA, Nickells RW, Kerrigan LA, et al. Retinal ganglion cell death in experimental glaucoma and after axotomy occurs by apoptosis. Invest Ophthalmol Vis Sci 1995;36:774–786.

57. Pearson HE, Thompson TP. Atrophy and degeneration of ganglion cells in central retina following loss of postsynaptic target neurons in the dorsal lateral geniculate nucleus of the adult cat. Exp Neurol 1993;119:113–119.

63. Quigley HA, Addicks EM. Chronic experimental glaucoma in primates. II. Effect of extended intraocular pressure elevation on optic nerve head and axonal transport. Invest Ophthalmol Vis Sci 1980;19:137–152.

74. Lieven CJ, Schlieve CR, Hoegger MJ, et al. Retinal ganglion cell axotomy induces an increase in intracellular superoxide anion. Invest Ophthalmol Vis Sci 2006;47:1477–1485.

84. Libby RT, Li Y, Savinova OV, et al. Susceptibility to neurodegeneration in a glaucoma is modified by Bax gene dosage. PLoS Genet 2005;1:e4.

87. Deckwerth TL, Johnson EM Jr. Neurites can remain viable after destruction of the neuronal soma by programmed cell death (apoptosis). Dev Biol 1994;165: 63–72.

88. Glass JD, Brushart TM, George EB, et al. Prolonged survival of transected nerve fibres in C57BL/Ola mice is an intrinsic characteristic of the axon. J Neurocytol 1993;22:311–321.

89. Beirowski B, Babetto E, Coleman MP, et al. The WldS gene delays axonal but not somatic degeneration in a rat glaucoma model. Eur J Neurosci 2008;28:1166–1179.

CHAPTER 43

Leber's hereditary optic neuropathy

Alfredo Sadun and Alice Kim

Clinical background

Historical development

Leber's hereditary optic neuropathy (LHON) is a maternally inherited disease that presents with sudden or subacute non-synchronous bilateral vision loss. Males in their second and third decade of life are typically affected. The classic visual field loss is a large and dense cecocentral scotoma usually associated with a decline of vision to greater than 20/200. LHON was first described by Von Graefe in 1858 and then characterized formally into a distinct clinical entity by Leber in 1871. Originally, it was believed to be X-linked and inherited with partial penetrance.[1] Erickson in 1972 was the first to propose that LHON could have a maternal inheritance pattern from a mitochondrial mutation.[2] Then in 1988, Wallace and colleagues confirmed the hypothesis by identifying a G to A mutation at nucleotide position 11778 in the mtDNA of nine pedigrees.[3]

Key symptoms and signs

LHON commonly manifests with acute or subacute painless central vision loss in one eye associated with dyschromatopsia. Within days, months, or rarely years, the second eye is similarly affected and the average interval time is 1.8 months.[4] A few months after onset, the vision loss will typically plateau at or below 20/200. Acutely on clinical examination, the optic discs may appear hyperemic with a characteristic circumpapillary telangiectatic microangiopathy (Figure 43.1). The nerve fiber layer will be swollen without evidence of leakage of dye on fluorescein angiography, leading to the term pseudopapilledema. Over time, axonal loss of the papillomacular bundle (PMB) leads to temporal pallor and eventually severe and diffuse optic atrophy and large absolute cecocentral scotomas are found on visual field testing (Figure 43.2).

Genetics

Approximately 95% of the LHON cases of northern European descent are caused by the three most common mtDNA mutations at nucleotide positions 3460, 11778, and 14484.[5] These three mutations all result in an amino acid substitution in complex I of the respiratory chain. To date, more than 37 point mtDNA mutations have been identified.[4] Of these point mutations, genes encoding for ND1 and ND6 appear to occur the most frequently. The ND1 and ND6 subunits are essential for mtDNA-encoded subunit assembly of complex I.[4]

However the presence of LHON mtDNA mutations does not necessarily correlate with vision loss. Only 50% of men and 10% of women who carry the LHON mtDNA mutation develop the optic neuropathy.[6] However, over 80% of affected patients are male.[7]

Epidemiology

Studies in the north-east of England found that the minimum point prevalence of visual failure due to LHON was 3.22 per 100 000 and the minimum point prevalence for the LHON mtDNA mutation was 11.82 per 100 000. Therefore, LHON has a population prevalence similar to many autosomally inherited neurological disorders.[8]

Differential diagnosis

There are other conditions of inherited optic neuropathies, such as Kjer's dominant optic atrophy (OPA1) and Wolfram syndrome (WFS1 gene on chromosome 4), that share similar clinical characteristics and hence must be differentiated from LHON. Though these inherited optic neuropathies are coded by somatic genes, it does not mean that they are not mitochondrial optic neuropathies. Indeed, we now know that their gene products do indeed interact in or with mitochondria. Metabolic optic neuropathies, including a large number of toxic and nutritional optic neuropathies, must also be considered in the differential diagnosis of LHON; nutritional deficiencies include insufficient levels of folic acid and vitamin B_{12} and toxic mitochondrial optic neuropathies such as ethambutol, chloramphenicol, and linezolid.[9] Combinations of nutritional deficiencies and toxic exposure include tobacco–alcohol amblyopia and the Cuban epidemic of optic neuropathy.[10–13]

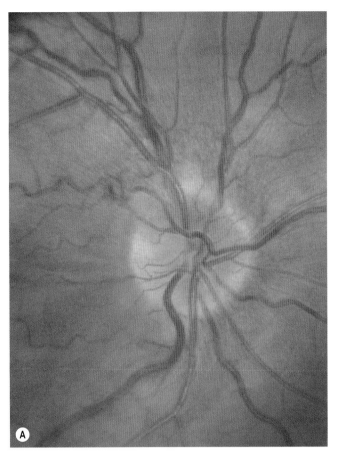 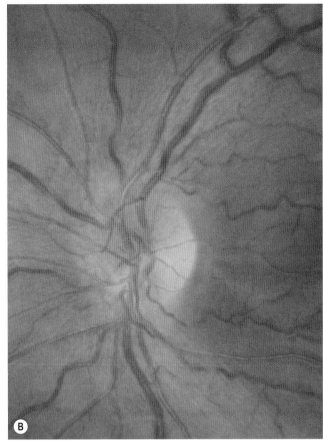

Figure 43.1 Fundus views revealing pseudopapilledema in acute Leber's hereditary optic neuropathy (LHON). (A) Right optic disc. (B) Left optic disc. Swelling is observed involving the retinal nerve fiber layer, particularly in the superior and inferior arcuate bundles, along with marked atrophy of the temporal fibers of the papillomacular bundle. This patient was a 15-year-old male with a family history of LHON mtDNA mutation 11778, who realized he was unable to see centrally in the week prior to presentation. His visual acuity was 20/400 in the right eye and counting fingers in the left eye.

Treatment

As yet, no treatment for LHON has been proven effective. Antioxidants, such as vitamins C, E, and coenzyme Q10, have been offered to patients with LHON. This is based on theoretical grounds related to the electron transfer chain of oxidative phosphorylation, but without any demonstration of clinical efficacy. A coenzyme Q10 analog (idebenone) seems slightly more promising; it offers the additional advantage of transport into mitochondria and a few anecdotal case reports have demonstrated some clinical improvement.[14,15]

Prognosis

Visual recovery has been reported up to several years after vision loss and it is dependent on the age of onset and the specific mtDNA mutation. 14484 mtDNA mutations tend to have the best prognosis, whereas 11778 mtDNA mutations have the worst.[16]

Pathology

A few cases of molecularly characterized LHON have been studied histopathologically; however these tissues were examined several decades after the clinical onset of disease.[17] The most striking finding was the dramatic loss of retinal ganglion cells (RGC) and their axons, which constitute the nerve fiber layer and optic nerve (Figure 43.3). The centrally located small-caliber fibers of the PMB were completely lost, whereas the larger axons of the periphery were spared.[18–20] Mitochondria tend to accumulate in the retinal nerve fiber layer (rNFL) and particularly just anterior to the lamina cribrosa.[9] In the retrolaminar optic nerve, damaged mitochondrial accumulations occurred in demyelinated fibers, with activated astrocytes, glial cells, and lipofuscin-laden macrophages being observed near areas of relative axonal sparing.[17,21] A wide variability in myelin thickness was seen along with evidence of some remyelination.[17]

As yet, no cases of histopathology of LHON have been obtained and examined during the acute phase of the disease. In this regard, rNFL analysis by optical coherence tomography (OCT) has been valuable and demonstrates significant thickening of the rNFL during the early and acute stages of LHON.[22] These findings were most evident in the superior quadrant, followed by the nasal and inferior quadrants. Consistent with the PMB rNFL loss, less significant thickening was observed in the temporal quadrant. In the late stages, OCT revealed that the rNFL was significantly thinned and atrophic, with the temporal fibers being the most severely affected and the nasal fibers being relatively spared.[23] Taken

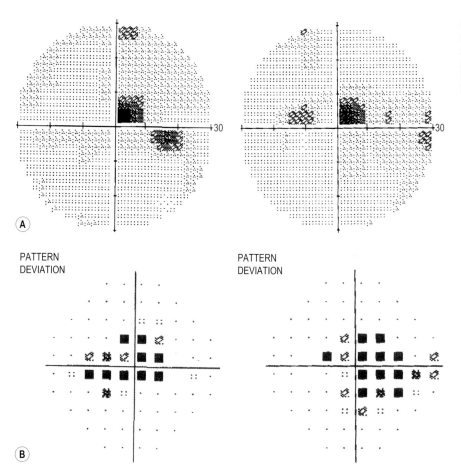

Figure 43.2 Humphrey visual field strategies 30-2. (A) In these gray-scale fields of both eyes, note the bilateral central scotomas. (B) In the pattern deviation images of the same fields, the bilateral cecocentral scotoma (involvement of the blind spots) becomes evident.

as a whole, these studies suggest that the pathophysiology of LHON in the rNFL begins in the PMB and is associated with axonal swelling of the arcuate bundles. As atrophy sets in, the smaller-caliber fibers of the PMB are affected first. Later, the larger-caliber fibers of the arcuate bundles become thinned with comparative sparing of the nasal periphery.

Etiology

As yet, parts of the pathogenesis of LHON remain unclear. However, the underlying inherited basis of this disorder is understood. Though the primary etiologic cause is a mitochondrial genome (mtDNA) mutation, the presence of the LHON mtDNA mutation is necessary but not sufficient to lead to serious visual loss. As this is not a somatic mutation, the term carrier has been applied to those with the mutation but without significant visual loss. Many patients who are asymptomatic carriers may demonstrate subclinical disease, manifested as subtle dyschromatopsia.[24] Affected patients are then said to have converted when they suffer abrupt and serious loss of vision. Thus, the penetrance of LHON is variable. Other genetic, epigenetic, and environmental factors appear to play a role in triggering the phenotypic expression of the disease. Studies of a large Brazilian pedigree of over 300 individuals have demonstrated this variable penetrance and the role of some environmental factors.[10] In particular, smoking tobacco and drinking alcohol seem to increase significantly the odds of conversion from carrier to affected status.[25,26]

Genetic factors

The three most common LHON mtDNA mutations are at nucleotide positions 3460, 14484, and 17788. Approximately 8–25% are due to the 3460 mutation, 10–15% account for the 14484, and 50–70% have the 17788 mutation.[27] A higher amount of Asian LHON patients have the 11778 mtDNA mutation.[28] In most LHON patients and family members, the mtDNA mutation is homoplasmic, containing only mitochondria with the pathogenic mutation. Approximately 14% of LHON patients carry both the mutant and wild-type DNA, a condition known as heteroplasmy. Studies have estimated that the heteroplasmy threshold for the phenotypic expression of LHON was 75–80%.[29] The prevalence of at least some heteroplasmy was 5.6%, 40%, and 36.4% for the 11778, 3460, and 14484 mtDNA mutations, respectively, in 167 unrelated LHON pedigrees.[30]

As stated earlier, approximately 50% of men and 10% of women who carry the LHON mtDNA mutation progress to develop the optic neuropathy.[5] This male bias would suggest that the X chromosome plays a nuclear modulating role in the phenotypic expression of the disease. A previous study of 100 European pedigrees harboring all three mtDNA mutations identified a susceptibility locus on chromosome

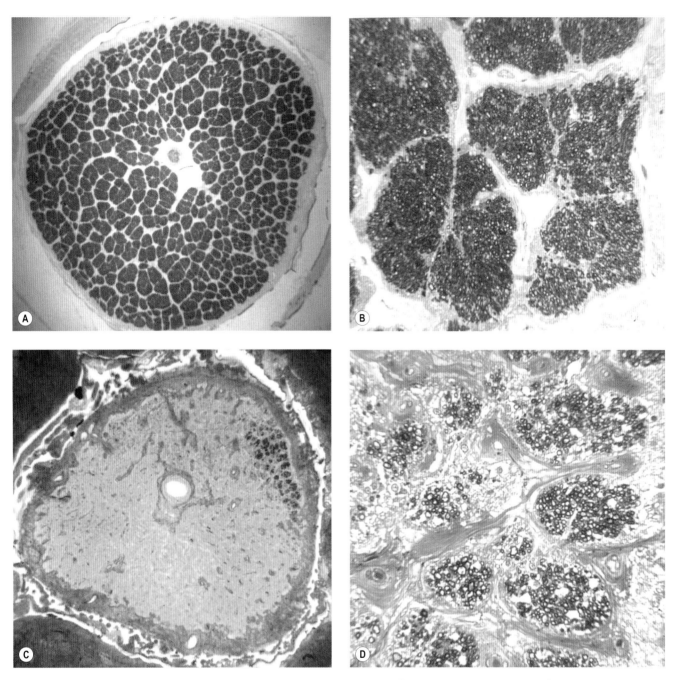

Figure 43.3 Cross-sections through human optic nerves: paraphenylene diamine staining of myelin. (A) Age-matched control of a normal optic nerve with myelinated axons (30×). (B) Higher magnifications (750×) reveal the myelinated bundles. (C) Leber's hereditary optic neuropathy mtDNA 3460 mutation with severe loss of myelinated axons (30×). (D) Higher magnifications (750×) are striking for the loss of myelinated bundles.

Xp21-q21.[31] An additive interaction was observed between this high-risk nuclear haplotype spanning markers DXS8090-DXS1068 and mtDNA haplogroups. It found that 100% of individuals with both this chromosome X haplotype and a nonhaplogroup J background were visually impaired. Another novel susceptibility locus on chromosome Xq25-27.2 has been identified in a large Brazilian pedigree that carry a homoplasmic 11778 mtDNA mutation on a haplogroup J background.[32]

Pathophysiology

Why are RGCs and their fibers in the optic nerve so vulnerable?

There are 1.2 million fibers of the optic nerve that arise from the RGCs of the retina.[33] These RGC are highly concentrated in the perifoveal region and decrease in number moving out to the periphery. From each RGC is derived an

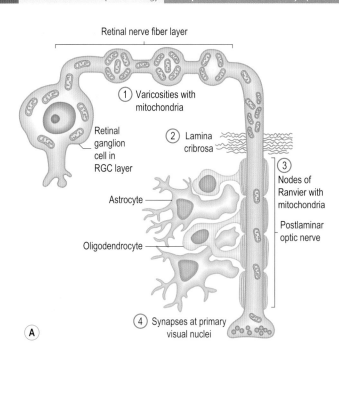

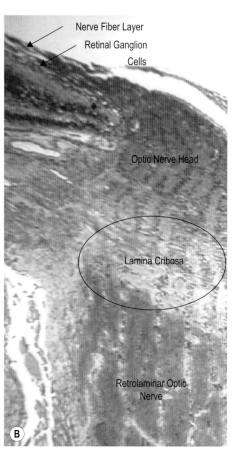

Figure 43.4 (A) Retinal ganglion cell diagram. Mitochondrial accumulations occur in the nerve fiber layer varicosities, the prelaminar and laminar optic nerve, at the nodes of Ranvier, and the axon terminals. (B) Sagittal section of a normal human eye with immunoperoxidase staining. It depicts the transition from the retina to the optic nerve head, passing through the lamina cribrosa to become myelinated retrolaminar optic nerve.

axon which merges into the overlying nerve fiber layer and eventually the optic nerve.[34] Over 90% of the RGC are smaller parvo (P) cells which perform the discriminatory visual functions of high spatial frequency contrast sensitivity, spatial resolution, and color vision. The number of P cells is greatest in the macula. The other 5–10% of the RGC is comprised of the larger magno (M) cells that subserve low spatial frequency contrast sensitivity, depth perception, and motion. The PMB is composed of the smallest rNFL axons, and is dominated by P cells.[35,36]

The mitochondrial genome is very small, comprising only 16 569 basepairs, and most of the protein products necessary for mitochondrial biogenesis are not encoded in its genome. Hence, mitochondria replicate by organelle splitting and budding in the soma, near the nucleus and its chromosomes. Newly made mitochondria are transported down the axon to the terminals, pausing in this passage to provide adenosine triphosphate (ATP) at highly energy-dependent locations. Since the rNFL is unmyelinated and energy-inefficient, mitochondria are plentiful in the prelaminar RGC axons, forming abundantly filled varicosities[37] (Figure 43.4). The prelaminar and laminar regions of the optic nerve head represent another site of high energy dependency.[38] Posterior to the lamina cribrosa, the axons are ensheathed by oligodendrocytes and become myelinated.[34] Because of energy and temporally efficient saltatory conduction, the

number of mitochondria in the retrobulbar optic nerve is dramatically less, though they still congregate in the unmyelinated gaps (nodes of Ranvier) and synaptic terminals. These unmyelinated areas require higher amounts of energy to restore the electrical potential. Thus, an inverse relationship exists between mitochondrial oxidative phosphorylation (OXPHOS) and myelination. Due to their high energy dependence, the unmyelinated rNFL and the prelaminar optic nerve are probably areas that remain the most vulnerable to mitochondrial dysfunction, whether in inherited conditions such as LHON or acquired metabolic disorders.

Mitochondria and oxidative phosphorylation

Mitochondria are double-walled organelles, found in all cells of the body except red blood cells. Located within the mitochondrial matrix are multiple copies of their own 16569-bp circular mtDNA.[39] It encodes for 13 proteins, which are essential subunits of the OXPHOS complexes I, II, IV, and V. The rest of the approximately 80 subunit components are derived and transported from the nuclear genome. Since the OXPHOS chain is under both nuclear and mitochondrial genetic control, diseases that result from mitochondrial dysfunction can be inherited by both mendelian and maternal mitochondrial genetics[40,41] (Figure 43.5).

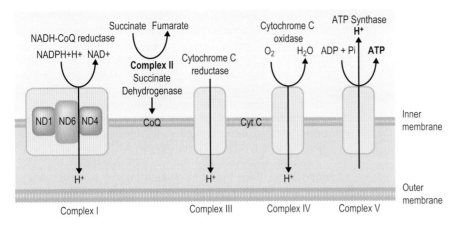

Figure 43.5 The mitochondrial chain of oxidative phosphorylation. The three most common pathogenic Leber's hereditary optic neuropathy mutations 3460, 11778, and 14484, respectively affect the ND1, ND4, and ND6 subunits in complex I. Complexes I and II deliver electrons in parallel to complex III, after which serial electron transfer occurs down the chain to complex V.

Reactive oxygen species

OXPHOS is a vital part of metabolism. Byproducts of this highly efficient generation of ATP are reactive oxygen species (ROS) that are capable of damaging cellular enzymes, mtDNA, and membranes. Excess free electrons primarily spill from complexes I and III to react with molecular oxygen forming superoxide anion (O_2^-). The superoxide anion can undergo several transformations: conversion into hydrogen peroxide (H_2O_2) by manganese superoxide dismutase (MnSOD) or a reaction with nitric oxide (NO) to produce peroxynitrite (ONOO). Hydrogen peroxide can be further transformed by glutathione peroxidase (GPx) into water or react with transition metals to produce the hydroxyl radical (OH) via the Fenton reaction.

The excess ROS may go on to injure the Fe-S centers of complexes I, II, and III and proteins of the tricarboxylic acid cycle enzymes.[42,43] Furthermore, ONOO can damage complex I through thiol-nitrosylation and via the addition of nitrate to tyrosine residues of complex I and MnSOD.[44,45] The ROS can damage the mtDNA itself, resulting in multiple gene deletions, and instigate lipid peroxidation of the mitochondrial membranes. It is likely that this toxic ROS-rich environment provided selection pressure eons ago, such that much of the original mtDNA derived from primitive prokaryotes "moved" to the nuclear chromosomes. For reasons having to do with transmitochondrial membrane transport, only mtDNA encoding for 13 protein products remained in the mitochondria still vulnerable to the damaging effect of the ROS.

Mitochondrial role in apoptosis

There are many parallel pathways that converge and diverge in the regulation of the execution of apoptosis. However, one important process appears to use mitochondria as a lynch pin that determines cellular death by apoptosis.[46] OXPHOS, ROS, the mitochondrial inner membrane potential, and calcium fluxes are all involved in the regulation of mitochondrial permeability. If circumstances allow a critical threshold to be reached, small gates called mitochondrial permeability transition pores can open, allowing the release of proapoptotic factors. These gates are also under nuclear control by proapoptotic signals such as Bax, Bak, Bim, and Bid and the anti-apoptotic protein Bcl-2, which blocks *cyt c*

release.[47,48] *Cyt c*, which functions as an electron carrier to complex IV, can then pass through the mitochondrial membrane into the cytosol to form a complex called "apoptosome." This cleaves procaspase 9 to become caspase 9, setting off a chain of caspase reactions that leads to the destruction of somatic DNA and apoptosis.[46]

Biochemical effects of the mtDNA mutations

Complex I of the respiratory chain is composed of 39 nuclear and seven mitochondrial encoded subunits.[49] The three most common pathogenic LHON mutations, 3464, 11778, and 14484, respectively affect the ND1, ND4, and ND6 subunits in complex I. Cellular models using transmitochondrial hybrids called cybrids have been widely used in order to study the effect of the mtDNA mutations on complex I activity. A significant reduction in complex I activity was observed with the 3460/ND1 mutation, whereas minimal reductions were noted with the 11778/ND4 and 14484/ND6 mutations.[50] Rotenone is a powerful complex I inhibitor that acts as a coenzyme Q intermediate antagonist and the mitochondrial activity of each LHON mtDNA mutations is variously affected by it. The 11778/ND4 and 14484/ND6 mutations seem to have decreased sensitivity to rotenone. The biochemical effect of other product inhibitors such as quinol and myxothiazol have also been evaluated and all three common mutations are observed to have increased sensitivity.[50] This suggests that LHON mutations impair the interaction of complex I with the Q substrate.

Proposed LHON pathogenesis that leads to RGC death

There are two main consequences of complex I dysfunction as evidenced in LHON: impaired efficiency of the respiratory chain manifested as a reduction in ATP synthesis and increased ROS production. In turn, the decreased ATP production may lead to slowed axoplasmic transport, particularly of mitochondria. Consequently, axonal swelling and stasis develop in the prelaminar unmyelinated portion at the optic nerve head. The mitochondria, which must make their way from the RGC soma down the long axons of the optic nerve to their synaptic terminals in the brain, have a short lifespan, in the order of a week or two. Thus, their failure to arrive in a timely fashion would ultimately lead to retrograde

---

Box 43.1 Key points

- The majority of Leber's cases are caused by three common mtDNA point mutations at nucleotide positions 3460, 11778, and 14484, which respectively affect the ND1, ND4, and ND6 subunits in complex I of the respiratory chain

- Leber's hereditary optic neuropathy has a variable penetrance. Other genetic, epigenetic, and environmental factors appear to play a role in triggering the phenotypic expression of the disease

- All mitochondrial optic neuropathies similarly manifest with cecocentral scotomas, dyschromatopsia, poor vision, and a loss of high spatial frequency contrast sensitivity. Leber's hereditary optic neuropathy is perhaps the best-studied model of mitochondrial deficiency

---

and result in the progressive decompensation of the RGC and optic nerve system. Hence, it is not so surprising that all mitochondrial optic neuropathies can manifest similarly with cecocentral scotomas, dyschromatopsia, poor visual acuity, and a loss of high spatial frequency contrast sensitivity. LHON is perhaps the best-studied model of mitochondrial deficiency and recent discoveries, such as the demonstration of subclinical disease, are likely to have applications in other related mitochondrial optic neuropathies of inherited (Kjer's), metabolic, and toxic etiologies.

Since the discovery of point mtDNA mutations in LHON, progress has been made in elucidating the pathogenesis of the disease (Box 43.1). However, much has yet to be clarified about the male predilection, incomplete penetrance, and abrupt age-related onset of vision loss. Cellular and animal models will likely pave the way for understanding the complex biochemical interactions, nuclear and mtDNA genomic factors, and pathologic progression of the disease. Future therapeutic modalities for LHON could be directed toward a genetic approach to prevent optic atrophy, the discovery of ROS scavengers, and antiapoptotic strategies once the onset of vision loss transpires. However since many of these therapies will require the resolution of complex biochemical and biological issues, currently we look forward to the development of serum biomarkers and psychophysical measures to identify patients with early disease or at least subclinical evidence that decompensation may be near.

wallerian degeneration of the optic nerve fibers. Compounding this loss of energy and axonal stasis, the impairment in complex I activity results in the accumulation of ROS which can, at a certain threshold, lead to RGC and axon death by apoptosis. The small fibers of the PMB are uniquely vulnerable to this process, responding with an early and rapid wave of cellular death.

These described mechanisms are likely to be critical in the different inborn and acquired impairments of mitochondria

Key references

A complete list of chapter references is available online at www.expertconsult.com. See inside cover for registration details.

3. Wallace DC, Singh G, Lott MT, et al. Mitochondrial DNA mutation associated with Leber's hereditary optic neuropathy. Science 1988;242:1427–1430.

4. Carelli V, Ross-Cisneros FN, Sadun AA. Mitochondrial dysfunction as a cause of optic neuropathies. Prog Retin Eye Res 2004;23:53–89.

5. Mackey DA, Oostra R-J, Rosenberg T, et al. Primary pathogenic mtDNA mutations in multigeneration pedigrees with Leber hereditary optic neuropathy. Am J Hum Genet 1996;59:481–485.

7. Newman NJ, Lott MT, Wallace DC. The clinical characteristics of pedigrees of Leber's hereditary optic neuropathy with the 11778 mutation. Am J Ophthalmol 1991;111:750–762.

9. Sadun AA, Carelli V, Salomao SR, et al. A very large Brazilian pedigree with 117 788 Leber's hereditary optic neuropathy. Trans Am Ophthalmol Soc 2002;100:169–178; discussion 178–179.

17. Carelli V. Leber's hereditary optic neuropathy. In: Schapira AHV, DiMauro

S (eds) Mitochondrial Disorders in Neurology, 2nd edn. Boston: Butterworth-Heinemann, 2002:115–142.

18. Sadun AA, Kashima Y, Wurdeman AE, et al. Morphological findings in the visual system in a case of Leber's hereditary optic neuropathy. Clin Neurosci 1994;2:165–172.

19. Sadun AA. Acquired mitochondrial impairment as a cause of optic nerve disease. Trans Am Soc 1998;XCVI:881–923.

20. Sadun AA, Win PH, Ross-Cisneros FN, et al. Leber's hereditary optic neuropathy differentially affects smaller axons in the optic nerve. Trans Am Ophthalmol Soc 2000;98:223–235.

22. Barboni P, Savini G, Valentino ML, et al. Leber's hereditary optic neuropathy with childhood onset. Invest Ophthalmol Vis Sci 2006;47:5303–5309.

23. Barboni P, Savini G, Valentino ML, et al. Retinal nerve fiber layer evaluation by optical coherence tomography in

Leber's hereditary optic neuropathy. Ophthalmology 2005;112:120–126.

24. Ventura DF, Quiros P, Carelli V, et al. Chromatic and luminance contrast sensitivities in asymptomatic carriers from a large Brazilian pedigree of 11778 Leber hereditary optic neuropathy. Invest Ophthalmol Vis Sci 2005;46:4809–4814.

25. Sadun AA, Carelli V, Salomao SR, et al. Extensive investigation of large Brazilian pedigree of Italian ancestry (SOA-BR) with 117788/haplogroup J Leber's hereditary optic neuropathy (LHON). Am J Ophthalmol 2003;136:231–238.

26. Sadun F, De Negri A, Carelli V, et al. Ophthalmologic findings in large pedigree of 11778/haplogroup J Leber's hereditary optic neuropathy. Am J Ophthalmol 2004;137:271–277.

46. Sadun AA, Carelli V. The role of mitochondria in health, aging, and diseases affecting vision. Br J Ophthalmol 2006;90:809–810.

CHAPTER 44

Optic atrophy

Nathan T Tagg and Randy H Kardon

Clinical background

Optic atrophy can be considered the wasting of a once-healthy optic nerve. This definition excludes conditions associated with optic nerve dysplasia, hypoplasia, or aplasia in which the optic nerve is developmentally and structurally abnormal. Optic atrophy is the final common result of injury to the retinal ganglion cells, nerve fiber layer, optic nerve, chiasm, or optic tract. Additionally, prenatal or perinatal injury of posterior structures including occipital cortex may result in transsynaptic degeneration of the optic nerves.[1] The range and variety of potential insults to these structures are vast and include: vascular, infectious, metabolic, traumatic, toxic, neoplastic/paraneoplastic, autoimmune/inflammatory, compressive, and inherited etiologies. The evolution of optic atrophy depends on the location and extent of injury as well as the nature of the insult (i.e., rapid progression in the case of traumatic section of the optic nerve versus slow progression in the case of optic nerve sheath meningioma). Because optic atrophy is a late marker of irreversible optic nerve injury and not a disease itself, visual symptoms are directly related to the underlying pathology.

Localizing value of optic atrophy patterns

Segmental or regional atrophy of the retinal nerve fiber layer (RNFL) or pallor of the optic disc, in concert with the clinical history and other exam findings, may have localizing value. Nonarteritic anterior ischemic optic neuropathy (NAION) often preferentially affects the superotemporal fibers, producing inferonasal visual field loss. Segmental pallor of the optic disc can often be appreciated after the acute swelling has resolved. Segmental pallor not preceded by optic disc edema may result from a nonischemic optic nerve lesion (Figure 44.1A) and may be indistinguishable from post-swelling NAION.

Segmental atrophy has localizing value in the case of band atrophy (Figure 44.2) or so-called "bowtie" atrophy,[2] such as in lesions of the optic chiasm or optic tract[3] (Box 44.1).

Temporal pallor may be seen when a disease processes preferentially affects the maculopapillary bundle, such as toxicity, vitamin deficiency, inherited optic neuropathy, and demyelination.[4] Apparent temporal pallor can be seen in normal individuals but does not represent atrophy; the nerve fiber layer coursing into the optic disc is thinnest in this region and so the neuroretinal rim may not be as pink in this sector. Additionally, there may be other factors such as an enlarged cup or a scleral temporal crescent that give the appearance of pallor when there is no atrophy.

Diffuse optic atrophy (Figure 44.1C) has less potential localizing value than segmental atrophy. If it is strictly unilateral, it localizes to the ipsilateral optic nerve. Bilateral diffuse optic atrophy has the least localizing value as it can be due to disorders of both optic nerves, optic chiasm, bilateral optic tracts or, in rare cases, bilateral postgeniculate visual structures occurring in the perinatal period (see discussion of transsynaptic degeneration, above).[1]

Segmental atrophy in the form of pathological cupping is seen in the case of glaucoma as notching of the neuroretinal rim (Figure 44.1D).

Mimics of optic atrophy

Any condition that causes the disc to appear pale in the absence of atrophy may lead to misdiagnosis of optic atrophy. A common condition is aphakic or pseudophakic pseudopallor (Figure 44.3E). This results after lens extraction because of loss of the light-attenuating properties of the natural lens. In a unilateral pseudophakic patient who has a nuclear cataract in the fellow eye, the difference in the color of the discs is even more pronounced because nuclear sclerosis causes the disc to appear redder than normal.[5]

Another condition which may mimic optic atrophy is the setting of resolved optic disc edema, in which there may be significant gliosis over the optic disc. The disc may look pale but there will be a normal or even thickened peripapillary RNFL by optical coherence tomography (OCT). Myelinated nerve fibers may also give the appearance of disc pallor (Figure 44.3A). This can be segmental (occurring in only one portion of the disc) or diffuse (covering the entire disc). Arteritic anterior ischemic optic neuropathy (AION) is occasionally associated with pallid swelling of the optic nerve during the acute stage due to optic nerve infarction (Figure 44.3B). Infiltrative diseases such as lymphoma may also present with a pale but not atrophic nerve. Buried drusen and retinitis pigmentosa (Figure 44.3C and 44.3D) are also occasionally associated with optic disc pallor, but not necessarily atrophy.

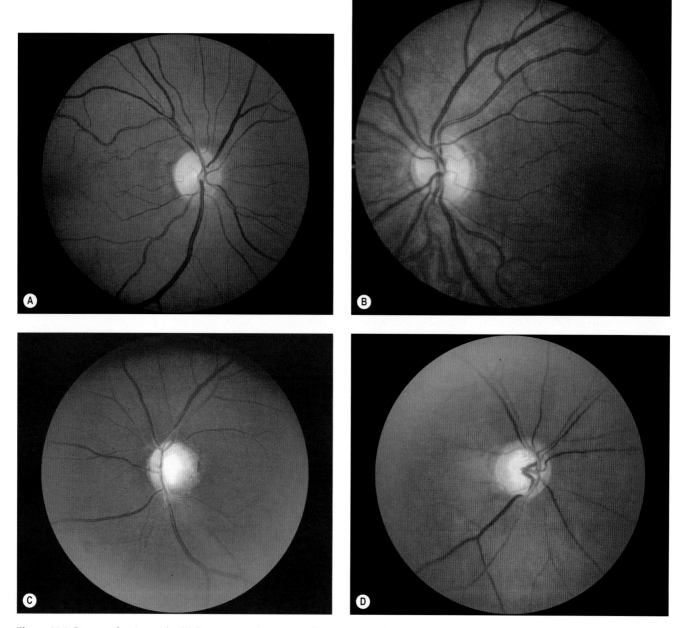

Figure 44.1 Patterns of optic atrophy. (A) Superotemporal sector atrophy in a 59-year-old woman with a supraclinoid internal carotid artery aneurysm compressing the optic nerve. (B) Band ("bowtie") atrophy in an 8-year-old boy with a craniopharyngioma compressing the optic chiasm. (C) Diffuse optic atrophy in a 41-year-old woman with neuromyelitis optica after a severe attack that left her with no light perception. (D) Glaucomatous cupping with atrophy of the superior and inferior neuroretinal rim appearing as "notching" of the neuroretinal rim and vertical elongation of the cup.

Box 44.1 Optic atrophy clinical pearls

- Band atrophy localizes to the contralateral optic tract if unilateral and the optic chiasm if bilateral
- Pallor of the temporal optic disc can be a normal finding; it should be judged in the context of all available clinical information
- Unilateral atrophy with optic disc edema in the fellow eye likely represents a subfrontal intracranial mass lesion or bilateral, nonsimultaneous nonarteritic anterior ischemic optic neuropathy
- "Pseudoatrophy" occurs when the optic disc appears pale without evidence of atrophy

Pathophysiology

Pathogenic mechanisms of optic atrophy

Under experimental conditions, atrophy of the optic nerve occurs as a predictable, reproducible, and irreversible response to injury of retinal ganglion cells or their axons. Injured axons degenerate in both a retrograde (toward the cell body) and antegrade (wallerian degeneration – away from the cell body) fashion. An eventual additional consequence of axon injury is apoptosis of retinal ganglion cells (RGCs).

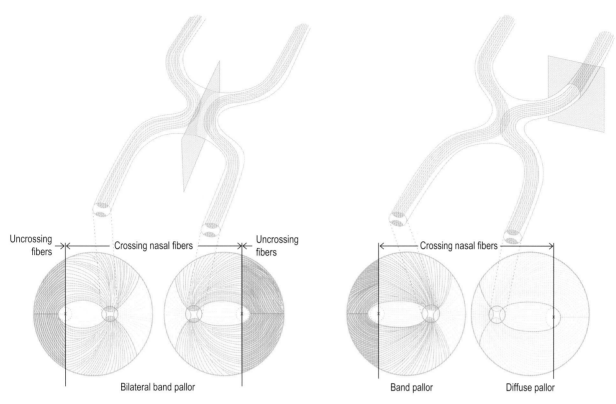

Uncrossing fibers | Crossing nasal fibers | Uncrossing fibers

Bilateral band pallor

Crossing nasal fibers

Band pallor | Diffuse pallor

Figure 44.2 The basis of band atrophy in optic chiasm and tract lesions. The maculopapillary and temporal wedge retinal nerve fiber layer bundles are disproportionately represented on the nasal (crossing) side of the fundus. Damage to these crossing fibers causes selective atrophy of the nasal and temporal segments of the disc and the pattern of "band" pallor results. Chiasmal lesions (left) cause bilateral band atrophy/pallor. Optic tract lesions (right) cause contralateral band atrophy/pallor and ipsilateral diffuse atrophy/pallor. (Modified from Hoyt WF, Rios-Montenegro EN, Behrens MM, et al. Homonymous hemioptic hypoplasia. Fundoscopic features in standard and red-free illumination in three patients with congenital hemiplegia. Br J Ophthalmol 1972;56:537–545.)

A murine model of antegrade degeneration has made use of a spontaneously occurring dominant mutation dubbed Wld[s] for "slow wallerian degeneration." Mice with this mutation have significantly delayed wallerian degeneration after a variety of insults, including traumatic, toxic, and genetic insults.[6] Studies indicate that important final common pathway features of antegrade degeneration include failure of antegrade axonal transport from the cell body followed by mitochondrial failure. These cause a rise in intra-axonal Ca^{2+} which activates calpain, a proteolytic enzyme whose activation results in degradation of the cytoskeleton and membrane proteins.[7] The genetic defect in the Wld[s] murine model appears to resist this series of events after an experimental crush injury, delaying but not preventing atrophy. A recent study by Wang et al[8] demonstrated that axon degeneration and RGC body death proceed via different cellular mechanisms. They showed that, after optic nerve axotomy, Wld[s] mice showed the expected delay in axonal degeneration but no delay in RGC body (retrograde) degeneration, even though the Wld[s] gene product appears to be located in the RGC nucleus.

While optic atrophy secondary to transsynaptic retrograde axonal degeneration (from an injury to the occipital cortex or lateral geniculate body) has been rigorously demonstrated in primates,[9] evidence that it occurs in humans is anecdotal and based only on case reports.[1,10] There are conflicting opinions regarding its occurrence in older children and adults[11]

but most authors believe this phenomenon only occurs in patients who have sustained perinatal or prenatal cerebral injuries.[11,12] The cellular mechanisms which underlie trans-synaptic degeneration are not well understood. In addition, there is evidence that prenatal cerebral injury results not in optic atrophy but in a specific pattern of optic nerve hypoplasia.[3]

Pathogenic mechanisms of optic disc pallor

The clinical hallmark of nonglaucomatous optic atrophy is pallor of the optic disc, seen ophthalmoscopically (Box 44.2). Strictly speaking, "pallor" is a subjective and comparative term that is somewhat ill-defined. To state that a disc is pale requires appreciation of "normal" disc color, which can vary widely among individuals. Furthermore, factors which may influence perception of the disc color include the color of the background fundus (a darkly colored fundus may make a normal optic disc appear relatively pale), the size of the physiologic optic cup (a larger cup shows more of the white lamina cribrosa), and the patient's refraction (a myopic eye may have a white scleral crescent adjacent to the disc, making it appear pale).[4] It is often helpful to compare the color of the disc in the fellow eye in cases of suspected unilateral optic atrophy. It is important to understand the mechanisms responsible for the development of optic disc pallor when making a diagnosis of optic atrophy.

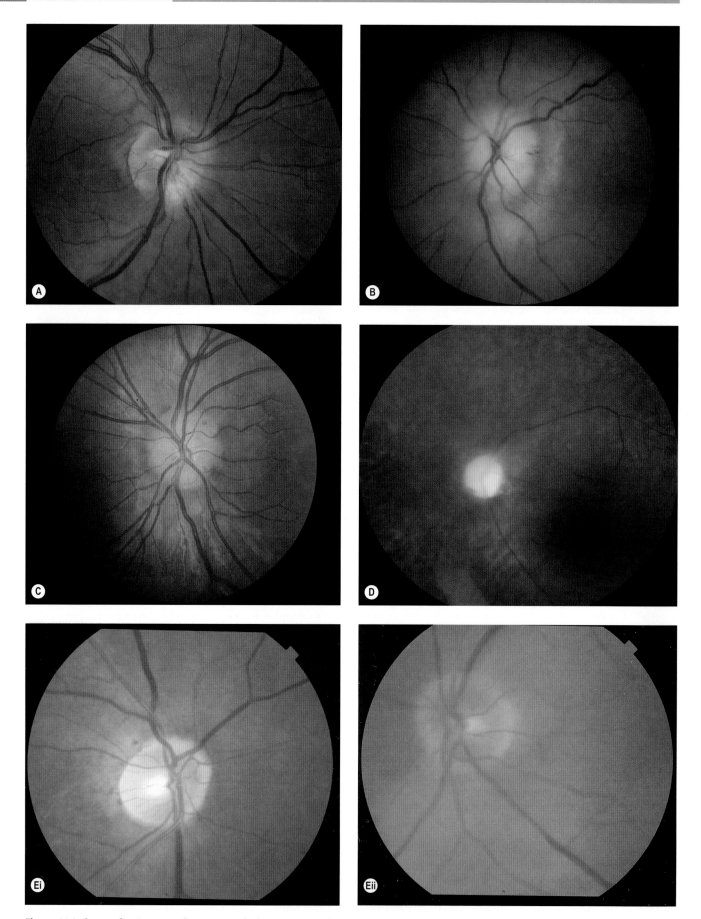

Figure 44.3 Causes of optic nerve pallor not primarily due to optic atrophy. (A) Segmental myelination of intraocular nerve fiber layer. (B) Acute arteritic anterior ischemic optic neuropathy (AAION). (C) Buried drusen. (D) Retinitis pigmentosa. (E) Pseudophakic pseudopallor: (i) right eye and (ii) left eye, same patient.

Box 44.2 Pallor of the optic disc

- The clinical hallmark of optic atrophy is pallor of the optic disc
- Optic disc pallor occurs as a result of astrocytic element rearrangement with collapse onto the optic disc
- Nerve fiber layer loss can be measured as early as 3 weeks after optic nerve injury whereas pallor is a later manifestation

In 1977, Quigley and Anderson[13] reported the results of an elegant study, entitled "The histologic basis of optic disk pallor in experimental optic atrophy." In this study, optic nerve axotomy was performed on 10 squirrel monkeys. The clinical appearance of the fundus and histological features of the optic nerve head were followed over time. They found that several factors contributed to the appearance of optic disc pallor, including loss of RCG axons and rearrangement of astrocytes at the disc head. They did not find significantly increased astrogliosis overlying the optic disc or loss of disc capillaries. The authors postulated that the normal appearance of the neuroretinal rim was due to light traveling into the substance of the disc via the bare ganglion cell axons (a "fiberoptic" effect). The incident light diffuses among the adjacent columns of glial cells and capillaries and the reflected light is tinted by the pink color of the capillaries within the light path. However, after damage, when axons disappear secondary to atrophy, the astrocytes collapse on to the disc head (Figure 44.4) and are no longer oriented in columns but are arranged at right-angles to the entering light, reflecting it back like a mirror. Thus, pallor results from decreased transmission of light into the cytoarchitecture of the atrophic nerve head and not from absence of capillaries[14] or from extensive astrocytic proliferation.[13]

Thus, mere loss of axonal mass at the disc head is a necessary but not sufficient condition for pallor. There must also be rearrangement and collapse of astrocytic elements onto the disc head. The time course of these changes may depend heavily on the nature and pace of the inciting injury.

Timing and evolution of optic atrophy

The development of optic atrophy in response to traumatic injury of the optic nerve has been well studied both clinically in humans and experimentally in primates and other animals. Because these studies involve sudden and complete nerve injury, they provide a framework for understanding the "worst-case scenario" of pathological and clinical changes in the optic nerve over time, i.e., the maximum rate at which changes occur.

Pathological studies of retrograde optic nerve degeneration in squirrel monkeys, involving complete axotomy of the optic nerve at the orbital apex, have shown that there is no significant change in the histologic appearance of the optic nerve proximal to the injury for up to 4 weeks after axotomy. After 6 weeks, there is definite axonal degeneration seen on histopathologic sections characterized by condensed mitochondria, crinkled lipoprotein membranes, and disintegration of microtubules. By 8 weeks, most axons proximal to the lesion were entirely disintegrated.[15]

Lundstrom and Frisen in 1975[16] described a patient who suffered complete, traumatic intracranial optic nerve transec-

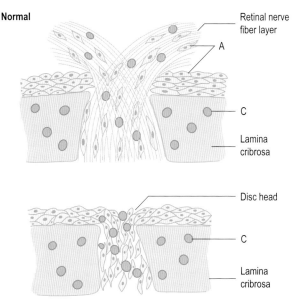

Figure 44.4 Histologic mechanism of the appearance of optic disc pallor. Top: normal: astrocytes (A) are interspersed among the axons of the optic nerve. Light is conducted into the substance of the disc by the nerve fiber bundles. Light then diffuses among the columns of astrocytes and capillaries (C) and the disc thus acquires its characteristic pink color. Bottom: atrophic state: when axons degenerate, astrocytes collapse on to the disc head at right angles to the incident light, reflecting it back. Histologically, there is no significant astrocytic gliosis that occurs, nor is there significant loss of disc capillaries. (Modified from Quigley HA, Anderson DR. The histologic basis of optic disk pallor in experimental optic atrophy. Am J Ophthalmol 1977;83:709–717.)

tion just anterior to the chiasm caused by a self-inflicted gunshot wound. The lesion resulted in no-light-perception vision with complete loss of the pupil light reflex in the ipsilateral eye and a superior temporal visual field defect in the contralateral eye . The patient was followed for 12 weeks with serial fundus photographs and ophthalmoscopy. After 25 days, there was no change in either the nerve fiber layer (assessed using red-free photography) or the appearance of the optic disc. At around 30 days, the nerve fiber layer started to show atrophy and by 47 days there was near complete loss of the nerve fiber layer. Interestingly, the optic disc still appeared normal, and without pallor at this time. Not until day 60 was there initial evidence of optic disc pallor and not until day 85 was there conspicuous pallor of the optic disc. A subset of nasal fibers from the fellow eye was also affected by the same lesion (just anterior to the chiasm) and demonstrated atrophy over the same time course. The authors concluded that retrograde atrophy occurring gradually affected the entire length of the nerve simultaneously and was not "length-dependent." This conclusion was drawn from the observation that affected axons from both eyes atrophied at the same rate, despite the fact that affected axons from the contralateral eye were longer, coursing through the chiasm.[16]

Newer, more sensitive methods have been used to measure earlier changes in the nerve fiber layer after traumatic injury. In a report by Medeiros et al,[17] a 14-year-old boy with traumatic optic neuropathy was studied using OCT to follow peripapillary RNFL thickness over time. As soon as 20 days after injury, the average nerve fiber layer thickness had

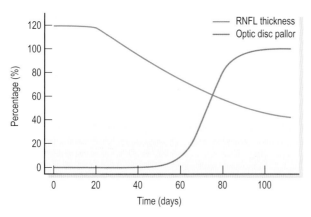

Figure 44.5 Time course of optic atrophy (measured) and pallor (hypothetical) after sudden intracanalicular or intracranial optic neuropathy. Shortly after the insult, there is a slight increase in the retinal nerve fiber layer (RNFL) thickness in some patients, presumably from axonal swelling at the level of the optic disc. Thereafter, the RNFL follows an exponential decline in thickness.[18] Pallor is not first appreciated until about 60 days after the insult and is maximal by about 85 days.[16]

decreased by 40%.[17] Meier et al[18] documented the time course of RNFL loss by scanning laser polarimetry in 5 patients with severe acute optic neuropathy and found that it followed a model of exponential decay (Figure 44.5).

These studies suggest that measurable atrophy occurs before pallor can be detected ophthalmoscopically and only after significant atrophy does the optic nerve appear pale. They also underscore the notion that mere axonal loss is not sufficient to produce pallor; there must be rearrangement of the astroglial elements over the optic disc. This should be kept in mind by the clinician who may rely too heavily on the optic nerve appearance to detect permanent optic nerve damage.

The extent and timing of axon loss in nontraumatic lesions may not correlate well with the degree and duration of dysfunction, since many causes of injury may interfere with optic nerve conduction without permanent axonal damage. However, once permanent axon damage occurs, measurable changes in the thickness of the RNFL proceed at a rate commensurate with the nature and degree of injury. For example, atrophy secondary to an optic nerve sheath meningioma may be quite gradual over years, whereas atrophy secondary to AION will be much more rapid. In practice, many insults to the optic nerve occur over long periods of time and do not reach the threshold for triggering axonal degeneration and cell death for weeks to months or longer. It may take even more time for pallor to be appreciated.

Structure/function relationships in optic atrophy

The relationship between optic atrophy and optic nerve function is only beginning to be elucidated (Box 44.3). Hood et al[19-21] demonstrated that, for certain optic neuropathies such as NAION and glaucoma, there is a strong linear correlation between RNFL thickness (measured by OCT) and visual field function (measured by standard automated perimetry). This relationship may not hold for other etiologies such as optic neuritis or compressive optic neuropathy.

On occasion, visual function is severely depressed out of proportion to the degree of RNFL axon loss. This occurs most often when conduction block is present, as in the case of chronic compressive lesions (i.e., pituitary adenoma compressing the chiasm) or demyelination (i.e., optic neuritis). It may also occur in the setting of subacute injury (i.e., not enough time has passed for atrophy or pallor to be appreciated). In the case of compression, the extent of damage is great enough to impair functioning but not (yet) great enough to induce axonal degeneration and ganglion cell apoptosis. This has important clinical implications because such patients can expect significant improvement in vision after decompression of the optic apparatus even after years of compression, providing there is preservation of the RNFL.

Conclusions

While the causes of irreversible optic nerve injury are myriad, the end result is universal: loss of RGC bodies and axons. This almost always results in pallor of the optic disc which may be diffuse or segmental, unilateral, or bilateral. When taken in context with other clinical parameters, the pattern of optic disc pallor can often help determine the localization and etiology of a problem. Absence of atrophy and pallor can be equally useful in cases of severe vision loss secondary to chronic optic nerve compression or demyelination. Recognition of common mimics of optic disc pallor is important in avoiding misdiagnosis.

Key references

A complete list of chapter references is available online at www.expertconsult.com. See inside cover for registration details.

2. Unsold R, Hoyt WF. Band atrophy of the optic nerve. The histology of temporal hemianopsia. Arch Ophthalmol 1980;98: 1637–1638.

6. Vargas ME, Barres BA. Why is Wallerian degeneration in the CNS so slow? Annu Rev Neurosci 2007;30:153–179.

7. Coleman M. Axon degeneration mechanisms: commonality amid diversity. Nat Rev Neurosci 2005;6: 889–898.

8. Wang AL, Yuan M, Neufeld AH. Degeneration of neuronal cell bodies following axonal injury in Wld(S) mice. J Neurosci Res 2006;84:1799–1807.

13. Quigley HA, Anderson DR. The histologic basis of optic disk pallor in experimental optic atrophy. Am J Ophthalmol 1977;83:709–717.

14. Radius RL, Anderson DR. The mechanism of disc pallor in experimental optic atrophy. A fluorescein angiographic study. Arch Ophthalmol 1979;97:532–535.

15. Anderson DR. Ascending and descending optic atrophy produced experimentally in squirrel monkeys. Am J Ophthalmol 1973;76:693–711.

16. Lundstrom M, Frisen L. Evolution of descending optic atrophy. A case report. Acta Ophthalmol (Copenh) 1975;53:738–746.

17. Medeiros FA, Moura FC, Vessani RM, et al. Axonal loss after traumatic optic neuropathy documented by optical coherence tomography. Am J Ophthalmol 2003;135:406–408.

18. Meier FM, Bernasconi P, Sturmer J, et al. Axonal loss from acute optic neuropathy documented by scanning laser polarimetry. Br J Ophthalmol 2002;86:285–287.

19. Hood DC, Anderson S, Rouleau J, et al. Retinal nerve fiber structure versus visual field function in patients with ischemic optic neuropathy a test of a linear model. Ophthalmology 2008;115:904–910.

20. Hood DC, Anderson SC, Wall M, et al. Structure versus function in glaucoma: an application of a linear model. Invest Ophthalmol Vis Sci 2007;48:3662–3668.

CHAPTER 45

Nystagmus

Frank Proudlock and Irene Gottlob

Introduction

Nystagmus is defined as a rhythmic oscillation of the eyes. The term "nystagmus" is a transliteration of a Greek word for "drowsy head-nodding movements," since the jerky eye movements seen in many types of nystagmus resemble the slow downward drift and upward-jerking head movements observed when sleepy. Nystagmus caused by pathology is essentially involuntary, although individuals may be able to modulate certain features of their nystagmus voluntarily. The appearance of the eye movements in nystagmus is extremely diverse.[1] They can be described using a number of characteristics which can also assist in the diagnosis[2,3] (Figure 45.1A):

- Intensity: the overall speed or intensity of the eye movements can be estimated by multiplying the amplitude (degrees) with the frequency (hertz) of the eye movements.
- Plane: nystagmus most commonly occurs along the horizontal axis, although nystagmus can also be vertical, torsional, or any combination of these, such as seesaw nystagmus (vertical with torsional) or cyclorotatory nystagmus (horizontal with vertical).
- Waveform: historically, nystagmus has been divided into jerk nystagmus, which exhibits a quick and slow phase, and pendular nystagmus, which is a sinusoidal-like oscillation without any obvious quick phase. Many nystagmus waveforms, however, are more complex, often consisting of an underlying pendular oscillation interrupted by regularly occurring quick phases.
- Conjugacy: with most nystagmus the eyes move in tandem and are described as conjugate or associated. Disconjugate or dissociated nystagmus occurs when the eye movements differ in amplitude, frequency, waveform, or when the oscillations of the two eyes are out of phase with each other.
- Foveation: many forms of congenital nystagmus show periods where the eyes move at a lower velocity allowing high-acuity vision at the fovea to function. The dynamics of these foveation periods can be related to visual acuity.[4]
- Dependence on other parameters: certain types of nystagmus waveform are not constant but vary with time (e.g., can be intermittent or reverse direction), monocular or binocular viewing, convergence or eccentricity of gaze (Figure 45.1B). Nystagmus may also be associated with head movements.

Nystagmus can be grouped into infantile nystagmus, which usually appears within the first few months of life, and acquired nystagmus. Acquired nystagmus is typically associated with oscillopsia, the perception that the world is in motion.[5,6] This can be extremely disabling, leading to worse visual function than is caused by low vision or age-related macular degeneration.[7] Nystagmus leads to deterioration in visual acuity mainly because of deterioration in foveal vision when images move across the retina rapidly.[4] The constant motion can also lead to reduced motion sensitivity.[8] Nystagmus can also have a significant psychological and social impact.[7]

A classification scheme for pathological nystagmus has been proposed by the National Eye Institute, USA, under the Classification of Eye Movement Abnormalities and Strabismus (CEMAS).[9] Nystagmus has been subdivided into: (1) infantile nystagmus syndrome; (2) fusion maldevelopment nystagmus syndrome; (3) spasmus nutans syndrome; (4) vestibular nystagmus; (5) gaze-holding deficiency nystagmus; (6) vision loss nystagmus; (7) other pendular nystagmus and nystagmus associated with disease of central myelin; (8) ocular bobbing (typical and atypical); and (9) lid nystagmus. Although the CEMAS classification is comprehensive and includes all forms of nystagmus it is mainly based on the nystagmus waveform observed using eye movement recordings which can be difficult to determine in routine clinical practice. It also pools together many forms of infantile nystagmus such as idiopathic infantile nystagmus (IIN), nystagmus associated with albinism, and achromatopsia.

The prevalence of nystagmus is 2.4 per 1000.[10] The main types of childhood nystagmus are IIN, associated with albinism, nystagmus secondary to retinal disease and low vision, manifest latent nystagmus (MLN), spasmus nutans, and nystagmus due to neurological syndromes (Figure 45.2). Acquired nystagmus can result from a range of neurological disorders, of which the most common are multiple sclerosis, disease of the vestibular apparatus and innervations, insult to the nervous system caused by stroke, tumours, or trauma, and as a result of drug toxicity.

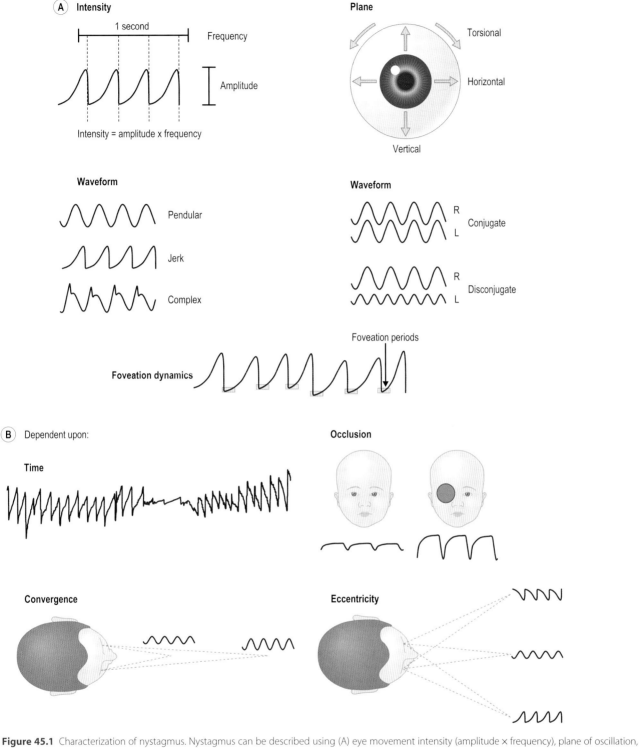

Figure 45.1 Characterization of nystagmus. Nystagmus can be described using (A) eye movement intensity (amplitude × frequency), plane of oscillation, waveform, conjugacy between right (R) and left (L) eyes, and duration and position of periods when the velocity of eye movements is slow enough to allow useful foveal vision (foveation). (B) Some of these characteristics can also vary with time, occlusion of one eye, convergence, and eccentricity of eye position.

Infantile nystagmus

Manifest latent nystagmus

Clinical background

MLN (classified as "fusion maldevelopment nystagmus syndrome" by CEMAS) is a predominantly horizontal, jerk nystagmus that becomes more apparent when one eye is covered (Box 45.1).[11] It is caused by a slow drift towards the covered eye with corrective quick phases towards the open fixing eye. In almost all patients, nystagmus is present with both eyes open: it is smaller in intensity and may be subclinical in size.[12] The manifest component describes the nystagmus observed when both eyes are open and the latent component

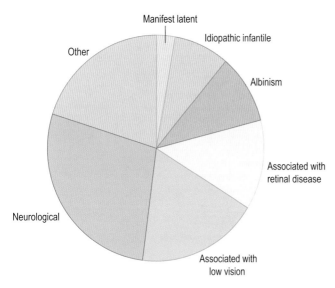

Figure 45.2 A breakdown of the types of nystagmus (taken from 357 patients attending clinics in Leicester Royal Infirmary, UK, between February 2002 and October 2007).

Box 45.1 Manifest latent nystagmus

Characteristics

- Predominantly a horizontal, jerk nystagmus with decelerating slow phases
- The manifest component of the nystagmus is evident when both eyes are open
- The latent component (increase in nystagmus amplitude) is revealed when one eye is occluded

Underlying cause

- Interruption of binocular visual development, through strabismus and amblyopia, leading to a nasalward bias of the eyes
- This leads to a drift towards the nonfixing (or covered) eye with the fast phases being corrective
- Due to reduced input from the visual cortical binocular motion areas leading to the domination of the direct retinal pathway which has a nasalward motion bias

Treatment

- Surgical correction of strabismus
- May also be combined with correction of a head posture used by some patients to suppress the nystagmus
- Treatment of amblyopia using occlusion therapy

---

when one eye is covered (Figure 45.3A). MLN is associated with congenital squint syndrome which leads to disrupted binocular vision. The manifest component of MLN is due to suppression of the image from one eye. In patients who show an alternating esotropia, the direction of drift and beating can change spontaneously depending on which eye is fixing.

Eye movements of MLN typically have "decreasing velocity" or "decelerating" slow phases and increasing intensity in abduction (Figure 45.3A). Patients with MLN can show a head turn to keep the fixating eye in adduction in order to reduce the nystagmus intensity[13] (Figure 45.3B). Patients may also show a head tilt which could be part of the congenital squint syndrome unrelated to MLN or may be to compensate for the cyclovertical (i.e., torsional and vertical) component often seen in MLN.[14] MLN can be treated by correcting the esotropia: this can be combined with correction of the head posture using eye muscle surgery.[15] Treating the underlying amblyopia using patching therapy can also reduce the nystagmus caused by MLN.[16]

Pathology

The underlying mechanism behind MLN is the disruption of binocular vision during visual development. Specifically, MLN appears to result when the motion-sensitive areas of the middle temporal and medial superior temporal (MT/MST) cortex do not develop binocular function.[11]

Etiology

Most commonly MLN is associated with congenital esotropia or congenital squint syndrome. A genetic component of concomitant strabismus is supported by twin studies. Inheritance does not follow mendelian patterns, however, but is more complex, with environmental risk factors contributing.[17] MLN can also result from conditions that cause unilateral loss of vision during visual development such as cataract[18] and optic nerve hyoplasia.[19] MLN is often associated with Down syndrome.[20]

Pathophysiology

Insights into the cause of MLN come from neurophysiological investigations in monkey models with strabismus induced using visual deprivation.[11,21,22] The nucleus of the optic tract (NOT), a subcortical structure, appears to have a pivotal role in the generation of MLN (Figure 45.3C). This structure receives two types of inputs[23] (indicated by right and left sides of Figure 45.3C). The NOT receives ascending projections directly from the contralateral retina and responds primarily to nasalward motion from that eye. Through this pathway a simple optokinetic response to global motion of the visual field is generated but demonstrates a monocular nasalward preference.[24,25] This pathway is complementary to the rotational vestibulo-ocular reflex driven by the semicircular canals. A second projection descending from motion-sensitive MT/MST cortex causes the NOT to be driven by moving images that have no disparity between the eyes. This is a more refined level of global motion processing generating optokinetic responses to moving stimuli at a particular depth[11] and requires normal binocular alignment. It drives more symmetrical horizontal optokinetic nystagmus (OKN) responses. It is complementary to the translational vestibulo-ocular reflex (horizontal), mediated by the otoliths, which has a gain dependent on viewing distance.

During early visual development, infants demonstrate a monocular nasalward preference to optokinetic stimulation due to the later development of pathways from the visual cortex causing the optokinetic response to be dominated by

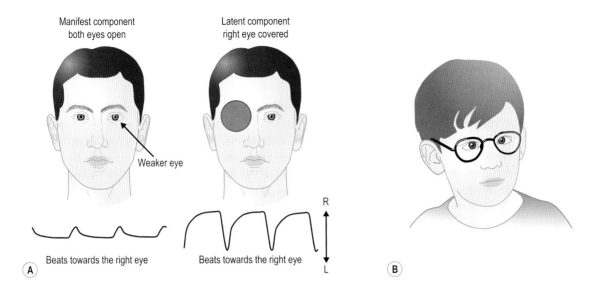

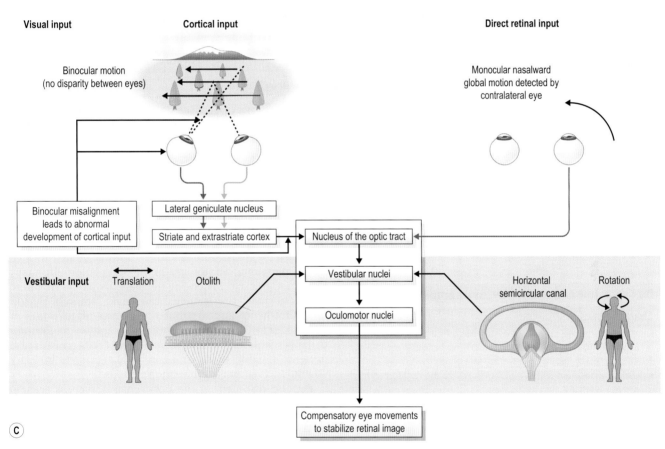

Figure 45.3 Manifest latent nystagmus (MLN). (A) Schematic of the typical pattern of eye movements seen in MLN associated with esotropia. When the right dominant eye is fixing the nystagmus beats to the right. When covering over the dominant eye, the nystagmus becomes larger and beats to the left. (B) Head posture adopted to reduce MLN. The boy has an amblyopic right eye and is fixing with his left eye. Since MLN dampens on adduction he adopts a head turn to the left. (C) The normal cortical and direct retinal inputs to the nucleus of the optic tract (NOT). MLN is thought to be caused by binocular misalignment leading to abnormal cortical development. The reduced cortical input to the NOT allows the direct retinal input to dominate, leading to nasalward drift of the eyes (based on reference 11).

the retinal pathway to the NOT.[26] With development of binocular vision OKN usually becomes symmetrical. If development of binocular function is interrupted in MT/MST then asymmetry persists[27] and can become exaggerated, leading to a nasalward drift under monocular conditions, i.e., MLN.[21,22] Since the NOT projects to the vestibular nuclei which integrate visual and vestibular inputs, MLN can be considered as an imbalance between visual and vestibular inputs caused by deficient binocular input from MT/MST cortex.

Idiopathic infantile nystagmus

Clinical background

IIN is an often hereditary condition that usually appears in the first few months of life. The oscillations are usually horizontal and conjugate but may also rarely appear as primarily vertical or even torsional nystagmus.[2,28] The term "idiopathic infantile nystagmus" is used in preference to "congenital idiopathic nystagmus" as the nystagmus is not always present at birth.[29] The waveform is typically a large slow pendular or triangular oscillation when the nystagmus first appears in infancy and develops into a smaller jerk waveform with age (Box 45.2).[30,31] This has led to the view that individuals with IIN develop a "foveation strategy" during visual development to improve vision.[32] The jerk nystagmus develops with age as individuals learn how to use "foveating saccades" to maximize the time periods when the eyes are moving slowly. Individuals use these slow periods (called foveation periods) to line up the fovea with targets of interest.

The intensity of the nystagmus will usually change with the direction of gaze, with the region of lowest nystagmus intensity and longest foveation periods being described as the "null region."[3] The patient will often prefer to take up fixation at the null region to improve vision and this may result in an anomalous head posture if the null region is eccentric.[13] Although IIN is often described in the literature as being a jerk nystagmus with accelerating slow phase, IIN may show different waveforms that usually vary with eccentricity. Often IIN consists of an underlying pendular oscillation interrupted by regularly occurring foveating saccades (quick phases). Typically, the oscillation drifts towards the null region with the drift becoming accentuated further away from the null region. This results in the quick phases usually beating away from the null region. At the null region the quick phases may beat in either direction or the nystagmus may be pendular. Twelve types of waveform have been described by Del'Osso and Daroff.[32] The majority of these are variations in the timing, amplitude, and direction of foveating saccades with respect to the underlying pendular oscillation.

Apart from the correction of head posture using eye muscle surgery the treatment of IIN has mainly been empirical with most previous research lacking placebo-controlled comparisons.[33] Since IIN dampens on convergence, artificial divergence introduced with eye muscle surgery or prisms has been used to treat patients with IIN and binocular vision.[15] Recession of all four horizontal muscles[15] and, more recently, tenotomy (disinsertion and reattachment on the original insertion) of the four horizontal muscles have been reported to improve visual function and eye movements in nystagmus.[34] Gabapentin and memantine, drugs which may both have an antiglutaminergic action, have also been recently shown to improve vision in IIN patients in a randomized-controlled trial.[35,36] The mechanism behind how these interventions improve nystagmus is unclear. Several treatments are now becoming available, although they are still at trial stage.

Pathology

The mechanisms underlying IIN are still unknown; however, the genetic basis of the most common form of inherited IIN is just beginning to emerge.

Etiology

IIN can be sporadic or inherited. The most common mode of inheritance is due to X-linked mutations.[37,38]

Pathophysiology

The cause of IIN is still unknown, with suggested mechanisms remaining in the realm of speculation. In many respects the visual system of IIN patients has been found to be normal. IIN patients can make smooth pursuit eye movements and vestibular responses if foveation is considered.[39,40] They show normal saccadic oculomotor dynamics, although latencies are delayed.[41] IIN patients also perceive a stable world and can localize targets in space accurately, even outside foveation periods.[42]

Because disorders of the optic chiasm such as seen in albinism lead to nystagmus with many similarities to IIN it has been suggested that the anatomical cause of IIN could be developmental miswiring of the visual system.[43] Physiologically, the sinusoidal-like oscillations commonly lying behind IIN suggest an unstable feedback loop of some sort. Various models have been proposed based around current knowledge of oculomotor circuitry. However, there is no consensus concerning the dysfunctional neuronal structure(s) in IIN, with suggestions including the fixational eye movement system,[44] the pursuit system,[45] and the saccadic system.[45] Recently, it has also been suggested that IIN is a developmental response to poor high-contrast foveal vision where contrast sensitivity to low spatial frequencies is enhanced by moving images across the retina.[46]

Tangible developments in understanding the pathophysiology of IIN have been made with respect to the genetic basis

---

Box 45.2 Idiopathic infantile nystagmus (IIN)

Characteristics

- Mainly horizontal conjugate nystagmus, often consisting of accelerating slow phases or an underlying pendular oscillation interrupted by regularly occurring fast phases
- Usually associated with a null region where the nystagmus has a lower intensity
- The nystagmus appears before 6 months of age and changes during childhood, possibly due to the development of a foveation strategy to improve vision

Underlying cause

- Recent developments have been made in establishing the genetic basis of IIN in locating the *FRMD7* gene (on chromosome Xq26.2) which is associated with a common form of X-linked nystagmus

Treatment

- Surgery can be used to correct head postures due to eccentrically placed null regions
- Treatment of the underlying IIN is empirical
- Future treatments with surgical and drug interventions look promising

of IIN. Recently, we described IIN associated with a frequently occurring X-linked recessive inheritance localized to various mutations on a single gene called *FRMD7* (Xq 26.2) (NYS1)[37] (Figure 45.4A). Although the exact function of this gene is still unknown, it is expressed in the retina, cerebellum, and lateral ventricles during development. The FRMD7 protein shows a close homology to the amino acid sequence seen in FARP1 and FARP2 proteins. These appear to modulate the length and degree of neurite outgrowth in the developing rat cortex.[47]

Individuals with mutations in the *FRMD7* gene have relatively good visual acuity and typically possess stereopsis. Waveforms associated with a single type of mutation on the *FRMD7* gene (as found in family members) can show a wide phenotypic variability (Figure 45.4). However, individuals with *FRMD7* mutations show a less anomalous head posture compared to individuals with IIN not caused by *FRMD7* mutations (Figure 45.4B). This appears to be caused by an increased likelihood of a central null region in individuals possessing mutations in the *FRMD7* gene.

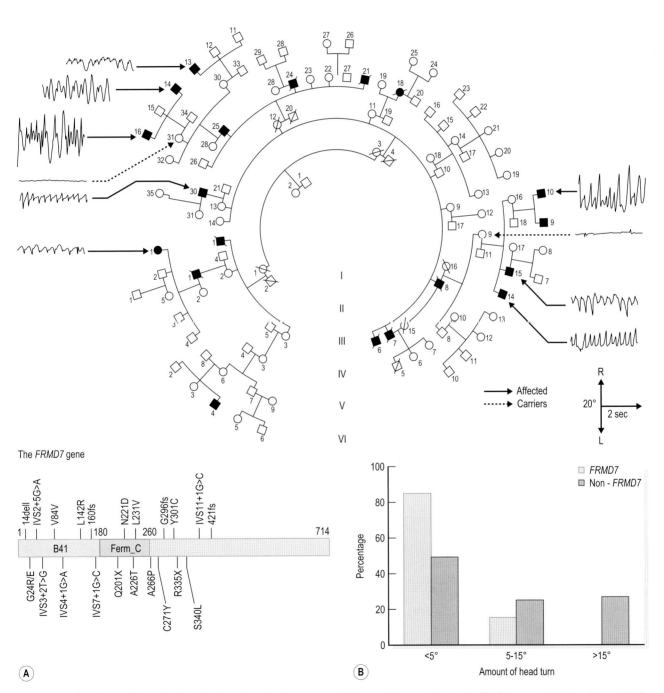

Figure 45.4 Family tree of a large family with idiopathic infantile nystagmus (IIN) caused by a mutation in the *FRMD7* gene. Individuals with an *FRMD7* mutation are shown as filled circles (females) or squares (males). Horizontal eye movements are also displayed for some representative individuals. There is a high degree of variability in the nystagmus waveform characteristics associated with this single mutation. Eye movements of unaffected female carriers are indicated by a dotted arrow. (Inset A) The *FRMD7* gene with location of mutations relative to B41 and FERM-C domains found by Tarpey et al.[37] (Inset B) IIN patients with mutations in the *FRMD7* gene showed less anomalous head posture than those without mutations in the gene.

Albinism

Clinical background

Oculocutaneous albinism (OCA) is characterized by a lack of pigmentation in the eyes, skin and hair (Figure 45.5A and Box 45.3) and is caused by disruption in the production of melanin due to a number of genetic mutations.[48] In certain forms of albinism there is no apparent lack of pigmentation in hair or skin (Figure 45.5B) and only disorders in the visual system are evident (listed below). This is described as ocular albinism (OA) and has a different genetic basis.

Various structures along the visual pathway are affected by albinism:

- Iris: lack of pigmentation causes transillumination of the iris, which is most clearly seen on slit-lamp examination (Figure 45.5Aii and Bii).
- Retina: hypopigmentation of the retinal pigmentary epithelial layer leads to greater reflection of light within the eye. The fovea does not develop fully, leading to a poorly demarcated foveal pit (foveal hypoplasia) (Figure 45.5 Aiii and Biii). Optical coherence tomography shows a spectrum of foveal development in albinism, sometimes with complete absence of development (Figure 45.5C) or with a central depression with thickened fovea. The abnormal foveal development frequently leads to reduced visual acuity. Also, optic discs can be small and dysplastic.
- Chiasm: the most distinguishable feature of albinism is abnormal crossing of axons at the chiasm.[49] This can be detected diagnostically as an asymmetry in the visual evoked potential when measuring the response of the two visual cortices to monocular light stimulation (flash) or checkerboard pattern (pattern-onset) (Figure 45.5D).
- Visual cortex: albinism is often associated with a loss of cortical stereoscopic vision due to misrouting of axons through to the cortex and also strabismus. This leads to reorganization of the visual cortex which can be measured using retinotopic mapping of visual cortex with functional magnetic resonance imaging[50] (Figure 45.6).
- Eye movements: albinism is associated with nystagmus and also strabismus. The nystagmus shows many similarities to that observed in IIN patients (Figure 45.5Aiv and Biv). It is usually horizontal, conjugate, with increasing slow-phase velocities and the nystagmus intensity and waveform changing with gaze direction.[3] These patients also typically show a null zone and often have an anomalous head posture.[13]

Just as with IIN, anomalous head postures can also be corrected using eye muscle surgery. The methods used to treat nystagmus associated with IIN, i.e., muscle tenotomy[34] and drug therapy,[35] have also been used to treat albinism. Although improvements in intensity of nystagmus have been shown to be effective, improvements in visual acuity are limited by the underdeveloped fovea in these patients.[35] Optimal refractive correction is particularly important in these patients to prevent amblyopia and assist visual development.

Pathology

OCA and OA are caused by disruption in melanin synthesis or transport due to mutations in a series of genes.

Etiology

To date four types of OCA have been found (not associated with syndromes) linked to mutations in four genes.[48,51] OCA1 is present in most populations except African-Americans and can present with either a complete lack of melanin production (OCA1A) or partial melanin production (OCA1B). It is caused by mutations in the tyrosinase gene (*TYR*). OCA2 and OCA3 are more common in African populations and are milder forms of albinism. OCA2 is linked to mutations in a gene involved in melanosome production (*OCA2* or *P* gene) and OCA3 is caused by mutations in a tyrosine-related gene (*TYRP1*). OCA4 is another mild form of albinism that has recently been found in Turkish, Japanese, German, and Korean patients. The OCA4 gene codes for a protein called MATP. The function of this protein is not entirely clear but it is thought it may have a role in the transport of melanosomes.

There are two known causes of OA: (i) due to mutations in the OA1 gene which follows an X-linked recessive inheritance or (ii) autosomal-recessive ocular albinism (AROA).[52] The OA1 gene codes for a transmembrane glycoprotein which appears to function as a G-protein-coupled receptor, although the exact function of the protein is unknown. In at least some cases AROA results from mutations in *TYR* and *OCA2* genes.

Pathophysiology

Melanin is the most common light-absorbing pigment in living organisms. It is synthesized from tyrosine to DOPA by the tyrosinase enzyme and subsequently to DOPAquinone. Consequently, mutations to the tyrosinase enzyme can render it either completely or partially functional, resulting in the two variants of the OCA1 form of albinism (OCA1A and OCA1B). Disorders of melanosome production, the organelles used to store melanin, also lead to the physical and visual abnormalities associated with albinism (OCA2). The mechanisms by which the visual system abnormalities arise in association with albinism are unclear. Several authors suggest that abnormal retinal development could lead to the incorrect axonal pathfinding which causes abnormal chiasmal crossing.[49,51]

Spasmus nutans

Spasmus nutans is a rare form of infantile nystagmus that is characterized by a triad of nystagmus, head nodding, and head torticollis. It appears around 1–3 years of age but abates to subclinical levels at around 5–12 years of age.[53] It is an intermittent, fine, high-frequency, pendular dissociated nystagmus. Spasmus nutans is not inherited and is more common in low socioeconomic classes.[54] Interestingly, head nodding suppresses nystagmus in spasmus nutans (Figure 45.7), whereas in other nystagmus forms head nodding has not been found to benefit the patient and might be an associated pathological phenomenon.[55] Spasmus nutans can be easily mistaken for nystagmus associated with retinal disease[56] or nystagmus caused by lesions to the anterior

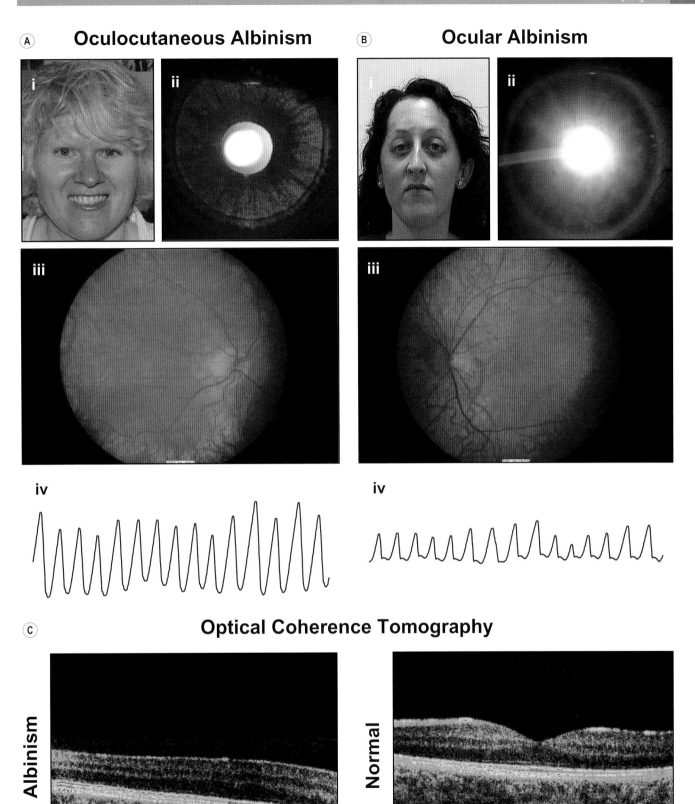

Figure 45.5 Oculocutaneous (A) and ocular (B) albinism. Albinism shows various degrees of iris transillumination (ii), foveal and optic nerve hypoplasia (iii). Nystagmus is similar to idiopathic infantile nystagmus (IIN) and shows a spectrum of intensities with increasing slow-phase velocity (iv). (C) Optical coherence tomography can demonstrate thickening of the macula.

(D)

Visual Evoked Potentials

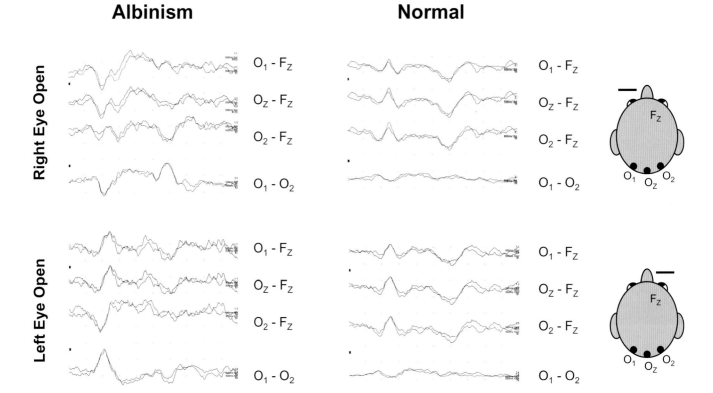

Figure 45.5, cont'd (D) There is increased crossing of optic fibers in the chiasm which can result in asymmetries in visual evoked potentials (O_1, O_2, and O_3 are electrodes placed over the back of the head near the occipital pole of the cortex) in left, central, and right positions, respectively; F_Z is the reference electrode. An asymmetry can be seen in the deflection of the O_1–O_2 trace.

Box 45.3 Albinism

Characteristics

- Oculocutaneous albinism (OCA) is a lack of pigmentation in the eyes, skin, and hair
- OCA is also associated with a series of visual disorders, including iris transillumination, foveal hypoplasia, retinal hypopigmentation, abnormal crossing of the optic nerves at the chiasm, reorganization of the striate cortex, and nystagmus
- The visual disorder without the lack of pigmentation in the skin and hair is described as ocular albinism (OA)
- The nystagmus shows similar characteristics to idiopathic infantile nystagmus

Underlying cause

- OCA is linked to mutations in four known genes and OA in one known gene
- All these mutations lead to dysfunctional melanin synthesis and storage
- The link between nystagmus and the role of melanin is unknown

Treatment

- As for idiopathic infantile nystagmus

---

visual pathway caused by tumors, for example, optic nerve and chiasmal gliomas.[57] Therefore, thorough neuro-ophthalmological (including electrophysiology), neuropediatric, and possibly neuroradiological workup of the patient is necessary.

Nystagmus associated with retinal diseases and low vision

Lesions at numerous locations along the sensory visual pathway are associated with nystagmus. The term "sensory nystagmus" has been used to describe these types of nystagmus, although in some diseases it is not entirely clear whether the sensory deficits cause the nystagmus or whether the nystagmus is intrinsic to the disease.[58] Deficits of rod and cone systems, such as congenital stationary night blindness, achromatopsia (complete or partial, e.g., blue-cone monochromatism) and Leber's amaurosis are all associated with nystagmus.[59] Congenital cataract can lead to nystagmus if not operated on early enough.[18] Aniridia, bilateral optic nerve hypoplasia, and retinopathy of prematurity are also associated with nystagmus. Achiasmatic subjects have been described to have congenital seesaw nystagmus.[60] Cortical visual impairments such as periventricular leukomalacia also lead to a range of oculomotor deficits, including nys-

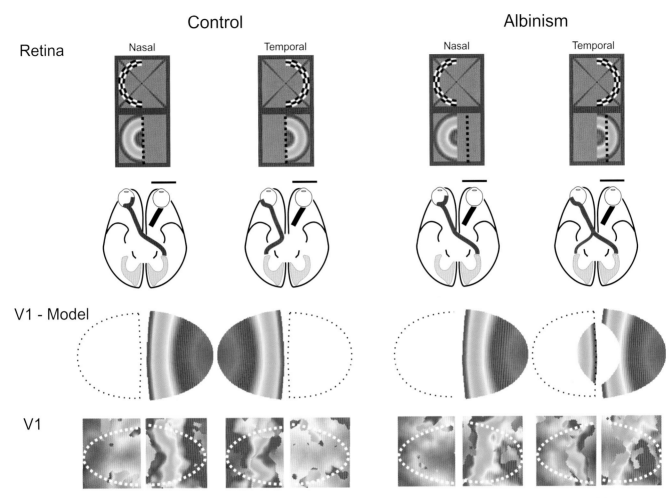

Figure 45.6 Retinotopic mapping of the primary visual cortex using functional magnetic resonance imaging (fMRI). Retinotopic mapping of the striate cortex can be achieved by progressively stimulating from the central through to the peripheral visual field using a flashing checkerboard annulus pattern. In the normal visual system (control), monocular stimulation in one hemifield should yield an ordered retinotopic map in the contralateral visual cortex, as indicated by the colors in the model. The representation of activity in the flattened primary visual cortex (V1) recorded using fMRI shows that this is a good approximation, with foveal stimulation yielding responses near the occipital pole. In an albino patient, because of the higher proportion of axons crossing at the chiasm, we might expect less obvious segregation, with both hemispheres responding to monocular stimulation of the temporal hemifield. Using fMRI, stimulation of the temporal hemifield yielded a less ordered retinotopic map in ipsilateral visual cortex and some stimulation of the contralateral cortex. Stimulation of the nasal hemifield causes stimulation of the contralateral visual cortex but is less well ordered compared to the control. (Reproduced with permission from Hoffmann MB, Tolhurst DJ, Moore AT, et al. Organization of the visual cortex in human albinism. J Neurosci 2003;23:8921–8930.)

tagmus.[61] Nystagmus associated with retinal diseases and low vision often consists of small horizontal or vertical movements superimposed on larger oscillations.[62]

Nystagmus associated with neurological syndromes

Nystagmus occurs in a number of neurological syndromes such as Down syndrome, Joubert syndrome, Pelizaeus–Merzbacher syndrome, fetal alcohol syndrome, and Cockayne's syndrome. These are usually related to abnormalities in the lower-level oculomotor circuitry in the brainstem and cerebellum. The underlying mechanisms and nystagmus characteristics are similar to those seen in many acquired nystagmus types.

Acquired nystagmus

Acquired nystagmus can result from both vestibular and/or neurological disorders and is often extremely disabling due to the associated oscillopsia.[1,63,64]

Nystagmus caused by disorders of vestibular sensory organs or nerves is characterized by a pure jerk waveform (linear slow phase) in a plane equivalent to that monitored by the defective sense organ(s). Causes include paroxysmal positional vertigo, vestibular neuronitis, and Ménière's disease.[65] Vestibular nystagmus is characterized by sensitivity to altering vestibular input through head movements.

A range of neurological disorders, including tumors and strokes, can cause acquired nystagmus, presenting in many

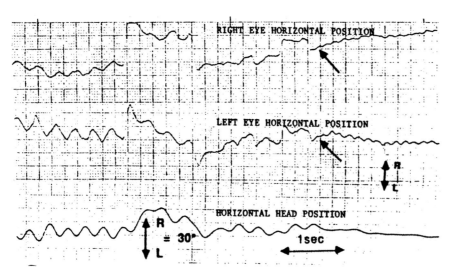

Figure 45.7 Original recordings of a patient with spasmus nutans. At the beginning of the trace head nodding dampens the high-frequency nystagmus which can be seen at the end of the trace, where little head nodding occurs. (Modified from Gottlob I, Zubcov AA, Wizov SS, et al. Head nodding is compensatory in spasmus nutans. Ophthalmology 1992;99:1024–1031.)

Box 45.4 Acquired nystagmus

Characteristics

- Due to neurological or vestibular conditions
- Associated with oscillopsia
- Acquired pendular nystagmus waveforms are commonly associated with multiple sclerosis and are often multivectoral and dissociated
- Vertical jerk nystagmus is frequently associated with disorders of the vestibulocerebellum

Underlying causes

- Hypothesized that acquired pendular nystagmus may be due to instability in the neural integrator
- Vertical jerk nystagmus may be due to insult of an inhibitory control mechanism by the cerebellar flocculus upon eye elevator muscles. The resulting nystagmus could be upbeat or downbeat depending on the pathology

Treatment

- Acquired pendular nystagmus forms are often responsive to certain drug treatments such as gabapentin, baclofen, and memantine

---

different forms. However, several forms of nystagmus are characteristic of acquired neurological nystagmus.

Acquired pendular nystagmus

Acquired pendular nystagmus (APN) is commonly associated with multiple sclerosis.[66] Here, the nystagmus is often disconjugate and may be a combination of horizontal, vertical, and torsional nystagmus (e.g., elliptical or oblique) (Box 45.4). APN also occurs in Whipple's disease, brainstem stroke, spinocerebellar degeneration, encephalopathy, and syndromes such as Pelizaeus–Merzbacher syndrome and Cockayne's syndrome.[1]

One hypothesis about the cause of APN in multiple sclerosis is that it is due to instability in the neural integrator,

the neural circuitry used to generate the tonic neural signal that allows the eyes to be held eccentrically. This was based on observations that saccades cause a phase shift, apparently resetting the integrator.[67] Also, the paramedian tracts, which form an important part of the neural integrator, frequently show plaques.[68] Several drugs have proved to be successful in treating APN in multiple sclerosis, including gabapentin, baclofen, and memantine.[69]

Vertical jerk nystagmus

Vertical jerk nystagmus is frequently associated with disorders of the vestibulocerebellum. A hypothetical scheme has been proposed to explain upbeat and downbeat jerk nystagmus based on specific pathological lesions in human and animal models[63,64,70] (Figure 45.8). The pathway from the anterior semicircular canal through to the eye elevators is under inhibitory control by the cerebellar flocculus at the level of the superior vestibular nucleus. Only upward movement of the eyes is under this inhibitory control with no direct equivalent for downward movements of the eyes. The level of inhibition is controlled by a feedback loop that synapses at the level of the caudal medulla. This mechanism appears to be prone to insult at various levels. Firstly, the pathway from the superior vestibular nucleus through to the motoneurons of the superior rectus in the third nerve (the ventral tegmental tract) can be injured through pontine lesions (Figure 45.8, arrow 1). Hypoactivity of eye elevator muscles leads to downward drift of the eyes with corrective upbeating, i.e., upbeat nystagmus. The inhibitory pathway can also be damaged, leading to hyperexcitability of eye elevator motoneurons causing upward drift of the eyes with corrective downbeating, i.e., downbeat nystagmus. This can result from lesions to the flocculus directly (Figure 45.8, arrow 3) or to the caudal medulla (Figure 45.8, arrow 2) affecting the integrity of the inhibitory feedback mechanism.

Vertical downbeat nystagmus is associated with abnormalities of the vestibulocerebellum and can be caused by cerebellar degeneration, tumor, stroke, Chiari malformation (downward displacement of cerebellar tonsils), multiple sclerosis, or head trauma. Downbeat nystagmus can also be

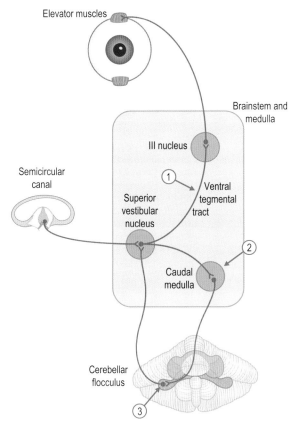

Figure 45.8 A hypothetical scheme to explain upbeat and downbeat nystagmus. Injury to (1) the ventral tegmental tract can lead to upbeat nystagmus. Damage to (2) the caudal medulla or the flocculus can cause downbeat nystagmus (based on data from references 59, 60, and 66).

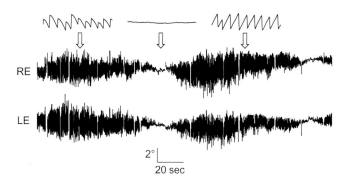

Figure 45.9 Acquired periodic alternating nystagmus (APAN). The lower traces indicate the change in nystagmus over the time course of several minutes for right (RE) and left (LE) eyes. The upper traces show expanded sections of data lasting 3 seconds (adapted from reference 72).

caused by intoxication through substances such as lithium or anticonvulsants, and depletion of substances such as thiamine (Wernicke's encephalopathy), vitamin B_{12} and magnesium.[1] Upbeat nystagmus is associated with disorders of the medulla, pons, midbrain, and cerebellum as caused by stroke, tumor, cerebellar degeneration or demyelination (multiple sclerosis).

Acquired periodic alternating nystagmus

Acquired periodic alternating nystagmus (APAN) consists of a horizontal jerk nystagmus that is modulated so that the nystagmus goes through cycles of left-beating and right-beating nystagmus, reversing about every 1–2 minutes (Figure 45.9). It appears to be caused by lesions of the cerebellar nodulus and uvula, which control the velocity storage mechanism.[63,64,71] This is a neural mechanism that effectively expands the time course of signal from the semicircular canals, which decay rapidly during sustained rotations. Experimental models in which the nodulus and uvula are ablated cause APAN in animals. This is thought to be caused by abnormally exaggerating the time constant of the velocity storage mechanism. Causes of APAN include Chiari malformation, cerebellum dysfunction due to tumor, infection (e.g., syphilis) or degeneration, multiple sclerosis, and toxic effects of anticonvulsants and lithium.[1]

Conclusion

Nystagmus can result from an array of conditions leading to diverse but characteristic eye oscillations. The nature of these oscillations provides clues concerning the underlying pathogenesis; however, the majority of nystagmus forms are still poorly understood. It is likely that disturbances to sensory systems have an important role in the genesis of many infantile nystagmus forms: MLN, albinism, and nystagmus associated with retinal disease and low vision are all strongly allied with visual loss in some way. Acquired nystagmus forms are more commonly associated with motor dysfunction due to lesions imposed on oculomotor circuitry in the cerebellum and brainstem. Our understanding of the genetic basis of nystagmus and the mechanisms underlying nystagmus is rapidly becoming clearer. Clinically proven treatments for nystagmus are now beginning to emerge.

Acknowledgments

We would like to acknowledge the contributions of Shery Thomas, Nagini Sarvananthan, Nitant Shah, Rebecca McLean, and Mervyn Thomas. We would like to thank the Nystagmus Network for their continued interest in and support for nystagmus research. We acknowledge the financial support of Ulverscroft Foundation, Medisearch, National Eye Research Centre and "Fight for Sight". We would also like to thank the many willing volunteers who have assisted in these studies.

Key references

A complete list of chapter references is available online at www.expertconsult.com. See inside cover for registration details.

1. Leigh RJ, Zee DS. The Neurology of Eye Movements, 4th edn. Oxford: Oxford University Press, 2006:x, 763.

2. Khanna S, Dell'Osso LF. The diagnosis and treatment of infantile nystagmus syndrome (INS). Scientific World J 2006;6:1385–1397.

3. Abadi RV, Bjerre A. Motor and sensory characteristics of infantile nystagmus. Br J Ophthalmol 2002;86:1152–1160.

8. Bedell HE. Sensitivity to oscillatory target motion in congenital nystagmus. Invest Ophthalmol Vis Sci 1992;33:1811–1821.

11. Brodsky MC, Tusa RJ. Latent nystagmus: vestibular nystagmus with a twist. Arch Ophthalmol 2004;122:202–209.

12. Dell'Osso LF, Schmidt D, Daroff RB. Latent, manifest latent, and congenital nystagmus. Arch Ophthalmol 1979;97:1877–1885.

28. Abel LA. Infantile nystagmus: current concepts in diagnosis and management. Clin Exp Optom 2006;89:57–65.

35. McLean R, Proudlock F, Thomas S, et al. Congenital nystagmus: randomized, controlled, double-masked trial of memantine/gabapentin. Ann Neurol 2007;61:130–138.

37. Tarpey P, Thomas S, Sarvananthan N, et al. Mutations in FRMD7, a newly identified member of the FERM family, cause X-linked idiopathic congenital nystagmus. Nat Genet 2006;38:1242–1244.

42. Bedell HE. Perception of a clear and stable visual world with congenital nystagmus. Optom Vis Sci 2000;77:573–581.

48. Gronskov K, Ek J, Brondum-Nielsen K. Oculocutaneous albinism. Orphanet J Rare Dis 2007;2:43.

59. Gottlob I. Nystagmus. Curr Opin Ophthalmol 2001;12:378–383.

63. Leigh RJ, Das VE, Seidman SH. A neurobiological approach to acquired nystagmus. Ann NY Acad Sci 2002;956:380–390.

70. Pierrot-Deseilligny C, Milea D. Vertical nystagmus: clinical facts and hypotheses. Brain 2005;128:1237–1246.

CHAPTER 46

Toxic optic nerve neuropathies

FT "Fritz" Fraunfelder and FW "Rick" Fraunfelder

The toxic optic neuropathies (TON) are caused by a widely varied group of insults that may include chemicals, drugs, nutritional defects, and vaccines (Box 46.1). The goal of this chapter is to introduce this subject with emphasis on a subgroup, mitochondrial optic neuropathies (MON) (Box 46.2), which probably have a common pathophysiologic pathway.[1,2] MON also have a nontoxic form, Leber's hereditary optic neuropathy (LHON), which causes mitochondrial dysfunction due to pathogenic mutations of the mitochondrial DNA (mtDNA). This affects complex I in the respiratory chain and causes biochemical changes that are not yet fully understood.[3,4] The importance of LHON to TON is that not only does it help us understand the pathophysiology of TON, but it also alerts us to possible genetic influences for some MON. Many abbreviations will be used in this chapter, and are reproduced in Box 46.3.

Clinical background

TON patients usually present with a history of exposure to a foreign substance. Except in a few cases of acute toxicities, e.g., methanol or cyanide toxicity, onset occurs only after several months of exposure. The acute toxicities usually cause irreversible damage to the visual system, while damage in subacute cases of TON is usually reversible, especially if exposure to the toxin is stopped. Both eyes are involved; however, in some cases it may be a number of weeks before the damage is clinically evident in the second eye. There are no pathognomonic features in the diagnosis of TON. The disease is painless, so if the patient experiences eye pain, clinicians should consider another diagnosis. The observant patient may note dyschromatopsia as an early complaint. This may present as certain colors not appearing as vivid or bright as usual, or as generalized suppression of overall color vision. Blurred vision followed by a generalized decrease, primarily of central vision, is an early symptom (Box 46.4).

Historical background

One of the first case studies of a suspected TON was of tobacco–alcohol amblyopia. This was described by Beer in 1817[5] with extensive follow-up studies by others in the late 1800s. However, the first to put the TON in perspective was George Edmund de Schweinitz in 1897.[6] de Schweinitz wrote the initial classic paper on "toxic amblyopia," helping ophthalmologists understand the importance of these adverse effects on the optic nerve and also expanding our knowledge of optic nerve pathology. He used the term "toxic amblyopia" as a general designation for diseases of visual loss secondary to exposure to external poisons.

Epidemic nutritional optic neuropathy (ENON) was best documented by physicians treating Allied prisoners during World War II[7,8] and in studies of Cuban epidemic optic neuropathy (CEON).[9,10] In both groups, signs and symptoms occurred in the undernourished only after roughly 4 months (or more) of poor diet. These studies, especially those of CEON, gave birth to the classic paper proposing nongenetic MON.[1]

Epidemiology

TON are rare except in epidemics, where the cause was initially unknown, such as in Cuba with CEON[9,10] or in the far East with the amebicides diiodohydroxyquin or iodochlorhydroxyquin.[11] However, once the causative factor or factors are suspected, the incidence of TON is small. Socioeconomics often play a role, especially in TON, which may be multifactorial since in these diseases syndrome malnutrition is often prominent. Also, as in CEON, home-brewed alcohol may be a factor, and home brew was more commonly consumed in the lower-income communities.[12] Age is important, as shown with cocaine optic neuropathy. This is only seen in newborns whose mothers were users of cocaine during pregnancy.[13] TON associated with home-brewed alcohol or tobacco use is seen more commonly in males.[12] In some cases, TON are caused by occupational exposure to toxins, as with arsenic or cyanide.[12]

To date, TON may not have clearcut subsets in which disease severity or protection from the disease is genetically driven. There are, however, case reports of "idiosyncratic" dramatic loss of vision (within days) whereas the usual history is of many months of toxin exposure. Dotti et al described a case of ethambutol-induced optic neuropathy possibly aggravated by a genetic predisposition to optic nerve pathology.[14] There are many ways that genetics can be involved, from how the toxin is absorbed to how it is metabolized or interacts with other factors. In time, we will

---

Box 46.1 Toxic optic neuropathies

- Amiodarone
- Chloramphenicol
- Cuban epidemic optic neuropathy
- Cyanide
- Disulfiram
- Epidemic nutritional optic neuropathy
- Ethambutol
- Ethylene glycol
- Folic acid
- Halogenated hydroxyquinolines
- Linezolid
- Methanol
- Streptomycin
- Tobacco
- Vaccines
- Vitamin B_{12}

Box 46.2 Probable mitochondrial optic neuropathies

- Leber's hereditary optic neuropathy
- Tobacco–alcohol amblyopia
- Vitamin deficiency
  - Vitamin B_{12}
  - Folic acid
- Arsenic
- Cyanide
- Methanol
- Cuban epidemic optic neuropathy
- Drugs
  - Ethambutol
  - Chloramphenicol
  - Streptomycin
  - Linezolid

Box 46.3 Abbreviations

- TON: toxic optic neuropathies
- MON: mitochondrial optic neuropathies
- LHON: Leber's hereditary optic neuropathies
- CEON: Cuban epidemic optic neuropathies
- ENON: epidemic nutritional optic neuropathies

---

probably find that there will be subsets of this disease in which genetics will play a role.

Diagnostic workup

The level of workup depends on the clinical findings and what tests are available in the medical community. At a minimum, the examination should include:

1. A suspicion that a toxin is involved and a careful history with inquiries about possible exposure, as well

---

Box 46.4

Optic neuropathy

Usually a reduction in vision associated with some ophthalmic observations of disc hyperemia and/or various degrees of disc edema, usually minimal. This may start unilaterally, but with time, if the toxin is continued, becomes bilateral.

Optic atrophy

The severe form of optic neuropathy in which ophthalmoscopic evidence of an abnormally white or pale appearance of the optic disc is associated with a decrease in the number of fine blood vessels on its surface. If due to toxin exposure, this is a bilateral condition, although the degree of atrophy may vary between the eyes.

This may occur slowly or, as in the acute form with methanol toxicity, within hours. In most of the toxic optic neuropathies (TON), the decrease in vision rarely becomes worse than 20/400. Central or central centrocecal scotomas with sparing of the peripheral vision are common. The optic discs may appear normal, hyperemic, or have minimal edema. Optic atrophy may be seen early, but only in the acute forms of TON. In long-term, unrecognized TON, it takes many months for the optic nerve atrophy to occur and this is a rare event. Usually a neuropathy occurs with the subacute form of TON.

---

as consideration of the probability of others who were exposed having a similar disease pattern.
2. An ophthalmic examination with dilation of the pupils, manifest refraction, Amsler grid, color vision testing, and detailed optic nerve evaluation.
3. Visual fields testing, e.g., Humphrey 24-2.

Depending on the suspected cause of disease and the availability of the tests, the examination may also include photographs of the optic disc, visual evoked potential testing, and contrast sensitivity tests using either Arden or Pelli–Robson contrast sensitivity plates.

Differential diagnosis

If there is bilateral uncorrected visual loss with otherwise normal findings, one should consider:

1. Toxic and nutritional optic neuropathies
2. Ruling out maculopathy. This may require fluorescein angiography or focal electroretinograms for diagnosis
3. Conversion disorder or malingering
4. MON
5. Kjer's optic neuropathy
6. Compressive or infiltrative optic chiasm lesion
7. Demyelinating, inflammatory, or infectious optic neuritis, which rarely affects both eyes
8. Nonarteritic ischemic optic neuropathy.

Treatment

The most effective treatment of TON is the recognition that a toxic product may be the cause of the abnormal signs and symptoms, and immediate withdrawal from the toxic agent.

Depending on the toxins, some specific therapy may be important.[11,15]

For example:

For ethambutol

1. No proven treatment to date. Treatment is controversial other than discontinuing the drug
2. 100–250 mg of oral zinc sulfate 3 times daily
3. If no improvement after 4 months, parenteral 40 mg hydroxocobalamin daily for 10–28 weeks.

For CEON

1. Stop drinking home-brewed rum
2. Stop smoking
3. Start vitamin B complex therapy
4. Start folic acid therapy
5. Improve diet.

For tobacco toxicity

1. Stop smoking
2. Decrease alcohol intake
3. Improve diet
4. Start taking multivitamins.

Prognosis and complications

Prognosis, for the most part, is totally dependent on the toxicity of the agent causing neuropathy, the amount the patient has ingested, and the length of exposure, plus individual compounding factors. Complications are primarily the degree of visual impairment or toxicity to the various organ systems.

For example:

Ethambutol

Once a visual abnormality is found, and even if the drug is discontinued, ocular signs and symptoms may continue to progress for 1–2 months. If the drug is discontinued when the visual changes first occur, the majority of patients will recover completely over a period of weeks to many months. There are, however, more than 200 well-documented cases of permanent visual loss.[16]

CEON

Prognosis is directly dependent on how soon vitamin therapy is started after visual symptoms first occur. If vitamin therapy is started within a few weeks after a decrease in vision or color vision occurs, prognosis is excellent. However, if treatment is delayed by 3 months or longer, prognosis is poor.[11]

Tobacco

If smoking is discontinued, slow improvement is expected. In occasional debatable cases, improvement has been hastened by injections of hydroxocobalamin.[15]

Pathology

In general, our overall knowledge of pathogenesis and even pathologic anatomy of these TON is inadequate. This is because, if the poisoning is acute and part of generalized central nervous system toxicity, e.g., methanol or cyanide poisoning, the outcome is fatal before significant pathology occurs, or advanced postmortem changes occur, limiting the findings of light or electron microscopic examinations before significant autolysis occurs. In the subacute toxic response there is a long time lapse before pathology is obtained. Therefore, very few acute or subacute specimens have been obtained.

In the acute forms of TON, optic nerve pathology is merely a part of the generalized central nervous system damage. However, in the vast majority of TON, the process is subacute, with exposure over many months before the disease manifests clinically. The papillomacular bundle is particularly vulnerable, probably in the nonmyelinated fibers anterior to the lamina cribrosa. Pathology is not uniformly the same, but similar in the TON. Much of the minimal human pathology has been supplemented by animal model studies. For example, in CEON, a scarcity of retinal ganglion cells in the macula has been found in addition to optic nerve changes. This scarcity is associated with various states of nuclear chromatolysis, thinning of the papillomacular bundle, and degenerating axons.[11]

Etiology

Cause of the disease

TONs are due to exposure to chemicals, poisons, drugs, and other agents that may affect the entire central nervous system, parts of the central nervous system, including the eye, or only the optic nerve, with or without the retina. While dose and length of exposure are the primary risk factors determining the extent and reversibility of the disease, many have multifactorial etiologies.

Course of the disease (risk factors)

Environmental factors

This varies with the toxic agent, but is important for many of the TON. For example, in CEON, poor socioeconomic circumstances can contribute to poor nutrition, or to consumption of home-brewed alcohol instead of purchase of commercially produced spirits. Some TON are worsened by occupational exposure to agents such as lead, organic solvents, or cyanide.[1]

Other diseases

Many TON are clearly worse in patients with diabetes, alcoholism, renal disease, or low plasma zinc levels.

Nutrition

The vitamin B-complex deficiency plays a role in a few of the TON, such as in CEON, ENON, and tobacco amblyopia. Folate deficiency may be due to fad diets, incorrect vegetarian diets, malnutrition, or alcoholism, all of which may cause or aggravate TON. In rarer cases, vitamins A and E can cause optic neuropathy, as seen in patients with extensive small-bowel disease or after surgical bowel resection. TON due to alcohol is now felt not to be due to the toxic effects of alcohol, but rather to poor nutrition, as the chronic alcoholic does not maintain an adequate diet. Nutritional factors are important in ENON due to war, famine, or major natural catastrophes.[15]

Genetic factors

Genetic factors are not well understood, but in all probability play a role in some subsets.

Age

The effects of some toxins are more severe in younger patients. For example, ethambutol has a greater effect in patients younger than 6 years old[15] and cocaine affects newborns, as previously mentioned.[13] Iodochlorhydroxyquin effect was the most devastating in children.[12] Tobacco optic neuropathy affects mainly middle-aged to elderly males. This is in large part due to the fact that men in this age group are primarily the pipe and cigar smokers.[16]

Tobacco use

In some TON, e.g., CEON, tobacco use may be a cofactor in the severity of the disease. Contaminants in the tobacco leaves have been implicated.[11]

Drugs

Various drugs have been implicated in causing TON. Using the World Health Organization (WHO) classification system, Box 46.5 provides a list of drugs that can cause optic nerve atrophy.[16]

Box 46.5 Drug-induced toxic optic neuropathy to the point of atrophy

Certain

- Aspirin
- Broxyquinoline
- Chloramphenicol
- Chloroquine
- Dapsone
- Diiodohydroxyquinoline
- Ethambutol
- Gentamicin
- Hexachlorophene
- Hydroxychloroquine
- Isoniazid
- Nitrous oxide
- Quinine
- Tobramycin
- Tryparsamide

Probable

- Cycloserine
- Linezolid

Pathophysiology

TON are caused by a variety of insults, but only recently has a significant subgroup been identified which crosses boundaries of drugs, chemicals, hereditary, and malnutrition. This group is called the MON (Box 46.2). They have a clinical pattern (Box 46.6). The primary interruption of normal physiology is at the site of the mitochondria. Mitochondria are double-membrane cytoplasmic organelles which carry multiple copies of their own 16569-bp circular mtDNA. MtDNA is located in the matrix, the internal compartment delimited by the inner mitochondrial membrane. The mtDNA encodes 13 proteins which host numerous metabolic pathways, including oxidative energy metabolism, which plays a major role in promoting and regulating the apoptotic death of a cell. Mitochondria are noted as traveling powerhouses that need to be located within the cytoplasm according to the local metabolic needs of the cell. While much has yet to be defined, MON may be due to a single factor or a combination of factors.

The classic example of a single insult causing MON is acute methanol poisoning. This neural toxin is well known and still seen. It is not a classic MON since it is of acute onset, often life-threatening, has severe systemic findings, and often causes irreversible optic neuropathy. The biochemical reaction which leads to acute visual toxicity occurs when methanol is converted to formate via formaldehyde (Figure 46.1). Formate directly interferes with the oxidative phosphorylation since it inhibits cytochrome oxidase. This acute buildup causes acute, irreversible systemic, neurologic, and optic nerve damage.[17,18] In the more typical MON there is a much slower process since the insult is less toxic and the offending toxin will only build up over time. As seen in CEON, patients who develop neuropathy in the course of long-term exposure to multiple possible toxins that enhance the toxic effects of low-dose methanol exposure then develop a chronic folic acid deficiency.[11] These mechanisms would at least initially deplete the levels of folic acid by shunting it away from formate detoxification. This inhibition of the cytochrome oxidase system over time would both disrupt the folic acid-mediated production of adenosine triphosphate (ATP) and inhibit electron transport. This diminished mitochondrial ATP production is the basic cause of impaired optic nerve function, probably in retinal ganglion cells as well as in the optic nerve axons. The mitochondria must move to the nodes of Ranvier and the distal axon terminals

---

Box 46.6 Typical findings of mitochondrial optic neuropathies

- Fairly symmetric visual losses
- Loss of visual acuity and high spatial frequency contrast sensitivity
- Early and profound loss of color vision
- Centrocecal visual field defects (with good preservation of the peripheral fields)
- Temporal pallor of the optic discs (delayed)
- Preferential loss of the papillomacular bundle of the retinal nerve fiber layer

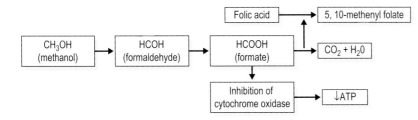

Figure 46.1 Methanol inhibits the production of adenosine triphosphate (ATP). (Redrawn with permission from Sadun AA. Acquired mitochondrial impairment as a cause of optic nerve disease. Trans Am Ophthalmol Soc 1998;96:881–923.)

where ATP production is needed. Since mitochondria only survive 7–10 days, delays in axonal transport may affect longer, smaller, or myelinated nerves, which are the most metabolically active. This is a possible explanation of why selective loss, i.e., the retinal ganglion cells and the maculo-papillary bundle of the optic nerve anterior to the cribiform plate, are initially affected. Sadun proposes a mitochondrial catastrophe theory (Figure 46.2).[12] Mitochondrial impairment leads to decreased ATP production, which in turn may lessen axoplasmic transport responsible for moving these mitochondria to the distal axon before they expire. In the beginning, the cells can compensate for mild insults without clinical impairment. However, with time a threshold is reached and the cells decompensate.

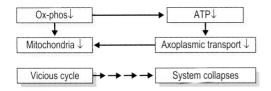

Figure 46.2 Mitochondrial catastrophe theory. ATP, adenosine triphosphate. (Redrawn with permission from Sadun AA. Acquired mitochondrial impairment as a cause of optic nerve disease. Trans Am Ophthalmol Soc 1998;96:881–923.)

The paradigm of MON is LHON, which is the best studied of the MON and clearly a genetic disease involving an abnormality of the mitochondria. LHON and the acquired non-acute MON all involve mitochondrial abnormalities which cause major optic nerve problems without evidence of other neurologic abnormalities. Neuman[15] points out that other diseases of the mitochondria, e.g., Kjer's or Wolfram's syndrome, cause significant systemic neurologic abnormalities but do not affect the retina or optic nerve. She feels that this is somewhat surprising. If the mitochondria are the major area of concern, then why is it so selective in one group (MON) without affecting the visual systems? While the above-mentioned systemic mitochondrial abnormalities cause major neurologic defects, they spare the eye. This may in part be answered by the variability of proposed mechanisms. The damage to the mitochondria may be genetic, as in LHON,[2] caused by chelation of copper- or zinc-containing enzymes within the mitochondria, or caused by ethambutol,[19] poor nutrition, or a defect in sulfur metabolism as in cyanide toxicity.[20] Regardless, TON is often a multifactorial pathophysiologic disease unless the agent is highly toxic. There is a subset of TON, MON, where single or multiple factors impede the mitochondria's ability to function and manifest varying degrees of optic nerve diseases.

Key references

A complete list of chapter references is available online at www.expertconsult.com. See inside cover for registration details.

1. Sadun AA. Mitochondrial optic neuropathies. J Neurol Neurosurg Psychiatry 2002;72:423–425.
2. Carelli V, Ross-Cisneros FN, Sadun AA. Mitochondrial dysfunction as a cause of optic neuropathies. Prog Retin Eye Res 2004;23:53–89.
4. Chalmers RM, Schapira AHV. Clinical biochemical and molecular genetic features of Leber's hereditary optic neuropathy. Biochim Biophys Acta 1999;1410:147–158.
5. Beer W. Lehre von den Augenkrakheiten, also Leitfaden zu seinen öffentlichen Vorlesungen entworfen. Vienna: Camesina, Heubner und Volke, 1813–1817.
8. Bloom SM, Merz EH, Taylor WW. Nutritional amblyopia in American prisoners of war liberated from the Japanese. Am J Ophthalmol 1946;29: 1248–1257.
9. Sadun AA, Martone JF, Muci-Mendoza R, et al. Epidemic optic neuropathy in Cuba: eye findings. Arch Ophthalmol 1994;112:691–699.
10. Sadun AA, Martone JF, Reyes L, et al. Optic and peripheral neuropathy in Cuba. JAMA 1994;271:663–664.
11. Tjalve H. The aetiology of SMON may involve an interaction between clioquinol and environmental metals. Med Hypotheses 1984;15:293.
15. Phillips PH. Toxic and deficiency optic neuropathies. In: Miller NR, Newman NJ, Biousse V, et al. (eds) Walsh and Hoyt's Clinical Neuro-ophthalmology, 6th edn. Philadelphia: Lippincott Williams and Wilkins, 2005:447–463.
16. Fraunfelder FW, Fraunfelder FT, Chambers WA. Clinical ocular toxicology. Philadelphia: WB Saunders, 2008.
18. Dethlefs R, Naraqi S. Ocular manifestations and complications of acute methyl alcohol intoxication. Med J Aust 1978;2:483–485.
19. Kozak SF, Inderlied CB, Hsu HY, et al. The role of copper on ethambutol's antimicrobial action and implications for ethambutol-induced optic neuropathy. Diagn Microbiol Infect Dis 1998;30:83–87.
20. Freeman AG. Optic neuropathy and chronic cyanide intoxication: a review. J R Soc Med 1988;81:103–106.

Uveal melanoma

Zélia MS Corrêa and J William Harbour

Clinical background

Uveal melanoma is a malignant neoplasm that arises from neuroectodermal melanocytes within the choroid, ciliary body, or iris, and it is the most common primary malignant intraocular neoplasm.[1,2] Uveal melanoma can cause flashes, floaters, and other visual symptoms, but it is most often asymptomatic and discovered on routine eye examination (Box 47.1). These tumors can range from minimally to darkly pigmented, usually grow slowly, and invade through the sclera to involve the orbit (Figure 47.1). Uveal melanomas have a strong tendency to metastasize hematogenously to the liver and other organs. Despite advances in diagnosis and treatment in recent decades, the mortality rates have not exhibited a commensurate improvement.[3] Uveal melanoma occurs in about 4–5 per million individuals in the USA, and it is much more common in Caucasians than in individuals of African and Asian descent.[4] Men are at slightly higher risk than women, and the peak incidence occurs in patients between the age of 50 and 60, although individuals of any age can be affected.

The differential diagnosis includes uveal nevus, melanocytoma, metastasis, congenital hypertrophy of the retinal pigment epithelium, circumscribed choroidal hemangioma, hemorrhagic detachment, and/or disciform scarring of the choroid or the retinal pigment epithelium, choroidal osteoma, choroidal detachment, uveal effusion, posterior nodular scleritis, choroidal granuloma, toxoplasmic retinochoroiditis, retinal detachment, retinoschisis, neurilemoma, leiomyoma, and combined hamartoma of the retina and retinal pigment epithelium, leiomyoma, intraocular foreign body, medulloepithelioma, pigment epithelial adenoma, or adenocarcinoma.[1]

Treatment options include observation, local microsurgical tumor resection, diode laser hyperthermia, plaque radiotherapy, charged particle radiotherapy, stereotactic radiotherapy, and enucleation.[1] Complications of radiotherapy, the most frequently used treatment option, include cataract, dry eye, radiation retinopathy and optic neuropathy, neovascular glaucoma, vitreous hemorrhage, and local tumor recurrence. Factors that influence therapeutic decision include patient age, overall health, visual status of the affected and unaffected eyes, tumor size and location, extrascleral tumor extension, systemic metastasis, and patient preference.

Pathology

Uveal melanomas are composed of transformed melanocytes arising from the uveal tract of the eye, which includes the choroid, ciliary body, and iris. The histopathologic classification originally proposed by Callender included six categories based on cell morphology: spindle A, spindle B, fascicular, mixed spindle and epithelioid, and necrotic.[5] Subsequently, a modified classification was developed in which tumors are classified as spindle, mixed, or epithelioid (Figure 47.2).[6] Tumors containing mostly spindle cells have a more favorable prognosis than those composed of epithelioid cells. Other histopathologic features associated with poor outcome include greater mean nuclear size, greater mean and standard deviation of the nucleolar area, scleral invasion, higher mitotic index, greater tumor pigmentation, and extracellular matrix patterns (Box 47.2).[7,8]

Etiology

Caucasian ancestry is the most important risk factor for uveal melanoma.[4] Skin freckling, light iris, and light hair color have been linked to uveal melanoma. However, iris freckles, iris nevi, and choroidal nevi have not been convincingly linked to uveal melanoma.[9] Another systemic risk factor is oculo(dermal) melanocytosis.[10] Although there have been reports of familial clustering of uveal melanoma, clear mendelian inheritance is rare. Germline BRCA2 mutations are present in up to 3% of uveal melanoma patients.[11] Mutations in the p16INK4a tumor suppressor are extremely rare in uveal melanoma.[12] There is a weak epidemiologic association between uveal melanoma and ultraviolet light.[13] Arc welding is one of few occupational exposures that is associated with uveal melanoma, but there have been too few reported cases to establish reliable risk estimates.[13]

Pathophysiology

The hallmark features of cancer cells include proliferation independent of normal growth signals, continued proliferation beyond normal replicative limits, resistance to apoptosis, recruitment of a tumor blood supply, and metastasis to other locations.[14] The molecular mechanisms governing

Box 47.1 Summary of clinical features

- Melanocytic tumor of choroid, ciliary body, or iris
- Choroidal and ciliary body tumors usually larger than iris tumors
- Often asymptomatic and discovered on routine eye exam
- Unilateral and unifocal in almost all patients
- Strong tendency to metastasize hematogenously to the liver and other organs
- Much more common in Caucasians
- Men are at slightly higher risk
- Common features include subretinal fluid, orange pigment (lipofuscin), and mushroom-like shape due to eruption through Bruch's membrane

Box 47.2 Clinical and pathologic prognostic factors

- Increased patient age
- Larger tumor size
- Ciliary body involvement
- Juxtapapillary location
- Extrascleral extension
- Epithelioid cell type
- Increased pigmentation
- Extracellular matrix patterns
- Lymphocyte infiltration
- Macrophage infiltration

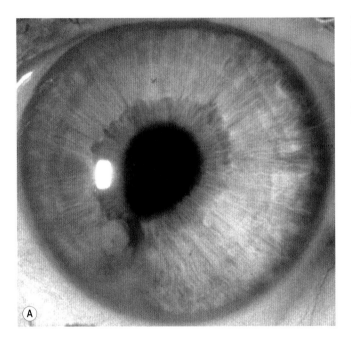

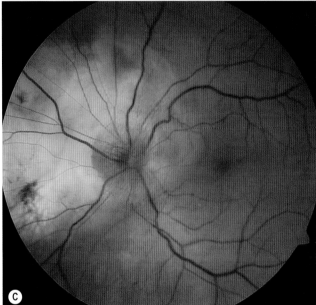

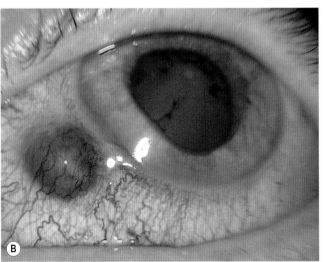

Figure 47.1 Clinical photographs of uveal melanoma. (A) Iris melanoma. (B) Ciliary body melanoma. (C) Choroidal melanoma surrounding and invading optic nerve head.

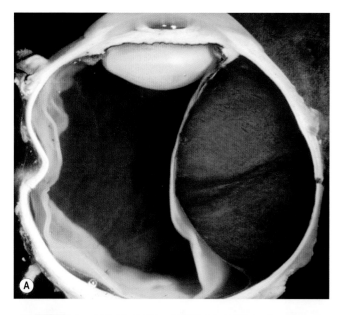

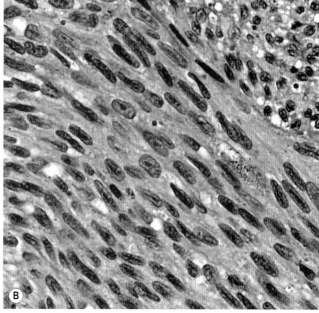

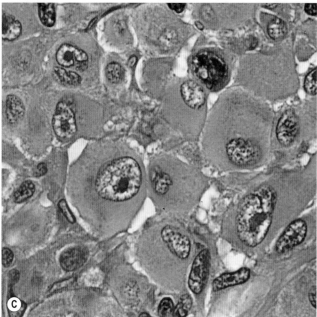

Figure 47.2 Photomicrographs of uveal melanoma. (A) Gross appearance of enucleated globe containing uveal melanoma. (B) Spindle cell melanoma. (C) Epithelioid melanoma.

these characteristics have been found to be defective in uveal melanoma (Box 47.3).

Proliferation independent of normal growth signals

Cell proliferation is normally regulated through extracellular signals, such as growth (mitogenic) factors and extracellular matrix interactions. Cell surface receptors transmit these signals to intracellular signaling cascades that converge upon the nucleus to activate the transcription of genes involved in cell cycle progression. Growth factors such as stem cell factor, transforming growth factor-β and hepatocyte growth factor/scatter factor, and growth factor receptors such as the

---

Box 47.3 Pathophysiologic events associated with tumor progression

- Abnormal proliferation resulting from mutations that circumvent normal cell cycle control
- Acquisition of immortality by overexpressing telomerase and derailing the DNA damage response
- Evasion of cell death by disrupting apoptotic pathways
- Recruitment of a blood supply by expressing angiogenic molecules
- Metastasis to distant organs

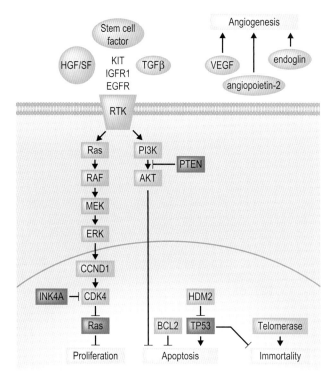

Figure 47.3 Pathway diagram of molecular defects in uveal melanoma leading to abnormal proliferation, resistance to apoptosis, immortality, and angiogenesis. Gene products in pink have been shown to be upregulated and those in teal downregulated in uveal melanoma. HGF/SF, hepatic growth factor/scatter factor; TGF-ß, transforming growth factor-ß; VEGF, vascular endothelial growth factor; RTK, receptor tyrosine kinase; MEK, mitogen extracellular kinase; ERK, extracellular signal-related kinase; CCND1, cyclin D1; CDK4, cyclin-dependent kinase-4; INK4A, inhibitor of CDK4; RB, retinoblastoma; PI3K, phosphoinositol triphosphate; PTEN, phosphatase with tensin homology; HDM2, human homolog of murine double minute-2; TP53, p53 tumor suppressor gene.

insulin-like growth factor receptor-1 (IGFR1), the KIT oncogene, and the epidermal growth factor receptor, have been shown to be aberrantly expressed in uveal melanoma (Figure 47.3).[15–20] The mitogen-activated protein kinase (MAPK)/ mitogen extracellular kinase (MEK)/extracellular signal-related kinase (ERK) signaling pathway, which is a major conduit for transfer of growth signals to the nucleus, is constitutively activated by oncogenic mutations in KIT, RAS, NRAS, or BRAF in cutaneous melanomas and many other cancers.[21] However, such mutations are extremely rare in uveal melanoma.[22–24] Nevertheless, this pathway is constitutively activated in uveal melanoma,[25,26] suggesting that unidentified mutations in this pathway are present. Alterations in nuclear cell cycle proteins provide further evidence for disrupted mitogenic signaling in uveal melanoma. The retinoblastoma tumor suppressor (Rb) is a key cell cycle inhibitor that couples cell cycle exit with differentiation in melanocytes.[27] Phosphorylation of Rb by cyclin-dependent kinase-4 (Cdk4), which is activated by its binding partner cyclin D, blocks the tumor suppressor activity of Rb.[28] Aberrant phosphorylation of Rb in differentiating melanocytes allows them to re-enter the cell cycle and proliferate.[27] Almost all uveal melanomas show evidence of such inappropriate phosphorylation of Rb, either through overexpression of cyclin D or silencing of the Cdk4 inhibitor

p16Ink4a.[29,30] The cyclin D overexpression appears to result from constitutive activation of the MAPK/MEK/ERK pathway.[26]

Sustained proliferation beyond normal replicative limits

Even in the context of abnormal proliferation, cells have a second level of defense against malignant transformation in the form of senescence.[31] With each cell division, the lengths of the telomeres at the ends of chromosomes become shorter. After a finite number of cell divisions, the telomeres become shorted to a critical length where they trigger a DNA damage response that drives the cell permanently out of the cell cycle and into a senescence state. This mechanism likely accounts for the arrest in growth that is observed in benign tumors. Tumors that progress to a fully malignant state must overcome this senescence mechanism. One way in which tumors do this is by stopping the erosion of telomeres through upregulation of telomerase, the enzyme that maintains telomere length. Telomerase activity is upregulated in at least 90% of uveal melanomas (Figure 47.3).[32,33] Another way that tumors can bypass the senescence mechanism is to disrupt the DNA damage response, such as by mutation of the p53 pathway, which triggers cell cycle arrest or apoptosis in response to DNA damage.[34] While p53 is rarely mutated in uveal melanoma,[35,36] the DNA damage response is defective in most tumors, as evidenced by defective downstream signaling to Bax, p21, Bcl-XL, and other p53 targets.[37] Functional inhibition of p53 is due at least in part to overexpression of HDM2, an inhibitor of p53 that targets it for degradation.[36] Targeted blockade of HDM2 induces apoptosis in uveal melanoma cells.[38]

Resistance to apoptosis

Since p53 can trigger apoptosis in response to DNA damage and other oncogenic insults, functional blockade of the p53 pathway described above also conveys resistance to apoptosis (Figure 47.3). The Bcl2 protein and IGFR1 are expressed at high levels in many uveal melanomas and provide additional antiapoptotic activity.[36,39,40] Constitutive activation of the phosphatidylinositol 3-kinase (PI3K) survival pathway is yet another mechanism commonly used by uveal melanoma cells to avert apoptosis. The phosphatase with tensin homology (PTEN) tumor suppressor protein, which is a negative regulator of the PI3K pathway, is silenced in over 76% of uveal melanomas.[41] Consistent with these findings, PTEN expression is associated with increased genomic aneuploidy.[42]

Recruitment of a tumor blood supply

Complex patterns of extracellular matrix deposition within uveal melanomas have been convincingly linked to metastasis and poor systemic outcome.[43] However, the biological nature of these patterns remains controversial. They have been suggested to represent "vasculogenic mimicry," a hypothetical phenomenon in which tumor cells may form embryonic-like blood-conveying channels.[43] While these structures can convey fluid,[44] they do not typically contain red blood cells, so it seems unlikely that they represent the major conduits for tumor blood flow. Another possibility is that these "vascular mimicry patterns" represent basement membrane-like extracellular matrix material deposited by highly aggressive uveal melanoma cells that have acquired epithelial-like characteristics.[45] It seems more likely that endothelial-lined neovasculature provides most tumor blood flow,[46] as supported by the expression of angiogenic factors such as vascular endothelial growth factor (VEGF), endoglin, and angiopoietin-2,[47–49] and the staining of tumor blood vessels with endothelial markers in uveal melanoma (Figure 47.3).[50]

Metastasis

There are many steps in the metastatic process, including disengagement from local cell–cell and cell–matrix adhesive restraints, resistance to anoikis (detachment-induced apoptosis), migration and invasion into nearby tissues, vascular intravasation, embolization and extravasation, and modulation of and proliferation at the secondary site. The relative importance of each step varies between cancer types. For example, disengagement from adhesive interactions is of paramount importance in the progression of cutaneous melanoma, because cutaneous melanocytes are enmeshed within the epithelium through E-cadherin-mediated cell–cell adhesions with surrounding keratinocytes. In order for these melanoma cells to metastasize, they must first downregulate E-cadherin to dissociate from the epithelium, then invade through the underlying basement membrane and migrate to lymphatics and blood vessels. Uveal melanoma cells do not face these boundaries to metastatic progression. They do not have to contend with an epithelium or basement membrane, nor do they have to migrate far to encounter blood vessels since they arise within the highly vascular uveal tract. Thus, the rate-limiting step in metastasis is likely to be different in cutaneous and uveal melanomas as a result of their differing local environments. The factors that determine whether a given uveal melanoma will spawn clinically significant metastatic disease are not known, but indirect evidence from clinical observations and genetic studies allows us to make some reasonable predictions.

Uveal melanomas metastasize almost exclusively by the hematogenous route, and the liver is the predominant secondary site.[51] Many patients develop fatal metastatic disease even after successful treatment of the ocular tumor, and this survival rate has not changed in the past four decades despite improvements in local treatment.[3] Most patients experience a delay of months to years from ocular diagnosis to the detection of metastatic disease,[3] suggesting the presence of subclinical micrometastasis and a period of dormancy following ocular treatment. Indeed, it has been calculated from tumor doubling times that most micrometastasis occurs up to 5 years prior to ocular diagnosis.[52] Circulating melanoma cells can be demonstrated in peripheral blood from about 90% of uveal melanoma patients, including many that never develop metastatic disease.[53] Taken together, these observations suggest that uveal melanoma cells commonly gain access to the circulation, so this is probably not rate-limiting in metastasis. Rather, the key events in metastasis appear to occur later, such as survival in the circulation, extravasation, and successful colonization of the secondary site. Uncover-

> ### Box 47.4 Molecular prognostic testing in uveal melanoma
>
> - The most accurate molecular prognostic feature currently is gene expression profiling of the primary tumor
> - Class 1 tumors have a low risk, and class 2 tumors have a high risk of metastasis
> - Gene expression profiling can now be performed rapidly and inexpensively on whole tumor samples, fine-needle biopsies, and archival paraffin-embedded tissue

ing the rate-limiting events in metastasis will shed light on the phenomenon of tumor dormancy and suggest novel treatment approaches in high-risk patients.

To date, most research on the metastatic process in uveal melanoma has been through indirect genetic studies. In recent years, these studies have led to a paradigm shift in our understanding of uveal melanoma and its propensity for metastasis. Clinical and pathologic risk factors for metastasis, such as tumor size, location, and cell type, form a continuous spectrum from low risk to high risk with no discrete stages,[54] which was assumed for many years to mean that the risk for metastasis is also a continuous scale from low risk to high risk.[55] However, it is now clear that there are two major forms of uveal melanoma based on molecular/genetic features that differ markedly in their metastatic capacity. Monosomy 3 (loss of one copy of chromosome 3) has been shown to be strongly associated with metastasis independently of other prognostic factors.[56–59] The dichotomous, rather than continuous, nature of this chromosomal abnormality supports the idea that metastatic risk represents a discontinuous, bimodal trait. This possibility has been further confirmed by high-density microarray-based gene expression profiling in primary tumor specimens. Whereas chromosomal analysis provides only a one-dimensional marker, gene expression profiling provides a highly dimensional biological "snapshot" of the transcriptional activity of the entire tumor. Based on gene expression profile, uveal melanomas form two distinct groups, which we refer to as class 1 and class 2.[60] About half of tumors fall into each class. This gene expression-based classification has been independently validated by other groups,[61,62] and it predicts metastasis more accurately than clinical and pathologic risk factors, and even monosomy 3.[63] We have identified a set of only three genes that accurately predicts metastatic risk and have optimized the testing platform for polymerase chain reaction-based assay that can be performed on a routine basis on primary tumor tissue and paraffin-embedded archival tissue.[64] An international study is now underway to validate the predictive accuracy of this state-of-the-art prognostic assay (Box 47.4).

Other nonrandom chromosomal alterations have been identified in uveal melanoma, such as 6p gain, 8p loss, and 8q gain.[65] These changes do not predict metastatic risk as well as gene expression profiling or monosomy 3, but recent studies on temporal sequence of chromosomal changes suggest that these chromosomal alterations may allow tumors to be further subgrouped according to metastatic risk.[42] Consequently, we have now expanded our original gene expression-based classification to include class 1A (minimal chromosomal changes), class 1B (6p gain), class

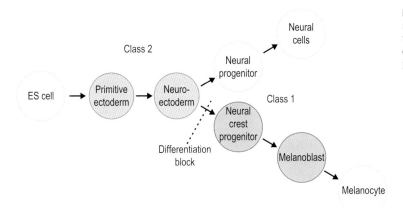

Figure 47.4 Schematic depiction of class 1 and class 2 uveal melanomas in relation to melanocyte development. Class 1 tumor cells closely resemble normal melanocytes in their gene expression profile, whereas class 2 tumor cells resemble more primitive, less differentiated cells.

2A (no 8p loss), and class 2B (8p loss). Although much attention has been focused on 8q gain as a prognostic factor, this change occurs so frequently in both class 1 and class 2 tumors that it does not appear to provide independent prognostic information.[42] Nevertheless, the frequent gain of 8q suggests that relevant genes on this chromosomal arm are targeted for upregulation during tumor progression. Several possible oncogenes on 8q that are upregulated in uveal melanoma have been identified, including MYC, DDEF1, and NBS1 (now called NBN).[66–68]

The identification of genes that are expressed differentially in class 1 versus class 2 uveal melanomas has provided an opportunity to explore biological differences between these tumors that may provide insights into the metastatic process. The gene expression signature of class 1 tumors is very similar to normal melanocytes, including the expression of genes involved in melanocyte specification from neural crest (e.g., EDNRB, ERBB3, CTNNB1) and genes involved in melanocyte differentiation and pigment production (e.g., MITF, DCT, TYR, TRP1). In contrast, class 2 tumors express genes involved in cell-cell adhesion (e.g., CDH1), basement membrane/extracellular matrix production (e.g., COL4A1, SPARC, LAMC1), and other epithelial-like functions (e.g., EMP1, EMP3, CITED1).[45] Recent work in our laboratory suggests that the class 2 tumors express a signature similar to neural/epithelial stem/progenitor cells, and it is these cells that are present in metastatic lesions (JW Harbour, unpublished data). Taken together, these findings suggest that class 1 tumors are composed mostly of melanoma cells that can traverse far down the melanocyte differentiation pathway, where they are resistant to metastatic progression. Class 2 tumors, on the other hand, contain melanoma cells that are less differentiated and more stem-like, and perhaps it is this property that conveys metastatic potential (Figure 47.4).

The epithelial-like phenotype of class 2 tumors may promote metastasis by allowing them to survive after detachment from surrounding extracellular matrix by substituting the survival signals emanating from cell–matrix interactions with ones from E-cadherin-mediated cell–cell interactions. Consistent with this possibility, E-cadherin expression is required for anchorage-independent growth of uveal melanoma cells in soft agar.[45] The primitive nature of class 2 melanoma cells may also promote the dissemination and

colonization of distant sites, which is reminiscent of the behavior of neural crest cells, from which melanocytes are derived.

Unifying concepts

Many clinical and pathologic features of uveal melanoma have been shown to be associated with metastatic risk, including advanced patient age, ciliary body involvement, larger tumor size, epithelioid cell type, and extracellular matrix patterns.[69] However, the pathogenetic relationships between these factors remain unclear. When viewed from the perspective of our current genetic understanding of uveal melanoma, many of these other features can be reconciled into a unifying concept of uveal melanoma pathobiology. For example, epithelioid cytology, looping extracellular matrix patterns, and monosomy 3 are all significantly associated with the class 2 gene expression signature.[60,63,70,71] Even though none of these features predicts metastasis as accurately as gene expression profiling, their association with the class 2 signature suggests that they may be biologically related. Perhaps epithelioid cytology and looping extracellular matrix patterns represent manifestations of the epithelial-like phenotype of class 2 melanoma cells.[45] It is tempting to speculate that one or more genes on chromosome 3 are required for melanocytic differentiation, and the loss of these genes in tumors with monosomy 3 inhibits differentiation and promotes primitive class 2 melanoma cells with stem/progenitor qualities.

Conclusions

We are entering a new era in the management of uveal melanoma. It will remain important to manage the primary ocular tumor with the most effective techniques available, but it is clear that this alone will not have an impact on future improvements in patient survival. Rather, such improvements will require the identification and preventative treatment of high-risk patients. As discussed herein, we now have highly accurate molecular tests for identifying patients at high risk of metastasis. The next step is to develop adjuvant treatments for high-risk patients that will delay or prevent the development of metastatic disease, such as by inducing sustained dormancy in micrometastatic lesions. Such progress will require a greater understanding of tumor dormancy and the mechanisms governing successful colonization of secondary sites by metastatic melanoma cells. A recent study has shed important light on this issue by comparing the gene expression profiles of primary and metastatic uveal melanoma cells.[72] This study identified the NF-κB pathway as potentially important in regulating the development of metastatic tumors. Such studies will be critically important for identifying "druggable" molecular targets for treating high-risk patients.

Acknowledgments

This work was supported by grants to ZMC from Quest for Vision, Research to Prevent Blindness, Inc., Mary Knight Asbury Chair of Ocular Pathology and E Vernon and Louise Smith Fund, and to JWH from the National Cancer Institute (R01 CA125970), Research to Prevent Blindness, Inc., Barnes-Jewish Hospital Foundation, the Kling Family Foundation, the Horncrest Foundation, and the Tumori Foundation.

Key references

A complete list of chapter references is available online at www.expertconsult.com. See inside cover for registration details.

2. Ramaiya KJ, Harbour JW. Current management of uveal melanoma. Exp Rev Ophthalmol 2007;2: 939–946.

7. Gamel JW, McLean IW, Foster WD, et al. Uveal melanomas: correlation of cytologic features with prognosis. Cancer 1978;41:1897–1901.

9. Harbour JW, Brantley MA Jr, Hollingsworth H, et al. Association between posterior uveal melanoma and iris freckles, iris naevi, and choroidal naevi. Br J Ophthalmol 2004;88: 36–38.

13. Egan KM, Seddon JM, Glynn RJ, et al. Epidemiologic aspects of uveal melanoma. Surv Ophthalmol 1988;32: 239–251.

17. Girnita A, All-Ericsson C, Economou MA, et al. The insulin-like growth factor-I receptor inhibitor picropodophyllin causes tumor regression and attenuates mechanisms involved in invasion of uveal melanoma cells. Clin Cancer Res 2006;12:1383–1391.

22. Rimoldi D, Salvi S, Lienard D, et al. Lack of BRAF mutations in uveal melanoma. Cancer Res 2003;63:5712–5715.

25. Zuidervaart W, van Nieuwpoort F, Stark M, et al. Activation of the MAPK pathway is a common event in uveal melanomas although it rarely occurs through mutation of BRAF or RAS. Br J Cancer 2005;92:2032–2038.

42. Ehlers JP, Worley L, Onken MD, et al. Integrative genomic analysis of aneuploidy in uveal melanoma. Clin Cancer Res 2008;14:115–122.

45. Onken MD, Ehlers JP, Worley LA, et al. Functional gene expression analysis uncovers phenotypic switch in aggressive uveal melanomas. Cancer Res 2006;66: 4602–4609.

54. Gamel JW, McLean IW. Quantitative analysis of the Callender classification of uveal melanoma cells. Arch Ophthalmol 1977;95:686–691.

59. Onken MD, Worley LA, Person E, et al. Loss of heterozygosity of chromosome 3 detected with single nucleotide

polymorphisms is superior to monosomy 3 for predicting metastasis in uveal melanoma. Clin Cancer Res 2007;13: 2923–2927.

60. Onken MD, Worley LA, Ehlers JP, et al. Gene expression profiling in uveal melanoma reveals two molecular classes and predicts metastatic death. Cancer Res 2004;64:7205–7209.

61. Tschentscher F, Husing J, Holter T, et al. Tumor classification based on gene expression profiling shows that uveal melanomas with and without monosomy 3 represent two distinct entities. Cancer Res 2003;63:2578–2584.

63. Worley LA, Onken MD, Person E, et al. Transcriptomic versus chromosomal prognostic markers and clinical outcome in uveal melanoma. Clin Cancer Res 2007;13:1466–1471.

72. Meir T, Dror R, Yu X, et al. Molecular characteristics of liver metastases from uveal melanoma. Invest Ophthalmol Vis Sci 2007;48:4890–4896.

CHAPTER 48

Genetics of hereditary retinoblastoma

Alejandra G de Alba Campomanes and Joan M O'Brien

Clinical background

Epidemiology

Retinoblastoma is a tumor of the developing retina. It is the most common malignant ocular tumor in childhood, affecting approximately 1 in 20 000 live births.[1–3] In the USA retinoblastoma is the 10th most common pediatric cancer,[4] with an incidence of 10.6 per million children under the age of 4, 1.53 per million in children between the ages of 5 and 9 years and only 0.27 per million in children over the age of 10.[5] Worldwide, retinoblastoma is responsible for 1% of childhood cancer deaths and 5% of childhood blindness.[6] No gender or race predilection and no significant environmental risk factors have been identified. However there may be an association between retinoblastoma and low socioeconomic status worldwide.[7]

Historical development

Knudson in 1971 provided critical insight into the genetic understanding of retinoblastoma by postulating the "two-hit" hypothesis.[8] He proposed that two mutational events were necessary for retinoblastoma tumorigenesis. Comings later expanded the theory by proposing that the mutations were in both alleles of a gene with a tumor-suppressive function.[9] The retinoblastoma gene (RB1) was later localized[10–12] and cloned[13–15] on chromosome 13q14, becoming the first tumor suppressor gene identified and laying the groundwork for great advances in the understanding of oncogenesis.

In this chapter we will briefly discuss the clinical presentation and management of retinoblastoma. We will also summarize the current understanding of the molecular pathophysiology and genetics of hereditary retinoblastoma.

Signs and symptoms

Patients usually present in the first year of life (average 7 months) for bilateral cases and at approximately 24 months for unilateral cases.[16] In patients without a family history, when retinoblastoma is not suspected, the most common clinical presentation is leukocoria or white pupil (Figure 48.1). The second most common presenting sign is strabismus, which is usually constant and unilateral and can manifest as an eso- or exodeviation. This is the result of macular involvement and represents an early sign of the disease, with higher survival rates and higher chances of globe preservation. In contrast leukocoria is a late sign and is associated with lower rates of globe salvage. A small proportion of patients have a more atypical presentation with consequent poor prognosis.[16] If the tumor spreads into the anterior chamber, the patient can develop hypopyon, rubeosis, or glaucoma or present with an apparent orbital cellulitis secondary to extensive tumor necrosis. Other presenting signs include unilateral mydriasis, heterochromia, hyphema, uveitis, and nystagmus. Extraocular extension of the disease may present with proptosis. Systemically, patients can present with signs of increased intracranial pressure secondary to an intracranial mass when affected by trilateral retinoblastoma.

Diagnostic workup

All patients with any clinical suspicion of retinoblastoma should have a complete ophthalmic exam and a careful family history. In the presence of hypopyon or orbital cellulitis, retinoblastoma should be ruled out before performing any surgical intervention such as a needle tap or biopsy. Exam under anesthesia is required for a thorough examination of the posterior pole and peripheral retina with scleral depression in infants and young children. A wide-angle camera (Ret-Cam) is commonly used and provides 130° imaging of the retina and the anterior segment.

On dilated fundus exam a round creamy yellow-white mass can be identified projecting into the vitreous cavity with large irregular blood vessels on the surface and penetrating the tumor (Figure 48.2). Vitreous or subretinal seeding of tumor cells can be observed. Calcification within the tumor mass is common. The localization of the tumor is variable but related to the age at presentation. Posterior pole masses tend to present at an earlier age. Patients can also present with a retinal detachment covering an underlying tumor mass. An irregular gray plaque on the retinal surface can be seen in the diffuse infiltrating form of this

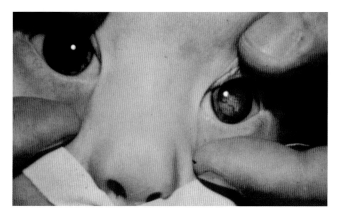

Figure 48.1 Leukocoria is the presenting sign of retinoblastoma in 60% of patients, as demonstrated here in a patient with unilateral disease. Strabismus is a presenting sign in 20% of patients with retinoblastoma. The remaining 20% of patients present with atypical clinical presentations like orbital cellulitis.

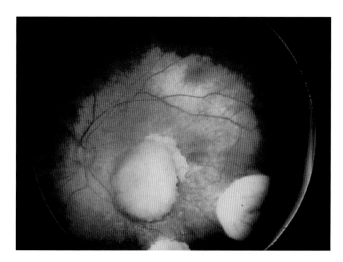

Figure 48.2 Fundus photograph showing multiple round elevated white masses projecting into the vitreous cavity.

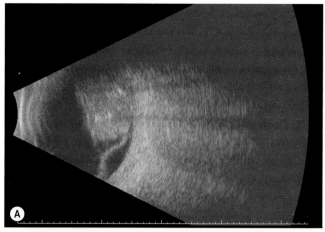

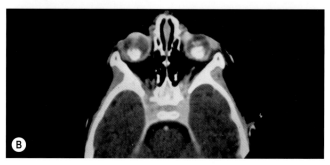

Figure 48.3 (A) B-scan ultrasonography demonstrating a high-reflectivity mass with characteristic shadowing. (B) Computed tomography can identify calcified masses.

disease. This is an uncommon presentation that is more difficult to diagnose; the presence of a hypopyon can sometimes alert the clinician to this unusual presentation.

In the presence of vitreous opacity or a retinal detachment, when visualization of the tumor mass is difficult, B-scan ultrasonography or computed tomography (CT) can identify calcifications (Figure 48.3). These tests should always be performed to exclude retinoblastoma before any surgical intervention is performed in a child with a restricted fundus exam.

B-scan ultrasonography characteristically demonstrates a high reflectivity mass with shadowing behind the tumor. Magnetic resonance imaging may be preferred to CT to reduce the risk of radiation-associated cancer in these pediatric patients.

Ultrasound biomicroscopy is useful to detect disease anterior to the ora serrata: this is an indication for immediate enucleation due to the increased risk for systemic metastasis. A biopsy of the tumor or vitreous is contraindicated due to the associated risk for tumor spread outside the eye. Bone

marrow aspiration and lumbar puncture should be performed to screen for metastasis in children who present late or with high-risk features of the disease.

Screening examinations of babies with a family history allow early detection of tumors even before they are clinically evident. Currrent recommendations for screening include: initial fundoscopic exam under anesthesia at birth and subsequently every 2–4 weeks for the first several months. The oldest age that a patient with a family history of retinoblastoma has presented is 48 months.[17]

Genetic testing for retinoblastoma

Genetic testing can characterize the specific mutation affecting an individual patient as well as identify the presence of a nonpenetrant mutation in a carrier parent. Karyotypic studies are less useful for clinical diagnosis because only 3–5% of retinoblastoma patients carry large deletions detectable by these methods.[18] Occasionally 13q deletions or translocations are evident through application of these techniques. In these cases, other systemic abnormalities, including severe developmental delay and dysmorphic features (13q deletion syndrome), can be clinically observed.

More sophisticated direct and indirect DNA analysis techniques are needed to detect smaller mutations. These techniques identify the initial germline mutation in approximately 85% of patients.[19] Direct methods involve extracting DNA from a fresh unfixed fragment of the tumor after enucleation. If this is not available, testing can be performed with leukocytes from peripheral blood. These techniques include single-strand conformation polymorphism (SSCP) analysis, gel electrophoretic analysis of synthetically amplified exons, and fluorescent in situ hybridization (FISH). Indirect methods can also be used in cases where the initial mutation cannot be found. These methods involve restriction fragment length polymorphism (RFLP) or variable number of tandem repeats (VNTR) analysis of parental and tumor DNA to detect the presence of a genetic marker that segregates along the retinoblastoma gene (RB1). Indirect techniques require the presence of two or more affected family members[20] and are in general less sensitive than direct techniques.

A recently described multistep testing strategy combines multiplex polymerase chain reaction (PCR) with double exon sequencing and promoter-targeted methylation-sensitive PCR to achieve a sensitivity of 89% in detecting the RB1 mutation.[21] Protein truncation testing has also been shown to be effective in screening for germline mutations.[22] New methodologies using microarray chips and robotic sequencing are currently on the horizon. In the future, knowing the specific gene mutation in a particular patient could be useful to predict disease severity and to provide prognostic and therapeutic guidance.

Genetic testing of affected patients and their families is extremely important, not only because patients with a germline mutation are at risk of developing secondary tumors, but also for genetic counseling. Occasionally, low-penetrance pedigrees can be identified where there is unilateral or even no detectable disease or family history. It is possible to perform preimplantation genetic diagnosis during in vitro fertilization. Therefore, screening for constitutional RB1 mutations should become an integral part of the management of patients with retinoblastoma, irrespective of tumor laterality or family background.

Differential diagnosis

The differential diagnosis of retinoblastoma includes lesions that simulate retinal tumors like *Toxocara canis* and astrocytic hamartoma, lesions that can cause retinal detachments such as retinopathy of prematurity, Coats disease, and persistent hyperplastic primary vitreous and other conditions like retinal dysplasia and medulloepithelioma (dikytoma).

Retinoma is a benign growth of the retina that is also produced by a mutation in the RB1 gene. It presents as a nonprogressive, elevated gray retinal mass that can have calcification and pigmentation. It may develop when the second mutation occurs in a nearly developed retinal cell and does not acquire the additional necessary mutations for full malignancy.

Treatment (Box 48.1)

Management algorithms for retinoblastoma have changed rapidly over the past few decades and continue to evolve. The goals of treatment are cure of the disease, globe salvage, preservation of vision, and early detection and treatment of secondary malignancies. A wide array of systemic and local treatments exists (Table 48.1).

Systemic chemotherapy protocols have replaced enucleation and radiation as the primary treatment for retinoblastoma. Chemotherapy reduces tumor volume

---

Box 48.1 Treatment key points

- Enucleation is still the most common form of treatment worldwide. In the developed world it is only used for advanced tumors
- External-beam radiation is used less commonly today due to associated increased secondary tumor risk and other complications
- Chemoreduction in combination with focal therapy is a highly effective treatment strategy
- Ongoing clinical trials will further elucidate the most appropriate treatment strategies
- New understandings in the pathogenesis of retinoblastoma will likely produce targeted molecular treatments with reduced systemic side-effects

---

Table 48.1 Treatment of retinoblastoma

Focal	Cryotherapy, laser photocoagulation, thermotherapy, brachytherapy, accelerated proton beam radiation
Whole eye	Subconjunctival/intravitreal chemotherapy, enucleation, external-beam radiation
Systemic	Intravenous chemotherapy

(chemoreduction) to permit application of focal techniques such as laser photocoagulation or cryotherapy to ablate remaining tumor mass. The choice of agents, combination, and dosage varies among treatment centers. The most commonly used chemotherapeutic agents include vincristine, carboplatin, etoposide, and teniposide. Ciclosporin A is sometimes used to combat multidrug resistance. Subtenon injections of carboplatin can be used as an adjunct to systemic chemotherapy. Intravenous carboplatin can also be used in conjunction with infrared diode laser radiation applied directly to the tumor through the pupil (transpupillary thermotherapy) because heat increases the permeability of the cellular membrane to antimitotics, reinforcing their cytotoxic effect. For small tumors (diameter less than 3 mm), transpupillary thermotherapy can be used alone, relying on the cytotoxic effect of heat by raising the temperature of the tumor above 45 °C. Complete tumor control can be achieved in 85% of appropriately selected patients.[23] Complications include iris atrophy, lens opacities, retinal traction, retinal detachment, and disk edema. Chemotherapy alone does not achieve permanent tumor control. When local therapy is applied in conjunction with chemotherapy, success rates approach 85%.[24] Systemic chemotherapy carries potentially serious systemic adverse effects, including hearing loss, cytopenia, neutropenia, infections, gastrointestinal toxicity, and neurotoxicity.

External-beam radiation is indicated in advanced bilateral cases or in cases of disease relapse. It may also be considered for small tumors located within the macula, because it offers a better chance for useful vision when compared to other focal treatments. Radiation increases the risk of secondary nonocular malignancies. Side-effects include cataract formation, dry eye, retinopathy, vitreous hemorrhage, growth retardation of the orbit, and resultant midface hypoplasia.

Brachytherapy uses radioactive plaques, like iodine-125 or ruthenium-106, on the sclera over the base of the tumor. The total dose of radiation is ~4000 cGy delivered at a rate of 1000 cGy daily. It can be used for medium-sized tumors (4–10 disk diameters) for consolidation or as a secondary method after treatment failure with localized relapse. Tumors involving the macula or optic disk are not optimal candidates for this treatment modality. The recurrence rate for this treatment is 12% at 1 year if used as primary treatment and 8–34% if used as salvage therapy after failure of other methods.[25] Radiation retinopathy, cataract, and neovascular glaucoma are reported complications of brachytherapy. Accelerated proton beam irradiation uses tantalum rings sutured to the sclera to mark the tumor edges in order to deliver an accelerated particle beam to active intraocular tumor. It can also be applied as an adjunct to enucleation with positive tumor margins in the optic nerve stump.

Focal treatments include transpupillary argon laser photocoagulation and transscleral cryotherapy. Small tumors (less than 3 mm in diameter and 2 mm in thickness) without vitreous seeding are good candidates for photocoagulation. Complications include retinal detachment, fibrosis, and vascular occlusions. Alternatively, cryotherapy can be used if a small tumor is located peripherally. Cryotherapy causes intracellular ice crystal formation, protein denaturation, pH changes, and cell membrane rupture. Circulation to the tumor is also disrupted. Cryotherapy can also be applied as a secondary treatment for tumor previously treated with laser, transpupillary thermotherapy, or external-beam radiation. Tumor destruction is usually achieved after one or two sessions of triple-freeze therapy at 1-month intervals. Complete destruction is achieved in 90% of tumors.[26] Complications include pain, intraocular inflammation, chemosis, lid edema, vitreous hemorrhage, and retinal detachment.

In the USA, enucleation is reserved for advanced cases of retinoblastoma with massive involvement of the retina and vitreous, rubeosis, glaucoma, or tumor invasion into the anterior segment or optic nerve. It remains the most common form of treatment worldwide.[16] Fortunately, enucleation is effective, achieving total cure in 99% of patients with no extraocular involvement.[7] During enucleation it is of utmost importance to avoid inadvertent perforation of the globe, since this carries a very high risk for extraocular tumor seeding. A long section of the optic nerve should be obtained for histopathological analysis. Enucleation is the only treatment modality that allows genetic analysis of fresh tissue. High-risk characteristics of enucleated specimens include massive choroidal infiltration, anterior-chamber seeding, tumor invasion beyond the lamina cribrosa, and scleral invasion. Children with these high-risk features are recommended to have adjunctive chemotherapy (Children's Oncology Group, Group E Prospective Trial).[27] Tumor at the surgical margin of the optic nerve has an associated mortality rate of 50–81%.[28] High-dose chemotherapy with autologous marrow transplantation is therefore indicated to prevent metastases in patients with tumor extending beyond the cut end of the optic nerve (Children's Oncology Group, Group F Concept Proposal).[27]

Novel treatment modalities under investigation include subconjunctival (Figure 48.4) and intravitreal delivery of chemotherapeutic agents,[29] injection of photosensitizing agents followed by selective laser treatment, gene therapy, and ophthalmic artery injection of chemotherapeutic agents. New understanding in the genetic alterations in retinoblastoma tumorigenesis will likely produce novel molecular targets to treat the tumors directly with reduced systemic side-effects.[30]

Prognosis and complications

When diagnosis is timely, local control is excellent and survival exceeds 85% in patients who present with disease confined to the globe. Survival has improved dramatically in the past century, approaching 96% in specialized centers where patients have access to modern therapeutic strategies. However in developing countries mortality is still as high as 50%.[31] Extraocular disease carries a significantly worse prognosis and is fatal in 50–85% of cases.[16] Visual prognosis depends on the size of the tumor, location, and multifocality, and the presence of retinal detachment, vitreous seeding, or subretinal seeding.

The most common route for metastasis is direct extension into the optic nerve with subsequent intracranial or meningeal involvement. Systemic metastasis can also occur through extensive involvement of the choroidal circulation. The bone marrow is the most common site for metastasis. Other less frequent sites for metastases include bone, lymph nodes, liver, and lungs. The greatest risk factor for metastasis is extensive invasion down the optic nerve or into the orbit.

Patients who carry an *RB1* germline mutation are at risk of developing other nonocular malignancies, such as midline intracranial tumors (also known as pinealoma, pinealoblastoma, ectopic intracranial retinoblastoma, trilateral retinoblastoma, or primitive neuroectodermal tumor), osteosarcoma, other soft-tissue sarcomas, and cutaneous melanoma. The cumulative incidence of second tumor development is 1% per year; after 50 years, 50% of patients would have developed another primary malignant tumor. The risk of developing osteosarcoma is increased by radiation, especially when administered within the first year of life.[32] Secondary primary tumors, rather than retinoblastoma itself, are the most common cause of death in retinoblastoma patients.[33]

Pathology

Different growth patterns can be identified on gross pathology: the endophytic form of retinoblastoma grows into the vitreous cavity, whereas the exophytic form grows into the subretinal space, producing an overlying retinal detachment (Figure 48.5). A mixed-growth pattern is a combination of these two endophytic and exophytic forms. Diffuse infiltrating or plaque-like retinoblastoma presents with no obvious mass or calcification.[34]

Histopathologically, retinoblastoma consists of poorly differentiated neuroblastic cells with large hyperchromatic nuclei and scant cytoplasm. Mitotic figures are common. More differentiated cells can form Flexner–Wintersteiner rosettes, a spherical structure of columnar cells arranged around a lumen composed of internal limiting membrane. Flexner–Wintersteiner rosettes are a unique histopathologic feature of retinoblastoma.

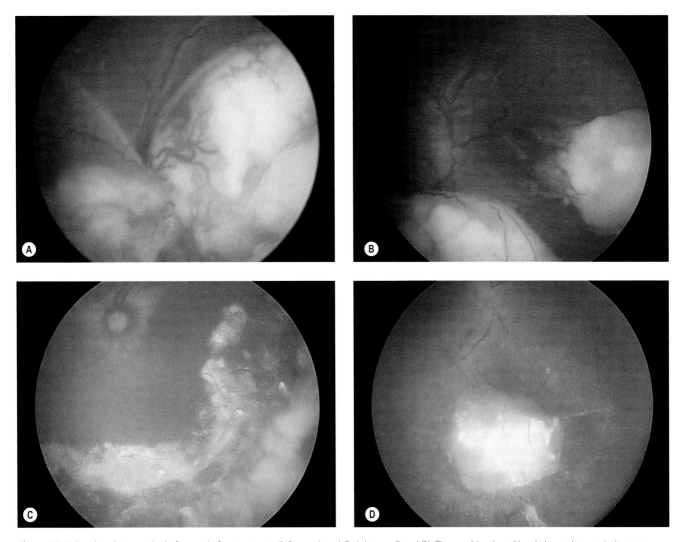

Figure 48.4 Fundus photographs before and after treatment (left eye, A and C; right eye, B and D). The combination of local chemotherapy (subtenon carboplatin) and local laser therapy (green laser photoablation) can often significantly improve a patient's outcome.

Etiology

Genetics

The retinoblastoma tumor arises from loss or mutation of both alleles of the *RB1* on the q14 band of chromosome 13.[13,14] Approximately 60% of affected children have the sporadic or nonheritable form of this disease.[1] Characteristically unilateral and unifocal, this form of the disease arises when both of the *RB1* alleles are inactivated somatically in a single developing retinal cell. The remaining 40% of patients have heritable or familial retinoblastoma (Table 48.2), where affected individuals carrying a predisposing germline mutation suffer an additional mutational event in the normal allele of the developing retinal cell (Figure 48.6). In general, heritable retinoblastoma is characterized by high

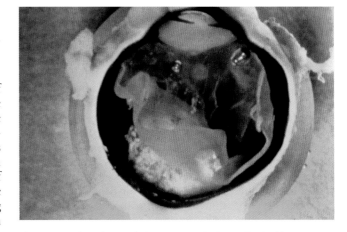

Figure 48.5 Gross histopathology section of advanced retinoblastoma demonstrating an exophytic tumor with overlying retinal detachment.

373

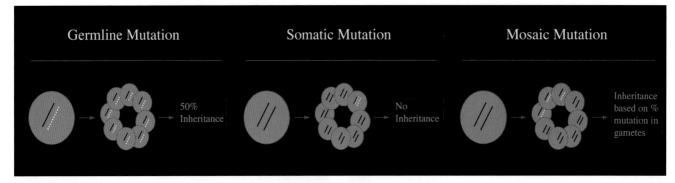

Figure 48.6 Inheritance patters for retinoblastoma. (A) Germline mutation (predisposing germline mutation plus additional mutational event in the normal allele of the developing retinal cell). (B) Somatic mutation (both of the *RB1* alleles are inactivated in a single developing retinal cell) and (C) mosaic mutation (aside from previously recognized germline and somatic forms of retinoblastoma, mosaicism for this gene mutation may also be responsible for heritable disease).

Table 48.2 In heritable retinoblastoma a germline mutation is present 100% of the time[1]

De novo mutation	75%
Inherited from affected/nonaffected parent	25%
Known family history	10–15%

Box 48.2 Mutational mechanisms

Germline mutations → first mutational event

- Point mutation (single base change)
- Small insertion or deletion
- Chromosomal translocation
- Large deletion or insertion

Somatic mutation → second mutational event[38]

- Distinct point mutation
- Allele-specific hypermethylation (40%)
- Loss of heterozygosity (60%) by mechanisms that include nondysjunction, duplication of the entire chromosome, mitotic recombination

penetrance (nearly 90% of carriers develop the disease) and high expressivity (bilateral and multifocal tumors). However least common mutations can result in a different pattern with reduced penetrance and expressivity ("low-penetrance retinoblastoma"). Approximately 11% of patients with unilateral tumors harbor a germline mutation (i.e., have the heritable form).[35] Heritable retinoblastoma is considered a genetic cancer predisposition syndrome since the presence of a germline mutation imposes an elevated risk for the development of cancer in other organ systems.

Mutations (Box 48.2)

In the majority of cases the first *RB1* mutation is a single nucleotide change (point mutation) or small deletion. In 60% of cases the second mutational event occurs following loss of heterozygosity (LOH) by nondisjunction followed by reduplication or mitotic recombination, resulting in homozygosity of the initial mutation in the susceptible retinal cell. Mutations occur throughout the *RB1* gene with no single mutational "hotspot." Ninety percent of clinically significant mutations are characterized by frameshift, nonsense, or splice mutations, which produce a premature stop codon and a truncated transcript.[36] These mutations involve the large pocket domain of the retinoblastoma protein (pRb) 98% of patients.[36] The high frequency of truncating mutations in retinoblastoma suggests that tumorigenesis is most favored by mutations that globally inactivate pRb. In contrast truncating mutations are absent in low-penetrance retinoblastoma. The mutations reported in these kindreds minimally alter the expression of the pRb, permitting residual protein function. Retinoblastoma in these low-penetrance kindreds often skips generations, is unilateral, has a delayed onset with few intraocular recurrences, and shows an early and complete response to therapy.[37]

Pathophysiology

The human *RB1* gene spans 180 kb of DNA[39] and contains 27 exons. It encodes a 4.8-kb mRNA.[40] Its protein product (pRb) is a 110-kDa phosphoprotein composed of 928 amino acids. This protein functions as a regulator at the cell cycle checkpoint between the G1 and S-phase. When inactivated, transcription of downstream genes that promote progression through the cell cycle occurs. Along with p107 and p130, pRb belongs to the pocket protein family.

Retinoblastoma likely arises from either a precursor cone photoreceptor or a multipotent retinoblast. The retinal cells in these patients develop and mature between the third month postconception and the age of 4 years, being susceptible to mutations at any point during this time.

Function of pRb

pRb inhibits cellular proliferation by altering the expression of genes that promote cellular division through an interaction with the E2F transcription factors. Of the six E2F members (E2F1–E2F6), pRb interacts preferentially with

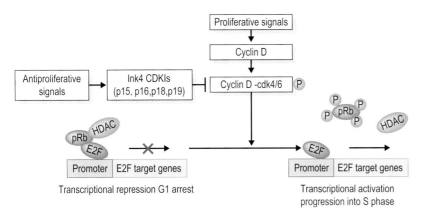

Figure 48.7 The role of the retinoblastoma protein (pRb) in the cell cycle. pRb is hyperphosphorylated (inactivated) by cyclin-dependent kinases in response to mitogenic signals, leading to its dissociation from E2F and enabling the cell to progress into the DNA synthesis phase.

E2F1–E2F4, whereas p107 and p103 interact with E2F4 and E2F5.[41] The activation of E2F1–E2F3[41] is required for cell proliferation, since these transcription factors activate the expression of genes required for G1/S-phase progression and for DNA replication.[42]

In its hypophosphorylated state, the active form of pRb binds to E2F in early G1,[43] blocking its transactivating function and inhibiting cell cycle progression.[44] This interaction may result in permanent or reversible cell cycle arrest (G0). Continuous mitogenic signaling is required to induce the cell out of G0 (quiescence) and allow it to progress through the cell cycle. pRb is hyperphosphorylated by cyclin-dependent kinases in response to mitogenic signals. Mitogenic stimuli induce the expression of cyclin D which in turn binds to cdk4 and cdk6 to form complexes. These complexes phosphorylate and inactivate pRb, leading to its dissociation from E2F and enabling the cell to progress into the DNA synthesis phase of the cell cycle (S) (Figure 48.7). The conformational changes that inactivate pRb can be mimicked by mutations in the *RB1* gene or by binding to viral proteins (adenovirus E1A, simian virus 40, large T-antigen, and human papillomavirus E7).[45,46] On the other hand, antiproliferative signals, such as DNA damage and senescence,[47] induce the expression of cyclin-dependent kinase inhibitors, which positively regulate pRb by inactivating the cyclin–cdk complexes through the upregulation of Ink4 and Cip/Kip family proteins. Data suggest that pRb is only partially inactivated at G1. During later phases of the cell cycle, pRb has a significant function, such as inducing cell cycle arrest at G2/M.[48]

Loss of pRb does not necessarily lead to tumor formation. In some tissues, the response to pRb loss is apoptosis.[49] This is because pRb plays a critical role in the terminal differentiation of many cell types, including neurons, muscle, bone, erythrocytes, and fibers of the crystalline lens.[50] In these cell types, loss of the pRb results in massive apoptosis or developmental defects.[51] In other tissues like the retina and bone, the loss of pRb initiates tumorigenesis.

Role of the pRb in the development of retinoblastoma

The precise manner in which loss of the retinoblastoma protein results in retinoblastoma tumor development is still unclear. Retinoblastoma presumably arises from the dependence of retinal cells on pRb for terminal differentiation

through a complex process involving the regulation of cell cycle progression, apoptosis, and the expression of differentiation genes. During organogenesis the retina begins as a single layer of neuronal stem cells (neuroblasts). Murine studies suggest that pRb plays an important role in the differentiation of these neuroblasts into ganglion cells, amacrine and horizontal cells, and cone photoreceptors. *RB1* expression is absent in bipolar cells and rod photoreceptors.[52] Knockout mice models (*RB1* -/-) suggest that in the absence of *RB1* there is ectopic proliferation and enhanced apoptosis in this inner retinal progenitor layer, indicating that pRb is required for terminal cell cycle arrest and for suppression of apoptosis.[53]

The biallelic loss of the *RB1* gene is a necessary and rate-limiting event in the development of retinoblastoma, but it is not sufficient. In humans, it has been proposed that a third mutational event is required to allow retinoblastoma cells to escape apoptosis and to proliferate.[52] However, studies from knockout and chimeric mouse models have shown intact apoptotic mechanisms.[53] In murine models, retinoblastoma only results when *RB1* loss is accompanied by at least another cell cycle regulatory gene alteration. The susceptibility in humans with *RB1* mutations to develop retinoblastoma is unexplained by these models. The inactivation of other pocket proteins and also of the tumor suppressor p53 has been extensively studied without conclusive evidence. In the mouse, combined loss of p107 and pRb appears to be a requirement for the development of retinoblastoma[54]; however, in humans, p130 appears to be more important as a tumor suppressor protein acting in conjunction with pRb.[55]

Human retinoblastoma tumor analysis has identified other chromosomal alterations and additional mutations. Frequently found genetic alterations include + 1q, + 2p, + 6p, − 16, −16q, − 17, and −17p. p53 is located on 17p13; however, the potential involvement of p53 in human retinoblastoma has been controversial. As mentioned earlier, p53 inactivation may be required for murine retinoblastoma, but no p53 mutation has ever been characterized in primary retinoblastoma and studies in retinoblastoma tumor specimens suggest the presence of normal p53 function.[56] MDM2 (mouse double minute 2 homolog) encodes a protein that inhibits transactivation by tumor protein p53. Overexpression of this gene can result in excessive inactivation of p53, diminishing its tumor suppressor function. *MDMX* is a gene related to MDM2, with the same p53 antagonistic properties.

p14 Arf (cyclin-dependent kinase inhibitor 2A) expression has been found to be increased in human retinoblastoma cells when compared to normal retina.[57] p14 Arf inactivates MDM2/MDMX, leading to apoptosis mediated by p53. However, a recent study found *MDMX* to be amplified in human retinoblastoma samples. In vitro, *MDMX* suppressed cell death in *RB1* deficient human retina and led to rosette formation similar to human retinoblastoma.[57] This recent evidence suggests that retinoblastoma does not bypass tumor surveillance mechanisms and that there is inactivation of the p53 pathway after loss of *RB1*, probably by subsequent amplification of the *MDMX* gene in the preneoplastic retinoblastoma cells.[57]

Conclusion

Retinoblastoma is a rare disease, but understanding of retinoblastoma gene derangements which underlie this condition has provided major insights in cancer research. The retinoblastoma gene was the first tumor suppressor gene to be identified, representing a new category of genes which have been found to be etiologic in a spectrum of tumor predisposition syndromes. As knowledge of the *RB1* gene and the pathway it regulates continues to emerge, so too will a greater understanding of mechanisms for carcinogenesis.

Key references

A complete list of chapter references is available online at www.expertconsult.com. See inside cover for registration details.

8. Knudson AG Jr. Mutation and cancer: statistical study of retinoblastoma. Proc Natl Acad Sci USA 1971;68:820–823.

14. Lee WH, Bookstein R, Hong F, et al. Human retinoblastoma susceptibility gene: cloning, identification, and sequence. Science 1987;235:1394–1399.

16. Balmer A, Zografos L, Munier F. Diagnosis and current management of retinoblastoma. Oncogene 2006;25:5341–5349.

18. Ejima Y, Sasaki MS, Kaneko A, et al. Types, rates, origin and expressivity of chromosome mutations involving 13q14 in retinoblastoma patients. Hum Genet 1988;79:118–123.

19. Lohmann DR. RB1 gene mutations in retinoblastoma. Hum Mutat 1999;14:283–288.

20. Smith BJ, O'Brien JM. The genetics of retinoblastoma and current diagnostic testing. J Pediatr Ophthalmol Strabismus 1996;33:120–123.

21. Richter S, Vandezande K, Chen N, et al. Sensitive and efficient detection of RB1 gene mutations enhances care for families with retinoblastoma. Am J Hum Genet 2003;72:253–269.

24. Shields CL, Mashayekhi A, Cater J, et al. Chemoreduction for retinoblastoma. Analysis of tumor control and risks for recurrence in 457 tumors. Am J Ophthalmol 2004;138:329–337.

32. Moll AC, Imhof SM, Schouten-Van Meeteren AY, et al. Second primary tumors in hereditary retinoblastoma: a register-based study, 1945–1997: is there an age effect on radiation-related risk? Ophthalmology 2001;108:1109–1114.

35. Brichard B, Heusterspreute M, De Potter P, et al. Unilateral retinoblastoma, lack of familial history and older age does not exclude germline RB1 gene mutation. Eur J Cancer 2006;42:65–72.

36. Harbour JW. Overview of RB gene mutations in patients with retinoblastoma. Implications for clinical genetic screening. Ophthalmology 1998;105:1442–1447.

39. Toguchida J, McGee TL, Paterson JC, et al. Complete genomic sequence of the human retinoblastoma susceptibility gene. Genomics 1993;17:535–543.

44. Weinberg RA. The retinoblastoma protein and cell cycle control. Cell 1995;81:323–330.

49. Corson TW, Gallie BL. One hit, two hits, three hits, more? Genomic changes in the development of retinoblastoma. Genes Chromosomes Cancer 2007;46:617–634.

57. Laurie NA, Donovan SL, Shih CS, et al. Inactivation of the p53 pathway in retinoblastoma. Nature 2006;444:61–66.

CHAPTER 49

Molecular basis of low-penetrance retinoblastoma

Katie Matatall and J William Harbour

Clinical background

Retinoblastoma is the most common intraocular malignancy in children and is the prototype inherited cancer predisposition syndrome. About 60% of new patients exhibit unilateral ocular involvement with familial inheritance pattern. The remaining patients have a heritable form of retinoblastoma, which is often associated with bilateral ocular involvement, germline transmission to offspring, and second primary tumors.[1] In most retinoblastoma families, the penetrance (the proportion of individuals with a germline mutation in the RB gene who develop clinical manifestations of the disease) is about 90%.[2] However, about one in seven families will exhibit reduced penetrance as low as 30–60%. This chapter will focus on features that are specific to low-penetrance retinoblastoma (Box 49.1). The features of retinoblastoma in general are covered in Chapter 48.

The diseased-eye ratio (DER), calculated by dividing the number of eyes containing tumors by the number of mutation carriers in a family, has been devised as a means of more precisely defining low-penetrance families.[3] A DER less than 1.5 is consistent with low-penetrance retinoblastoma. Retinoblastoma patients in low-penetrance families will often exhibit reduced expressivity (the extent to which an affected individual expresses the disease phenotype), such as unilateral ocular involvement, fewer ocular tumors, and benign retinal tumors called retinomas or retinocytomas.[2,4–6] The clinical appearance of retinoblastoma in low-penetrance patients is indistinguishable from that in full-penetrance retinoblastoma patients, which is described in Chapter 48.

Pathology

The pathologic appearance of retinoblastomas in low-penetrance patients is indistinguishable from that in full-penetrance retinoblastoma patients, which is described in Chapter 48.

Etiology

The rate-limiting event in the development of low-penetrance retinoblastoma, like that of full-penetrance retinoblastoma, is thought to be mutation of the retinoblastoma (RB) tumor suppressor gene on chromosome 13q. The existence of a putative tumor suppressor gene responsible for retinoblastoma was first suggested by Knudson in 1971,[7] and confirmed by the discovery of the RB gene.[8–10] RB gene mutation can be demonstrated in the vast majority of retinoblastomas, as well as some other types of cancer.[11,12] The mechanisms by which the RB gene is mutated, and how this leads to retinal tumors, is covered in more detail in Chapter 48.

Pathophysiology

Most retinoblastoma families demonstrate autosomal-dominant inheritance with almost complete penetrance and high expressivity, due to the transmission of an inactive copy of the RB gene and subsequent loss of the remaining copy in somatic retinal cells. However, about one in seven families displays decreased penetrance and reduced expressivity. Low-penetrance retinoblastoma has been recognized for many years,[2] and various mechanisms have been proposed, including immunologic factors, DNA methylation, epigenetic mechanisms, delayed mutation, host resistance factors, a second retinoblastoma locus, and "modulator genes."[2,13–16] However, recent advances in our understanding of the structure and function of the retinoblastoma protein (pRB) have shown that low-penetrance retinoblastoma results from special types of mutations at the RB gene that result in a reduced amount or activity of pRB.

Genetic mechanisms of low-penetrance retinoblastoma

In one of the first reports of low-penetrance retinoblastoma, a family was described that transmitted a constitutional chromosomal deletion involving the RB gene locus at chromosome 13q14 with unaffected carriers retaining a balanced insertional translocation.[17] Although chromosomal rearrangements now appear to be a rare cause of low-penetrance retinoblastoma, this study was important in demonstrating that low-penetrance retinoblastoma could be caused by alterations at the RB locus without invoking other nongenetic mechanisms. Subsequently, it was suggested that low-penetrance retinoblastoma may be caused by RB gene mutations that result in a "weak" copy (or allele) of the RB gene that can partially suppress tumorigenesis. In this theory, as long as one normal allele is present, an individual carrying a weak allele would be protected from retinoblastoma. In this same individual, a developing somatic retinal cell that lost the normal allele, such as by nondisjunction, and duplicated the weak allele, such as by reduplication or mitotic recombination, would have a low risk for retinoblastoma. However, if the normal allele is lost and the weak allele is not duplicated, the risk for retinoblastoma would be high (Figure 49.1). This theory appears to explain most low-penetrance retinoblastoma. Approximately 60% of second hits that would be tumorigenic with full-penetrance mutations would have a low risk for causing tumors with a weak, or low-penetrance, mutation.

In recent years, the molecular nature of many of these "weak" RB gene alleles has been elucidated (Box 49.2). At least 14 different RB gene mutations have now been described in low-penetrance retinoblastoma families (Tables 49.1 and 49.2).[3,6,16,18–21] These mutations fall into two functional classes: (1) mutations that reduce the level of expression of normal pRB; and (2) mutations that result in a mutant pRB that is partially inactivated. There may also be mutations that both reduce protein levels and partially inactivate the protein,[22] although these have not yet been convincingly proven.

Type 1 mutations that reduce the expression of normal retinoblastoma protein

Type 1 mutations that cause a reduction in the amount of functional pRB are less common than type 2 mutations and fall into two main subtypes: promoter mutations and splice site mutations. Promoter mutations presumably reduce the amount of RB mRNA produced by perturbing the interaction

between the transcriptional machinery and the promoter. For example, low-penetrance point mutations have been found in the binding sites for transcription factors, such as SP1 and ATF,[18,20] both of which are known to be required for normal pRB expression.[23] Another form of type 1

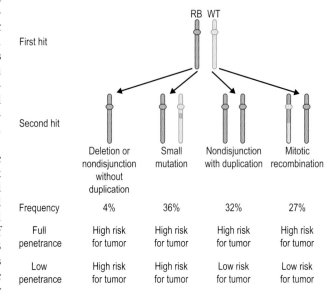

Figure 49.1 Chromosomal events leading to tumorigenesis in retinoblastoma according to the Knudsen "two-hit" hypothesis.[7] The first "hit" or mutation of the RB gene occurs either in the germline or in a somatic cell (i.e., retinoblast). The second hit, which is always a somatic event, disrupts the remaining RB allele by one of the indicated mechanisms (their approximate frequencies in retinoblastoma tumors are indicated).[61] The predicted result of the two hits (high versus low tumor risk) is indicated when the first hit involves a full-penetrance versus a low-penetrance mutation. These predictions are based on the assumption that two copies of a low-penetrance mutation may be sufficient to suppress tumorigenesis. Approximately 60% of second hits that are tumorigenic with full-penetrance mutations may not cause tumors with low-penetrance mutations. RB, chromosome 13q bearing mutant copy of RB; WT, chromosome 13q bearing wild-type (normal) copy of RB gene.

Box 49.1 Low-penetrance retinoblastoma

- Pathologically indistinguishable from full-penetrance retinoblastoma
- Displays decreased penetrance and expressivity
- Caused by distinct types of mutations in the retinoblastoma gene

Box 49.2 Low-penetrance retinoblastoma mutations

- Type 1 mutations result in decreased production of normal retinoblastoma protein
- Type 2 mutations result in the production of partially inactivated retinoblastoma protein

---

Table 49.1 Type 1 low-penetrance retinoblastoma mutations that reduce expression of normal retinoblastoma protein

Mutation number	Diseased-eye ratio	DNA alteration	Location	Functional significance	References
1	0.88	G > A at -198	Promoter	SP1 binding site	18
2	1.00	G > T at -189	Promoter	ATF binding site	18
3	0.83	G > A at -189	Promoter	ATF binding site	53
4	0.34	G > C at -149	Promoter	Transcription factor binding site	20
5	NR	A > G at 1331	Exon 13	Exon splice site	42, 56, 57
6	0.64	G > A at 2215	Exon 21	Exon splice site	6
7	NR	G > A at 2325	Exon 22	Exon splice site	42, 58

NR, not reported.

Table 49.2 Type 2 low-penetrance retinoblastoma mutations that partially inactivate the retinoblastoma protein

Mutation number	Diseased-eye ratio	Affect on protein	Domain affected	Nuclear localization	Phosphorylation	LxCXE binding	E2F binding	Colony suppression	Differentiation	Temperature-sensitive	References
1	0.4	Delete AA1–112	Amino terminus	Yes	Yes	NR	NR	Yes	NR	NR	22, 59
2	0.65	Delete AA127–166 (exon 4)	Amino terminus (G2/M Kinase-binding site)	Yes	Minimal	NR	Reduced	Yes	Yes	NR	21, 40
3	0.5	Delete AA287–313 (exon 9)	Amino terminus (lobe B)	NR	NR	NR	NR	NR	NR	NR	42, 53, 55
4	1	Delete AA480 (exon 16)	A box	Yes	Yes	Reduced	Minimal	Yes	NR	Yes	3,36, 40
5	1	Arg661 Trp (exon 20)	B box	Yes	Yes	Reduced	Minimal	Yes	Yes	Yes	3, 36, 39–41
6	0.5	Cys712Arg (exon 21)	B box (adjacent to LxCxE-binding site)	NR	Yes	Minimal	Minimal	NR	NR	Yes	36, 60
7	0.78	Delete AA830–887 (exon 24–25)	Carboxy terminus (NLS, E2F, MDM2-binding sites)	Reduced	NR	NR	Reduced	Minimal	NR	NR	2

AA, amino acid; NR, not reported.

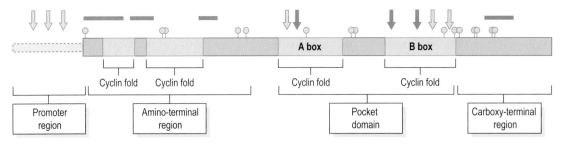

Figure 49.2 The structural map of the retinoblastoma protein and location of low-penetrance mutations. Open arrows, type 1 mutations; closed arrows and bars, type 2 mutations; open circles, phosphorylation sites.

Box 49.3 Structure of the retinoblastoma protein

- Pocket domain contains binding sites for chromatin remodeling proteins and E2F family transcription factors
- Carboxy terminal region contains regulatory phosphorylation sites, binding sites for oncoproteins such as Hdm2 and c-abl
- Amino terminal region is less well characterized and contains binding sites for proteins such as MCM7, EID-1, and RbK

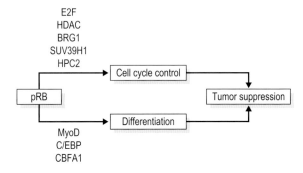

Figure 49.3 The complex role of the retinoblastoma protein (pRB) in tumor suppression. Initially, pRB was noted to inhibit cell cycle progression through binding to proliferative factors such as E2F. However, binding of pRB to chromatin remodeling proteins, such as histone deacetylases (HDAC), SWI/SNF ATPases (e.g., BRG1), histone methyltransferases (e.g., SUV39H1), and polycomb proteins (e.g., HPC2), is also critical for its ability to control the cell cycle. In addition, pRB can suppress tumorigenesis by inducing differentiation, which appears to be linked to its ability to interact with differentiation factors such as myoD (muscle differentiation), C/EBP (adipocyte differentiation), and CBFA1 (bone differentiation). Some low-penetrance mutations appear to result in the production of a mutant pRB that cannot control the cell cycle but can still induce differentiation.

mutation occurs when a mutation within a splice site reduces the efficiency of mRNA splicing and/or inconsistent intron excision. These mutations result in a reduced amount of correctly spliced mRNA and, consequently, a reduced amount of protein. An example of this is a G to A transition that is seen in the last base of exon 21 which causes a reduction in the match of the exon boundary acceptor site to the consensus.[6] This change from the consensus results in a 90% reduction in the production of normal mRNA.

Type 2 mutations that partially inactivate the retinoblastoma protein

Type 2 mutations partially inactivate the pRB protein by affecting the coding region of the protein. These mutations are usually small in-frame deletions or missense mutations (single nucleotide changes that do not result in a premature stop codon) that have subtle effects on the overall structure and function of the protein. A better understanding of the effects of type 2 mutations can be gained by understanding the detailed structure and function of each region of the pRB protein.

Structure of the retinoblastoma protein

The retinoblastoma gene encodes a 105-kDa nuclear phosphoprotein made up of three major regions: the amino terminus, the pocket domain, and the carboxy terminus (Box 49.3; Figure 49.2). pRB is able to function as a tumor suppressor primarily through its ability to inhibit the cell cycle at the G-to-S transition (Figure 49.3). This function of pRB is due to its ability to interact with, and inhibit, the transcription of cell cycle genes through the E2F family of transcription factors.[24] pRB interacts with E2Fs through both its pocket domain and its carboxy terminus, so mutations in either of these regions could affect tumor suppressor function.

Interaction with E2Fs directly blocks their transactivation domain, but pRB also suppresses transcription by recruiting chromatin remodeling proteins, such as histone deacetylases, SWI/SNP ATPases, DNA methylases, histone methylases and polycomb proteins, to remodel local chromatin into an inactive, closed state.[24-28] The tumor suppressor function of pRB may also derive from its ability to cooperate with differentiation factors, such as myoD, C/EBP, and CBFA1, to promote terminal differentiation and cell cycle exit, which protects cells from malignant transformation (Figure 49.3).[29,30] Similarly, pRB can bind and inhibit differentiation inhibitors such as Id2.[31]

The pocket domain

The pocket domain (amino acids 379–792) is perhaps the most well-studied region of pRB, since much of its tumor suppressor activity maps to this domain. The pocket is made up of two highly conserved regions known as the A and B boxes, which are separated by a less conserved spacer region.[32] The importance of the pocket domain is due, at least in part, to its ability to bind to many different proteins, some of which contain an LxCxE motif (e.g., HDACs, BRG1, EID-1, and the viral oncoproteins simian virus-40 large T antigen, human papillomavirus E7, and adenovirus E1A).

The binding site within the pocket for the LxCxE-containing proteins is made up of at least five highly conserved amino acids that are separated within the linear polypeptide sequence.[32] The crystal structure of the pocket bound to the LxCxE-containing protein E1A showed that there were as many as 20 residues within the pocket that were mediating the interaction.[33] Mutations in any of these or surrounding residues could potentially reduce binding efficiency and, thus, inhibit key functions of pRB. Although the majority of the key residues for these interactions are located in the B box, mutations in the A box could also potentially disrupt binding of the B box to other proteins, since the A and B box exhibit a complex interaction with each other that is required for proper conformation and function of the B box.[34]

One low-penetrance mutation has been shown to involve a missense nucleotide alteration that affects Cys712 in the LxCxE-binding site.[23,35] The residue directly next to this mutation site, Lys713, is one of the key residues in the LxCxE-binding site.[32] Mutations in this site result in reduced binding to HDAC and E2F.[26,36]

The pocket domain is also responsible for binding non-LxCxE proteins, such as E2Fs, which bind to the pocket domain at a highly conserved groove that is formed at the interface between the A and B boxes.[37] When key residues within this groove are mutated, the resultant pRB protein has a marked reduction in binding affinity for E2F1.[37] The crystal structure of pRB bound to E2F1 showed a total of 17 pocket residues involved in their interaction,[38] and some of these residues include the binding sites for LxCxE proteins.[33]

One mutation seen in low-penetrance families involves amino acid substitution at Arg661.[3,36,39–42] This residue is in exon 20 within the B box of the pocket and is in close proximity to Lys653, which is located within the A–B groove and is critical for E2F1 binding. The Arg661 mutant protein can interact through hydrogen bonds with residues in the A box, which may help to stabilize the A–B interface, yet it can be inactivated in a temperature-dependent manner.[36,40,43] This suggests that the mutant protein is not completely inactive but is subject to subtle changes in structure that affect binding efficiency.

The carboxy terminal region

In addition to the pocket domain, the carboxy terminus (amino acids 793–928) also plays an important role in the tumor suppressor activity of pRB.[43] This region contains binding sites for the oncoproteins Hdm2 and c-abl,[44,45] seven phosphorylation sites that regulate protein activity, and docking sites for cyclin-dependent kinases that phosphorylate pRB.[46] This region also contains a nuclear localization signal that is critical for pRB to reach the nucleus, where its function is carried out.[23] The carboxy terminus also contains sites that are important for binding to E2Fs.[47,48]

One example of a low-penetrance mutation within this region is an in-frame deletion of exon 24 and 25, which removes amino acids 830–887.[16] This mutant protein lacks one of the two E2F-binding sites, as well as the binding site for HDM2 and c-abl, and the nuclear localization signal. This mutant protein is unable to bind HDM2 and has reduced binding to E2F, but still has some residual nuclear localization due to sequences within the pocket that can mediate nuclear entry.[49]

The amino terminal region

The amino terminal region of pRB (amino acids 1–378) has largely been ignored in functional studies of pRB, but a recent crystal structure of the region has helped to shed light on its potential importance. The domain is made up of tandem cyclin-like folds that form two lobes that are reminiscent of the pocket region of pRB.[50] There are also binding sites for several proteins, including a replication licensing factor (MCM7),[51] an E1A-like inhibitor of differentiation (EID-1),[50] and a G2/M kinase (RbK).[52]

The amino terminus appears to interact directly with the pocket and may contribute to the overall structure and stability of the pRB protein. The crystal structure showed that the amino acids encoded by exons 4, 7, and 9 form integral parts of the core of the amino terminus, and deletion of these exons was predicted to cause misfolding and increased turnover of the protein.[50] Among these three key exons that make up the core of the amino terminus, two have been shown to be mutated in low-penetrance retinoblastoma. One of these is a mutation that causes an in-frame deletion of exon 4 that removes the G2/M kinase binding site.[21] The mutant protein retains some tumor suppressor functions, but it would be predicted to be unstable and to have decreased affinity for its binding partners.[40,41] Another low-penetrance mutation in the amino terminus involves residues encoded by exon 9.[42,53–55] This mutation affects the polypyrimidine tract of the 5′ acceptor splice site of intron 8, causing an in-frame deletion in exon 9. As this is another of the key domains in the amino terminus, the deletion of exon 9 would be predicted to have detrimental effects on tertiary protein structure and binding affinity.

Conclusions

Low-penetrance retinoblastoma mutations have yielded important new insights into the molecular structure and cellular function of pRB. These studies have already led to improved diagnostic testing and family counseling for retinoblastoma families. We propose a classification scheme modified from Otterson et al[40] that accounts for virtually all low-penetrance mutations reported to date. The common theme in all of these mutations is a reduction in the quantity or quality of cellular pRB. Insufficient quantity of normal pRB may result from mutations in the promoter or splice site sequences, whereas pRB may be partially disabled by subtle mutations that reduce the stability and binding affinity of the protein. The tumor suppressor activity of pRB derives both from its ability to arrest the cell cycle and to induce differentiation. Some low-penetrance mutations appear to compromise preferentially one or the other of these functions, suggesting that regulation of the cell cycle and differentiation may play cooperative roles in tumor suppression by pRB. Further studies are needed to understand more clearly the mechanism of low-penetrance mutations and to apply this knowledge to improved care of patients with retinoblastoma.

Acknowledgments

This work was supported by grants (to JWH) from the National Eye Institute (R01 EY13169-01), Research to Prevent Blindness, Inc., Barnes-Jewish Hospital Foundation, the Kling Family Foundation, and a training grant (to KM) from the Cancer Biology Pathway of the Siteman Cancer Center at Barnes-Jewish Hospital and Washington University.

Key references

A complete list of chapter references is available online at www.expertconsult.com. See inside cover for registration details.

1. Harbour JW. Retinoblastoma: pathogenesis and diagnosis. In: Char DH (ed.) Tumors of the Eye and Orbit. Philadelphia: BC Decker, 2001:253–265.

2. Matsunaga E. Hereditary retinoblastoma: delayed mutation or host resistance? Am J Hum Genet 1978;30:406–424.

3. Lohmann DR, Brandt B, Hopping W, et al. Distinct RB1 gene mutations with low penetrance in hereditary retinoblastoma. Hum Genet 1994;94:349–354.

7. Knudson AG Jr. Mutation and cancer: statistical study of retinoblastoma. Proc Natl Acad Sci USA 1971;68:820–823.

17. Strong LC, Riccardi VM, Ferrell RE, et al. Familial retinoblastoma and chromosome 13 deletion transmitted via an insertional translocation. Science 1981;213:1501–1503.

24. Harbour JW, Dean DC. The Rb/E2F pathway: emerging paradigms and expanding roles. Genes Dev 2000;14:2545–2562.

32. Lee JO, Russo AA, Pavletich NP. Structure of the retinoblastoma tumour-suppressor pocket domain bound to a peptide from HPV E7. Nature 1998;391:859–865.

35. Harbour JW. Overview of RB gene mutations in patients with retinoblastoma. Implications for clinical genetic screening. Ophthalmology 1998;105:1442–1447.

40. Otterson GA, Chen WD, Coxon AB, et al. Incomplete penetrance of familial retinoblastoma linked to germ-line mutations that result in partial loss of RB function. Proc Natl Acad Sci USA 1997;94:12036–12040.

41. Sellers WR, Novitch BG, Miyake S, et al. Stable binding to E2F is not required for the retinoblastoma protein to activate transcription, promote differentiation, and suppress tumor cell growth. Genes Dev 1998;12:95–106.

CHAPTER 50

Vasculogenic mimicry

Robert Folberg and Andrew J Maniotis

Overview and clinical context

By the mid-1980s, many uveal melanoma patients were electing treatment by vision-sparing radiation therapy, avoiding surgical removal of the affected eye (enucleation). The Collaborative Ocular Melanoma Study eventually demonstrated no significant difference in survival between patients treated by radiation therapy and enucleation.[1] Although fine-needle aspiration biopsies (FNAB) were used in selected cases to help to discriminate between uveal melanomas and lesions that clinically simulated melanoma (such as metastases to the eye), such procedures were not typically used to grade the melanoma, to assign risk of metastasis to the patients.

At this time, the only parameter of risk that could be assessed from tumor cells extracted by FNAB was cell type, assigned by the Callender classification.[2,3] The Callender classification of uveal melanomas had been known to be strongly associated with outcome, but the assignment of risk based on the morphological assessment of cells was challenging for two reasons: (1) Callender classification had been shown to be poorly reproducible between pathologists; and (2) epithelioid cells – those cells most strongly associated with adverse outcome – were distributed heterogeneously throughout these tumors. Discrepancies between FNAB-based cytological classifications and the assignment of cell type on the subsequent enucleation were reported, and in one case, the FNAB needle track was traced through the tumor and was found to have missed a pocket of epithelioid cells, leading to an erroneous classification on the FNAB sample.[3,4] Discrepancies were also reported between the more objective assignments of risk based on the morphometric measurements of nucleolar size between FNAB samples and matched enucleation specimens.

Some experts began to question why it was necessary to assign patients into risk categories if no effective treatments were available to administer to patients with metastatic uveal melanoma. Sadly, even to this day, there is no effective regimen to treat patients with metastatic uveal melanoma. The development of new classification schemes to assign risk was justified then, and is justifiable today, on the basis of

two observations: (1) many patients simply want to know the risk to their life expectancy so that they can either make plans to put their affairs in order, or to make longer-term financial and personal commitments[5]; and (2) there is hope that with intensive research into the molecular basis of metastasis in uveal melanoma, new treatment strategies will emerge and, when this happens, it will be helpful to be able to stratify patients into risk categories to design meaningful clinical trials. Vasculogenic mimicry was therefore discovered in the context of a search to develop a noninvasive substitute for biopsy of uveal melanomas.

In 1992 a pilot study[6] reported the association between death from metastatic uveal melanoma and the presence of histological patterns that stained positive with the periodic acid–Schiff (PAS) reagent. This was followed by a description of nine patterns, including the incorporation of pre-existing choroidal vessels, incomplete circles (arcs) around packets of tumor cells, arcs that bifurcated (arcs with branching), circles around packets of tumor cells (loops), back-to-back loops (three back-to-back loops were designated as networks), parallel linear patterns, and parallel patterns that cross-linked. A subsequent study of the association of these patterns and outcome disclosed that the detection of loops and networks – and the parallel with cross-linking pattern – were associated independently with death from metastatic melanoma in multivariate statistical models.[7] Most patients whose tumors lacked these patterns were long-term survivors of uveal melanoma after enucleation, and fewer than half of the patients whose tumors contained these patterns survived disease-free after enucleation. These patterns, when detected histologically, were interpreted as markers of the risk for metastasis. The association between the detection of these patterns and metastasis was confirmed by multiple independent laboratories[8–10] and the patterns were subsequently identified in cutaneous melanoma[11] and other cancers.[12]

Investigators eventually discovered a number of important associations between the detection of these patterns and other markers of metastatic behavior, including the presence of epithelioid cells, location in the ciliary body,[13] monosomy 3,[14] and gene expression profiles.[15] Because many markers – cytological, molecular, and cytogenetic – are distributed heterogeneously throughout tumors, a healthy skepticism began to surface about the use of FNAB to extract material from which tumors could be graded on the basis of these markers. Thus, attention was directed to the detection of PAS-positive patterns by noninvasive means as a surrogate marker for more sensitive molecular and cytogenetic markers.

Two approaches were taken to image PAS-positive patterns clinically. A strong association was demonstrated between the analyses of raw radiofrequency ultrasound data and the histological detection of PAS-positive patterns,[16] but the equipment to image and analyze these patterns was never made available commercially. Using indocyanine green angiography and laser scanning confocal ophthalmoscopy, perfusion channels, corresponding to the histologically detected PAS-positive patterns could be imaged clinically for tumors in the posterior pole,[17] and the detection of these patterns was found to be predictive of growth of indeterminate-sized lesions in a prospective trial.[18] Nevertheless, the practice of imaging tumors to detect these patterns clinically by noninvasive means never became part of the clinical ophthalmic oncology workup. However, the detection of fluid within these patterns through angiography strengthened the suspicion that PAS-positive patterns were part of the microcirculation.

Indeed, in histological sections, PAS-positive patterns were associated with blood vessels and red blood cells were detected within the patterns. It was assumed that these patterns were remodeled blood vessels, and the patterns were initially designated as "microcirculatory patterns."[19] No one had any reason to challenge this assumption until the histogenesis of these patterns was studied in vitro.

The histogenesis of PAS-positive patterning: vasculogenic mimicry

Because PAS-positive patterns were thought to represent remodeled blood vessels, the histogenesis of these patterns was first explored in vitro in co-cultures of uveal melanoma cells, endothelial cells, and fibroblasts. However, looping patterns, identical to those seen in tissue sections, were generated by highly invasive uveal melanoma cells, in the absence of endothelial cells and fibroblasts in three-dimensional culture conditions. Interestingly, poorly invasive uveal melanoma cells did not generate these patterns under any culture condition, thus establishing a functional relationship between the in vitro observations and the association between the identification of these patterns in tissue sections and death from metastatic melanoma. Moreover, these patterns – formed in vitro exclusively by highly invasive uveal melanoma cells – conducted fluid after direct injection and after iontophoresis, strengthening the hypothesis that these patterns conducted fluid in vivo. The histogenesis of these patterns was described as vasculogenic mimicry[20] – vasculogenic because, although these pathways do not form from pre-existing vessels, they distribute plasma and may contain red blood cells; and mimicry because the pathways are not blood vessels and merely mimic vascular function by functioning as a "fluid-conducting meshwork."[21]

Questions asked about vasculogenic mimicry

Are vasculogenic mimicry patterns blood vessels?

Looping PAS-positive patterns are not blood vessels. The patterns do not stain with endothelial cell markers[22] and they are composed ultrastructurally of sheets of electron-dense material in which tumor cells are embedded.[23] The patterns are composed of laminin, fibronectin, collagens IV and VI, and possibly heparan sulfate proteoglycan.[24] Three-dimensional reconstructions have shown these patterns to represent sleeves of extracellular matrix material wrapped around branching cylindrical projections of melanoma cells.[25] Plasma and some red blood cells are conducted by the patterned extracellular matrix which connects focally to blood vessels.[23] Thus, vasculogenic mimicry patterns are not blood vessels by composition, ultrastructure, or topology, although they do conduct fluid.

Investigators have described the formation of tubes by melanoma cells and have identified tubular structures in tissue sections of melanomas and other tumors that are lined by tumor cells and not endothelial cells. One group has advanced the hypothesis that highly invasive and genetically dysregulated melanoma cells undergo transdifferentiation into an endothelial cell genotype (because of the upregulation of genes such as VE-cadherin).[26] There are several challenges to this approach. First, vascular spaces in tissue may be formed by tumor cells replacing endothelial cells – a "complete" manifestation of mosaic tumor vessels. Second, even if transdifferentiation does provide a mechanism for the generation of tubes of tumor cells mimicking the appearance of blood vessels, the transdifferentiation is incomplete because tumor cells do not form cobblestone monolayers in vitro as do endothelial cells and because angiogenesis inhibitors do not block the formation of tumor cell-generated cords.[23]

The generation of the highly patterned fluid-conducting meshwork has been designated as vasculogenic mimicry of the patterned matrix type, and the formation of tubes by tumor cells has been called vasculogenic mimicry of the tubular type.[12] The material that follows in this chapter refers only to vasculogenic mimicry of the patterned matrix type.

Are vasculogenic mimicry patterns a stromal response to the tumor (i.e., are these patterns fibrovascular septa)?

Before the histogenesis of PAS-positive patterns was described, some investigators assumed that these patterns represented fibrovascular septa.[9] Even after it had been shown that tumor cells generated these patterns, some investigators persisted in describing these patterns as stromal response to the tumor.[27] Although fibrovascular septa have been identified in uveal melanomas, their prevalence is low and fibrovascular septa do not have any prognostic associations with outcome.[24] Perhaps the most convincing evidence in support of the tumor cell generating these patterns comes from a set of experiments in which human uveal melanoma cells were injected into the livers of immunosuppressed mice. Polyclonal antibodies to laminin, not species-specific, labeled vasculogenic mimicry patterns generated by the tumor cells as well as mouse liver structures. However, a monoclonal antibody that was species-specific for human laminin labeled only vasculogenic mimicry patterns within the tumor and not the mouse liver. Thus, the laminin within the tumor was not co-opted from the mouse stroma and vasculogenic mimicry patterns are therefore not a stromal response by host tissue to the tumor.[28]

Does fluid flow through vasculogenic mimicry patterns?

It is clear from animal model studies that intravenous tracers co-localize to vasculogenic mimicry patterns. In a recent clinical study, patients with posterior uveal melanomas were injected with indocyanine green in the antecubital vein of one arm, and shortly after injection, blood was phlebotomized from the contralateral arm while a confocal angiogram was being taken. The blood removed after injection continued to fluoresce weeks after the injection, while fluorescence within intratumoral vasculogenic mimicry patterns was extinguished within 15 minutes after injection, thus demonstrating indirectly that fluid flows through vasculogenic mimicry patterns.[29] It is possible that leaky intratumoral vessels permit blood to enter into the tumor cell-generated extracellular matrix, but that once in the matrix, plasma and red blood cells circulate throughout the patterns.

What is the relationship between vasculogenic mimicry and angiogenesis?

In the early 1990s, an association was demonstrated between increased microvascular density in breast cancer and adverse outcome,[30] and a large series of papers then followed demonstrating similar associations in other cancers, including uveal melanoma.[31] Although it was intuitive that increased risk of metastasis should accompany angiogenesis, these associations were somewhat paradoxical because highly invasive cancers are typically destructive of the host microenvironment: by what mechanisms would new blood vessels be able to penetrate into the cellular compartment of highly malignant tumors when these tumors were simultaneously elaborating a variety of substances leading to the degradation of stroma? Indeed, a careful examination of angiogenesis in breast cancer revealed that angiogenic blood vessels were situated in the fibrous connective tissue surrounding tumor cells and were not in direct contact with the tumor cell compartment, consistent with the notion of the tumor stroma representing a form of scar tissue.[32] Furthermore, when endothelial cells were co-cultured with highly invasive uveal melanoma cells, the uveal melanoma cells destroyed the endothelial cells on contact.[23]

It was known that highly invasive uveal melanoma cells are genetically dysregulated and express markers that are inappropriate for cells of neural crest lineage (like fetal cytokeratins[33] and endothelial cells such as VE-cadherin[34]). Therefore, the relationship of microvascular density to adverse outcome in uveal melanoma was studied by double-labeling histological sections with CD34 (a nonspecific endothelial cell marker found by one group to provide for the highest microvascular density measurements), and with S100 protein (a nonspecific marker of cells of neural crest lineage such as melanocytes that do not label vascular endothelial cells). A high level of co-expression of CD34 and S100 protein was identified, and as "microvascular density" – as measured by CD34 labeling – increased, so did co-expression of this protein by melanoma cells. Therefore, the association between high microvascular density and metastasis in uveal melanoma may be explained on the basis of a population of highly invasive and genetically dysregulated tumor cells rather than angiogenesis.[35] Aberrant expression of CD34 in cutaneous melanoma was discovered subsequently.[36]

The microcirculation of uveal melanoma is therefore complex, including normal choroidal vessels that are incorporated into tumors, angiogenic vessels (especially next to zones of necrosis or in tumors previously treated by radiation therapy), mosaic vessels (lined by tumor cells and endothelial cells), and vasculogenic mimicry patterns.[12] Vasculogenic mimicry patterns provide at least 11-fold increased perfusion surface area in comparison to incorporated tubular vessels or angiogenic vessels.[37]

One might speculate that vasculogenic mimicry patterns facilitate metastasis, functioning like lymphatic channels in a location devoid of lymphatic vessels. However, there is no direct evidence implicating vasculogenic mimicry in the dissemination of tumor cells. Because vasculogenic mimicry patterns are formed by highly aggressive melanoma cells, it is possible that the detection of these patterns is merely a marker for the presence of an aggressive tumor phenotype and therefore has little or nothing to do with the actual spread of tumor.

Similarly, one might speculate that plasma and red blood cells circulating through vasculogenic mimicry patterns provide sufficient oxygen and nutrients to prevent necrosis. Most uveal melanomas lack zones of necrosis: the architecture of most uveal melanomas is far different from highly angiogenic retinoblastomas which feature zones of necrosis beyond a narrow cuff of tumor cells surrounding blood vessels. However, plasma flowing through vasculogenic mimicry patterns is not likely to be well oxygenated, and only scattered red blood cells – most often in a rouleaux formation – are identified histologically within these patterns. Is it possible, therefore, that uveal melanomas may not require a high degree of oxygenation? Might vasculogenic mimicry patterning serve a function other than perfusion or the facilitation of metastasis? Indeed, there is evidence that vasculogenic mimicry patterning regulates the behavior of tumor cells.

Vasculogenic mimicry as a tumor biofilm: therapeutic implications

When vasculogenic mimicry patterns form in vitro, some highly invasive and genetically dysregulated melanoma cells become entrapped within the extracellular matrix that they generate. Typically, spindle A melanoma cells are entrapped within vasculogenic mimicry patterns while the patterns themselves surround packets of epithelioid melanoma cells.[38] The mechanisms underlying this observation were explored in a series of in vitro studies.

In general, the chromatin of cancer cells is more sequestered than chromatin of noncancerous cells. However, laminin in the extracellular matrix microenvironment can induce chromatin sequestration of benign cells, and can increase the sequestration of chromatin in malignant cells through a novel mechanical signaling pathway mediated by the cytoskeleton (mechanogenomic signaling).[39] Dramatic shifts in gene expression have been shown to accompany the sequestration of uveal melanoma cells in vitro, especially during the formation of vasculogenic mimicry patterns by the highly invasive melanoma cells that generate these patterns. Paradoxically, when vasculogenic mimicry patterns form, genes that are typically associated with invasive behavior (such as CD44) are downregulated while genes associated with differentiation and suppression of the cell cycle (such as p21) are upregulated. Indeed, after highly invasive uveal melanoma cells form vasculogenic mimicry patterns, their ability to proliferate and migrate is significantly compromised. When highly invasive epithelioid uveal melanoma cells are seeded over discrete zones of laminin that have been stenciled on to plastic surfaces, the cells retain their epithelioid morphology on plastic, but after contact with the edge of the laminin stencil, these cells elongate, the nucleolus diminishes in size, and a nuclear fold appears – morphologic evidence of a dramatic change in morphology from epithelioid to spindle A morphology. That these in vitro observations are clinically relevant is reflected in tissue microarray studies of human uveal melanoma samples in which the proliferation index (measured by Ki67 labeling) was significantly decreased in melanoma cells adjacent to vasculogenic mimicry patterns compared with melanoma cells located where vasculogenic mimicry patterning is absent.[38]

Therefore, in addition to any role that vasculogenic mimicry patterns may play in tumor perfusion or the dissemination of tumor cells, these patterns regulate higher-order chromatin structure, gene expression, phenotypic behavior, and morphology. The generation of extracellular matrix proteins, especially laminin, by highly invasive melanoma cells provides a microenvironment in which these cells generate vasculogenic mimicry patterns. In the formation of these patterns, tumor cells become entrapped within the matrix and revert to an indolent (spindle A) phenotype, and the proliferation rate of melanoma cells in the vicinity of these patterns decreases. Thus, paradoxically, although vasculogenic mimicry patterns are histological features associated with metastatic behavior because the generation of these patterns requires the presence of highly invasive tumor cells, the generation of these patterns dampens malignant behavior.

Thus, vasculogenic mimicry itself mimics another biological phenomenon: the formation of microbial biofilms.[40] The generation of an extracellular matrix by certain microbial organisms entraps these potential pathogens and renders them phenotypically quiescent as long as they are within the biofilm. Disruption of the biofilm can disperse the organisms and increase their pathogenicity. Interestingly, the organisms in a microbial biofilm may be highly drug-resistant.

Vasculogenic mimicry may therefore provide at least one explanation for the well-documented latency between the detection of the primary tumor and the development of clinically detectable metastases in the liver. Ophthalmic oncologists seldom encounter patients who have evidence of metastatic uveal melanoma when the primary tumor is detected, and it is well known that metastases may emerge many years after treatment of the primary tumor. The formation of vasculogenic mimicry in hepatic metastases may render these subclinical metastases biologically quiescent and it is possible that clinically relevant metastatic disease emerges when vasculogenic mimicry patterning in hepatic micrometastases is disrupted, allowing for the phenotypically indolent melanoma cells entrapped within the vasculogenic mimicry patterning to emerge from "hibernation." There is some experimental evidence supporting this hypothesis. When primary uveal melanoma cells are placed directly into the liver of severe combined immunodeficient (SCID) mice, the earliest lesions – only a few cells in diameter – are typically encased in looping matrices rich in laminin, suggesting that vasculogenic mimicry may be an early response to the colonization of the liver by tumor cells. Over a period of time in these experiments, large masses of melanoma cells develop in the mouse liver, and in highly invasive tumors; vasculogenic mimicry patterning may not be easily identified in these large experimental tumors. However, in animals with large intrahepatic masses, secondary micrometastases to the lungs are identified, and almost without exception, these micrometastases feature looping patterns rich in laminin, characteristic of vasculogenic mimicry.[28] These observations are consistent with the study of vasculogenic

---

Box 50.1 Vasculogenic mimicry: key points

- Vasculogenic mimicry as seen in uveal melanoma and many other cancers consists of extracellular matrix proteins that are generated by highly invasive tumor cells
- Therefore, the histological detection of these patterns is associated with an adverse outcome
- Vasculogenic mimicry patterns, generated by melanoma cells, are not fibrovascular septa and are not derived from the surrounding stroma
- Vasculogenic mimicry patterns actively transport fluid through the tumor, even though the patterns are not blood vessels
- Vasculogenic mimicry patterns may be detected by noninvasive imaging techniques such as laser scanning confocal angiography with indocyanine green and by specialized ultrasonography
- Vasculogenic mimicry patterns are strongly associated with molecular markers of aggressive tumor behavior such as monosomy 3 and gene expression signatures. Thus, the clinical detection of vasculogenic mimicry patterns may be a noninvasive substitute for biopsy to assign risk of metastasis to patients
- Although vasculogenic mimicry patterns are generated by invasive tumor cells, those cells in contact with the patterns revert to a more indolent phenotype and genotype, thus drawing an analogy between these matrix-rich, tumor cell-generated patterns and microbioal biofilms
- Vasculogenic mimicry patterning may contribute to drug resistance

mimicry in human liver specimens. Although vasculogenic mimicry patterns may be identified in nearly every location to which uveal melanoma disseminates, including the liver,[13] their presence in advanced human hepatic metastases is variable.

Thus, vasculogenic mimicry may help to keep hepatic uveal melanoma micrometastases biologically "in check," at least for a period of time, and when the dampening effect of vasculogenic mimicry on aggressive tumor cell behavior is overridden, clinically significant and lethal hepatic metastases emerge. Additional investigations into the mechanisms by which vasculogenic mimicry dampens tumor cell behavior in the liver and identification of those events that suppress the microenvironmental dampening of aggressive tumor cell behavior are indicated. If ophthalmic oncologists can identify patients at high risk for metastasis when the primary tumor is first diagnosed and treated, these patients can be assumed already to have subclinical micrometastatic disease and therapeutic intervention targeted to maintaining the dampening effects of vasculogenic mimicry on aggressive tumor cell behavior can be implemented. A therapeutic strategy of maintaining patients on chronic therapy to suppress the emergence of clinically significant and lethal metastatic disease from subclinical micrometastases – the chemoprevention of clinically overt metastases – may be a viable clinical approach to achieving long-term survival in uveal melanoma patients now without hope of cure.

Vasculogenic mimicry may, by analogy, play a key role in the well-known resistance of uveal melanoma to most forms of conventional chemotherapy. If the most malignant cells in a tumor can generate a tumor biofilm, then cells entrapped within the biofilm may evade targeting by drugs, and the chromatin sequestration induced by contact with the biofilm may also contribute to a novel form of drug resistance. It is of interest that the malignancies most susceptible to chemotherapy are the leukemias, planktonic malignancies lacking a stroma and the opportunity to develop a tumor biofilm. Molecular targeting of the tumor cell-generated microenvironment – the tumor biofilm known as vasculogenic mimicry – may therefore provide a novel approach to the treatment of metastatic uveal melanoma, a condition for which no effective therapy currently exists (Box 50.1).

Conclusion

Highly invasive melanoma cells generate a patterned extracellular matrix around packets of these cells. The histologic

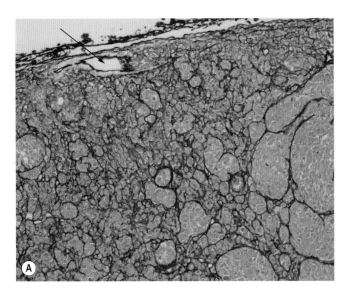

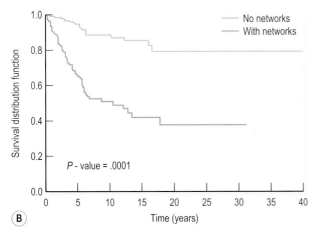

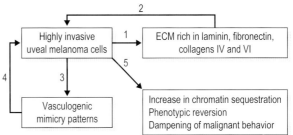

Figure 50.2 This schematic diagram illustrates the functional pathways by which highly invasive tumor cells generate an extracellular matrix microenvironment – vasculogenic mimicry patterns – that, in turn, modulate the behavior of the tumor cells. Highly invasive uveal melanoma cells generate an extracellular matrix rich in laminin, collagens IV and VI, fibronectin, and other extracellular matrix molecules (1). In the presence of this microenvironment, the phenotypic behavior of tumor cells is modulated (2) such that the cells generate the characteristic looping patterns of vasculogenic mimicry (3). However, the vasculogenic mimicry patterns themselves modulate the behavior of the melanoma cells (4): chromatin in tumor cells that are in contact with vasculogenic mimicry patterns becomes sequestered, tumor cells entrapped within the matrix undergo phenotypic reversion to phenotypically indolent spindle A melanoma cells, and the malignant properties of tumor cells in contact with the patterns are dampened. For example, the proliferation index of tumor cells in the vicinity of vasculogenic mimicry patterns is diminished (5). Thus, the matrix produced by highly invasive uveal melanoma cells functions in a manner analogous to microbial biofilms. The generation of vasculogenic mimicry patterns may contribute to drug resistance in this tumor system. The histologic or angiographic detection of these patterns is nevertheless strongly associated with aggressive biological behavior because only highly invasive tumor cells generate vasculogenic mimicry patterns.

Figure 50.1 (A) Vasculogenic mimicry patterns stained with an antibody to fibronectin. The looping patterns surround packets of uveal melanoma cells. The patterns connect to blood vessels (arrow). The patterns have been shown to contain laminin, collagens IV and VI, fibronectin, and heparan sulfate proteoglycan. (B) Kaplan–Meier survival curve showing that patients whose tumors contain vasculogenic mimicry patterns have a significantly worse prognosis than patients whose tumors lack these patterns. (Redrawn with permission from Folberg R, Rummelt V, Parys-Van Ginderdeuren R, et al. The prognostic value of tumor blood vessel morphology in primary uveal melanoma. Ophthalmology 1993;100:1389–1398.)

detection of these vasculogenic mimicry patterns is associated with an aggressive clinical course. Pattern generation is also very strongly associated with other markers of tumor progression, such as monosomy 3 and gene expression signatures. Therefore, the detection of these patterns clinically by noninvasive means such as indocyanine green angiography or specialized ultrasonography may serve as a noninvasive substitute for biopsy. The patterns have been shown to conduct fluid in vitro, in animal models, and in patients and may contribute to the tumor microcirculation independent of angiogenesis. Angiogenesis inhibitors are not effective in preventing the formation of vasculogenic mimicry patterns. However, vasculogenic mimicry provides novel targets for therapy because after the tumor cells generate these patterns, the invasive behavior of these cells is diminished and chromatin is sequestered. The generation of this "tumor biofilm" may provide a new explanation for drug resistance in uveal melanoma, and the molecular interactions between the extracellular matrix and the tumor cells may constitute novel approaches to nontoxic therapies for the chemoprevention of hepatic metastases and the treatment of established clinical metastatic disease (Figures 50.1 and 50.2).

Acknowledgment

This work was supported by grant R01 EY10457, National Institutes of Health, Bethesda, Maryland, USA.

Key references

A complete list of chapter references is available online at www.expertconsult.com. See inside cover for registration details.

1. The COMS randomized trial of iodine 125 brachytherapy for choroidal melanoma: V. Twelve-year mortality rates and prognostic factors: COMS report no. 28. Arch Ophthalmol 2006;124:1684–1693.

2. McLean IW, Foster WD, Zimmerman LE, et al. Modifications of Callender's classification of uveal melanoma at the Armed Forces Institute of Pathology. Am J Ophthalmol 1983;96:502–509.

3. Augsburger JJ, Shields JA, Folberg R, et al. Fine needle aspiration biopsy in the diagnosis of intraocular cancer cytologic–histologic correlations. Ophthalmology 1985;92:39–49.

4. Folberg R, Augsburger JJ, Gamel JW, et al. Fine-needle aspirates of uveal melanomas and prognosis. Am J Ophthalmol 1985;100:654–657.

5. Damato B. Current management of uveal melanoma. Ejc Suppl 2005;3:433–435.

6. Folberg R, Pe'er J, Gruman LM, et al. The morphologic characteristics of tumor blood vessels as a marker of tumor progression in primary human uveal melanoma: a matched case-control study. Hum Pathol 1992;23:1298–1305.

7. Folberg R, Rummelt V, Parys-Van Ginderdeuren R, et al. The prognostic value of tumor blood vessel morphology in primary uveal melanoma. Ophthalmology 1993;100:1389–1398.

8. Sakamoto T, Sakamoto M, Yoshikawa H, et al. Histologic findings and prognosis of uveal malignant melanoma in Japanese patients. Am J Ophthalmol 1996;121:276–283.

9. McLean IW, Keefe KS, Burnier MN. Uveal melanoma: comparison of the prognostic value of fibrovascular loops, mean of the ten largest nucleoli, cell type and tumor size. Ophthalmology 1997;104:777–780.

10. Makitie T, Summanen P, Tarkannen A, et al. Microvascular loops and networks as prognostic indicators in choroidal and ciliary body melanomas. J Natl Cancer Inst 1999;91:359–367.

11. Thies A, Mangold U, Moll I, et al. PAS-positive loops and networks as a prognostic indicator in cutaneous malignant melanoma. J Pathol 2001;195:537–542.

12. Folberg R, Maniotis AJ. Vasculogenic mimicry. APMIS 2004;112:508–525.

13. Rummelt V, Folberg R, Rummelt C, et al. Microcirculation architecture of melanocytic nevi and malignant melanomas of the ciliary body and choroid. A comparative histopathologic and ultrastructural study. Ophthalmology 1994;101:718–727.

14. Scholes AGM, Damato BE, Nunn J, et al. Monosomy 3 in uveal melanoma: correlation with clinical and histologic predictors of survival. Invest Ophthalmol Vis Sci 2003;44:1008–1011.

15. Onken MD, Lin AY, Worley LA, et al. Association between microarray gene expression signature and extravascular matrix patterns in primary uveal melanomas. Am J Ophthalmol 2005;140:748–749.

CHAPTER 51

Treatment of choroidal melanoma

Aimee V Chappelow and Andrew P Schachat

Overview

Choroidal melanoma is the most common primary malignant intraocular tumor with an annual incidence in the USA of 0.8 cases per 100 000 population.[1] Once metastasis becomes clinically apparent, the 1-year mortality rate approaches 80%.[2] Given this poor prognosis, enucleation was historically considered the only appropriate management for choroidal melanoma. However, in recent decades there have been many new developments in management, with a trend toward more conservative therapeutic methods. The impetus for this shift in paradigm was the proposition by Zimmerman et al[3] that enucleation may in fact promote metastasis by intraoperative dissemination of tumor emboli. The transient rise in post-therapeutic mortality that prompted this theory has been validated over the ensuing 25 years, but is now believed to be attributable to prediagnosis and treatment micrometastasis in uveal melanoma. Therapeutic options have since expanded to include transpupillary thermotherapy (TTT), plaque radiotherapy, charged-particle irradiation, local resection, and observation.

The Collaborative Ocular Melanoma Study (COMS)[4] is the first set of randomized clinical trials designed with sufficient power to detect a difference in survival outcomes between treatment modalities. Between 1986 and 1994, investigators screened 6078 patients at 43 clinical centers, placing each eligible subject into one of three categories: small, medium, or large choroidal melanoma (Figure 51.1). Specifically, small tumors were defined as less than 2.5 mm in apical height. Tumors between 2.5 and 10 mm in apical height and no more than 16 mm in basal diameter were classified as medium, and those greater than 16 mm in basal diameter were classified as large. Herein, we review management options for each of these size classifications, as evaluated by the COMS and other clinical studies.

Small choroidal melanoma

Of the three sizes of choroidal melanoma, treatment of small-sized tumors is most controversial. This is due in large part to the inability to differentiate reliably suspicious nevi from true cancers, with consequential limited understanding of the natural history and metastatic potential of such tumors.

Natural history

Five risk factors for growth were identified in a retrospective review of 1329 patients with choroidal tumors less than 3 mm in thickness.[5] By multivariate analysis each of these clinical features (greater tumor thickness, orange pigment, symptoms of blurred vision or flashes/floaters, subretinal fluid, posterior margin touching the optic disc) was found independently to increase the relative risk of growth (Box 51.2). Further, documented growth was predictive of metastasis. Another retrospective series found not only tumor thickness, orange pigment, and presence of symptoms but also hot spots on fluorescein angiogram and internal quiet zone on B-scan to be significant predictors of growth.[6] Stratification of treatment based upon risk factors has been suggested to optimize management, but studies have failed to show a treatment benefit with respect to mortality.

Small choroidal melanocytic lesions will exhibit growth in 18–36% of cases and metastasis in 2–5% of cases when followed for at least 5 years.[5,6] Given a lack of tumor-related mortality in cases that failed to exhibit growth,[5,6] it has been argued that indeterminate lesions may be observed and treated only if growth is documented.

Transpupillary thermotherapy (TTT)

TTT is a technique by which a 3 mm diode laser beam introduced through the pupil heats the tumor to 60–65°F for 1 minute. In contrast to photocoagulation, which has been abandoned due to inadequate tumor control, TTT raises the tumor to a lower temperature but achieves a greater depth of tumor necrosis. Tumor necrosis is due primarily to the direct thermal effect of the laser, with secondary effect from ischemia due to vascular occlusion. TTT is contraindicated in patients with media opacity, peripheral tumor, significant subretinal fluid, and small pupil.

Originally introduced as monotherapy for choroidal melanoma in 1994,[7] TTT was designed to spare patients the visual morbidity that plaque brachytherapy was known to impart. Early results were encouraging, with tumor control achieved in 91% of cases after a mean of three treatment sessions.[8] However, Kaplan–Meier estimates revealed recurrence rates of 4% at 1 year, 12% at 2 years, and 22% at 3 years of follow-up. Further, a lack of benefit with respect to visual outcomes was demonstrated in a case-matched retrospective comparison of TTT monotherapy with plaque

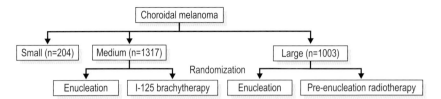

Figure 51.1 Collaborative Ocular Melanoma Study (COMS) design and randomization scheme.

brachytherapy, which has more reliable tumor control rates.[9] Clinicopathologic examination of eyes enucleated after failed TTT suggests high rates of extrascleral extension, in most cases undetectable on ultrasonography.[10] Minor degrees of extraocular extension are expected to be locally controlled by brachytherapy. TTT is thus best employed as an adjunct to plaque brachytherapy, with TTT necrosing superficial tumor and plaque radiation necrosing tumor adjacent to and invading sclera. One study reported 93.8% local tumor control rate with combination therapy with brachytherapy and adjunctive TTT over a mean follow-up period of 5 years.[11]

COMS small tumor trial

As part of the COMS, an observational study of small choroidal melanomas was undertaken with the goal of assessing tumor growth (defined as increase from small to either medium or large) and its impact on survival. Probability of growth by Kaplan–Meier analysis was 11%, 21%, and 31% at 1, 2, and 5 years following enrollment (Figure 51.2A; Box 51.1).[12] Clinical features associated with tumor growth included prominent orange pigment, absence of drusen, absence of retinal pigment epithelium changes adjacent to the tumor, tumor thickness of at least 2 mm, and largest basal diameter of 12 mm or more (Box 51.2). Though only 16 of the 204 patients received treatment, the risk of death was low, with the authors reporting a Kaplan–Meier melanoma-related mortality of 1% at 5 years (Figure 51.2B).[13] All-cause mortality was higher, with patients are three to four times more likely to die of some competing cause than of their melanoma.

Medium choroidal melanoma

A large body of literature attests to the efficacy of radiotherapy (either external-beam radiation therapy (EBRT) or episcleral plaque therapy) in the treatment of medium-sized choroidal melanoma. The COMS trial for medium-sized melanomas (discussed in detail below) concluded that sight-conserving brachytherapy does not adversely affect survival outcomes when compared with enucleation. Since the globe and some vision can usually be maintained, radiotherapy has become the mainstay for sight-preserving treatment of medium- and large-sized choroidal melanoma.

Plaque brachytherapy

Brachytherapy is the most commonly used radiation modality for the treatment of choroidal melanoma. A bowl-shaped heavy-metal plaque implanted with a radioactive isotope (Figure 51.3), sized to exceed tumor margins by 2 mm, is

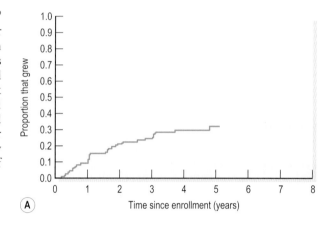

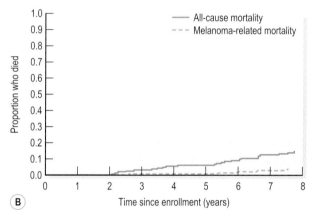

Figure 51.2 Collaborative Ocular Melanoma Study small melanoma observational study. (A) Kaplan–Meier plot of growth of small tumors. (B) All-cause (solid line) and small melanoma-related (dashed line) mortality. (Reproduced with permission from Singh AD, Kivela T. The Collaborative Ocular Melanoma Study. Ophthalmol Clin North Am 2005;18:129–142.)

Box 51.1 Small choroidal melanoma (Collaborative Ocular Melanoma Study definition)

- < 2.5 mm in apical height
- At 5-year follow-up, probability 31% of growth is 18–36% and metastasis is 2–5%
- Decision to treat or observe is controversial
- Monotherapy with transpupillary thermotherapy (TTT) lacks benefit with respect to local tumor recurrence or visual outcomes
- Favorable local recurrence rates have been achieved with brachytherapy (±TTT)

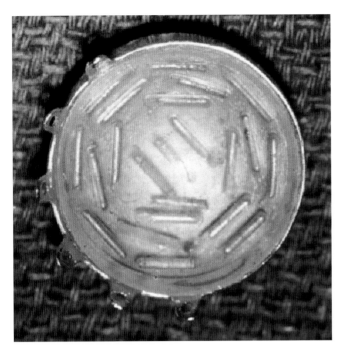

Figure 51.3 Episcleral brachytherapy plaque with radioisotope seeds.

have noted 82–84% overall (all-cause) 5-year survival rates with ruthenium-106.[15,16] Strontium-90[17] and palladium-103[18] have been shown to produce local tumor control rates of 92% and 96% at 5-year follow-up. Due to the large sample size required to detect a difference between treatment outcomes with different isotopes, no randomized trials have been undertaken. Figure 51.4 shows a medium melanoma before and 1 year after treatment with iodine brachytherapy.

Brachytherapy versus enucleation

The COMS randomized 1317 patients with choroidal melanoma classified as medium-sized to receive either I-125 brachytherapy or enucleation (Figure 51.1 and Box 51.3). Eligible patients were free of metastasis at enrollment. Follow-up is ongoing via periodic queries to the National Death Index, though formal clinical follow-up has ended. The 5-, 10-, and 12-year rates of death with histopathologically confirmed melanoma metastasis were similar for I-125 brachytherapy (10%, 18%, and 21%) and enucleation (11%, 17%, and 17%) (Figure 51.5).[19] Further, a trend towards increased 5-year risk of death for patients who were eligible for the COMS but deferred treatment when compared with COMS trial patients suggested a life-extending effect of treatment of medium- and large-sized melanomas.[20]

When a subset of patients in each treatment group were questioned regarding difficulty driving, anxiety, near vision, and other quality of life measures, patients treated with brachytherapy were more likely to have symptoms of anxiety and those treated with enucleation reported poorer visual function.[21] However, difference in visual function between treatment groups declined by 3–5 years following treatment, in accordance with decrease in visual acuity due to radiation-induced side-effects. Given no significant difference in survival between brachytherapy and enucleation, treatment choice should be made on an individual basis based upon patient preference.

The vast majority of patients with medium-sized melanoma will not have detectable metastasis at the time of diagnosis; nonetheless, a preoperative systemic evaluation should be undertaken. The presence of clinically detectable metastasis could shorten life expectancy and deem local treatment inappropriate; further, treatment for metastatic disease may be indicated depending on location and extent. In all, 60–89% of patients with metastatic choroidal melanoma will have hepatic involvement.[2,22] Other common sites of metastasis include lung, bone, subcutaneous tissues,

sutured to episclera for a period of up to 1 week with the goal of delivering 80–100 Gy to the tumor apex. Plaques implanted with cobalt-60 were introduced in the 1960s; however, visual morbidity was high due to substantial radiation dosage to surrounding ocular structures by virtue of the high-energy emission properties of Co-60 which do not permit adequate shielding. Favorable long-term tumor control rates and improved visual outcomes have since been demonstrated with several other isotopes. Iodine-125 brachytherapy was evaluated by the COMS (discussed below) and as a result has become the most common isotope used in North America. One-half millimeter of gold can shield the I-125 source whereas equivalent shielding of Co-60 requires 2 meters or 6 foot of lead. Ruthenium-106, a beta-emitter, was concurrently popularized in Europe during the Cold War, and has since been adopted by some centers in the USA due to the theoretical decreased risk in visual morbidity suggested by dosimetry studies. A total of 579 patients in Sweden treated with ruthenium-106 for choroidal melanoma less than 7 mm in diameter (9.2% classified as "large" by COMS standard) enjoyed a 5-year tumor-specific survival rate of 94.9%.[14] Other large studies

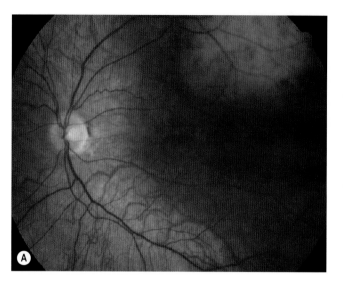
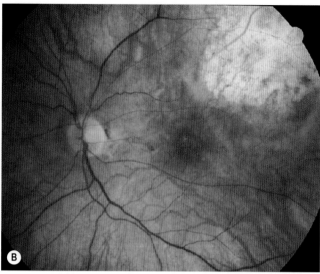

Figure 51.4 Medium choroidal melanoma before (A) and approximately 1 year after (B) iodine-125 brachytherapy. Tumor regression is observed.

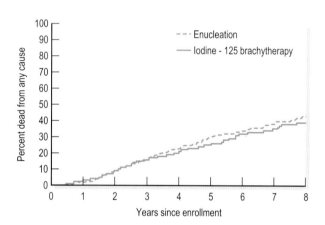

Figure 51.5 Collaborative Ocular Melanoma Study medium melanoma randomized trial. Kaplan–Meier plot of all-cause mortality following brachytherapy (solid line) or enucleation (dashed line). Note similar outcomes.

> **Box 51.4   Large choroidal melanoma (Collaborative Ocular Melanoma Study (COMS) definition)**
>
> - >16 mm in basal diameter
> - Treatment with pre-enucleation radiotherapy versus enucleation results in similar melanoma-specific mortality (COMS)
> - Favorable local recurrence rates are achievable with local resection and external-beam radiation therapy (EBRT)

lymph node, and brain. Thus, evaluation should include a complete physical exam, a complete blood count, serum liver function studies, and a chest X-ray or computed tomography. Therapeutic regimens administered to patients enrolled in COMS who developed metastasis included chemotherapy (23%), radiation (4%), immunotherapy (2%), and a combination of these (5%).[2] Of the 793 patients who developed metastatic disease, only 8 survived 5 years or longer.

Large choroidal melanoma

Choroidal melanomas classified as large by the COMS standard are most commonly managed by enucleation. However, radiation therapy (either as monotherapy or adjunct therapy) and local resection may be viable treatment options in some cases.

External-beam radiation therapy (EBRT)

EBRT (charged-particle beams of proton or helium ions) allows for a high dosage of radiation to be delivered to a tumor, regardless of size or proximity to fovea or optic nerve (Box 51.4). At most centers, patients undergo preradiation surgery during which tumor borders are delineated by transillumination and tantalum rings subsequently sutured to the sclera at the tumor borders. EBRT is then administered with the assistance of a sophisticated treatment planning program that utilizes a three-dimensional model of the tumor based on fundus photographs, ultrasound measurements, and location of tantalum rings on roentgenogram.

Though its use is limited by the cost and limited availability of proton facilities, with less than 50 worldwide, outcomes with respect to local control, eye loss, and vision loss have been favorable for EBRT. Of 1922 patients with choroidal melanoma treated with proton therapy at the Harvard Cyclotron over the course of 20 years, local recurrence was documented in only 45 (3.2%) at mean follow-up of 5.2 years.[23] Of note, large tumor size (>15 mm in diameter and >5 mm in height) imparted more than double the risk of recurrence in multivariate analysis. Another series of patients treated at the Biomedical Cyclotron Centre (Nice, France) reported a 4.5% rate of local recurrence at 5 years.[23] Helium

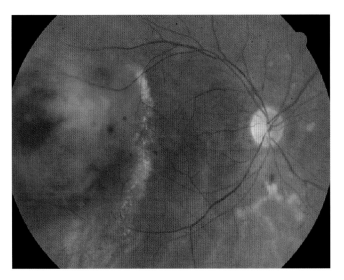

Figure 51.6 Fundus phototograph illustrating radiation retinopathy 2 years following iodine brachytherapy for a medium choroidal melanoma.

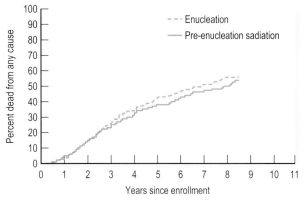

Figure 51.7 Collaborative Ocular Melanoma Study large melanoma randomized trial. Kaplan–Meier plot of all-cause mortality following enucleation (dashed line) or pre-enucleation external beam radiation (solid line). Note similar outcomes.

ion irradiation has been shown to produce similar local tumor control (4.6% at 10 years).[24]

As with brachytherapy, adverse effects of EBRT are substantial and include radiation retinopathy (Figure 51.6) and optic neuropathy, neovascular glaucoma, and posterior subcapsular cataract. One series reported at least one ocular complication (maculopathy, optic neuropathy, vascular occlusion, retinal detachment, or neovascular glaucoma) in 57% of patients treated with proton therapy at 5-year follow-up.[25] Neovascular glaucoma has been reported in 35% of patients treated with helium ion therapy, with 49% of these patients eventually requiring enucleation.[24] The 5-year rate of vision loss at 5 years is 52–68%,[26,27] with tumor location within 2 disc diameters of the optic nerve and macula being the strongest predictor of poor visual outcome.[26] A randomized controlled trial has established a dose of 50 GyE (Gray equivalents) as providing comparable local tumor control (versus 70 GyE), while imparting a lesser degree of visual loss.[28]

Enucleation after EBRT may be indicated if the patient experiences tumor recurrence or radiation-related complications. Neovascular glaucoma is the most common complication leading to enucleation after EBRT. The probability of enucleation 2 years after proton beam radiation is 5%, and increases to 9% and 12% by 5 years and 10 years after irradiation, respectively.[29]

Enucleation versus pre-enucleation radiation treatment (PERT)

In the third part of the COMS, 1003 patients with a large choroidal melanoma were randomly assigned to enucleation with and without prior radiation (Figure 51.1), based on the finding that preoperative radiation reduces metastasis in other malignancies. The study found no difference between the two treatment arms with respect to mortality[30] and local complications.[31] Specifically, the death rate at 10 years due to histopathologically confirmed metastases was 40% for enucleation alone and 45% for pre-enucleation radiation.[30]

Kaplan–Meier estimates of 5-year all-cause mortality were also similar for enucleation and pre-enucleation arms (57% and 62%, respectively; $P = 0.32$) (Figure 51.7). The hazard ratio for death for patients enrolled in the COMS PERT trial (versus eligible but not enrolled) was 1.12, after adjusting for prognostic covariates and stratifying by clinical center.[32] This finding suggests that, while treatment for large choroidal melanoma may not be beneficial with respect to mortality outcomes, it does not appear to accelerate metastasis and death, as suggested by Zimmerman et al.[3]

Local resection

Foulds[33] pioneered transscleral local resection as a method for conservation of the eye and vision in patients with choroidal melanoma deemed too large for radiotherapy. It has been argued that the procedure is time-consuming and requires more complicated postoperative care. It is a technically difficult procedure and is performed by only a few skilled surgeons; however, in experienced hands outcomes are favorable. Of 310 tumors with mean diameter of 13 mm and thickness of 7 mm resected by either Foulds[33] or Damato et al[34] between 1970 and 1994, 24 had residual tumor postoperatively and 57 developed delayed local recurrence over a median follow-up of 36 months. Further, 39% retained vision between 6/6 and 6/36 at the time of final visit.[34]

Future directions

Stereotactic radiotherapy

Stereotactic radiotherapy involves using gadolinium-enhanced magnetic resonance imaging scans to aid in the precise delivery of high-energy X-ray or gamma-ray radiation to the tumor from multiple directions either concurrently or sequentially. During the treatment, the patient lies supine and the head and eye are immobilized. Radiation is delivered with a safety margin of approximately 2 mm in all directions, and a dose–volume histogram analysis is performed to determine probability of complications. Local tumor control rates ranging between 84 and 98% have been reported.[35–37] However, radiation-induced side-effects, including retinopathy, cataract, and optic neuropathy are problematic, with 44%, 23%, and 41% prevalence at 33-month follow-up in one series.[35]

Adjuvant/targeted therapy

At this time, there is no chemotherapy with proven efficacy against choroidal melanoma. Recent meta-analysis of several randomized trials has shown a significant survival benefit of adjuvant treatment with interferon-α for cutaneous melanoma.[38] Ocular melanoma behaves differently and has different cell surface markers than cutaneous melanoma; thus such studies need to be repeated for the eye tumor. However, given a significantly lower incidence of choroidal (versus cutaneous) melanoma, randomized prospective trials with sufficient power to detect a difference between two treatment groups are not feasible. Regardless, systemic chemotherapy offers perhaps the greatest hope for improvement in survival outcomes in a disease entity in which hematologic micrometastases are often detectable at presentation.[39]

Cytogenetic studies of choroidal melanomas have revealed common nonrandom cytogenetic aberrations affecting chromosomes 3, 6, and 8. Monosomy 3, the most common chromosomal abnormality found in choroidal melanoma, has been implicated as a significant predictor of poor prognosis and metastatic disease[40] (Figure 51.8). Other abnormalities observed more often in metastasizing tumors include loss of 6q and gain of 8q.[41] Extra copies of 6p have been correlated with better prognosis.[42] It has also been reported that certain chromosomal aberrations become more frequent as the tumor progresses.[43] Further investigation into the exact contributions of various chromosomal abnormalities to the pathogenesis and progression of choroidal melanoma may provide opportunity for customized therapy for different chromosomal subtypes.

An important current opportunity for research involves the management of small ocular melanoma. Most patients do not die of their tumor and treatment damages vision, so deferral of treatment is common. Yet, if the tumor grows to medium tumor size, the mortality rate increases significantly. Randomized trials comparing prompt treatment versus treat-

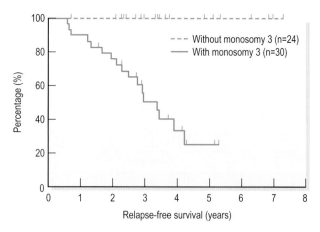

Figure 51.8 Monosomy 3 as a poor prognostic factor. Kaplan–Meier relapse-free survival of patients with and without monosomy 3. Note decrease in survival in patients with tumors exhibiting monosomy 3. (Reproduced with permission from Prescher G, Bornfeld N, Hirche H, et al. Prognostic implications of monosomy 3 in uveal melanoma. Lancet 1996;347:1222–1225.)

ment if growth is detected should be undertaken if an adequate sample size of eligible subjects becomes available.

Conclusion

A shift in paradigm towards more conservative treatment of choroidal melanoma in recent decades was initially spurred by the Zimmerman hypothesis and later substantiated by the COMS. Whereas medium-sized melanomas were once treated by enucleation, in the post-COMS era patients enjoy similar all-cause mortality and perhaps improved quality of life with sight-conserving brachytherapy. Large choroidal melanomas are still largely managed by enucleation; however, EBRT (either as primary or adjunct therapy) and local resection may be effective alternative treatment options. Whether small melanomas should be observed or treated with brachytherapy (with or without adjunctive TTT) remains controversial. Future development of targeted adjuvant chemotherapy guided by tumor cytogenetic studies holds promise for improvement in mortality rates, which have remained unchanged for decades despite improvement in local recurrence rates.

Key references

A complete list of chapter references is available online at www.expertconsult.com. See inside cover for registration details.

1. Singh AD, Topham A. Incidence of uveal melanoma in the United States: 1973–1997. Ophthalmology 2003;110: 956–961.
2. Diener-West M, Reynolds SM, Agugliaro DJ, et al. Development of metastatic disease after enrollment in the COMS trials for treatment of choroidal melanoma: Collaborative Ocular Melanoma Study group report no. 26.

Arch Ophthalmol 2005;123:1639–1643.
3. Zimmerman LE, McLean IW, Foster WD. Does enucleation of the eye containing a malignant melanoma prevent or accelerate the dissemination of tumour cells? Br J Ophthalmol 1978;62:420–425.
4. Design and methods of a clinical trial for a rare condition: the Collaborative Ocular Melanoma Study. COMS report

no. 3. Control Clin Trials 1993;14:362–391.
12. Factors predictive of growth and treatment of small choroidal melanoma: COMS report no. 5. The Collaborative Ocular Melanoma Study Group. Arch Ophthalmol 1997;115:1537–1544.
13. Mortality in patients with small choroidal melanoma. COMS report no. 4. The Collaborative Ocular Melanoma

Study Group. Arch Ophthalmol 1997; 115:886–893.

19. The COMS randomized trial of iodine 125 brachytherapy for choroidal melanoma: V. Twelve-year mortality rates and prognostic factors: COMS report no. 28. Arch Ophthalmol 2006;124:1684–1693.

20. Straatsma BR, Diener-West M, Caldwell R, et al. Mortality after deferral of treatment or no treatment for choroidal melanoma. Am J Ophthalmol 2003;136:47–54.

21. Melia M, Moy CS, Reynolds SM, et al. Quality of life after iodine 125 brachytherapy vs enucleation for choroidal melanoma: 5-year results from the Collaborative Ocular Melanoma Study: COMS QOLS report no. 3. Arch Ophthalmol 2006;124:226–238.

30. The Collaborative Ocular Melanoma Study (COMS) randomized trial of pre-enucleation radiation of large choroidal melanoma II: initial mortality findings. COMS report no. 10. Am J Ophthalmol 1998;125:779–796.

31. The Collaborative Ocular Melanoma Study (COMS) randomized trial of pre-enucleation radiation of large choroidal melanoma III: local complications and observations following enucleation COMS report no. 11. Am J Ophthalmol 1998;126:362–372.

32. Gilson MM, Diener-West M, Hawkins BS. Comparison of survival among eligible patients not enrolled versus enrolled in the Collaborative Ocular Melanoma Study (COMS) randomized trial of pre-enucleation radiation of large choroidal melanoma. Ophthalm Epidemiol 2007;14:251–257.

CHAPTER 52

Sebaceous cell carcinoma

Alon Kahana, Jonathan T Pribila,
Christine C Nelson, and Victor M Elner

Overview

Sebaceous cell carcinomas account for 1–5% of all eyelid malignancies and primarily affect older adults with a slight female gender bias.[1] Despite representing a small fraction of all eyelid tumors, proper identification and treatment of these tumors are critical because the rate of misdiagnosis has been estimated to be as high as 50%, with a mortality rate of at least 20% (Box 52.1). Sebaceous cell carcinomas typically arise from the meibomian glands, but can also develop within the pilosebaceous glands of the eyelid cilia (glands of Zeis) and the caruncle.[2,3] Although the clinical science of diagnosing and treating sebaceous cell carcinomas of the eyelid has advanced significantly in the past two decades, treatment is still surgical and hampered by poor understanding of the biology of these tumors. Given that cell biology and molecular signaling are intimately related to the function and development of these glands, this chapter will: (1) review the functional role of the sebaceous glands on the eyelid and normal sebaceous gland biology; (2) discuss the clinical and pathologic features of sebaceous cell carcinoma; and (3) summarize the important genetic, molecular, and cellular regulators of sebaceous cell carcinoma and demonstrate how these might shed light on the clinical behavior of these tumors.

Sebaceous gland physiology

Sebaceous glands can be grouped based on their location, association with hair follicles, and function. Although sebaceous glands are found throughout the body, certain areas are particularly rich in sebaceous gland content. While most sebaceous glands are associated with hair follicles (i.e., pilosebaceous glands), free glands can be found throughout the body, and some of them have evolved to perform specialized functions such as hormone signaling and odor production.[4] The meibomian glands of the eyelids are one type of specialized sebaceous gland. While this chapter will focus on the biology of sebaceous cancer of the eyelids, much of the science of sebaceous glands and sebaceous cell carcinoma is based on studies of the common pilosebaceous glands.

The evolutionary origins of pilosebaceous glands are not clear, and their function in humans is controversial. Sebaceous glands are holocrine glands which release sebum via the disintegration of mature, lipid-laden cells and, as a result, require continual cellular proliferation, differentiation, and maturation. These processes and, hence, the kinetics of sebum secretion, are regulated by a complex set of signals under both endocrine and neuroregulatory control.

The function of human sebum is controversial. One interesting hypothesis suggests that sebum assumes unique functions at different temperatures. At temperatures below 30°C, the sebum of pilosebaceous glands serves to create a water-repellent skin cover. At temperatures above 30°C, human sebum assumes the characteristics of a surfactant. Sweat with high surface tension that drips off skin will cause dehydration without contributing to evaporative cooling.[5] By acting as a surfactant for eccrine secretions, sebum lowers the surface tension of sweat and allows the sweat to be retained on the skin to achieve its thermoregulatory function. The meibomian glands of the eyelid have a similar function, namely to stabilize the tear film. The normal evaporation rate of the tear film is 25 μg/cm²/min. This increases 4–20-fold in the absence of the lipid layer.[6] However, the makeup of sebum is quite different from that of meibomian secretions. The main lipids in human sebum are triglycerides, wax esters, and squalene.[4] In contrast, meibomian lipids are composed of sterols and wax esters, with only minor amounts of triglycerides, hydrocarbons, polar lipids, and free fatty acids. In addition, the chains of meibomian lipids are longer and contain unique fatty acids and alcohols. Cutaneous sebum was shown to disrupt the tear film, suggesting that the unique composition of meibomian gland lipids is important to the maintenance of the tear film and likely prevents the spread of cutaneous sebum on to the ocular surface.[7]

Clinical background

The diagnosis of sebaceous cell carcinoma is difficult as it often masquerades as more common processes. This can lead to critical delay in the diagnosis and contribute to the morbidity and mortality associated with the disease.[8,9] Therefore, understanding the demographics and risk factors as well as recognizing the key clinical features of sebaceous cell carcinoma may allow prompt diagnosis and therapy, to reduce mortality and ocular morbidity.

Demographics

Sebaceous cell carcinoma mostly affects older adults with an estimated mean age at diagnosis between 63 and 77 years.[10-13] However, it may occur at a much younger age in people with prior history of facial irradiation.[14,15] Asia and the Indian subcontinent have a high incidence of sebaceous cell carcinoma. In North America, sebaceous cell carcinoma is primarily seen in people of European descent.[3] A possible association with the autosomal–dominant Muir–Torre syndrome with mutations in the mismatch repair genes hMLH-1 and hMLH-2 has been shown in some cases.[16]

Clinical presentation

Theoretically, sebaceous cell carcinoma can occur anywhere in the body where sebaceous glands are found. However, the ocular adnexa is by far the most common location for this neoplasm, with a vast majority occurring in the meibomian glands and fewer developing in the pilosebaceous glands of Zeis and caruncle.[9,17]

The most common presentation of sebaceous cell carcinoma is a solitary lid nodule with yellowish discoloration and madarosis, a key clinical feature differentiating it from more common benign lesions such as a chalazion or hordeolum. A recurrent chalazion in an older patient should raise

---

Box 52.1 Presentation

- Sebaceous cell carcinomas account for 1–5% of all eyelid malignancies
- The eyelids contain at least two major anatomic structures that can degenerate into sebaceous cell carcinomas: the cilia-associated glands of Zeis and the meibomian glands
- Proper identification and treatment of these tumors are critical because the rate of misdiagnosis has been estimated to be as high as 50%, with a mortality rate of at least 20%
- The diagnosis of sebaceous cell carcinoma is difficult as it often masquerades as more common processes

---

the suspicion for sebaceous cell carcinoma.[3] Madarosis is not a requisite, however (Figure 52.1), so a high level of suspicion must be maintained in the proper clinical setting.

The second most common pattern for sebaceous cell carcinoma development is a diffuse pattern with unilateral lid thickening and reactive inflammation which is often mistaken for blepharitis (Figure 52.2). Refractory and unilateral cases should raise suspicion for sebaceous cell carcinoma. A recent discussion of the varied clinical presentations of sebaceous cell carcinoma and the differential diagnosis has been published.[3]

Pathology

The histopathologic patterns of sebaceous cell carcinoma vary among tumors, making the disease challenging to diagnose (Box 52.2). However, there are certain characteristics that should be looked for in making the diagnosis. Sebaceous carcinoma cells are pleomorphic: they commonly exhibit enlarged nuclei and basophilic cytoplasm that is foamy in appearance due to the presence of fat. Mitotic figures, often with unusual appearance, are common. In well-differentiated carcinomas, vacuolization is common (Figure 52.3), and a comedo pattern can often be seen, showing the tumor cells attempting to reiterate the normal holocrine architecture of sebaceous glands (Figure 52.4). Poorly differentiated carcinomas have large cells, greater pleomorphism, higher mitotic rates, and disorganized architectures (Figure 52.5). Intraepithelial spread, also called pagetoid invasion – an important hallmark of sebaceous cell carcinoma – is known to occur in 44–80% of cases[18,19] (Figure 52.6). It is characterized by invasion of tumor cells, individually or in clusters, within the epithelium of the conjunctiva and skin, often eliciting subepithelial chronic inflammation.[18,19] Pagetoid invasion often results in skip lesions in which normal epithelial tissue may be found between nests of tumor cells, raising the need for map biopsies to sample the ocular surface.[3]

The level of differentiation appears to correlate well with the aggressiveness of the tumor: well-differentiated tumors

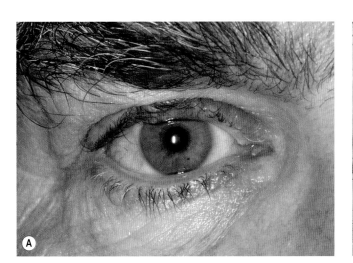
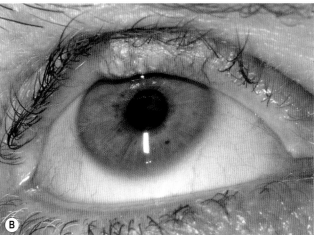

Figure 52.1 Wide (A) and closeup (B) view of sebaceous cell carcinoma presenting as a solitary lid margin nodule with the appearance of an internal hordeolum. Note the presence of lashes but the abnormal lid margin architecture and notching/ulceration.

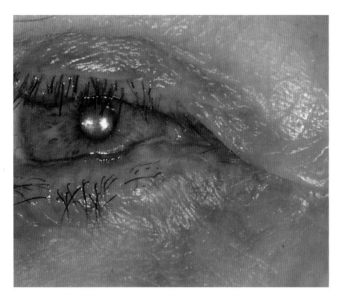

Figure 52.2 Sebaceous cell carcinoma presenting as diffuse thickening and inflammation, which can lead to misdiagnosis of blepharitis.

Box 52.2   Histology

- The histopathologic patterns of sebaceous cell carcinoma vary among tumors
- The level of differentiation appears to correlate well with the aggressiveness of the tumor
- Given the likelihood of pagetoid invasion, map biopsies of the skin and conjunctiva are essential to determining the extent of the disease and treatment options

---

are typically less aggressive than poorly differentiated tumors. The cytologic appearance of low-grade sebaceous cells is characterized by a cytoplasm containing many vacuoles, little nuclear pleomorphism, and rare mitoses (Figures 52.3 and 52.4). High-grade tumors are more intensely basophilic, exhibiting fewer cytoplasmic vesicles, prominent nucleoli, and more mitotic figures (Figure 52.5).[20] Unfortunately, both well- and poorly differentiated sebaceous tumor cells can be found within the same tumor (Figures 52.3–52.5 are from the same patient as shown in Figure 52.1). A recent publication attempted to classify histological patterns of sebaceous cell carcinoma into lobular, comedocarcinoma, papillary, and mixed.[3] However, the clinical value of such a classification is unclear. In addition, the term seboapocrine carcinoma has been proposed to describe sebaceous tumors with focal glandular pattern of apocrine glands (decapitation secretion).[2,21] Such a variety of architectures and tumor configurations highlights the likelihood that these tumors arise from stem cells associated with sebaceous and pilosebaceous glands (see below), but have not been shown to alter prognosis.

The pathologic diagnosis of poorly differentiated sebaceous cell carcinomas can be difficult because epidermal and sebaceous cells are derived from a common precursor and may display sebaceous and epidermal characteristics. For instance, sebaceous cell carcinomas may show areas with keratin pearls, intracellular bridges, and dyskeratosis, leading to a misdiagnosis as a poorly differentiated squamous cell carcinoma. In addition, there are spindle cell and basaloid variants of sebaceous cell carcinoma which mimic spindle cell squamous cell carcinoma and basal cell carcinoma, respectively.[20] The roles of the Wnt and Notch signaling systems and of the transcriptional regulator Lef-1 in cell type specification will be discussed below.

Given the difficulty in correctly identifying poorly differentiated sebaceous cell carcinomas, several immunohistochemical markers and special stains have been used to aid in diagnosis. Like normal sebaceous cells, the tumor cells contain lipid, which stains red with the oil red-O stain, a histochemical stain which has been performed with frozen sections of tumors for many years.[3] Immunohistochemistry staining for human milk fat globule-1 (HMFG1) and epithelial membrane antigen (EMA) has also been used as these antigens are strongly expressed on sebaceous cells.[22] Other studies have demonstrated that low-molecular-weight cytokeratins such as Cam5.2 and anti breast carcinoma-associated antigen-225 (BRST-1) are expressed in sebaceous cell carcinoma, but not in basal or squamous cell carcinomas, and may be useful in differentiating these tumors.[23–25]

Regional metastasis to preauricular, parotid, submandibular, and cervical lymph nodes is known to occur in approximately 30% of cases. Distant metastases of sebaceous cell carcinoma are rare, occurring in the lungs, liver, brain, and bone.[3] There are current studies on the usefulness of sentinel lymph node biopsy for assessing regional metastasis, followed by treatment with local lymph node dissection and/or adjuvant chemotherapy.[26–28] In the largest study to date, 10 patients with sebaceous cell carcinoma underwent sentinel lymph node biopsy and two of the 10 demonstrated microscopic evidence of tumor metastasis.[28] It remains to be determined whether detection and treatment of lymph node micrometastases will alter the clinical course of the disease.

Disease management

The initial management of sebaceous cell carcinoma depends on several factors, including the index of clinical suspicion and the size of the tumor (Box 52.2). Small tumors for which there is high clinical suspicion should be excised with margin control as the first intervention. In contrast, a full-thickness biopsy of the eyelid is considered a better approach for the initial assessment of large lesions requiring extensive eyelid reconstruction following excision.[3,29,30] At the present time there is still considerable controversy as to whether Mohs micrographic surgery, serial excisions with frozen section control, or serial excisions with permanent section control are most effective.[31–33] Based on retrospective studies, there is a suggestion that, in experienced hands, traditional excision with permanent section control of the margins provides the best chance of avoiding recurrence.[32–34] With pagetoid spread, wide surgical margins are advisable, although the ideal width of clear margins is controversial.[35]

Given the likelihood of pagetoid invasion, map biopsies of the skin and conjunctiva are essential to determining the extent of the disease and treatment options.[36] Historically, extensively positive map biopsies have been an indication for orbital exenteration. However, the development of new

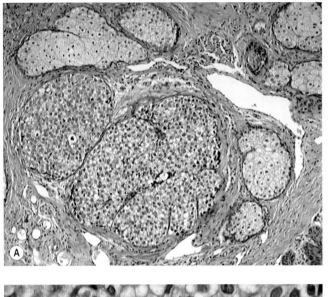

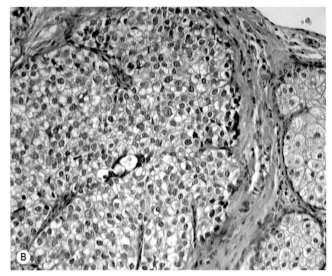

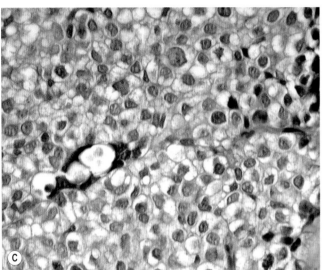

Figure 52.3 Well-differentiated sebaceous cell carcinoma with lacy, foamy, basophilic cytoplasm and vacuolization. Note the normal sebaceous gland above and on the side for comparison. (A) 100×. (B) 200×. (C) 400×.

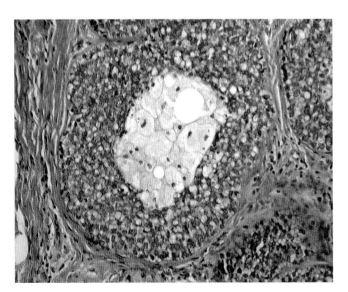

Figure 52.4 Well-differentiated sebaceous cell carcinoma attempting to reiterate the normal sebaceous gland architecture, leading to comedo pattern with holocrine secretion centrally. Note the vacuolization. 200×.

surgical techniques and materials for reconstructing the eyelid and conjunctiva following extensive excision have prompted more localized tumor excision.[3,31] In addition to surgery, a number of adjuvant techniques have been employed to supplement surgical excision or to treat local recurrences. Cryotherapy has been used with success as an adjuvant to surgical excision to treat pagetoid invasion of the conjunctiva.[31,37] More recently, topical mitomycin C, an alkylating agent that inhibits DNA synthesis, has been advocated as an adjuvant agent to treat pagetoid invasion on the conjunctiva and cornea in a small number of patients.[38,39] Further studies are needed to determine the efficacy of these treatments, particularly as pagetoid invasion may extend into adnexal structures, including the lacrimal gland ducts and drainage system.

Orbital exenteration remains the definitive treatment in cases of extensive conjunctival involvement and where there is orbital invasion without evidence of metastases.[3,31] In patients with orbital extension who are unable or unwilling to undergo orbital exenteration or who have advanced disease and are seeking palliative measures, irradiation with

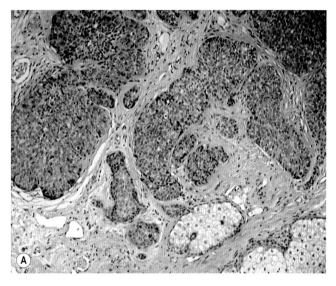

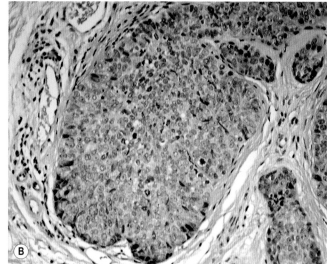

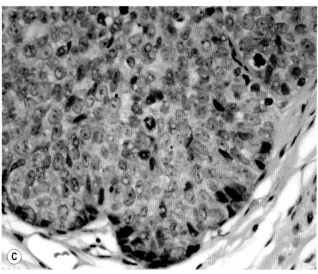

Figure 52.5 Poorly differentiated sebaceous cell carcinoma from the same patient from which Figures 52.1, 52.3, and 52.4 were obtained. Note the lack of vacuolization, the lack of coherent architecture, and the presence of mitotic figures. A normal sebaceous gland is to the side. (A) 100×. (B) 200×. (C) 400×.

at least 55 Gy of radiation has been used with some success.[31,40,41] However, the use of radiotherapy for this neoplasm is controversial and surgical excision is preferred.[31] Finally, some authors advocate brachytherapy, in which a radioactive plaque is inserted close to the tumor and delivers 150 Gy directly to the area as an alternative to orbital exenteration while protecting much of the surrounding tissue from additional exposure.[42] Additional studies will be required to assess its efficacy.

Pathophysiology

The pilosebaceous gland, the bulge, and the role of hair follicle stem cells

The skin and its appendages are critical for animal survival. Among its many biological functions, skin protects animals from dehydration, radiation, trauma, temperature changes, and microbial infections. The adult skin is composed of varied groups of cells from diverse embryologic origins. The surface ectoderm forms a layer of progenitor cells that goes on to form stratified epidermis, hair follicles, as well as sebaceous and apocrine glands. The mesoderm contributes the collagen-producing fibroblasts of the dermis, the skin vasculature, the erector pili muscles of the hair follicles, the subcutaneous fat, and immune cells. Neural crest cells contribute melanocytes, sensory nerve endings, and the dermis of the head and face.[43]

Sebaceous cell carcinomas of the ocular adnexa can derive from both pilosebaceous glands of Zeis and the specialized sebaceous glands of the eyelid margin – the meibomian glands (Box 52.3). Our understanding of the biology of the pilosebaceous gland is significantly greater than that of the meibomian glands, but this understanding can be extrapolated to shed some light on the origins, genetics, and cell biology of eyelid sebaceous carcinomas in general. This extrapolation is based on the self-renewal properties that the holocrine cells of all sebaceous glands share with the progenitor cells of the hair follicle and skin.

The epidermis and hair follicles are renewed throughout life. Hair follicle renewal is achieved through a cycle comprising a growth phase (anagen), a regression phase

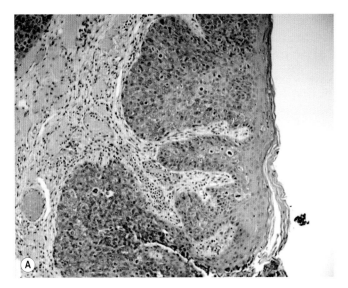

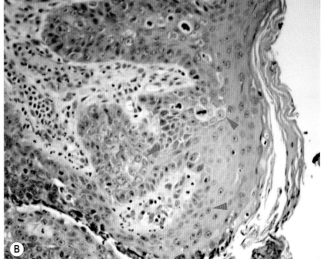

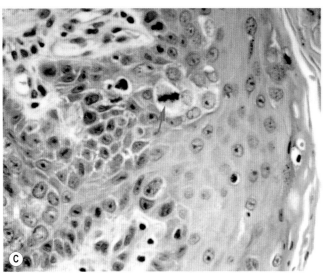

Figure 52.6 Pagetoid spread. Sebaceous carcinoma cells have replaced the basal layer and are seen spreading along the epithelium. These cells are notable for the basophilic foamy cytoplasm (arrowhead). Occasional mitotic figures are also seen. Pagetoid spread is a critical feature of sebaceous cell carcinoma, and has important clinical implications. (A) 100×. (B) 200×. (C) 400×.

Box 52.3 Pathophysiology

- Normal holocrine function requires the presence of a multipotent stem cell population that serves to regenerate the cells of holocrine glands
- These populations of multipotent stem cells are responsible for the malignant degeneration that results in eyelid cancer
- Signaling pathways are involved in the malignant process, including the Hedgehog, Notch, and Wnt pathways
- The association between Lef-1 mutations and sebaceous hyperplasia and tumorigenesis is intriguing because of the apparent dual roles of Lef-1 in activating squamous cell differentiation and concurrently serving as an activator of tumor suppressor genes such as p53 and p21

(catagen), and a resting phase (telogen). This renewal depends on the presence of progenitor stem cells in an area referred to as "the bulge" in both rodents and humans. The bulge region contains undifferentiated stem cells that maintain a high proliferative capacity and multipotency (similar to intestinal, corneal, and other clustered stem cell populations; Figure 52.7). It should be noted that the stem cell population of the bulge may have been experimentally overestimated by label-retaining techniques, since rigorous studies of stem cell behavior and label retention revealed that this presumed stem cell characteristic is not universal.[44] On the other hand, the multipotency of epidermal stem cells is well established, and use of epidermal stem cells for generating cells with embryonic pluripotency has been published.[45,46]

The morphology of the bulge is different between mouse and human hair follicles. The murine bulge is a discrete protuberance of the outer root sheath, while the human bulge is in fact just a subtle swelling. However, the biology of the human and murine epidermal and bulge stem cells appears to be quite similar.[47] The adult skin epithelium is composed of the pilosebaceous unit and the surrounding interfollicular epidermis (IFE) and its associated apocrine glands. The IFE relies on its own source of progenitor cells to provide for tissue renewal in the absence of injury, while the pilosebaceous bulge contains multipotent stem cells that

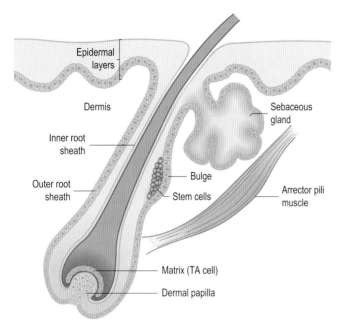

Epidermal layers

Dermis

Inner root sheath

Outer root sheath

Sebaceous gland

Bulge

Stem cells

Arrector pili muscle

Matrix (TA cell)

Dermal papilla

Figure 52.7 Epithelial stem cells are often clustered where they can supply cellular renewal to tissues that require it. These cells are multipotent, and capable of differentiating into a variety of cell types within the proper milieu. Label-retaining cells of the hair follicle reside below the sebaceous gland in a region known as the bulge, which is connected to the arrector pili muscle. During periods of rest, bulge stem cells form the base of the follicle, which is adjacent to the specialized new hair germ. As the germ grows, a proliferative compartment of transient amplifying (TA: matrix) cells engulfs the dermal papilla (DP) at the base. These cells progress to differentiate to form seven concentric shells of discrete cell lineages, which are from outer to inner: the companion layer, the three layers of the inner root sheath, and the three layers of the hair shaft. These differentiated layers are surrounded by the outer root sheath, which extends below the bulge and is thought to contain stem cells that continue to migrate down to the follicle base during the growth phase of the hair cycle. The interfollicular epidermis is a stratified epithelium with a basal layer that contains unipotent progenitor cells and TA cells. Basal cells differentiate upward to form the spinous, granular, and stratum corneum layers of the epidermis. (Modified from Blanpain C, Horsley V, Fuchs E. Epithelial stem cells: turning over new leaves. Cell 2007;128:445–458.)

are activated at the start of each new hair cycle, at the time of injury, and as needed to supply the holocrine cells of the sebaceous gland. During the hair cycle, bulge stem cells are stimulated to migrate out of the stem cell niche, proliferate, and differentiate into the various cell types of the pilosebaceous unit. Although the bulge stem cells are relatively quiescent, they can also be induced to migrate and proliferate by mitogenic stimuli such as phorbol esters (12-O-tetradecanoylphorbol-13-acetate (TPA)). Bulge stem cells appear to be in continuous flux throughout the growth phase of the hair cycle, migrating from the bulge along the basal layer of the outer root sheath where they proliferate and differentiate. The ability of these stem cells to differentiate into multiple cell types of the epidermis, sebaceous glands, and hair follicles has been shown by elegant in vivo and in vitro experiments, including transplantation experiments and clonal analysis.[43] In addition, even when bulge cells detach from the basal lamina and undergo early commitment to the hair follicle lineage, the process is reversible, at least in vitro.[48]

Genetic and molecular regulation of sebaceous cell carcinoma

Genetic profiling of bulge stem cells using microarray analysis has identified many genes which are expressed at higher levels within this population. Interestingly, 14% of these genes are also expressed at higher levels in other stem cell types such as hematopoietic, neuronal, and embryonic stem cells.[48–50] The most interesting of these are genes that belong to the Wnt-β-catenin and the transforming growth factor-β/bone morphogenic protein (BMP) genetic signaling pathways.[48,51] In addition, microarray analysis demonstrated decreased expression of many genes that inhibit proliferation in bulge stem cells, consistent with their relatively quiescent state.[48,51] Both the Wnt and the BMP signaling pathways play very important roles in hair follicle morphogenesis and cycling.[52–59] Hence, upregulation of Wnt and BMP regulatory components in bulge stem cells strongly suggests that these pathways are critical for proper stem cell function.

The Wnt/β-catenin signaling pathway is conserved throughout the eukaryotic kingdom and has repeatedly been shown to be critical to embryonic and postnatal development.[60] It is often referred to as the canonical Wnt pathway and is involved in a variety of human cancers (Figure 52.8). An effector of intercellular adhesion, β-catenin is usually stabilized at the plasma membrane through association with cadherin at adherens junctions via armadillo repeats. Under basal conditions, free cytoplasmic β-catenin is rapidly degraded by the proteosome in a ubiquitin-dependent manner. β-catenin is normally bound by two scaffolding proteins, adenomatous polyposis coli (APC) and axin, which leads to the phosphorylation and ubiquitination of β-catenin, resulting in the subsequent proteosomal degradation.[60] Wnts are a large family of cysteine-rich secreted glycoproteins which bind members of the frizzled family of serpentine receptors and a member of the low-density lipoprotein receptor family, Lrp5/6. The binding of Wnt to a frizzled receptor inactivates axin by a mechanism that may involve the binding of disheveled. This inactivates the phosphorylation and ubiquitination of β-catenin, leading to β-catenin stabilization. Stable, free β-catenin is then translocated to the nucleus, where it binds the N-termini of DNA-binding transcription factors of the T-cell factor/leukocyte enhancer factor (Tcf/Lef) family.

There are important lines of evidence showing a direct link between the Wnt system and sebaceous cell carcinomas. The history of the research that revealed this link can provide important insights into the scientific process that will continue to tease out the genetic and cellular processes underlying human adnexal tumors. The first clue for the importance of the Wnt system was the finding that lymphoid enhancer factor Lef-1 is critically important for ectodermal commitment to hair follicle differentiation and the required epithelial–mesenchymal interactions.[61] Next, mice carrying a stabilized β-catenin were shown to undergo de novo hair morphogenesis, including the formation of new ectopic sebaceous glands in the adult mouse.[62] The clinical relevance of this was revealed by studies that identified β-catenin-stabilizing mutations in human pilomatricomas, a common skin tumor.[63] Concurrently, Lef-1 and Tcf-3 were found to form transcriptional complexes with β-catenin that were

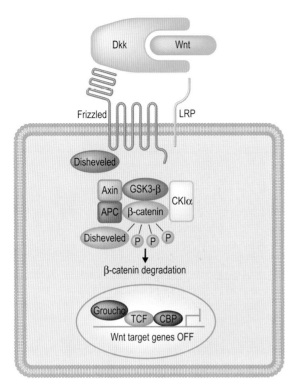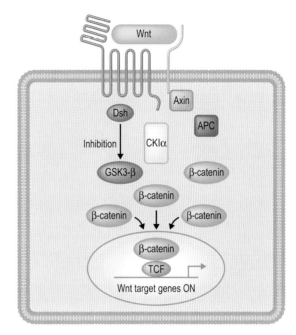

Figure 52.8 Schematic of the canonical Wnt pathway. In the absence of a Wnt signal, the excess of cytoplasmic ß-catenin is targeted for degradation through its association with a multiprotein complex. Upon binding Wnt, its activated receptor complex recruits certain key components of the ß-catenin degradation targeting machinery. Stabilized free cytoplasmic ß-catenin is now translocated to the nucleus, where it can associate with transcription factors of the leukocyte enhancer factor (LEF)/T-cell factor (TCF) family to transactivate the expression of their target genes. LRP, lipoprotein receptor-related protein; APC, adenomatous polyposis coli; GSK3-ß, glycogen synthase kinase. (Modified from Blanpain C, Fuchs E. Epidermal stem cells of the skin. Annu Rev Cell Dev Biol 2006;22:339–373.)

critically important in regulating cell fate and differentiation commitment during hair follicle development.[64] Indeed, when β-catenin is selectively deleted from the developing epidermis and hair follicles using Cre/loxP technology with the keratin-14 promoter driving Cre-recombinase, hair follicle development was aborted in wide patches, and hair follicles that did develop failed to regenerate after the first hair cycle.[52] Specifically, skin stem cells failed to develop into hair keratinocytes and associated cells, and instead differentiated into epidermal keratinocytes. In addition, ectopic expression of the diffusible Wnt inhibitor Dickkopf-1 resulted in failure of hair follicle development.[54] Hence, the canonical Wnt system was found to be critical for both morphogenesis and maintenance of cell fate commitment. The role of the canonical Wnt pathway in pilosebaceous differentiation and cell fate commitment was further elucidated by experiments showing that dominant negative Lef-1 mutations lead to suppression of hair follicle differentiation while promoting sebocyte differentiation.[65]

The association of Lef-1 activity, epidermal differentiation, and skin tumors was further revealed by studies of a Lef-1 mutant lacking the amino terminus (ΔN-Lef-1). This mutant cannot bind to translocated β-catenin, and functions as a disruptor of skin differentiation. Overexpression of ΔN-Lef-1 under the control of the keratin 14 promoter resulted in the formation of dermal cysts and spontaneous skin tumors, most of which exhibited sebaceous differentiation.[66] This association between sebaceous differentiation and Lef-1

mutations led to a key study in which human sebaceous tumors were tested for the presence of Lef-1 mutations. The finding that 30% of human sebaceous adenomas carried somatic Lef-1 mutations that interfere with Wnt signaling and act as dominant-negative alleles to reduce Wnt-driven gene expression provided critical links among: (1) the genetic pathways that regulate normal skin development; (2) the genetic signals that control stem cell lineage determination and differentiation in the bulge; and (3) the genetic underpinnings of human sebaceous tumors.[67] Further research revealed that Lef-1 has two complementary roles that together promote the development of sebaceous tumors. First, it is involved in lineage specification, and can determine whether randomly mutagenized skin cells will develop into squamous or sebaceous tumors (Figure 52.9). Second, normal Lef-1 function is important for the activation of the checkpoint tumor suppressor genes p53 and p21 via p14ARF induction. Therefore, Lef-1 inactivation can cause failure of tumor suppression activity when progenitor cells accumulate mutations (Figure 52.9).[68] It can be concluded that the Wnt pathway in general, and the transcriptional regulator Lef-1 in particular, are likely to be intimately involved in the generation of human sebaceous cell carcinomas of the ocular adnexa.

Like the Wnt signaling pathway, the Hedgehog pathway is a critical regulator of metazoan development and differentiation, often acting in concert with the Wnt-β-catenin pathway. The details of the Hedgehog signaling pathway are

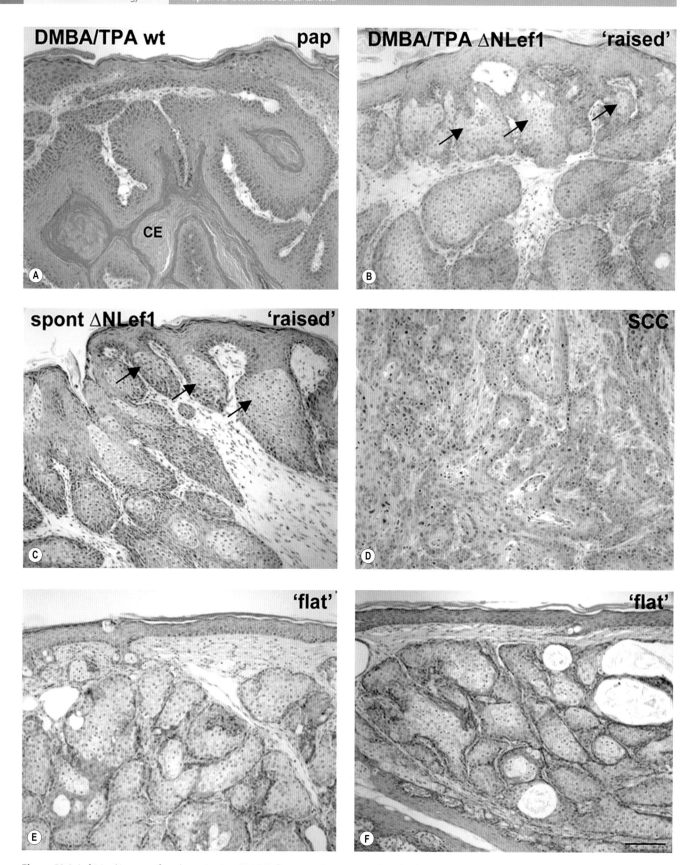

Figure 52.9 Lef-1 in skin tumor fate determination. K14ΔNLef1 transgenic mice were found to be much more sensitive to mutationally induced carcinogenesis than transgene-negative mice. In response to dimethylbenzanthracene (DMBA) and tetradecanoylphorbol acetate (TPA)-induced mutations, wild-type mice develop papillomas, some of which progress to squamous cell carcinoma with interfollicular epidermal differentiation and accumulation of cornified layers. In contrast, tumors induced in K14ΔNLef1 transgenic mice exhibited a high degree of sebocyte differentiation. Hematoxylin and eosin-stained sections of tumors from wild-type (wt; A) and K14ΔNLef1 transgenic mice (ΔNLef1; B and C). A and B, chemically induced tumors; C, spontaneous tumors. Pap, papilloma; SCC, squamous cell carcinoma. Sebaceous tumors (B and C) were macroscopically raised or flat. Arrows, regions of extensive sebaceous differentiation. CE, accumulation of cornified layers, indicating squamous differentiation. Bar, 100 μm. (Reproduced with permission from Niemann C, Owens DM, Schettina P, et al. Dual role of inactivating Lef1 mutations in epidermis: tumor promotion and specification of tumor type. Cancer Res 2007;67:2916–2921.)

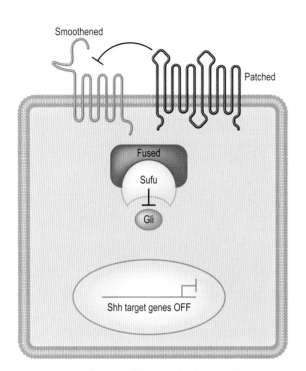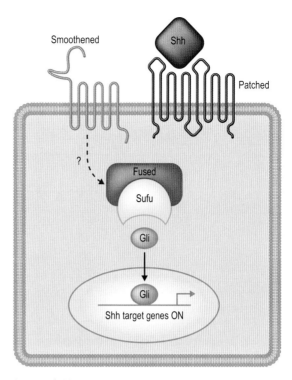

Figure 52.10 Schematic of the Sonic hedgehog (Shh) pathway. In the absence of Shh, its receptor Patched (Ptch) inhibits Smoothened (Smo) activity. Upon Shh binding, Ptch can no longer repress Smo, which activates the translocation of Gli into the nucleus, allowing it to transactivate its target genes. (Modified from Blanpain,C, Fuchs E. Epidermal stem cells of the skin. Annu Rev Cell Dev Biol 2006;22:339–373.)

beyond the scope of this chapter, and the literature includes several excellent reviews.[69-74] Briefly, Sonic hedgehog (Shh) is a secreted factor that binds the transmembrane receptor Patched (Figure 52.10). In a simplified model of Hedgehog signaling, the absence of Shh ligand activity allows Patched constitutively to inhibit Smoothened (Smo), which results in the ubiquitin-dependent proteolysis of the zinc-finger activator/repressor proteins of the Gli family. In the proteolized form, Gli proteins function as transcriptional repressors. Once Shh binds to Patched, Smoothened is no longer inhibited, leading to stabilization and nuclear translocation of the full-length activator form of Gli. This results in the induction of specific gene expression.

The Hedgehog signaling pathway has essential roles in the proliferation and differentiation of epidermal stem cells,[69,75-78] and sebaceous gland development.[79,80] In addition, the Hedgehog pathway plays critical roles in the pathogenesis of skin cancer.[72,81-84] Specifically, mutations in the Patched and Smoothened genes have been demonstrated in sporadic basal cell carcinomas. Moreover, basal cell nevus syndrome is an autosomal-dominant condition caused by a mutation in the Patched gene, which results in the development of multiple basal cell carcinomas.[85,86] The Hedgehog and Wnt signaling pathways share many commonalities, and are also known to interact with and regulate one another, including in the regulation of skin development and disease.[53,80,87]

Another signaling pathway that likely participates in the pathogenesis of sebaceous tumors is the Notch pathway. Notch signaling is involved in a variety of cellular processes: cell fate specification, differentiation, apoptosis, proliferation, migration, adhesion, angiogenesis, and the epithelial–mesenchymal transition.[88-90] The pathway consists of several Notch receptors that contain extracellular epidermal growth factor (EGF) repeats that bind to transmembrane ligands of the Delta-Serrate-Lag2 (DSL) family (Figure 52.11). Notch receptors also contain negative regulatory regions and a heterodimerization domain that are important in inhibiting Notch activity. As with the Wnt and Hedgehog pathways, canonical Notch signaling requires regulated, ubiquitin-mediated proteolysis. The Notch pathway is a complex array of interrelated cellular processes, and for greater detail, the interested reader is directed to one of many outstanding reviews.[88-90] The ability of Notch to function as either a tumor suppressor or an oncogene in various contexts reflects the plasticity of this signaling pathway. The clearest example of oncogenic Notch signaling is found in acute lymphoblastic T-cell leukemia (T-ALL), an aggressive neoplasm of T cells. However, Notch can also function as a tumor suppressor, since Notch knockout mice develop basal cell carcinoma with increased levels of both Wnt and Hedgehog signaling,[91] and overexpression of the Notch inhibitor MAML1 in mice results in squamous cell carcinoma.[92] Finally, both oncogenic and tumor suppressor activities may be related to the roles of Notch in establishing and maintaining a variety of stem cell populations.[88,90]

In the epidermis, Notch has a critical role in the normal development and regeneration of adnexal tissues. The literature on this subject is growing rapidly and supports a clear interaction between the Notch and Wnt signaling cascades in epidermal growth and differentiation.[93] After the initial discoveries showing that Notch is important in skin differentiation,[94] Notch expression was found to be modified in basal cell carcinoma.[95] Subsequent studies demonstrated

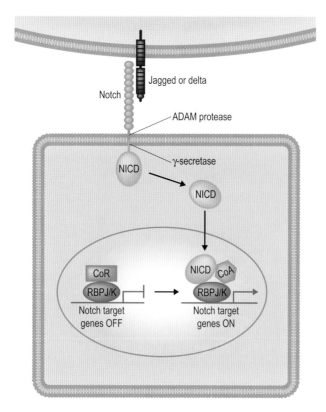

Figure 52.11 Schematic of canonical Notch signaling. Upon ligand (Jagged or Delta) binding, the Notch transmembrane receptor is cleaved by proteases (ADAM protease and γ-secretase), releasing the Notch intracellular domain (NICD), which can then translocate into the nucleus and associate with the DNA-binding protein RBP-Jk to permit transcription of target genes. (Modified from Blanpain C, Fuchs E. Epidermal stem cells of the skin. Annu Rev Cell Dev Biol 2006;22:339–373.)

that disruption of Notch signaling in mice results in epidermal and corneal hyperplasia followed by the development of skin tumor and heightened sensitivity to mutagenesis.[91] Interestingly, these tumors were found to express elevated levels of the Hedgehog transcription factor Gli2 as well as the activation of β-catenin signaling which maintained cells in a poorly differentiated state. Shortly thereafter, Notch was found to regulate the differentiation and commitment of the multiple skin layers. As proliferating cells leave the basal layer, migrate outwardly, and terminally differentiate into spinous, granular, and stratum corneum skin layers, Notch signaling, mediated by the RBP-J and Hes1, pushes cells toward terminal differentiation and induces spinous-specific gene expression.[96]

More recently, the Notch ligand, JAG1, was identified as an important target of the Wnt/β-catenin signaling pathway, and its expression was particularly localized to stem cells and progenitor cells, where it is important in maintaining the self-renewal properties of these cells.[97] Finally, both Notch and Wnt pathways are highly active in precommitment hair follicle cells, and the deletion of JAG1 resulted in the inhibition of the hair growth cycle and the activation of epidermal differentiation. Conversely, activation of Notch resulted in expansion of the pilosebaceous progenitor cell population along with enlargement of sebaceous glands.[98] Interestingly, induction by β-catenin of ectopic pilosebaceous development in the adult mouse was blocked by Notch inhibition

through either JAG1 deletion or by treatment with the Notch inhibitor N-[N-(3,5-difluorophenacetyl)-l-alanyl]-S-phenylglycine t-butyl ester (DAPT).

The recent discovery of increased retinoic acid receptor expression in sebaceous cell carcinoma[99,100] adds another layer of complexity to an already complex picture. Retinoid receptors are members of the superfamily of nuclear receptors that include steroid hormone, vitamin D, and thyroid hormone receptors. These receptors serve to regulate gene expression through complex dimerization DNA binding and recruitment of other gene expression regulators. Retinoic acid is a well-known regulator of cell proliferation and differentiation, and vitamin D was found to be particularly important for maintenance of the stem cell population of the hair follicle bulge. Mutations in the vitamin D receptor result in alopecia in both mice and humans, which is caused by the inability of bulge stem cells to regenerate. Vitamin D receptor ablation is associated with biasing hair follicle stem cells toward the sebaceous differentiation pathway, which is strikingly similar to the phenotype seen with impaired Wnt signaling. Indeed, the absence of vitamin D receptor activity results in the inhibition of Lef-1 activity, suggesting that vitamin D, and possibly other member of the nuclear receptor superfamily, are important regulators of the Wnt/Notch/Hedgehog pathways in skin.[101]

Summary

From careful and productive research into the normal biology of skin development, we have gained important insights into the processes that are responsible for generating sebaceous cell carcinomas of the ocular adnexa.[102] The eyelids contain at least two major anatomic structures that can degenerate into sebaceous cell carcinomas: the cilia-associated glands of Zeis and the meibomian glands. In both cases normal holocrine function requires the presence of a multipotent stem cell population that serves to regenerate the cells of these structures. It is likely that these populations of multipotent stem cells are responsible for the malignant degeneration that results in eyelid cancer. Maintaining a population of poorly differentiated and multipotentiated cells is tenuous and hence tightly regulated by an incredible array of cellular and genetic pathways. Nevertheless, the three critical signaling pathways in this process appear to be: (1) the Hedgehog pathway, which controls cellular proliferation; (2) the Notch pathway, which controls cell commitment and differentiation to maintain the cellular balance as skin adnexa develop and mature, and, most importantly; (3) the Wnt pathway, which appears to serve as a master regulator of stem cell maintenance and cell fate, particularly in the case of sebaceous differentiation. It is likely that the natural accumulation of mutations in adnexal stem cells is coupled with the proliferative burden that is placed on these cells by the nature of their functions. It also appears possible that sebaceous-like differentiation is a default fate when progenitor cells are signaled to proliferate, and triggers for epidermal differentiation are lacking. The association between Lef-1 mutations and sebaceous hyperplasia and tumorigenesis is intriguing because of the apparent dual roles of Lef-1 in activating squamous cell differentiation and concurrently serving as an activator of tumor suppressor genes such as p53 and p21. The concurrent loss of squamous potential and loss of tumor suppressor activity can push mutant multipotent cells toward sebaceous tumorigenesis. The regulatory roles of the nuclear receptors for retinoic acid, vitamin D, and other nuclear receptor ligands are unknown, but they are likely to interact genetically with the major transcriptional signaling pathways to regulate proliferation and differentiation. It is important to note that, while sebaceous cells are distributed across the entire body, the eyelids give rise to far more sebaceous cell carcinomas than any other locations. It is tempting to speculate about the reasons for this propensity, with a likely explanation being the high concentration of sebaceous cells in the eyelids, along with the anatomic exposure to mutagenic solar radiation, which combine to create the environment in which sebaceous cell carcinomas can arise. We now have substantial tools to dissect carefully the molecular pathways and cellular environments to shed light on the processes involved in dermatologic carcinogenesis, and to permit the development of diagnostic and therapeutic strategies for the successful medical treatment of sebaceous cell carcinoma.

Conclusion

Sebaceous cell carcinomas account for 1–5% of all eyelid malignancies and proper identification and treatment of these tumors are critical because the rate of misdiagnosis has been estimated to be as high as 50%, with a mortality rate of at least 20%. The diagnosis of sebaceous cell carcinoma is difficult as it often masquerades as more common processes. This can lead to critical delay in the diagnosis and contribute to the morbidity and mortality associated with the disease. Sebaceous cell carcinomas result from dysregulation of glandular stem cells, involving the Hedgehog, Notch, and Wnt signaling pathways. Poorly differentiated carcinomas have large cells, greater pleomorphism, higher mitotic rates, and disorganized architectures. Intraepithelial spread, also called pagetoid invasion – an important hallmark of sebaceous cell carcinoma – is known to occur in 44–80% of cases. The level of differentiation appears to correlate well with the aggressiveness of the tumor. At the present time there is a suggestion that, in experienced hands, traditional excision with permanent section control of the margins provides the best chance of avoiding recurrence. Given the likelihood of pagetoid invasion, map biopsies of the skin and conjunctiva are essential to determining the extent of the disease and treatment options.

Acknowledgment

The authors would like to acknowledge the generosity of Research to Prevent Blindness to the Department of Ophthalmology and Visual Sciences at the University of Michigan. Figure 52.9 was kindly provided by Professor Fiona Watt, Wellcome Trust Centre for Stem Cell Research, University of Cambridge, UK. Alon Kahana and Victor Elner gratefully acknowledge research support from the National Institutes of Health, USA.

Key references

A complete list of chapter references is available online at www.expertconsult.com. See inside cover for registration details.

3. Shields JA, Demirci H, Marr BP, et al. Sebaceous carcinoma of the ocular region: a review. Surv Ophthalmol 2005;50:103–122.

4. Thody AJ, Shuster S. Control and function of sebaceous glands. Physiol Rev 1989;69:383–416.

5. Porter AM. Why do we have apocrine and sebaceous glands? J R Soc Med 2001;94:236–237.

12. Chao AN, Shields CL, Krema H, et al. Outcome of patients with periocular sebaceous gland carcinoma with and without conjunctival intraepithelial invasion. Ophthalmology 2001;108: 1877–1883.

22. Johnson JS, Lee JA, Cotton DW, et al. Dimorphic immunohistochemical staining in ocular sebaceous neoplasms: a useful diagnostic aid. Eye 1999;13: 104–108.

23. Murata T, Nakashima Y, Takeuchi M, et al. The diagnostic use of low molecular weight keratin expression in sebaceous carcinoma. Pathol Res Pract 1993;189:888–893.

24. Sinard JH. Immunohistochemical distinction of ocular sebaceous carcinoma from basal cell and squamous cell carcinoma. Arch Ophthalmol 1999;117:776–783.

28. Ho VH, Ross MI, Prieto VG, et al. Sentinel lymph node biopsy for sebaceous cell carcinoma and melanoma of the ocular adnexa. Arch Otolaryngol Head Neck Surg 2007;133: 820–826.

30. Yeatts RP, Waller RR. Sebaceous carcinoma of the eyelid: pitfalls in diagnosis. Ophthalm Plast Reconstr Surg 1985;1:35–42.

32. Folberg R, Whitaker DC, Tse DT, et al. Recurrent and residual sebaceous carcinoma after Mohs' excision of the primary lesion. Am J Ophthalmol 1987;103:817–823.

36. Putterman AM. Conjunctival map biopsy to determine pagetoid spread. Am J Ophthalmol 1986;102: 87–90.

37. Lisman RD, Jakobiec FA, Small P. Sebaceous carcinoma of the eyelids. The role of adjunctive cryotherapy in the management of conjunctival pagetoid spread. Ophthalmology 1989;96:1021–1026.

38. Shields CL, Naseripour M, Shields JA, et al. Topical mitomycin-C for pagetoid invasion of the conjunctiva by eyelid sebaceous gland carcinoma. Ophthalmology 2002;109:2129–2133.

48. Blanpain C, Lowry WE, Geoghegan A, et al. Self-renewal, multipotency, and the existence of two cell populations within an epithelial stem cell niche. Cell 2004;118:635–648.

51. Ohyama M, Terunuma A, Tock CL, et al. Characterization and isolation of stem cell-enriched human hair follicle bulge cells. J Clin Invest 2006;116:249–260.

CHAPTER 53

Neurofibromatosis

Robert Listernick and David H Gutmann

Neurofibromatosis type 1 (NF1) is an autosomal-dominant tumor predisposition syndrome in which affected children are prone to the development of low-grade astrocytic (glial) neoplasms along the optic pathway (optic pathway glioma, OPG). In this regard, 30% of OPGs are found in children with NF1, making NF1 the most common genetic cause for this visual pathway tumor. The protean manifestations and unpredictability of the clinical course of an individual with NF1 often make this complex condition challenging to manage for the practitioner.

Clinical background

Historical development

Historical depictions of individuals who clearly display manifestations of NF1 can be found in art dating back to as early as the 15th century. Frederick Daniel von Recklinghausen provided the first complete pathologic description of NF1 (1881), reporting both the gross and histologic features, and demonstrating for the first time that the cutaneous masses contained neural elements. Although Crowe (1953)[1] emphasized the importance of the café-au-lait spot in the diagnosis of "von Recklinghausen disease," the recognition of NF1 as a distinct clinical entity did not occur until 1981. Finally, in 1987 the National Institutes of Health Consensus Development Conference[2] defined the seven diagnostic criteria for NF1, of which two must be present to confirm the diagnosis (Box 53.1).

Key signs and symptoms of NF1

Café-au-lait spots and intertriginous freckling (Figure 53.1A)

Café-au-lait spots are flat, pigmented macules, and are generally the first cutaneous manifestation of NF1. Often present at birth, they become apparent during the first few years of life. As many as 97% of children who are eventually diagnosed with NF1 will have six or more café-au-lait spots by the time they are 6 years of age.[3] Patients with greater numbers of café-au-lait spots are not at risk for the development of more severe disease. While freckling is common in sun-exposed areas of individuals without NF1, smaller café-au-lait spots or freckling may be seen in areas not directly exposed to the sun in individuals with NF1, and constitutes the second most common diagnostic criterion found in young children. These freckles typically occur in skinfolds, including the axilla, inguinal creases, submammary regions, and the neck.

Dermal neurofibromas (Figure 53.1B)

Neurofibromas, the hallmark lesion of NF1, are benign nerve sheath tumors arising from peripheral nerves. These tumors are composed of neoplastic Schwann cells as well as numerous stromal cell types (i.e., mast cells, fibroblasts, and perineural cells). Cutaneous neurofibromas arise from small superficial nerves; they are soft, protrude just above the skin's surface, and often display a violaceous hue. In contrast, subcutaneous neurofibromas arise from deeper nerves and are generally firm. Deep visceral neurofibromas may cause symptoms by compressing vital structures, such as is seen in spinal cord compression from dorsal root neurofibromas. Although young children may have some neurofibromas, these tumors tend to appear with the onset of puberty and increase in both size and number with advancing age.

Plexiform neurofibromas (Figure 53.1C)

Although plexiform neurofibromas are histologically similar to dermal neurofibromas, they are clinically quite distinct. They are often present at birth or develop in the first several years of life, undergoing a phase of rapid growth during childhood. Although these tumors are generally soft, the observer can often feel multiple firmer thickened nerves within the tumor, described as a "bag of worms." Overlying hyperpigmentation or fine hair growth may be a clue to the presence of an underlying plexiform neurofibroma. Often arising from branches of major nerves, they can become large and cause significant dysfunction. Plexiform neurofibromas involving the eyelid or orbit may lead to visual loss from associated glaucoma, amblyopia secondary to proptosis, or optic nerve damage. Internal plexiform neurofibromas can cause morbidity as a result of spinal cord compression, erosion of contiguous bone, or ureteral/bladder outlet obstruction.

Box 53.1 Neurofibromatosis type 1 (NF1) diagnostic criteria

Two or more of the following must be present to establish the diagnosis of NF1:

- Six or more café-au-lait macules >5 mm in prepubertal individuals, or >15 mm in postpubertal individuals
- Two or more neurofibromas, or one plexiform neurofibroma
- Freckling in the axillary or inguinal region
- Optic glioma
- Two or more Lisch nodules
- A distinctive osseous lesion (sphenoid dysplasia or thinning of long bone cortex with or without pseudarthrosis)
- A first-degree relative with NF1 by above criteria

Lisch nodules (Figure 53.1D)

Lisch nodules are dome-shaped melanocytic hamartomas of the iris, and are virtually pathognomonic of NF1. Not associated with any visual abnormalities, they are present in 90–95% of adults with NF1. They are best visualized using a slit lamp by an experienced ophthalmologist.

Optic pathway gliomas

Although children 6 years of age and younger with NF1 are at greatest risk for the development of an OPG, new symptomatic OPGs may also arise in older children and adults.[4] If neuroimaging is performed on all children with NF1 at the time of diagnosis, 15–20% of these children will harbor an OPG. However, only half of these tumors will ever become symptomatic, giving an overall incidence of symptomatic OPGs of 7%.[5]

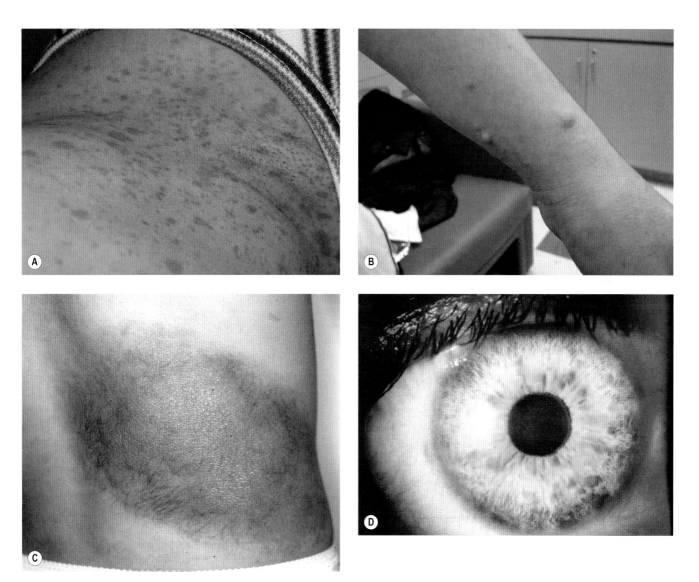

Figure 53.1 Clinical features of neurofibromatosis type 1. (A) Café-au-lait spots. (B) Dermal neurofibromas. (C) Plexiform neurofibroma. (D) Lisch nodules.

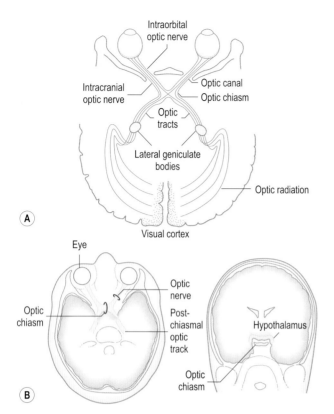

Figure 53.2 Visual pathway anatomy. (A) Visual information is transmitted from the retina by the optic nerves whose fibers cross at the optic chiasm and proceed to the lateral geniculate bodies before coursing to the visual cortex. (B) Optic pathway gliomas in individuals with neurofibromatosis type 1 may involve the optic nerves, optic chiasm, postchiasmatic optic tracks, and hypothalamus (highlighted in yellow) in sagittal (left) and coronal (right) orientations.

NF1-associated OPGs are usually to the anterior visual pathway, including the intraorbital optic nerve, intracranial optic nerve, and the optic chiasm (Figure 53.2). In contrast, sporadic OPGs not associated with NF1 commonly involve the optic tracts and postchiasmatic optic radiations as well. Bilateral intraorbital OPGs are virtually pathognomonic of NF1 (Figure 53.3A).

Symptomatic OPGs may become apparent in one of several ways. Approximately 30% of such tumors will present with the rapid onset of unilateral proptosis and significantly decreased visual acuity secondary to large intraorbital tumors. An additional 30% of patients will have an abnormal ophthalmologic examination without any visual symptoms, since young children rarely complain of gradual visual loss. Abnormal ophthalmologic signs may include optic nerve atrophy or pallor, an afferent pupillary defect, uncorrectable decreased visual acuity, strabismus, or papilledema.[5] The remaining 40% of children will present with signs of precocious puberty, usually with accelerated linear growth. Such children invariably harbor chiasmatic tumors which can affect the hypothalamic–pituitary–gonadal axis (Figure 53.3B). Thus, it is essential that all young children with NF1 have annual assessments of linear growth plotted on standardized pediatric growth charts.[6]

Natural history of OPG

Predicting the natural history of an individual OPG is impossible. For example, rapidly progressive intraorbital tumors

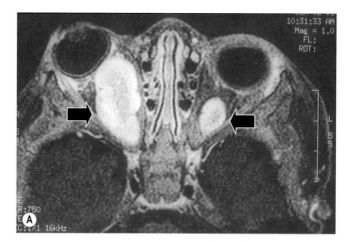

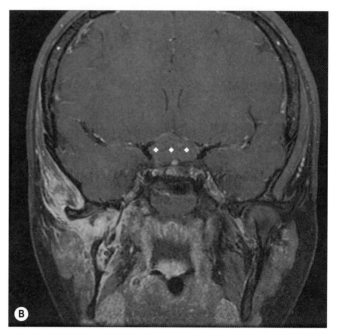

Figure 53.3 Optic pathway gliomas (OPGs) in children with neurofibromatosis 1. (A) Representative bilateral orbital OPG (denoted by the arrows). (B) Representative chiasmatic OPG (denoted by the dotted line).

which cause proptosis and significant visual loss may stop growing following initial presentation. While progressive disease following the diagnosis of a symptomatic OPG occurs in 35–52% of cases, OPGs found by screening neuroimaging of asymptomatic individuals with NF1 rarely progress.[5,7] Most importantly, the natural history of NF1-associated OPGs is markedly different from that of sporadic OPG. The latter are significantly more likely to progress radiographically and clinically, leading to the development of increased intracranial pressure and hydrocephalus with substantially greater ophthalmologic morbidity.[8]

Diagnostic evaluation of asymptomatic children with NF1

All young children with NF1 should undergo complete yearly ophthalmologic examinations in order to identify the earliest manifestations of a symptomatic OPG. Complete examinations including ocular alignment and rotations, assessment of color vision, pupillary light response, refractive status, and fundoscopic evaluation should be performed. Visual acuity should be measured using age-appropriate testing (i.e., preferential looking tests in infants, Lea figure, or HOTV matching in preliterate children, Snellen charts in older children). Routine measurement of visual fields is unnecessary as clinically important visual field compromise without concomitant loss of visual acuity is rare. There is no reliable evidence supporting the routine use of visual evoked potentials in the diagnosis of NF1-associated OPG.[7]

There has been considerable debate as to the role of neuroimaging of asymptomatic children with NF1. Routine "screening" neuroimaging would be important if it led to the early detection of OPG which, in turn, led to significantly decreased ophthalmologic morbidity. However, there are substantial data showing that such a strategy would fail; in previous studies, many tumors were detected that never progressed and some children developed symptomatic OPG after a normal visual screening examination. Thus, there is no conclusive evidence that the early detection of OPGs leads to improved outcome. For these reasons, screening "baseline" neuroimaging of asymptomatic children with NF1 is not recommended.[7]

Follow-up of an asymptomatic OPG

Once an asymptomatic NF1-associated OPG has been identified, close follow-up is warranted, as the natural history of an individual tumor cannot be predicted. Generally, ophthalmologic examinations should be performed every 3 months during the first year following diagnosis. Magnetic resonance imaging should also be performed at frequent intervals; the exact protocols vary among institutions. As the child gets older without evidence of either clinical or radiographic progression, the intervals between examinations can be progressively lengthened.

Treatment

There are scant data as to what constitutes sufficient clinical or radiographic progression to warrant treatment. Radiographic progression without a concomitant change in the child's visual examination may not be sufficiently compelling to mandate treatment. Additionally, the appearance of clinical signs, such as the development of precocious puberty, does not constitute in itself a reason for treatment. However, once the decision to undergo treatment has been made, certain truths exist.

There is a limited role for surgery in the management of NF1-associated OPG. Partial removal of an intraorbital optic nerve glioma is usually reserved for cosmetic purposes only. On occasion, surgical decompression of a hypothalamic glioma may be necessary to treat hydrocephalus secondary to third ventricular compression. Biopsy is only recommended in very atypical cases as NF1-associated OPG are most often low-grade juvenile pilocytic astrocytomas.[7] Similarly, radiotherapy in children with NF1 is not recommended, because of the unacceptable neurovascular (cerebral occlusive vasculopathy), endocrinologic, and neuropsychologic sequelae. Moreover, recent evidence suggests that children with NF1 treated with radiation therapy develop secondary brain malignancies later in life.[9]

Chemotherapy has become the mainstay of treatment for NF1-associated OPGs. The most commonly used chemotherapeutic regimen is the combination of carboplatin and vincristine. This combination is effective in controlling the growth of most NF1-associated OPGs, and is typically well tolerated in this age group. Other chemotherapies have also been used; however, there is no consensus on which second-line therapy is most effective for these tumors.[7]

Pathology

The vast majority of NF1-associated OPGs are classified by the World Health Organization (WHO) as grade I astrocytic neoplasms (pilocytic astrocytomas). Similar to pilocytic astrocytomas arising in other brain regions in individuals with NF1, these low-grade gliomas are characterized by a biphasic histologic pattern of more cellular areas alternating with looser cystic regions.[10] Within the less compact areas, there are Rosenthal fibers (tapered corkscrew-shaped hyaline masses) and eosinophilic granular bodies (globular aggregates). These tumors exhibit low mitotic indices with rare mitoses and occasional hyperchromatic nuclei. Despite their benign nature, pilocytic astrocytomas are rather infiltrative tumors with significant microvascular proliferation and the presence of microglia. Immunohistochemical analyses of these tumors reveal robust staining with glial fibrillary acidic protein antibodies, characteristic of astrocytic neoplasms.

Etiology

NF1 is caused by a germline mutation in the *NF1* gene; however, only 50% of all individuals with NF1 have an affected parent.[11] These individuals without a family history of NF1 represent new mutations, which presumably arise from a mutation in the *NF1* during spermatogenesis in the male.[12] Since NF1 is an autosomal-dominant disorder with complete penetrance, the risk of transmitting NF1 is 50% with each pregnancy. Children who inherit a mutated (nonfunctional) copy of the *NF1* gene have NF1, yet the clinical manifestations may be variable. In this regard, a child with NF1 with the identical *NF1* gene mutation as a parent or sibling can be more severely or more mildly affected. Moreover, there are no obvious genotype–phenotype correlations that predict disease severity, with the exception of children with large chromosomal deletions surrounding the *NF1* gene. These children frequently have mental retardation and distinctive facial features, and may be at risk for the development of malignancy.[13,14] Finally, there are no known environmental risk factors and NF1 has been described in all ethnic and racial groups worldwide.

Pathophysiology

With the identification of the *NF1* gene and its protein product, neurofibromin, there is renewed excitement that future therapies for NF1-associated OPG might involve treatments that target the pathways deregulated in these tumors. The *NF1* gene is classified as a tumor suppressor gene, since patients affected with NF1 develop benign and malignant

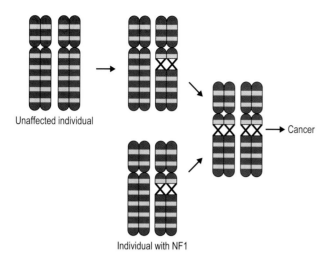

Figure 53.4 Knudson two-hit hypothesis. Individuals with neurofibromatosis type 1 (NF1) begin life with one functional and one nonfunctional (denoted by the X) copy of the *NF1* gene. Tumors result from somatic mutation of the remaining functional copy of the *NF1* gene.

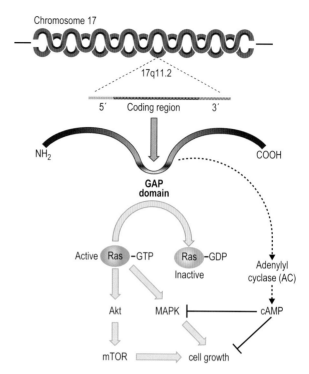

Figure 53.5 Neurofibromin growth regulation. The *NF1* gene is located on chromosome 17q and codes for a large cytoplasmic protein, neurofibromin. A small region of the neurofibromin protein contains the GTPase-activating protein (GAP) domain which serves to inactivate Ras by converting it from its active, guanosine triphosphate (GTP)-bound form to an inactive, guanosine diphosphate (GDP)-bound conformation. Active Ras promotes cell growth by activating its downstream effectors, Akt and mitogen-activated protein kinase (MAPK). Akt, in turn, activates the mammalian target of rapamycin (mTOR) protein. In addition to negative Ras regulation, neurofibromin serves to regulate intracellular cyclic adenosine monophosphate (cAMP) levels positively, likely by stimulating adenylyl cyclase (AC) activity. cAMP inhibits cell growth either by reducing MAPK signaling or through other mechanisms.

tumors at an elevated rate. Consistent with Knudson's two-hit hypothesis for inherited cancer syndromes,[15] individuals with NF1 start life with one functional and one mutated copy of the *NF1* gene in every cell of their body. Tumors form when the remaining functional *NF1* gene undergoes somatic mutation and is rendered nonfunctional (Figure 53.4). Examination of tumors from patients with NF1, including OPGs,[16] has demonstrated biallelic inactivation of the *NF1* gene and loss of *NF1* gene expression.

Function of the NF1 protein

The *NF1* gene resides on chromosome 17q and encodes a large cytoplasmic protein (neurofibromin) of 220–250 kDa.[17-20] Examination of the predicted protein sequence of neurofibromin revealed that a small region of the protein shares striking sequence similarity with the catalytic domain of a family of proteins known to regulate the RAS proto-oncogene negatively (Figure 53.5).[21-23] RAS is an intracellular signaling molecule that exists in an active guanosine triphosphate (GTP)-bound conformation and an inactive guanosine diphosphate (GDP)-bound state. Active GTP-bound RAS provides a strong mitogenic growth signal, such that constitutive RAS activation as a result of mutation in cancer leads to unregulated cell growth and tumor formation. Neurofibromin as a negative RAS regulator functions to maintain RAS in an inactive form and inhibit cell growth. Loss of neurofibromin expression, such as seen in NF1-associated OPG tumors, leads to high levels of active GTP-bound RAS and increased tumor growth.[24-27]

RAS imparts its growth signal through the sequential activation of other signaling intermediates, including mitogen-activated protein kinase (MAPK), protein kinase B (Akt), and the mammalian target of rapamycin (mTOR) protein (Figure 53.5). In this regard, loss of neurofibromin in tumor cells leads to high levels of MAPK, Akt, and mTOR activity, which promote cell growth, cell survival, cell motility, and increased protein translation.[28-33] Inhibition of RAS or mTOR activity using pharmacologic inhibitors, including farnesyltrans-

ferase inhibitors (RAS) and rapamycin analogs (mTOR), are logical targets for future antineoplastic biologically based drug therapies for NF1-associated OPG.

In addition to its ability to regulate RAS negatively, neurofibromin also functions to generate intracellular cyclic AMP (cAMP) positively.[34-36] Although less is known about the role of cAMP in growth control, several studies have shown that increased cAMP levels inhibit cell growth in glioma cells.[37,38] In primary mouse astrocytes, loss of *Nf1* expression results in decreased levels of intracellular cAMP, likely at the level of adenylyl cyclase,[36] and elevated cAMP reduces cell growth by inhibiting MAPK signaling.[39] Recent studies on neurofibromin cAMP control in astrocytes have shown that specific cells in the brain (e.g., neurons, microglia, and endothelial cells) produce chemokines (e.g., stromal-derived growth factor-α; CXCL12) that uniquely promote *Nf1*-deficient astrocyte survival in a cAMP-dependent fashion.[40]

Small-animal models of NF1-associated OPG

As we move into an era of targeted therapeutics, it is important to develop robust and tractable small-animal models of NF1-associated OPG.[41] Over the past several years, genetically engineered *Nf1* optic glioma mice have been generated

Box 53.2 Use of small-animal models

- Discovery platform to identify new targeted therapies for neurofibromatosis type 1 (NF1)-associated tumors
- Preclinical platform to evaluate new therapies for NF1-associated tumors
- Define the cell populations within the tumors sensitive to targeted therapies
- Determine why therapies succeed or fail
- Identify the molecular and cellular pathogenesis of tumor formation and growth
- Pinpoint genetic risk factors for NF1-associated tumors

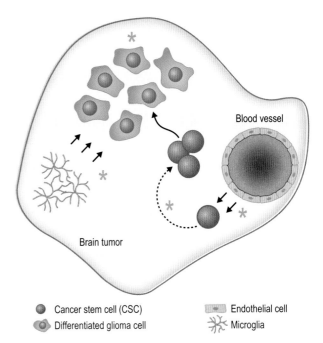

- ● Cancer stem cell (CSC)
- ◉ Differentiated glioma cell
- ▦ Endothelial cell
- ✳ Microglia

Figure 53.6 Anatomy of a glioma. Neurofibromatosis type 1-associated optic pathway gliomas are likely composed of a diverse collection of cell types, including microglia, endothelial cells, differentiated glioma cells, and cancer stem cells. Each of these cell types participates in glioma formation and continued growth. Moreover, each cell type represents a logical target for future antiglioma therapy (denoted by the asterisks).

by inactivation of *Nf1* gene expression in glial cells. Interestingly, *Nf1* mutant mice lacking neurofibromin expression in glial cells exhibit increased numbers of astrocytes, but do not develop brain tumors.[42] Since individuals with NF1 are born with one functional and one nonfunctional copy of the *NF1* gene in each cell of their body (*NF1+/−* cells), two groups developed *Nf1+/−* mice lacking neurofibromin expression in glial cells to model the human condition more accurately.[43,44] Similar to the human tumors, these *Nf1* mutant mice developed low-grade astrocytic (glial) tumors affecting the optic nerves and chiasm. Examination of the optic gliomas in these genetically engineered mice demonstrated low proliferative indices, microvascular proliferation, and microglial infiltration. In addition, these tumors demonstrated maximal proliferation between 2 and 4 months, with significantly less proliferation observed thereafter.[45] However, unlike their human counterparts, they lack Rosenthal fibers and eosinophilic granular bodies, and cannot be strictly classified as pilocytic astrocytoma. Lastly, small-animal magnetic resonance imaging has been successfully employed to detect these tumors and follow their growth in vivo.[46]

These small-animal *Nf1* optic glioma mouse models have been useful for several purposes (Box 53.2). First, they can be used as platforms for the discovery and evaluation of new therapies against NF1-associated OPG. In this regard, *Nf1* mutant mice can be treated with promising therapies as an initial screen prior to evaluation in children with NF1. The availability of such preclinical filters should greatly facilitate the translation of basic science discoveries to clinical practice. Second, these mice can be employed to discover predictive markers of tumor formation, growth, and response to treatment. Researchers have used these mice to identify body fluid proteins whose expression might correlate with disease activity.[47] In addition, *Nf1* mutant mice have allowed scientists to pinpoint genetic risk factors for brain tumors, which might facilitate the identification of children at greatest risk for developing OPGs. Studies using glioma-prone mice on different genetic backgrounds have identified several genetic regions that harbor genes that strongly influence tumor formation.[48] The identification of similar "modifier" genes in humans might lead to the development of predictive genetic tests that allow physicians to counsel patients more accurately about their risk of glioma formation.

Lastly, *Nf1* mutant mice are currently being exploited to understand why brain tumors form in children with NF1.

These studies have shown that NF1-associated OPGs are composed of a number of different cell types that each contribute to tumor formation (Figure 53.6). In this respect, immune system cells (microglia) found in NF1-associated OPG produce specific growth signals that promote tumor growth. The microglia in both human and mouse tumors harbor one mutated *NF1* gene (*Nf1+/−* cells) and exhibit functional properties distinct from normal microglia.[49] The observation that *Nf1+/−* microglia increase *Nf1−/−* astrocyte and glioma growth in vitro and in vivo raises the intriguing possibility that future NF1 optic glioma therapies might target microglia or microglia-produced growth signals.

Finally, within both human pilocytic astrocytomas and *Nf1* mouse optic gliomas are rare progenitor (stem) cells.[44,45] These cancer stem cells (CSCs) have been proposed to represent cancer-generating cells within the tumor.[50,51] In addition, these CSCs have unique cellular and biochemical properties, and therefore respond differently to conventional treatments compared to the more differentiated glioma cells within the tumor.[52] Recent studies have shown that neurofibromin plays a critical role in stem cell function relevant to tumorigenesis.[53,54] Future studies on these CSCs may lead to the development of future therapies for NF1-associated OPG that target this unique cell type.

As we enter into an age of targeted therapeutics, the development and refinement of robust mouse models of NF1-associated OPG provide novel platforms for evaluating new anticancer drugs, assessing therapeutic index, identifying surrogate markers of tumor progression, and defining epigenetic and environmental influences on tumorigenesis. These advances show great promise for more targeted and effective treatments for these tumors.

Conclusion

OPGs in children with NF1 represent both diagnostic and management challenges for clinicians. Whereas considerable progress has been made over the past decade in both our clinical and basic science understanding of these tumors, several key areas deserve future investigation. First, we need to be able to identify efficiently children at greatest risk for developing a symptomatic OPG. Second, these at-risk children require age-appropriate visual assessment tools to determine when they should be treated. Third, symptomatic children should be treated with agents that have maximal therapeutic efficacy against the tumor with minimal effects on the developing brain. Lastly, improved therapeutic strategies need to be developed for those children who fail initial treatment. With the advent of preclinical and clinical consortia focused on NF1, we are uniquely positioned to improve the future management of these children.

Key references

A complete list of chapter references is available online at www.expertconsult.com. See inside cover for registration details.

2. Neurofibromatosis. National Institutes of Health Consensus Development Conference Consensus Statement 1987;6:1–7.

4. Listernick R, Ferner RE, Piersall L, et al. Late-onset optic pathway tumors in children with neurofibromatosis 1. Neurology 2004;63:1944–1946.

6. Habiby R, Silverman B, Listernick R, et al. Precocious puberty in children with neurofibromatosis type 1. J Pediatr 1995;126:364–367.

7. Listernick R, Ferner RE, Liu GT, et al. Optic pathway gliomas in neurofibromatosis-1: controversies and recommendations. Ann Neurol 2007;61:189–198.

9. Sharif S, Ferner R, Birch JM, et al. Second primary tumors in neurofibromatosis 1 patients treated for optic glioma: substantial risks after radiotherapy. J Clin Oncol 2006;24:2570–2575.

16. Gutmann DH, Donahoe J, Brown T, et al. Loss of neurofibromatosis 1 (NF1) gene expression in NF1-associated pilocytic astrocytomas. Neuropathol Appl Neurobiol 2000;26:361–367.

43. Bajenaru ML, Hernandez MR, Perry A, et al. Optic nerve glioma in mice requires astrocyte Nf1 gene inactivation and Nf1 brain heterozygosity. Cancer Res 2003;63:8573–8577.

45. Bajenaru ML, Garbow JR, Perry A, et al. Natural history of neurofibromatosis 1-associated optic nerve glioma in mice. Ann Neurol 2005;57:119–127.

53. Dasgupta B, Gutmann DH. Neurofibromin regulates neural stem cell proliferation, survival, and astroglial differentiation in vitro and in vivo. J Neurosci 2005;25:5584–5594.

54. Hegedus B, Dasgupta B, Shin JE, Emnett RJ, et al. Neurofibromatosis-1 regulates neuronal and glial cell differentiation from neuroglial progenitors in vivo by both cAMP- and Ras-dependent mechanisms. Cell Stem Cell 2007;1:443–457.

Phthisis bulbi

Ingo Schmack, Hans E Völcker, and Hans E Grossniklaus

Clinical background

Key symptoms and signs

Phthisis bulbi represents an ocular end-stage disease of various causes and is defined by atrophy, shrinkage, and disorganization of the eyeball and intraocular contents (Box 54.1).[1,2] Subjective complaints depend on the etiology and severity of phthisis bulbi. Typical clinical symptoms and signs include chronic ocular hypotension (5 mmHg), a shrunken globe, pseudoenophthalmos, intraocular tissue fibrosis and scarring, vision loss, and recurrent episodes of intraocular irritation and pain.[3]

Historical development

The term phthisis bulbi derives from the Greek word *phthiein* or *phthinein*, meaning shrinkage or consuming, and was first used by Galen.[3] Over the last 200 years, the clinical interpretation of phthisis bulbi has often been modified according to the underlying disease and structural changes; a clear distinction from ocular atrophy was often difficult and controversial.[4] Hogan and Zimmerman[1] were the first ones who stated that both terms – atrophy and phthisis bulbi – refer to consecutive stages in the degeneration process of a severely damaged eye. Their descriptive classification system including three different stages – (1) ocular atrophy without shrinkage; (2) with shrinkage; and (3) with shrinkage and disorganization – has been further modified by Yanoff and Fine[2] (Table 54.1).

Epidemiology

Epidemiological data on phthisis bulbi are mainly based on retrospective clinicopathological studies on enucleated eyes.[5-10] Enucleations are usually the result of failed ocular treatment or end-stage diseases (i.e., phthisis bulbi) associated with blind, painful, or cosmetically unacceptable eyes. The incidence of enucleation in general has slightly decreased during the last decades because of improved diagnostic and therapeutic approaches, and the trend towards globe-preserving procedures; however, information on the incidence of phthisis bulbi is limited.[10,11] In contrast, the prevalence of phthisis bulbi in enucleated eyes is well documented, ranging from 11.2% to 18.7% with an average of 13.7%, and has remained fairly stable over the last 60 years (Table 54.2).[5-9] However, statistical evaluations indicate a slight increase in the number of enucleations for phthisis bulbi during the last two decades.[9,10,12]

In general, phthisis bulbi involves elderly patients, usually 65–85 years of age.[9,12] Children and adolescents (≤20 years of age) are only rarely affected (3.7–6.4%), mainly due to ocular trauma and congenital malformations. Right and left eyes are almost equally affected. The initial insult usually takes place 20–30 years prior to enucleation. Two age peaks at 35 and 75 years of age were found in 69 phthisical eyes with previous trauma.[3] Overall, phthisis bulbi occurs more often in males than in females.[3,5,6,8,9] The imbalance in sex distribution, at least in part, can be explained by predominance of ocular trauma (i.e., concussion, perforation) in the past ocular history of patients with phthisis bulbi, which occurs more often in men than women.[6,9,13]

Genetics

A possible relationship between myotonic dystrophy and ocular hypotony has been described by Kuechle and co-workers.[14] The examined eyes displayed a diminished blood–aqueous barrier (BAB) function and diffuse choroidal edema, presumably due to elevated follicle-stimulating hormone and luteal hormone serum levels.

Diagnostic workup

Phthisical eyes are usually easily accessible for slit-lamp examination, which allows evaluation of the periocular region and structures of the anterior segment. In less advanced stages of the disease with a lack of significant corneal opacification, intraocular fibrosis (i.e., cyclitic membranes) or cataractous changes of crystalline lens, gonioscopy, direct and indirect ophthalmoscopy, fluorescein angiography, and optical coherence tomography may be useful for evaluation of the anterior-chamber angle, choroid, and retina.[15] Once optical visualization of the intraocular structures is obscured, ultrasound biomicroscopy and other noninvasive diagnostic imaging techniques such as computed tomography (CT) and magnetic resonance imaging (MRI) may be applied to validate morphologic abnormalities of the anterior chamber and ciliary body as well as to exclude intraocular ossification, or possibly foreign bodies (Box 54.2).[16,17] However, the differential diagnostic utility of these imaging techniques is often limited based on the severe structural changes seen in phthisical eyes.

Although phthisis bulbi is defined as ocular shrinkage and ocular hypotony, intraocular pressure (IOP) readings using applanation or impression tonometry devices (i.e., Goldmann, Schiotz), may be inaccurate because of the anatomical changes of the anterior segment (i.e., corneal edema, scarring, shrinkage) and the sunken location of the eyes in the orbit.

Differential diagnosis

Although the underlying diseases and the clinical course of phthisis bulbi are quite variable, the end-stage disease is rarely missed because of characteristic clinical features (i.e., small, soft, atrophic eyes), which are often associated with

decreased or lost vision. However, clinicians should be aware of any potential disease entity which, if not treated properly, may result in a blind, often painful phthisical eye. Intraocular malignancies (i.e., retinoblastoma, malignant uveal melanoma) should be taken into consideration if the ocular history is limited and an obvious cause for phthisis is missing.[6] In addition, congenital abnormalities like microphthalmos and microcornea should be kept in the differential diagnosis of phthisis bulbi.[18]

Treatment

Therapeutic approaches are very limited in phthisical eyes; symptomatic treatment (i.e., artificial tears, ointments, topical corticosteroids, nonsteroidal eye drops, antiinfectious agents) may be recommended in patients with mild ocular symptoms (i.e., irritation, pain). Contact lenses or scleral shells can be used for cosmetic purposes. Once phthisical eyes become chronically irritated and painful, enucleation or evisceration with implantation of an intraocular or orbital implant should be performed, especially with regard to potential long-term complications (i.e., sympathetic ophthalmia, ulceration, perforation) and to exclude intraocular malignancies.[19,20]

Prognosis and complications

The diagnosis of phthisical eyes implies a frustrating clinical situation demonstrating the result of failed previous ocular therapy in which restoration of the morphologic and func-

---

Box 54.1 Definition–phthisis bulbi

Phthisis bulbi represents an ocular end-stage disease characterized by:

- Atrophy
- Shrinkage
- Disorganization of the eyeball and its intraocular contents

---

Box 54.2 Diagnostic workup of phthisical eyes

Useful diagnostic tools in the evaluation of phthisis bulbi include:

- Indirect/direct ophthalmoscopy
- Gonioscopy
- Fluorescein angiography
- Optical coherence tomography
- Ultrasound (A- and B-scan)
- Computed tomography (CT) and magnetic resonance imaging (MRI)

Table 54.1 Grading system of atrophia and phthisis bulbi

I	Atrophy bulbi without shrinkage
II	Atrophia bulbi with shrinkage
III	Atrophia bulbi with shrinkage and disorganization (phthisis bulbi)
IV	Phthisis bulbi with intraocular ossification
V	Phthisis bulbi with intraocular calcium deposition

Modified from Yanoff M, Fine BS. Nongranulomatous inflammation: uveitis, endophthalmitis, panophthalmitis, and sequelae. In: Yanoff M, Fine BS (eds) Ocular Pathology, 5th edn. St. Louis, MO: Mosby, 2002:72–73.

Table 54.2 Prevalence of phthisis bulbi in enucleated eyes

Publication		Enucleated eyes			Initial insult resulting in phthisis bulbi					
	Observation period	Overall	Phthisical		Trauma		Surgery		Inflammation	
Authors	(years)	(n)	(n)	(%)	(n)	(%)	(n)	(%)	(n)	(%)
Naumann and Portwich[5]	1969–1974	1000	118	11.8	77	65.3	24	20.3	9	7.6
de Gottrau et al[6]	1980–1990	1146	214	18.7	137	64.0	46	21.5	6	2.8
Gassler and Lommatzsch[7]	1980–1990	817	97	11.9	23	23.7	62	64.0	5	5.2
Guenlap et al[8]	1945–1995	3506	587	16.7	N/A	N/A	N/A	N/A	N/A	N/A
Kitzmann et al[9]	1990–2000	523	61	11.7	22	36.1	8	13.1	3	4.9
Saeed et al[10]	1994–2003	285	32	11.2	N/A	N/A	N/A	N/A	N/A	N/A

tional integrity of the eye is not possible. Most phthisical eyes eventually become blind, painful, and cosmetically unacceptable for the patient. Potential harmful complications include corneal ulceration and perforation with the risk of ocular and periocular inflammation (i.e., panophthalmitis), sympathetic ophthalmia, and malignant transformation.[3,20]

Pathology

Clinical and pathologic findings of phthisical eyes are variable and depend on the underlying disease and time interval between primary lesion and enucleation. The following section describes the main clinicopathological ocular features commonly seen phthisis bulbi.

Clinical features

Phthisical eyes are usually easy to detect by inspection of the patient's face and are summarized in Table 54.3. The diagnosis is simplified due to the unilaterality of the disease with asymmetry of the eyeballs and interpalpebral fissures. Additional indirect clinical signs include narrow lid fissures (pseudoptosis), lagophthalmos, pseudoenophthalmos, small-sized and soft, hypotonic (IOP 5 mmHg) eyes (Figure 54.1A; Box 54.3). Axial displacement in relation to the surrounding structures may occur in advanced stages, which are often associated with vision loss. The conjunctiva may be swollen (chemotic) and hyperemic. The appearance of cornea is variable displaying corneal haze, scarred, vascularization, and dystrophic calcification (Figure 54.1B). The anterior chamber is usually shallow, demonstrating a narrow to closed chamber angle. Synechia (peripheral, posterior), neovascularization of the iris surface and chamber angle (rubeosis iridis), fibrotic or fibrovascular membranes at the pupil may be present, often as a result of intraocular hypoxia or recurrent episodes of intraocular inflammation (uveitis).[21,22] The lens

usually undergoes cataractous changes and may become floppy (lentodonesis) because of anterior displacement of the ciliary body. The choroid and retina are often detached by retrolenticular or epiretinal membranes.[23–25]

Macroscopic and microscopic features

Gross pathology of the external eye

External examination of enucleated phthisical eyes typically shows a soft and partially collapsed globe. The shape and size of the eyes may vary depending on the nature and dura-

---

Box 54.3 Clinical signs of phthisical eyes

Phthisical eyes can be characterized clinically by:

- Small and soft eyes
- Pseudoptosis and pseudoenophthalmos
- Corneal opacification and scarring
- Shallow anterior chambers and neovascularization of the iris and chamber angle
- Cataract formation
- Ciliochoroidal and retinal detachment

Table 54.3 Clinicopathological features of phthisical eyes

Microphthalmos
Enophthalmos
Reduced eyelid fissure
Strabism
Corneoscleral scarring, thickening, and shrinkage
Flattening of the anterior chamber
Intraocular inflammation (uveitis/endophthalmitis)
Synechia (peripheral/posterior)
Cyclitic/epiretinal membranes (fibrous/fibrovascular)
Cataract formation
Choroidal/ciliary body and retinal detachment
Choroidal/ciliary body, retinal, and optic nerve degeneration/atrophy
Intraocular hemorrhages
Dystrophic calcification and heterotopic ossification

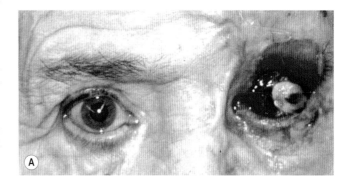

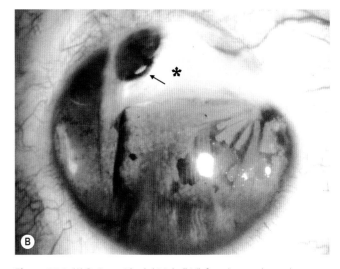

Figure 54.1 (A) Patient with phthisis bulbi (left eye) secondary to herpes zoster infection. (B) Phthisical eye of a 49-year-old man with history of perforating trauma to his right eye displaying corneal scarring (asterisk) and dystrophic calcification.

tion of the underlying disease as well as the age of the patient at the initial event. Phthisical eyes usually demonstrate a squared-off shape with scleral buckling behind the insertion line of the horizontal and vertical extrinsic rectus muscles. Other specimens seem to maintain their "normal" spherical shape despite marked shrinkage and decreased volume. On average, phthisical eyes are about 20% smaller in dimension compared to "normal"-sized adult eyes (24 × 24 × 24 mm).[3] The cornea is usually flattened, smaller in diameter (≥20%), and hazy due to edema, scarring, or dystrophic calcification.[3]

Gross pathology of the internal eye

The cornea and sclera are usually markedly thickened, on average by 80% (cornea) to 50% (sclera) (Figure 54.2).[3] The

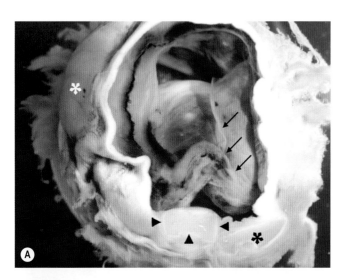

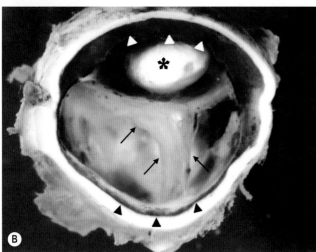

Figure 54.2 (A) Phthisical eye of a 73-year-old male with a history of penetrating trauma. The cornea (white asterisk) is vascularized and scarred; the retina is detached (arrows) and the sclera partially thickened and thrown in folds. An encircling band (arrowheads) and a scleral buckle (black asterisk) indicate previous retinal surgery. (B) Horizontal section through a 23 × 22 × 22 mm phthisical eye demonstrates a cataractous crystalline lens (asterisk) and hemorrhage of the anterior chamber (white arrowheads) and ciliochoroidal tract The retina is completely detached (arrows) and torn anterior by a retrolenticular fibrovascular membrane.

anterior chamber is often shallow or collapsed; iris defects (partial, complete) from previous trauma or surgery may be present. The lens is usually thickened and cataractous. The ciliary body and retina are often detached and displayed anteriorly by a retrolenticular or epiretinal fibrotic tissue; the optic nerve head may be pulled into the vitreous cavity. Intraocular hemorrhages may be present in the anterior chamber, vitreous, or choroid.

Histopathology

All intraocular structures may be involved in phthisical eyes (Table 54.3). The cornea is usually thickened, edematous, scarred, and vascularized (57%); a fibrovascular tissue and areas of dystrophic calcification may be present in the anterior stroma next to the epithelium.[3] The posterior stroma and Descemet membrane are thrown into folds by a fibrous tissue proliferation at the inner surface of Descemet membrane (stromal downgrowth) (Figure 54.3A). The endothelium, if present, may display cystic changes of its cytoplasm. Additional pathologic findings of the anterior chamber may include epithelialization and vascularization of the chamber angle and iris surface (24%), peripheral and posterior synechia with secondary angle closure, and fibrous or fibrovascular cyclitic membranes at the pupillary margin (Figure 54.3A).[3] The lens usually displays epithelial proliferation,

Figure 54.3 (A) Photomicrographs showing secondary angle closure (arrows) by a retrocorneal fibrous tissue (asterisk). The posterior corneal stroma and Descemet membrane are thrown in folds (arrowheads). Original magnification: 4× (main image) and 10× (inset). (B) The crystalline lens (inset; periodic acid–Schiff) displaying cataractogenous changes including artificial clefting of the lens cortex, differential staining between the nucleus (white asterisk) and the cortex (black asterisk), and hydropic degeneration of lens epithelial cells (arrows). Occasionally, phthisical eyes demonstrate calcification of the cortical fibers next to the lens capsule (main image). Original magnification: 20× (main image) and 10× (inset). (C) Phthisical eyes often demonstrate an almost complete separation of the ciliary body from the sclera by proliferative fibrovascular membranes pulling the ciliary body into the anterior vitreous cavity. The ciliary muscle (black asterisk) usually remains attached at the scleral spur (arrows). Secondary findings include a tubular-like proliferation of the nonpigmented ciliary body epithelium (arrowheads). Original magnification: 4× (main image) and 20× (inset). (D) The retina of phthisical eyes often exhibits a funnel-shape appearance (inset bottom left) due to perpendicular and circumferential traction by epiretinal and retrolenticular membranes (asterisk, inset top right). In advanced stages it loses its normal structure and displays gliosis and cystoid degeneration (arrows, main image). Original magnification: 10× (main image) and 4× (insets). (E) Image demonstrating a section of thickened sclera. Chronic ocular hypotony results in loss of tension on the sclera with subsequent wrinkling and shortening of the collagen lamellae. (F) Photomicrographs showing heterotopic secondary ossification of the retinal pigment epithelium (RPE) in an eye with long-standing phthisis bulbi (asterisk, main image). Pigment-laden cells and lacunae (arrows, inset bottom right) containing fatty or hematopoietic bone marrow can often be detected within the bony structures. Additional degenerative changes of the RPE include large (pathologic) drusen formation (white asterisk, inset top right).

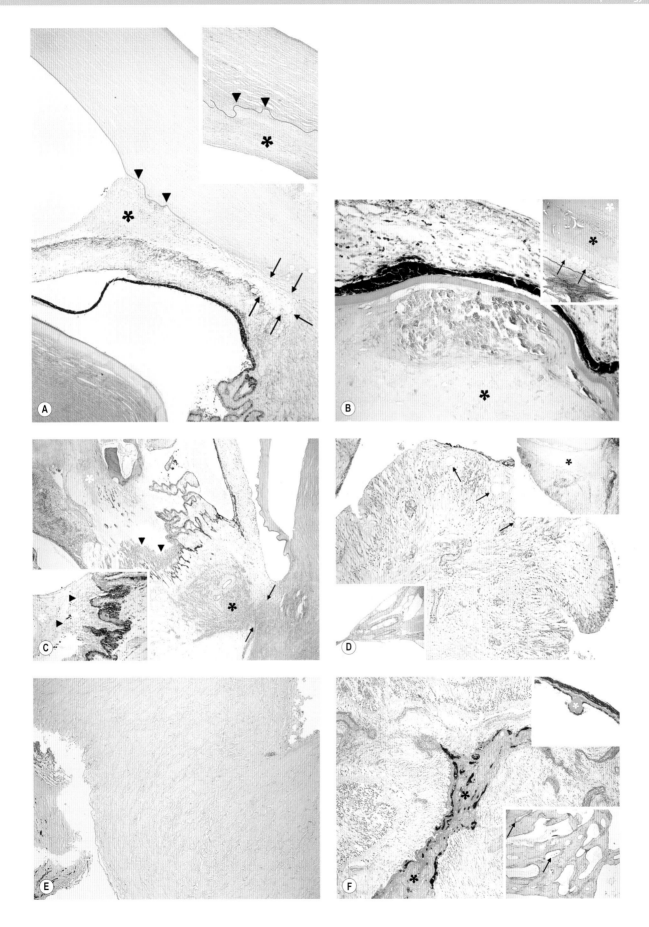

differential staining of nucleus and cortex, and clefting of the lens fibrils. Occasionally, calcification can be seen adjacent to the anterior lens capsule; ossification is rare and always associated with capsular breaks (Figure 54.3B). The ciliary body usually shows atrophy and fibrous shortening of the ciliary processes, thickening of the basal laminar, proliferation of nonpigmented epithelium, and is often separated from the sclera, mainly close to the scleral spur; posterior extension towards the optic disc is also possible (Figure 54.3C).[21] Pathologic changes of the choroid include vasodilatation and focal vascular compression of small vascular channels as well as areas of choroidal thinning and atrophy. The retina may display full-thickness folds, fibrous epiretinal membranes, cystic degeneration of the inner nuclear layer with and without proteinaceous exudates, loss of photoreceptor cells, gliosis, and funnel-shaped retinal detachments; calcification of retinal blood vessels is occasionally seen (Figure 54.3D).[26] The optic nerve is atrophic and shows proliferation of the glial cells. The sclera is thickened, mainly posterior to the insertion of the external muscles, and displays folding of the collagen lamellae due to decreased intra-ocular tension and increased water-binding to mucopolysaccharides (Figure 54.3E). Cholesterol crystals as signs of previous hemorrhage may occur in the anterior chamber, vitreous, and suprachoroidal space. Areas of heterotopic ossification, containing lacunas of fatty and hematopoietic bone marrow, are common in eyes with long-standing phthisis bulbi (Figure 54.3F).[23,24] They mainly form in pre- and subretinal fibrovascular membranes in association with proliferating retinal pigment epithelium (RPE) cells and within the choroid; lens and sclera are rarely involved.[24,27]

Etiology

Phthisis bulbi cannot be understood as a specific clinical entity; rather, it is considered the endpoint of a number of ocular diseases with various stimuli. Potential risk factors contributing to phthisis bulbi include failed surgical procedures (i.e., cataract, glaucoma, retina surgery), infections and inflammation (i.e., keratitis, uveitis, endophthalmitis), intraocular malignancies (i.e., choroidal melanoma, retinoblastoma) as well as systemic cardiovascular diseases (i.e., diabetes, hypertension) (Table 54.1).[3,19,28,29] Although it is not known how long an individual eye will tolerate a specific ocular damage, virtually all diseased eyes will finally become atrophic if therapeutic treatment fails.

Pathophysiology

Aqueous humor dynamics and blood–ocular barrier functions

The aqueous humor that fills the anterior and posterior chambers is important in the physiology of the mammalian eye. It provides oxygen and nutrients for the avascular tissues of the anterior segment such as cornea, trabecular meshwork, and lens and subsequently removes metabolic waste products. In addition, it maintains an IOP of about 15 mmHg that is required for the functional and morphological integ-

rity of the eye. The aqueous humor is derived from the blood plasma and secreted in an energy-consuming process (approximately 2–3 µl/min) by a monolayer of nonpigmented epithelial cells at the inner surface of the ciliary body. Compared to the plasma, the aqueous has a low protein level (about 0.02 g/ml compared to 7 g/ml), mainly composed of albumin and transferrin.[30] Other components include various growth and neurotrophic factors such as transforming growth factor-ß (TGF-ß), acidic and basic fibroblastic growth factor (aFGF, bFGF), vascular endothelial growth factor (VEGF), and pigment epithelial-derived factor (PEDF).[31]

To maintain an appropriate environment in the eye by restricting entry of cellular and soluble plasma components, the aqueous humor is separated from the blood by two functional barriers, the BAB and the blood–retinal barrier (BRB).[32] The BAB is supported by the nonpigmented epithelium of the ciliary body, the endothelium of the iris vasculature, and the endothelium of Schlemm's canal next to the trabecular meshwork. In contrast, the posteriorly located BRB is composed of the RPE (outer level) and the endothelial membrane of the retinal vasculature (inner level). Any perturbations of the blood–ocular barriers by trauma, disease, or drugs result in an inward movement of blood plasma constituents and may cause a plasmoid aqueous formation with disruption of the balance among the various growth factors and induce subretinal exudates and retinal edema.

Ocular hypotony and phthisis bulbi

Ocular hypotony, a key feature of phthisical eyes, is defined as IOP of $\geq$5 mmHg at consecutive measurements in an individual eye.[28] While clinical signs and symptoms are usually reversible in acute and transient stages, chronically decreased IOP can have deleterious effects on intraocular tissue morphology and function, eventually leading to phthisis bulbi (Table 54.2).[28,33,34] Although the underlying pathologies and mechanisms of ocular hypotony may be quite variable, they all work together, inducing an imbalance of aqueous production and outflow (trabecular, uveoscleral) (Figure 54.4).[21,28,35,36] Subsequent alterations of aqueous flow dynamics associated with compromised oxygen supply, nutrition, and metabolic exchange within the anterior chamber are main points of concern. In particular, intraocular hypoxia has been shown to contribute to BAB breakdown associated with invasion of serum components (i.e., proteins, growth factors), inflammatory cells, and tissue edema.[26]

Common causes of ocular hypotony in phthisis bulbi (i.e., trauma, filtration or vitreoretinal surgery, long-standing uveitis) are characterized by defects in the corneoscleral coat (i.e., external and internal fistulation), ciliary body insufficiency (i.e., cyclodialysis, cyclodestruction), choroidal and retinal detachment, or inflammation (primary and secondary) (Box 54.4).[26,28,36] Intraocular inflammation in particular represents a common pathway in the pathophysiology of ocular hypotony and phthisis bulbi. Inflammation-based IOP reduction is likely mediated by prostaglandins (i.e., prostaglandin-2α), which facilitate decreased aqueous production and increased uveoscleral outflow.[37,38] While in normal, nondiseased eyes, entry of

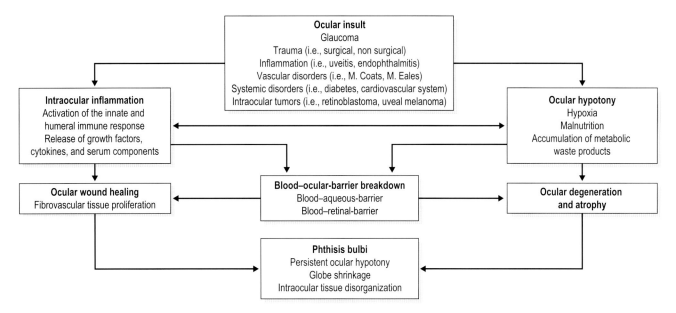

Figure 54.4 Diagram illustrating possible pathways resulting in phthisis bulbi.

aqueous humor into the suprachoroidal space is restricted by connective tissue strands between choroid and sclera, inflammation of the ciliary body results in stromal edema and breakdown of the functional barrier between the anterior chamber and the suprachoroidal space. Fluid transudation into the suprachoroidal space and increased uveal capillary fluid permeability lead to ciliochoroidal detachment.[36,37,39] The process becomes further facilitated since only minor amounts of suprachoroidal fluid will be drained through the emissary vessels secondary to low transscleral hydrostatic pressure differences. Thus, inflammation combined with hypotony creates a self-perpetuating cycle. Similar effects with decreased aqueous production can be seen in patients with traumatic cyclodialysis secondary to perforation or glaucoma surgery.[21,28] In addition, intraocular inflammation results in BAB breakdown with release of plasma proteins, cytokines, chemotactic, and angiogenic factors (i.e. TGF-ß, tumor necrosis factor-α (TNF-α), VEGF, angiopoietin-1, -2) that can contribute to migration, transformation, and proliferation of resident cells such as RPE, nonpigmented epithelial cells and Müller cells, fibrovascular tissue proliferation (i.e., cyclitic, epiretinal membranes), ocular neovascularization, and ocular hypotony.[22,25,40] In

particular, cyclitic and epiretinal membranes have the potential to lower IOP by traction and forward displacement of the ciliary processes (increased uveoscleral outflow) as well as direct damage to the ciliary body epithelium (decreased aqueous production).[21,39] Finally, all the processes described above may result in sclerosis and atrophy of the ciliary body and/or the adjacent intraocular tissues.[37,41]

Ocular wound healing in phthisis bulbi

Fibrovascular and fibrous tissue proliferation can also be observed after trauma (i.e., concussion, perforation) or complicated vitreoretinal surgery. Similar to proliferative vitreoretinopathy (PVR), it represents a specific ocular wound-healing response, which, if not treated properly, contributes to ocular hypotony and subsequent atrophy of the globe (Figure 54.4).[25,42–44] Potent predisposing risk factors include long-standing retinal detachment and retinal breaks with release of RPE cells into the vitreous.

Briefly, ocular injury results in breakdown of the blood–ocular barrier with release of serum components and chemotactic factors such as fibronectin (FN), TGF-ß, and platelet-derived growth factor (PDGF) into the anterior chamber and vitreous cavity. These factors accelerate migration, proliferation, and transformation of inflammatory cells and RPE.[31] Later cells are able to secrete additional growth factors and cytokines like interleukins (IL-1, -6), TNF-α, and TGF-ß, contributing to proliferation and transformation of RPE and glial cells into fibroblast- and myofibroblast-like cells with subsequent granulation tissue formation (i.e., fibrous, fibrovascular membranes).[25,31,42–45] Membrane composition varies depending on their location within the eye (i.e., RPE, nonpigmented ciliary body epithelium, fibroblasts, myofibroblasts, inflammatory cells, collagen, and fibronectin). They can be observed adjacent to perforation wounds, anterior and posterior to the lens, as well as at the inner side (preretinal) and outer side (subretinal) of the retina. Mem-

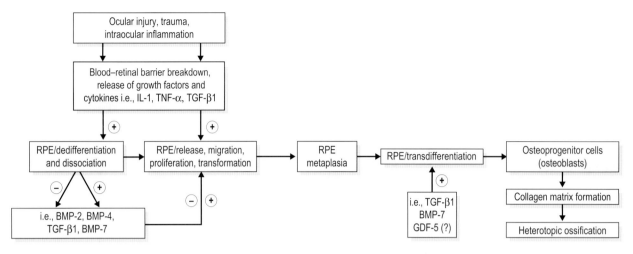

Figure 54.5 Diagram illustrating potential pathways of intraocular bone formation (heterotopic ossification). Intraocular inflammation primary or secondary to ocular trauma and surgical injury stimulates inflammatory cells (monocytes, macrophages) to release various cytokines such as interleukin 1 (IL-1), tumor necrosis factor-α (TNF-α), and transforming growth factor-ß$_1$ (TGF-ß$_1$), which are involved in retinal pigment epithelium (RPE) cell proliferation, transformation, and transdifferentiation. The processes are further facilitated by RPE-mediated bone morphogenic proteins (BMP-2 and -4 and -7) and growth differentiation factor 5 (GDF-5) expression. (Modified from Toyran S, Lin AY, Edward DP. Expression of growth differentiation factor-5 and bone morphogenic protein-7 in intraocular osseous metaplasia. Br J Ophthalmol 2005;89:885–890.)

brane contraction, mainly induced by RPE and Müller cells, will finally result in retinal and ciliary body detachment.[45,46] Of particular note is anterior PVR. The progressive stages of anterior PVR include traction, incorporation of ciliary body elements, and cellular proliferation.[47] It is felt that surgical intervention (vitrectomy) must be performed some time during or before the incorporation phase, as there will be no chance to re-establish the ciliary epithelium's ability to produce aqueous humor, thus leading to phthisis bulbi.[47] Anterior PVR has been previously classified as a cyclitic membrane.

Dystrophic calcification and heterotopic ossification in phthisis bulbi

Calcification and ossification are frequent end-stage changes of degenerating tissues. Both can be observed in phthisical eyes, often associated with chronic inflammation, multiple traumas, long-standing retinal detachment, or PVR.[23,24,48,49] Intraocular calcium deposits are mainly composed of calcium phosphate and carbonate and typically occur in the cornea (band keratopathy), lens, RPE (drusen), and retina, "depending on low carbon dioxide tension due to metabolic inactivity."[50] In contrast, bone formation usually involves the choroid and fibrovascular or fibrocellular cyclitic membranes external to the neurosensory retina. The time between original insult and bone formation is quite variable, ranging from a few months to several years, with an average of approximately 20 years.[23,48] While trauma seems to be more common in young patients with formation of compact bone tissue, inflammation is often associated with an older age group of ≥50 years, resulting in spongy bone tissue.[49] Fibrous and osseous metaplasia of RPE plays a central role in the pathogenesis of heterogenic ossification, as illustrated in Figure 54.5 (Box 54.5).[24,49–51] RPE cells, stimulated by inflammatory cytokines such as TNF-α, IL-1, and TGF-ß, undergo

Box 54.5 Function of the RPE in the pathophysiology of phthisis bulbi

The retinal pigment epithelium (RPE) is a pluripotent tissue, which plays a central role in the pathophysiology of:

- Ocular wound healing (migration, proliferation, transformation)
- Heterotopic ossification (osseous metaplasia) in phthisis bulbi

mesenchymal transformation into fibroblast-like cells and subsequent transdifferentiation into osteogenic progenitor cells, finally resulting in ectopic bone tissue.[44,50] Proliferating RPE cells can often be seen adjacent to intraocular bones structures. In addition, heterotopic ossification can also be observed in tissues with abundant blood supply such as the posterior peripapillary choroid, probably because of vascular delivery of osteoblasts.[23,49] These osteoblasts may be derived from circulating hematopoietic stem cells and be related to changes in choroidal blood flow that occurs during phthisis bulbi.

Conclusion

Phthisis bulbi represents an ocular end-stage disease that results from wound healing secondary to various causes such as severe trauma, inflammation, necrotizing tumors, and/or vascular diseases. It results in vision loss and continues to be an important cause of blindness. The clinical diagnosis of phthisis bulbi, which is characterized by atrophy, shrinkage, and disorganization of the globe, is a frustrating situation since therapeutic approaches are limited to symptomatic or cosmetic treatment options. Prophylactic procedures and close follow-up visits are required in patients at high risk for the development of phthisis bulbi.

Key references

A complete list of chapter references is available online at www.expertconsult.com. See inside cover for registration details.

3. Stefani FH. Phthisis bulbi – an intraocular florid proliferative reaction. Dev Ophthalmol 1985;10:78–160.

5. Naumann GOH, Portwich E. [Etiology and final clinical cause for 1000 enucleations: a clinicopathologic study.] Klin Mbl Augenheilkd 1976;168:622–630.

21. Chandler PA, Maumenee AE. A major cause of hypotony. Am J Ophthalmol 1961;52:609–618.

25. Elner SG, Elner VM, Diaz-Rohena R, et al. Anterior proliferative vitreoretinopathy. Clinicopathologic, light microscopic, and ultrastructural findings. Ophthalmology 1988;95:1349–1357.

26. Voelcker HE, Naumann GOH. [Histopathology of persistent ocular hypotension syndrome.] Berl Dtsch Ophthalmol Ges 1978;75:591–595.

28. Schubert HD. Postsurgical hypotony: relationship to fistulation, inflammation, choroidal lesions, and the vitreous. Surv Ophthalmol 1996;41:97–125.

31. Klenkler B, Sheardown H. Growth factors in the anterior segment: a role in tissue maintenance, wound healing, and ocular pathology. Exp Eye Res 2004;79:677–688.

38. Kim HC, Hayashi A, Shalash A, et al. A model of chronic hypotony in the rabbit. Graefes Arch Clin Ophthalmol 1998;236:69–74.

40. Dorrell M, Uusitalo-Jarvinen H, Aguilar E, et al. Ocular neovascularization: basic mechanisms and therapeutic approaches. Surv Ophthalmol 2007;52:S3–S19.

43. Pastor JC. Proliferative vitreoretinopathy: an overview. Surv Ophthalmol 1998;43:3–18.

44. Hiscott P, Sheridan C, Magee RM, et al. Matrix and the retinal pigment epithelium in proliferative retinal disease. Prog Retin Eye Res 1999;18:167–190.

45. Grisanti S, Guidry C. Transdifferentiation of retinal pigment epithelial cells from epithelia to mesenchymal phenotype. Invest Ophthalmol Vis Sci 1995;36:391–405.

47. Lopez PF, Grossniklaus HE, Aaberg TM, et al. Pathogenetic mechanisms of anterior proliferative vitreoretinopathy. Am J Ophthalmol 1993;100:415–422.

48. Zeiter HJ. Calcification and ossification in ocular tissue. Am J Ophthalmol 1962;53:265–274.

CHAPTER 55

Myopia

Terri L Young

Definition and prevalence

Myopia is the most common human eye disorder in the world. For this refractive state, the retina is located behind the focal plane so that a concave (negative-power) lens is needed to move the focal plane back to the retinal plane, restoring a focused, clear image. Definitions of myopia vary, but generally an eye is considered myopic if a negative spherical equivalent correction of at least 0.50 diopters (D) is needed to restore emmetropia, the refractive state in which images are focused on the retina. Because of varying definitions, the reported prevalence of myopia varies. In the US adult population an estimated prevalence of 25–30% is supported by multiple studies.[1–6] Females are reported to have an earlier onset and a slightly higher prevalence than males.[4,5,7,8] US Asians and Hispanics have a higher prevalence than whites or African-Americans.[9] Chinese and Japanese populations have very high myopia prevalence rates of > 50–70%.[5,8,10,11] Ashkenazi Jews, especially orthodox Jewish males, have shown a higher prevalence than other white US and European populations.[11] Comparative prevalence rates from different countries show considerable variability, but confirm that myopia affects a significant proportion of the population in many countries.[2,6,12–18] Worldwide, there may be as many as one billion myopic individuals (Box 55.1).[19] Uncorrected myopia is an important cause of correctable low vision in developed and underdeveloped countries.[20] A priority of refractive error correction is part of the World Health Organization's global initiative, Vision 2020.[21]

Myopia is typically divided into two basic types. "Juvenile-onset" or moderate myopia (also called "simple" or "school" myopia) most often develops and progresses between the ages of 8 and 16 years, and generally does not require a correction stronger than −5 D.[1,7,22–24] In contrast, "pathologic" or high-grade myopia usually begins to develop in the perinatal period, and is associated with rapid refractive error myopic shifts before 10–12 years of age due to axial elongation of the vitreous chamber.[1,7,12,23,25]

Whether it occurs from continued progression of juvenile-onset myopia, or from early-onset high-grade myopia, a high level of axial myopia (spherical equivalent refractive correction of −5 D or greater) is a major cause of legal blindness in many developed countries.[4,11–15,26] High myopia has a prevalence of 1.7–2% in the general population of the USA[1,3]

and is especially common in Asia.[13,14,16] In Japan, high myopia reportedly affects 6–18% of the myopic population and 1–2% of the general population.[13]

The public health and economic impact of myopia is considerable.[1–5,7,8,10–12,23–25] Costs associated with optical corrections for adults were over US $26 billion in 2005 for glasses, contact lenses, and refractive surgery. Of this, at least 61% ($14.6 billion) was for myopic correction, and did not include costs for correcting myopia in children.

Ocular morbidities associated with myopia

Many investigators have reported on the association of high myopia with premature cataract development,[27] glaucoma,[28] severe retinal thinning with eventual retinal detachment (RD), and posterior staphyloma with retinal degenerative changes.[1,29–45] High myopia is associated with progressive and excessive elongation of the globe, which may be accompanied by degenerative changes in the sclera, choroid, Bruch's membrane, retinal pigment epithelium (RPE), and neural retina. Various fundoscopic changes within the posterior staphyloma develop in highly myopic eyes. These changes include geographic areas of atrophy of the RPE and choroid, lacquer cracks in Bruch's membrane, subretinal hemorrhage, and choroidal neovascularization (CNV). Among these various fundus lesions, macular CNV is the most common vision-threatening complication of high myopia.[33–37,39] Clinical and histopathologic studies have documented CNV in 4–11% of highly myopic eyes. Relative to emmetropic eyes, an approximately twofold increased risk of CNV was estimated for eyes with 1–2 D of myopia, a fourfold increase with 3–4 D, and a ninefold increase with 5–6 D.[32,39,45,46] Poor visual outcome following CNV in myopic eyes is not uncommon, and often affects relatively young patients.

The risk of RD is estimated to be 3–7 times greater for persons with greater than 5 D of myopia, compared with those with a lower amount of myopia.[42,45,47] Myopia of 5–10 D was associated with a 15–35-fold greater risk of RD relative to that associated with low levels of hyperopia.[42,45,47] The lifetime risk for RD was estimated to be 1.6% for patients with myopia less than 3 D and 9.3% for those with more

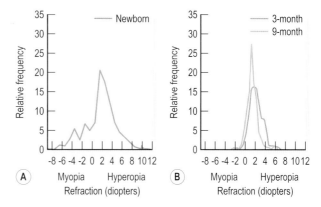

Figure 55.1 (A) Refractive error distribution at birth. Data from Cook and Glasscock.[52] (B) Refractive distribution at 3 months (dashed line) and 9 months of age. Approximately 25% of infants are myopic at birth. By 9 months, nearly all children are emmetropic or slightly hyperopic. (Reproduced from Mutti et al.[58])

than 5 D.[42,43] A subgroup with lattice degeneration and more than 5 D of myopia had an estimated lifetime risk of 35.9%.[43] The prevalence of lattice degeneration increases with increasing amounts of myopia, as measured by axial length.[45,47–49] Glaucoma was observed in 3% of individuals with myopia with axial lengths of less than 26.5 mm, in 11% with axial lengths between 26.5 and 33.5 mm, and in 28% of those with longer lengths.[44]

Myopia is the most studied refractive error due to the high prevalence and the increased risk of associated blinding complications. Research pursuits include why and how myopia develops, and whether treatments can be developed to prevent this refractive error, or prevent progression to high amounts. A fundamental question is whether myopic development is a result of predetermined genetic[50] or environmental factors[51] such as excessive near work. Both appear to play a role in human myopia.

Human emmetropization process

Although myopia is highly prevalent, the majority of eyes are emmetropic in childhood. The normal postnatal development of emmetropia has been examined for clues about possible underlying mechanisms by which this is achieved. At birth (Figure 55.1A), the refractive distribution of human newborns is very broad. The mean is approximately 2 D of hyperopia, but the standard deviation is great and nearly 25% of newborns are myopic.[52] The major determinants of the focal plane are the cornea and lens, while the axial length (vitreous chamber depth) determines whether the retina is located at the focal plane.[53] At birth, the size, shape, and power of all are determined largely by inheritance,[54] although conformational factors such as intrauterine environment and the bony orbits and eyelids can also influence eye shape and growth.[55]

During the first postnatal weeks and months, the ocular components and refractive state undergo rapid changes. The corneal diameter of the infant is 9–10 mm compared to the adult size of 12 mm. Due to the steep curvature, corneal power averages 51 D at birth and flattens to approximately 44 D by 6 weeks of age.[56,57]

Mutti et al[58] found the average corneal power at 3 months of age to be 43.9 D. By 9 months it decreased to 42.8 D. Between 6 and 14 years of age, corneal power is stable.[59] Lenticular power averages 34 D at birth and decreases to 28 D by 6 months of age, and to 21 D by adulthood.[56] Mutti et al[58,60] found the average lens power (Gullstrand–Emsley indices) showed a continual decline with age from 21.5 D at age 6 years to 19.8 D at age 14 years.

In addition to the changes in corneal and lens powers, the distribution of refractive errors narrows dramatically in the postnatal months (Figure 55.1B).[7,56,58,61,62] In the infantile growth period the eyes grow from around 16 mm axial length at birth[63] to an average of 19 mm at 3 months of age and over 20 mm by 9 months.[58] During this time the axial length changes in a manner that moves the retina to the focal plane.[63,64] As described by Mutti et al,[58] "modulation in the amount of axial growth in relation to initial refractive error appeared to be the most influential factor in emmetropization of spherical equivalent refractive error." Eyes that are initially hyperopic increase their axial length rapidly to move the retina to the focal plane. Eyes that are initially myopic have a slower axial elongation rate so that, as the cornea and lens powers decrease, the focal plane moves to the retina. The result of the controlled growth of the axial length is that nearly all eyes become emmetropic with the majority being slightly (0.5–1 D) hyperopic when measured with cycloplegia.

There is little change in refractive status in most eyes during the rest of childhood, even though there is continued change in anterior-chamber depth, lens power, and axial length. Because of the continued decreases in corneal and lens power during childhood, control of the axial elongation rate to maintain a match to the focal plane is needed until the eyes are fully mature. Refractive error distribution in the adult population has a narrow peak with most people between emmetropia and +1.0 D. This amount of hyperopia is readily compensated for by accommodation of the crystalline lens, so that most eyes are functionally emmetropic. The human eye normally maintains an axial length of within 2% of its optimal focal point.[1,53,54] In an adult (~24 mm) eye, a deviation from optimal of 0.2 mm in axial length would produce a refractive error of more than 0.5 D.[65]

Although the individual refractive components of the corneal and lenticular dioptric powers and anterior-chamber depth follow a bell-shaped (normal) distribution, several studies have shown that the refractive status of the eye is determined primarily by variation in axial length, which does not display a normal distribution.[1,22,47,54,55] Spherical refractive error usually represents a mismatch between axial length and the combined dioptric powers of the cornea and lens. Moderate myopia results from a "failure of correlation" of these components where all components fall within normal limits, but are borderline high or low. For example, an eye with a relatively steep cornea and normal axial length could be myopic even though none of the ocular component dimensions is abnormal. Low myopia (smaller than 6 D) is usually the result of this lack of correlation. In children whose myopia is progressing the amount of progression is closely related to the increase in vitreous chamber length.[66] Higher levels of myopia are due to "component ametropia," in which the axial length exceeds normal values.[53,55] "Correlational" and "component" myopia may have different genetic etiologies.

To some extent, narrowing of the distribution of refractive errors during the first postnatal months could be explained by the "passive proportional" growth of the eye.[67] However, more eyes are emmetropic than would be expected from a random combination of the optical elements and the axial length.[68,69] This has led to the suggestion that an active feedback mechanism coordinates the axial length with the optical elements to produce emmetropia.[52,54,68-72] However, based on clinical observations, it was not possible to test this suggestion.

Animal models of emmetropization

In the 1970s, studies with animal models (primarily monkeys,[73,74] chicks,[75] and tree shrews[76,77]) demonstrated that an emmetropization mechanism exists. It has been shown in animals that this emmetropization mechanism normally controls the axial elongation rate of the eye to achieve and maintain a match of the axial length to optical power so that the photoreceptors are in focus for distant objects.[78-80] Vision plays a critical role in this process (Box 55.2).

Form deprivation myopia

Animal models of the emmetropization process began with "form deprivation myopia" (see recent reviews[78-82]). Form deprivation was initially produced by tarsorrhaphy or by the placement of a translucent diffuser over the eye, held in place by a goggle or mask. This eliminates higher spatial frequencies and decreases the contrast of the retinal image, while still allowing limited transmission of light to the retina. It is now recognized that form deprivation removes the visual feedback needed to guide the eye growth to an emmetropic state and to maintain emmetropia. Form deprivation during the juvenile postnatal period causes the vitreous chamber elongation of chicks, tree shrews, macaque monkeys, and other species. The axial growth continues from a standard, slightly hyperopic state extending past a set point that would produce emmetropia to become myopic.[73,75,76] Degenerative retinal fundus changes typical of human myopia were noted in monkey[83,84] and tree shrew.[85] A decrease in choroidal thickness also occurs in the

monkey[86,87] and tree shrew,[88,89] and is prominent in the chick.[90] The "induced myopia" occurs only monocularly in form-deprived eyes, and not in the paired eye which serves as an untreated within-animal control. Thus, the myopia is clearly environmental in nature. The observation that eyelid closure myopia could not be induced in dark-reared animals further suggests that visual experience is required.[91,92] Form deprivation myopia occurs consistently across species, including the grey squirrel,[93] cat,[94] and mouse.[95]

Compensation for negative lenses

Form deprivation myopia demonstrates that the visual environment plays a role in establishing and maintaining emmetropia. Recognition that the emmetropization mechanism uses visual feedback to match the axial length to the focal plane emanates from studies that used negative-power (and positive-power) lenses to shift the focal plane of the eye.[96-98] As shown in Figure 55.2B, a monocular negative lens shifts the focal plane posteriorly, away from the cornea. This consistently produces a compensatory increase in the axial elongation rate of the growing eye, such that the retinal location is shifted to match the shifted focal plane (Figure 55.2C.) When measured with the lens in place, the refractive state matches the untreated fellow control eye.[96,99,100] Thus, in compensating for the negative lens the eye is, in fact, restoring optical emmetropia.

With the lens removed, the eye is myopic (Figure 55.2D). Compensation can be quite accurate[101-103] and negative lenses of different powers produce different axial elongation appropriate to move the retina to compensate for the lens power. Some strains of mice can develop negative lens-induced myopia, even though mice are not strongly

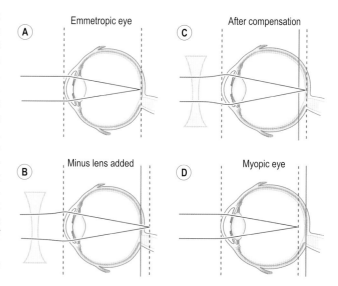

Figure 55.2 Compensation for a minus lens. In an emmetropic eye (A), the focal plane for distant objects, without accommodation, is coincident with the retina. Placing a negative-power lens in front of one eye (B) displaces the focal plane posteriorly, assuming accommodation is set by the control eye. The emmetropization mechanism produces elongation that moves the retina to the displaced focal plane (C) so that the eye's refractive state is emmetropic with the lens in place. When the lens is removed (D), the eye is myopic.

Box 55.2 Myopia animal models

Animal model studies of myopia provide the best source of biologically similar tissue types to test various eye growth paradigms. Their relationship to human myopia remains unclear however

---

dependent on vision.[104] Fish (*Tilapia*), which are more vision-dependent, display this modulation characteristic.[105]

Interestingly, for negative lens compensation to occur in animals, the lens must be worn almost constantly. Removing the negative lens and allowing normal unrestricted vision (or plano-lens wear) for as little as 2 hours per day is sufficient to block negative lens compensation in monkeys,[106] tree shrews,[107] and chicks.[108]

Plus lenses

Plus lenses shift the focal plane anteriorly, converting an emmetropic eye into one that is myopic. In examining the effect of plus lenses in animal studies, it is important to note that they are applied to juvenile eyes that are still undergoing normal axial elongation. If the axial elongation rate is slowed below normal while the optical components continue to mature normally, the eye gradually becomes emmetropic while wearing the plus lens. With the lens removed it is hyperopic. Thus, to respond to a plus lens, the eye must not only be able to detect that it is myopic, but also be able to slow its elongation rate. In a young, growing chick eye, plus lens wear quickly causes a decrease of the elongation rate such that the eye becomes emmetropic while wearing the lens and hyperopic when the lens is removed.[96,98] Even short exposures to myopic defocus have a potent slowing effect.[108-112]

The response to plus lenses differs somewhat in monkeys and tree shrews. When plus lenses are applied to tree shrews that have achieved emmetropia, little effect is noted.[113] However, if plus lenses are applied early in the emmetropization process in younger, hyperopic tree shrews and monkeys, the elongation rate of the eyes decreases, and emmetropia is maintained while wearing the lens.[99,114-116] With lens removal, the eye remains hyperopic. The lack of a response to plus lenses in older tree shrews and monkeys may be due to an inability to slow axial elongation rate substantially below normal once the eyes have achieved emmetropia. The source of this difference in the chick is unknown, but may be related to different sclera composition in the avian eye relative to that of the mammalian. The chick eye sclera has an inner cartilaginous layer in addition to the fibrous sclera layer present in humans, monkeys, and tree shrews. Controlling the growth of the cartilage may be a more powerful way of controlling axial elongation than can be achieved with a fibrous sclera alone.

Recovery from induced myopia

Further evidence for active control of axial length growth comes from the effect of removing form deprivation or negative lens wear after an induced myopia has developed. In the several species that have been studied, "recovery" from induced myopia occurs. Restoration of unrestricted vision causes the axial elongation rate to decrease below normal. As the focal plane moves posteriorly due to continued corneal flattening and lens maturation the induced myopia dissipates.[67,103,117-119] It has been suggested that recovery occurs for two reasons: first, the eye is myopic, and second, it is elongated relative to normal. These factors together produce a stronger response than is produced by plus lens wear alone.[120] In animals with monocular induced myopia, the refractive state of the recovering eye eventually matches that of the untreated fellow control eye at emmetropia, suggesting that active guidance occurs moving towards a "target" of emmetropia. The emmetropization mechanism is thus capable of acting to control axial elongation to achieve emmetropia from the myopic, as well as the hyperopic, direction. The consistency of responses to form deprivation, negative lens wear, and recovery provides evidence that an active emmetropization mechanism exists and is conserved across phyla. Together with the rapid development in human infants of a very narrow refractive error distribution, these data argue strongly that an emmetropization mechanism exists in humans.

The emmetropization feedback loop

The signaling cascade

How does the retina control the axial elongation rate to match the retina to the focal plane and maintain that match throughout the juvenile developmental period? The broad outline of a feedback loop has emerged from studies of animal models. The starting place is the visual stimulus (1 in Figure 55.3). Although it is not precisely known what aspect of the images on the retina stimulates elongation, there is general agreement that hyperopic defocus (image plane behind the retina) serves as a stimulus for eyes to increase the axial elongation rate ("go" signal). Myopic defocus, or perhaps clear images projected on the retina,

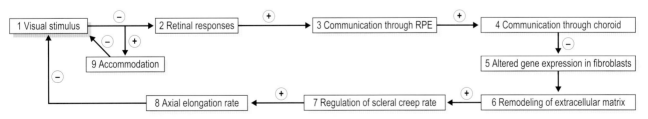

Figure 55.3 An emmetropization model. When the axial length is shorter than the focal plane, hyperopic defocus (1) occurs on the retina unless fully cleared by accommodation (9). Hyperopic defocus reduces the amplitude of responses (variability in response) of retinal neurons (2), altering the communication of signals (3) through the retinal pigment epithelium (RPE) and (4) choroid. This is communicated to the sclera where (5) gene expression in fibroblasts is altered. Remodeling of the scleral extracellular matrix (ECM) occurs (6), increasing the creep rate of the sclera (7) which increases the axial elongation rate (8) of the eye. Axial elongation moves the retina closer to the focal plane, reducing the amount of defocus. With reduced retinal defocus, responses increase, altering communication to the sclera. Scleral remodeling is altered such that the creep rate is decreased and axial elongation is slowed. Accurate accommodation (9) is important, as it reduces defocus.[187]

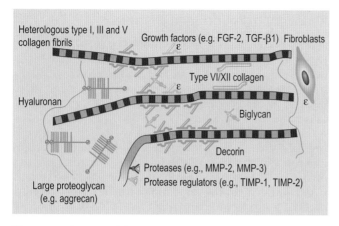

Figure 55.4 Structure of the mammalian sclera. Model illustrating the likely biochemical structure of the extracellular matrix of the mammalian sclera. FGF-2, fibroblast growth factor-2; TGF-β₁, transforming growth factor-β₁; MMP, matrix metalloproteinase; TIMP, tissue inhibitors of metalloprotease. (Adapted from Fransson et al.[157])

produces signals that slow axial elongation ("stop" signal). Defocus, or its absence, is detected by the retina (2 in Figure 55.4), presumably at the level of center-surround bipolar cells or later.[121,122] As has been established by single-unit studies of retinal ganglion cells,[123] defocused images produce weaker responses from cells with center-surround receptive fields than do sharply focused images. Thus, as the eyes move from target to target, with varying retinal image stimulation, focused images will produce large changes in the retinal cell activity level.

In chicks, a class of amacrine cells that contain glucagon are involved in sending a "stop" signal to slow the eye elongation rate of the eye.[124-126] Without these cells, eyes elongate and become myopic. With them, and with additional glucagon administered intravitreally,[126] eyes resist becoming myopic with form deprivation. It has also been reported that the protein apolipoprotein A1 provides a retinal "stop" signal in chicks.[127]

Perhaps surprisingly, the emmetropization mechanism persists after sectioning of the optic nerve,[128] or blocking the output from the retina to central visual structures with tetrodotoxin,[129,130] leading to the conclusion that there is direct communication across the RPE and choroid (3 and 4 in Figure 55.3) to the sclera of the eye. The communication to the sclera must also be spatially local. When form deprivation or negative lens treatment is applied to half of the visual field (either nasal or temporal) using specially designed goggles, only the treated half of the eye elongates and becomes myopic.[131-134] More surprisingly, the fovea is neither necessary nor sufficient to establish and maintain emmetropia. Macaque monkeys that underwent laser destruction of the entire macular region maintain emmetropia.[135] Monkeys that wear form-depriving diffuser goggles with a clear central 30° to allow foveal vision develop form deprivation myopia.[135,136]

How the visually derived signals pass through the RPE is unknown. It has been suggested[137] that changes in retinal activity produce changes in ionic concentrations across the RPE that in turn affect the tissues of the choroid. This part of the emmetropization signaling cascade is under active investigation. Mertz and Wallman[138] suggested that all-trans-retinoic acid in the choroid may serve as a signaling molecule to the sclera. Rada et al[139] have suggested that ovotransferrin might also serve a similar role.

Visual response remodeling of the sclera

As the structural outer coat of the eye, the sclera controls the location of the retina. The sclera in eutherian mammals is a soft, but tough, fibrous viscoelastic connective tissue comprised of an extracellular matrix (ECM) produced by fibroblasts that are of neural crest origin.[140-142] It consists of layers, or lamellae, composed of collagen (85–90% of the scleral total protein), associated proteoglycans, hyaluronan, and other extracellular proteins produced by the fibroblasts. Type I collagen is the primary subtype (>99%)[143] but types III, V, and VI are present in tree shrew sclera.[115,144] Unlike the corneal stroma, the diameter and spacing of the collagen fibrils vary widely, so that the sclera is not transparent. In addition to collagen, elastic fibrils comprised of elastin and laminin have been reported in the human sclera.[145] The proteoglycans aggrecan, biglycan, and decorin are also present in the adult human sclera[146] and in tree shrew sclera.[147] Austin et al[148] suggested that another proteoglycan, lumican, is important in the formation of scleral collagen fibrils.

Glycosaminoglycans (GAGs) constitute a small (~0.2%), but potentially important, fraction of the scleral dry weight. Functionally, GAGs have been suggested to stabilize the spacing of collagen fibrils[149] and to affect the hydration levels of ECM.[150,151]

In addition to these structural components, the sclera contains several growth factors (e.g., transforming growth factor-ß, fibroblast growth factor-2)[152] as well as degradative enzymes (matrix metalloproteinases and tissue inhibitors of metalloproteinases).[153,154] A simplified scleral structure is provided in Figure 55.4.

After completion of the infantile growth period, there is little evidence in mammals for continued scleral remodeling.[143] Rather than modulating cartilage growth (as occurs in chicks[155,156]), the visual environment controls remodeling of the scleral ECM. This discussion will focus on mammalian sclera, with particular emphasis on tree shrew because it has been the subject of considerable research.

When "go" signals reach the sclera, changes in expression for some genes occur (5 in Figure 55.3), along with remodeling (6 in Figure 55.3) of the scleral ECM.[158] In tree shrews, and perhaps in mammals generally, these biochemical changes appear to control the biomechanical property of sclera, creep rate (6 in Figure 55.3). The creep rate is the extension of the sclera over time when a constant tension is applied. Normally in juvenile tree shrew eyes, scleral extensibility is low. As a result of the remodeling of the sclera, the creep rate rises.[100] Loosely speaking, the sclera becomes more readily extensible. The changes in creep rate in turn allow normal intraocular pressure to increase the axial elongation rate of the eye (8 in Figure 55.3), moving the retina away from the cornea. In a hyperopic eye an increased axial elongation rate reduces the hyperopia, decreasing the defocus on the retina. Through this emmetropization feedback system, a hyperopic eye elongates until the visual signals (1 in Figure 55.3) that drive the feedback loop diminish and the eye stabilizes at emmetropia.

Scleral changes during myopia development and recovery

Many of the details of how the visual environment controls scleral remodeling summarized in the model shown in Figure 55.3 emanate from studies using form deprivation or negative lenses to induce the eyes to become myopic. Both interventions ("treatments") produce a visual signal that stimulates the feedback loop, raising the amount of scleral remodeling, increasing the creep and axial elongation rates. Changes observed during recovery are generally the reverse of those found during myopia development.

When myopia is induced, the sclera becomes thinner, due in part to a reduction in the amount of type I collagen.[141,157-159] Reductions of dry scleral weight of 3–5% develop after a few days of form deprivation or negative lens wear in tree shrews.[159] Long-term form deprivation in tree shrew leads to a more substantial thinning, similar to that seen in humans with moderate myopia.[160] Humans with pathological myopia have a marked scleral thinning, particularly at the posterior pole.[161] In addition to scleral thinning, the collagen fibrils often show altered architecture in high human myopia, with a reduction in diameter, loss of longitudinal fibril striations, and a derangement of the growth and organization of the fibrils.[162] Following long-term form deprivation in tree shrews, Norton and Rada[158] noted a reduction in hydroxyproline (−11.8%) which suggests a loss of collagen. McBrien et al found similar changes: a reduction in median fibril diameter and misshapen collagen fibrils in tree shrews.[153]

One advantage of animal models, in contrast to examination of human donor eyes, is that it is possible to examine the sclera and other tissues during the time an induced myopia is developing, rather than studying the postmortem endpoint of a longstanding myopic condition. After short-term form deprivation, although the sclera is thinner, the collagen fibrils appear normal in morphology, diameter, and spacing.[153,163] During recovery, there is an increase in collagen synthesis and in mRNA expression level for type I collagen.[115] These findings suggest that more subtle remodeling of scleral tissue occurs rather than destruction of structural elements, causing axial elongation and myopia development immediately after the onset of form deprivation or negative lens wear.

Animal model form deprivation study in relation to human myopia

Although animal models have provided information about how environmentally induced myopia can develop, questions have been raised about the applicability of animal studies to human myopia. For instance, form deprivation myopia has been reported to develop in young children with obstructive visual axis conditions such as ptosis or cataract.[164-167] The myopic shift from form deprivation is inconsistent in humans, however.[168]

An important similarity between animals and humans was noted by Gwiazda et al,[169] who reported that progressing myopes (children with increasing myopia) underaccommodate to near visual targets more than do emmetropic children. The resulting hyperopic defocus resembles the hyperopic defocus that is produced by minus lens wear, which causes axial elongation in many animal species. This observation led to the "blur hypothesis," which suggests that the eyes of children also elongate in response to the hyperopic defocus that occurs when the child underaccommodates to near targets. To the extent that accurate accommodation occurs, the defocus is reduced, which may be why the children with more accurate accommodation remained emmetropic in the Gwiazda et al study.[169] The blur hypothesis is attractive as it not only relates animal studies to the human experience, but is also consistent with studies that have associated myopia development with near work.[3,11] It contrasts with the suggestion, never supported by direct measurement, that accommodation itself is a cause of myopia[170,171] by increasing tension on the sclera, stretching it so the eye elongates.[53] The alternative provided by the blur hypothesis is that accommodation is beneficial, because it provides clear images on the retina and thereby removes the visual stimuli for increased axial elongation that can lead to myopia.

Human molecular genetics of myopia

Ocular refractive component genetics

The refractive state is determined by the relative contributions of the optical components, primarily corneal curvature, anterior-chamber depth, and lens thickness – all of which determine the location of the focal plane, and the axial length (primarily the vitreous chamber depth) – which determines whether the retina is located at the focal plane (Box 55.3). Separately, these may be assessed as quantitative traits intimately related to the clinical phenotype of myopia. Multiple reports have examined familial aggregation and heritability of ocular components.[172-181]

As expected from the previous sections, axial length is the largest contributor to the determination of refractive error. Several studies have reported an inverse relationship of axial length to refraction (the longer the eye, the more myopic the refractive error).[174-178] Axial length of a myopic adult population may show a bimodal distribution with a second peak of increased axial length relating to high myopia (< −6 D at 24 mm, > −6 D at 30 mm) when plotted as a distribution curve.[54] This suggests that myopia of −6 D or greater represents a deviation from the normal distribution of axial length and is not physiologic.

Estimates of heritability for axial length range from 40% to 94%.[172,179-184] A study of three large Sardinian families found modest evidence for linkage on chromosome 2p24 with a likelihood of the odds (LOD) score of 2.64.[181] Overall

---

Box 55.3 Human myopia molecular genetic studies

Molecular genetics studies of human myopia provide a relatively new translational possibility for determining genetic variants associated with myopia. The groundwork from these types of studies may enable the development of new therapies for treatment or prevention, or provide genetic tests for predicting those at greater risk for accompanying ocular morbidities of myopia

axial length includes anterior-chamber depth, and studies have shown that increased anterior-chamber depth has an inverse relationship as well to refractive error.[178] The heritability reports for anterior-chamber depth range from 70% to 94%,[173,179–181] and the same Sardinian study found modest linkage evidence to chromosome 1p32.2 with a LOD score of 2.32.[181]

The steeper the corneal curvature, the more likely the resulting refractive error is myopic – eyes with hyperopia are more likely to have flatter corneal curvature readings by keratometry.[174,185,186] Heritability estimates for corneal curvature range from 60% to 92%.[173,179–181] The Sardinian family study noted modest linkage evidence of corneal curvature to chromosomes 2p25, 3p26, and 7q22 with LOD scores ranging from 2.34 to 2.50.[181] Increased lens thickness correlates with increased myopia.[178] A di- and monozygotic twin study reported 90–93% heritability for lens thickness.[179]

Role of environment in myopic development

The prevalence of myopia in some populations appears to have increased dramatically from one generation to the next in progressively industrialized settings, or with increased level of educational achievement.[45,187–189] Assessing the impact of inheritance on myopic development may be confounded by children adopting parental behavioral traits associated with myopia, such as higher-than-average near-work activities (i.e., reading).[190] Observational studies of this risk factor do not fully explain the excessive familial clustering of myopia, however. A detailed assessment of confounding effects and interactions between hereditary and environmental influences in juvenile-onset myopia has shown that near work describes very little of the variance in refractive error compared to parental myopia.[191] Additionally, near work exerted no confounding influence on the association between parent and child myopia, indicating that children do not become myopic by adopting parental reading habits. More importantly, there was no significant interaction between parental myopia and near work; reading was weakly and equally associated with myopia regardless of the number of myopic parents. This indicates that children could inherit myopia as a trait from parents. Of late, it has been proposed and accepted that relatively decreased outdoor activity, rather than near work, has a greater impact on myopic refractive error development.[192]

Hereditary factors in myopic development

Multiple familial aggregation studies report a positive correlation between parental myopia and myopia in their children, indicating a hereditary factor in myopia susceptibility.[193–196] Children with a family history of myopia had on average less hyperopia, deeper anterior chambers, and longer vitreous chambers even before becoming myopic. Yap and colleagues noted a prevalence of myopia in 7-year-old children of 7.3% when neither parent was myopic, 26.2% when one parent was myopic, and 45% when both parents were myopic. This implies a strong role for genetics in myopia.[182]

Multiple familial studies support a high hereditary basis for myopia, especially higher degrees.[183,184,197,198] Naiglin and colleagues performed segregation analysis on 32 French multiplex families with high myopia, and determined an autosomal-dominant (AD) mode of inheritance.[199] The l_s for myopia (the increase in risk to siblings of a person with a disease compared to the population prevalence) has been estimated to be approximately 4.9–19.8 for sibs for high myopia (–6.00 spherical D or greater), and approximately 1.5–3 for low or common myopia (approximately –1.00 to –3.00 spherical D), suggesting a definite genetic basis for high myopia, and a strong genetic basis for low myopia.[200,201] A high degree of familial aggregation of refraction, particularly myopia, was reported in the Beaver Dam Eye Study population after accounting for the effects of age, sex, and education.[202] Segregation analysis suggested the involvement of multiple genes, rather than a single major gene effect.

Twin studies provide the most compelling evidence that inheritance plays a significant role in myopia.[55,172,179,184,203] Multiple studies note an increased concordance of refractive error as well as refractive components (axial length, corneal curvature, lens power) in monozygotic twins compared to dizygotic twins.[55,179,184,204] Sorsby et al noted a correlation coefficient for myopia of 0 for control pairs, 0.5 for dizygotic twins, and almost 1.0 for monozygotic twins in a study of 78 pairs of monozygotic twins and 40 pairs of dizygotic twins.[204] Twin studies estimate a notable high heritability value for myopia (the proportion of the total phenotypic variance that is attributed to genetic variance) of between 0.5 and 0.96.[172,179,184,203,204]

Molecular genetic studies of human high-grade myopia

Several highly penetrant genetic loci for moderate and high myopia have been mapped (reviewed by Young et al).[205] These loci are primarily AD or X-linked. They have been mapped in either large, isolated pedigrees, or populations derived from a limited number of founders that have experienced limited migration. Except for the X-linked MYP1 gene, none of the causative mutations has yet been found.[206–209]

Much of the current information on human myopia molecular genetics can be drawn from studies of familial high-grade myopia, usually defined as spherical refractive error > – 5.00 D. An X-linked recessive form of myopia, named the Bornholm (Denmark) eye disease (BED), was designated the first myopia locus (MYP1: OMIM 310460) on chromosome Xq28.[86,206] Collaborating with BED researchers, we made comparative molecular genetic haplotype and sequence analyses of a large Minnesota family of Danish descent that showed significant linkage of myopia to chromosome Xq27.3-q28. The phenotype of both families appears to be due to a novel cone dysfunction, and not simple myopia.[207] The genetic etiology of each family appears to be distinct, as the haplotypes were different.[207] A report by Michaelides et al confirms the different X-linked cone dysfunction syndrome with an associated high myopia phenotype as distinct from the BED in four families.[208] The first identified myopia gene – CXorf2 at the MYP1 locus – has a distinct sequence mutation in the promoter region, and is a copy number variant.[209]

Loci identified to date for isolated nonsyndromic high-grade myopia are primarily AD and highly penetrant. The first AD locus for nonsyndromic high-grade myopia was mapped within a 7.6-cm region on chromosome 18p11.31 (MYP2: OMIM 160700) in seven US families.[210] This locus was confirmed in Chinese Hong Kong and Italian Sardinian cohorts.[211,212] Using the Hong Kong cohort, investigators identified transforming growth-induced factor-β (TGIF-β) as the implicated gene for MYP1 using limited single-nucleotide polymorphism (SNP) association studies and exonic sequencing.[213] Our group fully sequenced TGIF-β in our cohort of original MYP1 families, and found no associations with high myopia affected status.[214] An Australian lab also investigated the association of TGIF with refraction and ocular biometric measurements in a Caucasian case-control population, and found no association.[215] No association of TGIF to high-grade myopia case-control studies was found in Japanese and Chinese cohorts.[216,217]

A second locus for AD high myopia mapped to a 30.1 cM region on chromosome 12q21-23 (MYP3: OMIM 603221) in an American family of German–Italian descent also in our laboratory.[218] This locus was confirmed in a high-myopia Caucasian British cohort, and in a large German family.[219,220] A statistically suggestive third locus for AD high myopia was reported on chromosome 7q36 in a Caucasian French cohort (MYP4: OMIM 608367).[221] A fourth AD locus on chromosome 17q21-23 (MYP5: OMIM 608474) was determined in a large multigenerational English–Canadian family in our laboratory.[222] We identified a locus for AD high-grade myopia on chromosome 2q37 (MYP12: OMIM 609994) in a large, multigenerational US Caucasian family.[223] This locus was replicated in an Australian study of three multigenerational AD moderate myopia families.[224] We determined a new locus (MYP17) on chromosome 10q21.2 in a Hutterite (Austrian/German) colony.[225] Loci on chromosomes Xq23-25[226] (MYP13: OMIM 300613) and 4q22-27[227] (MYP11: OMIM 609994) were identified by Zhang et al in ethnic Chinese families. Other high-grade myopia loci have been recently mapped to chromosomes 15q12-13, 5p15.33-p15.2, and 21q23.3.[228–230] The first locus implicated in ocular axial length, which is a major endophenotype for refractive error, was identified on chromosome 5q.[231]

Juvenile-onset myopia genetics

At least two studies have shown nominal or no linkage of low to moderate myopia to many of the known high myopia loci. Mutti et al genotyped 53 common myopia families (at least one child with more myopia than −0.75D in each meridian) using the highest intrainterval LOD score microsatellite markers for the chromosome 18p and 12q loci and did not establish linkage.[232] Ibay et al found no strong evidence of linkage to the chromosomes 18p, 12q, 17q, and 7q in a cohort of 38 Ashkenazi Jewish families with mild/moderate myopia (−1.00 D or more).[233] These studies suggest that different genes account for mild/moderate myopia susceptibility or development, or that the gene effects are too small to be detected with the relatively small sample sizes. However, a recent study showed replication of the chromosome 2q37 (MYP12) locus in a cohort of Caucasian Australians with moderate to low myopia.[224]

Three whole-genome mapping studies have identified several candidate gene intervals for common, juvenile-onset myopia using spherical refractive error data. The results of these studies demonstrate the potential for determining

molecular genetic factors implicated in myopia at all levels of severity. These studies used microsatellite genotyping technology and a limited cohort sample size, and two used homogenous isolated populations. One study was a genome screen of 44 families of Ashkenazi Jewish descent.[234] Individuals with at least −1.00 D of myopic spherical refractive error were classified as affected. Their strongest signal localized to chromosome 22q12 (MYP6: OMIM 608908) (heterozygous linkage of the odds = 3.56; nonparametric linkage = 4.62). Eight additional regions (14q, 4q22-q28, 8q22.2, 10q22, 11q23, 13q22, 14q32, and 17qter) had nominal linkage evidence. The same group replicated the same locus with additional Ashkenazi Jewish families.[235] Hammond et al evaluated 221 dizygotic twin pairs with moderate myopia and found significant linkage to four loci, with a maximum LOD score of 6.1 on chromosome 11p13 (MYP7: OMIM 609256).[173] Other identified loci mapped to chromosomes 3q26 (MYP8: OMIM 609257: LOD 3.7), 4q12 (MYP9: OMIM 609258: LOD 3.3), and 8p23 (MYP10: OMIM 609259: LOD 4.1). This group found that the PAX6 gene at the chromosome 11p13 locus showed linkage with 5 SNPs, but no association. They suggested that PAX6 (a major eye development gene) may play a role in myopia development, possibly due to genetic variation in an upstream promoter or regulator. This group later reported that neither of the master control genes PAX6 or SOX2 was implicated in common myopia in a large population study cohort.[236] A report replicated the chromosome 8p23 myopia locus (MYP10) in an isolated Pennsylvania Amish population of 34 families.[237] Other loci identified include chromosomes 1p36, 1q, 7p15, and 3q26.[238–242]

Gene associations

High myopia also occurs as a feature of several ocular or systemic disease syndromes in which the causative disease gene is known (Table 55.1). Candidate gene association studies have led to the identification of a number of high-myopia-susceptibility genes (Table 55.2). These findings await replication in independent cohorts.

Mouse models of myopia

Factors that regulate rate and duration of eye growth in mice have revealed two loci (Eye1 and Eye2) that may be respon-

Table 55.1 Selected syndromic disorders featuring high myopia

Disorder	Disease gene
Stickler syndrome, type I (OMIM 108300)	COL2A1
Stickler syndrome, type II (OMIM 604841)	COL11A1
Marfan syndrome (OMIM 154700)	FBN1
Åland Island eye disease (OMIM 300600)	CACNA1F
Knobloch syndrome (OMIM 267750)	COL18A1
Congenital stationary night blindness, type I (OMIM 310500)	NYX
Cone–rod dystrophy, X linked, type III (OMIM 300476)	CACNA1F

Table 55.2 High-myopia-susceptibility genes

Genes	Locus
Myocilin (*MYOC*)[243]	1q23
Hepatocyte growth factor (*HGF*)[244]	7q21
Paired box gene 6 (*PAX6*)[245]	11p13
Collagen, type II alpha 1 (*COL2A1*)[246]	12q13
Lumican (*LUM*)[247]	12q21
Collagen, type I alpha 1 (*COL1A1*)[248]	17q21
Transforming growth-induced factor (*TGIF*)[213]	18p11
Transforming growth factor beta 1 (*TGFB1*)[249]	19q13

sible for larger eye size.[250,251] Human syntenic homologous regions are chromosomes 6p, 16q13.3, and 19q13 for Eye2, and chromosome 7q for Eye1.

The first knockout mouse model for relative myopia[131] was based on form deprivation experiments in chickens, mice, and rhesus macaque monkeys.[252] The immediate early gene transcription factor ZENK (also known as Egr-1) is implicated in the feedback mechanisms for visual control of

axial eye growth and myopia development.[253–255] ZENK is upregulated in retinal amacrine cells when axial eye growth is inhibited by positive lens wear, and is downregulated when axial growth is enhanced by negative lenses, suggesting that ZENK is linked to an axial eye growth-inhibitory signal. ZENK knockout mice had longer eyes and a relative myopic shift relative to heterozygous and wild-type mice with identical genetic background.[253]

Conclusions

The field of myopia science continues to expand with newer techniques of both assessing myopic development and determining molecular shifts. This chapter details research findings for the most common refractive error, myopia, describes human eye growth patterns, describes how animal models have advanced our understanding of the visually guided mechanism that matches the eye's axial length to its optical power, and discusses the genetic basis of human myopia. Understanding the molecular mechanism that controls axial length in humans is an important step toward developing customized treatments to control axial elongation.

Key references

A complete list of chapter references is available online at www.expertconsult.com. See inside cover for registration details.

2. Vitale S, Ellwein L, Cotch MF, et al. Prevalence of refractive error in the US, 1999–2004. Arch Ophthalmol 2008;126:1111–1119.

20. McCarty CA, Taylor HR. Myopia and vision 2020. Am J Ophthalmol 2000;129:525–527.

63. Fledelius HC, Christensen AC. Reappraisal of the human ocular growth curve in fetal life, infancy, and early childhood. Br J Ophthalmol 1996;80:918–921.

66. Hyman L, Gwiazda J, Hussein M, et al. Relationship of age, sex, and ethnicity with myopia progression and axial elongation in the correction of myopia evaluation trial. Arch Ophthalmol 2005;123:977–987.

95. Tejedor J, de la Villa P. Refractive changes induced by form deprivation in the mouse eye. Invest Ophthalmol Vis Sci 2003;44:32–36.

106. Kee C-S, Hung L-F, Ying QG, et al. Temporal constraints on experimental emmetropization in infant monkeys. Invest Ophthalmol Vis Sci 2007;48:957–962.

147. Siegwart JT Jr, Norton TT. Proteoglycan mRNA Levels in tree shrew sclera during minus lens treatment and during recovery. Invest Ophthalmol Vis Sci 2005;46:e-abstract 3335.

190. Wallman J. Parental history and myopia: taking the long view. JAMA 1994;272:1255–1256.

191. Mutti DO, Mitchell GL, Moeschberger ML, et al. Parental myopia, near work, school achievement, and children's refractive error. Invest Ophthalmol Vis Sci 2002;43:3633–3640.

192. Jones LA, Sinnott LT, Mutti DO, et al. Parental history of myopia, sports and outdoor activities, and future myopia. Invest Ophthalmol Vis Sci 2007;48:3524–3532.

202. Klein AP, Duggal P, Lee KE, et al. Support for polygenic influences on ocular refractive error. Invest Ophthalmol Vis Sci 2005;46:442–446.

205. Young TL, Metlapally R, Shay AE. Complex trait genetics of refractive error. Arch Ophthalmol 2007;125:38–48.

253. Schippert R, Burkhardt E, Feldkaemper M, et al. Relative axial myopia in Egr-1 (ZENK) knockout mice. Invest Ophthalmol Vis Sci 2007;48:11–17.

CHAPTER 56

Pathogenesis of Graves' ophthalmopathy

A Reagan Schiefer and Rebecca S Bahn

Clinical background

Graves' disease (GD) was named for the Irish physician, Sir Robert James Graves (1797–1853), who first described the triad of hyperthyroidism, goiter, and exophthalmos.[1] Graves' hyperthyroidism is caused by targeting and stimulation of the G protein-coupled thyroid-stimulating hormone receptor (TSHR) by TSH receptor autoantibodies, leading to the overproduction of thyroid hormones (Box 56.1).[2] After the cloning of the TSHR in 1989, insight regarding pathogenesis of GD grew markedly.[3–5] However, while recent strides have been made, the pathophysiology of Graves' ophthalmopathy (GO) remains less well understood.[2]

GD has an annual incidence in women of one per 1000 population; the annual incidence of GO in women is 16 in 100 000 and in men 3 in 100 000.[6] Approximately 25–50% of patients with Graves' hyperthyroidism have clinical eye involvement.[7] A temporal relationship exists between the onset of Graves' hyperthyroidism and the onset of GO. In 80% of affected patients, regardless of which condition occurs first, the other condition develops within 18 months.[8]

GO patients characteristically display symptoms of a dry, gritty sensation in their eyes, blurry vision, photophobia, excessive tearing, diplopia, or a pressure sensation behind the eyes.[9] The clinical signs of GO include ophthalmoplegia, lid lag, proptosis, chemosis, corneal ulceration, and conjunctival erythema (Figure 56.1). Computed tomographic scans of the orbits in 90% of GD patients reveal characteristic orbital modifications indicating eye involvement, whether or not clinical signs are present.[10] While the majority of GO patients have only mild congestive ocular symptomatology, in 3–5% severe eye disease is present, and compressive ischemic optic neuropathy with vision loss develops in the rare patient.[11]

Although the majority of GO patients have an increase in both the orbital fat and extraocular muscle volumes, some exhibit primary involvement of only one of these tissue compartments.[12] The age of the patient appears to influence the tissues involved as increased orbital fat is more commonly seen in patients younger than 40 years, and enlarged extraocular muscles predominate in patients over 70 years.[13] In early disease stages, enlargement of the extraocular muscles is caused by edema and excessive accumulation of

hyaluronic acid, leading to intermittent or inconstant diplopia. In later stages of the disease, the muscles may atrophy and become fibrotic due to the chronic inflammatory process, with resultant ocular malalignment and restrictive, constant diplopia.[6]

Pathology

Histologic examination of orbital adipose and extraocular muscle tissues in GO shows an overabundance of complex carbohydrates termed glycosaminoglycans (GAGs), in which hyaluronic acid predominates. Orbital fibroblasts are the major source of these molecules and these cells are thought to be the autoimmune target in GO.[14] In early stages of GO, muscle fibers are grossly intact, but are widely separated by edematous perimysial connective tissues resulting from accumulation of hydrophilic GAGs.[15] Similarly, expansion of the orbital adipose tissue compartment is in part attributed to accumulation of GAGs. In addition, the expansion of orbital fat results from the differentiation of a population of preadipocytes within the orbit into mature lipid-laden adipocytes.[2]

In addition to the excess of GAGs, histologic examination of orbital tissues in GO shows diffuse infiltration of lymphocytes. While these cells are predominantly T lymphocyte, occasional B cells are present as well.[2] The existence of activated lymphocytes and cytokines in GO orbital tissues suggests that the disease is autoimmune in nature.[16] The major cellular constituents are T lymphocytes showing an increase in both CD4+ and CD8+ cells, with a slight predominance of the latter. In early GO, cell-mediated T helper cell type 1 cells predominate and produce the cytokines interleukin-2 (IL-2), interferon-gamma (IFN-γ), and tumor necrosis factor-α (TNF-α). In more long-standing disease, T helper type 2 cells that participate in humoral responses are dominant and produce IL-4, IL-5, and IL-10.[17] The resident macrophages and fibroblasts release additional inflammatory mediators including IL-1α, IL-6, IL-8, IL-16, tumor growth factor-β (TGF-ß), RANTES, and prostaglandin 2 (PGE$_2$). These inflammatory mediators and chemokines incite local inflammation and activate T-cell migration across primed endothelium (Box 56.2).[18,19] The stimulatory effects of proinflammatory cytokines result in high production of

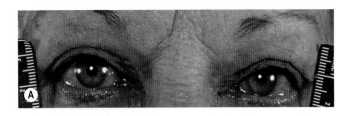

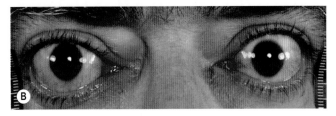

Figure 56.1 (A, B) Patients with severe Graves' ophthalmopathy demonstrating proptosis, lid retraction, conjunctival erythema, and periorbital edema.

Box 56.1 Clinical background of Graves' ophthalmology

- Graves' hyperthyroidism is caused by stimulation of thyroid-stimulating hormone (TSH) receptor by TSH receptor autoantibodies
- Approximately 25–50% of patients with Graves' disease have clinical eye involvement
- The majority of Graves' ophthalmology patients have an increase in both the orbital fat and extraocular muscle volumes

---

Box 56.2 Pathology of Graves' ophthalmology

- The expanded orbital fat compartment in Graves' ophthalmology contains excess glycosaminoglycans and a diffuse infiltration of lymphocytes
- Orbital fibroblasts produce glycosaminoglycans and a subset have the ability to differentiate into mature adipocytes
- Orbital fibroblasts are thought to be the autoimmune target in Graves' ophthalmology

---

hyaluronan by orbital fibroblasts[20]; a 50% increase in hyaluronan production has been demonstrated in these cells following exposure to IFN-γ.[21]

Etiology

Genetic contributions

Several genes, including various human leukocyte antigen (HLA) alleles,[22-25] cytotoxic T-lymphocyte antigen 4 (CTLA4),[26] T-cell receptor (TCR) ß-chain,[27] and immunoglobulin heavy chain, confer susceptibility to GD with low relative risk. However, while a number of candidate genes have been studied, including some HLA alleles, TNF-ß,

CTLA4, and TSHR, none has been shown to be associated with the development of GO in patients with GD. This suggests that environmental factors may play a more significant role than genetic factors in the development of the ocular manifestations of GD.[11]

Mechanical factors and trauma

The signs and symptoms of GO are attributable to mechanical pressures within the noncompliant, unyielding bony orbit owing to the presence of expanded orbital fat and increased extraocular muscle volume. The increased orbital tissue volume within the confines of the bony orbit leads to proptosis, or anterior displacement of the globe, which may be seen as a type of "natural" orbital decompression. The limited space for volume expansion within the bony orbit may impair venous and lymphatic outflow and result in chemosis and periorbital edema.[7] Individual variations in the orbital contour or the vascular vessels may make some patients with GD more prone to the development of clinically significant GO.[6]

The trauma delivered by orbital tissue expansion within a noncompliant bony orbit may aggravate the underlying inflammatory process. This could further stimulate release of proinflammatory cytokines and chemokines and lead to increased presentation of antigen within the orbit and augmentation of the autoimmune response.[28]

Tobacco smoking

Smoking is the primary risk factor known for the development of GO in patients with GD. The odds ratio, relative to controls, has been reported to be as high as 20.2 for current smokers and 8.9 for ex-smokers, suggesting a direct and immediate effect of smoking.[29,30] Smoking is highly associated with more severe GO[31] with failure of immunosuppressive therapy,[32] and with worsening of GO after radioiodine treatment.

Mechanisms underlying this association between smoking and GO are unclear. Smoking has been associated with other autoimmune diseases, such as rheumatoid arthritis[33] and Crohn's disease,[34] suggesting that the autoimmune process may be activated in smokers. However, circulating levels of cytokines do not appear to differ between smokers and non-smokers, except for the presence of higher levels of IL-6 receptor in the former.[35] Patients with both Graves' hyperthyroidism and GO have higher levels of circulating IL-6 receptor than do hyperthyroid GD patients without clinical GO.[36] In spite of this, there appears to be no difference in IL-6 receptor concentrations in the sera of smoking and nonsmoking GO patients.[37] In vitro studies have demonstrated that orbital fibroblasts cultured under hypoxic conditions produce increased amounts of hyaluronic acid.[38] In addition, exposure to cigarette smoke extract appears to stimulate both adipogenesis and secretion of hyaluronic acid by orbital fibroblasts.[39]

Radioiodine therapy for Graves' disease

Studies have suggested that treatment with radioiodine may worsen eye manifestations in patients with GD who have pre-existing, active GO.[40-42] In one study, 443 patients with

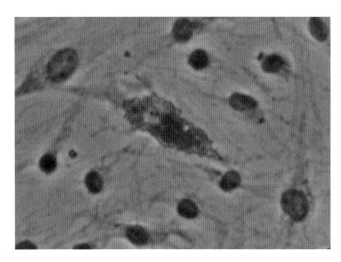

Figure 56.2 Cultured orbital fibroblasts following 10-day exposure to the PPAR-γ agonist rosiglitazone. Adipogenesis is evidenced by oil red O staining of a mature adipocyte.

GO were prospectively treated with radioiodine, methimazole, or the combination of radioiodine and prednisone.[40] The percentages of smokers and patients having GO at baseline in each group were comparable. Within 6 months of treatment, mild progression of ocular disease was seen in 15% of patients treated with radioiodine alone, in 2.7% of patients treated with methimazole, and in none of the patients treated with the combination of radioiodine and prednisone. Patients who experienced progression of ocular disease after receiving radioiodine were most commonly smokers and individuals having existing active GO.[40] It appears that progression of GO owing to radioiodine therapy does occur in some patients. However, it is generally mild and can be prevented by concurrent administration of corticosteroids. Patients with pre-existing eye disease, or those who smoke or have severe thyrotoxicosis, appear to be more likely to experience this complication (Box 56.3). In addition, ocular disease progression was not seen in another study in which postradioiodine hypothyroidism was prevented, suggesting that hypothyroidism itself might play a role and should be avoided.[43] Mechanisms responsible for ocular disease progression following radioiodine are unclear but might include increased TSHR autoantibody production, release of autoantigen from the thyroid, or destruction of radiosensitive suppressor T cells within the thyroid.

Pathophysiology

Orbital fibroblasts

Orbital fibroblasts are phenotypically heterogeneous multipotent cells that can be divided into subpopulations even within a single tissue. These subpopulations are distinguishable on the basis of the cell surface marker Thy-1.[6] A minority of fibroblasts originating from the orbital adipose/connective tissue compartment do not express this antigen (Thy-1⁻) and are "preadipocyte fibroblasts" capable of differentiating into adipocytes in the presence of PPAR-γ agonist (Figure 56.2). In contrast, perimysial fibroblasts uniformly express Thy-1 (Thy-1+) and lack the ability to undergo adipogenesis. Differences in orbital fibroblast phenotype and the distribution of these cells with orbital compartments may help to explain why some GO patients have predominant eye muscle disease while others have increased orbital adipose tissue volume as the predominant feature.[44]

Orbital fibroblasts from patients with GO appear to display amplified responses to proinflammatory cytokines compared with fibroblasts from other anatomic sites.[11] For

example, while orbital fibroblasts treated with IFN-γ or leukoregulin produce high levels of hyaluronic acid, dermal fibroblasts are only modestly stimulated by these same factors.[47] In addition, orbital fibroblasts are capable of initiating lymphocyte recruitment via their secretion of proinflammatory cytokines which, in turn, stimulate the production of chemoattractant molecules by T cells. Two such molecules, IL-16 and RANTES, account for more than 90% of T lymphocyte migration initiated by orbital fibroblasts. This suggests that these two chemoattractants act as important molecular triggers within the orbit, directing lymphocytes to areas of tissue injury and repair. Other cytokine-induced responses with potential relevance to GO include the inhibition of adipogenesis in orbital fibroblasts by TGF-ß, IFN-γ, and TNF-α, and its promotion by IL-6.[45,46] Orbital fibroblasts not only respond to cytokines, but also produce cytokines, including IL-1, IL-6, and IL-8, as well as prostaglandins, in response to ligation of their CD40 receptors by CD154 on T cells (Box 56.4).[48–50]

Orbital autoantibodies

TSHR autoantibodies

It is well accepted that autoantibodies directed against the thyroidal TSHR (TRAb) are responsible for Graves' hyperthyroidism. Due to the close clinical and temporal associations between Graves' hyperthyroidism and GO, it has been hypothesized that TRAb directed against TSHR expressed in the orbit may underlie the pathogenesis of GO. Indeed, the occurrence of GO is greatest in GD patients with the highest levels of circulating TRAbs,[51] and the clinical activity of the disease correlates with serum levels of these autoantibodies.[52]

A qualifying requirement to link TRAbs to the pathogenesis of GO is that the TSHR be expressed in orbital tissues. Recent studies have shown this to be the case as TSHR mRNA and protein have been demonstrated both in GO orbital adipose tissue and in normal orbital adipose tissue specimens.[52–54] Further, TSHR expression levels are higher in orbital fat tissues from GO patients than in those from normal individuals.[55] Additional support for this hypothesis lies in the positive correlation found between patients' clinical activity scores and TSHR mRNA levels measured in their orbital tissues removed during decompression surgery.[56]

Studies in vitro show that orbital preadipocyte fibroblasts can be induced to differentiate into mature adipocytes, and in doing so increase their expression of TSHR. When cultured in the presence in adipogenic PPAR-γ agonists, levels of TSHR mRNA, as well as mRNA encoding various adipocyte-associated genes, increase roughly 10-fold in these cells.[57,58] Studies of uncultured orbital fat specimens obtained from GO patients also show high levels of these genes compared with normal orbital fat specimens, suggesting that adipogenesis is increased within the orbit in GO.[59] Whether this is directly caused by TRAb targeting TSHR on these cells is an area of active investigation.

Gene array studies comparing GO and normal orbital adipose tissues also reveal increased expression of adipocyte-related genes in GO tissues. In addition, these studies demonstrate high expression of secreted frizzled-related protein-1 (sFRP-1), a known inhibitor of wingless type (Wnt) signaling (Box 56.5).[60] As active Wnt signaling inhibits adipogenesis, it is possible that sFRP-1 acts within the GO orbit to turn off this signaling system and thereby stimulate adipogenesis within these tissues.

IGF-1 receptor autoantibodies

Recent studies have implicated insulin-like growth factor-1 receptor (IGF-1R) as another important autoantigen in GO. Evidence for this includes that human orbital fibroblasts display high-affinity IGF-1 binding sites and that immunoglobulin G (IgG) extracted from the sera of GD patients

interacts with these sites.[61] No such effect was seen using IgG of normal patients. GD IgG has been shown to stimulate orbital fibroblasts to produce the chemokines IL-16 and RANTES, to increase production of cytokines, and to augment their synthesis of hyaluronic acid.[62,63] Evidence has been presented that these effects may be mediated through the IGF-1R, suggesting a possible role for autoantibodies directed against this receptor in the pathogenesis of GO.[61–63]

Novel approaches to therapy

Current medical management of GO is inadequate, generally imparting only modest benefit to patients as they await spontaneous improvement in the disease. While orbital decompression surgery has proven beneficial to patients with severe disease,[64] the prevention of this intervention is the goal of medical management. Recent progress in the understanding of GO pathogenesis has led to the identification of several potential targets for novel therapeutic agents (Figure 56.3). As discussed above, both the production of autoantibodies by B cells and the release of proinflammatory cytokines by activated T cells play a role in the development of GO. Therefore, targeting the initial stages of both B- and T-cell activation using costimulation inhibitors (CTLA4-Ig or alefacept) could be of therapeutic benefit (Box 56.6).[65]

Box 56.6 Novel approaches to therapy of Graves' ophthalmology (GO)

- Current medical management of GO is inadequate
- Specific monoclonal antibodies and pharmaceuticals aimed at the initial stages of both B- and T-cell activation and adipogenesis may be of therapeutic benefit
- Results of uncontrolled trials of rituximab in the treatment of GO are promising and have paved the way for randomized controlled trials which are now under way

---

Box 56.5 Autoantibodies in Graves' ophthalmology (GO)

- Orbital preadipocyte fibroblasts can be induced to differentiate into mature adipocytes with increased expression of thyroid-stimulating hormone receptors
- Gene array studies reveal increased expression of adipocyte-related genes in GO orbital tissues
- High expression of secreted frizzled-related protein-1 (sFRP-1), a known inhibitor of wingless type (Wnt) signaling, may stimulate adipogenesis in GO orbit

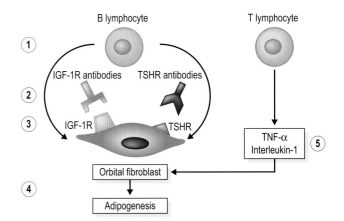

Figure 56.3 Potential targets for novel therapeutic agents in Graves' ophthalmopathy. (1) Costimulation inhibitors (CTLA4-Ig, alefacept); (2) anti-B-cell monoclonal antibody (rituximab); (3) specific novel anti-insulin-like growth factor-1 receptor (anti-IGF-1R) and anti-thyroid-stimulating hormone receptor (anti-TSHR) antibodies; (4) inhibitors of early phases of adipogenesis (PPAR-γ antagonists); and (5) biological agents that block tumor necrosis factor-α (TNF-α) (infliximab, adalimumab, etanercept) or interleukin-1R (anakinra).

Growing evidence for the involvement of TSHR and IGF-1R autoantibodies in the pathogenesis of GO has led to the concept that rituximab may be an attractive therapeutic agent to consider in the treatment of GO. This anti-B-cell monoclonal antibody targets the CD20 antigen and impacts antigen presentation and early steps in B-cell maturation.[6] Trials of rituximab in the treatment of systemic lupus erythematosus and rheumatoid arthritis have shown significant improvement in active disease concomitant with decreases in serum activity markers.[66,67] Results of uncontrolled trials of this agent in GO are promising and have paved the way for randomized controlled trials now underway.[68,69]

The participation of proinflammatory cytokines and chemokines in the development of GO suggests that monoclonal antibodies targeting these molecules might hold therapeutic promise. In particular, biological agents that block TNF-α (infliximab, adalimumab, etanercept) or IL-1 receptor (anakinra) are attractive theoretical choices that should be evaluated in randomized controlled trials.

Other approaches to GO therapy might include targeting early phases of adipogenesis in orbital preadipocytes to prevent the disease manifestations resulting from increased adipose tissue volume within the orbit. PPAR-γ ligation plays an important role in the initiation of adipogenesis and PPAR-γ agonists have been shown to stimulate both adipogenesis and TSHR expression in cultured orbital preadipocytes.[58] Therefore, agents that specifically block PPAR-γ ligation may be of benefit in GO.

Useful information regarding the efficacy of any drug (or combination of therapeutic agents) in the treatment or prevention of GO can be gained only through randomized controlled trials, several of which are currently under way. Equally important will be the continued study of GO pathogenesis and mechanisms of immune dysregulation. Information gained through these studies will be important in the development of novel approaches to prediction, prevention, and treatment of this debilitating condition.

Conclusion

Graves' hyperthyroidism is an autoimmune disease in which unregulated production of thyroid hormone results from the stimulation of the TSHR on thyroid follicular cells by circulating autoantibodies. While the pathophysiology of GO is less well understood, the condition likely stems from an autoimmune process directed against the TSHR within the orbit. Environmental factors, including mechanical pressures within the nonyielding bony orbit, smoking, and radioiodine treatment for hyperthyroidism, may also play a role in disease development. The mechanical pressures result from an increase in both the orbital fat and extraocular muscle volumes due to new fat cell development and excess accumulation of hydrated GAG, respectively. Orbital fibroblasts are thought to be the primary target cell in GO; these cells express TSHR, produce GAG, and a subset have the ability to differentiate into mature adipocytes. Novel therapies aimed at abrogating the initial stages of both B- and T-cell activation or the initiation of adipogenesis within the orbit may be of therapeutic benefit in the disease.

Key references

A complete list of chapter references is available online at www.expertconsult.com. See inside cover for registration details.

1. Khoo TK, Bahn RS. Pathogenesis of Graves' ophthalmopathy: the role of autoantibodies. Thyroid 2007;17:1013–1018.

2. Bahn RS. Pathophysiology of Graves' ophthalmopathy: the cycle of disease. J Clin Endocrinol Metab 2003;88:1939–1946.

6. Garrity JA, Bahn RS. Pathogenesis of Graves' ophthalmopathy: implications for prediction, prevention, and treatment. Am J Ophthalmol 2006;142:147–153.

32. Eckstein A, Quadbeck B, Meuller G, et al. Impact of smoking on the response to treatment of thyroid associated ophthalmopathy. Br Ophthalmol 2003; 87:773–776.

40. Bartalena L, Marcocci C, Bogazzi F, et al. Relation between therapy for hyperthyroidism and the course of Graves' ophthalmopathy. N Engl J Med 1998;338:73–78.

42. Wiersinga WM, Bartelena L. Epidemiology and prevention of Graves' ophthalmopathy. Thyroid 2002;12:855–860.

43. Perros P, Kendall-Taylor P, Frewin S, et al. A prospective study of the effects of radioiodine therapy for hyperthyroidism in patients with minimally active Graves' ophthalmopathy. J Clin Endocrinol Metab 2005;90:5321–5323.

44. Smith TJ, Koumas L, Gagnon A, et al. Orbital fibroblast heterogeneity may determine the clinical presentation of thyroid-associated ophthalmopathy. J Clin Endocrinol Metab 2002;87:385–392.

52. Heufelder AE, Dutton CM, Sarkar C, et al. Detection of TSH receptor RNA in cultured fibroblasts from patients with Graves' ophthalmopathy and pretibial dermopathy. Thyroid 1993;3:297–300.

54. Starkey KJ, Janezic A, Jones G, et al. Adipose thyrotrophin receptor expression is elevated in Graves and thyroid eye diseases ex vivo and indicates adipogenesis in progress in vivo. J Mol Endocrinol 2003;30:369–380.

59. Kumar S, Coenen MJ, Scherer PE, et al. Evidence for enhanced adipogenesis in the orbits of patients with Graves' ophthalmopathy. J Clin Endocrinol Metab 2004;89:930–935.

60. Kumar S, Leontovich A, Coenen MJ, et al. Gene expression profiling of orbital adipose tissue from patients with Graves' ophthalmopathy: a potential role for secreted fizzled-related protein-1 in orbital adipogenesis. J Clin Endocrinol Metab 2005;90:4730–4735.

Duane syndrome

Joseph L Demer

Clinical background

Duane retraction syndrome is a congenital cranial dysinnervation disorder characterized by uni- or bilateral abduction deficit, narrowing of the palpebral fissure on adduction, and globe retraction with occasional upshoot or downshoot in adduction (Box 57.1).[1] Unlike the large esotropia in abducens paralysis with which Duane syndrome shares the typical feature of abduction deficit, in Duane syndrome there is typically little to no esotropia in central gaze.

Huber's commonly used clinical classification of Duane syndrome consists of three groups: type 1, with limitation of abduction only; type 2, with limitation of adduction only; and type 3, with limitation of both ab- and adduction.[2,3] Type 1 Duane syndrome is most commonly encountered (Figure 57.1), followed by type 3. Type 2 Duane syndrome is rare, and often associated with exotropia. While there is wide agreement that unilateral Duane syndrome is more common than bilateral, the former is inconsistently reported to be more common sometimes on the left, and other times on the right, and sometimes with an inconsistent gender preponderance. Taken together, asymmetries of laterality and gender are probably artifacts of sampling and ascertainment in small studies.

An essential element of Duane syndrome is globe retraction in adduction, which is best recognized by examining the patient in profile view (Figure 57.2). As the globe translates posteriorly in the orbit, the lids slide passively together over the curvature of the globe, narrowing the palpebral fissure. The degree of globe retraction and palpebral fissure narrowing varies among affected individuals with Duane syndrome.

Pathology

The key element in the pathogenesis of Duane syndrome is abnormal innervation of the lateral rectus muscle. Limited abduction in Duane syndrome types 1 and 3 is associated with slowing of the abducting saccade,[4] a sign of deficiency in lateral rectus force generation. Normal saccades are brief, high-velocity eye movements reaching 400–700 degree/second; abducting saccades in Duane syndrome types 1 and 3 have reduced peak velocities, are visibly prolonged on physical examination, and have a lengthy terminal decelera-

tion to final position. Electromyographic studies suggest that this abduction deficiency in Duane syndrome type 1 is due to absence of normal abducens innervation to the lateral rectus muscle, and suggest that the retraction is due to paradoxical lateral rectus innervation in adduction.[2,5] Thus, in adduction, the paradoxical lateral rectus contraction counters the physiologic medial rectus contraction, increasing net posterior muscle force that causes the globe to retract against the elasticity of the orbital connective tissues. It seems plausible that the limitation of both abduction and adduction in type 3 Duane syndrome may simply be due to greater paradoxical lateral rectus contraction in attempted adduction, overcoming physiologic medial rectus contraction altogether. Duane syndrome of relatively rare type 2 may be explained by co-innervation of the lateral rectus by a normal abducens nerve, plus a strong projection of the medial rectus motor nerve to the lateral rectus that substantially or completely opposes the adducting effect of the medial rectus.

Absence of the abducens nerve and motor neurons has been confirmed in one sporadic unilateral[6] and another bilateral autopsy case of Duane syndrome.[7] Parsa et al[8] first used magnetic resonance imaging (MRI) to demonstrate absence of the subarachnoid portion of the abducens nerve in Duane syndrome, a finding that has been confirmed in six of 11 additional cases,[9] and later correlated with the presence of residual abduction in multiple cases.[10,11] Kim and Hwang have emphasized the frequent absence of the subarachnoid abducens nerve ipsilateral to Duane syndrome type 1[11,12] and type 3,[11] but the presence of the subarachnoid abducens nerve ipsilateral to type 2.[11] Examples of absence of the subarachnoid portion of the abducens nerve are illustrated in Figure 57.3. Innervation of the lateral rectus muscle by the abducens nerve is deficient in both type 1 Duane syndrome and abducens palsy, although, unlike abducens palsy, the eyes in central gaze are frequently aligned in Duane syndrome.[13] This evidence for contractile tonus in the lateral rectus muscle suggests that the involved lateral rectus is either solely, or co-innervated by a branch of the oculomotor nerve, as supported by the autopsy studies.[6,7]

Etiology

Most cases of Duane syndrome are sporadic. Some of these are clearly teratogenic, associated with intrauterine exposure to drugs such as thalidomide.[14] Other cases have well-characterized genetic causes. Dominant Duane syndrome has been linked to chromosome 2, the DURS2 locus.[15] Individuals with DURS2 exhibit unilateral or bilateral Duane syndrome types 1 or 3, or sometimes Duane syndrome type 1 in one eye and type 3 in the fellow eye.[16] This phenotypic variability indicates that the mutation causing DURS2 has variable expressivity or is modified by another genetic or environmental factor.

Duane radial ray syndrome (DRRS, also known as Okihiro syndrome, online mendelian inheritance in man 607323) is the dominant association of uni- or bilateral Duane syndrome with uni- or bilateral dysplasia of the radial bone, artery, and thumb[17] (Figure 57.4). DRRS results from heterozygous mutations in *SALL4*, a zinc finger transcription factor.[17,18] The developmental expression profile and func-

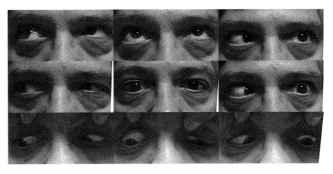

Figure 57.1 Versions in left Duane retraction syndrome type 1, showing limited abduction, with palpebral fissure narrowing in adduction.

> **Box 57.1 Clinical features of Duane retraction syndrome**
>
> - Limited ab- and/or adduction
> - Globe retraction on adduction
> - Palpebral fissure narrowing on adduction
> - Up- and downshoots in adduction (common but not universal)

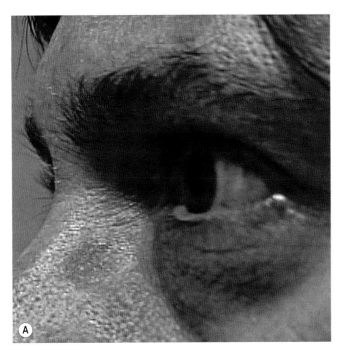

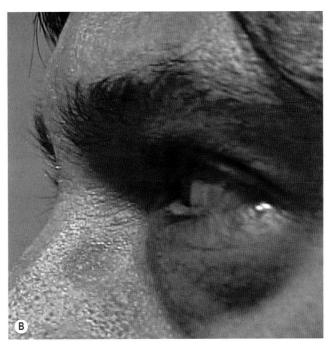

Figure 57.2 (A, B) Left globe retraction in Duane syndrome.

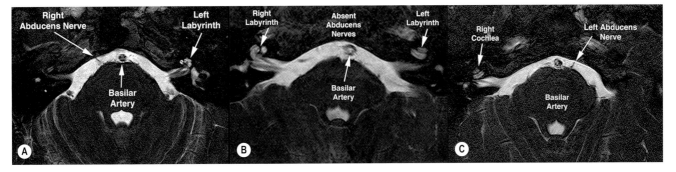

Figure 57.3 Magnetic resonance image in plane 0.8 mm thick parallel to plane of optic chiasm, obtained using fast imaging employing steady-state acquisition (FIESTA) technique, in Duane syndrome, demonstrating the subarachnoid portion of the abducens nerve. (A) Absence of the left abducens nerve. (B) Bilateral absence of the abducens nerve. (C) Absence of the right abducens nerve.

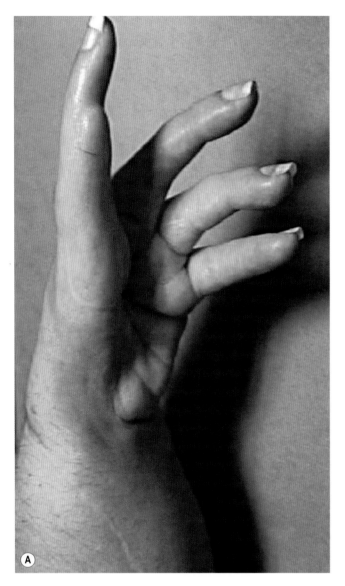

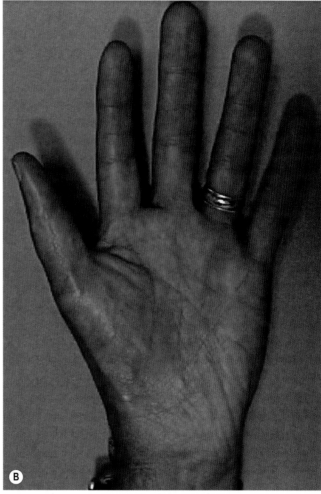

Figure 57.4 Hand abnormalities in two related patients (A) and (B) showing thenar hypoplasia in Duane radial ray syndrome.

tional role of *SALL4* in normal and abnormal ocular motor development are not yet elucidated, and *SALL4* mutations have not been identified in individuals with isolated sporadic Duane syndrome.[19] However, investigation of the role of *SALL4* in this rare form of Duane syndrome may provide important clues to its pathogenesis generally.

Pathophysiology

Imaging evidence of dysinnervation

High-resolution MRI enables direct demonstration of the size and contractility of extraocular muscles,[20] as well as their peripheral and subarachnoid motor innervation[16,21,22] (Figure 57.5A). Such MRI has shown that a branch of the inferior division of the oculomotor nerve abuts and probably enters the inferior zone of the lateral rectus muscle in dominant Duane syndrome linked to chromosome 2, the DURS2

> **Box 57.2 Peripheral neuroanatomy of Duane retraction syndrome**
>
> - Abnormality of abducens innervation to superior zone of lateral rectus muscle
> - Misrouting of inferior division of oculomotor nerve to inferior zone of lateral rectus muscle

locus.[16] The lateral rectus muscle in such cases frequently exhibits a prominent longitudinal fissure (Figure 57.5B), extending the anteroposterior length of the muscle, that divides it into superior and inferior zones.[23] When the abducens nerve is present, it innervates the superior zone of the lateral rectus muscle; innervation of the lateral rectus muscle by the oculomotor nerve is limited to the inferior zone only (Box 57.2).[16]

Other abnormalities of orbital motor innervation may be present in Duane syndrome, and may explain coexisting

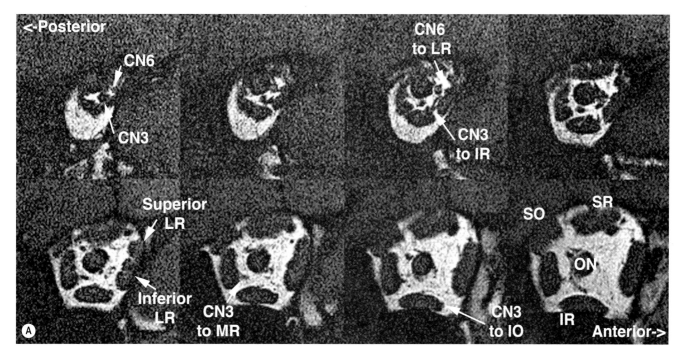

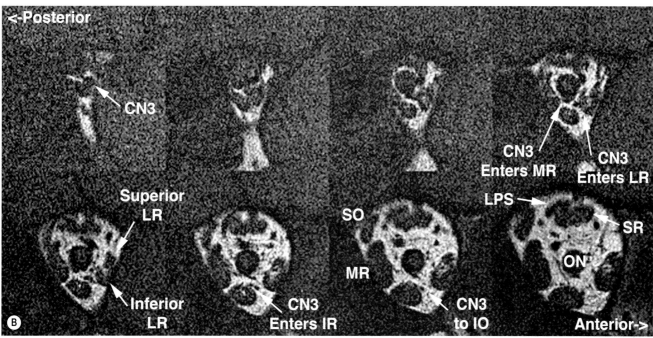

Figure 57.5 Magnetic resonance images in contiguous planes 2 mm thick, perpendicular to the long axis of the left orbit, arranged from posterior to anterior. (A) Normal orbit demonstrating innervation of the lateral rectus (LR) muscle by the abducens nerve (cranial nerve (CN) 6). The LR exhibits superior and inferior zones. IO, inferior oblique muscle; IR, inferior rectus muscle; MR, medial rectus muscle; ON, optic nerve; SO, superior oblique muscle; SR, superior rectus muscle. (B) Orbit with Duane syndrome type 1 demonstrating misinnervation of the inferior zone of the LR muscle by the inferior division of CN3. LPS, levator palpebrae superioris muscle.

vertical pattern strabismus, as well as up- or downshoots in adduction.[16] The foregoing are common in DURS2, where MRI shows that orbital motor nerves are typically small, and the abducens nerve often undetectable. Hypoplasia of the superior oblique, superior rectus, and levator is variably observed within the same families. Only the medial and inferior rectus and inferior oblique muscles have consistently normal structure.

Most cases of DURS2 exhibit evidence of oculomotor nerve innervation from axons normally targeting vertical rectus muscles leading to A or V patterns of strabismus. While MRI cannot directly image this innervation, paradoxical contractile changes in the deep belly of the lateral rectus muscle with vertical gaze changes allow secure inferences about sources of anomalous lateral rectur innervation. For example, contractile thickening of the lateral rectus muscle

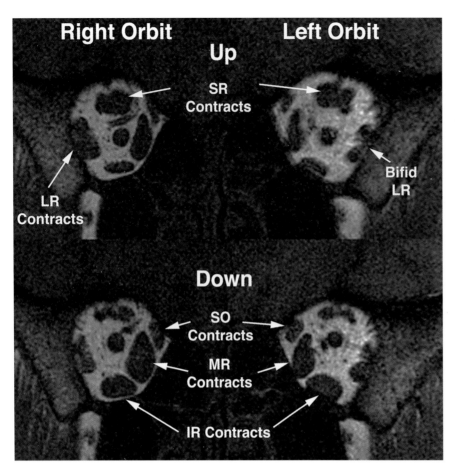

Figure 57.6 Magnetic resonance images in planes 2 mm thick, perpendicular to the long axis of the orbit, in subject with bilateral Duane syndrome type 3 demonstrating contractile thickening of the right lateral rectus (LR) muscle in upgaze, and bilateral contraction of both medial rectus (MR) muscles in downgaze. Note the prominent longitudinal fissuring of the left LR. The superior oblique (SO) and inferior rectus (IR) muscles exhibit bilateral contractile thickening in downgaze.

in upgaze associated with V-pattern exotropia allows the inference that the lateral rectus muscle is innervated or co-innervated by an oculomotor branch normally targeting the superior rectus muscles (Figure 57.6). In DURS2, the misrouted oculomotor nerve may also be hypoplastic in its subarachnoid segment, perhaps reflecting more generalized oculomotor nerve pathology.

Horizontal rectus co-contraction

While up- and downshoots of the affected eye in Duane syndrome may be due to misdirection of oculomotor nerve branches to vertically acting extraocular muscles in some cases, in other cases these phenomena are the mechanical consequences of medial and lateral rectus muscle co-contraction leading to a bridle effect mechanism (Box 57.3).[24] Normally, connective tissue pulleys prevent significant vertical sideslip over the globe of the horizontal rectus muscles, resisting muscle tendency to follow the shortest path over the globe.[25–27] In the bridle effect mechanism, the connective tissue suspensions of these pulleys presumably become weakened by aging and the abnormal forces chronically generated by horizontal rectus co-contraction. Horizontal rectus muscle paths then tend toward shortest paths, which are displaced superiorly in upgaze, and inferiorly in downgaze, relative to the normal situation. The forces exerted by horizontal rectus muscles thus vertically displaced include vertical components in the direction of displacement.

Box 57.3 Pathophysiology of Duane retraction syndrome

- Types 1 and 3: insufficient or absent abducens innervation to lateral rectus muscle limits abduction
- Type 2: oculomotor misinnervation causes lateral rectus contraction to oppose medial rectus in attempted adduction
- Medial and lateral rectus co-contraction causes globe retraction and narrows palpebral fissure
- Up- and downshoots in adduction may be due to vertical sideslip of co-contracting horizontal rectus muscles, or misinnervation of vertical rectus muscles

---

Duane syndrome with superimposed neuropathy

Binocular alignment in central gaze is nearly normal in many cases of Duane syndrome, or can be made normal by a small face turn toward the unilaterally affected side. Affected individuals frequently do not seek medical attention for this condition. Due to facultative strabismic suppression in deviated gaze positions, affected individuals seldom complain of diplopia. In infants and toddlers, Duane syndrome may go unnoticed for an extended interval before recognition. When Duane syndrome is suspected in this setting, it is important to distinguish it from the potentially ominous condition of abducens palsy. The hallmark signs of globe retraction and palpebral fissure narrowing in adduction may either not be developed in early infancy, or be unrecognizable due to the child's limited cooperation. If near orthotropia in central gaze is not present or clinically convincing in the young child with an abduction defect, orbital imaging can distinguish Duane's syndrome from abducens palsy. Chronic abducens palsy is reliably associated with lateral rectus muscle atrophy, whereas Duane syndrome is not.[20]

In patients suspected of having Duane syndrome, large angles of esotropia should motivate alternative consideration of abducens palsy, an entity in which abducens innervation to the lateral rectus muscle by the abducens nerve is also deficient and abducting saccades also slowed. However, while Duane syndrome is congenital and benign, abducens palsy may be progressive due to a growing structural lesion. A progressive mass lesion may have clinically grave consequences. Orbital imaging, by MRI or by computed X-ray tomography, may be valuable in distinguishing abducens palsy from Duane syndrome. Palsied extraocular muscles develop prominent denervation atrophy that is not observed in Duane syndrome.[20] Presumably even oculomotor innervation of the lateral rectus muscle in Duane syndrome prevents denervation atrophy in typical cases. In rare cases in which a mass compresses the oculomotor nerve, the lateral rectus will develop atrophy diagnostic of denervation.[28]

Associations with Duane syndrome

Duane syndrome may occasionally be associated with hearing defects, perhaps indicating abnormality of cochlear nerve or central hearing function.[29] A plethora of other neurological and somatic abnormalities, syndromic and nonsyndromic, has been occasionally reported in association with Duane syndrome.[30]

Duane radial ray (Okihiro) syndrome

Duane syndrome may have other syndromic associations. As noted above, DRRS due to *SALL4* mutation is associated with uni- or bilateral dysplasia of the radial bone, artery, and thumb, as well as pectoral musculature.[17,31] Despite these prominent extraocular abnormalities, DRRS is not associated with a high frequency of A- or V-pattern strabismus, structural abnormality of extraocular muscles, oculomotor nerve hypoplasia, optic nerve hypoplasia, or significant amblyopia.[31] One case of DRRS was associated with vertical saccade initiation failure, historically termed oculomotor apraxia, and is a central finding associated with metabolic disease and structural lesions of the cortex, brainstem, and cerebellum.[32]

Heritable forms of Duane syndrome

While the mutation or mutations causative for DURS2 has not been identified, its syndromic associations clearly differ from DRRS. In contrast to its relative absence in DRRS, DURS2 is associated with frequent A or lambda strabismus[31] similar to that observed in another congenital cranial dysinnervation disorder, congenital fibrosis of the extraocular muscles type 1 (CFEOM1)[21] resulting from heterozygous missense mutations in *KIF21A*.[33] In DURS2, optic nerve

cross-sections are subclinically reduced about 25% from normal,[16] while CFEOM1 due to *KIF21A* mutation is associated with 30–40% reduction in optic nerve cross-section.[21] In contrast, optic nerve size is normal in DRRS, suggesting that *SALL4* is not involved in optic nerve development or maintenance. There is little or no significant amblyopia associated with DURS2.

Moebius syndrome

Moebius syndrome is a heterogeneous clinical disorder whose clinical definition has evolved in the recent literature. The minimum criteria include congenital facial palsy with impairment of ocular abduction consistent with Duane syndrome type 1.[34–36] Thus Moebius syndrome may be considered minimally to consist of congenital facial palsy plus Duane syndrome. Other cranial nerves, orofacial malformations, limb malformations, and gross motor disturbance are also often present.[34,36] A family has been reported exhibiting complete ophthalmoplegia and bilateral facial paralysis consistent with autosomal-recessive inheritance.[37] In all three cases from that family, MRI of the brainstems and contiguous cranial nerves 3, 6, 7, and 8 exiting the brainstem were normal. All motor nerve branches, however, were abnormally small in the orbit, and the extraocular muscles were all hypoplastic. These findings suggest that Moebius syndrome includes some aspects of the pathophysiology of Duane syndrome.

Pathophysiology influences treatment of Duane syndrome

Indications for surgical treatment of Duane syndrome include central gaze strabismus, unacceptable compensatory head posture, and severe globe retraction. Since Duane syndrome is mainly due to peripheral misinnervation in the affected orbit, Hering's law of equal central innervational effort is not applicable, so strabismus surgery on the unaffected orbit of unilateral cases is generally useless in altering the innervation to the affected orbit. In cases of Duane syndrome type 1 with mild central gaze esotropia, ipsilateral medial rectus muscle recession (retroplacement on the sclera) often provides satisfactory reduction of esotropia, compensatory face turn, and may also reduce globe retraction and up- or downshoot in adduction. The affected medial rectus muscle is uniformly stiff and relatively inelastic, consistent with limited stretching due to the limited abduction. However, medial rectus recession may limit adduction to the degree that a postoperative exotropia may occur in extreme adduction of the unilaterally affected eye. Patients may develop a new and potentially disturbing diplopia when such consecutive exotropia occurs. Furthermore, medial rectus recession does little to increase the range of abduction of the affected eye.

An alternative approach to treating Duane syndrome type 1 may be particularly appropriate when a larger esotropia is present in central gaze. The superior and inferior rectus tendons may be partially or completely transposed to the edges of the affected lateral rectus insertion, along with posterior fixation of the transposed tendons to the underlying sclera to displace the vertical rectus pulleys further temporally.[38] Such an approach can increase the degree of abduction and the field of single binocular vision, but may require additional medial rectus recession simultaneously or as a later procedure if the medial rectus is excessively stiff. To avoid anterior-segment ischemia, caution may be appropriate in avoiding simultaneous disinsertion of three rectus muscles of the same eye in adults.

Surgical treatment of up- and downshoots, as well as pattern strabismus, is more complex and must be individualized to the clinical situation. Some of these signs may be due to significant structural abnormalities that may be impossible to recognize preoperatively without high-resolution orbital imaging by MRI or computed X-ray tomography. Structural abnormalities commonly include extraocular muscle dysplasia, rectus and oblique muscle hypoplasia or aplasia, and pulley heterotopy causing abnormal rectus muscle pulling directions. Surgery in such cases is tailored to the individual pathologic functional anatomy.

Up- and downshoots due to the bridle effect may respond to medial rectus recession alone. Resection of any rectus muscle is generally to be avoided, as this will increase total forces causing lid retraction, palpebral fissure narrowing, and the bridle effect. Up- and downshoots and patterns due to anomalous lateral rectus innervation will not respond to medial rectus recession. Some of these cases may respond to Y-splitting of the lateral rectus insertion, shifting the superior half superiorly on the sclera, and the inferior half inferiorly.[39]

Summary

Duane retraction syndrome is a congenital cranial dysinnervation disorder of the extraocular muscles in which the inferior zone of the lateral rectus muscle is misinnervated by the oculomotor nerve, with or without innervation of the superior zone of the lateral rectus muscle by the abducens nerve. The trochlear and optic nerves may also be abnormal, and the deep bellies of the extraocular muscles may exhibit structural anomalies. While most cases of Duane syndrome are sporadic, genetic evidence supports the concept that the condition is a developmental cranial neuropathy, leading secondarily to abnormalities of extraocular muscle structure and function.

Acknowledgment

This work was supported by NEI grants EY08313 and EY13583. Joseph L Demer is Leonard Apt Professor of Ophthalmology.

Key references

A complete list of chapter references is available online at www.expertconsult.com. See inside cover for registration details.

1. Duane A. Congenital deficiency of abduction associated with impairment of adduction, retraction movements, contraction of the palpebral fissure and oblique movements of the eye. Arch Ophthalmol 1905;34:133–159.

2. Huber A. Electrophysiology of the retraction syndromes. Br J Ophthalmol 1974;58:293–300.

6. Miller NR, Kiel SM, Green WR, et al. Unilateral Duane's retraction syndrome (type 1). Arch Ophthalmol 1982;100: 1468–1472.

11. Kim JH, Hwang JM. Presence of abducens nerve according to the type of Duane's retraction syndrome. Ophthalmology 2005;112:109–113.

13. DeRespinis PA, Caputo AR, Wagner RS, et al. Duane's retraction syndrome. Surv Ophthalmol 1993;38:257–288.

14. Miller MT. Thalidomide embryopathy: a model for the study of congenital incomitant horizontal strabismus. Trans Am Ophthalmol Soc 1991;89:623–674.

15. Engle EC, Andrews C, Law K, et al. Two pedigrees segregating Duane's retraction syndrome as a dominant trait linked to the DURS2 genetic locus. Invest Ophthalmol Vis Sci 2007;48:189–193.

16. Demer JL, Clark RA, Lim KH, et al. Magnetic resonance imaging evidence for widespread orbital dysinnervation in dominant Duane's retraction syndrome linked to the DURS2 locus. Invest Ophthalmol Vis Sci 2007;48:194–202.

21. Demer JL, Clark RA, Engle EC. Magnetic resonance imaging evidence for widespread orbital dysinnervation in congenital fibrosis of extraocular muscles due to mutations in KIF21A. Invest Ophthalmol Vis Sci 2005;46:530–539.

28. Silverberg M, Demer JL. Duane's syndrome with compressive denervation of the lateral rectus muscle. Am J Ophthalmol 2001;131:146–148.

29. Chung M, Stout T, Borchert MS. Clinical diversity of hereditary Duane's retraction syndrome. Ophthalmology 2000;107: 500–503.

31. Demer JL, Clark RA, Lim K-H, et al. Magnetic resonance imaging of innervational and extraocular muscle abnormalities in Duane-radial ray syndrome. Invest Ophthalmol Vis Sci 2007;48:5505–5511.

36. Verzijl HT, van der Zwaag B, Cruysberg JR, et al. Mobius syndrome redefined: a syndrome of rhombencephalic maldevelopment. Neurology 2003; 61:327–333.

38. Britt MT, Velez FG, Velez G, et al. Vertical rectus muscle transposition for bilateral Duane syndrome. J AAPOS 2005;9:416–421.

39. Rao VB, Helveston EM, Sahare P. Treatment of upshoot and downshoot in Duane syndrome by recession and Y-splitting of the lateral rectus muscle. J AAPOS 2003;7:389–395.

CHAPTER 58

Amblyopia

Robert F Hess and Nigel Daw

Clinical background

Classification

From a traditional clinical perspective, amblyopia is defined as a loss of visual acuity of three lines or more on a clinical letter chart that is not optically correctable and is not due to an ophthalmoscopically observable pathological cause. Amblyopia is classified by its underlying etiologic association with one or more of the following: strabismus, anisometropia, or form deprivation. Approximately one-third of amblyopes have a strabismus (eye deviation), one-third have anisometropia (unequal refractive error), and one-third have a mixture of the two. Deprivation amblyopia is rare (incidence 0.1%).

Initially amblyopia was conceptualized as a single condition resulting from one of these three types of disruption to normal visual development (Figure 58.1). Since then two more complicated classifications have been suggested, one based on the detailed properties of the behavioral deficit in small samples of amblyopes[1] that suggested a classification in terms of the presence or absence of a strabismus and the other based on a few summary measures conducted on a large sample of around 400 amblyopes, suggesting a classification based on whether binocular function has been preserved.[2] According to the summary measures of McKee et al,[2] only around 10% of strabismics have binocular function as opposed to 80% of anisometropes, so these two different dichotomies are very similar. However, what is neglected by all these classifications is that there is considerable variation from patient to patient even within one class. Amblyopia can be associated with disrupted vision at a variety of different ages and it is known from animal models that there are different critical periods for different visual functions.

Even if one were to consider amblyopia simply in terms of a monocular visual loss (which would be misleading, as argued above) it is still much more than simply a loss in visual acuity. Amblyopia is a complex syndrome in which many seemingly unrelated visual functions are impaired. Letters presented in a row with other letters adjacent are much harder to discriminate than isolated letters, a phenomenon known as crowding. Subtle spatial distortions are also a part of an amblyope's perception: the edges of letters close to the fovea are less blurred[3] and simple repetitive patterns

with a fine structure (i.e., high spatial frequencies) are seen to be distorted within central vision.[4,5] Further anomalies for spatial and motion processing are detailed below. In addition, under normal binocular viewing conditions, the two eyes of an amblyope do not work together correctly. Therefore, with both eyes open amblyopes are effectively monocular as most of the information seen by the fellow amblyopic eye is suppressed. The site and nature of this suppressive mechanism, thought to be cortical, are largely unknown but its importance, from both etiologic and treatment perspectives, is immense. Indeed, the visual deficit in the amblyopic eye that occurs under binocular viewing may include several components, including full monocular amblyopia, reduced peripheral function of the amblyopic eye's visual field in a region corresponding to the fovea of the fellow fixing eye (anomalous retinal correspondence owing to the strabismus), and suppression or masking from the fellow fixing eye (Box 58.1).[6]

Treatment

The traditional treatment for amblyopia has been to occlude the good eye with the intention of forcing the amblyopic eye to function.[7] If the child has a significant amount of hyperopia, atropine penalization can be used to blur the good eye by paralyzing its accommodation. In the case of emmetropia, an opaque occluder can be worn in front of the good eye. In the late 1980s it was generally accepted that such occlusion had to be complete and fulltime for it to be effective. This produced great psychological and social hardship for young children, most of whom were of school age, and consequently the compliance was never what it should have been.[8] Owing to a number of innovative treatment approaches,[9–13] it is now generally accepted that part time occlusion, if associated with an intensive, attention-demanding task, can be just as successful as fulltime occlusion with none of the associated psychosocial side-effects. The recovery of vision is believed to be age-dependent, with little recovery possible from occlusion beyond 12 years,[14] but see PEDIG.[15] However, active training regimes[11] based on the principle of perceptual learning have recently been shown to be effective in restoring at least some visual function in adult amblyopes.[16]

Interestingly, the rationale behind both the standard treatment for amblyopia and perceptual training approaches is that amblyopia is a monocular problem and, until the

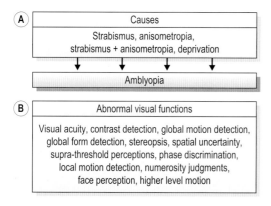

Figure 58.1 (A) Causes of amblyopia. (B) Various visual properties that are disrupted as a result.

Box 58.1 Binocular deficit

- Monocular amblyopia
- Reduced peripheral function suppression

Box 58.2 Causes of binocular loss

- Loss of binocular connections
- Interocular suppression

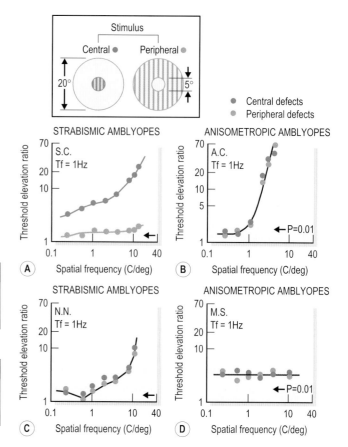

Figure 58.2 Contrast sensitivity measurements from the central and peripheral visual field for a representative strabismic amblyope and nonstrabismic anisometropic amblyope showing the selective loss of foveal function in the case of the former. (Redrawn with permission from Hess R, Campbell F, Zimmerman R. Differences in the neural basis of human amblyopias: the effect of mean luminance. Vis Res 1980;20:295–305.)

---

monocular function of the amblyopic eye is restored, one cannot expect the two eyes to work together in a binocular and/or stereoscopic sense.[17] What has been ignored[10–13] is that the monocular loss could be the consequence of disrupted binocular mechanisms that have to be rectified prior to monocular recovery and that the amblyopia per se may not be the limiting impediment to binocular function.[18] Accordingly, any therapeutic approach should involve binocular stimulation and an attempt to reduce not only the monocular acuity loss, but also any additional suppressive influences exerted by the good eye on the amblyopic eye.[6] Recent results suggesting that a reduction of intracortical inhibition in animals deprived of vision early in life leads to acuity improvement further highlight the importance of cortical suppressive mechanisms (Box 58.2).[19]

Laboratory perspective

Psychophysics

One observation[20–22] that has stood the test of time is that amblyopes require more contrast to detect stimuli with their amblyopic eyes, particularly those at higher spatial frequencies. Peak contrast sensitivity is often reduced to some extent but contrast sensitivity at higher spatial frequencies shows a more pronounced reduction. Unfortunately this has little diagnostic utility because similar losses are seen for all types of amblyopes as well as for many different types of optical, retinal, and cortical pathology. It does, however, provide a more sensitive way of monitoring recovery from treatment than the more conventional acuity measures simply because

of the steeper than unity slope of the contrast sensitivity fall off. On log/log axes this is usually between 3 and 4, giving a corresponding contrast sensitivity magnification.

The way that the contrast deficit is distributed across the visual field has some diagnostic value and suggests an important difference in the underlying mechanisms responsible for strabismic and nonstrabismic amblyopia.[1] The contrast sensitivity deficit is confined to central vision for strabismics, whereas it is more evenly distributed across the visual field in nonstrabismic anisometropes (Figure 58.2). This provides an explanation for another curious finding, that the contrast sensitivities of the two eyes of a strabismic amblyope normalize (i.e., are equated in sensitivity) under conditions of low light levels whereas those of nonstrabismic anisometropes do not.[23]

At suprathreshold levels, contrast is perceived normally by the amblyopic eye, as the deficit is confined to threshold. Again strabismics and nonstrabismic amblyopes show subtle differences in the way their visual systems go from obvious contrast deficits at threshold to normal contrast perception above threshold. For strabismics, this transition is abrupt, whereas for nonstrabismic anisometropes it is gradual.[24] For suprathreshold conditions, even though contrast is perceived normally, visual perception is quite abnormal for amblyopes for two other, possibly related, reasons that seem to have nothing to do with the aforementioned threshold deficit. The first of these reasons involves spatial distortions that mainly affect central vision and high spatial frequencies. These distortions predominantly affect strabismic amblyopes.[4] Their basis is not well understood but their presence has led to the suggestion that there may be a disruption to the retinotopic map provided by the amblyopic eye input (Box 58.3).[25] Another suggestion is that spatial distortions are a result of anomalous interactions between cells with different orientation preferences subserved by the amblyopic eye.[26] A possibly related finding is that strabismic amblyopes are more uncertain of the spatial position of objects when using their amblyopic eye.[27] Nonstrabismic anisometropes do not have such a deficit.[28] This has nothing to do with the poorer vision of the strabismic eye and it shows the unexpected property (i.e., compared with the contrast threshold deficit) of being spatial scale-invariant.[29] What this means is that the positional uncertainly of large objects is just as pronounced as that for small objects. This is shown in Figure 58.3 (left panel) where spatial accuracy in a three-element alignment task for the fixing eye is compared to that of the fellow amblyopic eye for stimuli of a number of spatial scales (i.e., sizes). Sensitivity for both eyes varies with spatial scale, being better at finer spatial scales. Importantly, the deficit in amblyopia is similar for large and fine scales. Therefore a deficit in spatial accuracy does not provide a good explanation for spatial distortion since the former is spatial scale-invariant and the latter is not. Apart from an inaccuracy there is also, in most cases, a standing distortion (measured as a bias in alignment tasks) that may well relate to the perceived distortions.[30–35] A number of attempts have been made to make this connection; both deficits could reflect different aspects of the fidelity of the retinotopic map. Animals with amblyopia secondary to a strabismus or lid suture experience exactly the same scale-invariant positional uncertainty as found in humans.[29,36] The size (often an order of magnitude or more) and spatial scale invariance of this deficit are shown in Figure 58.3 (middle and right panel). The fact that such an anomaly occurs not only in cases of strabismus but also as a consequence of lid suture suggests that a basic, but hitherto unknown, aspect of visual development has been disrupted, rather than it simply being the consequence of an adaptation to the strabismus, such as anomalous retinal correspondence.[37]

So far we have only considered the detection or appearance of stimuli in local regions of the visual field, regions small enough that they could be potentially explained in terms of single cells in V1. There are also reported deficits in amblyopia involving the processing of stimuli across much larger regions of visual space. Such tasks are considered to be "global" if information in very different regions of space has to be interrelated in some way. Cells with sufficiently large receptive fields and the processing properties required to accomplish the combination of information across space are found in the ventral and dorsal streams of the extrastriate cortex. Although local motion sensitivity (i.e., V1) is thought

to be normal in amblyopia (but see Ho and Giaschi[38]), global motion sensitivity has been shown to be anomalous in both eyes of strabismic amblyopes. The form of the deficit suggests it is not due to the visibility problem (i.e., V1) but to the "global processing" of local motion thought to occur in the dorsal stream of the extrastriate cortex.[39] Optic flow is also affected, suggesting a site beyond middle temporal area along the dorsal processing stream.[40] A similar deficit occurs for global form processing, suggesting an extrastriate deficit along the ventral processing stream.[41] There are two processes involved in the global processing of information, one involving integration and the other differentiation. The former involves the utilization of local signals distributed in different parts of the stimulus field, whereas the latter involves the segregation of signal from noise in the same parts of the field. Both operations must occur together in global signal/noise tasks (i.e., coherence measures) of the type that have revealed deficits in amblyopic processing. In similar tasks without noise where only signal integration is required, amblyopes perform normally on both a global form[42] and global motion tasks.[43] Since it is the introduction of noise to a global task that results in reduced performance for amblyopes, one is led to believe that signal/noise segregation is the main problem rather than signal integration per se.[44] Until we know more about the physiological basis for this important operation in normal vision, it is premature to discuss its physiological basis in amblyopia. However, a starting point would be the suppressive surrounds that have been shown to be an important part of extrastriate receptive fields (e.g., MT) and thought to play a role in signal/noise segregation.[45]

There are also suggestions that the deficits in amblyopia extend to visual cognition (Box 58.4). It has been shown that numerosity judgments are deficient,[46] that higher-order motion[38] is defective, and that the perception of faces is impaired.[47]

Models

Models of visual loss in amblyopia are not well developed and tend to apply only to separate aspects of the dysfunction. They have tried to explain the contrast sensitivity deficit and the binocular vision deficit in terms of the function of single cells in area V1. None has been completely successful. For example, the loss of contrast sensitivity in amblyopia that affects mainly high spatial frequencies and central vision, at least for strabismics, is thought to be located in area V1 because some centrally located neurons display reduced contrast sensitivity and anomalous spatial properties.[48] The fact that there is such variability from animal to animal and that the magnitude of the single-cell deficit is not enough to explain adequately the full extent of the behavioral deficit has led people to think that there is more to the story than is gleaned from the responses of single cells

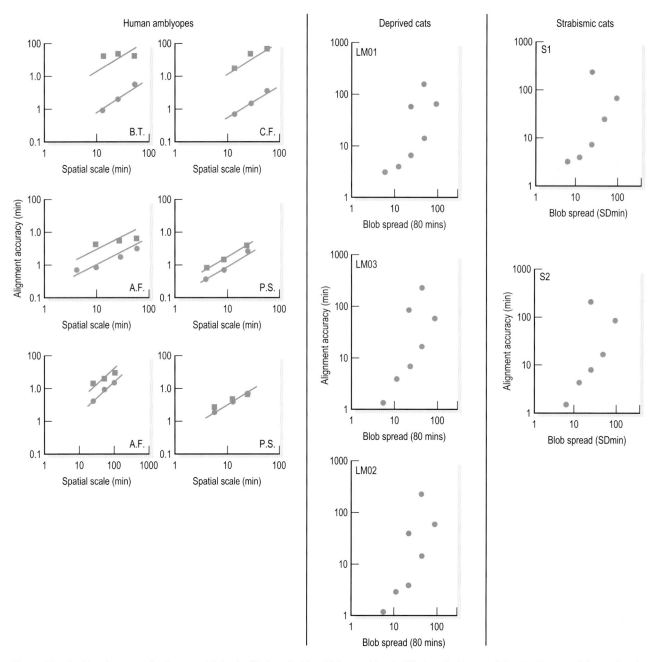

Figure 58.3 Positional accuracy for the normal fixing (unfilled symbols) and fellow amblyopic (filled symbols) eyes of deprived humans (left panel) and cats (middle and right panels) for a three-element alignment task where all the stimuli were of equal suprathreshold contrast for both eyes. The results are plotted against the spatial scale or size of the stimuli to be aligned. The deficit is the same at all spatial scales (i.e., spatial scale invariant). (Redrawn with permission from Hess R, Holliday I. The coding of spatial position by the human visual system: effects of spatial scale and contrast. Vision Res 1992;32:1085–1097; Gingras G, Mitchell DE, Hess RF. The spatial localization deficit in visually deprived kittens. Vision Res 2005;45:975–989.)

in V1.[49] In strabismic animals with a mild to moderate amblyopia there do not appear to be fewer neurons subserving the amblyopic eye, but some of these neurons do show a reduced sensitivity.[49] In strabismic animals where the amblyopia is severe, there is a suggestion that fewer neurons (i.e., as determined by the encounter rate) might subserve amblyopic function.[50,51] What is generally agreed is that fewer neurons appear to have binocular connections in amblyopic animals.[52]

The binocular vision deficit in amblyopia has traditionally been thought to be the result of loss of binocular connections in area V1.[52] However, a recent study[53] has shown that binocular summation can be normal in strabismic amblyopes once the sensitivity difference between their eyes is taken into account, suggesting that substantial binocular connections may be intact. It remains a possibility that the connections at the single-cell level are in fact intact and that this can only be revealed by first equating the contrast of the

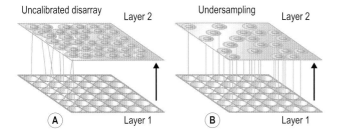

Figure 58.4 Two competing models to explain the spatial accuracy deficit in amblyopia. (A) A normal complement of cells with disordered connections. (B) Fewer cells with normal connections.

inputs to the two eyes, or observing the influence of one eye's input on the other, rather than the response from each eye alone. Another important aspect of the physiology is that strabismic animals display interocular inhibitory interactions[54] that may underlie the reduced binocular function in strabismic amblyopia and which may be amenable to treatment. There is good evidence that binocular function, including stereo, can be restored in strabismic and anisometropic amblyopes under suitable treatment regimes.[9,10,12,13,55] The key issue for the future is to understand the nature of these suppressive interactions that prevent normal binocular and stereoscopic function in amblyopia.

The positional uncertainty deficit that is an important feature of the vision of strabismic amblyopes (Figure 58.3) has been explained in two related ways. Levi and Klein[27] suggested that there were fewer cells driven by the amblyopic eye and as a consequence of the less than adequate sampling of space, positional accuracy is reduced (Figure 58.4B). The scale invariance of the deficit (Figure 58.3) would then imply that this undersampling occurs equally at all scales. The other proposal (Figure 58.4A) is that there is an uncalibrated neural disarray, implying not fewer cells, but rather a disarray in the retinotopic map. The idea is that at birth our visual systems are broadly accurate in their retinotopy but during visual experience this is refined or calibrated by functional Hebbian rules. A strabismus disrupts this calibration and results in a positionally uncalibrated cortex for the input from the deviated eye. While both proposals are able to explain the inaccuracy problem, the disarray hypothesis can account for the fixed spatial distortions reported by amblyopes.[56,57] The physiology suggests that there are a number of explanations including a loss of cells, modified cellular properties, and aberrant nerve connections.

The global motion and global form deficits in amblyopia have been investigated more extensively psychophysically. It has been proposed that the deficits are not due to poor contrast sensitivity or indeed poor local motion or local orientation discrimination, as might occur in area V1, but rather are due to impaired segregation of signal and noise,[58] a property of extrastriate cortex.

Brain imaging

The use of functional brain imaging in amblyopia is still at an early stage and the expectation that it will provide the

link between the behavioral picture of the dysfunction and the single-cell models has not yet been realized. What researchers have been able to show is that the cortical dysfunction extends well beyond V1, involving a substantial region of extrastriate cortex.[59-61] This is shown in Figure 58.5, where functional activation is displayed on a flattened region of cortex, comparing the fixing and fellow amblyopic eye stimulation. The solid lines demark the boundaries of the different retinotopically distinct visual areas.

The deficit is extensive, involving a substantial region of extrastriate cortex. This is not surprising given the now well-documented behavioral deficits for global form,[62] global motion,[39,40] higher-level motion and tracking,[38,63] numerosity,[46] positional uncertainty,[28,57] and face perception.[47] The single-cell models have concentrated on the V1 deficit in order to explain the contrast sensitivity deficit which is only a part, and possibly not that important a part, of the amblyopic syndrome. However, even the contrast sensitivity deficit may not be able to be adequately explained by considering V1 alone.[48]

An interesting result is that the retinotopic map supplied by the amblyopic eye is not as accurate as that from the fellow normal eye, at least in some strabismic amblyopes.[64] This finding is not related to the reduction in acuity, or the magnitude of activation for that matter, but may play a role in the increased positional uncertainty and/or the spatial distortions known to be a property of the vision of strabismic amblyopes. It may reflect a human analog of the small adaptive shift in retinal coordinates found for cells in the lateral suprasylvian cortex of strabismic cats[65] and postulated to be the neural basis of anomalous retinal correspondence.[66]

Critical periods

It has been known for a long time that there is a critical period for the creation of amblyopia. This comes out most clearly in studies of strabismus in humans, where the onset of strabismus after the age of 7–8 years does not cause amblyopia.[66] The time course of the critical period for the production of ocular dominance shifts by monocular deprivation has been worked out for several species (Figure 58.6). It starts a short time after opening, peaks at a young age, and declines from then until puberty.

Experiments in both animals and humans have shown that there is not a single critical period, but several. Amblyopia can be reversed after the critical period for its creation is over; there are different critical periods for different visual functions; the duration of the critical period depends on the severity of its cause and the previous visual history of the animal; and in some circumstances a deficit can be created in the adult.[67]

The ability to reverse amblyopia after the end of the critical period emerges most clearly in studies of human anisometropia. A regime of full refractive correction, lenses, or prisms to improve alignment, 2–5 hours/day of occlusion, and active vision therapy over 10–20 weeks improves acuity by 75–100% in patients 8–49 years of age.[68] The success appears to be due to the time and efforts of both eye care practitioners and patients. In addition, there are several cases showing recovery from strabismic amblyopia, in particular

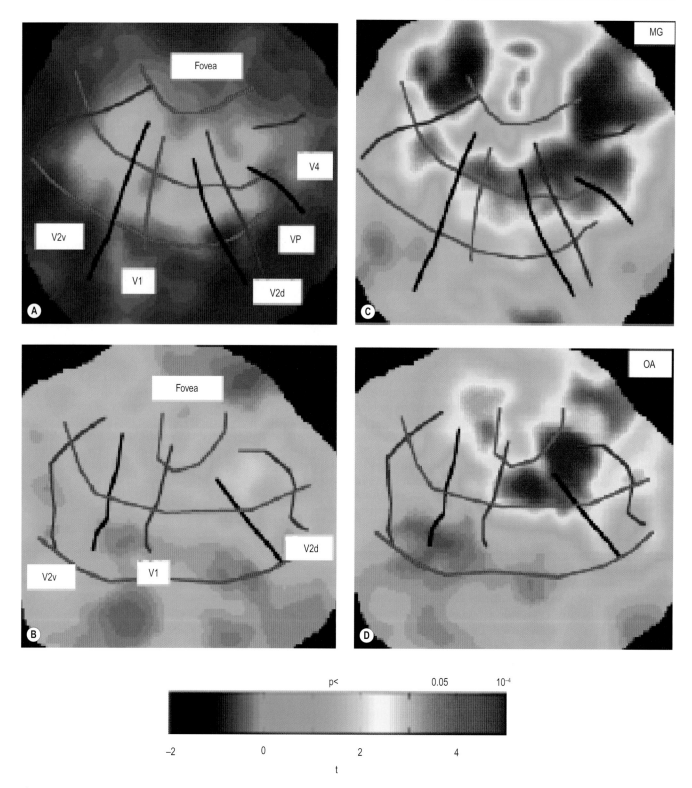

Figure 58.5 (A–D) Functional activity in the occipital lobe of two amblyopes in response to stimulation of either the fellow or amblyopic eye. The amblyopic eye produces substantially less functional activity than the fellow eye. The solid lines demark the different retinotopically distinct areas of the visual cortex and the color bar denotes the magnitude of activation in T value. The extent of the amblyopic activation deficit extends well beyond V1, involving much of the extrastriate visual cortex. (Redrawn with permission from Barnes GR, Hess RF, Dumoulin SO, et al. The cortical deficit in humans with strabismic amblyopia. J Physiol 2001;533:281–297.)

Table 58.1 Major syndromes/conditions associated with strabismus

Genetic/developmental

Congenital fibrosis of the extraocular muscles

Down syndrome

Marfan syndrome

Albinism

Sotos syndrome

Duane retraction syndrome

Brown syndrome

Moebius syndrome

Prader–Willi syndrome

Chiari malformation

Craniofacial dysostoses

Mitochondrial myopathies

Charcot–Marie–Tooth disease/centronuclear myopathy

Acquired

Fetal alcohol syndrome

Fetal hydantoin syndrome

Premature birth/perinatal hypoxia

Hydrocephalus/Sylvian aqueduct syndrome

Cerebral palsy

Myasthenia gravis

Graves disease

Multiple sclerosis

Stroke

Table 58.2 Treatment options for strabismus/amblyopia

Type	Purpose	Chapter references
Corrections of refractive error	Sharpen retinal image to promote fusion	2
	Relieve accommodative convergence	9
Extraocular muscle exercises	Strengthen convergence Reduce suppression	2
Eye patch, penalization	Reduce suppression/treat amblyopia	2, 9
Pharmacological treatment		
Botulinum toxin	Weaken the overacting muscle	16, 17, 19, 20, 44
Trophic factors	Strengthen the underacting muscle	41, 42, 44
Surgical treatment		
Resection	Strengthen extraocular muscle	2, 25
Recession	Weaken extraocular muscle	2, 25
Transposition	Treatment of paralytic strabismus	21, 22

pathway, which deals with fine detail and acuity.[70] In cats, the critical period for sensitivity to direction of movement ends earlier than the critical period for ocular dominance.[71] In human strabismus, it is difficult to produce improvement in stereopsis after 2 years of age, notwithstanding the case of stereo Sue, whereas improvement in acuity can be obtained after operations up to 7–8 years of age.[66] The production of amblyopia in adults has been found so far in mice with monocular deprivation and a light anesthetic[72] – monocular deprivation being a more severe form of deprivation than strabismus, which in turn is more severe than anisometropia (Tables 58.1–58.4).

Pathophysiology

Experiments on animals have demonstrated some of the physiological mechanisms involved in amblyopia, mostly from models of deprivation amblyopia. Axons coming from the deprived eye retract, and axons from the nondeprived eye expand, with corresponding changes in the dendrites of the postsynaptic cells. In addition to these anatomical changes, there are physiological changes in the neural connections leading to the strengthening of active synapses and the weakening of inactive ones. The afferent signals activate receptors, second messengers, and various genes and proteins involved in these changes. Several of these substances are more abundant, or more active, during the critical period, accounting for the ability of the visual cortex to adapt to strabismus, anisometropia, and deprivation in infants and children.[69] These are called plasticity factors.

The reduced ability of the adult visual cortex to make similar adaptations can be attributed partly to the lack of these plasticity factors. In addition, the neurons become less

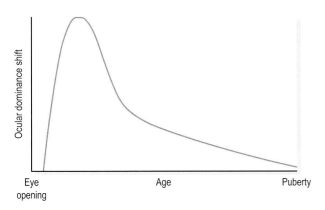

Figure 58.6 Critical period for ocular dominance shifts produced by monocular deprivation. The critical period starts shortly after eye opening, peaks a few weeks (rodents and higher mammals) or months (humans) after that, and declines until near puberty. At the peak, several days of monocular deprivation can produce a large ocular dominance shift.

the interesting case of stereo Sue, with recovery of stereoscopic vision in her 40s.[55]

The point that there are different critical periods for different visual functions emerges most clearly from experiments with animals.[69] In macaques, the critical period for the magnocellular pathway, which deals with movement, occurs earlier than the critical period for the parvocellular

Table 58.3 Causes of strabismus

Cause	References
Abnormal orbital pulleys (fibroelastic sleeves)	46–48
Orbital fibrosis/inflammation	Chapter 54
Mitochondrial myopathies	29
Orbital trauma/skull fracture	
Imbalance of extraocular muscle contractile force generation	
Abnormal tonic myofibers (multiply innervated fibers)	
Dysfunction of proprioceptive feedback (?)	6, 31
Abnormal neuromuscular junctions on extraocular muscles (myasthenia gravis)	29, 32
Cranial nerve palsies or dystrophies	
Cranial nerve nuclei agenesis or axonal misrouting	8, Chapter 58
Faulty afferent motor commands	
Internuclear ophthalmoplegia	9, 36
Abnormal motor command processing in midbrain/pons/cerebellum/brainstem	
Abnormal binocular processing in frontal eye field/extrastriate cortex	3
Abnormal binocular circuits/ocular dominance columns in visual cortex	3
Deficiencies in optic radiations/tract/optic nerve (hypoplasia) or thalamus	
Abnormal retinal circuitry/ retinoblastoma	
Defects (refractive errors) in the optic apparatus (lens/cornea): cataract/astigmatism	

Table 58.4 Animal models for strabismus and extraocular muscle (EOM) research

Animal	Advantages	Disadvantages	Chapter references
Monkeys	Human-like, frontal-eyed	Expensive	3, 5, 6, 24, 29, 35
Cats	Frontal-eyed, developmental model		6, 29, 35
Rabbits	Large EOMs, trophic factors	Lateral-eyed	41, 44
Rodents	Probes for gene expression		
Rats	Standard model	Poor vision, small EOMs	29
Mice	Genetic model	Poor vision, small EOMs	8, 29
Chicken	Developmental model, large EOMs	Lateral-eyed	6, 50

the end of the critical period.[74] This is a very active area of research, but none of these findings is close to leading to a therapy in humans.

Summary

Amblyopia is not one condition but many. In each, a number of basic visual functions are disrupted, ranging from contrast sensitivity to positional uncertainty to higher cognitive functions such as numerosity. The deficit is mainly cortical and extends well beyond V1 to include large areas of processing in the dorsal and ventral streams of the extrastriate cortex. It is produced by imbalancing the visual input to the two eyes during the critical period of early visual development. Since there are different critical periods for different visual functions, the timing of this early visual disruption may be critical for the type of amblyopic produced and may account for the heterogeneity of the condition.

plastic for structural reasons. For example, they become myelinated, so that in mice mutant for the myelin NoGo receptor, plasticity is maintained beyond the end of the critical period.[73] Moreover, there is a condensation of extracellular proteins into perineuronal nets, so that mutants that affect these processes also have increased plasticity beyond

Key references

A complete list of chapter references is available online at www.expertconsult.com. See inside cover for registration details.

1. Hess RF, Pointer JS. Differences in the neural basis if human amblyopias: the distribution of the anomaly across the visual field. Vis Res 1985;25:1577–1594.

4. Hess RF, Campbell FW, Greenhalgh T. On the nature of the neural abnormality in human amblyopia; neural aberrations and neural sensitivity loss. Pflugers Arch Eur J Physiol 1978;377:201–207.

24. Hess RF, Bradley A. Contrast coding in amblyopia is only minimally impaired above threshold. Nature 1980;287:463–464.

28. Hess RF, Holliday IE. The spatial localization deficit in amblyopia. Vis Res 1992;32:1319–1339.

29. Gingras G, Mitchell DE, Hess RF. The spatial localization deficit in visually deprived kittens. Vis Res 2005;45:975–989.

30. Bedell HD, Flom MC. Monocular spatial distortion in strabismic amblyopia. Invest Ophthalmol Vis Sci 1981;20:263–268.

39. Simmers AJ, Ledgeway T, Hess RF, et al. Deficits to global motion processing in human amblyopia. Vis Res 2003;43:729–738.

48. Kiorpes L, Kiper DC, O'Keefe LP, et al. Neuronal correlates of amblyopia in the visual cortex of macaque monkeys with

experimental strabismus and anisometropia. J Neurosci 1998;18:6411–6424.

53. Baker DH, Meese TS, Mansouri B, et al. Binocular summation of contrast remains intact in strabismic amblyopia. Invest Ophthalmol Vis Sci 2007;48:5332–5338.

54. Sengpiel F, Jirmann K-U, Vorobyov V, et al. Strabismic suppression is mediated by interactions in the primary visual cortex. Cerebral Cortex 2006;16:1750–1758.

59. Barnes GR, Hess RF, Dumoulin SO, et al. The cortical deficit in humans with strabismic amblyopia. J Physiol (Lond) 2001;533:281–297.

67. Daw NW. Critical periods and amblyopia. Arch Ophthalmol 1998; 116:502–505.

68. Wick B, Wingard M, Cotter S, et al. Anisometropic amblyopia: is the patient ever too old to treat? Optom Vis Sci 1992;69:866–878.

73. McGee AW, Yang Y, Fischer QS, et al. Experience-driven plasticity of visual cortex limited by myelin and Nogo receptor. Science 2005;309:2222–2226.

74. Pizzorusso T, Medini P, Berardi N, et al. Reactivation of ocular dominance plasticity in the adult visual cortex. Science 2002;298:1248–1251.

CHAPTER 59

Strabismus

Christopher S von Bartheld, Scott A Croes,
and L Alan Johnson

Evolution has bestowed humans and other frontal-eyed foveate animals with considerable overlap of the visual fields from the right and left eye. This allows for binocular vision and stereopsis. The three-dimensional appearance of fused binocular objects and depth perception are major perceptual advances in evolution with adaptive value.[1] Unfortunately, the advantages of binocular fusion and resulting correspondency of fused objects come with a price: they allow for the possibility of diplopia (double vision). Diplopia arises when the two eyes are misaligned – a condition called strabismus (Greek for squint). Strabismus has different consequences, depending on whether the misalignment occurs in a developing infant or in a mature adult. The successful formation of neural (and especially cortical) circuits for binocular vision is intricately linked to eye alignment and proper visual processing during development. This chapter provides an overview of strabismus with emphasis on the circular nature of interactions between the eye and the brain, and discusses current knowledge of pathophysiological mechanisms as well as treatment options.

Clinical background

Key symptoms and signs

Strabismus is a misalignment of the eyes which may occur in the horizontal or vertical direction (Figure 59.1), or along a torsional axis.[2] This misalignment may be constant, intermittent, or present only when normal binocular vision is interrupted. The term strabismus derives from the Greek *strabizein*, meaning to squint, to look obliquely or askance. Depending on age of onset, the individual may be asymptomatic, or may experience diplopia (double vision) or asthenopia (eyestrain).[2] Diplopia is rarely a symptom in childhood strabismus, due to the development of suppression – the brain actively "turns off" one cortical image, usually that from the deviated (weaker) eye. Thus, strabismus in children can cause amblyopia (loss of visual acuity not directly attributable to a structural abnormality of the eye or visual pathways: see Chapter 58). In both children and adults, strabismus results in a partial or complete degradation of the quality of binocular vision. Infantile esotropia (inward turning of one or both eyes) is more common than exotropia (an outward deviation of the eye) by a ratio of about 10:1.[3] Many genetic and other syndromes are associated with strabismus (Table 59.1).

Historical development

Strabismus has a history in European, but not other cultures,[4] as the "evil eye" of mythology and primitive folklore, as exemplified by Flotsam and Jetsam, the creepy, cross-eyed servants of the sea witch, Ursula, in Disney's animated feature film, *The Little Mermaid*. Hippocrates noticed that strabismus frequently affects parents and their children. Paulus of Aegina (Alexandria, 625–690) developed the use of a perforated mask to guide the squinting eye.[4] Al-kindi ("Alkindius") from Baghdad (813–873) advocated occlusion therapy and ocular exercises. A malposition of the lens or cornea was held responsible in the 18th century. In 1743, Buffon realized that the squinting eye had poorer vision and corrected refractive anomalies with glasses. Surgical treatment became common in the 19th century. Famous persons with squint include Michelangelo's sculpture of David, and the 16th American president, Abraham Lincoln. The history of strabismus was comprehensively reviewed[4] and modern research and hypotheses about major causes of strabismus summarized.[5]

Epidemiology

The prevalence of strabismus among humans and other primates is approximately 4–6% with little geographic variation.[3,6] Thus, the number of people affected by strabismus worldwide in 2008 was about 330–350 million. Males and females are equally affected. The risk of infantile esotropia increases significantly in infants with prematurity, neonatal intraventricular hemorrhage, Down syndrome, or hydrocephalus.[3] The importance of strabismus is reflected by the fact that four professional vision journals are devoted to strabismus: *Journal of Pediatric Ophthalmology and Strabismus* (since 1978); *Strabismus* (1993); *Binocular Vision and Strabismus Quarterly* (1996); and *Journal of American Association for Pediatric Ophthalmology and Strabismus* (1997).

Genetics

There is a genetic predisposition to strabismus. With the exception of some specific strabismus syndromes, the inher-

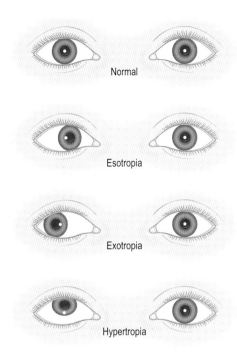

Normal

Esotropia

Exotropia

Hypertropia

Figure 59.1 Deviation of the eyes in strabismic humans. The Hirschberg test ("corneal light reflex") assesses eye alignment by the location of the light reflex. Note the light reflex centered in the straight, but not the deviated eyes. (Modified from Wright KW. Pediatric Ophthalmology and Strabismus. St. Louis: Mosby, 1995.)

Table 59.1 Major syndromes/conditions associated with strabismus

Genetic/developmental
Congenital fibrosis of the extraocular muscles
Down syndrome
Marfan syndrome
Albinism
Sotos syndrome
Duane retraction syndrome
Brown syndrome
Moebius syndrome
Prader–Willi syndrome
Chiari malformation
Craniofacial dysostoses
Mitochondrial myopathies
Charcot–Marie–Tooth disease/centronuclear myopathy
Acquired
Fetal alcohol syndrome
Fetal hydantoin syndrome
Premature birth/perinatal hypoxia
Hydrocephalus/sylvian aqueduct syndrome
Cerebral palsy
Myasthenia gravis
Graves' disease
Multiple sclerosis
Stroke

itance pattern appears to be multifactorial. Approximately 20–30% of children born to strabismic parents will develop strabismus.[3] Twin studies have shown a 70–80% concordance in monozygotic twins, but 30–40% in dizygotic twins.[7] The cause of several congenital strabismus syndromes was localized to mutations in genes required for the development and connectivity of motoneurons that innervate extraocular muscles.[8]

Diagnostic workup

Both sensory and motor factors must be assessed. Ocular alignment can be grossly evaluated by the position of the corneal reflection of a light held in front of a patient's eyes – in normally aligned eyes the light reflection is positioned symmetrically in each pupil (Figure 59.1). In the cover test, movement of the eyes is examined first with vision in both eyes, and then the eyes are alternately blocked by an occluder as the patient maintains visual fixation on a target. Movement of the unoccluded eye indicates strabismus[9] (Figure 59.2). Variations of the cover and prism test more accurately assess and quantify the angle of deviation which is important for treatment and follow-up[10] (Figure 59.2). Sensory evaluation determines the presence of diplopia, suppression, anomalous retinal correspondence, and stereopsis.[2,11,12] High-resolution orbital imaging (e.g., by dynamic magnetic resonance imaging) can reveal additional pathophysiological mechanisms relevant for treatment.[13] These measures – and the patient's history – contribute to determine the likely etiology and appropriate treatment (see below).

Differential diagnosis

Two conditions can be confused with true strabismus. In pseudostrabismus a wide, flat nasal bridge and epicanthal folds contribute to an esotropic appearance.[9] Abnormalities of "angle kappa" reflect an increased disparity between the visual axis and the anatomic pupillary axis.[9] In both conditions, cover testing will reveal the lack of actual strabismus.

Treatment

The treatment of strabismus varies with the type and cause. The correction of refractive errors with glasses is important. Appropriate hyperopic spectacle correction may be the only treatment needed for accommodative esotropia (overconvergence in response to a hyperopic refractive error). Types of strabismus that are due to weakness of the fusional reflexes can be treated with occlusion of one eye to reduce the suppression response and to increase the brain's fusional response,[2] or with exercises to strengthen the convergence reflex. Some optometrists advocate visual training more generally, but the effectiveness for other types of strabismus is controversial.[14,15] Botulinum toxin can be injected into overacting extraocular muscles to reduce their contractility.[16–19] This approach is used in small-angle esotropia and in paretic strabismus where the toxin is injected into the overacting

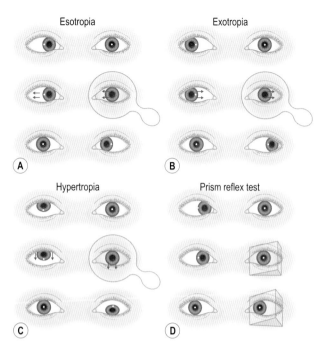

Esotropia

Exotropia

Hypertropia

Prism reflex test

(A)   (B)   (C)   (D)

Figure 59.2 Cover and prism tests for the diagnosis of strabismus. In the normal individual (shown in Figure 59.1), the eyes remain straight when covered. (A) Esotropia: outward movement indicates that the right eye is esotropic. (B) Exotropia: inward movement indicates a right exotropia. (C) Hypertropia: movement of the right eye indicates a right hypertropia. (D) Measuring the angle of deviation with the Krimsky test: prisms of increasing power are placed before the strong (fixating) eye until the light reflex is centered in the weak (deviating) eye. Prisms of increasing power can also be placed before one eye until the shift of the eyes with alternating cover is neutralized (prism/alternate cover test). (Modified from Wright KW. Pediatric Ophthalmology and Strabismus. St. Louis: Mosby, 1995 and von Noorden GK. Atlas of Strabismus, 4th edn. St. Louis: Mosby, 1983.)

Box 59.1 Importance of early treatment

Early treatment – within months of recognition – is advised for optimal outcome in infantile strabismus

---

antagonist muscle to the paretic muscle.[20] The main techniques of strabismus surgery consist of recession to weaken an extraocular muscle (physically shortening it by moving its normal insertion), resection to strengthen a muscle (by removing a portion of the muscle), or transposition (by moving a muscle out of its original plane of action to assume the action of a paretic muscle).[21,22]

Early treatment is advised in infantile esotropia to allow for the potential development of binocular vision and to decrease the risk of amblyopia and abnormal binocular vision as the visual system matures (Box 59.1). A short interval between symptoms and alignment is a powerful predictor of treatment success. The eyes should be aligned within months upon recognition of the misalignment.[3,11,12,23,24]

Sensory deficiencies such as a cataract, refractive error, or amblyopia have to be addressed, because sensory fusion is needed to maintain eye alignment and prevent postsurgical drift. In adults with acquired strabismus from trauma or cranial nerve palsy, a period of observation for spontaneous improvement is often indicated. In adults, small deviations may be managed with prism glasses, but larger deviations

Table 59.2 Treatment options for strabismus/amblyopia

Type	Purpose	References
Correction of refractive error	Sharpen retinal image to promote fusion	2
	Relieve accommodative convergence	9
Extraocular muscle exercises	Strengthen convergence	2
	Reduce suppression	
Eye patch, penalization	Reduce suppression/treat amblyopia	2, 9
Pharmacological treatment		
Botulinum toxin	Weaken the overacting muscle	16, 17, 19, 20, 44
Trophic factors (experimental)	Strengthen the underacting muscle	41, 42, 44
Surgical treatment		
Resection	Strengthen extraocular muscle	2, 25
Recession	Weaken extraocular muscle	2, 25
Transposition	Treatment of paralytic strabismus	21, 22

usually require eye muscle surgery[25] or botulinum injections (Table 59.2).

Prognosis and complications

Strabismus treatment reduces the likelihood of amblyopia and potentially restores binocular vision. The potential to relieve diplopia and improve binocularity ("fusional potential") is present in both children and adults.[9,26] Strabismus carries a stigma and psychosocial burden, i.e., strabismic patients may be regarded as less intelligent and can face discrimination in job hiring and promotion.[27] Strabismus treatment should be considered restorative, rather than purely cosmetic.[2,3] The most frequent complication of strabismus surgery or botulinum injection is an over- or undercorrection which may require further treatment. Success rates after single botulinum injections are lower (30–40%) than after initial surgery (90%), but final results after multiple botulinum injections can be comparable. Success rates differ between studies, based on the type of strabismus being treated.[17–20,33]

Pathology

Pathologies of strabismus vary greatly with the particular primary etiology (see below) and secondary adaptations that occur in response to the disturbance of binocular vision. At the level of the extraocular muscles, primary pathological conditions may involve inflammation, infiltration, fibrosis, scarring after trauma, as well as secondary adaptations due to altered usage of the muscle.[28,29] Tissue from congenitally strabismic human eye muscles was examined for alterations in ultrastructure. Damaged myofibers were found, particularly at the scleral aspect, and damaged myofibers were lacking palisade endings (potential proprioceptive innervation).[6,30,31] In general, lack of representative muscle samples from human surgery hampers progress.[29] Primary pathologies may also be found at the level of the motor nerve, e.g., neuropathies or disorders of the neuromuscular junction. Within the brain, specific pathologies may reflect developmental (agenesis of motor nuclei) or acquired conditions (brain lesions due to stroke, trauma, or disease such as multiple sclerosis). The cortex may show alterations due to abnormal circuitry for binocular vision, making it difficult to distinguish between primary cause and secondary adaptation. In Graves' disease (hyperthyroidism), shared epitopes between orbital fibroblasts, extraocular muscles, and the thyroid may lead to interstitial edema and enlarged extraocular muscles that are infiltrated with inflammatory cells (see Chapter 56). In Duane retraction syndrome, the abducens nucleus and nerve are absent or hypoplastic, and the lateral rectus muscle is innervated by a branch of the oculomotor nerve (see Chapter 57). In the autoimmune disease myasthenia gravis, circulating antibodies lead to a reduced number of acetylcholine receptors in neuromuscular junctions, reducing the safety factor and extraocular muscle function.[32]

Etiology

Environmental and genetic risk factors

Fetal alcohol syndrome and fetal hydantoin syndrome[22] as well as prematurity and perinatal hypoxia are risk factors for infantile esotropia.[33] Major risks are listed in Table 59.1 and include Down syndrome, Duane's retraction syndrome, and congenital fibrosis of the extraocular muscles (CFEOM), caused by mutations of genes that regulate oculomotor neuron development and axonal transport or guidance.[8] Nevertheless, the etiology and pathophysiology of strabismus are unclear in the large majority of cases.

Other causes

Major categories of conditions that cause strabismus along the sensorimotor loop are compiled and illustrated in Figure 59.3. It is important to emphasize the circular nature and interdependencies between the motor and sensory loops: any disruption along this circle may cause derailment of binocular vision (Box 59.2). Disruption at multiple sites may have additive effects to surpass a critical threshold, possibly explaining the multifactorial inheritance pattern. Strabismus may result from etiologies that can be broadly grouped as "developmental" or "acquired" (Table 59.1). Developmental or early-onset forms of strabismus may be caused by abnormal maturation of binocular horizontal connections in the striate visual cortex.[3,5,24] Later-onset forms of childhood strabismus may be caused by uncorrected hyperopia (far-sightedness) or weak fusional reflexes. Acquired strabismus may result from damage to the brainstem (internuclear ophthalmoplegia) or damage to the cranial nerves as a result of trauma, tumor, or strokes (paretic strabismus), interference with neuromuscular synaptic transmission (myasthenia gravis), alteration of the extraocular muscles (thyroid ophthalmopathy), or direct damage to the extraocular muscles, orbital tissues, or pulley systems (orbital

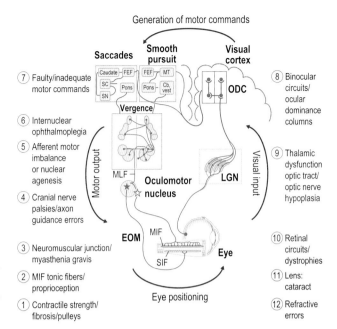

Figure 59.3 Synopsis of the circular, sequential flow of information between the eye and the brain for eye alignment and binocular vision. Eye positioning, visual input, generation of motor commands, and motor output constitute an interdependent circle that can be disrupted at each of the locations, as listed from 1 to 12. Cb, cerebellum; EOM, extraocular muscle; FEF, frontal eye field; LGN, lateral geniculate nucleus; MIF, multiply innervated fiber; MLF, medial longitudinal fasciculus; MT, medial temporal area; ODC, ocular dominance column; SC, superior colliculus; SIF, singly innervated fiber; SN, substantia nigra; Vest, vestibular nuclei. (Modified from Tychsen L. Infantile esotropia: current neurophysiologic concepts. In: Rosenbaum AL, Santiago AP (eds) Clinical Strabismus Management. Philadelphia: Saunders, 1999:117–138; Büttner-Ennever JA. Anatomy of the oculomotor system. Dev Ophthalmol 2007;40:1–14; and Goldberg ME. The control of gaze. In: Kandel ER, Schwartz JH, Jessell TM (eds) Principles of Neural Science, 4th edn. New York: McGraw-Hill, 2000:782–800.)

> **Box 59.2 Multiple causes of strabismus**
>
> Strabismus can be caused by a large number of primary causes along an interdependent sensorimotor loop that operates in a circular fashion

fractures). Major specific causes of strabismus are listed in Table 59.3.

Pathophysiology

Biological basis of the disease

Strabismus has unique pathophysiological features. Multiple, highly diverse primary causes contribute to strabismus. The resulting visual misalignment interferes, especially in the developing infant, with the reinforcing intrinsic mechanisms that normally lead to fused images and binocular vision. Finally, this vicious cycle invokes secondary, generally maladaptive responses that lock in the disturbance of binocular vision. We will discuss the presumptive sequence of events in detail, with an emphasis on trophic feedback mechanisms of circuit development and maintenance.

Table 59.3 Causes of strabismus

Cause	References
Abnormal orbital pulleys (fibroelastic sleeves)	46–48
Orbital fibrosis/inflammation	See Chapter 56
Mitochondrial myopathies	29
Orbital trauma/skull fracture	
Imbalance of extraocular muscle contractile force generation	
Abnormal tonic myofibers (multiply innervated fibers)	
Dysfunction of proprioceptive feedback (?)	6, 31
Abnormal neuromuscular junctions on extraocular muscles (myasthenia gravis)	29, 32
Cranial nerve palsies or dystrophies	
Cranial nerve nuclei agenesis or axonal misrouting	8, Chapter 57
Faulty afferent motor commands	
Internuclear ophthalmoplegia	9, 36
Abnormal motor command processing in midbrain/pons/cerebellum/brainstem	
Abnormal binocular processing in frontal eye field/extrastriate cortex	3
Abnormal binocular circuits/ocular dominance columns in visual cortex	3
Deficiencies in optic radiations/tract/optic nerve (hypoplasia) or thalamus	
Abnormal retinal circuitry/retinoblastoma	
Defects (refractive errors) in the optic apparatus (lens/cornea): cataract /astigmatism	

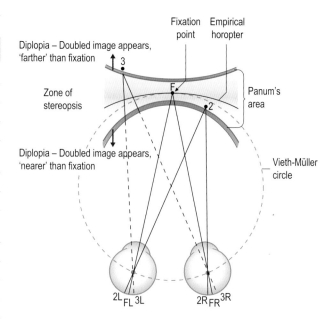

Figure 59.4 The empirical horopter shows the range of binocular fusion, visual fixation points, and the optical basis of physiological and, by extension, pathophysiological double vision (diplopia). Panum's fusional area (yellow) defines the zone of stereo vision. When images fall outside Panum's area, diplopia results (green). The mathematically determined Vieth–Müller circle passes through the optical centers of each eye and the points of fixation. (Modified from American Academy of Ophthalmology. Pediatric Ophthalmology and Strabismus, Section 6, Basic and Clinical Science Course. San Francisco, CA: American Academy of Ophthalmology, 2007.)

Alignment of the eyes for binocular vision requires that each of the crucial relays and links in a complex series of neural circuits works smoothly and precisely, from the eye to the visual cortex (sensory loop), and via motor relay stations to the eye muscles (motor loop) (Figure 59.3). Any imbalance or disruption along this pathway can cause the system to malfunction, resulting in strabismus. Naturally, the system is most vulnerable during its development, when during a critical period stereoacuity develops[34] and the crucial binocular neuronal connections form in the visual cortex.[35] The normal retinal disparity can be used for depth perception. Whether images on the fovea of each eye are interpreted as a fused image or give rise to diplopia depends on the precise visual optics (whether the fixation points fall within Panum's area; Figure 59.4) and the visual projections to cortex. A small deviation in the highly complex eye-positioning feedback system can disrupt the fine balance and place the image "out of range," giving rise to diplopia and suppressing the image from the weaker eye in the developing visual system.

Primary causes and secondary adaptations

It is often stated that malfunction of one or more eye muscles causes strabismus. However, the reason for such malfunc-

tion can have a variety of primary causes. It may be a deficit that is intrinsic to that muscle, or the muscle may not receive proper commands from motor neurons, or there may be defects further upstream in the brain that compromise afferent input to the "phasic" and/or "tonic" motor neurons.[36,37] There has been much controversy about the primary causes of strabismus (Table 59.3).[4,5]

Due to the circular processing (Figure 59.3), it can be difficult to assess which defect is primary, and which processes represent secondary (mal)adaptations, since muscles are altered in response to demand.[28,29] To some extent, the brain can even reorganize its retinal orientation to compensate for ocular misalignment ("anomalous retinal correspondence").[9] Some investigators emphasize cortical lesions and their association with strabismus and suggest that such dysfunctional cortical development is causative.[3,5] On the other hand, the fact that manipulations of the periphery (surgery of the eye muscles without any direct effect on the brain) can cure strabismus suggests that the brain circuits are principally intact and points to the eye muscles as the primary site.[6] Minor, but important manipulations along the circular processing route may suffice to nudge – and subsequently maintain – the fused images within Panum's area, thus restoring the system to work within a functional range (Figure 59.4).

A trophic theory of strabismus

We emphasize an interdependency and multilevel communication between the motor command centers, the motor

Box 59.3 Strabismus and trophic signals

A unifying link of some strabismus syndromes may be defects in the processing of trophic signals that regulate muscle strength as well as neural circuit development and maintenance

Table 59.4 Animal models for strabismus and extraocular muscle (EOM) research

Animal	Advantages	Disadvantages	References
Monkeys	Human-like, frontal-eyed	Expensive	3, 5, 6, 24, 29, 35
Cats	Frontal-eyed, developmental model		6, 29, 35
Rabbits	Large EOMs, trophic factors	Lateral-eyed	41, 44
Rodents	Probes for gene expression		
Rats	Standard model	Poor vision, small EOMs	29
Mice	Genetic model	Poor vision, small EOMs	8, 29
Chicken	Developmental model, large EOMs	Lateral-eyed	6, 50

pathway (to eye muscles) and the sensory pathway (from the eye), and the binocular visual processing in the cortex (Figure 59.3). We propose that this interdependency between neural circuits and their effector organ is mediated, at least in part, by trophic factors or trophic signals that move both anterogradely and retrogradely along axons.[38–40] Such trophic mechanisms regulate the development of ocular dominance columns in visual cortex,[39] and appear to affect binocular visual circuitry as well as regulation of contractile force of extraocular muscles.[41,42] We postulate that these trophic signals are an essential part of a feedback system that precisely regulates eye movements which ultimately allow the fusion of the images from both eyes in the cortex (Box 59.3). Interestingly, several congenital forms of strabismus are linked to molecules involved in either the internalization (dynamins) or transport (kinesins) of proteins along axons, including the transport of trophic factors.[8,43] Thus, a unifying link of strabismus syndromes may be defects in the processing, transport, and delivery of plasticity signals (trophic factors) that regulate muscle strength,[41,42,44] motor neuron survival,[43] afferent motor commands, ocular dominance columns, binocular circuits, and synaptic plasticity.[39]

Biological basis of the treatment

Multiple conditions along the motor and sensory routes can contribute to derail the alignment of images from the two eyes (Figure 59.3). If the alignment is near threshold, a small additional dysfunction may prevent fusion (Figure 59.4). Without fusion, there may be no "trophic reward" or reinforcement to maintain the connectivity between binocular neurons at the cortical level, and as a result, the downstream pathways are not strengthened or stabilized, exacerbating the vicious cycle (Figure 59.3). When the system is manipulated at the level of the eye muscles to restore normal eye alignment, then fusion may be achieved. The system can then acquire and stabilize the single fused image within the normal range of binocular vision (Panum's area) and maintain the new alignment (Figure 59.4). Despite their limitations, research studies using animal models have rendered valuable new insights (Table 59.4).

How does surgery work?

By classical explanation, the surgeon creates either slack (recession) or increased tension (resection) in the muscle that is operated on. However, altering the length–tension relationship of the muscle does not account for all observed effects.[45] Many quantitative characteristics of recessions are better explained by a torque vector model, instead of the classical length–tension model, consistent with the relevance of muscle pulleys (fibroelastic sleeves).[46–48] This new understanding of the mechanics of ocular motility mechanics has implications for surgical techniques to correct ocular motility disorders.[45,46]

How does botulinum toxin work?

Botulinum toxin acts by transient chemical denervation. This weakens an overacting muscle. The apparent paradox is that the therapeutic effect can be permanent, even though the effect of the toxin and the denervation lasts only 3–4 months. Initial studies indicated that the toxin's long-term beneficial effects were due to a permanent alteration of one specific type of (developing) extraocular myofiber.[6,49] However, developing extraocular muscles fully recover within 3–4 months after botulinum toxin treatment, without any residual loss of contractile force or any permanent structural alteration.[19,50] The new data favor a central "reset" hypothesis which postulates that, once the system is realigned (by muscle lengthening[19]), even for a brief period, then the altered feedback can reinforce and engage the intrinsic brain mechanisms that support and stabilize visual alignment, achieving binocular fusion in the long term.[50]

How does orthoptics/vision therapy work?

Nonsurgical management of strabismus seeks to sharpen the retinal image by prescribing the appropriate spectacle correction and treating amblyopia. This provides an improved stimulus for fusion and reduces accommodative convergence. Orthoptics (eye exercises) can increase fusional amplitudes. This technique is especially effective for convergence insufficiency.[2] Vision therapy can reduce suppression and make the patient aware of diplopia, potentially increasing fusional control. However, this increases the risk of making a patient permanently diplopic if fusional potential is lacking.[2]

Mutations

Genetics has an important role in identifying pathophysiological processes at the molecular level. Some gene mutations are responsible for defects in development and connectivity of oculomotor neurons[8] (Figure 59.3, Box 59.4). If a crucial circuit (such as a population of cranial

---

> ### Box 59.4 Strabismus and gene mutations
>
> Several congenital strabismus syndromes are caused by mutations of genes that regulate the development of motoneurons which innervate extraocular muscles

nerve nuclei) is missing (rather than simply malfunctioning because of inappropriate input or stimulation), then that defect is much more difficult to rectify.

Conclusion

Considerable progress has been made with new imaging techniques[13] and with the identification of some of the molecular players responsible for congenital strabismus.[8]

Screening for such risk factors (inherited genes) will be possible in the future. Since the importance of early diagnosis and rapid treatment has been established, systematic early-childhood screening, including genetic testing, will be beneficial. Combined use of multiple treatment modalities such as botulinum toxin and trophic factors along with surgery may improve the precision of strabismus surgeries and predictability of outcome, potentially improving sensory fusion and reducing the need for reoperations. Larger-scale studies are needed that compare the long-term success and outcomes of different treatment options.

Acknowledgments

Our own research was supported by NIH grants EY 12841, EY 14405, NS 35931, and HD 29177.

Key references

A complete list of chapter references is available online at www.expertconsult.com. See inside cover for registration details.

2. von Noorden GK, Campos EC. Binocular Vision and Ocular Motility. Theory and Management of Strabismus, 6th edn. St. Louis: Mosby, 2002.

3. Tychsen LF. Strabismus: the scientific basis. In: Taylor DH, Hoyt CS (eds) Pediatric Ophthalmology and Strabismus, 3rd edn. Edinburgh: Elsevier-Saunders, 2005:836–848.

4. von Noorden GK. The History of Strabismology. Hirschberg History of Ophthalmology: The Monographs, vol. 9. Ostend, Belgium: JP Wayenborgh, 2002.

5. Tychsen L. Infantile esotropia: current neurophysiologic concepts. In: Rosenbaum AL, Santiago AP (eds) Clinical Strabismus Management. Philadelphia: Saunders, 1999:117–138.

6. Porter JD, Baker RS, Ragusa RJ, et al. Extraocular muscles: basic and clinical aspects of structure and function. Surv Ophthalmol 1995;39:451–484.

8. Engle EC. The genetic basis of complex strabismus. Pediatr Res 2006;59:343–348.

9. Wright KW. Pediatric Ophthalmology and Strabismus. St. Louis: Mosby, 1995.

10. von Noorden GK. Atlas of Strabismus, 4th edn. St. Louis: Mosby, 1983.

19. McNeer KW, Magoon EH, Scott AB. Chemodenervation therapy: technique and indications. In: Rosenbaum AL, Santiago PS (eds) Clinical Strabismus Management. Philadelphia: WB Saunders, 1999:423–432.

21. Parks MM. Atlas of Strabismus Surgery. Philadelphia, PA: Harper and Row, 1983.

22. American Academy of Ophthalmology. Pediatric Ophthalmology and Strabismus, Section 6, Basic and Clinical Science Course. San Francisco, CA: American Academy of Ophthalmology, 2007.

23. Wright KW, Edelman PM, McVey JH, et al. High-grade stereoacuity after early surgery for congenital esotropia. Arch Ophthalmol 1994;112:913–919.

25. Wright KW. Color Atlas of Strabismus Surgery. Philadelphia: JB Lippincott, 1991.

29. Spencer RF, Porter JD. Biological organization of the extraocular muscles. Prog Brain Res 2006;151:43–80.

33. Rosenbaum AL, Santiago PS. Clinical Strabismus Management. Philadelphia: WB Saunders, 1999.

CHAPTER 60

Albinism

Gerald F Cox and Anne B Fulton

Albinism refers to a heterogeneous group of hypopigmentation disorders that share an absolute or relative inherited deficiency of the pigment melanin that leads to characteristic changes in the skin, hair, and visual system (eyes and optic tracts). Melanin is produced and contained within melanosomes, intracellular organelles that are present in the stratum basale of the epidermis, hair bulbs, and intraocular epithelia. Most individuals with albinism have a simple, or nonsyndromic, form that affects the visual system, hair, and skin (oculocutaneous albinism, OCA) or mainly the visual system (ocular albinism, OA). Less commonly, individuals may have a complex, or syndromic, form of albinism that includes a distinctive pattern of organ involvement in addition to OCA. In recent years, much progress has been made in understanding the clinical features, pathophysiology, and molecular basis of albinism (Box 60.1).

Clinical background

Individuals with albinism are typically fair of skin and hair and have hypopigmentation of ocular structures (Figure 60.1). The degree of cutaneous hypopigmentation can vary greatly, ranging from the classic image of the albino with white hair, white skin, and pink-red irides to one in which no apparent cutaneous hypopigmentation is present. More constant are the effects that albinism has on the eye and visual pathways. Consequently, examination of the eyes remains an essential step for the diagnosis of albinism.

The key ocular symptoms and signs are intimately related (Table 60.1). Deficits in iris pigmentation typically impart a gray or blue color to the irides, which transilluminate light (Figure 60.2A and B). Foveal hypoplasia and mild optic nerve hypoplasia are typical (Figure 60.2C), as is nystagmus. The foveal reflex is almost always absent. The ocular fundi appear pale with the choroidal vasculature visible through the neurosensory retina and retinal pigment epithelium (Figure 60.2D). Strabismus and high refractive errors are common (Box 60.2).[1]

Acuity is low, ranging from a legal blind level to only mild acuity deficits; median acuity is often cited as approximately 20/60. The low acuity is secondary to foveal hypoplasia[2,3]; nystagmus may also degrade acuity. Anomalous head posture is used to counteract the effects of the nystagmus. Depth perception may be poor; typically no stereopsis is demonstrated. Strabismus is common, with esotropia more frequent that exotropia. High refractive errors are common in albinism,[1] apparently from failure of emmetropization.[4] In children with albinism, the ophthalmologist must be alert to amblyopia superimposed on the acuity deficit directly related to the foveal hypoplasia. In a child with albinism, as in other children, asymmetric acuity should alert the ophthalmologist to possible amblyopia associated with strabismus or with difference in refractive error between right and left eye, anisometropia.

The lack of the protective effect of melanin in the eye underlies photophobia. The individual with albinism is also at risk for sunburn rather than tanning, and for malignancies of the skin, especially if exposed unprotected to intense tropical sun.

History

From biblical times albinism has been recognized; it has been argued that Noah was an albino (Box 60.3).[5] There is a long, anecdotal history of albinism throughout the animal kingdom with notable ocular features.[6] Foveal hypoplasia was recognized and documented histologically by Elschnig[7] and a paucity of nondecussated fibers at the chiasm was reported in classical studies of the visual system in albino animals.[8] In human subjects with albinism, electrophysiological[9,10] and, more recently, functional magnetic resonance imaging[11,12] studies have demonstrated anomalous organization of the visual pathways.

For many years albinism was classified on a biochemical basis as tyrosinase-positive or tyrosinase-negative in the hair bulb incubation test. However, this test is seldom performed today because of its lack of sensitivity and specificity, giving rise to many false negatives and false positives; for example, patients with OCA1B and OCA2 have different genetic bases for their albinism, but both yield tyrosinase-positive results in the hair bulb test. Conversely, OCA1A and OCA1B are caused by the same gene but give rise to tyrosinase-negative and tyrosinase-positive results, respectively.

Gradually the genetic foundation for the simple forms of albinism has been established.[13] Four autosomal-recessive genes for OCA and one gene for X-linked OA have been

Box 60.1 Overview

- Albinism is a heterogeneous group of disorders
- Melanin pigment is deficient in all forms of albinism
- Hypopigmentation affects the eyes, skin, and hair to varying degrees
- Identification of ocular features is essential for the diagnosis of albinism

Table 60.1 Ocular features of albinism

Low acuity
Nystagmus
High refractive errors
Strabismus
Irides that transilluminate light
Foveal hypoplasia
Fundus hypopigmentation
Photophobia

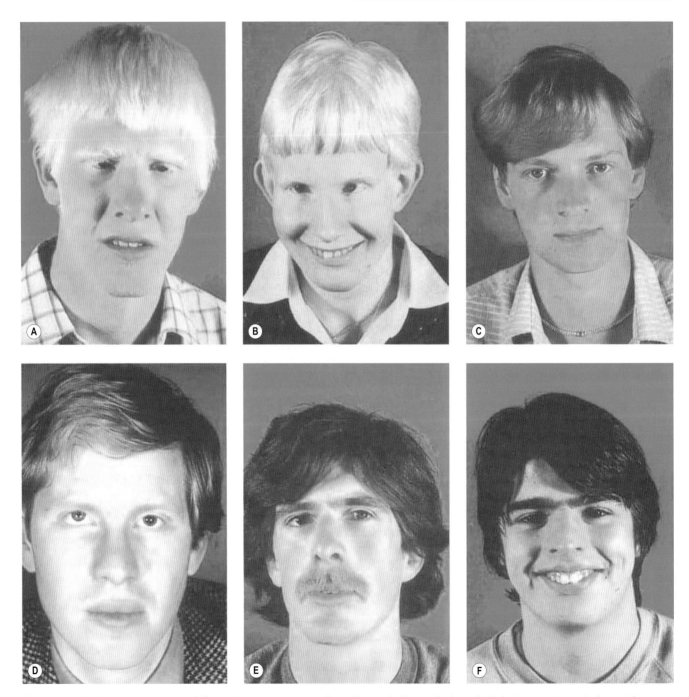

Figure 60.1 The phenotypic spectrum of albinism. Pigmentation ranges from white to dark hair with photophobia being conspicuous in those with the most marked deficits in pigment. Each of these individuals has ocular features of albinism. (Reproduced with permission from Spekreijse H, Apkarian P. The use of a system analysis approach to electrodiagnostic (ERG and VEP) assessment. Vis Res 1986;26:195–216.[55])

Box 60.2 Common ocular features

- Low visual acuity
- Nystagmus
- Iris sites that transilluminate light
- Foveal hypoplasia
- Hypopigmented fundi
- Strabismus
- High refractive errors

Box 60.3 History

- Albinism has been recognized since biblical times
- Structural and functional anomalies of the visual pathways have been substantiated
- Molecular genetic basis for simple and complex forms of albinism has been delineated

Box 60.4 Diagnostic workup

- Identify ocular features
- Evaluate visual pathways
- Genetic testing
- If clinically indicated, evaluate for complex forms

Box 60.5 Differential diagnosis

Simple forms of albinism

- OCA1
- OCA2
- OCA3
- OCA4
- OA1

Complex forms of albinism

- Hermansky–Pudlak syndrome
- Prader–Willi syndrome
- Angelman syndrome
- Chédiak–Higashi syndrome

Other disorders with hypopigmentation

- Waardenburg syndrome
- Piebaldism
- Vitiligo
- Griscelli syndrome

identified (Table 60.2). OCA types 1–4 are inherited with equal frequency in males and females. The recurrence risk to couples with an affected child is 25% with each pregnancy. The ophthalmic characteristics of OCA1–4 are listed in Table 60.1. OA1 follows an X-linked pattern of inheritance with affected hemizygous males, and female carriers who have healthy eyes, normal vision, and uneven fundus pigmentation (Figure 60.2E). Males with OA share essentially the same ophthalmic characteristics of those with OCA. All daughters of fathers with X-linked OA are obligate carriers, and carriers have a 50% chance of having an affected son (or carrier daughter) with each pregnancy.

The genetic basis has also been determined for a number of complex forms of albinism that have systemic comorbidities (Table 60.2). In contrast, the simple forms of albinism (Table 60.2) do not lead to systemic comorbidities.

The overall frequency of albinism in the general population is estimated to be 1 in 17 000, and about 1 in 65 individuals is a carrier for OCA. The frequency varies with specific type (Table 60.2) and with ethnicity. An estimated 18 000 individuals in the USA have a form of albinism. OCA1 and OCA2 are the two most common forms of albinism and occur with similar frequencies.

Diagnostic workup

A history of nystagmus, decreased visual acuity, and fair skin and hair within the family group raises the suspicion for albinism (Box 60.4). Inspection of the ocular structures adds diagnostic information. Typically, the irides transilluminate light (Figure 60.2A and 60.2B). Foveal hypoplasia and albinotic fundi (Figure 60.2C and 60.2D) are the main fundus features; mild optic nerve hypoplasia may also be present.[14] The optic nerve head in children with albinism is significantly smaller than in normally pigmented, age-similar children, being about 80% of the normal mean diameter (AB Fulton, personal observation).

We favor an attempt at genotyping to secure a specific diagnosis of albinism, which is important for genetic counseling and anticipatory guidance. Complex forms of albinism, e.g., Hermansky–Pudlak syndrome, can be mistaken for OCA but have important medical complications. These syndromic forms are virtually excluded if a genetic diagnosis of OCA or OA is secured (Table 60.2). Other hypopigmentation syndromes that do not share all of the cardinal features of albinism (e.g., eye and optic tract) can also be excluded with a genetic diagnosis. However, even in dedicated laboratories, a genetic diagnosis of albinism is currently achieved in only about half of the patients who have a well-substantiated clinical diagnosis.[15] This may improve with the recent availability of more comprehensive clinical testing for OCA1 and OCA2. In individuals with nystagmus and foveal hypoplasia, the diagnosis of albinism may pertain even if there is no obvious hypopigmentation.[16] Thus, there is no ignoring the importance of the ophthalmic examination.

Differential diagnosis

Differentiation of the several types of albinism depends on history, and ideally, a genetic diagnosis (Table 60.2; Box 60.5). The ocular features are similar across the various types; OCA1A has the most pronounced hypopigmentation, but there is considerable overlap of the phenotype among

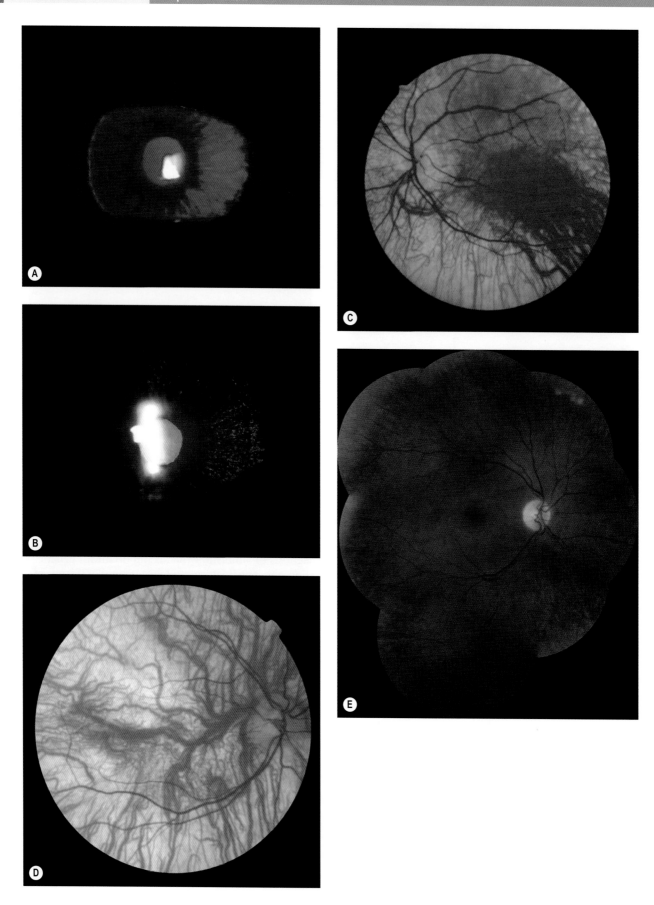

Figure 60.2 Typical ocular features in individuals with albinism. (A and B) The irides have sites that transilluminate light. At times the sites that lack pigment are punctate, microscopic areas which are visualized only by using high magnification of the slit lamp with the beam adjusted to fill the pupil with a reddish glow. (C) In albinism, the foveal pit is blunted or not identifiable. Normally the pit appears like a dimple made by a pebble hitting the shiny surface of a car. In this eye there is sufficient normal pigment to obscure the choroidal vasculature at the center of the macula. The optic nerve head is clinically normal although measurement of the diameter indicates that there is mild but statistically significant hypoplasia of the optic nerve head, consistent with the results of a structural magnetic resonance imaging study of the optic nerve and chiasm in albinism.[14] The retinal vasculature is of normal caliber although, as pointed out by Neveu et al,[56] the temporal arcades have a wider arch than seen in nonalbinotic fundi. The extramacular fundi are albinotic. (D) This photograph shows the posterior pole of another individual with albinism. Throughout the macula, the choroidal vasculature is visible through the neural retina and pigment epithelium as there is insufficient normal pigment. (E) Composite fundus photograph of a woman who is a carrier for X-linked ocular albinism. The pigmentation is uneven in the extramacular retina with scattered geographic areas of hypopigmentation. This woman had healthy eyes with superb visual acuity and no nystagmus.

Table 60.2 Genetic forms of albinism

Albinism type	OMIM	Gene symbol	Historical name	Protein	Estimated frequency	Chromosomal location	Cellular defect	Clinical features
OCA1A OCA1B	203100 606952	TYR	Tyrosinase-negative Tyrosinase-positive	Tyrosinase	1/40 000	11q14-q21	Synthesis of melanin Retention in endoplasmic reticulum	1A: White hair and skin at birth, no freckling, poor acuity 1B: Cream skin and yellow-tinged hair at birth; some progressive pigmentation over time; improved vision over time
OCA2	203200	OCA2	Tyrosinase-positive	P-protein	1/36 000	15q11.2-q12	Melanosome membrane protein involved in processing and transport of tyrosinase and other melanosomal proteins in small vesicles immediately post-Golgi	Cream skin and yellow-tinged hair; some progressive pigmentation over time; improved visual acuity over time. High prevalence in Africa
OCA3	203290	TYRP1	Rufous albinism	Tyrosinase-related protein	Unknown	9p23	Binds to tyrosinase, function unclear. Retention in endoplasmic reticulum	Red hair and red-brown skin. High prevalence in sub-Sahara Africa and New Guinea
OCA4	606574	SLC45A2		MATP	Rare outside Japan	5p13.3	Processing and transport of tyrosinase to melanosomes	Similar to OCA2
OA, type 1	300500	OA1	Nettleship–Falls	GRP143	1/50 000	Xp22.3	Regulation of melanosome number and size	Ocular features of albinism with normal skin and hair pigmentation. Female carriers have uneven pigmentation in retina and megamelanosomes in skin

Table 60.2 Genetic forms of albinism—cont'd

Albinism type	OMIM	Gene symbol	Historical name	Protein	Estimated frequency	Chromosomal location	Cellular defect	Clinical features
Hermansky–Pudlak syndrome	604982 608233 606118 606682 607521 607522 607145 609762	HPS1 HPS2 HPS3 HPS4 HPS5 HPS6 HPS7 HSP8	Same	HPS1 AP3B1 HPS3 HPS4 α-Integrin BP63 HPS6 DTNBP1 BLOC1S3	1/1800 among Puerto Ricans	10q23.1 5q14.1 3q24 22q11.2-22.2 11p15-13 10q24.32 6p22.3 19q13	Biogenesis of specialized organelles of endosomal lysosomal system, including melanosomes and platelet-dense bodies	Bleeding diathesis, restrictive lung disease, pulmonary fibrosis, inflammatory bowel disease
Chédiak–Higashi syndrome	214500	CHS1	Same	LYST	Rare	1q42.1-q42.2	Lysosomal trafficking regulator	Immunodeficiency, neutropenia, malignant lymphoma, large lysosomal granules
Prader–Willi syndrome	176270	Absence of paternally expressed genes at 15q11-13, including SNRPN, Necdin, P-gene	Same	SNRPN, Necdin, P-protein, possibly others	1/15 000 (1% have albinism)	15q11-13	P-gene-related and possibly other pigmentary genes	Obesity, hypotonia, mental retardation, short stature, hypogonadotrophic hypogonadism, almond-shaped eyes, narrow bifrontal diameter of skull, small hands and feet, food obsession, skin-picking behavior, sleep apnea
Angelman syndrome	105830	Absence of maternally expressed genes at 15q11-13, including UBE3A, P-gene	Happy puppet syndrome	UBE3A, P-protein, possibly others	1/15 000 (1% have albinism)	15q11-13	P-gene-related and possibly other pigmentary genes	Ataxia, mental retardation, absent speech, inappropriate laughter, seizures, microcephaly, prognathism, widely spaced teeth, poor sleep

the several types of albinism (Table 60.2). Complex forms of albinism share ocular features of albinism but also include other systemic findings such as bleeding diatheses (Hermansky–Pudlak syndrome), severe cognitive impairment (Prader–Willi and Angelman syndromes), and immunodeficiency (Chédiak–Higashi syndrome). Other individuals with syndromic hypopigmentation are not clinically considered albinos because they do not have the requisite ocular features. These include Waardenburg syndrome, piebaldism, vitiligo, and Griscelli syndrome.

Some previously described forms of albinism now appear to be related to unusual presentations of OCA or OA. For example, autosomal-recessive OA has in most cases been shown to be due to a mild form of OCA with inconspicuous cutaneous involvement. In one study, 56% of 36 unrelated Caucasian individuals diagnosed with autosomal-recessive OA were found genetically to have OCA1 or OCA2, and almost all of the OCA1 cases were heterozygous for one severe mutation and one temperature-sensitive R402Q mutation.[17] Autosomal-recessive OA and deafness have been shown in one extended family to be caused by digenic inheritance of mutations in the microphthalmia-associated transcription factor (MITF) gene (causing Waardenburg syndrome type II) and in the tyrosinase gene (causing OCA1), whose expression MITF controls.[18] Autosomal-recessive OCA and deafness were shown to be coincidental in one family, caused by co-inheritance of mutations in the connexin 26 gene and the OCA4 gene.[19] X-linked OA and late-onset neurosensory deafness map to the same locus as the OA1 gene and likely represent an allelic variant or a contiguous gene syndrome.

Treatment

Management is supportive rather than curative. Protection of the skin and eyes from excessive light reduces the risk of photic damage to these organs (Box 60.6). For eye protection, hats or caps with visors and dark glasses are advisable.

Box 60.6 Treatment

- Protect skin and eyes from excessive light
- Correct refractive errors
- Low-vision support
- Social support (www.positivexposure.org)

Box 60.8 Pathology

- Melanosomes with paucity of melanin granules
- Megamelanosomes (X-linked ocular albinism and Chédiak–Higashi syndrome)
- Reduced number of ganglion cells in the central retina
- Foveal hypoplasia
- Subclinical hypoplasia of optic nerve
- Small chiasm
- Relative deficit in nondecussated fibers at the chiasm

Box 60.7 Prognosis

- Gradual improvement in vision through infancy and childhood
- Stable vision thereafter

Not only is protection important, but it is in moderate light that vision is the best. Optimal correction of refractive errors is indicated. In early childhood, we favor full optical correction for refractive errors that are outside the prediction interval for normal[20]; this advice is modified if the child's head position to damp the nystagmus precludes using the glasses lenses close to the optical center. Strabismus surgery may be considered when improvement in ocular alignment and anomalous head position is sought.[21,22] Low-vision support, including use of optical and electronic devices, is needed to facilitate education and communication. Strategies for safe independent orientation and mobility may require specialized instruction. This is especially important outdoors in daylight hours when photophobia is an added impairment. The importance of social support cannot be overestimated (www.positivexposure.org) to counteract the negative press that albinism has suffered at times.

Prognosis

In general, individuals with OCA1A have more impaired vision than those with OCA1B, OCA2, and OA1. Newborns with OCA1A have very white skin and hair at birth, whereas newborns with OCA2 have more of a cream-colored complexion with yellow-tinted hair and those (males) with OA1 generally have normally pigmented skin and hair. During childhood, the developmental increases in acuity and visual performance that ordinarily occur may be further improved by a slight, gradual increase in pigmentation that is generally seen in many children with albinism. Vision is otherwise stable, although with the passing years, supports need modification to match demands of school and life (Box 60.7).

Pathology

Albinism is characterized by foveal hypoplasia, which clinicians attempt to identify by ophthalmoscopy (Box 60.8). Optical coherence tomography (OCT) performed by a number of groups supports the clinical impression of an absent or blunted foveal dimple.[23–25] There has been a paucity of anatomic specimens and each has had limited generalizability due to comorbidities or advanced age of the donors.[2,3,26] High-resolution OCT with eye-tracking capability may be the most promising approach to contemporary analysis of the neurovascular elements[27] that must define the anomalies of the albino fovea.

Anomalies, that is, misrouting of the visual pathways, are commonly considered to be specified in the retina during development and are related to the deficiency in melanin. Fundus pigmentation, graded on a five-point scale, predicts the shift in the nasotemporal line of decussation in humans with albinism.[28] Furthermore, the number of ganglion cells in the central retina is reduced in albinism, and anomalies of the visual pathway are limited to those brain regions representing the central retina.[29,30] The mechanisms, however, by which melanin induces the spatial temporal defects in the immature ganglion cells that might give rise to the anomalous pathways, classically described as a paucity of nondecussated fibers, remain unknown.[29,31,32] Another perspective is based on careful observations of well-pigmented patients with foveal hypoplasia who also had misrouting of the visual pathways demonstrated using visual evoked potential procedures.[33] Thus, not only do foveal hypoplasia and misrouting of the visual pathways exist distinct from albinism, but they call into question the retinal specification of the misrouting. The fovea has a protracted course of development from approximately 24 weeks' gestation to well into childhood. The decussation at the chiasm is established earlier. van Genderen and colleagues raise the possibility that retrograde processes govern the development of foveal hypoplasia in general, perhaps even in albinism.[33]

The photoreceptors, the last retinal cells to mature, are also abnormal in animal models of albinism. The rods are too few in number,[34] rhodopsin content is low,[35] and sensitivity is low.[36] Each of these reports presents evidence that light damage to the rods does not account for the abnormalities of the photoreceptors. In some children with albinism there is an anecdotal report of mild deficits in rod sensitivity, as derived from analysis of the electroretinogram a-wave.[37] Although the mechanisms leading to the reported changes in the rod photoreceptors[34–37] have not been delineated, we note that signaling pathways involved in melanization appear to modulate oxygen consumption by the photoreceptors and the rate of photoisomerization in the rod outer segments. Furthermore, low melanin is associated with increased phagocytosis of rod outer segments by the retinal pigment epithelium.[38]

Alterations in physics of tissues or cells

Melanin, which has maximum absorbance of light at ~340 nm, blocks ultraviolet wavelengths that are damaging to tissues; melanosomes are positioned within the cell to protect the nuclear DNA. The low amount of protective pigment in albino ocular tissues allows light to enter and then scatter within the eye. This is the basis for photophobia, and potentially, for damage to the retina.

Light damage of the photoreceptors, theoretically a risk in unprotected humans with albinism, has been documented in albino animals. Melanin is one of the best sound-absorbing materials known and its position in the stria vascularis of the inner ear may afford protection of that neurosensory organ. Individuals with light pigmentation appear to be more susceptible to hearing loss in noisy environments (Box 60.9).

Box 60.9 Alterations in physics of tissues or cells

- Melanin blocks ultraviolet light
- Melanosomes protect nuclear DNA from damaging ultraviolet light
- Skin and retina at risk for photic damage
- Intraocular light scatter and glare
- Melanin absorbs sound; protects stria vascularis in the ear

---

Specific cellular features

Melanosomes are specialized pigment-containing organelles that are derived from the endosomal-lysosomal system.[39] Stage I, or premelanosomes, are spherical organelles that originate from the smooth endoplasmic reticulum and contain an amorphous matrix (Figure 60.3). Stage I melanosomes contain a transmembrane protein, gp100, which is proteolytically cleaved to form an internal fibrillar matrix that gives rise to the stage II melanosome with an ovoid structure. Stage III melanosomes are characterized by the beginning of melanin deposition, while stage IV melanosomes are completely filled with melanin.

All forms of albinism are characterized by a reduction in the amount of melanin in melanosomes, stemming either from a defect in its biosynthesis or an abnormality in melanosome biogenesis (Figure 60.3). In OCA, the melanosomes have a normal size and number, whereas in OA1 and Chédiak–Higashi syndrome the melanosomes are unusually large (megamelanosomes) and fewer in number (Box 60.10). Animal models of albinism and in vitro studies of cultured melanocytes from these animal models have helped to elucidate the various steps in the melanin biosynthetic pathway and melanosome biogenesis.

OCA1 and OCA3

Tyrosinase is the enzyme that catalyzes the rate-limiting step in melanin biosynthesis, converting tyrosine to DOPA in stage II–IV melanosomes. Tyrosinase is involved in at least two additional steps in the synthetic pathway. Tyrosinase-related protein, also known as catalase B and gp75, is a

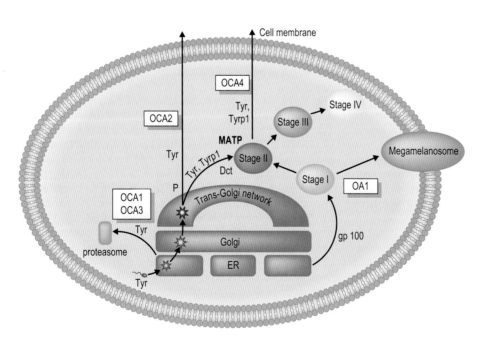

Figure 60.3 Melanosomal protein trafficking and aberrant processing seen in various types of albinism. Disruption of tyrosinase trafficking may occur at the level of the rough endoplasmic reticulum (ER: OCA1 and OCA3), in small vesicles immediately post-Golgi (OCA2), and in vesicles before delivery to early melanosomes (OCA4). Disruption in melanosome biogenesis may result in unusually large melanosomes (megamelosomes) that are reduced in number (OCA4). MATP, membrane-associated transporter protein. (Modified from Costin GE, Valencia JC, Vieira WD, et al. Tyrosinase processing and intracellular trafficking is disrupted in mouse primary melanocytes carrying the underwhite (uw) mutation. A model for oculocutaneous albinism (OCA) type 4. J Cell Sci 2003;116:3203–3212.).

Box 60.10 Specific cellular features

Melanosomes are derived from the endosomal lysosomal system

Stage I (premelanosomes)

- Spherical
- Originate from smooth endoplasmic reticulum
- Contain transmembrane protein, gp 100

Stage II

- Ovoid
- Internal fibrillar matrix, arising from cleavage of gp100

Stage III

- Beginning of melanin deposition

Stage IV (mature)

Filled with melanin

In albinism, low amount of melanin in melanosomes due to:

- Defect in melanin biosynthesis
- Abnormal biogenesis of melanosome

OCA1, OCA3

- Tyrosinase (OCA1) and tyrosinase-related protein (OCA3) retained in rough endoplasmic reticulum

OCA2

- Abnormal P-protein prevents targeting of tyrosinase and other proteins to the melanosome immediately post-Golgi

OCA4

- Membrane-associated transporter protein (MATP) interferes with processing and trafficking of tyrosinase to the melanosome and results in secretion of early melanosomes

---

melanocyte-specific protein whose precise function is not well understood. Various roles may include stabilizing tyrosinase, regulating melanin production through peroxide levels, and determining the shape of melanosomes. Normally, tyrosinase and tyrosinase-like protein are synthesized in the rough endoplasmic reticulum, transported through the Golgi apparatus, and targeted to small vesicles that pass through the endosomal–lysosomal compartment and fuse with melanosomes (Figure 60.3). In OCA1 and OCA3, the abnormal proteins are instead largely retained within the rough endoplasmic reticulum and targeted for disposal in the proteosome.[40–42]

OCA2

The P-gene (human homolog of the murine pink-eyed dilution gene, *p*), is located on chromosome 15q11-13 and encodes a transmembrane protein of the melanosome membrane. In cultured primary melanocytes from mice with *p*-gene mutations, abnormal p-protein prevents the efficient targeting of tyrosinase and other melanosomal proteins immediately post-Golgi from small vesicles to melanosomes (Figure 60.3).[43–45] Instead, the proteins are retained in small vesicles and mainly secreted from melanocytes, such that only 20% of the synthesized tyrosinase is localized in melanosomes. Another and perhaps related role of the

P-protein is the acidification of melanosomes and their precursors, which is required for melanin biosynthesis and possibly the sorting and localization of tyrosinase.[46]

Approximately 1% of patients with Angelman and Prader–Willi syndromes have a form of albinism related to OCA2. This low frequency is consistent with the carrier frequency of P-gene mutations in the general population. These two neurodevelopmental disorders are caused by the loss of either maternally expressed genes (Angelman) or paternally expressed genes (Prader–Willi) within imprinted regions of chromosome 15q11-13. Since imprinted genes are expressed from only one parental chromosome, the presence of a deletion on that chromosome leads to the total lack of expression of the imprinted genes from both chromosomes. In a few such individuals with albinism, it has been shown molecularly that one copy of the P-gene is lost as part of the chromosome 15q11-13 deletion responsible for Angelman or Prader–Willi syndrome, while the other copy of the P-gene carries a mutation by chance.[47,48] Even individuals with Angelman or Prader–Willi syndrome who do not have a second P-gene mutation often appear less pigmented than their relatives, suggesting that there are other pigment-modifying genes located in this chromosomal region.

OCA4

Like the P-protein, membrane-associated transporter protein (MATP) contains 12 membrane-spanning domains and shares homology with transport proteins. In a cultured primary murine melanocyte model of OCA4 containing the *underwhite* (*uw*) mutation, lack of MATP interfered with the processing and intracellular trafficking of tyrosinase to melanosomes (Figure 60.3).[49] Tyrosinase was abnormally secreted from cells in immature melanosomes, thereby disrupting the normal maturation process of these organelles.

OA1

Abnormalities in the OA1 protein, GRP143, lead to a defect in melanosome biogenesis and the regulation of melanosome size; consequently, stage III and IV melanosomes are decreased in number and unusually large (megamelanosomes). They are found in most carrier females in a mosaic pattern in tissues because of random X-linked inactivation, which allows for only one X chromosome to be expressed in a given cell.

Most of the complex forms of albinism involve not only melanosomes, but other organelles as well. Hermansky–Pudlak syndrome is a genetically heterogeneous group of disorders, all of which involve abnormalities of vesicles of the lysosomal lineage that form melanosomes, lysosomes, and platelet dense bodies. Decreased or absent platelet dense bodies can be demonstrated by electron microscopy of fresh blood. Chédiak–Higashi syndrome is caused by a defect in the CHS1 (*LYST*) gene, which is thought to play a role in vesicular formation and transport. As in OA1, megamelanosomes are present in Chédiak–Higashi syndrome.

Pathophysiology

In patients with OCA1, two mutations are identified in less than 50% of cases, suggesting that noncoding and regulatory regions of the gene harbor a substantial proportion of the mutations.[50] Most patients are compound heterozygotes, with only a few mutations being common (e.g., T373R and P81L in Caucasians). Patients with OCA1A have mutations that cause complete absence of tyrosinase activity, whereas mutations that cause OCA1B encode tyrosinase that has 5–10% residual enzymatic activity. R402Q is a temperature-sensitive mutation that renders tyrosinase partially active at 31°C and completely inactive above 37°C. These individuals typically have ocular features of albinism (because of high core body temperature) but then develop some pigmentation in skin of the extremities and their hair. Patient mutations tend to cluster near functional domains of the enzyme, specifically near the copper-binding regions in proximity to the active site, the N-terminus that is important for targeting to the rough endoplasmic reticulum, and the C-terminus that is important for sorting to melanosomes. Many of the mutations cause misfolding or instability of the nascent protein with retention in the rough endoplasmic reticulum and rerouting to the proteosome.

Less is known about mutations that cause OCA2 because of the large size of the gene; this should change with gene sequencing becoming available clinically. Of the approximately 200 individuals who have been genotyped, most have missense mutations that are spread throughout the gene, often present in the loops between the membrane-spanning domains.[50] A 2.7-kb deletion accounts for 75–80% of P-gene mutations in sub-Saharan Africans, where the frequency of OCA2 is as high as 1 in 1400 in Tanzania and 1 in 3900 in South Africa.

OCA3, rufous or red albinism, is associated with red hair and reddish-brown skin and has been reported mainly in South Africa and New Guinea. Of the small number of patients who have been genotyped, a variety of mutations has been observed (http://albinismdb.med.umn.edu/oca3mut.html).

OCA4, which is clinically similar to OCA2, appears to be an uncommon form of OCA except in the Japanese population, where it accounts for 24% of OCA patients.[51] A common missense mutation, D157N, was present in 39% of alleles, and the mutation was present on the same haplotype in both Japanese and Korean patients, indicating a founder effect in Asia.[52]

A variety of mutations have been identified in the OA1 gene, and of note, large intragenic deletions appear to be particularly common.[53] The high rate of deletions is partly explained by the presence of Alu-repeat sequences within the first two introns, which makes these regions prone to unequal recombination during meiosis. Curiously, the rate of large deletions in patients varies by geographic region, accounting for more than 50% of North American mutations but less than 10% of European mutations. Given the heterogeneous breakpoints of the deletions, this difference cannot be due to a single founder mutation, nor, given the lack of genotype–phenotype correlations, can the difference be attributed to environmental selection; the different frequencies may simply be incidental.[53] While genetic testing of the OA1 gene by the polymerase chain reaction is straightforward in males, deletions cannot be reliably detected in carrier females because of the presence of the second X chromosome. In suspected carriers, the presence of megamelanosomes on skin biopsy and uneven pigmentation in the retina is useful for clinical diagnosis.

Hermansky–Pudlak syndrome has its highest prevalence in Puerto Rico (1 in 1800 individuals), but is rare elsewhere in the world. Of the eight known genetic causes, HPS1 is the most common. HPS1 has two common founder mutations: a 16-basepair duplication mutation in Puerto Rican patients and a splice-site mutation (IVS5+5G>A) in Japanese patients.[50] HPS3 also has a founder mutation in Puerto Rican patients, involving a deletion of exon 1.

Chédiak–Higashi syndrome is caused by mutations in the CHS1 (*LYST*) gene. Genotype–phenotype correlations in a limited number of patients suggest that childhood disease is associated with null mutations, while juvenile and adult forms are associated with missense mutations that retain some residual functional activity.[54]

Conclusion

Albinism refers to a group of genetic conditions that are characterized by reduced melanin levels leading to hypopigmentation of the eyes, hair, and skin, and importantly, all affect vision. Simple or nonsyndromic forms of albinism affect melanosomes only, whereas complex or syndromic forms of albinism include systemic features caused by disturbances in both melanosomes and other intracellular organelles. While the eponymous syndrome names are useful clinically, genetic classification is recommended. For further information, there are excellent web resources on the disease (National Organization for Albinism and Hypopigmentation at www.albinism.com; Gene Reviews at www.genereviews.com), the laboratories that perform genetic testing (www.genetests.com), and the albinism gene mutation database at the International Albinism Center located at the University of Minnesota (http://albinismdb.med.umn.edu/).

Key references

A complete list of chapter references is available online at www.expertconsult.com. See inside cover for registration details.

1. Taylor WO. Edridge-Green lecture, 1978. Visual disabilities of oculocutaneous albinism and their alleviation. Trans Ophthalmol Soc UK 1978;98:423–445.

8. Guillery RW. Visual pathways in albinos. Sci Am 1974;230:44–54.

12. von dem Hagen EA, Hoffmann MB, Morland AB. Identifying human albinism: a comparison of VEP and fMRI. Invest Ophthalmol Vis Sci 2008;49:238–249.

13. Sturm RA, Teasdale RD, Box NF. Human pigmentation genes: identification, structure and consequences of polymorphic variation. Gene 2001; 277:49–62.

17. Hutton SM, Spritz RA. A comprehensive genetic study of autosomal recessive ocular albinism in Caucasian patients. Invest Ophthalmol Vis Sci 2008;49:868–872.

23. Seo JH, Yu YS, Kim JH, et al. Correlation of visual acuity with foveal hypoplasia grading by optical coherence tomography in albinism. Ophthalmology 2007;114:1547–1551.

28. von dem Hagen EA, Houston GC, Hoffmann MB, et al. Pigmentation predicts the shift in the line of decussation in humans with albinism. Eur J Neurosci 2007;25:503–511.

32. Rachel RA, Dolen G, Hayes NL, et al. Spatiotemporal features of early neuronogenesis differ in wild-type and albino mouse retina. J Neurosci 2002;22:4249–4263.

33. van Genderen MM, Riemslag FC, Schuil J, et al. Chiasmal misrouting and foveal hypoplasia without albinism. Br J Ophthalmol 2006;90:1098–1102.

41. Toyofuku K, Wada I, Valencia JC, et al. Oculocutaneous albinism types 1 and 3 are ER retention diseases: mutation of tyrosinase or Tyrp1 can affect the processing of both mutant and wild-type proteins. Faseb J 2001;15:2149–2161.

44. Manga P, Boissy RE, Pifko-Hirst S, et al. Mislocalization of melanosomal proteins in melanocytes from mice with oculocutaneous albinism type 2. Exp Eye Res 2001;72:695–710.

46. Puri N, Gardner JM, Brilliant MH. Aberrant pH of melanosomes in pink-eyed dilution (p) mutant melanocytes. J Invest Dermatol 2000;115:607–613.

49. Costin GE, Valencia JC, Vieira WD, et al. Tyrosinase processing and intracellular trafficking is disrupted in mouse primary melanocytes carrying the underwhite (uw) mutation. A model for oculocutaneous albinism (OCA) type 4. J Cell Sci 2003;116:3203–3212.

50. King RA, Oetting WS, Summers CG, et al. Abnormalities of pigmentation. In: Rimoin DL, Conner JM, Pyeritz RE, et al. (eds) Emery and Rimoin's Principles and Practice of Medical Genetics, vol. 3, 5th edn. Philadelphia: Elsevier, 2007:3380–3427.

53. Bassi MT, Bergen AA, Bitoun P, et al. Diverse prevalence of large deletions within the OA1 gene in ocular albinism type 1 patients from Europe and North America. Hum Genet 2001;108:51–54.

CHAPTER 61

Aniridia

Elias I Traboulsi

Clinical background

Aniridia refers to a bilateral malformation of the eye in which the most prominent clinical finding is variable to near-total absence of the iris.[1,2] The word aniridia is a misnomer since the iris is not totally absent (Figure 61.1) and there are in fact a number of other accompanying ocular abnormalities that result from the underlying genetic defect in one of the master ocular developmental genes, *PAX6*. Even in the more severe cases, a stump of tissue is invariably present at the base of the iris, and gonioscopy may be required for its adequate visualization. Careful ocular examination will reveal other abnormalities that include persistent strands of the fetal pupillary membrane, congenital lens opacities that could be cortical, anterior polar, or of other types, ectopia lentis or subluxation of the crystalline lens as a result of poor zonular development, developmental glaucoma, a superficial keratopathy referred to as corneal pannus, persistence of the retina over pars plana, and foveal hypoplasia that is almost universal and leads to decreased visual acuity and nystagmus.[3]

Congenital poor visual function in aniridia results from macular, foveal, and optic nerve hypoplasia.[4] Acquired causes of visual loss in aniridia include the development or progression of cataracts, optic nerve damage from glaucoma,[5,6] corneal opacification, and anisometropic or strabismic amblyopia. The keratopathy/corneal pannus of aniridia appears late in the first decade of life and is presumably due to insufficient/absent limbal stem cells that depend on the presence of normal *PAX6* complement for their development and maintenance.[7] Nystagmus is most likely due to congenital poor visual acuity, although underlying central nervous causes may exist that have not been adequately investigated. There are at least two families in which some members have classical aniridia and other members have atypical iris defects ranging from radial clefts or atypical colobomas and relatively good vision.[8,9] We have recently described four patients with aniridia, preserved vision, little or no foveal hypoplasia and no detectable mutations in *PAX6*.[10] Vascular anomalies of the iris have also been described.[9] Aniridia can also occur in association with malformations of the globe such as Peters' anomaly or congenital anterior staphyloma or with microcornea and subluxated lenses.

Aniridia is associated with systemic abnormalities when it occurs in the context of the well-defined contiguous gene syndrome of "Wilms' tumor–aniridia–genitourinary abnormalities–retardation" (WAGR) or Miller syndrome (Box 61.1). This type of aniridia is of the nonheritable variety and is always associated with a deletion of band 13 on the short arm of chromosome 11.[11,12]

Aniridia can also occur in the context of multisystem malformation syndromes and chromosomal abnormalities such as a ring chromosome 6,[13] pericentric inversion of chromosome 9,[14] the syndrome of multiple ocular malformations, and mental retardation described by Walker and Dyson[15] and Hamming et al,[16] and the syndrome of aniridia and absence of the patella.[17] When iris hypoplasia is not severe, aniridia may be confused with conditions such as Rieger anomaly (Figure 61.2), ectopia lentis et pupillae, atypical coloboma of the iris, or essential iris atrophy (Chandler syndrome).

PAX6 is widely expressed in the central nervous system. Sisodiya et al[18] performed magnetic resonance imaging (MRI) and smell testing in patients with aniridia and showed absence or hypoplasia of the anterior commissure and reduced olfaction in a large proportion of cases, demonstrating that *PAX6* haploinsufficency causes more widespread human neurodevelopmental anomalies[18]; Mitchell et al[19] demonstrated widespread structural abnormalities of the brain, including absence of the pineal gland and unilateral polymicrogyria on MRI of 24 patients heterozygous for defined *PAX6* mutations. Thompson et al[20] studied 14 patients with *PAX6* gene mutations and MRI abnormalities for defects in cognitive functioning. None were found except in a subgroup of patients with agenesis of the anterior commissure who performed significantly more poorly on measures of working memory than those without this abnormality. In another study, brain MRI, central auditory testing, and a questionnaire were administered to a group of 11 children with aniridia.[21] The corpus callosum area was significantly smaller on brain volumetry in patients compared with controls. The anterior commissure was small in 7 cases and was normal in 3 cases on visual inspection of brain MR images. Audiograms showed no abnormalities in any of the children. Central auditory test results were normal in all the controls and were abnormal in all the cases, except for 1 case with a pattern of abnormalities consistent with reduced auditory interhemispheric transfer. The cases had greater difficulty

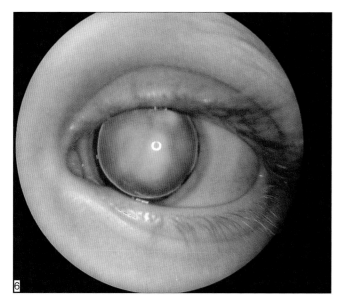

Figure 61.1 Classic aniridia phenotype with almost total absence of iris tissue. Only a small rim of iris is present. The edge of the lens is visible.

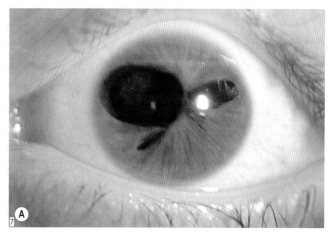

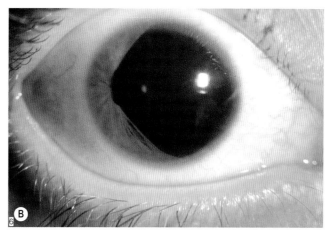

Figure 61.2 (A, B) Variable degrees of absence of iris tissue in aniridia. The phenotype can simulate Rieger anomaly.

> **Box 61.1 Clinical findings in aniridia**
>
> - Aniridia is an autosomal-dominant panocular malformative disorder in which the most prominent clinical abnormality is absence of iris tissue
> - Poor vision in aniridia results mostly from foveal hypoplasia
> - Aniridia results from mutations in the *PAX6* gene on 11p13
> - The WAGR syndrome of Wilms' tumor, aniridia, genitourinary malformations and retardation results from deletions of chromosome 11p13

---

localizing sound and understanding speech in noise than the controls. These findings indicate that, despite normal audiograms, children with *PAX6* mutations may experience auditory interhemispheric transfer deficits and have difficulty localizing sound and understanding speech in noise.

Aniridia with cerebellar ataxia and mental retardation is a very rare condition inherited in an autosomal-recessive fashion and known as Gillespie syndrome.[22,23] Gillespie syndrome is not caused by mutations in *PAX6*.[24]

Most recently glucose intolerance and diabetes mellitus have been described in some patients with aniridia and are possibly due to the importance of *PAX6* in pancreatic development and function.[25-27] *PAX6* plays an indispensable role in islet cell development. Yasuda et al performed oral glucose tolerance tests in patients with *PAX6* mutations and found glucose intolerance characterized by impaired insulin secretion.[26]

Etiology and distribution

Aniridia occurs in 1/50 000 live births. Shaw et al[1] estimated the prevalence of aniridia in the lower peninsula of Michigan in 1960 to be about 1 in 64 000. Approximately two-thirds

to three-fourths of patients have at least one other affected family member; the remainder are sporadic.

In one large series of 125 patients, 74 cases were sporadic, 24 were familial, and 14 had the WAGR syndrome, or other malformations.[28] Two cases had chromosome rearrangements involving 11p13, 16 cases had visible deletions, and 16 cases had cryptic deletions identified by fluorescent in situ hybridization (FISH). The frequency of cryptic deletions in familial aniridia was 27% and in sporadic isolated aniridia was 22%. Of the 14 cases referred with WAGR syndrome, 10 (71%) had chromosomal deletions, 2 cryptic, and 8 visible. Of the 13 cases with aniridia and other malformations, 5 (38%) had a chromosomal rearrangement or deletion. In 37 cases with no karyotypic or cryptic chromosome abnormality, sequence analysis of the *PAX6* gene was performed. Mutations were identified in 33 cases: 22 with sporadic aniridia, 10 with familial aniridia, and 1 with aniridia and other non-WAGR syndrome-associated anomalies. Overall, 67 of 71 cases (94%) undergoing full mutation analysis had a mutation in the *PAX6* genomic region.

Aniridia is caused in most cases by mutations in *PAX6*, a homeobox transcription factor on 11p13.[29,30] There appears to be a correlation between the type of mutation and the clinical phenotype. A classic severe phenotype results from mutations that lead to stop codons and protein haploinsufficiency.[31] Missense mutations cause aniridia as well as other

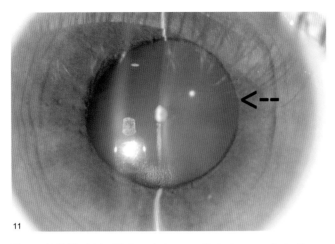

Figure 61.3 The iris in this figure is from a patient who presented with nystagmus. She had a small defect in the papillary sphincter (arrow) and poorly delineated limbus. She had a mutation in *PAX6*.

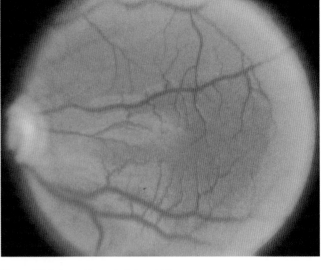

Figure 61.5 Foveal hypoplasia in aniridia.

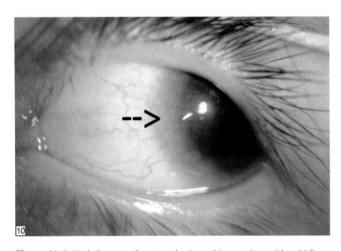

Figure 61.4 Limbal pannus/keratopathy (arrow) in a patient with aniridia.

> **Box 61.2 Management of patients with aniridia**
>
> - The workup of patients with aniridia includes mutation analysis of the *PAX6* gene. If a mutation is found in sporadic patients, a deletion of 11p13 is ruled out and the risk of Wilms tumor becomes that of the general population
> - Patients with aniridia are at high risk of developing glaucoma. Intraocular pressure needs to be checked frequently
> - Cataracts are common and should only be extracted if vision is expected to improve
> - Other family members should be carefully examined, especially in families where the clinical manifestations are mild

phenotypes, including cataracts, Peters' anomaly, other types of anterior-segment dysgenesis, and occasionally a clinical picture predominated by keratopathy (Figure 61.3).[32] Rarely, the iris is so well preserved (Figure 61.4) that the phenotype is one of isolated foveal hypoplasia (Figure 61.5).[33] Some patients with mutations in *PAX6* have microphthalmia.

Prognosis, prevention, and treatment

Once the clinical diagnosis of aniridia is made, it becomes imperative to determine whether the patient has a mutation inside the *PAX6* gene or whether he/she carries a deletion that involves the adjacent Wilms' tumor gene *WT1*. Clinical molecular genetic testing is available and will identify a mutation in more than 75% of cases. Karyotyping has been superseded by microarray analysis, a test that will detect small deletions or chromosomal rearrangements of 11p13 where the *PAX6* gene is located. FISH analysis can also be used to detect submicroscopic deletions of 11p13. As a general rule, familial cases have intragenic mutations, while sporadic cases may be due to either *PAX6* mutations or to

chromosomal deletions that may include adjacent genes and cause the WAGR syndrome. In any patient with aniridia and a negative family history, the risk of developing Wilms' tumor is 20%. About 1 in 70 patients with Wilms' tumor have aniridia. The presence of other systemic abnormalities in a sporadic case of aniridia should raise the suspicion of a chromosome 11p deletion or rearrangement. If access to genetic testing is not possible, careful, repeated examination and imaging of the renal system should be performed. Ultrasound examination of the kidneys is done at 6-month intervals supplemented with intravenous pyelography, computed tomography, or MRI to evaluate further any suspicious finding.

Other family members should be examined for the presence of mild degrees of iris hypoplasia as this may indicate dominant inheritance with variable expressivity and circumvent the worries about the potential occurrence of Wilms' tumor.

The management of ocular problems in patients with aniridia can be very challenging (Box 61.2). Visual acuity is less than or about 20/200 in most patients, but may be as good as 20/20 in patients with aniridia and preserved ocular function.[10] The main cause of acquired visual loss in aniridia is glaucoma, and patients are screened for its presence at regular intervals.[5] The glaucoma in aniridia typically develops in late childhood or in adulthood; however, it may be present in the first year of life. Aniridic glaucoma may be due to trabeculodysgenesis, but a more likely mechanism is occlusion of the filtering angle by an up-pulling of the iris stump. Goniotomy or trabeculotomy may be successful in controlling or preventing aniridic glaucoma[34]; however, filtering surgery or cyclocryotherapy may be required. Medical therapy should be tried in older individuals with aniridic glaucoma. Cataracts, which develop in most aniridic patients, are extracted if they produce significant further decrease in visual acuity. Some patients have congenital anterior polar cataracts while others have acquired cataracts that usually develop in early adulthood. Ectopia lentis is occasionally found in aniridic eyes and should be looked for before a lensectomy is performed. Finally, penetrating keratoplasty may be required in some instances if progressive keratopathy leads to corneal opacification and to further loss of vision.

Pathology

There are very few histopathologic studies of the eye in aniridia, some of which are from eyes blind with advanced glaucoma.[35] In typical cases, the iris is rudimentary and there is an absence of dilator and pupillary sphincter muscles. Grant and Walton[6] reported their observations of the angle in a large number of patients with aniridia. They noted that the peripheral stump of the iris gradually extended anteriorly to cover the filtration portion of the angle as patients got older. They also noted that this correlated with worsening of glaucoma. The lens may be subluxated from underdeveloped zonular apparatus, and the ciliary processes may be small.

Etiology

Mutations in *PAX6* account for a majority of cases of aniridia (Box 61.3). There is evidence of genetic heterogeneity and some cases with aniridia do not have detectable mutations in *PAX6*.[10]

Using positional cloning and DNA samples from patients with aniridia and deletions involving the 11p13 aniridia locus, Ton and coworkers cloned a cDNA which they presumed to be complementary to AN2.[29] This gene was found

to be the human homolog of the murine *Pax6* gene that, when mutated, results in the small-eye (*Sey*) phenotype. Homozygous *Sey/Sey* mice are anophthalmic, lack nasal structures, and die shortly after birth.[36] Hemizygous Sey/+ mice are microphthalmic and have a range of anterior-segment abnormalities ranging from colobomas to iris hypoplasia and lenticulo-irido-corneal adhesions. A neuropathological study of *Small eye* mice showed that there was a delay of premigratory neurons and an impairment of axonal growth and differentiation. This eventually results in a broad spectrum of neuronal migration disorders of the neocortical roof.[37] The murine *Pax6* gene mapped to a region of chromosome 2 in the mouse which is syntenic to the aniridia locus on chromosome 11 in humans, giving further support that *Sey* is the murine homolog of the aniridia gene. *PAX6* is expressed in the fetal eye, forebrain, cerebellum, and olfactory bulbs.[29,38] In the developing eye *Sey* is expressed first in the optic sulcus and subsequently in the eye vesicle, in the lens, in the differentiating retina, and finally in the cornea. Glaser and coworkers described the complete genomic structure of the human *PAX6* gene and discovered mutations in familial and sporadic cases.[30] Using mutation analysis of the *PAX6* gene, investigators from around the world identified numerous mutations in patients with aniridia (http://pax6.hgu.mrc.ac.uk/).

The human *PAX6* gene spans 22 kb and consists of 14 exons (Figure 61.6). It belongs to the Pax family of developmental control factors that possess the paired domain originally identified in the *Drosophila melanogaster* segmentation gene *paired*. The encoded PAX6 protein contains two DNA-binding domains: the paired box of 128 amino acids and a paired-type homeobox of 61 amino acids, separated by the linker region. The paired domain has two functional sub-domains, the 74-amino-acid N-terminal domain which is relatively conserved among paired domains, and the less well conserved 54-amino-acid C-terminal domain. PAX6 is alternatively spliced and inclusion of exon 5a (PAX6-5a) alters the DNA-binding properties resulting in DNA contact by the C-terminal domain instead of the N-terminal domain. In the C-terminal part of the protein there is a proline, serine, and threonine-rich (PST) domain of 152 amino acids which resembles the activation domain of transcription factors, and has been shown to possess transcriptional activity in vitro. Pax6 is involved in the transcriptional regulation of the crystalline genes and interacts closely with a number of genes essential in embryonic eye development. A striking amino acid identity is observed of PAX-6 proteins between species, especially in the functional domains, with only one amino acid difference between the mouse and the human gene located in the alternatively spliced exon. The expression patterns of Pax-6 are also conserved throughout the vertebrates and transcripts have been detected in the developing eye, the

---

Box 61.3 Mutations in *PAX6* cause aniridia

- More than 300 mutations in *PAX6* have been reported to date, most of which result in protein truncation and haploinsufficiency
- Rare cases of Peters' anomaly and cataracts have resulted from *PAX6* mutations
- Insect and animal models of aniridia have been discovered and result from mutations in *Pax6* in the mouse and rat for example, and in *eyeless* in *Drosophila*. These models have been very important in studying the function of the gene

---

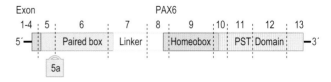

Figure 61.6 Organizational diagram of the *PAX6* gene. PST, proline, serine, and threonine-rich.

brain, spinal cord, and pancreas. It has been shown in the bovine eye that the 5a isoform predominates in the iris in contrast to the lens and retina where PAX6 and PAX6-5a seem to be equally represented, indicating that the PAX6-5a isoform is important for iris development.

In the human *PAX6* database there are now more than 300 mutations and over 100 sequence variations (http://pax6.hgu.mrc.ac.uk/). Most of the mutations cause premature truncation of the protein and relatively few missense mutations have been reported, some with aniridia and others with congenital cataracts, Peters' anomaly, and foveal hypoplasia. Autosomal-dominant keratitis has been associated with a splice site mutation (IVS10-2A>T) in *PAX6*. Missense mutations are generally associated with milder phenotypes.

Some *PAX6* mutations give rise to panocular effects with signs that are less severe or different from classic aniridia. For example, a missense mutation (R26G) caused a heterogeneous syndrome of anterior-segment malformations, including iris hypoplasia and Peters' anomaly. A nonsense mutation in codon S353 produces a truncated protein in the PST domain and is associated with normal irides, cataracts, and late onset of cone dystrophy.[39] These two truncated PST domains have partial transcriptional activity, possibly accounting for the milder phenotype. An exon 11 splice acceptor mutation caused autosomal-dominant keratitis in a family.[32] Yanagisawa and colleagues[40] reported a missense mutation at nucleotide 799, a C to T transition associated with a phenotype dominated by foveal hypoplasia and, according to the authors, no iris defects.

The *Drosophila* gene *eyeless* (*ey*) is the homolog of *PAX6* in humans and *Pax6* in the mouse. Eyeless flies have partial or total absence of their compound eyes. Hypomorphic (weak) alleles lead to the reduction or absence of compound eyes but do not affect the ocelli or simple eyes. Null alleles are not available now but presumably affect all eyes and are lethal when homozygous. The proteins encoded by *ey*, *Sey*, and AN2 share 94% sequence identity in the paired domain and 90% identity in the homeodomain. Furthermore, there are similarities in the flanking sequences and some of the splice sites in the paired box and in the homeobox are conserved between the fly and mammalian genes, indicating that the genes are orthologous.[41]

Grove et al[42] reported two matings of aniridic patients in a large family. One couple had no children. A second couple had a total of six children: one girl with aniridia lived to 11 months and died of central nervous system problems; three boys died at less than 24 hours of age; there was also one spontaneous abortion at 3 months of gestation and one near-term intrauterine fetal death. Elsas and coworkers[8] also reported one mating between aniridics. The couple had four living children: three had aniridia and one was normal; there was a stillborn child with unknown phenotype. Other cases are those reported by Hodgson and Saunders,[43] who described the necropsy findings in a stillborn girl whose mother and father had aniridia. There were two previous miscarriages at 10 weeks of gestation. The fetus had absence of the palpebral fissures and eyes. The nasal bones were completely absent and the nasal cavity was small. Both parietal bones had elliptical defects at their posterior medial aspects and overlapped the occipital bone. The adrenals were absent. The skeletal, urogenital, alimentary, cardiovascular,

and respiratory systems appeared normal. The thyroid and thymus were normal. The brain was macerated. Glaser et al reported a family where two mutations of the *PAX6* gene segregated independently, causing either aniridia or a syndrome of cataracts and late-onset corneal dystrophy.[39] A compound heterozygote for the mutations at codons 103 and 353 had severe craniofacial and central nervous system defects and no eyes. This study demonstrates a dosage effect of the *PAX6* gene and its critical role in the development of eye and brain structures.

Pathophysiology

PAX6 is widely expressed in the neurectoderm and the surface ectoderm of the developing eye, and in their derivatives with specific dosage requirements of the transcription factor in these tissues.[44] *PAX6* activity is essential in the ectoderm for lens placode formation (Box 61.4).

Ashery-Padan and coworkers showed that several independent, fully differentiated neuroretinas developed in a single optic vesicle in the absence of a lens from a mutation in Pax6, demonstrating that the developing lens is not necessary for the differentiation of the neuroretina but is required for the correct placement of a single retina in the eye.[45] *PAX6* continues to be expressed in the adult retina, lens, and cornea. The progressive nature of the aniridia phenotype with corneal and lens changes over time reflects the maintenance functions of *PAX6* in the adult eye.[46] *PAX6* is also expressed in the olfactory system, from the earliest nasal placode to the mature olfactory bulb and the olfactory epithelium. It is also expressed in the developing telencephalon, thalamus, pituitary, pineal, cerebellum, spinal cord, and pancreas. *PAX6* plays a key role in the development of the brain where it affects cell fate, cell proliferation, and patterning. The paired domain is necessary for the regulation of neurogenesis, cell proliferation, and patterning effects of *PAX6*, whereas the homeodomain plays a lesser role in the brain. Splicing of one or the other exon 5 appears to play a pivotal role in neurogenesis.[47]

The *Drosophila* gene *eyeless* (*ey*) is homologous to the mouse *Small eye* (*Pax6*) gene and to the aniridia gene in humans. By targeted expression of the *ey* complementary DNA in various imaginal disc primordia of *Drosophila*, Halder et al induced ectopic eye structures on the wings, legs, and antennae. The ectopic eyes appeared morphologically normal and consisted of groups of fully differentiated

---

Box 61.4 Functions of *PAX6*

- *PAX6* is a master control gene that is expressed in the developing eye and brain
- *PAX6* is essential in lens placode formation and other early developmental stages of the eye
- *PAX6* interacts with a large number of other transcription factors that are essential in normal ocular development
- *PAX6* continues to be expressed in ocular surface cells such as the limbal epithelium, where it plays a vital role in corneal epithelial cell maintenance and regeneration

ommatidia with a complete set of photoreceptor cells. These findings support the concept that *PAX6* is a master control gene of eye development.[41]

Heterozygous intragenic mutations in *PAX6* have been identified in more than 80% of classical aniridia patients tested (http://pax6.hgu.mrc.ac.uk/), suggesting that *PAX6* is the predominant gene implicated in this condition. The majority of classical aniridia cases are due to *PAX6* haploinsufficiency, resulting from heterozygous null mutations. The homozygous null phenotype in mice and human cases reflect more closely the wide expression pattern of the gene, with perinatal lethality associated with absence of eyes, nasal structures, and pancreas, and with severe brain defects. Overexpression of Pax6 is also deleterious, leading to reduced eye size in mice transgenic for five copies of a human PAX6-bearing yeast artificial chromosome, suggesting that correct Pax6 dosage is critical for eye development.[48]

Conclusions

Aniridia is only one of a complex of ocular malformations that results from mutations in the *PAX6* gene. Molecular testing is now available and circumvents the need for Wilms' tumor screening in patients with nonfamilial aniridia. Patients should be followed carefully and checked for elevation in intraocular pressure that can lead to additional vision loss. Animal, insect, and invertebrate models have allowed a good understanding of the functions of *PAX6* in embryogenesis and in ocular tissues after birth.

Key references

A complete list of chapter references is available online at www.expertconsult.com. See inside cover for registration details.

2. Nelson LB, Spaeth GL, Nowinski TS, et al. Aniridia. A review. Surv Ophthalmol 1984;28:621–642.

5. Walton DS. Aniridic glaucoma: the results of gonio-surgery to prevent and treat this problem. Trans Am Ophthalmol Soc 1986;84:59–70.

7. Koroma BM, Yang JM, Sundin OH. The Pax-6 homeobox gene is expressed throughout the corneal and conjunctival epithelia. Invest Ophthalmol Vis Sci 1997;38:108–120.

10. Traboulsi EI, Ellison J, Sears J, et al. Aniridia with preserved visual function: a report of four cases with no mutations in PAX6. Am J Ophthalmol 2008;145:160–164.

12. Turleau C, de Grouchy J, Tournade MF, et al. Del 11p/aniridia complex. Report of three patients and review of 37 observations from the literature. Clin Genet 1984;26:356–362.

18. Sisodiya SM, Free SL, Williamson KA, et al. PAX6 haploinsufficiency causes cerebral malformation and olfactory dysfunction in humans. Nat Genet 2001;28:214–216.

22. Gillespie FD. Aniridia, cerebellar ataxia, and oligophrenia in siblings. Arch Ophthalmol 1965;73:338–341.

28. Robinson DO, Howarth RJ, Williamson KA, et al. Genetic analysis of chromosome 11p13 and the PAX6 gene in a series of 125 cases referred with aniridia. Am J Med Genet A 2008;146A: 558–569.

29. Ton CC, Hirvonen H, Miwa H, et al. Positional cloning and characterization of a paired box- and homeobox-containing gene from the aniridia region. Cell 1991;67:1059–1074.

30. Glaser T, Walton DS, Maas RL. Genomic structure, evolutionary conservation and aniridia mutations in the human PAX6 gene. Nat Genet 1992; 2:232–239.

32. Mirzayans F, Pearce WG, MacDonald IM, et al. Mutation of the PAX6 gene in patients with autosomal dominant keratitis. Am J Hum Genet 1995;57:539–548.

36. Hill R, Favor J, Hogan B, et al. Mouse small eye results from mutations in a paired-like homeobox-containing gene. Nature 1991;354:522–525.

39. Glaser T, Jepeal L, Edwards J, et al. PAX6 gene dosage effect in a family with congenital cataracts aniridia anophthalmia and central nervous system defects. Nat Genet 1994;7:463–469.

41. Halder G, Callaerts P, Gehring W. Induction of ectopic eyes by targeted expression of the eyeless gene in *Drosophila*. Science 1995;267:1788–1792.

46. Van Heyningen V, Williamson KA. PAX6 in sensory development. Hum Mol Genet 2002;11:1161–1167.

Color vision defects

Maureen Neitz and Jay Neitz

Clinical background

Key symptoms and signs

"Normal" color vision refers to the form of trichromatic color vision shared by most humans. It is mediated by three types of retinal cone photoreceptors, designated long- (L), middle- (M), and short- (S) wavelength cones. Each cone type is maximally sensitive to a different region of the visible spectrum (Figure 62.1). The neural circuitry for color vision compares the outputs of the three cone types and generates neural signals that give rise to the percepts of six basic colors: blue, yellow, red, green, black, and white, and to their mixtures. Color vision defects can either be inherited as the consequence of gene defects that affect the function of one or more cone type, or they can be acquired secondary to disease or through exposure to neurotoxins. The hallmark feature of color vision defects is a reduction in the number of different colors that are seen as distinguishable from each other. The terms "protan" and "deutan" refer to color vision defects that result from abnormalities in the L and M cones and are collectively termed red–green color vision deficiency. These are characterized by diminished sensations of red and green, and this translates to a difficulty with several color combinations: (1) confusion between colors in the middle-to-long-wavelength region of the spectrum, which include green, yellow, orange, and red, particularly the pale versions of those colors and their very dark counterparts, olive, brown, and brick; (2) confusion between greenish and reddish colors, and gray, especially turquoise and gray and magenta or pink and gray; and (3) confusion between blue, violet, and purple. The term "tritan" refers to color vision deficits that result from abnormalities in the S cones and they are characterized by diminished sensations of blue and yellow difficulty, resulting in confusions between dark blue and black, yellow and yellow–green and white and also confusions among colors in the short-wavelength region of the spectrum: violet, purple, blue, and blue–green. Achromatopsia refers to complete or nearly complete absence of color perception (see glossary, below).

Quick reference for terminology for inherited color vision defects

- Protan: from the Greek for "the first": defective color vision mediated by S cones and M cones with no L-cone function. A category of red–green color vision deficiency.
- Deutan: from the Greek for "the second": color vision mediated by S cones and L cones with no M-cone function. A category of red–green color vision deficiency.
- Tritan: from the Greek for "the third": color vision mediated by L and M cones with abnormal or no S-cone function. Blue–yellow color vision deficiency.
- Achromatopsia: vision mediated either by S cones and rods (blue-cone monochromacy) or rods only (rod monochromacy)

Glossary of official gene designations

- *OPN1LW*: X-chromosome gene encoding the opsin for the L-cone photopigment.
- *OPN1MW*: X-chromosome gene encoding the opsin for the M-cone photopigment.
- *OPN1SW*: chromosome 7 gene encoding the opsin for the S-cone photopigment.
- *CNGA3*: gene encoding the alpha subunit of the cyclic nucleotide gated ion channel that photoreceptors use to modulate membrane potential in response to light.
- *CNGB3*: gene encoding the beta subunit of the cyclic nucleotide gated ion channel that photoreceptors use to modulate membrane potential in response to light.
- *GNAT2*: gene encoding the alpha subunit of transducin, the G-protein to which the cone photopigments, which are G-protein-coupled receptors, are coupled.

Historical development

The mechanisms of inherited color vision defects are far better understood than those of acquired defects, largely

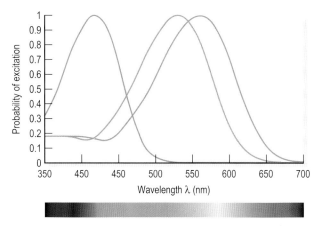

Figure 62.1 Relative spectral sensitivities of the three cone types that mediate normal human color vision expressed as a function of the probability (*y*-axis) that an individual cone type will absorb light a specified wavelength (*x*-axis). The S cone has peak sensitivity at 415 nm, the M cone has peak sensitivity at ~530 nm, and the S cone has peak sensitivity at ~560 nm. Below the graph of the spectral sensitivity functions is a representation of the color appearance of the wavelengths on the *x*-axis, as they would appear to a person with normal trichromatic color vision.

because inherited color vision deficiencies are extremely common and they are more tractable to investigation. The first recorded description of color vision deficiency was a report by John Dalton describing his own red–green defect,[1] hence "daltonism" is the accepted term for inherited red–green color vision deficiency in many languages. Dalton hypothesized that his color vision defect was caused by blue tinted vitreous, which was disproven after his death in 1844, and in 1995, a molecular genetic study of Dalton's preserved retinas allowed the basis of his defect to be identified: this was the deletion of the gene encoding the M-cone photopigment.[1] Although the tendency for color vision defects to run in families and to skip generations has long been recognized, the underlying genetics has only been well characterized within the last 100 years. In the 1920s Waaler used results he collected from nearly 20 000 schoolchildren in Oslo to form the basis for his hypothesis that two separate genes on the X chromosome – one for L-cone sensitivity and another for M-cone sensitivity – accounted for the inheritance patterns of normal and defective color vision (2 1457), and over the next few decades his ideas were developed into a two-locus model of red–green color vision in which a series of alleles of the L-pigment gene were proposed to account for the range of protan red–green color vision defects and a separate set of alleles of the M-pigment gene accounted for the range of deutan red–green defects.

The next big breakthrough in understanding the biological basis of color vision and its defects came when Jeremy Nathans and colleagues cloned and sequenced the genes encoding the S-, M-, and L-cone opsins (see glossary above for definition), and demonstrated that the L- and M-opsin genes are, in fact, adjacent on the X chromosome. From his observations, Nathans hypothesized that color vision defects were not the result of independent mutations at separate L and M pigment gene loci, as had previously been believed, but were instead a consequence of genetic recombination between the L and M genes. Another outcome of the tandem arrangement of the photopigment genes as observed by

Nathans is that expression of both the L and M genes is controlled by a by a shared DNA-regulatory element that, when deleted, causes blue-cone monochromacy. Finally, Nathans observed that there was variability in the number of X-linked opsin genes among people with normal color vision, and this presumably arose from unequal crossing over between X-chromosome pigment gene arrays.[3–6]

Subsequently, point mutations in the S opsin gene were found to underlie inherited tritan defects.[7–9] (Gunther 2006 #1115). The advent of methods for efficient genetic linkage analysis, which has been applied to families and populations affected by rod monochromacy, allowed the discovery of gene defects underlying these disorders.[10]

Epidemiology

Inherited color vision defects

In the USA and western Europe, red–green color vision defects are extremely common, but the prevalence is about 19 times greater in males than in females because it is X-linked recessive. An estimated 1 in 12 males and 1 in 230 females is affected. The prevalence of red–green color vision defects varies with ethnicity.[11] Caucasian populations in the USA and western Europe are reported to have the highest prevalence, with about 8% of males being affected. Native Fijians have the lowest, with fewer than 1% of males affected, and African and Japanese males have intermediate frequencies, with an estimated 4% of African and ~2% of Japanese males being affected (reviewed in reference 12). All other color vision defects are relatively rare.

Inherited blue–yellow color vision defects affect males and females equally. Prevalence values reported in the literature range from 1 in 500 to 1 in 65 000.[10,13] Estimating the prevalence has been challenging because most commonly used clinical color vision tests do not adequately test for color discrimination in the blue–yellow region of the spectrum. Achromotopsias are also extremely rare, and include both blue-cone monochromacy and rod monochromacy. The prevalence of blue-cone monochromacy, which is an X-linked trait and therefore preferentially affects males, has been estimated to be about 1 in 100 000, whereas rod monochromacy affects males and females equally, with prevalence estimates ranging from 1 in 20 000 to 1 in 50 000.[10]

Genetics

Inherited color vision defects

The vast majority of inherited color vision defects are caused by mutations that affect the expression or function of the cone photopigments. Photopigments are comprised of a protein, termed opsin, attached to an 11-*cis* retinal chromophore. The cone photopigments all use the same chromophore, but different opsins. Three opsins corresponding to each cone type, L, M, and S, are encoded by three genes designated *OPN1LW*, *OPN1MW*, and *OPN1SW*, respectively. *OPN1LW* and *OPN1MW* are located on the X chromosome at Xq28, and *OPN1SW* resides on chromosome 7 at 7q32.

Blue–yellow color vision deficiency is inherited as an autosomal-dominant trait caused by mutations in the *OPN1SW* gene. Both the common red–green color vision defects and the relatively uncommon blue-cone mono-chromacy are X-linked, being caused by mutations and gene rearrangements of the X-chromosome opsin genes, *OPN1LW* or *OPN1MW*. For red–green defects the gene rearrangements result in the absence of one cone type, L or M, but for blue-cone monochromacy the mutations result in the absence of both L and M cones. Rod monochromacies are autosomal recessive and causative mutations have been identified in the three genes: the *CNGA3* and *CNGB3* genes encoding the α and β subunits, respectively, of the cyclic nucleotide gated ion channel that is essential for cone photoreceptors to modulate membrane potential in response to light absorption,[14–18] and in the *GNAT2* gene that encodes the α subunit of cone transducin.[19] These gene defects result in the loss of function for all three cone types.

Diagnostic workup

There are a large number of different tests used in the diagnosis of color vision defects. Pseudoisochromatic plates are the most familiar color vision tests. The most widely used examples are Ishihara's test of color vision and the Hardy, Rand and Rittler (HRR) pseudoisochromatic plates. These tests each consist of a book containing a series of printed colored plates. Each plate is designed to conceal a hidden figure that can be seen by a person with normal color vision but is obscured for people with particular color vision deficiencies.

Arrangement tests – the best examples are the Farnsworth–Munsell 100 hue test and its abridged version, the Farnsworth–Munsell dichotomous D-15 test – consist of a series of colored disks in which the color changes from one to the next in small steps. The caps are mixed up and the task is to "arrange" the disks "in order" so that each disk is next to the color closest to it in appearance. Color vision defects are diagnosed by the misordering of the disks.

The anomaloscope is an instrument that contains an optical system that produces two side-by-side lighted fields, one monochromatic amber and the other a mixture of red and green light. The subject adjusts the ratio of red-to-green light in the mixture until it exactly matches the amber monochromatic light. People who have inherited red–green color anomalies in which either the L or M pigment is shifted in spectral peak compared to normal will require either a higher or lower ratio of red-to-green light in the mixture. This test is extraordinarily sensitive to genetic alterations in the spectral sensitivities of the photopigments and will detect them even in individuals in whom the alteration in the photopigment has little or no effect on the person's ability to discriminate between different colors. Because of its extreme sensitivity in detecting the presence of anomalous photopigments, the anomaloscope is often referred to as the "gold standard" for diagnosing inherited red–green color vision deficiencies. However, while an abnormal result on this test does indicate a photopigment abnormality, some mild photopigment abnormalities are associated with little or no loss in color discrimination ability.

Differential diagnosis

Acquired color vision defects are usually not present from birth, are often accompanied by other visual problems

---

Box 62.1 Color vision defects

Inherited color vision defects

Red–green color vision defects

- X-linked
- Very common
- More common in males than females
- Most often caused by deletions and rearrangements of the genes encoding the long- and middle-wavelength-sensitive cone opsins on the X chromosome

Blue–yellow color vision defects

- Autosomal dominant
- Relatively rare
- Caused by mutations in gene encoding short-wavelength cone opsin that produces amino acid substitutions

Acquired color vision defects

- Caused by diseases that affect nerve function or by exposure to neurotoxins
- Because red–green color vision defects are so common, it is not unusual for a person with an acquired color vision defect also to have an inherited color vision defect, making diagnosis of the acquired defect more challenging

---

including decreased acuity and visual field defects, can affect one or both eyes, and usually become progressively worse.[20–22] Common causes are optic neuropathies (e.g., toxic, inflammatory, nutritional) or retinopathies (e.g., toxic, paraneoplastic, degenerative). These are discussed at length in other chapters. Inherited color vision deficiencies are suggested by congenital onset, stability, and a compatible family history (Box 62.1). They are most reliably distinguished from acquired deficiencies by genetic testing, which is not commercially available at present.

Treatment

Inherited color vision defects

The ability of some red–green color-deficient individuals to name colors correctly and to pass standard color vision tests can be improved by placing a broadband red filter over one eye. A contact lens with a red tint, known as the X-chrom lens, was developed for this purpose; however, such lenses do not cure color vision deficiency, and have been reported to cause visual distortions.[23]

Gene therapy as a cure for ocular diseases has been an area of intense investigation over the last decade. Successful rescue of achromatopsia in a mouse model of rod monochromacy caused by *GNAT2* mutations has been reported.[24] At present, there is no cure for red–green color vision deficiency; however, in the majority of cases the cone photoreceptors are healthy and viable, and viral-mediated gene therapy is a viable option for delivering the missing cone opsin gene to photoreceptors to rescue the defect.

Acquired color vision defects

Color vision defects acquired through exposure to toxins can frequently be treated by removing exposure to the toxin. If done soon enough, the loss in color vision is, in some cases,

Table 62.1 Inherited red–green color vision defects

Photoreceptors*	Percentage of red–green color vision defects	Term for the color vision phenotype	Term for affected person
Deutan defects (6%)			
S L₁ L₂	5%	Deuteranomaly, anomalous trichromacy	Deuteranomalous, anomalous trichromat
S L	1%	Deuteranopia, dichromacy	Deuteranope, dichromat
Protan defects (2%)			
S M₁ M₂	1%	Protanomaly, anomalous trichromacy	Protanomalous, anomalous, trichromat
S M	1%	Protanopia, dichromacy	Protanope, dichromat

*L₁ and L₂ cones differ in spectral sensitivity, as do M₁ and M₂ cones.

reversible. If a patient is to be administered a drug associated with loss in color vision, a baseline color vision test should be given prior to beginning drug treatment to establish the presence or absence of an inherited color vision defect. Once drug treatment has started, patients should be monitored for changes in color vision so that drug treatment can be stopped before irreversible nerve damage occurs. Similarly, workers exposed to neurotoxins in industry should have baseline color vision testing done, followed by periodic color vision testing to monitor for changes that would indicate neurotoxic effects.

Pathology

Inherited color vision defects

Red–green color vision defects are present from birth, almost always affect both eyes, are not usually accompanied by other vision problems, and are stable throughout life. As will be discussed in more detail below, under pathophysiology, red–green color vision defects are most often caused by deletions of X-chromosome opsin genes such that only one category of X-chromosome-encoded opsin, L or M, is expressed. Protan defects are caused by the absence of functional L cones and protan defects are caused by the absence of functional M cones. Deutan-type defects are more prevalent than protan types, with about 6% of color-deficient males having a deutan type and 2% having a protan-type defect (Table 62.1). Both protan and deutan defects are subcategorized according to the degree of color vision loss.[25–27] Deutan color vision is mediated by S cones and L cones and accounts for about 6% of red–green color vision deficiency. Deutan males can either be dichromatic, having only S cones and one type of L cone, or they can be anomalous trichromats, having S cones and two different L-cone subtypes (Table 62.1). Protan color vision is mediated by S cones and M cones, and accounts for about 2% of red–green color vision defects. Protan males can also either be dichromatic, having only S cones and one type of M cone, or anomalous trichromatic, having S cones and two different M-cone subtypes (Table 62.1).

Usually in protan and deutan defects, the cones are healthy and viable without significant loss of photoreceptors. For example, deutans have only S cones and L cones, but the cells that would normally have become M cones are not usually lost; instead they become L cones. Likewise, protans are not usually missing the photoreceptors that would normally have become L cones; instead they become M cones. However, there are examples of protan and deutan defects in which cone photoreceptors are lost. Adaptive optics imaging has been used to examine the retinas of several red–green color-defective males, one of whom was estimated to have lost 30% of his cones. The individual was a dichromat (deuteranope), and cone-classing experiments using retinal densitometry plus adaptive optics showed that he had only S and L cones. His retina contained large dark (cone-less) areas, presumably where his M cones had been.[28]

Although relatively rare, red–green color vision defects arise from mutations in either the *OPN1LW* or *OPN1MW* gene that result in an amino acid substitution (missense mutations) that inactivates the encoded opsin.[28,29] The most common such mutation is a substitution of arginine for cysteine at position 203 (C203R) of either the L or M opsin. Cysteine 203 participates in a highly conserved disulfide bond that is critical for proper folding of the cone opsin.[30] Mutation of the corresponding cysteine in the rod pigment rhodopsin results in retinal degeneration.[31] It is not known what happens to the cone photoreceptors expressing a C203R mutant photopigment, but this question will likely be addressed in the near future as high-resolution adaptive optics imaging techniques become more available to examine affected patients.

Tritan defects are caused by missense mutations in the *OPN1SW* gene, and five such mutations have been reported to date.[7–9,32] Although the disorder is inherited, the color vision deficit is not always present from birth; instead it exhibits incomplete penetrance, meaning that not everyone who has a causative gene mutation has the color vision defect. A recent study using adaptive optics to image the retinas of a father and daughter, both with a tritan defect, revealed an absence of S cones in the father, but the presence of S cones in the daughter.[9] These results suggest that some tritan defects may be associated with a progressive loss of S cones, and this would account for the incomplete pentrance. That is, patients with the gene mutation may not exhibit a color vision deficiency until loss of S cones has progressed to a critical level at which the color defect manifests. The S-cone dystrophy hypothesized for tritan defects is analogous to rod dystrophy caused by rhodopsin mutations.

Inherited monochromatic color vision defects, termed achromatopsias, are associated with reduced (incomplete achromatopsia) or absent (complete achromatopsia) cone function. Blue-cone monochromacy is an inherited form of incomplete achromatopsia characterized by the absence of functional L and M cones, with normal functional rods and S cones. Rod monochromacy is a form of complete achromatopsia characterized by the absence of all normal functioning cones.[14,33] Achromatopsias are bilateral defects accompanied by photophobia, nystagmus, and poor visual acuities, usually 20/200 or worse.[5,18,34] The majority of cone photoreceptors in the human retina are L and M cones, with only about 5% being S cones.[35,36] Since cones serve high-acuity vision the loss of function of 95–100% of cones in achromatopsia accounts for the severe visual acuity deficits.

Etiology

Inherited color vision defects

X-linked traits such as protan and deutan defects and blue-cone monochromacy are passed from mothers to sons. Females have two X chromosomes and each X chromosome has 50% chance of being passed to each of her offspring.

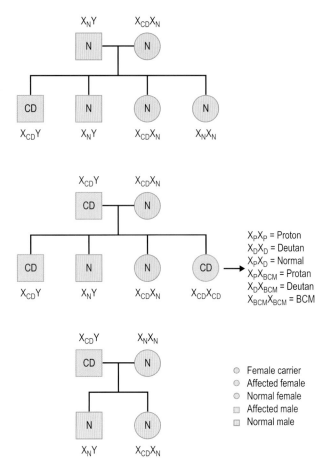

Figure 62.2 Inheritance of X-linked color vision deficiencies. X_{CD}, X chromosome carrying a color vision defect; X_N, X chromosome carrying normal color vision; X_{BCM}, X chromosome carrying blue-cone monochromacy. Squares indicate males; circles indicate females; the letters inside the squares and circles indicate the color vision phenotype of the individual with CD for color-deficient and N for normal color vision. Top pedigree: possible offspring from a normal father and a mother that is a carrier of a color vision defect. Middle pedigree: possible offspring from an affected father and a carrier mother. Indicated to the right of the CD daughter are the possible color-deficient phenotypes of a female with color deficiency on both X chromosomes depending on the type of color defect carried by each of her X chromosomes. Bottom pedigree: possible offspring from an affected father and a normal, noncarrier mother.

Males have one X chromosome, which they pass on to their daughters, and a Y chromosome, which they pass on to their sons. If a female carries an X-linked color vision defect, her sons will have 50% chance of getting the X chromosome with the defect, and thus of being affected by a color vision deficiency (Figure 62.2). A daughter of a female carrier will also have 50% chance of receiving the X chromosome with the defect. If a daughter receives the X chromosome with the defect from her mother and a normal X chromosome from her father, she will not be affected, because the normal X chromosome will ensure that she will have both L and M cones. The daughter of a color-defective father and a carrier mother may or may not be affected by a color vision defect (Figure 62.2). If her mother is a carrier of the same category of color vision defect that affects her father, then she will have the same category of defect. However, if her mother carries a different category of red–green color vision defect

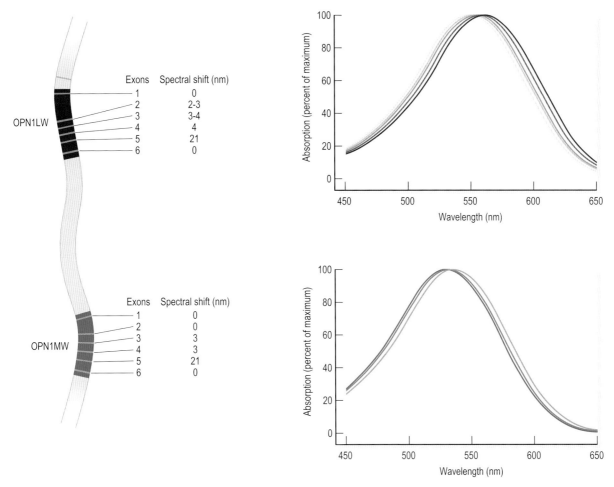

Figure 62.3 Genes and photopigments for red–green color vision. The structures of the *OPN1LW* and *OPN1MW* gene are drawn to scale with the exons (protein coding regions) indicated by number. The column labeled "spectral shift" gives the magnitude of the shift produced by polymorphic amino acid positions specified by individual exons. The absorption spectra of the L-class photopigments encoded by *OPN1LW* and the M-class photopigments specified by *OPN1MW* are shown to the right.

compared to the defect her father has, the daughter will have normal color vision because, between her two X chromosomes, the daughter will have genes that specify opsins for both L and M cones. If a female is a carrier of both blue-cone monochromacy and a red–green color vision defect, she will be affected by the red–green color vision defect (Figure 62.2). The offspring of an affected male and a normal, non-carrier female will not have the color vision defect; however, all of the daughters will be carriers of the color vision defect, and thus will have 50% chance of passing it on to their sons.

Tritan color vision defects are autosomal dominant, and most affected people are heterozygous for the defect, having only one defective copy of the *OPN1SW* gene and one normal copy. In order to be homozygous for an *OPN1SW* mutation, the defect must be inherited from both the mother and from the father. Due to rarity of the defect, this generally only occurs when there is consanguinity in a family. Heterozygotes have 50% chance of passing the defect on to their offspring.

Rod monochromacies are autosomal-recessive traits: individuals will only be affected if they receive a gene defect from both their mother and from their father. Affected individuals have 50% chance of passing a defective gene on to their offspring.

Acquired color vision defects

People who suffer from diabetes, glaucoma, muscular dystrophy, multiple sclerosis, and optic neuropathies are all at risk for color vision loss as a secondary consequence of the disease. Occupational exposure to chemicals including solvents and metals is another risk factor for developing acquired color vision deficiency. Finally, a variety of drugs, including those used to treat tuberculosis, epilepsy, and heart disease, can cause losses in color vision. Medications that have been reported to cause color vision loss are acetaminophen, ethanol, chloroquine, digoxin, erythromycin, ethambutol, ibuprofen, indometacin, nitroglycerin, oral contraceptives, quinine, salicylate, sildenafil citrate (Viagra), sulfonamides, thiazides, and tobacco.[37]

Pathophysiology

Both *OPN1LW* and *OPN1MW* have six exons each. The encoded pigments share 98% amino acid sequence identity, and whether a pigment is of the L class versus M class is determined by amino acids encoded by exon 5, which collectively produce a spectral difference of about 21 nm (Figure 62.3).

Table 62.2 Genetic mechanisms for the common color vision defects

Cross-over	Recombination product	Color vision phenotype
	L M NE	Deutan (deuteranope or deuteranomalous)
	M	Protanope
	L M NE	Normal
	L	Deuteranope
	M M	Protan (protanope or protanomalous)
	L L NE	Deutan (deuteranope or deuteranomalous)

L, L opsin; M, M opsin; NE, not experienced.

L-class pigments have peak sensitivities near 560 nm; M-class pigments have peak sensitivities near 530 nm (Figure 62.3). In L-class pigments, exons 2, 3, and 4 encode amino acid differences that produce spectral shifts of 2–3, 3–4, and 4 nm, respectively. In M-class pigments, exons 3 and 4 each encode amino acids that produce about a 3-nm spectral shift. Thus, L-class pigments have peak sensitivities spanning a range of about 10 nm, but M-class pigments have peak sensitivities spanning a range of only about 6 nm (Figure 62.3).

Protan and deutan color vision defects are most often caused by deletions and rearrangements that affect the *OPN1LW* and *OPN1MW* genes, as illustrated in Table 62.2. *OPN1LW* and *OPN1MW* share greater than 98% nucleotide sequence identity over a span of about 40 000 basepairs of DNA.[4,38] As a consequence, during meiotic cell division in females, misalignment of two X chromosomes allows unequal homologous recombination that produces new opsin gene arrays that differ in the number of opsin genes compared to the parental arrays and that contain chimeric genes that have segments from both parental *OPN1LW* and *OPN1MW* genes. The absorption spectra of the pigments encoded by the chimeric genes are determined by the complement of amino acids encoded at the spectral tuning sites.[39–41]

As illustrated in Table 62.2 (top row), a cross-over between an L gene on one X chromosome and an M gene on another X chromosome produces an array in which the parental L and M genes are separated by a chimeric gene that encodes an L-class pigment. Despite the presence of a normal *OPN1MW* gene, a male inheriting this array will have a deutan color vision defect because the *OPN1MW* gene has been displaced to a nonexpressed position. Only the first two genes in the array are usually expressed. Males with a deutan color vision deficiency who have two different L-class pigments have color vision ranging from quite good (approaching normal) when the underlying pigments differ in peak sensitivity by about 10 nm, to dichromatic when the underlying pigments do not differ in peak sensitivity.[25] Spec-

tral separations intermediate between 0 and 10 nm give rise to the variation in phenotypes among deuteranomalous males.[25,26] The other product of the recombination is an array with a single gene that encodes an M-class pigment, thus a male inheriting this array will be a protanope (Table 62.2 top row).

The region downstream of the last gene in the X-chromosome opsin gene array is nearly identical to the region separating two adjacent opsin genes, and thus misaligned X chromosomes can cross over in this region. As illustrated in Table 62.2 (middle row), such a cross-over produces two new arrays that differ in gene number compared to the parental arrays. The single-gene array will confer dichromacy – protanopia in the illustrated case – on a male, while the three-gene array will confer normal color vision. In the human population, there is variation in the number of opsin genes on the X chromosome, primarily in the number of *OPN1MW* genes. Cross-overs that occur between arrays with different gene numbers are responsible for producing two new arrays, both of which confer a color vision defect in males, as illustrated in Table 62.2 (bottom panel). When an *OPN1LW* and an *OPN1MW* gene in arrays with different gene numbers undergo a recombination, one product is an array in which the first gene is a chimera and encodes an M-class pigment, followed by an intact parental *OPN1MW* gene. Both genes encode M-class pigments, and the phenotype of a male inheriting such an array depends on the spectral separation between the two pigments, with better color vision being correlated with larger spectral separations. The other array contains two genes encoding L-class pigments and an *OPN1MW* gene in a nonexpressed position, thus producing a deutan defect, the severity of which is determined by the spectral separation between the L-class pigments.

Mixing of the *OPN1LW* and *OPN1MW* genes by recombination has produced combinations of the amino acids at the polymorphic positions that appear to be "poison combinations" that inactivate the photoreceptors that express them.[42] For example, the deuteranope described above, in the section on pathology, for whom adaptive optics revealed large patches of dark areas where cones should have been, had an intact *OPN1MW* gene that encoded an unusual combination of amino acids at the polymorphic positions encoded by exon 3. The same "poison combination" was also identified in blue-cone monochromats as the cause of photoreceptor dysfunction.[43]

Two genetic mechanisms have been identified as the cause of blue-cone monochromacy. One mechanism is a combination of gene deletions and mutations that results in the absence of a gene on the X chromosome that encodes a functional opsin.[5,6] The second mechanism is the deletion of a regulatory DNA element termed the locus control region that lies upstream of the X-chromosome opsin genes and that plays a critical role in the expression of both *OPN1LW* and *OPN1MW* genes.

In rod monochromacy, there is evidence that cone photoreceptors are present and contain photopigments[5]; however, the gene defects prevent the cones from signaling that light has been absorbed because they cannot effectively open and close ion channels in response to light.

Key references

A complete list of chapter references is available online at www.expertconsult.com. See inside cover for registration details.

4. Nathans J, Piantanida TP, Eddy RL, et al. Molecular genetics of inherited variation in human color vision. Science 1986;232: 203–210.

5. Nathans J, Davenport CM, Maumenee IH, et al. Molecular genetics of blue cone monochromacy. Science 1989;245:831–838.

6. Nathans J, Maumenee IA, Zrenner E, et al. Genetic heterogeneity among blue-cone monochromats. Am J Hum Genet 1993;53:987–1000.

7. Weitz CJ, Miyake Y, Shinzato K, et al. Human tritanopia associated with two amino acid substitutions in the blue sensitive opsin. Am J Hum Genet 1992;50:498–507.

8. Weitz CJ, Went LN, Nathans J. Human tritanopia associated with a third amino acid substitution in the blue sensitive visual pigment. Am J Hum Genet 1992;51:444–446.

9. Baraas RC, Carroll J, Gunther KL, et al. Adaptive optics retinal imaging reveals S-cone dystrophy in tritan color vision deficiency. J Optic Soc Am A Optics Image Sci Vision 2007;24:1438–1447.

12. Sharpe LT, Stockman A, Jägle H, et al. Opsin genes, cone photopigments, color vision, and color blindness. In: Gegenfurtner KR, Sharpe LT (eds) Color Vision: From Genes to Perception. New York: Cambridge University Press, 1999:3–52.

25. Neitz J, Neitz M, Kainz PM. Visual pigment gene structure and the severity of human color vision defects. Science 1996;274:801–804.

28. Neitz M, Carroll J, Renner A, et al. Variety of genotypes in males diagnosed as dichromatic on a conventional clinical anomaloscope. Vis Neurosci 2004;21: 205–216.

39. Neitz M, Neitz J, Jacobs GH. Spectral tuning of pigments underlying red–green color vision. Science 1991;252:971–974.

41. Asenjo AB, Rim J, Oprian DD. Molecular determinants of human red/green color discrimination. Neuron 1994;12:1131–1138.

42. Carroll J, Neitz M, Hofer H, et al. Functional photoreceptor loss revealed with adaptive optics: an alternate cause of color blindness. Proc Natl Acad Sci USA 2004;101:8461–8466.

CHAPTER 63

Acute retinal vascular occlusive disorders

Sohan Singh Hayreh

Overview

Acute retinal vascular occlusive disorders collectively constitute a major cause of serious visual impairment. Despite the fact that retinal artery occlusion (RAO) and retinal vein occlusion (RVO) have been known for about almost 150 years,[1,2] their pathogenesis, clinical features, and particularly their management have been plagued by controversy and misconceptions. RAO and RVO in fact comprise about a dozen separate clinical entities, and there is a voluminous literature on their pathogenesis and management. The following represents an abbreviated discussion of the salient aspects of the pathogenesis and management of these diseases.

RETINAL ARTERY OCCLUSION

Central RAO (CRAO), branch RAO (BRAO), and cilioretinal artery occlusion have different clinical characteristics, etiologies, pathogenesis, and management. Therefore, they constitute distinct clinical entities. Of the three, CRAO is usually associated with the most extensive visual loss.

Pathogenesis

From the etiologic, pathogenetic, clinical characteristics, and management point of view, CRAO consists of nonarteritic CRAO, arteritic CRAO, transient CRAO, and nonarteritic CRAO with cilioretinal artery sparing.[3]

Nonarteritic CRAO

This is the most common type, and studies[4] have shown that embolism is a far more common cause than thrombosis. Rarely, vasculitis or trauma can cause CRAO. A detailed anatomical study of 100 human central retinal arteries showed that the narrowest lumen of the artery is where it pierces the dura mater of the optic nerve sheath before entering the optic nerve (Figures 63.1 and 63.2).[5-7] Therefore, the chances of an embolus becoming impacted at this site are much higher than at any other site in the artery. In contrast,

histopathological studies show that the site of occlusion in thrombosis of the CRA is at the lamina cribrosa.

The site of occlusion is an important factor in determining the amount of residual retinal circulation. When the site of occlusion is in the dural sheath, multiple anastomoses established by all the pial and intraneural branches of the CRA[6,8] distal to the occlusion site are left intact, and play a major role in determining the amount of residual retinal circulation.[9-14] Also in this type of CRAO, fluorescein angiography shows the CRA trunk slowly filling from within the optic nerve. By contrast, when the site of occlusion is at the lamina cribrosa, no collaterals are available to establish retinal circulation; in these eyes, angiography shows only filling of capillaries on the surface layer of the optic disc from deeper posterior ciliary artery circulation,[9-14] without any filling of the CRA trunk itself. Thus, angiography can provide useful information about the site of occlusion. The frequent presence of residual circulation in the retina in eyes with CRAO, and the belief that the site of occlusion is in the lamina cribrosa, has resulted in a prevalent misconception that there is usually incomplete occlusion of the artery in CRAO. (This misconception and its visual implications are discussed at length elsewhere.[3,5]) Briefly, in experimental CRAO studies in rhesus monkeys, where the CRA was completely occluded by clamping the artery, immediate postocclusion fluorescein fundus angiography showed a variable amount of slow filling of the retinal circulation in the vast majority of eyes.[9-14] The basis for various treatments for CRAO and the visual improvement associated with those has often been erroneously attributed to this misconception of "incomplete CRAO."

Arteritic CRAO

In this type, giant cell arteritis (see Chapter 40) is the cause of development of CRAO. Giant cell arteritis has a special predilection for involvement of the posterior ciliary arteries and only very rarely involves the CRA directly. CRA not infrequently arises from the ophthalmic artery by a common trunk with the posterior ciliary artery.[6,7] When giant cell arteritis involves that common trunk, it results in occlusion of both the CRA and posterior ciliary artery, and consequently development of both arteritic CRAO and arteritic anterior ischemic optic neuropathy.[15-17] Clinically, these

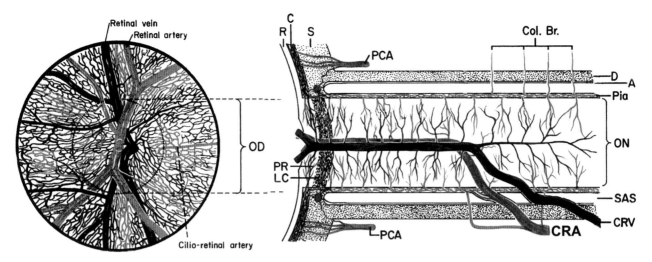

Figure 63.1 Schematic representation of blood supply of the optic nerve on the right and the retinal vascular pattern on the left. A, arachnoid; C, choroid; CRA, central retinal artery; Col. Br., collateral branches; CRV, central retinal vein; D, dura; LC, lamina cribrosa; OD, optic disc; ON, optic nerve; PCA, posterior ciliary artery; PR, prelaminar region; R, retina; S, sclera; SAS, subarachnoid space. (Modified from Hayreh SS. Anatomy and physiology of the optic nerve head. Trans Am Acad Ophthalmol Otolaryngol 1974;78:OP240–OP254.)

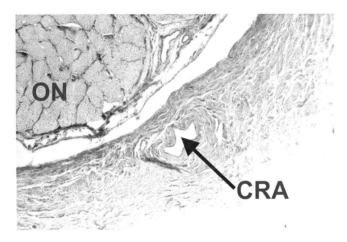

Figure 63.2 Histological transverse section of a normal human optic nerve (ON) at the level of site of penetration of the central retinal artery (CRA) into the sheath of the optic nerve, showing the CRA lying within the substance of the dural sheath of the nerve. (Reproduced with permission from Singh (Hayreh) S, Dass R. The central artery of the retina I. Origin and course. Br J Ophthalmol 1960;44:193–212.)

eyes have the classical fundus findings of CRAO with or without optic disc edema, but, most importantly, on fluorescein angiography there is evidence of a posterior ciliary artery occlusion in addition to CRAO,[15,16] which is a diagnostic feature of this type of CRAO. Since giant cell arteritis is a blinding disease and a prime medical emergency in ophthalmology, it is essential to rule out the presence of associated posterior ciliary artery occlusion by fluorescein angiography in all these eyes, as well as giant cell arteritis, in patients >50 years.

Transient nonarteritic CRAO

This can be produced by:

1. Transient impaction of an embolus in the CRA. The most common type of embolus to cause this is a thrombotic or platelet-fibrin embolus and, less frequently, a cholesterol embolus; calcific emboli tend to remain impacted at one site because of their irregular texture.

2. Vasospasm of the CRA. This is a rare cause of transient CRAO. There is evidence to suggest that platelets stick and aggregate on atherosclerotic plaques in the carotid arteries and release vasoactive substances, including serotonin and thromboxane. Serotonin can cause transient vasospasm of the CRA and result in transient CRAO.[18]

3. Fall of perfusion pressure below the critical level in the retinal vascular bed. Factors that produce fall of perfusion pressure below the critical level in the retinal vascular bed can result in transient CRAO. The perfusion pressure in the CRA is equal to the mean blood pressure in the artery minus the intraocular pressure (IOP). Therefore, a fall of perfusion pressure can be due to either a marked fall in mean arterial blood pressure or a rise of IOP, or a combination of the two. A marked fall in arterial blood pressure can occur for several reasons, including nocturnal arterial hypotension (Figure 63.3A), particularly in patients who take blood pressure-lowering medicines in the evening or at bedtime (Figure 63.3B),[19,20] severe shock, during hemodialysis, spasm of the CRA, marked stenosis or occlusion of the internal carotid or ophthalmic artery, or ocular ischemia.[4,21] A rise in IOP may be due to several causes, including ocular compression during certain surgical procedures or marked orbital swelling, acute angle closure glaucoma, or neovascular glaucoma (NVG) in association with ocular ischemia.[4,21,22] The extent of retinal ischemia and consequent visual loss depends upon the duration of the transient CRAO (see below). In transient nonarteritic CRAO, fluorescein fundus angiography always shows normal or almost normal filling of the retinal vascular bed.[3]

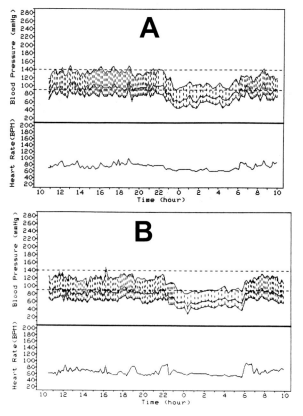

Figure 63.3 Ambulatory blood pressure and heart rate-monitoring records (based on individual readings) over a 24-hour period in two individuals. (A) A 58-year-old woman on no medication. (B) A 63-year-old woman who was taking verapamil (a calcium ion influx inhibitor) at bedtime. This shows a marked degree of nocturnal hypotension, which improved markedly on stopping the bedtime dose.

Nonarteritic CRAO with cilioretinal artery sparing

This type of nonarteritic CRAO only develops in eyes with a cilioretinal artery. The cilioretinal artery may vary in size from a minute one to one supplying a large part of the retina.[23–25] The visual outcome[3] and fundus findings[26] in this type of CRAO are different from the classical nonarteritic CRAO.

Branch retinal artery occlusion

Most frequently, BRAO is caused by embolism, and only occasionally by vasculitis.[27] When BRAO is due to embolism, the most common site is where the branch retinal arteries bifurcate because the embolus is not large enough to enter the smaller branches. That is not the case in BRAO due to vasculitis.

Cilioretinal artery occlusion

This is the least common type of RAO. Pathogenetically it can be divided into three types:

1. Embolic: since the cilioretinal artery is supplied by the posterior ciliary artery, emboli going to the latter can result in cilioretinal artery occlusion.

2. Giant cell arteritis: giant cell arteritis has a predilection for posterior ciliary artery involvement. If giant cell arteritis causes occlusion of the posterior ciliary artery supplying the cilioretinal artery, this results in cilioretinal artery occlusion. In such an eye there is almost invariably associated arteritic anterior ischemic optic neuropathy[15–17,28] since the optic nerve head is mainly supplied by the posterior ciliary artery circulation.[11,29] That combination is diagnostic of giant cell arteritis.[28,30] Cilioretinal artery occlusion in these eyes has been misdiagnosed as BRAO caused by giant cell arteritis; the branch retinal artery is in fact an arteriole and giant cell arteritis is a disease of medium and large arteries and not of arterioles, therefore giant cell arteritis cannot cause BRAO.[17] Since giant cell arteritis is a blinding disease and a prime medical emergency in ophthalmology, it is essential to rule out the presence of associated posterior ciliary artery occlusion by fluorescein angiography in all eyes with cilioretinal artery occlusion, as well as giant cell arteritis, in patients >50 years.

3. Central or hemicentral RVO: this type of occlusion of cilioretinal artery is invariably due to hemodynamic blockage.[25]

Retinal tolerance time to acute retinal ischemia

The chance of recovery of vision only exists as long as the retina has reversible ischemic damage. Experimental study of CRAO in elderly, atherosclerotic, and hypertensive rhesus monkeys (similar to most patients with CRAO) showed that the retina suffers no detectable damage with CRAO of up to 97 minutes, but after that, the longer the CRAO, the more extensive the irreversible ischemic retinal damage.[10,31] CRAO lasting for about 240 minutes results in ischemic retinal damage that is massive and irreversible.[10,31] Contrary to prevalent impression, the retinas of old, atherosclerotic, hypertensive rhesus monkeys could tolerate ischemia for much longer than younger, normal rhesus monkeys.[10,32,33] In eyes where the retinal circulation was restored to normal after CRAO of more than 2 but less than 4 hours' duration, retinal function did not show signs of major improvement until many hours or even a day or more after restoration of circulation – the longer the ischemia, the longer the lag before any improvement of function started.

Clinical background

CRAO is an ophthalmic emergency associated with a catastrophic visual loss. In one study,[3] central scotoma was the most common visual field defect in CRAO. Following is the mechanism of selective development of central scotoma without any peripheral visual field defect in CRAO. Unlike the rest of the retina, the macular region has more than one layer of retinal ganglion cells, which are maximum close to the foveola, making that region the thickest part of the retina. Experimental[9,10] and clinical[3,34] CRAO studies showed that CRAO results in ischemic swelling of the inner retina,

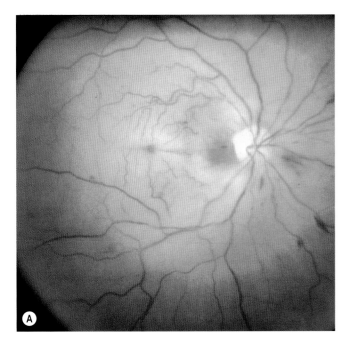

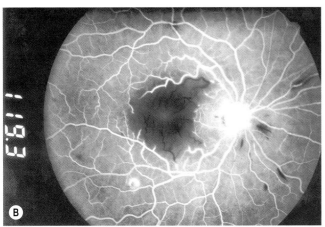

Figure 63.4 At initial visit, fundus and fluorescein angiogram of right eye that had developed transient nonarteritic central retinal artery occlusion 10 days earlier. (A) Fundus photograph shows cherry red spot, retinal opacity of posterior fundus, most marked in the central macular region, and a small area of normal retina temporal to the optic disc corresponding to a patent cilioretinal artery. (B) Angiogram 120 seconds after injection of the dye, showing complete filling of the retinal vascular bed except in the central macular region with marked retinal swelling (see (A); due to "no-reflow phenomenon"). (Reproduced with permission from Hayreh SS. Prevalent misconceptions about acute retinal vascular occlusive disorders. Prog Retin Eye Res 2005;24:493–519.)

and this is maximal in the perifoveolar region (Figure 63.4A). If there is restoration of circulation in the CRA, as in transient CRAO, the retinal capillaries in the central, markedly swollen part of the macular region cannot fill (Figure 63.4B) because of compression by the surrounding swollen retinal tissue, resulting in the "no-reflow phenomenon."[10,32] Consequently, there is ganglion cell death in the nonperfused central retina. The area of central retinal capillary nonfilling may vary from eye to eye, depending upon the severity of retinal swelling in the macular region. This results in the variable size of the permanent central scotoma.[3] The oxygen

supply and nutrition from the choroidal vascular bed to the thinner peripheral retina help in its much longer survival, and the maintenance of peripheral visual fields.

Treatment

Since Von Graefe first described CRAO as a clinical entity in 1859,[1] a voluminous literature has accumulated on its management, but no treatment has stood the test of time. Treatments include ocular massage in an effort to dislodge the embolus in the CRA, a reduction of IOP by various medical and surgical means to increase retinal perfusion pressure, vasodilatation of the CRA, antiplatelet therapy, heparin therapy, thrombolysis by administering a thrombolytic agent intravenously or local intra-arterial fibrinolysis by superselective administration of thrombolytic agent directly into the ophthalmic artery, isovolumic hemodilution, hyperbaric oxygen, and embolectomy. However, there are important considerations when evaluating claims of visual improvement associated with CRAO treatment:

1. Experimental CRAO lasting for about 240 minutes results in massive, irreversible retinal damage.[10,31] Thus, no treatment restoring CRA circulation instituted much longer than 4 hours after the onset of CRAO would be expected to restore vision.

2. Most CRAO treatment studies do not demonstrate restoration or significant improvement of retinal circulation with fluorescein angiography, immediately after the treatment.

3. It is usually claimed that visual improvement is due to treatment, when it may simply represent the natural history of the disease. For example, the claim of a 66% success rate for visual improvement with local fibrinolysis using tissue plasminogen activator in CRAO[35] actually represented the natural history of the disease.[36]

4. In almost all CRAO studies, visual outcome is based on evaluation of visual acuity only. However, visual acuity is a function of the fovea only while CRAO involves the entire retina. Visual fields performed with a Goldmann perimeter provide information about the function of the entire retina, a far better measure than visual acuity alone. Furthermore, visual field information is essential to evaluate visual disability in any severely blinding disease, including CRAO. The constant tracking provided by the peripheral visual fields is essential for sensory input in our day-to-day activity, e.g., in routine "navigation."[5]

Thrombolysis is currently the most popular therapy and success has been enthusiastically claimed. However, a meta-analysis[37] of studies of local intra-arterial fibrinolysis in CRAO concluded that, outside a randomized clinical trial, the use of superselective fibrinolytic therapy for CRAO cannot be recommended based on current evidence, because all studies were retrospective and nonrandomized and their methodology was often unsatisfactory.

In conclusion, none of the claimed treatments for CRAO produced a visual outcome better than that seen in the natural history of the disease.[3] Treatments similar to those advocated in CRAO have also been advocated for BRAO, with similar problems.

In contrast, patients with arteritic CRAO (from giant cell arteritis) require immediate attention because there is a risk of developing irreversible bilateral visual loss if the patient is not immediately treated with high doses of corticosteroid therapy. (This is discussed further in Chapter 40.) Similarly, patients with cilioretinal artery occlusion, for which giant cell arteritis is an important cause, should be worked up for the latter.

Diagnostic workup

Since embolism is the most common cause of nonarteritic CRAO and BRAO, an important part of the management of all patients is evaluation for the source of embolism by doing carotid and cardiac evaluation, to prevent further vascular accidents. However, one should be aware of the limitations of those tests in evaluation of embolism.[5] In an eye with transient CRAO, evaluation of IOP and arterial hypertensive therapy are also essential.

Prognosis

Visual outcome in CRAO depends on the type. A natural history study[3] showed that a significant improvement in visual acuity and visual field can occur without any treatment. Visual acuity improvement occurred primarily within the first 7 days. In eyes with vision of counting fingers or worse, visual acuity improved within 7 days in 82% of transient nonarteritic CRAO, 67% of nonarteritic CRAO with cilioretinal artery sparing, 22% of nonarteritic CRAO, and little in arteritic CRAO. The central visual field improved in 39% of transient nonarteritic CRAO, 25% of nonarteritic CRAO with cilioretinal artery sparing, and 21% of nonarteritic CRAO. The peripheral visual field was normal at initial visit in 63% of eyes with transient nonarteritic CRAO, 22% in those with nonarteritic CRAO, and in none of the other two types. Peripheral fields improved in nonarteritic CRAO (39%) and in transient nonarteritic CRAO (39%). When the junction between the infarcted and normal retinal artery passes through the foveal zone (Figure 63.5), there is a marked spontaneous visual improvement within a few days to weeks, which has erroneously been attributed to various treatments.

RETINAL VEIN OCCLUSION

RVO is divided into the following six distinct clinical entities[38,39]:

- Central RVO (CRVO): experimental[40-45] and clinical[38,39,46-52] studies have shown that CRVO consists of two distinct clinical entities: (1) nonischemic CRVO (or venous stasis retinopathy); and (2) ischemic CRVO (or hemorrhagic retinopathy).
- Hemicentral RVO (HCRVO): this is a variant of CRVO where, as a congenital anomaly, the central retinal vein (CRV) has two trunks in the optic nerve instead of one, and only one of those is occluded.[53] Like CRVO, this can also be nonischemic or ischemic.

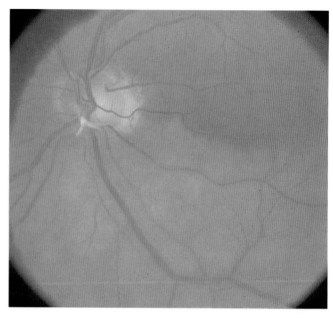

Figure 63.5 Fundus photograph of the left eye with inferior branch retinal artery occlusion, with an embolus (white) impacted at its origin on the optic disc. Note the junction of the normal (upper half) and infarcted (lower half) parts of the retina, passing through the fovea. (Reproduced with permission from Hayreh SS. Prevalent misconceptions about acute retinal vascular occlusive disorders. Prog Retin Eye Res 2005;24:493–519.).

- Branch RVO (BRVO): this consists of: (1) major branch RVO when one of the major branch retinal veins is occluded, usually near, or rarely at, the optic disc; and (2) macular branch RVO, when only one of the macular venules is occluded.

Risk factors

Like all ocular vascular occlusive disorders, almost all types of RVO are multifactorial in origin; that is, there is rarely any one single factor that causes the occlusion[54,55]; there may be a whole host of local and systemic risk factors acting in different combinations and to different extents. The risk factors can be divided into two types, predisposing and precipitating, and they may play one role in one group and the other in another. CRVO and HCRVO are pathogenetically similar but very different from BRVO. In conclusion, all types of RVO cannot be explained by one common pathogenetic mechanism.

Local risk factors

CRVO and HCRVO

The CRA and CRV lie side by side in the center of the optic nerve, enclosed in a common fibrous tissue envelope[7,56] (Figure 63.6). Klien and Olwin[57,58] postulated the following

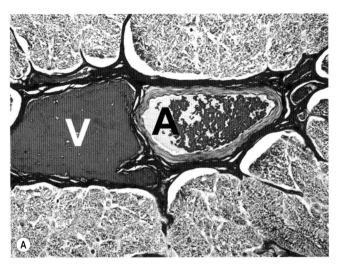
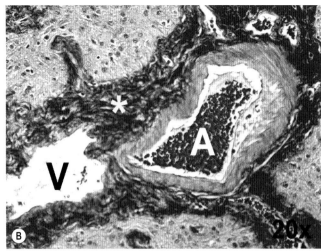

Figure 63.6 Histological sections of the central retinal vessels and surrounding tissues, as seen in transverse sections of the central part of the retrolaminar region of the optic nerve in two rhesus monkey eyes (Masson's trichrome staining). (A) Control monkey eye. (B) Monkey with experimental arterial hypertension, atherosclerosis, and glaucoma. The figure shows marked thickening of the perivascular fibrous tissue envelope (*), with secondary central retinal vascular changes and marked narrowing of the central retinal vein. A, central retinal artery; V, central retinal vein. (Reproduced with permission from Hayreh SS. Central retinal vein occlusion. Ophthalmol Clin North Am 1998;11:559–590.)

three occlusive mechanisms in CRVO: (1) occlusion of the vein by external compression by sclerotic adjacent structures (i.e., CRA and surrounding fibrous tissue envelope) (Figure 63.6 right) and secondary endothelial proliferation; (2) occlusion by primary venous wall disease (degenerative or inflammatory in nature); and (3) hemodynamic disturbances produced by a variety of factors (e.g., subendothelial atheromatous lesions in the CRA, sudden reduction of blood pressure, blood dyscrasias, and further aggravated by arteriosclerosis or unfavorable anatomic relations). These produce stagnation of the blood flow in the vein. According to the Virchow's triad for thrombus formation – (1) slowing of blood flow; (2) changes in vessel wall; and (3) changes in the blood – the stagnation finally results in primary thrombus formation in susceptible eyes.

CRVO is significantly more common in patients with ocular hypertension and glaucoma.[59] Stasis in the CRV may be produced by several factors, including the following three factors in glaucoma/ocular hypertension:

1. Blood pressure in the CRV at the optic disc depends upon the IOP, the former always being somewhat higher than the latter to maintain retinal blood flow. A rise of IOP could produce stasis and sluggish blood flow in the CRV, and may also collapse the vein on the optic disc.[60–62] Hence, elevated IOP may be one of several predisposing factors in the etiology of CRVO and not the sole cause, except perhaps in eyes with a sudden increase of IOP to very high levels, e.g., acute angle closure.
2. A histopathologic study[56] of experimentally produced glaucomatous optic neuropathy in hypertensive and atherosclerotic rhesus monkeys showed a marked thickening of the fibrous tissue envelope around the central retinal vessels in the center of the optic nerve, as compared with age-matched controls (Figure 63.6), that resulted in marked stenosis of the CRV during its

intraneural course, which would consequently cause stasis of circulation.
3. In some eyes, optic disc cupping may predispose to CRVO, either directly through a local mechanical effect or because of the secondary morphologic changes in the optic nerve in marked glaucomatous optic neuropathy associated with cupping.[59] However, there is no strong evidence of a cause-and-effect relationship between cupping and development of CRVO/HCRVO.

Glaucoma or ocular hypertension does not influence the conversion rate between nonischemic CRVO and ischemic CRVO.[59]

The site of occlusion of the CRV within the optic nerve (see below) has important implications, because that determines the number of venous collateral channels anterior to the site of occlusion which are available to restore circulation (Figure 63.1); that in turn would determine the type and severity of the CRVO: the farther back the occlusion in the optic nerve, the more collaterals are available and the less severe the CRVO.

BRVO

Local risk factors in BRVO are discussed in the section on site of occlusion in BRVO, below.

Systemic risk factors

CRVO and HCRVO

A cross-sectional study[63] of 197 patients with CRVO found a significantly higher prevalence of arterial hypertension and diabetes mellitus when compared to that in the National Health Interview Survey. The Eye Disease Case-Control Study Group[64] found a significant association of diabetes mellitus, cardiovascular disease, and arterial hypertension in ischemic CRVO and arterial hypertension and fibrinogen levels in nonischemic CRVO. The odds ratio for ischemic CRVO was 4.8 for hypertension, 2.7 for diabetes mellitus, 2.1 for cardiovascular disease, and 2.1 for α_1-globulin. The odds ratio for nonischemic CRVO was 1.8 for arterial hypertension and 1.8 for diabetes mellitus.

Hayreh et al[54] prospectively investigated several risk factors in patients with CRVO (612 patients), HCRVO (130 patients), and BRVO (348 patients). The prevalence of systemic diseases was similar between CRVO and HCRVO – evidence that they are pathogenically identical. The combined group of CRVO and HCRVO patients had a higher prevalence of arterial hypertension, diabetes mellitus (in ischemic-type CRVO), peptic ulcer, and thyroid disorder relative to the control population. Arterial hypertension and diabetes mellitus were more common in ischemic CRVO than nonischemic CRVO. None of the systemic diseases had any significant effect on the rate of conversion of nonischemic to ischemic CRVO.

Compared to CRVO and HCRVO, patients with BRVO showed a higher prevalence of arterial hypertension, cerebrovascular disease, peripheral vascular disease, systemic venous disease, gastrointestinal disease, and peptic ulcer. Compared to the control population, patients with BRVO showed a greater prevalence of arterial hypertension, ischemic heart disease (in major BRVO only), cerebrovascular disease, chronic obstructive pulmonary disease, peptic ulcer, and thyroid disorder. Arterial hypertension and ischemic heart disease were more prevalent in major BRVO than in macular BRVO.

The presence of a particular disease may or may not be one of the risk factors in a multifactorial scenario predisposing an eye to develop a particular type of RVO, or may be just a coincidence. Apart from a routine medical evaluation, extensive and expensive workup for systemic diseases in patients with RVO is not cost-effective and not warranted in the vast majority of cases.

Hematological risk factors

There is no definite evidence of a cause-and-effect relationship between hematologic abnormalities associated with thrombosis and the development of various types of RVO in the vast majority of RVO patients; a chance occurrence of some of these hematologic abnormalities in RVO cases or the possibility of the findings due to unrelated associated systemic disease cannot be ruled out.[55]

In young persons, although CRVO may be associated with any of the systemic diseases mentioned in the above studies,[54,55] all the available evidence suggests that phlebitis of the CRV is probably the most common cause of thrombosis.[65] CRVO due to phlebitis has been given different eponyms, including "papillophlebitis," "retinal vasculitis," "mild retinal and papillary vasculitis," and "optic disc vasculitis type II."[66]

Nocturnal arterial hypotension in CRVO

Nocturnal arterial hypotension may play an important role in: (1) development of CRVO; and (2) conversion of nonischemic CRVO to ischemic CRVO. Retinal blood flow depends upon perfusion pressure. Nocturnal arterial hypotension is a physiological phenomenon (Figure 63.3A).[19,20]

Thus, a combination of very low mean blood pressure at night with a very high venous pressure from CRV narrowing (see above) would cause a precipitous fall of perfusion pressure → reduction of retinal blood flow to below the critical levels during sleep → retinal hypoxia/ischemia. This would explain why visual loss in CRVO is frequently discovered on waking up from sleep. With retinal ischemia, there is also ischemic capillaropathy. As the blood pressure returns to normal or even hypertensive levels during waking hours, there is an increase in retinal blood flow and associated rise in intraluminal pressure in ischemic retinal capillaries; this ruptures the weakened ischemic capillaries and produces extensive retinal hemorrhages. In some patients, this mechanism may also result in conversion of nonischemic CRVO to ischemic CRVO either overnight or gradually.[19,67] The other mechanism for such a conversion (usually slow) may be a gradual extension of the thrombotic process in the CRV forward in the optic nerve, involving and eliminating many of the available venous collaterals in the optic nerve which previously protected these eyes from developing ischemic CRVO (Figure 63.1).

BRVO

Systemic risk factors have already been discussed above. An increased risk of BRVO is associated with arterial hypertension, cardiovascular disease, and higher serum levels of α_2-globulin.[68]

Site of occlusion

CRVO and HCVO

This is an important issue because the rationale for various surgical procedures of "decompression of the CRV" for management of CRVO relies on this concept, which is based solely on histological examination of blind CRVO eyes, enucleated because of painful NVG. The histopathologic study by Green et al[69] on CRVO is usually cited in support. In that study, 82.8% of the eyes had ocular neovascularization and most of the eyes were enucleated because of NVG – all definite signs of ischemic CRVO.[38,70] Since nonischemic CRVO eyes never develop NVG,[38] those are never enucleated. Thus, the study was essentially based on ischemic CRVO eyes, which must have skewed the sample. Clinical studies[38,71] have shown that only about 20% of eyes with CRVO are of the ischemic type. In ischemic CRVO eyes, the maximum risk of developing NVG is only about 45%[38] (Figure 63.7); that means the overall risk of CRVO eyes developing NVG is only about 9%. Of the eyes that develop NVG, only a rare one is enucleated for pain or secondary phthisis bulbi – that means 1% or even less. Therefore, histopathological findings from less than 1% of CRVO eyes cannot be applied to more than 99% of CRVO eyes. Most importantly, the eyes enucleated for painful NVG have the most severe form of ischemic CRVO and are likely to have occlusion in the CRV at or close to the lamina cribrosa; therefore, they do not represent the vast majority of CRVO eyes; that provides a distorted impression about the site of occlusion in all CRVO eyes. This fact is critical when considering options for management of CRVO.

All the available anatomical, experimental, and clinical evidence in CRVO shows that the actual site of occlusion in

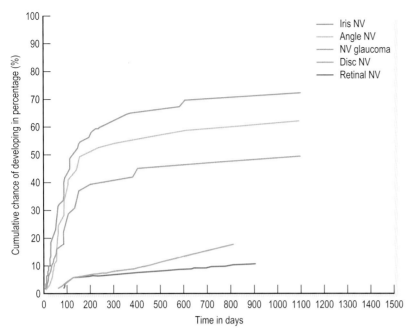

Figure 63.7 A graphic representation of cumulative chances (as a percentage) of developing various types of ocular neovascularization (NV) in ischemic central retinal vein occlusion, in relation to time from onset of the disease. (Modified from Hayreh SS, Rojas P, Podhajsky P, et al. Ocular neovascularization with retinal vascular occlusion III. Incidence of ocular neovascularization with retinal vein occlusion. Ophthalmology 1983;90:488–506.)

the CRV is typically in the optic nerve at a variable distance posterior to the lamina cribrosa, and not at the lamina cribrosa. Fluorescein fundus angiography proves that almost all eyes with CRVO show retinal circulation on angiography, although sluggish. If the site of occlusion were at the lamina cribrosa, there would be no outlet for the retinal blood, which would result in complete stoppage of retinal circulation, because if the blood cannot get out, it cannot get in. All the available evidence indicates that in nonischemic CRVO the site of occlusion is usually farther back in the optic nerve, so that multiple collaterals are available anterior to the site of occlusion, to drain the blood away (Figure 63.1). Compared to nonischemic CRVO, in most ischemic CRVO eyes, the site of occlusion is most probably immediately posterior to the lamina cribrosa, with only a few small collaterals left to drain away the blood (Figure 63.1).

BRVO

A number of studies have shown that the retinal arteriole lies anterior to the vein at the site of occlusion in 93–100% of cases, and that such an arrangement is significantly more common in BRVO than in control groups.[72–76] Since the first report by Ammann in 1899,[77] it has also been known that BRVO is more common in the temporal than nasal part of the retina, and of the temporal retina, more frequently in the superior than inferior quadrant. The arteriovenous crossings have been shown to be more frequent in the superotemporal quadrant than elsewhere,[75,78] and situated closer to the optic disc in the superotemporal than inferotemporal quadrant.[78]

Seitz[79] in histological studies of hypertensive patients found thickening of walls and narrowing of the lumen of both retinal arteriole and vein. At the arteriovenous crossing, the vessels shared a common vascular wall and a common, thickened, adventitial and glial sheath, irrespective of which

vessel was anterior. He found no compression of the underlying vessel, and attributed the indentation and obscuration of the underlying vein, when the arteriole crossed over the vein, to the deeper position of the vein, rather than to any true compression of the vein. In a histopathologic report on BRVO,[80] of four BRVOs in three eyes, the lumen of the vein at the arteriovenous crossing was "fully patent" in three of the four, with complete occlusion in the fourth. The authors found a marked degree of arteriolar changes in all. In a histopathologic examination[81] of an eye 7 years after development of BRVO, at the arteriovenous crossing the lumen of the vein was occluded except for several very small recanalized channels with moderate sclerosis and narrowing of the arteriole there.

These findings suggest that: (1) the arteriovenous crossing plays an important role in the pathogenesis of BRVO, and the anterior position of the arteriole at the crossing somehow renders the underlying vein vulnerable to occlusion; and (2) the clinical picture and fluorescein angiography in most eyes with acute BRVO do not show a complete occlusion at the site of obstruction; this is in agreement with the findings of the histopathologic study by Rabinowicz et al.[80] From this information, it would seem logical to conclude that the sclerotic retinal arteriole probably compresses the accompanying vein because of a common thickened, adventitial, and glial sheath. Moreover, the very low incidence of BRVO in spite of the very high incidence of anterior location of the arteriole at the arteriovenous crossing in patients with arteriosclerosis and hypertension clearly indicates that, in the multifactorial etiology of BRVO, factors other than simple anatomical arrangement and sclerotic changes in the retinal arterioles must play important roles. In addition to all that, focal phlebitis is a well-known cause of BRVO. Unlike CRVO and HCRVO, glaucoma and ocular hypertension play no role in the pathogenesis of BRVO.

Pathogenesis

CRVO

In elderly persons, sclerotic changes in the CRA and the fibrous tissue envelope around the central retinal vessels within the optic nerve (Figure 63.6B), and secondary compression of the CRV and endothelial proliferation in it[57,58] cause narrowing of the lumen of the CRV. This produces circulatory stasis and stagnation thrombosis. In addition, hemodynamic disturbances on the arterial side may play an important role in the development of this thrombosis. This is because blood flow in the retinal vessels depends upon the perfusion pressure. With venous stasis, secondary to narrowing of the lumen of the CRV from whatever cause, the venous pressure proximal to the site of narrowing rises, and that results in a fall of perfusion pressure and sluggish circulation in the CRV. A fall in systemic arterial blood pressure would further lower the perfusion pressure in the retinal vascular bed. Recent studies with 24-hour ambulatory blood pressure monitoring have established that during sleep there is a physiological fall in blood pressure (Figure 63.3A).[19,20] This may convert a partial thrombus in the CRV to a complete thrombus because of poor, sluggish circulation during sleep (i.e., Virchow's triad). The fact that many CRVO patients complain of discovering visual blurring on waking up from sleep strongly suggests that nocturnal arterial hypotension plays an important role as the final insult precipitating CRVO in persons who are already susceptible.[19,20] Some CRVO patients initially complain of episodes of amaurosis fugax when they wake up from sleep or during the day – in both cases the vision clears after a short interval – before they finally develop permanent visual deterioration. My explanation for this phenomenon is the following three sequences of events.

1. As the thrombus initially progresses and finally suddenly occludes the CRV completely → leaves no outlet for the retinal blood → sudden stoppage of blood flow in the closed loop retinal circulatory system → transient retinal ischemia → visual blurring.
2. At the same time, CRA is still pumping in blood in the closed-loop retinal circulation with no outlet for the retinal blood to flow out → sudden rise in blood pressure to the arterial level in the entire retinal vascular bed and proximal to the site of thrombus in the CRV.
3. Since the thrombus is freshly formed and not firmly adherent to the venous wall, it cannot withstand the force of this sudden rise of blood pressure to high arterial level anterior to it in CRV → the thrombus popping out like a champagne cork → restoration of retinal circulation → normal visual function.

A gradual and progressive increase in the size of the thrombus in the CRV and nocturnal arterial hypotension for many hours during sleep (Figure 63.3A) then finally produces permanent, irreversible occlusion of the CRV; however, in the meantime some venous collaterals have developed in the optic nerve so that the venous stasis is not as severe as discussed above.

HCRVO

The pathophysiology is similar to that in CRVO. This is because, during the third month of intrauterine life, there are always two trunks of the CRV in the optic nerve, one on either side of the CRA.[53] The two trunks are united with each other by numerous anastomoses. As the two venous channels pass back from the eyeball, they approach one another and finally coalesce at a variable distance behind the optic disc into one – the main trunk of the CRV. One of the two trunks usually disappears before birth; however, in 20.5% of eyes a dual-trunked CRV persists as a congenital anomaly.[82] In HCRVO, usually only one of the two trunks of the CRV is involved by occlusion within the optic nerve[53]; occasionally, however, both trunks may be involved, presumably because the site of occlusion is in the main trunk of the CRV after the union of the two trunks, or the two trunks may be involved independently, one after the other, and this would appear on routine examination to be ordinary CRVO; however, one can see two venous trunks entering the optic disc.

Nonischemic CRVO associated with cilioretinal artery occlusion

If an eye has a cilioretinal artery (Figure 63.8), sudden occlusion of the CRV can produce transient hemodynamic blockage of the cilioretinal artery circulation.[25] The mechanism of cilioretinal artery occlusion in these eyes is discussed in detail elsewhere.[25] Briefly, perfusion pressure is normally higher in the CRA than in the choroidal vascular bed (and consequently in the cilioretinal artery).[83–85] When there is sudden stoppage of blood flow by a thrombus in the CRV, the blood pressure in the entire retinal capillary bed transiently rises to the level of CRA blood pressure. Since the blood pressure in the cilioretinal artery is lower than that in

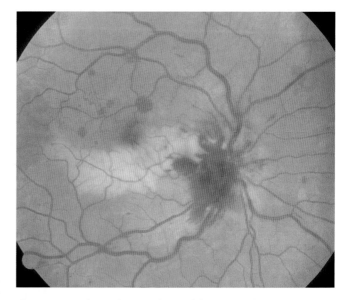

Figure 63.8 Right eye shows occlusion of the cilioretinal artery (and associated retinal infarct in a narrow strip below the foveola) in an eye with nonischemic central retinal vein occlusion. (Reproduced with permission from Hayreh SS, Podhajsky PA, Zimmerman MB. Branch retinal artery occlusion: natural history of visual outcome. Ophthalmology 2009;116:1188–1194.)

the CRA, and the blood pressure in the retinal capillary bed is at about the level of the CRA, the cilioretinal artery cannot pump in blood into the high-pressure system of the retinal capillary bed, resulting in a transient hemodynamic block in the cilioretinal artery circulation. Within a day or two, with the development of venous collaterals by the CRV in the optic nerve (Figure 63.1), the blood pressure in the retinal vascular bed falls to below the level of the blood pressure in the cilioretinal artery, resulting in restoration of the blood flow in the cilioretinal artery once again. However, in the meantime, the retina supplied by the cilioretinal artery has usually been irreversibly damaged by ischemia, resulting in visual loss – the severity of retinal ischemia in the area supplied by the cilioretinal artery and the associated visual loss depend upon the length of time elapsed before the circulation was re-established (see above).

Clinical background

Diagnostic workup

Inadequate differentiation between nonischemic and ischemic CRVO is a primary cause of controversy, resulting in misleading information.[5] A "10-disc area of retinal capillary obliteration" on fluorescein fundus angiograph is an inadequate criterion.[51,70] The Central Vein Occlusion Study Group[70] showed that eyes with less than 30 disc diameters of retinal capillary nonperfusion and no other risk factor are at low risk for developing iris/angle neovascularization (i.e., ischemic CRVO), "whereas eyes with 75 disc diameters or more are at highest risk."

Hayreh et al[51] evaluated four functional and two morphological tests to determine their sensitivity and specificity in differentiating ischemic from nonischemic CRVO (Table 63.1). Fluorescein angiography during the early stages of CRVO provides reliable information about retinal capillary nonperfusion in at best only 50–60% of cases. Ophthalmoscopy is the least reliable and most misleading test. Combining a relative afferent pupillary defect with electroretinography is effective in differentiating 97% of the CRVO cases reliably.

Table 63.1 The sensitivity and specificity of the four functional tests

Functional tests	Sensitivity	Specificity
Visual acuity:		
≤ 20/400	91%	88%
Peripheral visual fields*:		
No I-2e	97%	73%
Defective I-4e	92%	87%
Defective V-4e	100%	100%
Relative afferent pupillary defect:		
≥ 0.9 log units	80%	97%
Electroretinography:		
b-wave amp.≤60%	80%	80%

*Visual field plotted with a Goldmann perimeter.

Treatment

Although CRVO has been known as a clinical entity since 1878,[2] its management remains highly controversial.[71,86–88] What follows is a brief account of the main treatments: medical, surgical or invasive, and panretinal photocoagulation (PRP). Overall, there is little evidence to support most of them over observation alone.

Medical therapies

There is no scientific rationale for antiplatelet aggregation agents and anticoagulants, ocular hypotensive therapy, or systemic antihypertensive therapy.[86] Available evidence indicates that anticoagulants and antiplatelet agents are contraindicated in RVO, because they result in marked increase in retinal hemorrhages with associated destructive effect on the retinal neural tissue.[55,87]

Oral[66] or intravitreal[89–91] corticosteroids help to reduce macular edema only and improve visual acuity in nonischemic CRVO; however, a long-term maintenance dose is always required, until the macular edema resolves as a part of natural history. Both oral and repeated intravitreal steroids have multiple ocular/systemic side-effects and complications.

There is so far insufficient definite information about the long-term role of anti-vascular endothelial growth factor (VEGF) therapy in RVO. Repeated intravitreal injections of anti-VEGF therapy (required to maintain its effectiveness) are not without complications.

Oral acetazolamide may help to reduce macular edema associated with nonischemic CRVO and improve visual acuity in some patients; however, macular edema is under control only so long as the patient is taking the drug.[71,86,88]

Surgical or invasive treatments

Surgical decompression of the CRV in CRVO is ill-conceived, has no scientific rationale, and is hazardous.[92,93] A modified form of the procedure called "radial optic neurotomy"[94] has no beneficial effect in CRVO.[95–97] Laser-induced chorioretinal venous anastomosis for the treatment of nonischemic CRVO has been advocated,[98,99] but is associated with a large number of unacceptable, serious complications.[86,87]

Fibrinolytic agents (streptokinase or tissue plasminogen activator) have been administered intravenously,[100–103] intravitreally,[104,105] into the ophthalmic artery,[106,107] and into a branch retinal vein.[108] Some report a variable amount of improvement in visual acuity, others report no beneficial effect, and still others consider this risky. In spite of various claims of beneficial effects, there is little scientifically valid evidence of its effectiveness.[86,87] Thrombolytic agents are only effective if administered within the first few hours of thrombus formation, but the vast majority of CRVO patients are not seen until much later, when the thrombus is organized and cannot be dissolved.

Hemodilution therapy in CRVO is based on the assumption that hyperviscosity is the cause of CRVO; however, no significant difference has been reported between patients with RVO and normal subjects in plasma viscosity[109,110] or hematocrit[110,111] and there is not much scientific evidence of beneficial effects from this therapy.

Photocoagulation

PRP is almost universally considered the treatment of choice for CRVO, to prevent development of ocular neovascularization, and macular grid photocoagulation for the management of macular edema. Various aspects of this mode of treatment are discussed in detail elsewhere.[86–88] However, ocular neovascularization is only seen in ischemic CRVO.[38] Therefore, there is no indication for PRP in nonischemic CRVO. In ischemic CRVO, the theoretical justification advanced for PRP is to prevent development of ocular neovascularization and associated blinding complications of NVG and/or vitreous hemorrhage. A critical review of the literature on the subject reveals serious flaws in most of the studies claiming beneficial effects.[112–114]

The study which is considered as the "gold standard" for PRP in ischemic CRVO is that by "The Central Vein Occlusion Study" group.[70] The study found that "prophylactic PRP

does not totally prevent" development of iris/angle NV. The authors recommended "careful observation with frequent follow-up examinations in the early months (including undilated slit-lamp examination of the iris and gonioscopy) and prompt PRP of eyes in which 2 o'clock iris/angle NV develops." However, Hayreh[113] found some fundamental flaws in the design of this study which invalidate its claims.

In NVG from ischemic CRVO, the most important consideration is control of high IOP, the primary factor causing marked loss of vision in the vast majority of these eyes. Therefore, if NVG develops but the IOP is satisfactorily controlled by any means,[22] the eye will maintain reasonably good peripheral visual fields once the retinopathy burns itself out in due course, and the stimulus for neovascularization diminishes, resulting in spontaneous regression of neovascularization. Thus, overall PRP results in marked loss of peripheral visual field (Figure 63.9), and does more visual

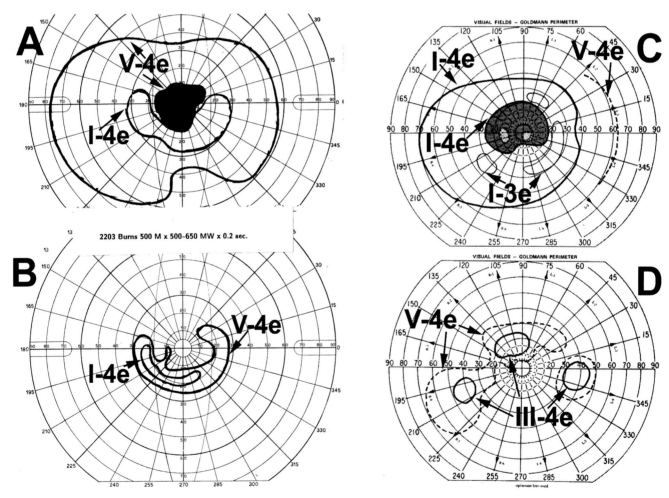

Figure 63.9 Visual field loss in two eyes with ischemic central retinal vein occlusion caused by panretinal photocoagulation (PRP). (A and B) Visual fields of left eye of a 60-year-old man that had 2203 argon laser burns, starting 71 days after onset of ischemic central retinal vein occlusion. (A) Pre-panretinal photocoagulation (PRP) visual field with V-4e was almost normal, with an inferior island field with I-4e, and an absolute central scotoma. (B) Post-PRP visual field 27 days after PRP was reduced to a tiny crescentic island only with both V-4e and I-4e. (C and D) Visual fields of left eye of a 63-year-old man that had 1754 argon laser burns, starting 81 days after onset of ischemic central retinal vein occlusion. (C) Pre-PRP peripheral field was normal with I-4e and V-4e and also had some intact island fields with I-3e, and a large central scotoma with I-4e. (D) Post-PRP fields 6 months after PRP showed marked deterioration and constriction of the visual field. This eye, in spite of having had PRP, developed iris neovascularization 2 months after PRP and that lasted for almost 4½ years. (Reproduced with permission from Hayreh SS, Klugman MR, Podhajsky P, et al. Argon laser panretinal photocoagulation in ischemic central retinal vein occlusion – a 10-year prospective study. Graefes Arch Klin Exp Ophthalmol 1990;228:281–296.)

harm than good, especially when it does not confer a statistically significant protection against development of ocular neovascularization, or offer any other significant benefit in NVG.[112]

The Central Retinal Vein Occlusion Group found that macular grid photocoagulation for macular edema resulted in no difference in visual acuity between treated and untreated eyes.[115]

BRVO and HCRVO

Most of the information on medical management of CRVO also applies to BRVO and HCRVO.

For management of macular edema, the Branch Vein Occlusion Study Group[116] advocated doing macular grid laser photocoagulation to reduce edema. The study found visual acuity improvement in two-thirds of cases but the improvement was usually small and only occasionally significant. Complications of macular grid laser photocoagulation include development of multiple microscotomas corresponding to the sites of laser burns, which may be visually bothersome, so that, in spite of somewhat improved visual acuity in the treated eye, patients might prefer not to use that eye; occasionally retinal fibrosis may develop.

For management of retinal and disc neovascularization associated with BRVO, the Branch Vein Occlusion Study Group[117] advocated scatter photocoagulation in the ischemic fundus area. The study showed that it reduces the likelihood of neovascularization development by 50%, and if neovascularization is already present, it reduces the likelihood of vitreous hemorrhages by 50%. The study did not recommend doing photocoagulation until neovascularization develops.

Another study[118] of sectoral scatter photocoagulation in major BRVO showed a significant reduction of development of retinal neovascularization (but not optic disc neovascularization) and vitreous hemorrhage in lasered eyes compared to untreated eyes. As in ischemic CRVO,[112] it also showed that photocoagulation resulted in significant worsening of the peripheral visual fields in the involved sector in lasered eyes compared to untreated eyes. The authors therefore recommended doing photocoagulation only when neovascularization develops and not otherwise, because in the latter case, the detrimental effects may outweigh the beneficial ones.

Prognosis

In RVO, the retinopathy spontaneously resolves after a variable length of time. There is marked interindividual variation in the time it takes to resolve – usually faster in younger than older people. Thus, RVO is a self-limiting disease, although during the period of activity the various types may produce diverse complications.

Natural history of visual outcome

CRVO

There is little firm information on the natural history of visual outcome in CRVO in the literature and, when described, that is based on either use of invalid criteria to differentiate the two types of CRVO[119] or lumping the two types together.[120] A recent preliminary report[93] described final visual acuity and visual fields in a prospective study of 155 consecutive eyes with nonischemic CRVO in which the retinopathy and macular edema had completely resolved during follow-up. It showed that the final visual acuity in the entire group was 20/25 or better in 65%, 20/40 or better in 77%, 20/50–20/70 in 7%, 20/80–20/200 in 9%, and 20/400 to counting fingers in 7%. A permanent central scotoma, varying in size from tiny to large, was present in 30%, with normal peripheral visual fields in all eyes. By contrast, in ischemic CRVO, during the initial stages, the ganglion cells in the macular retina are irreversibly damaged by ischemia, causing a permanent central scotoma, and thus little chance of improvement of visual acuity in such an eye.

HCRVO

This is reported in a series of 41 eyes (27 with nonischemic HCRVO and 14 with ischemic HCRVO).[53] The final visual acuity in eyes with nonischemic HCRVO was 20/25 or better in 40%, 20/30–20/80 in 29%, 20/100–20/200 in 18.5%, and 20/400 to counting fingers in 11%. In ischemic HCRVO, it was 7%, 14%, 43%, and 36%, respectively.

BRVO

The only study available so far is that of the Branch Vein Occlusion Study Group.[116] In that study, in eyes with intact retinal capillaries in the macular region, one-third of eyes with visual acuity of 20/40 or worse showed improvement over 3 years on follow-up. Another study of 229 major BRVO showed that older patients had more visual acuity deterioration than younger patients.[118]

Long-term complications of CRVO

Nonischemic CRVO is a comparatively benign disease; the main long-term complications are: (1) development of permanent central scotoma (with normal peripheral visual fields) if chronic macular edema produces secondary macular changes[93]; and (2) some eyes may convert to ischemic CRVO (12.6% within 18 months of onset[39]). By contrast, ischemic CRVO is a malignant disease, with a high risk of development of ocular neovascularization and NVG (Figure 63.7) and other blinding complications. In our prospective study[38] of 721 eyes with RVO, the risk of developing anterior-segment neovascularization was only in eyes with ischemic CRVO and occasionally ischemic HCRVO, while the risk of developing posterior-segment neovascularization was in ischemic CRVO, ischemic HCRVO, and major BRVO. Eyes with nonischemic CRVO/HCRVO per se do not develop ocular neovascularization, unless there is associated diabetic retinopathy or ocular ischemia.

Key references

A complete list of chapter references is available online at www.expertconsult.com. See inside cover for registration details.

3. Hayreh SS, Zimmerman B. Central retinal artery occlusion: visual outcome. Am J Ophthalmol 2005;140:376–391.

5. Hayreh SS. Prevalent misconceptions about acute retinal vascular occlusive disorders. Prog Retin Eye Res 2005;24:493–519.

10. Hayreh SS, Zimmerman MB, Kimura A, et al. Central retinal artery occlusion. Retinal survival time. Exp Eye Res 2004;78:723–736.

20. Hayreh SS, Podhajsky PA, Zimmerman B. Role of nocturnal arterial hypotension in optic nerve head ischemic disorders. Ophthalmologica 1999;213:76–96.

25. Hayreh SS, Fraterrigo L, Jonas J. Central retinal vein occlusion associated with cilioretinal artery occlusion. Retina 2008;28:581–594.

37. Beatty S, Au Eong KG. Local intra-arterial fibrinolysis for acute occlusion of the central retinal artery: a meta-analysis of the published data. Br J Ophthalmol 2000;84:914–916.

38. Hayreh SS, Rojas P, Podhajsky P, et al. Ocular neovascularization with retinal vascular occlusion. III. Incidence of ocular neovascularization with retinal vein occlusion. Ophthalmology 1983;90:488–506.

39. Hayreh SS, Zimmerman MB, Podhajsky P. Incidence of various types of retinal vein occlusion and their recurrence and demographic characteristics. Am J Ophthalmol 1994;117:429–441.

51. Hayreh SS, Klugman MR, Beri M, et al. Differentiation of ischemic from non-ischemic central retinal vein occlusion during the early acute phase. Graefes Arch Clin Exp Ophthalmol 1990;228:201–217.

53. Hayreh SS, Hayreh MS. Hemi-central retinal vein occlusion. Pathogenesis, clinical features, and natural history. Arch Ophthalmol 1980;98:1600–1609.

86. Hayreh SS. Management of central retinal vein occlusion. Ophthalmologica 2003;217:167–188.

94. Opremcak ME, Bruce RA, Lomeo MD, et al. Radial optic neurotomy for central retinal vein occlusion. Retina 2001;21:408–415.

112. Hayreh SS, Klugman MR, Podhajsky P, et al. Argon laser panretinal photocoagulation in ischemic central retinal vein occlusion – a 10-year prospective study. Graefes Arch Clin Exp Ophthalmol 1990;228:281–296.

113. Hayreh SS. The CVOS group M and N reports. Ophthalmology 1996;103:350–352.

116. The Branch Vein Occlusion Study Group. Argon laser photocoagulation for macular edema in branch vein occlusion. Am J Ophthalmol 1984;98:271–282.

CHAPTER 64

Retinal photic injury: laboratory and clinical findings

Daniel Organisciak and Marco Zarbin

Overview

Retinal photoreceptors are paradoxically efficient in their ability to capture photons for visual transduction while being vulnerable to cellular damage from excess light. Although the molecular mechanism of visual transduction is now relatively well understood, our understanding of retinal phototoxicity, or retinal light damage, is less complete. Nonetheless, based to a degree on comparable end-stage morphology, retinal photic injury in laboratory animals has served as a model of retinal degenerations of genetic origin, aging, and from light-induced trauma during ocular surgery for over 40 years.[1,2] Likewise, a long-standing clinical interest in the potential for interactions between diet, light environment, and retinal injury has prompted studies with animal models. But are animal models of light-induced retinal degeneration appropriate models for human retinal disease? Furthermore, although high levels of light accelerate some forms of inherited retinal degeneration and might influence the incidence of age-related macular degeneration (AMD), what role does light environment play in retinal disease?

Clinical background

Light duration and intensity

Visible light-mediated photoreceptor cell damage is a photochemical process with a well-known inverse time and intensity relationship. This effect, often referred to as reciprocity, implies that a longer-duration light exposure can be shortened by the use of higher-intensity light, and vice versa. This concept is well recognized in anterior-segment surgery and during vitrectomy where light intensity and time-dependent phototoxic lesions have been reported.[3,4] These lesions appear hours to days after surgery and are often seen in or near the cone-rich foveal region of the eye. The outcome for most phototoxic lesions found outside the fovea is generally good while the prognosis for repair of foveal damage, more often seen following vitrectomy, is less favorable.[3,4] Solar retinitis also presents with foveal damage. It is well known to occur in patients deliberately sungazing for extended periods, but a few cases have been reported following relatively short periods of sunbathing in high (often reflective) light environments.[5] Likewise, photic injury from an indirect ophthalmoscope following relatively brief exposure has been reported.[6] There are limits on photochemical damage in the retina and reciprocity, however, in that short-duration high-intensity coherent light actually results in thermal damage. Discussion of laser light-induced damage, sometimes employed in treating choroidal neovascularization and routinely used in the treatment of retinal breaks, is beyond the scope of this chapter.

Spectral characteristics of damaging light

Retinal light damage is also wavelength-dependent, with green light most effectively causing damage in rod photoreceptors. In other words, the action spectrum for light damage closely approximates the absorption spectrum for rhodopsin.[1,7,8] (Figure 64.1). However, blue light as well as full-spectrum white light also causes retinal damage by bleaching rhodopsin, albeit less efficiently. Blue light has a shorter wavelength than green light and is therefore more energetic (Planck's relation: $E = h/\lambda$, where E = energy, h = the Planck constant, and λ = wavelength). Accordingly, blue light is capable of photoisomerizing free all-trans retinal, the aldehyde form of vitamin A, into the 11-cis stereoisomer required for rhodopsin regeneration.[9] This reaction may short circuit the normal postrhodopsin-bleaching vitamin A cycle, involving migration of all-trans retinol into the retinal pigment epithelium (RPE) and enzymatic reisomerization to the 11-cis form.[10] In primates, cone cells undergo damage from short intermittent pulses of blue light, which has also been attributed to rapid bleaching and regeneration of blue-cone visual pigment.[11] RPE cell damage from blue light exposure probably involves different chromophores. For example, mitochondrial cytochrome proteins have been suggested as one chromophore, and a potential source for the generation of reactive oxygen species.[12] Another potential source of blue light-mediated reactive oxygen in RPE is photosensitization of bis-retinaldehyde-phosphatidylethanolamine (A2E), a lipophilic molecule that accumulates with age.[13] Epidemiological studies indicate that chronic light exposure may be a risk factor for the development of AMD, but this effect seems to be small compared to the risk factors of age (>70 years), race (caucasian), and smoking.[14-16] Light exposure might indirectly predispose to AMD through a variety of mecha-

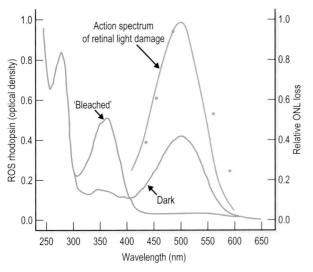

Figure 64.1 Absorption spectrum of rod outer segment (ROS) rhodopsin and the action spectrum of retinal light damage. Rhodopsin was extracted from rat ROS with a nonionic detergent[61] and absorption spectra recorded in darkness (Dark) and after light exposure in vitro (Bleached). The Dark spectrum shows a rhodopsin absorption maximum at 500 nm and a peak of protein absorbance at 278 nm. Following light, rhodopsin absorbance is reduced to baseline while a new peak of absorbance appears at 367 nm. There is no change in 278-nm absorbance, indicating no loss of protein from the detergent extract. The 367-nm peak arises from free *all*-trans retinal released during rhodopsin bleaching. The action spectrum for retinal light damage (green line), superimposed on the rhodopsin absorption spectra, shows a nearly identical 500-nm maximum for the pathological effect of light. The light damage action spectrum was determined by morphological measurements of the outer nuclear layer in rat retinas several days after exposure to narrow band width visible light. (Light damage spectrum redrawn from Williams TP, Howell WL. Action spectrum of retinal light damage in albino rats. Invest Ophthalmol Vis Sci 1983;24:285–287, with permission from the Association for Research in Vision and Ophthalmology.)

Box 64.1 Features of retinal light damage

- Light damage is a photochemical process: exposure duration and light intensity inversely affect the degree of damage (reciprocity)
- Action spectrum for light damage closely approximates the absorption spectrum for rhodopsin
- Green light causes damage most efficiently in rod photoreceptors
- Blue light can cause retinal damage by inducing photoisomerization of free retinaldehyde, which promotes more rapid rate of rhodopsin regeneration and subsequent rebleaching
- Blue light-mediated retinal pigment epithelium damage may involve mitochondrial cytochrome proteins and/or photosensitization via *bis*-retinaldehyde phosphatidylethanolamine (A2E)

Box 64.2 Pathological findings in retinal photic injury

- Loss of rod photoreceptors with relative sparing of cones
- Inner retina (bipolar, horizontal, amacrine, ganglion cells) initially spared
- Extensive photoreceptor cell loss leads to changes in inner retina neuron morphology, location, and synaptic function

---

nisms (see Chapter 68). For example, Zhou and coworkers have suggested that products of the photo-oxidation of *bis*-retinoid lipofuscin pigments in RPE cells may serve as a trigger for the complement system[17] (Box 64.1).

Pathology

Photoreceptor cells are differentiated postmitotic retinal neurons that normally function throughout the life of an individual. Some visual cell dropout occurs naturally as a result of aging, but rod and cone survival into the seventh decade and beyond is normally more than sufficient to preserve vision. A higher rate of visual cell loss is seen in many genetic conditions, but the rate of loss is still relatively slow compared to most experimental animal models of retinal degeneration. At the same time the morphological endpoints of both genetic and experimental retinal degenerations are so similar that they invite comparisons and inferences into etiology and prevention based primarily on studies with animals. In the case of photic injury in animal models, one sees loss of rod photoreceptors, with a relative sparing of cones.[18,19] Rod cell loss is graded, most pronounced in the central superior hemisphere, and often particularly severe in the region 1–2 mm superior to the optic nerve head.[20] At least initially, Müller cells and the inner

retinal neurons, consisting of horizontal, bipolar, amacrine, and ganglion cells, appear to be immune to light. The reasons for this dichotomy are unknown; however, it is not a simple lack of cellular chromophores, as light-absorbing proteins such as melanopsin and cryptochromes are present in the inner retinal layers.[21,22] Recently, it was suggested that the tripeptide glutathione may be absent, or nearly so, from photoreceptor cells while present in sufficient quantities in the inner retinal layers to prevent oxidative damage.[23] As in some animal models, rod cell degeneration precedes that of cone cells in the early stages of AMD. However, in AMD the loss of both rods and cones appears to result from RPE dysfunction in the parafoveal/macular region.[24] Irrespective of the reasons for their susceptibility, when photoreceptor cell loss is extensive remarkable changes in inner retinal neuron morphology, location, and synaptic function soon follow[25] (Box 64.2).

Etiology

Genetic risk factors

Under ordinary conditions, eye pigmentation and pupil size play major roles in preventing photic injury. By constricting pupil diameter during high light (photopic) conditions much of the light entering the eye is focused on the cone-rich fovea, which is relatively resistant to damage. Because melanin in the RPE absorbs light that passes entirely through the retina, its presence may help to reduce light scatter and photosensitized reactions in the choriocapillaris or in Bruch's membrane.[26,27] In addition, because the RPE cell layer covers the entire globe of the eye and melanin pigments are present in the iris, ciliary body, and choroid, extraneous light is largely prevented from entering the eye through the sclera. In fact, melanin is such an effective filter that, for photic damage to occur in pigmented animals, mydriatics are usually required. In low light (scotopic) conditions the pupils are also dilated, allowing a larger area of the retina to be illuminated, but the intensity of light is much reduced, as is the chance of retinal injury. Pigmented animals have the same action spectrum for retinal light damage (Figure 64.1) and exhibit the same morphological characteristics as nonpigmented animals.[2,28] However, because albino strains lack melanin, they are approximately twofold more sensitive to photic injury.[1,28]

Other genetic mutations also exacerbate the effects of light exposure on the rate of retinal degeneration. For example, the most common form of autosomal-dominant retinitis pigmentosa (RP) involves a histidine for proline substitution at amino acid position 23 in rhodopsin (P23H). In patients having the P23H mutation, external factors appear to affect the rate of functional loss of both scotopic and photopic vision.[29] Heckenlively et al found that patients working in bright light environments lost vision sooner than others working in dim light environments.[30] In transgenic animal models with the P23H mutation, rod cell loss also precedes that of cone cells, and the rate of loss also depends on lighting conditions.[31,32] While the P23H animal model does not mimic all of the electrophysiological findings in RP,[31] it correctly predicts the effects of light environment on the rate of retinal degeneration and has provided insights into the mislocalization of mutated rhodopsin in rod outer-segment disks. Similarly, Royal College of Surgeons (RCS) rats exhibit a retinal degeneration that depends on environmental light. Dark rearing delays the onset of photoreceptor cell loss, while normal light exposure greatly accelerates that loss.[33,34] As they age, RCS rats also accumulate a partially degraded cellular "debris" layer between the RPE and retina, which results from an inability of RPE to phagocytose rod outer-segment material.[33,34] This debris layer forms a barrier that impedes the exchange of metabolites and the flow of nutrients from choroid to retina, leading to cell death. Morphologically, the end-stage RCS retina resembles that of several human retinal diseases, but whether the inhibition of nutrient flow is an appropriate model for human disease is currently unknown. A number of mouse strains also present with variable light damage sensitivities.[35] In several strains, their susceptibility to retinal photic damage has been shown to correlate with a mutation in RPE 65, an enzyme involved in vitamin A (retinol) processing.[36,37] Mice having the RPE 65 Leu 450 variant are more easily damaged, while mice with the RPE 65 Met 450 variant are more resistant to the phototoxic effects of light[38] (Box 64.3).

Dietary factors

Animal models lend themselves particularly well to understanding the role of diet on retinal development and disease progression. The effects of dietary retinol on rhodopsin levels and retinal light damage have been described for vitamin A-deficient rats[39] and after inhibition of the visual cycle with 13-*cis* retinoic acid.[40] In each case, a reduced level of available 11-*cis*-retinaldehyde leads to an increase in

> ### Box 64.3 Genetic and dietary factors influence light damage
>
> - Melanin acts as screening pigment to reduce light effects on the retina
> - Genetic animal models mimic some aspects of human retinal disease
> - Vitamin A metabolism and dietary fatty acids affect retinal development and susceptibility to light damage
> - The polyunsaturated fatty acid docosahexaenoic acid can be converted into two different oxidative products

opsin levels and to reduced light damage susceptibility. A similar decrease in rhodopsin levels and increase in opsin in patients treated for acne with 13-*cis* retinoids is thought to lead to the development of deficits in scotopic vision.[40] Insufficient dietary linolenic acid (18:3n-3), the essential fatty acid precursor of docosahexaenoic acid (22:6n-3; DHA), leads to a decrease in retinal DHA and to a decrease in susceptibility to photic damage.[41–43] The amount of DHA in the retina is species-specific, but in rat rod outer segments it may represent as much as 50 mol% of the total.[41–43] In other words, one of every two fatty acids found in rod outer-segment lipids can be a polyunsaturated DHA. Rod outer segments from transgenic P23H rats contain lower levels of DHA than normal, but unpredictably these animals are more sensitive to the damaging effects of light than normal rats.[44,45] Furthermore, feeding P23H rats diets high in omega-3 fatty acids has not proven to be effective in delaying photoreceptor cell loss.[44,45] Some forms of RP are associated with low DHA levels in red blood cells,[46] but in these cases dietary DHA seems to be beneficial. Thus, a link between the reduced levels of DHA in rod outer segments of transgenic animal models and the low circulating levels of DHA in some RP patients[46] has not yet been established.

The importance of dietary omega-3 fatty acids during visual system development, however, has been established, for rats[47] and for primates,[48] and, more recently, for preterm infants.[49] Following clinical trials with full-term infants,[50] DHA is now routinely added to infant formulas, along with the omega-6 fatty acid, arachidonic acid. Dietary supplementation with these fatty acids has a positive outcome on the development of vision and, although total dietary fat intake is associated with AMD,[51] omega-3 fatty acids appear to slow disease progression.[51] Accordingly, as a part of the ongoing Age-Related Eye Disease Study (AREDS) II, DHA supplementation is now being tested in patients. A rationale for this clinical trial appears to be based on the neuroprotective effects of this omega-3 polyunsaturated fatty acid. In the RPE, small amounts of DHA are enzymatically converted to neuroprotectin D1 (NPD-1), which has been shown to be effective in reducing apoptotic cell death.[52] However, DHA is also capable of being oxidized by molecular oxygen,[53] leading to the formation of carboxyethylpyrrole (CEP) protein adducts.[54] NPD-1 is a 22-carbon DHA derivative containing two hydroxyl groups, while CEP is a 7-carbon DHA oxidation fragment, with a pyrrole ring adducted to the amine side chain of amino acids such as lysine (Figure 64.2). Crabb and associates analyzed drusen dissected from the RPE layer of AMD and age-matched controls and found

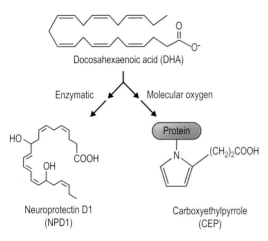

Figure 64.2 Structures of docosahexaenoic acid (DHA) and two products formed by oxidative processes. The polyunsaturated fatty acid DHA is oxidized by an enzymatic process to produce neuroprotectin D1, a 22-carbon hydroxylated fatty acid derivative. The reactions occur in retina, but are particularly active in the retinal pigment epithelium.[52] Molecular oxygen leads to the truncation of DHA[53] to produce a 7-carbon derivative which is capable of forming covalent adducts with free amino groups in proteins.[54]

higher than normal levels of these covalent adducts in AMD eyes.[54] Recently a mouse model of AMD, prepared by immunization with CEP adducted to albumin, has been shown to exhibit RPE deposits and pathology.[55] This model and others may be useful in preclinical studies to help sort out the protective and damaging effects of dietary DHA and its derivatives.

Pathophysiology

Initiation of retinal light damage

Mechanistically, the principal utility of the photic injury animal model resides in the synchronous involvement of rod photoreceptors. Unlike genetic or age-related conditions, where small numbers of visual cells are typically involved at any one time, nearly the entire complement of photoreceptors is affected by intense light. Noell et al were the first to report that extensive rhodopsin bleaching is the trigger for retinal light damage.[1] Genetic modification of photoreceptor cell proteins also points to rhodopsin as the key mediator of retinal damage by light. Rhodopsin knockout (KO) and RPE-65 KO mice are both protected against photic injury.[36,37,56] Because opsin, but not rhodopsin, is present in RPE-65 mice and rhodopsin KO mice lack the protein altogether, the rate of rhodopsin regeneration during light has been implicated in the damage mechanism. Ironically, whole-body hyperthermia during light exposure also accelerates rhodopsin regeneration and greatly exacerbates retinal light damage.[1,57] Photic injury occurs under ordinary room light in arrestin KO mice and rhodopsin kinase KO mice, while dark rearing prevents damage.[58,59] Arrestin and rhodopsin kinase both interact with light-activated rhodopsin and are involved in attenuating the photo response, implicating two additional visual transduction proteins in the damage mechanism. Young RCS rats are genetically pre-

disposed to retinal light damage, which correlates with the relative expression levels of arrestin and transducin.[60] In both RCS and normal rats, dark rearing leads to increases in transducin mRNA and protein levels and enhances light damage, while a normal cyclic light environment increases arrestin levels and reduces susceptibility to damage.[60-62] Other genetic evidence suggests that two distinct pathways of retinal damage may exist, one involving transducin and relatively low light exposure levels and a second pathway involving high light levels and the transcription factor activator protein-1.[63]

Antioxidants and oxidation

Compelling evidence exists that oxidative stress is an integral part of the light damage process, as both natural and synthetic antioxidants prevent photoreceptor cell damage and loss.[64-66] Oxidation also appears to be a relatively early event in the damage process. Light-induced oxidation occurs within minutes in isolated photoreceptor cells,[67] and the rapid appearance of blue light-induced reactive oxygen species, originating from mitochondria, has been reported.[68] Lipid hydroperoxides in retina were found to be elevated in normal rats exposed to green light, as well as in an oxidatively susceptible, drug-induced rat model of Smith–Lemli–Opitz syndrome.[69,70] The synthetic antioxidant dimethylthiourea (DMTU) was effective in preventing light damage when administered before lights on,[70] but is ineffective when given after the onset of light[71] (Figure 64.3). Retinal protein markers of oxidative stress are also altered by light and impacted by antioxidants. The expression of retinal heme oxygenase (HO-1) increases after intense light exposure.[71,72] HO-1 is a 32-kDa inducible stress protein and the first enzyme in a pathway involved in converting a prooxidant heme into bilirubin, an antioxidant. Retinol dehydrogenase (RDH), an oxidatively sensitive rod outer-segment enzyme that converts retinaldehyde into retinol, is partially inhibited by light exposure.[73] However, pretreatment of rats with DMTU prevents both the light-driven increase in HO-1 expression and the decrease in RDH activity.[72,73] In mice, inhibition of nitric oxide formation has been shown to reduce retinal light damage,[74] further implicating oxidative stress in retinal phototoxicity (Box 64.4).

Humans and nonhuman primates appear to be the only species with a well-developed capacity to accumulate carotenoids in the foveal-macular region of the retina. The primary carotenoids found there are lutein (L) and zeaxanthin (Z), which are dihydroxylated derivatives of beta-carotene.[75] The overall level of L and Z is affected by dietary intake,[76] and together they give rise to a yellowish (macular pigment) appearance in the central retina. L and Z both absorb blue light, effectively reducing the level of high-energy photons reaching photoreceptors and the RPE, but they are also potent antioxidants.[75] Accordingly, these carotenoids may function in two ways: (1) by preventing blue light stimulation of A2E in the RPE; and (2) by decreasing light-induced oxidative insult in photoreceptors. In either case, protection is concentration-dependent, and the highest concentrations of L and Z are found at the level of photoreceptor cell synapses in the cone-rich macular region.[75] The amount of macular pigment decreases with eccentricity from the center of the macula, reaching near-baseline levels in the

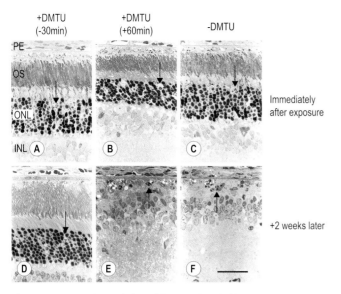

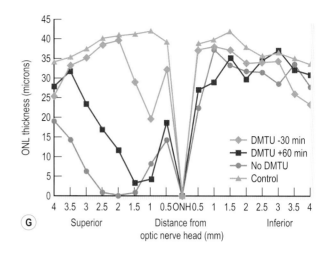

Figure 64.3 Retinal morphology following dimethylthiourea (DMTU) treatment and intense light exposure. Rats were given a single dose of DMTU 30 minutes before light treatment, or 1 hour after the start of light.[71] Immediately after an 8-hour light exposure both the antioxidant-treated (+DMTU) and untreated (–DMTU) animals have relatively intact outer segments (OS) and retinal pigment epithelium (RPE) cells (A, B, and C). Photoreceptor cell loss is almost complete when –DMTU retinas are examined 2 weeks later. An occasional rod cell nucleus and cone cell nuclei (arrowhead) appear adjacent to the RPE (F). The retina is compressed with the inner nuclear layer (INL) now in close proximity to the RPE. The retinal section from a +DMTU-treated rat exhibits an intact RPE and photoreceptor cell layer, with a normal rod inner segment and outer nuclear layer (ONL) (D), when the antioxidant is given before the start of light (compare D with E and F). Morphometric measurements of ONL thickness, along the vertical meridian (G), show that visual cell loss is extensive in the superior hemisphere and severe in the area 1–2 mm from the optic nerve head (ONH). The periphery and inferior hemisphere are least damaged by light. DMTU reduces visual cell loss when given before light treatment, but is much less effective when given after the onset of light. (Reproduced with permission from Vaughan DK, Nemke JL, Fliesler SJ, et al. Evidence for a circadian rhythm of susceptibility to retinal light damage. Photochem Photobiol 2002;75:547–553.)

Box 64.4 Mechanisms of retinal light damage

- Extensive rhodopsin bleaching is the trigger for retinal light damage
- Rate of rhodopsin regeneration during light exposure influences degree of damage
- Arrestin and rhodopsin kinase attenuate light damage
- Hyperthermia and transducin enhance light damage
- Oxidative stress is an integral part of the light damage process; antioxidants prevent light-induced photoreceptor damage
- Photoreceptor cell loss occurs via an apoptotic process; BCL-2 overexpression and a variety of neurotrophic factors reduce genetic as well as light-induced photoreceptor cell death
- Retinal pigment epithelium cell dysfunction is linked to photoreceptor cell degeneration, either as the initiating event or subsequent to toxic reactions in the retina

---

parafoveal region where AMD-associated photoreceptor (rod) loss is first observed.[24,75,77] Macular pigment levels are also decreased by pro-oxidants present in cigarette smoke, a well-established risk factor in AMD,[16,51,78] while high levels of carotenoids and other antioxidants in the circulation appear to reduce the probability of developing neovascular AMD.[79]

Photoreceptor and RPE cell death

Visual cell loss resulting from acute intense light exposure, chronic high light environments, or because of genetic inher-

itance occurs largely through an apoptotic process.[80] RPE cell dysfunction is linked to photoreceptor cell degeneration, either as the initiating event or subsequent to toxic reactions in the retina. The intimate metabolic and morphologic relationships between retina and RPE, their high oxygen tension, and the rate and duration of photon flux are all reasons why reactive oxygen species generated in one tissue can lead to degeneration in the other. One of the hallmarks of apoptotic cell death is double-strand cleavage of DNA by endonucleases.[80,81] The resulting DNA fragments appear within hours of lights on[80] and continue to accumulate for several days after acute intense light exposure.[63,80,82] Light-induced DNA fragmentation is prevented by antioxidants,[82] suggesting that oxidation also initiates the apoptotic process.[83] In addition, photoreceptor cell death from light is prevented by overexpression of the antiapoptotic protein BCL-2 and a variety of neurotrophic factors.[84,85] However, while antioxidants have not proven effective in preventing genetic retinal degenerations,[86] BCL-2 overexpression and neurotrophins are at least partially effective.[87]

Relationship between retinal light damage and macular degeneration

The pathogenesis of AMD is described in greater detail in Chapter 68. However, some relevant concepts are as follows. Lipofuscin accumulates in RPE cells over time, and A2E is the major photosensitizing chromophore in lipofuscin. When RPE cells are exposed to light in vitro A2E, conjugated to low-density lipoprotein, causes a loss of lysosomal integrity[88] and inhibition of phagolysosomal degradation of photoreceptor phospholipids.[89] RPE cells with excessive A2E exhibit membrane blebbing and extrusion of cytoplasmic material into Bruch's membrane. Epidemiological studies, AMD histochemistry, and drusen biochemistry indicate that oxidative reactions play a central role in AMD pathophysiology. AREDS demonstrated that among selected patients supplementation with vitamins (ascorbic acid, vitamin E, and beta-carotene) and minerals (zinc oxide, cupric oxide) reduces the risk of developing advanced AMD and the rate of at least moderate vision loss.[79] The AREDS data may mean that oxidative damage plays a role in the progression of AMD in its clinically evident intermediate and late stages and that disease progression can be altered with antioxidant supplementation. However, zinc also affects the complement system by inhibiting C3 convertase activity,[90] and C3a des Arg (a cleavage product of C3a that reflects complement activation) levels are higher in patients with AMD versus controls.[91] Zhou and coworkers have suggested that products of the photo-oxidation of *bis*-retinoid lipofuscin pigments in RPE cells may also trigger the complement system.[17] Given the relative abundance of lipofuscin in the submacular RPE, this trigger would predispose the macula to chronic inflammation and AMD. These experiments link RPE lipofuscin, oxidative damage, drusen, and inflammation, all of which have been implicated in the pathogenesis of AMD.[17,92,93]

Prolonged actinic light exposure can cause rod and cone degeneration in albino rats through a pathway that involves photoreceptor cell rhodopsin, retinoid metabolism, and the formation of reactive oxygen species in RPE cells.[27,71] Light-induced retinal damage kills three classes of cells almost concurrently: photoreceptors, RPE, and choriocapillary endothelium.[25] Light-induced retinal degeneration mimics important features of retinal remodeling observed in inherited retinal degenerations, including glial hypertrophy and reorganization of the neural retina. In contrast to retinal degenerative diseases (e.g., RCS rat, P23H rat), however, light-induced retinal damage is associated with eruption of processes from retinal neurons and eventual emigration of Müller cells and neurons from the retina into the choroid.[25] Marc and coworkers noted a striking parallel between atrophic zones in human geographic atrophy and severely damaged retina in light-induced retinal damage.[25] Specifically, the gradient between apparently functional surviving retina and severely damaged retina is steep in both conditions, which indicates that similar neuronal migration events might be involved in the late stages of geographic atrophy (Box 64.5).

Retinal remodeling in retinal degenerative conditions (e.g., light damage, RP-like disease, retinal detachment, and AMD) occurs in three phases.[25] In phase 1, photoreceptor outer-segment truncation, disease-dependent opsin mislocalization, and changes in synaptic architecture often lead to disconnection of bipolar and photoreceptor cells before photoreceptors die.[94–99] In phase 2, photoreceptor death and active debris removal attenuate the outer nuclear layer in association with microglial activation.[100–102] In phase 3, new processes from remaining neurons form neurite fascicles as well as novel synaptic tufts (termed microneuromas by Marc

> ## Box 64.5 Light-induced retinal degeneration versus geographic atrophy in age-related macular degeneration (AMD)
>
> - Gradient between apparently functional surviving retina and severely damaged retina is steep in both cases
> - Phase 1 (changes in photoreceptor outer segments and synapses) and phase 2 (photoreceptor cell death, outer nuclear layer attenuation, microglial activation) remodeling occurs quickly in light damage but slowly in AMD
> - Phase 3 (formation of new processes, novel synaptic tufts from remaining neurons) remodeling progresses with similar kinetics in light damage and AMD once cone photoreceptor death occurs
> - Both conditions exhibit spatially delimited areas of photoreceptor–retinal pigment epithelium–choriocapillaris atrophy, glial and neuron emigration from the retina, and are associated with oxidative stress

et al[25]) that develop outside the normal lamination of the inner plexiform layer. Neuron migration across the retina occurs, often near hypertrophic Müller cells.[98] In contrast to conditions such as RP or AMD, phase 1 and 2 remodeling occurs relatively quickly (weeks) in light-induced retinal damage, while phase 3 remodeling seems to progress with similar kinetics in all conditions, once cone photoreceptor death has occurred.[25]

Although the pathogenesis of light-induced retinal damage and of AMD are clearly distinct, light-induced retinal damage has several similarities to atrophic AMD that are not shared with RP-like diseases.[25] First, both conditions exhibit spatially delimited areas of photoreceptor–RPE–choriocapillaris atrophy. In contrast to RP, both light-induced retinal damage and geographic atrophy exhibit phase 1/phase 3 borders (versus phase1/phase2 and phase 2/phase 3 borders in RP). Choriocapillaris degeneration in both conditions is severe in affected areas but not in adjacent survivor areas.[103,104] Second, both conditions seem to exhibit glial and neuron emigration from the retina.[105,106] Third, both light-induced retinal damage and AMD are associated with oxidative stress.[86,107,108] Thus, some biochemical features and morphological changes found in light-induced retinal damage may be useful models of the changes that occur in late atrophic AMD.

In conclusion, the morphological end-stages of human retinal degenerations often bear a striking resemblance to those found in experimental light-induced retinal damage. Laboratory animal models have also provided insights into the role of nutrition in retinal development and potential therapies to slow the progression of retinal disease. Questions remain about basic mechanisms and whether animal models of photic injury are really appropriate as models for human retinal degeneration. This chapter has highlighted the similarities and differences that do exist, with a focus on comparisons between genetic, environmental, dietary, and age-related factors.

Key references

A complete list of chapter references is available online at www.expertconsult.com. See inside cover for registration details.

1. Noell WK, Walker VS, Kang BS, et al. Retinal damage by light in rats. Invest Ophthalmol 1966;5:450–473.

9. Grimm C, Reme CE, Rol PO, et al. Blue light's effects on rhodopsin: photoreversal of bleaching in living rat eyes. Invest Ophthalmol Vis Sci 2000;41:3984–3990.

15. Klein R, Klein BE, Jensen SC, et al. The five-year incidence and progression of age-related maculopathy: the Beaver Dam eye study. Ophthalmology 1997;104:7–21.

17. Zhou J, Jang YP, Kim SR, et al. Complement activation by photooxidation products of A2E, a lipofuscin constituent of the retinal pigment epithelium. Proc Natl Acad Sci 2006;103:16182–16187.

20. Vaughan DK, Nemke JL, Fliesler SJ, et al. Evidence for a circadian rhythm of susceptibility to retinal light damage. Photochem Photobiol 2002;75:547–553.

25. Marc RE, Jones CB, Vazquez-Chona F, et al. Extreme retinal remodeling triggered by light damage: implications for age related macular degeneration. Mol Vis 2008;14:782–806.

30. Heckenlively JR, Rodriguez JA, Daiger SP. Autosomal dominant sectoral retinitis pigmentosa: two families with a transversion mutation in codon 23 of rhodopsin. Arch Ophthalmol 1991;109:84–91.

31. Machida S, Kondo M, Jamison JA, et al. P23H rhodopsin transgenic rat: correlation of retinal function with histopathology. Invest Ophthalmol Vis Sci 2000;41:3200–3209.

40. Sieving PA, Chaudry P, Kondo M, et al. Inhibition of the visual cycle in vivo by 13-cis retinoic acid protects from light damage and provides a mechanism for night blindness in isoretinoin therapy. Proc Natl Acad Sci 2001;98:1835–1840.

50. Birch EE, Hoffman DR, Castaneda YS, et al. A randomized controlled trial of long-chain polyunsaturated fatty acid supplementation of formula in term infants after weaning at 6 wk of age. Am J Clin Nutr 2002;75:570–580.

52. Mukherjee PK, Marcheselli VL, Serhan CN, et al. Neuroprotectin D1: a docosahexaenoic acid-derived docosatriene protects human retinal pigment epithelial cells from oxidative stress. Proc Natl Acad Sci 2004;101:8491–8496.

54. Crabb JW, Miyagi M, Gu X, et al. Drusen proteome analysis: an approach to the etiology of age-related macular degeneration. Proc Natl Acad Sci 2002;99:14682–14687.

71. Organisciak DT, Darrow RM, Barsalou L, et al. Circadian dependent retinal light damage in rats. Invest Ophthalmol Vis Sci 2000;41:3694–3701.

79. AREDS #8. A randomized, placebo-controlled, clinical trial of high-dose supplementation with vitamins C and E, beta carotene, and zinc for age-related macular degeneration and vision loss. Arch Ophthalmol 2001;119:1417–1436.

92. Zarbin MA. Current concepts in the pathogenesis of age-related macular degeneration. Arch Ophthalmol 2004;122:598–614.

CHAPTER 65

Vascular damage in diabetic retinopathy

Timothy S Kern and Suber Huang

Overview

Diabetic retinopathy remains a major cause of morbidity in diabetic patients. To date, the retinopathy has been defined based on lesions that are clinically demonstrable, and all of those have been vascular in nature, including degeneration or nonperfusion of the vasculature, and excessive leakage of the vasculature (retinal edema, cottonwool spots, hemorrhage, hard exudates). Available clinical evidence strongly suggests that the late, clinically meaningful stages of the retinopathy are a direct consequence of the earlier changes. This chapter is an overview of the vascular changes associated with diabetic retinopathy. Macular edema is the specific focus of Chapter 67 and neovascularization of Chapter 66.

Clinical background

Clinical findings in nonproliferative diabetic retinopathy (NPDR) arise from progressive capillary cell damage, loss of blood–retina barrier integrity, and leakage of vascular components into adjacent retinal tissue.[1] Clinical signs of microaneurysms, retinal edema, retinal exudate, and retinal hemorrhage are all associated with increased capillary permeability and worsening vasculopathy. Yellow-white precipitates (hard exudates) may accompany leaking microaneurysms. Increased permeability of the blood–retinal barrier is known to occur in patients with diabetes, and this defect contributes to retinal edema and visual impairment in diabetic patients. Macular edema is the most common cause of visual loss in diabetic retinopathy (Figure 65.1A).

Larger microaneurysms and diffuse microvascular damage result in retinal hemorrhage. Focal areas of ischemia further damage the inner retina. Cottonwool spots describe opaque yellow-white lesions and represent areas of inner retinal infarction. The term soft exudate is now seldom used but describes the soft, ill-defined borders of these lesions. Retinal fluorescein angiography reveals progressive enlargement of areas of nonperfusion in diabetic retinopathy[2-4] (Figure 65.1B).

Proliferative diabetic retinopathy (PDR) occurs when progressive cell dysfunction, vascular nonperfusion, and/or ischemia stimulate the development of retinal neovascularization. Progressive growth of abnormal vessels may lead to vitreous hemorrhage, preretinal hemorrhage, and iris neo-

vascularization. Neovascular glaucoma is painful and arises as neovascular iris vessels block aqueous outflow. Contraction of fibrovascular proliferation may lead to retinal tears, vitreous hemorrhage, and traction retinal detachment.

It has long been appreciated that vascular permeability is increased in diabetic retinopathy.[5-7] In early NPDR, hyperpermeability arises primarily from well-defined microaneurysms and results in focal areas of edema. Capillary fenestration and gaps in the vascular wall allow egress of serum, serum proteins, lipoproteins, and cellular components of peripheral blood. Macular edema is defined as retinal edema involving or threatening the macula. Distortion of normal macular architecture results in visual symptoms of blurring. Moderate leakage is often accompanied by the presence of yellow-white intraretinal deposits – hard exudates. Exudate results from precipitation of soluble lipoproteins at the junction of edematous and nonedematous retina. This is discussed further in Chapter 67.

The prevalence of diabetic retinopathy varies widely depending on the population studied, but data from about 20 years ago indicate that nonproliferative stages of the retinopathy were almost universal after 20 years of diabetes, and PDR affected about half of the people with type 1 diabetes after 30 years' duration.[8] More recent assessments suggest that this may be changing.[9] The retinopathies of type 1 and type 2 diabetes are fundamentally similar (Box 65.1).[10]

Studies have shown that familial predispositions to diabetic retinopathy can be detected,[11] and there has been appreciable effort to identify the genetic component.[12-14] Current knowledge on the genetics of diabetic retinopathy has come from family studies, population studies, or studies using candidate genes focused primarily on genes related to vascular complications. There are problems with many of the studies reported, however, because many use small sample sizes that are often limited to specific ethnic groups, or have detected only weak associations.

Current means of inhibiting development or progression of diabetic retinopathy

Clinical studies of diabetic retinopathy have primarily focused on sequelae of vascular lesions (microaneurysms,

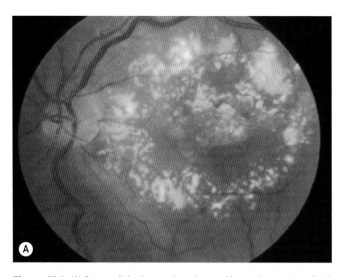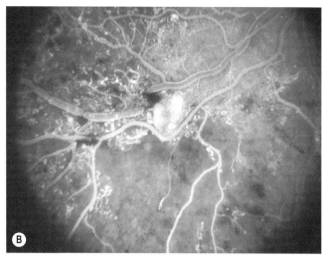

Figure 65.1 (A) Severe diabetic macular edema with massive circinate lipid accumulation in neural retina. (B) Severe capillary nonperfusion, retina ischemia, and early retinal neovascularization.

Box 65.1 Retinopathy in type 1 and type 2 diabetes

- Diabetic retinopathy seems not to be different in type 1 and type 2 diabetes
- The severity of lesions seems directly related to the severity of hyperglycemia, but the type of lesions that develop are not different between type 1 and type 2 diabetes

Table 65.1 Therapies and their effects on diabetic retinopathy in patients

Therapy	Effect of therapy	Reference
Insulin	Significant inhibition of capillary lesions	25
Laser photocoagulation	Significant inhibition of retinopathy progression	164
Aldose reductase inhibitor	No beneficial effect	165
Aspirin	No beneficial effect	166
Protein kinase C inhibitor	Preserved vision, but no effect on vascular lesions	167,168
Antivascular endothelial growth factor therapy	Significant correction of retinal edema	169–171
Steroids	Significant correction of retinal edema	172–174
Calcium dobesilate	Corrected permeability defect	175
Fibrates	Reduced need for retinal photocoagulation	47
Blood pressure medication	Inhibition of retinopathy progression	42,43

capillary nonperfusion, vascular leakage, and hemorrhage) to date (Table 65.1), although attention has also been paid to function of the neural retina.[15–24] There have been fewer attempts to inhibit the retinopathy in diabetic patients than there have been in diabetic animals, undoubtedly due to the long durations and significant costs required to demonstrate any effect, and those attempts have been far less successful compared to the animal studies (described below). Pharmacologic studies of histopathology lasting about 3 years or less have not been successful (whether this is due to a faulty hypothesis or insufficient study duration is not clear) to date. The Diabetes Control and Complications Trial (DCCT) did demonstrate efficacy of insulin therapy on development or progression of histopathology after about 5 years,[25] suggesting that 5 or more years may be required for an objective test of drug therapies in clinical studies for these parameters. Effects on retinal edema (secondary to vascular leakage) and retinal function have required lesser durations of study.

Advanced retinopathy can currently be treated by laser photocoagulation or intravitreal steroids. Panretinal (scatter) photocoagulation, which is performed using a relatively high-energy laser, ablates relatively large areas of retina, presumably to reduce the hypoxia of the remaining retina. It results in a decrease in the formation of proliferative vessels, intravitreal hemorrhage, and retinal detachment, and can significantly reduce the risk for severe vision loss.[26] Focal/grid laser photocoagulation to the retina can reduce the risk of loss of vision by nearly 50% in patients with clinically significant diabetic macular edema.[27–29] Intravitreal steroids likewise are having dramatic effects on visual impairments

due to macular edema.[30,31] Nevertheless, vision loss continues in some patients, and these approaches do not address the underlying etiology of the retinopathy.

Intensive insulin therapy has been shown to inhibit development of vascular lesions of diabetic retinopathy in patients,[25] dogs,[32,33] and rats transplanted with exogenous islets.[34] DCCT[25] showed that intensive control of blood glucose inhibited the progression of existing retinopathy by 54% in patients with type 1 diabetes. Likewise, both the UK

Prospective Diabetes Study (UKPDS)[35] and the Kumomoto study[36] demonstrated a protective effect of glycemic control on the development of retinopathy in type 2 diabetes. Nevertheless, the DCCT and the follow-up Epidemiology of Diabetes Interventions and Complications (EDIC) studies have shown that instituting tight glycemic control in diabetic patients does not immediately inhibit the progression of retinopathy (Box 65.2). Adverse effects of prior poor glycemic control continue to progress even if hyperglycemia is reduced or eliminated in diabetic patients,[25] in diabetic dogs[33] and rats,[37] and the benefits of good control persist even if the good glycemic control is not maintained: benefits of a few years of modestly improved glycemic control continued to be apparent for the decade after the glycemic control was relaxed.[38] This phenomenon, commonly referred to as "metabolic memory," has also been observed in diabetic dogs and rats.[33,39,40] The molecular basis of this memory is not yet known, but it is initiated early in the course of diabetes. Apparently, the level of glycemia results in a long-term imprinting on the cell.

Studies have also demonstrated that blood pressure medications, notably ß-blockers and inhibitors of angiotensin-converting enzyme, slow the development of capillary degeneration in diabetic animals,[41] and the progression of advanced stages of diabetic retinopathy in diabetic patients.[42,43] In the UKPDS[43,44] type 2 diabetics allocated to tight control of blood pressure had a 34% reduction in risk in the proportion of patients with deterioration of diabetic retinopathy by two steps, and a 47% reduced risk of deterioration in visual acuity. Likewise, lipid levels have been shown to influence the development or progression of the retinopathy in diabetic animals.[45,46] Lipid-lowering therapy using fenofibrate reduced the need for laser treatment for diabetic retinopathy,[47] although the mechanism of this effect was not regarded as secondary to plasma concentrations of lipids.

Pathology

Histologically, vascular lesions in the early stages of diabetic retinopathy in humans and animals are characterized by the presence of saccular capillary microaneurysms, pericyte-deficient capillaries, and obliterated and degenerate capillaries. These degenerate capillaries are not perfused,[2,3] and so increases in their frequency represent reductions in retinal perfusion. Capillary occlusion and degeneration initially occur in single, isolated capillaries, and have no clinical importance when only few capillaries have become nonperfused. As more and more capillaries become occluded, however, retinal perfusion likely decreases, at least locally (Figure 65.2). No one of these lesions is totally specific for diabetic retinopathy, but in combination, they are quite unique.

The clinically demonstrable changes to the retinal vasculature in diabetes have led to the general assumption that the retinopathy is solely a microvascular disease. Nevertheless, diabetes can also damage nonvascular cells of the retina, resulting in alterations in function,[23,24,46,48–50] loss of ganglion cells, horizontal cells, amacrine cells, and photoreceptors,[20,51–62] and activation[52,54,56–58,63–68] or death of Müller glial cells in some,[52,59] but not all, studies.[16,66,69,70] Findings in diabetic mice have not necessarily been in agreement with findings in rats.[57,60,68,71,72] These important topics exceed the breadth of the present review, and are covered elsewhere.

Box 65.2 "Inertia" of diabetic retinopathy

- Diabetic retinopathy develops slowly, and resists arrest after the process has begun
- "Metabolic memory" describes a poorly understood process by which cells are changed as a function of their previous exposure to hyperglycemia. In the Diabetes Control and Complications Trial/Epidemiology of Diabetes Interventions and Complications trial, beneficial effects of previous good glycemic control are maintained for many years (even if glycemia is no longer as good), but, likewise, adverse effects of previous poor glycemic control continue even after re-establishing relatively normal glycemia

---

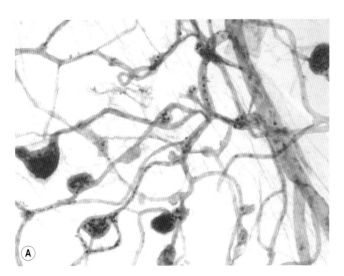

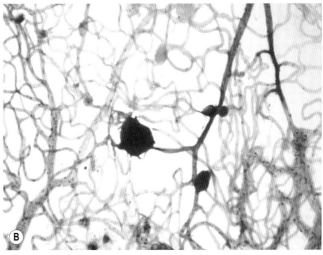

Figure 65.2   Isolated retinal vasculature from two diabetic patients. Both photomicrographs show capillary microaneurysms and capillary degeneration, and the photo on the right shows foci of degenerate capillaries (center) and also dilated, hypercellular capillaries (bottom right).

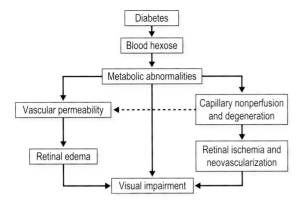

Figure 65.3 Schematic summarizing the postulated pathogenesis of diabetic retinopathy.

Pathophysiology

Diabetic retinopathy is an important cause of visual impairment in diabetes, but the pathogenesis of the condition remains unclear. A current working model of diabetic retinopathy is that the clinically significant (proliferative) phase of the retinopathy is a direct consequence of earlier changes, especially increased leakage and degeneration of retinal capillaries (Figure 65.3). Efforts to inhibit the development of the early stages of diabetic retinopathy have focused to a great extent on histologic endpoints (degeneration of retinal capillaries and neurons), and these studies have provided considerable insight into the pathogenesis of the retinopathy. Table 65.2 summarizes a number of therapies reported to inhibit retinal vascular histopathology in diabetes, grouped by their presumed mode of action. Most of the research focus to date has been on the role of hyperglycemia and its sequelae in the pathogenesis of the retinopathy. Also, most of these studies have been conducted in rodents, and accordingly, the histologic parameters of diabetic retinopathy that develop in those species (degeneration of retinal capillaries and pericyte loss) are the endpoints for most of these studies.

Other biochemical or metabolic abnormalities, including impaired insulin signaling,[55,73,74] have been postulated to contribute to the retinopathy, but effects of correcting these abnormalities have not been demonstrated histologically to date.

Hyperglycemia is strongly associated with development of diabetic retinopathy, and this has been strongly supported by clinical and animal studies showing that reduction in the severity of hyperglycemia significantly inhibited development of the retinopathy.[25,32,35] Nevertheless, this evidence does not prove that hyperglycemia per se is the critical abnormality, because intensive insulin therapy can normalize defects also related to lipids and proteins in diabetes. The strongest evidence that hyperglycemia is sufficient to initiate the vascular lesions of diabetic retinopathy is the evidence that lesions that are morphologically identical to those of diabetic retinopathy also develop in nondiabetic animals made experimentally hyperglycemic by feeding a galactose-rich diet.[75-80]

Although one would assume that all vascular cells should be exposed to the same concentration of blood glucose in a given individual, there is unexplained regional variability in susceptibility to diabetes-induced microvascular disease even within the same retina. Microaneurysms and acellular capillaries have been found to develop in a nonuniform distribution even within the same retina in diabetic patients[81-84] and in experimentally diabetic or galactosemic dogs.[85] In both species, lesions were most common in the superior and temporal portions of the retina. Likewise, neovascularization in diabetic patients has been noted to be more common in the superior and temporal portions of the retina than in other regions.[86]

Diabetic retinopathy is not made up of a single lesion (Box 65.3). It is a spectrum of abnormalities, none of which is totally unique to diabetic retinopathy, but which in combination offer a clinical picture that is relatively unique to diabetes. Whether or not these individual lesions share a common pathogenesis or differ in aspects remains to be determined. Thus, the individual lesions of early diabetic vascular disease in the retina are discussed individually below.

Capillary nonperfusion and degeneration

In its simplest form, mechanisms postulated to contribute to the nonperfusion and degeneration of retinal capillaries in diabetes include abnormalities that have developed within the vascular cells themselves (intrinsic abnormality) and those which have developed outside the vascular cells, but then stimulate a change in the cells of the retinal vasculature. These mechanisms, some of which are listed below, are not mutually exclusive.

Capillary cell death caused by metabolic abnormalities within capillary cells

Metabolic sequelae of hyperglycemia that may damage the vasculature have been the most extensively studied mechanism for development of diabetic retinopathy. Numerous of these postulated metabolic abnormalities are summarized below. Initiator and effector caspases have been found to become activated in the vasculature of the retina of diabetic animals or in retinal vascular cells incubated in elevated glucose concentration.[87] A variety of therapies have reduced the number of terminal uridine deoxynucleotidyl transferase dUTP nick end labeling (TUNEL)-positive capillary cells or degenerate capillaries compared to control,[24,41,57,88-98] suggesting that related metabolic abnormalities also contribute to the capillary cell death.

The rate of capillary cell showing evidence of apoptosis (TUNEL-positive at any given moment) is very small com-

Table 65.2 Experimental therapies and their effects on early lesions of diabetic retinopathy in diabetic animals

Presumed action	Therapy	Defect corrected by therapy	Species	Reference
Blood pressure	Captopril	Capillary degeneration	Rat	41
Inflammation	CD-18$^{-/-}$	Capillary degeneration, pericyte loss, permeability	Mouse	93
Inflammation	ICAM-1$^{-/-}$	Capillary degeneration, permeability	Mouse	93
Inflammation	IL-1β receptor$^{-/-}$	Capillary degeneration	Mouse	118
Inflammation	Minocycline	Capillary degeneration, permeability, neurodegeneration	Mouse	118,154
Inflammation	Nepafenac	Capillary degeneration, pericyte loss	Rat	24
Inflammation	PARP inhibitor	Capillary degeneration, pericyte loss	Rat	95
Iinflammation	Salicylates	Capillary degeneration, pericyte loss, neurodegeneration	Rat, dog	96,98,153,155
Metabolic abnormality	sRAGE	Capillary degeneration, retinal function	Mouse	46
Metabolic abnormality	Aldose reductase inhibitor	Capillary degeneration, neurodegeneration	Rat but not dog	57,151,152,156
Metabolic abnormality	Benfotiamine	Capillary degeneration	Rat	157
Metabolic abnormality	Pyridoxamine	Capillary degeneration	Rat	92
Metabolic abnormality, inflammation	Aminoguanidine	Capillary degeneration, pericyte loss	Rat, dog	89,153,158
Metabolic abnormality, inflammation	iNOS$^{-/-}$	Capillary degeneration	Mouse	97
Metabolic abnormality, inflammation	5-Lipoxygenase$^{-/-}$	Capillary degeneration	Mouse	160
Metabolic abnormality	Tenilsetam	Capillary degeneration but not pericyte loss	Rat	161
Oxidative stress	Antioxidants	Capillary degeneration, pericyte loss	Rat	91,94,162
Oxidative stress	Mn superoxide dismutase	Capillary degeneration, pericyte loss	Mouse	163
Oxidative stress, neuroprotection,	Nerve growth factor	Capillary degeneration, neurodegeneration	Rat, mouse	52, Kern, unpublished

ICAM-1, intercellular adhesion molecule 1; IL-1β, interleukin-1β; PARP, poly (ADP-ribose) polymerase; sRAGE, soluble receptor for advanced glycation endproducts; iNOS, inducible isoform of nitric oxide synthase.

pared to the total number of capillary cells. Apoptosis may not be the only form of cell death occurring in diabetic retinopathy. Joussen and coworkers[90,99,100] have reported that only 9 days of diabetes caused an increase in intracellular accumulation of propidium iodide (commonly used as a marker of necrosis) in the retinal vasculature. Thus, focusing solely on apoptotic cell death may underestimate the total number of cells dying at any time. On the other hand, propidium iodide may overestimate necrosis, since it can enter even viable cells having impaired membrane integrity.[101,102]

Capillary cell death due to extrinsic abnormalities
Vaso-occlusion by white blood cells or platelets
Attraction and adhesion of leukocytes to the vascular wall are significantly increased in retinas of diabetic animals,[90,93,100,103–112] and may contribute to the capillary nonperfusion or death of retinal endothelial cells in diabetic retinopathy.[90] Leukocyte stiffness is increased in diabetes (decreased filterability) and contributes to the occlusion of retinal vessels.[104,113] Each instance of occlusion by a blood cell is likely to be short-lived, but cumulative effects of such repeated ischemia/reperfusion injuries over a prolonged

interval are not known. Abnormal leukocyte adherence to retinal vessels in diabetes occurs via adhesion molecules, including intercellular adhesion molecule 1 (ICAM-1). Diabetes increases expression of ICAM-1 in retinas of animals and humans,[95,100,106,114,115] and interaction of this adhesion molecule on retinal endothelia with the CD18 adhesion molecule on monocytes and neutrophils contributes to the diabetes-induced increase in adherence of white blood cells to the vascular wall in retinal vessels.[106] Using in situ perfusion methods, changes consistent with capillary occlusion secondary to leukostasis have been observed in occasional retinal vessels. Diabetic mice lacking ICAM-1 and CD18 are protected from development of diabetes-induced increase in leukostasis, vascular permeability, and degeneration of retinal capillaries.[93] Whether the development of the retinal disease in diabetes results from ICAM-1-mediated capillary occlusion or some other mechanism, however, has not been explored.

Increased platelet aggregation has also been postulated to contribute to capillary nonperfusion in diabetes. Platelet microthrombi are present in the retinas of diabetic rats and humans, and have been spatially associated with apoptotic endothelial cells.[116,117] Nevertheless, the selective antiplatelet drug clopidogrel did not prevent neuronal apoptosis, glial reactivity, capillary cell apoptosis, or degeneration of retinal capillaries in diabetic rats,[96] suggesting that platelet aggregation does not play a critical role in the development of the vascular lesions of early diabetic retinopathy.

Abnormalities initiated by binding to extracellular receptors

In addition to physical obstruction of capillaries by nonvascular cells, binding of external stimuli such as advanced glycation endproducts (AGEs) or cytokines (such as interleukin (IL)-1ß) to extracellular receptors on vascular cells may damage or kill those cells. Interfering with signaling from the receptor for advanced glycation endproducts (RAGE) or the IL-1ß receptor has been found to inhibit diabetes-induced degeneration of retinal capillaries in diabetic mice,[46,118] demonstrating their role in the pathogenesis of the capillary degeneration.

Contribution of outer retina to degeneration of retinal capillaries in diabetes

The outer retina has also been implicated as a source of an unidentified extrinsic abnormality that contributes to diabetes-induced degeneration of retinal capillaries. Since photoreceptors are a major consumer of oxygen in the retina, it was postulated that photoreceptors may deprive a marginally oxygenated retina of needed oxygen or other products. This hypothesis was tested in mice having photoreceptor degeneration (rhodopsin knockout mice) that were made experimentally diabetic.[119] Hypoxia-specific immunostain increased in the retina of wild-type diabetic animals compared to that in nondiabetic controls, but this diabetes-induced change was absent in the diabetic animals having retinal degeneration. As expected, vascular density was subnormal in diabetic wild-type controls, but, remarkably, this capillary degeneration did not develop in the diabetics lacking photoreceptors. Thus, loss of the outer retina seems to reduce the severity of diabetes-induced degeneration of retinal capillaries, possibly via less consumption of oxygen.

Postulated effect of retinal neurodegeneration on capillary degeneration in diabetes

Retinal neuroglial cells have been observed to begin to degenerate in diabetic rats after only about 1 month of diabetes.[53] This is considerably before capillary degeneration has been detected, and consequently it was postulated that the neurodegeneration may play some role in the later development of capillary degeneration. Data to support this postulate are still only speculative, and evidence that topical nepafenac inhibited the diabetes-induced degeneration of retinal capillaries without any beneficial effect on neurodegeneration[24] does not support this hypothesis.

Invasion of retinal vessels by processes from glial cells

Cellular processes from retinal glial cells have been found inside occasional degenerate capillaries (identified from the basement membrane tube that surrounds vessels)[120-122] (Figure 65.4). It is not clear whether this glial invasion precedes and causes the capillary to degenerate, or is a result of the capillary cells dying (glial cells filling empty spaces in tissues).

Several gaps exist in our knowledge of capillary degeneration and its significance. Specifically, does capillary degeneration cause subretinal oxygenation or ischemia of retina in diabetes? Does neurodegeneration develop especially in areas having a compromised vasculature? How does the outer retina contribute to capillary degeneration in diabetes? Does neurodegeneration contribute to capillary degeneration in diabetic retinopathy?

Capillary permeability

Breakdown of the blood–retinal barrier in diabetes, resulting in increased vascular permeability, has been attributed to increases in leukostasis, cytokines, and growth factors, to

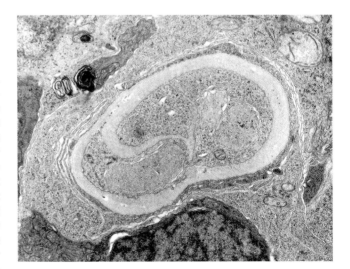

Figure 65.4 Degenerate retinal capillary is filled with processes of glial cells. Endothelial cells and pericytes are no longer present, but the basement membrane that remains clearly indicates that this was previously a functional capillary. This obliterated capillary (from a diabetic dog) is from the outer retina, indicating that these glial processes are from Müller cells. × 29 100.

name a few causes.[90,123–126] Molecular alterations, such as in proteins of the tight junction complex, have also been demonstrated to play a significant role in the diabetes-induced increase in capillary permeability.[127] Controversy remains as to how fast the permeability defect develops in retinas of diabetic rodents, with reports ranging from 8 days to more than 6 months after onset of diabetes.[100,125–132] Permeability was also increased in dogs diabetic for several years.[133] A number of therapies have been found to inhibit the diabetes-induced increase in vascular permeability within the retina, including aldose reductase inhibitors, protein kinase C inhibitors, tyrosine kinase inhibitors, aspirin, a cyclooxygenase-2 inhibitor, steroids, vascular endothelial growth factor (VEGF) antagonist, tumor necrosis factor-α receptor antagonists, and peroxisome proliferator-activated receptors (PPAR) gamma ligands.[100,112,129,130,134–144]

Microaneurysms

Microaneurysms, or dot hemorrhages, are detectable ophthalmoscopically, and the presence and number of microaneurysms have strong predictive value with respect to progression of the retinopathy.[145,146]

The capillary outpouchings have been identified as being predominantly around areas of occluded capillaries. Minute red-color lesions typically measuring 10–100 μm in diameter are located primarily in the posterior pole in early disease but may become widespread with disease duration and severity. Focal damage results in alveolar bulging of the capillary wall and loss of endothelial cell tight junction integrity. Areas of capillary leakage frequently have a microaneurysm at the center, suggesting that they leak more than other adjacent areas. Despite being one of the strongest predictors of progression of diabetic retinopathy, we know very little about the pathogenesis of microaneurysm in diabetes, the extent to which they contribute visual complications of diabetes, and the basis for their prognostic power.

As suggested by Ashton[147] and consistent with findings of Aguilar et al,[148] microaneurysms may be aborted attempts at neovascularization due to focal retinal ischemia. Since pericytes have been demonstrated to inhibit endothelial proliferation,[149] and microaneurysms have been regarded as relatively free of pericytes, it was postulated that microaneurysm formation may result from loss of endothelial growth suppression following pericyte loss.[150]

Why numerous therapies seem to inhibit the early stages of diabetic retinopathy in animals, but seem less effective in diabetic humans is an important question. Many of the pharmacologic approaches studied in animal models have not been studied also in patients, but when similar drug

types have been studied in both humans and animals, the animal data have both agreed[32,33,41,151] and disagreed[98,152,153] with results obtained in human trials. It is possible that the pathogenesis of the lesions is different in animals than in humans, but evidence that such differences play a critical role in the development of retinopathy is lacking. Other differences stand out, however. In hindsight, many studies of diabetic retinopathy in humans have been conducted for too short a duration, started too late (when appreciable retinopathy is already present), and using undesirably low levels of drug. In addition, the endpoints of human and animals studies are not usually the same: color fundus photography (the main method used for quantitation of retinopathy in human clinical trials) is far less able to demonstrate capillary degeneration than the high-resolution, microscope-based techniques to analyze the isolated retinal vasculature routinely used in animal studies.

Proliferative diabetic retinopathy

Neovascularization is a major contributor to visual dysfunction in diabetes, and accordingly has been a major therapeutic target in recent years. Success is being achieved using laser photocoagulation, and more recently using anti-VEGF therapies. These approaches are described in Chapter 66.

Conclusions and summary

We have learned much about the pathogenesis and how to treat diabetic retinopathy. Vascular abnormalities are still believed by many to account for most of the clinically meaningful visual consequences of diabetes, but the possible contribution of changes in the neural retina continues to be explored. Attention rightfully has focused on inhibiting clinical meaningful causes of visual impairment, such as neovascularization and retinal edema, but focusing on the later stages of the disease means that retinal vascular damage will have already occurred. Success is now being made also in the earlier stages of the retinopathy, with hopes that inhibiting the early damage (such as capillary degeneration) will inhibit development of the more advanced stages of the retinopathy. Unexplained observations about the retinopathy, however, demonstrate that there is still a considerable amount to learn about the retinal disease. Studies to date have offered statistical insight on efficacy of a given therapy towards a given population of patients or animals, but these studies offer little insight as to how an individual patient will respond to a given therapy.

Key references

A complete list of chapter references is available online at www.expertconsult.com. See inside cover for registration details.

11. Diabetes Control and Complications Trial Research Group. Clustering of long-term complications in families with diabetes in the diabetes control and complications trial. The Diabetes Control and Complications Trial Research Group. Diabetes 1997;46: 1829–1839.

25. Diabetes Control and Complications Trial Research Group. The effect of intensive treatment of diabetes on the development of long-term

complications in insulin-dependent diabetes mellitus. N Engl J Med 1993;329:977–986.

53. Barber AJ, Lieth E, Khin SA, et al. Neural apoptosis in the retina during experimental and human diabetes. Early onset and effect of insulin. J Clin Invest 1998;102:783–791.

70. Bresnick GM, Palta M. Predicting progression of severe proliferative diabetic retinopathy. Arch Ophthalmol 1987;105:810–814.

75. Engerman RL, Kern TS. Experimental galactosemia produces diabetic-like retinopathy. Diabetes 1984;33:97–100.

83. Niki T, Muraoka K, Shimizu K. Distribution of capillary nonperfusion in early-stage diabetic retinopathy. Ophthalmology 1984;91:1431–1439.

88. Mizutani M, Kern TS, Lorenzi M. Accelerated death of retinal microvascular cells in human and experimental diabetic retinopathy. J Clin Invest 1996;97:2883–2890.

93. Joussen AM, Poulaki V, Le ML, et al. A central role for inflammation in the pathogenesis of diabetic retinopathy. Faseb J 2004;18:1450–1452.

133. Wallow IH, Engerman RL. Permeability and patency of retinal blood vessels in experimental diabetes. Invest Ophthalmol 1977;16:447–461.

165. Sorbinil Retinopathy Trial Research Group. A randomized trial of sorbinil, an aldose reductase inhibitor, in diabetic retinopathy. Arch Ophthalmol 1990;108:1234–1244.

168. Effect of ruboxistaurin in patients with diabetic macular edema: thirty-month results of the randomized PKC-DMES clinical trial. Arch Ophthalmol 2007; 125:318–324.

CHAPTER 66

Neovascularization in diabetic retinopathy

Corey B Westerfeld and Joan W Miller

Clinical background

Introduction

Diabetes mellitus is a metabolic disorder caused by defects in insulin secretion (type 1), insulin action (type 2), or both. It is characterized by chronic hyperglycemia which ultimately may result in dysfunction and damage to various organ systems, including the brain, kidneys, eyes, and peripheral nerves. Diabetic retinopathy may be broadly classified in terms of the presence or absence of retinal neovascularization. The term nonproliferative diabetic retinopathy (NPDR) is used to describe intraretinal microvascular changes that occur in the early stages of diabetic retinopathy. The etiology and pathogenesis of NPDR are discussed in Chapters 65 and 67. Proliferative diabetic retinopathy (PDR) is used to indicate the presence of newly formed vessels, fibrosis, or both, arising from the retina or optic disc and extending along the inner retinal surface and/or into the vitreous cavity. PDR may be characterized by neovascularization of the iris (NVI) as well. The focus of this chapter will be on the proliferative changes seen in these advanced stages of diabetic retinopathy.

Epidemiology

Diabetic retinopathy is the leading cause of new cases of blindness in people aged 20–74 years in the USA.[1] The incidence of diabetic retinopathy increases with the duration of diabetes mellitus, and it is found in the vast majority of patients who have had diabetes for 20 years or more.[2] After 20 years of diabetes, PDR affects about 50% of patients with type 1 diabetes, 5–10% of patients with noninsulin-dependent type 2 diabetes, and 30% of patients with insulin-dependent type 2 diabetes[3] (Box 66.1). In the USA, African Americans and Hispanics have a higher prevalence of diabetes, approximately 25%, compared with 6.2% in the remainder of the population.[4] The major risk factors for progression of diabetic retinopathy are the duration of diabetes mellitus, poor glucose control, high blood pressure, and elevated cholesterol.[2] The Diabetes Control and Complications Trial (DCCT) and the UK Prospective Diabetes Study (UKPDS) have demonstrated the efficacy of intensive glucose control in reducing the incidence and progression of diabetic retin-

opathy.[5,6] However, results of these studies have also confirmed the difficulty of achieving and maintaining appropriate glycemic control over a long period. As such, recent attention has been given towards further elucidating the pathogenesis of diabetic retinopathy in an attempt to develop better, more targeted therapies for this prevalent and visually disabling condition.

Clinical features

Diabetic retinopathy is characterized by the appearance of microaneurysms, increased vascular permeability, occlusion of capillaries, and formation of new, abnormal vessels.[7] There are two primary pathological features in diabetic retinopathy responsible for vision loss: diabetic macular edema (DME) and retinal neovascularization. DME is the most common cause of vision loss in diabetes and is generally associated with other nonproliferative changes.[8] NPDR is characterized by microaneurysms, small "dot and blot" hemorrhages, "flame" hemorrhages, intraretinal microvascular abnormalities, and "cottonwool" spots. Later stages of diabetic retinopathy are characterized by the formation of new vessels on the optic nerve or in the retina which may extend along the surface of the retina and/or into the vitreous cavity. These proliferative changes occur as a programmed response to ischemia in the inner retina in an effort to improve tissue oxygenation. However, the new vessels are weak and may break, resulting in vitreous hemorrhage. Furthermore, the combination of neovascularization, fibrous tissue proliferation, and recurrent vitreous hemorrhage may lead to tractional retinal detachment (Box 66.2).

Etiology

The development of diabetic retinopathy is primarily related to the duration of diabetes, severity of hyperglycemia, and the existence of contributing factors such as hypertension and hyperlipidemia.[2] Hyperglycemia is the primary pathogenic factor in the development of diabetic retinopathy.[2,5] However, diabetic retinopathy may occur at higher rates in some patient groups in spite of relatively good glucose control and vice versa, suggesting that there are other contributing factors.

Genetics

Siblings of individuals with diabetic retinopathy have a higher risk of developing diabetic retinopathy themselves. This risk is in addition to the baseline risk of diabetes and is greater than the expected rate of diabetic retinopathy, indicating that there is a genetic component.[9] A variety of candidate genes have been investigated in diabetic patients and animal models, but large studies have not yet proven any direct correlation with diabetic retinopathy. The development of diabetic retinopathy is multifactorial, and as such, relevant genetic factors are probably modulated by many environmental factors as well. Recent studies have shown that polymorphisms in genes coding for intracellular adhesion molecule-1 (ICAM-1) and transforming growth factor-β are risk factors for diabetic retinopathy.[10,11] The authors propose that mutations result in leukocyte activation and adhesion to the retinal vascular endothelium, leading to the development of vascular leakage and capillary closure. Larger studies are needed to evaluate further these and other possible genetic components of diabetic retinopathy.

Box 66.1 Epidemiology

- Diabetic retinopathy is the leading cause of new cases of blindness in persons aged 20–74 in the USA
- Incidence of diabetic retinopathy increases with duration of disease
- After 20 years of diabetes, proliferative diabetic retinopathy affects:
  - 50% of type 1 diabetes
  - 5–10% of noninsulin-dependent type 2 diabetes
  - 30% of insulin-dependent type 2 diabetes

Box 66.2 Clinical features

Nonproliferative diabetic retinopathy

- Microaneurysms
- Dot-blot hemorrhages, flame hemorrhages, intraretinal microvascular abnormalities
- Cottonwool spots

Proliferative diabetic retinopathy

- Neovascularization on the optic nerve, retina, iris
- Vitreous hemorrhage
- Traction retinal detachment

Pathology

The earliest histologic change in diabetic retinopathy is the loss of pericytes. Pericytes line the retinal vascular endothelium and provide structural support to the retinal vasculature. Loss of pericytes leads to progressive dilation of capillaries and the formation of microaneurysms. A complete discussion of the classic histologic features of NPDR can be found in Chapter 65. PDR is characterized by the formation of new vessels which are evident histologically as thin-walled vessels devoid of pericytes.

Pathophysiology

Pathologic mechanisms in diabetic retinopathy

Several biochemical mechanisms may be responsible for the progression of diabetic retinopathy (Figure 66.1). Hyperglycemia causes the formation of reactive oxygen intermediates (ROIs) and advanced glycation endproducts (AGEs). ROIs and AGEs may cause direct damage to pericytes and vascular endothelial cells and also stimulate the release of vasoactive factors.[12] Chronic hyperglycemia also causes activation of the polyol pathway leading to increased glycosylation of cell membranes and extracellular matrix as well as the accumulation of sorbitol by increased aldose reductase expression.[13] Glycosylation and sorbitol accumulation cause further vascular endothelial damage and dysfunction of endothelial enzymes.[14] It is likely that activation of these pathways in association with vascular damage produces inflammation which further exacerbates the condition. Hyperglycemia may also impair autoregulation of retinal blood flow causing perfusion-related damage to endothelial cells.[15] The ultimate effects of glucose toxicity on pericytes and endothelial cells cause impaired circulation, hypoxia, inflammation, and further activation of angiogenic stimuli. Finally, hyperglycemia also causes activation of the protein kinase C (PKC) intracellular signaling pathway.[16] PKC influences progression of diabetic retinopathy in two ways. First, it directly promotes the activation of VEGF and other growth factors.[7] Second, binding of VEGF to its target receptors requires the presence of the PKC signaling protein.[17] Clinical trials investigating PKC inhibitors have demonstrated efficacy in the treatment of NPDR and further studies are ongoing.[18]

Production of vasoactive factors

The combined effects of these pathways lead to the production of vasoactive factors such as vascular endothelial growth factor (VEGF), nitric oxide, prostacyclin, insulin-like growth

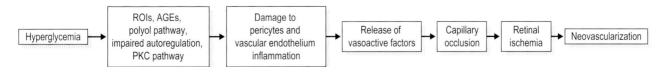

Figure 66.1 Pathologic mechanisms in proliferative diabetic retinopathy. ROIs, reactive oxygen intermediates; AGEs, advanced glycation endproducts; PKC, protein kinase C.

factor (IGF)-1, and endothelin (ET). These vasoactive factors act in concert with hyperglycemia to produce dysfunction of pericytes and vascular endothelial cells. One mechanism by which this occurs is via VEGF stimulation of ICAM-1 expression in the retinal vasculature. ICAM-1 promotes leukocyte binding to the vascular endothelium which triggers a Fas/Fas ligand-mediated endothelial cell death and breakdown of the blood–retinal barrier.[19] The culmination of these events leads to thrombosis and closure of retinal capillaries. Occlusion of capillaries gives rise to focal retinal ischemia and hypoxia. Local hypoxia induces further overexpression of angiogenic stimuli. In response, new vessels begin to form. However, the new vessels have reduced structural integrity including a fragile basement membrane, deficient tight junctions between endothelial cells, and lack of pericytes.[20] The walls of the vessels are porous, allowing leakage of plasma proteins and even hemorrhage into the retina or vitreous.

Advanced PDR

In advanced PDR, the new vessels are accompanied by fibrous tissue and grow from the retinal surface into the vitreous cavity to form fibrovascular membranes. Several studies have demonstrated that the vitreous plays a role in the pathogenesis of PDR.[21] Hyperglycemia causes changes in type 2 collagen in the vitreous, leading to liquefaction and vitreous syneresis.[22] Additionally, hypoxia and resultant abundance of growth factors lead to a thickening of the posterior vitreous cortex.[23] The resulting vitreous instability due to loss of the gel state without dehiscence at the vitreoretinal interface may induce retinal traction. Such traction may not only lead to retinal tears but may also contribute to the neovascular process. In support of this theory, the development of PDR is rare if the vitreous has detached completely, presumably since the scaffold for proliferating cells is removed.[24] Liberated serum proteins such as fibronectin accumulate at the junction of attached retina and vitreous[25] and mediate the migration and adhesion of proliferating endothelial cells.[26] In later stages of PDR, contraction of the posterior hyaloid causes rupture of proliferating vessels, vitreous hemorrhage, and traction and/or rhegmatogenous retinal detachment.

Iris neovascularization

NVI may also occur in PDR. The stimulus for the formation of NVI is the release of vasoactive factors by ischemic retina. The most common causes of NVI are central retinal vein occlusion, diabetes, and ocular ischemic syndrome. Angiogenic factors such as VEGF diffuse anteriorly into the aqueous and stimulate growth of new vessels.[27] The new vessels begin as capillary buds at the inner circle of the iris and then extend radially forming a fine vascular network.[28] The vessels may cross the trabecular meshwork of the angle and block aqueous outflow causing neovascular glaucoma.

Angiogenic factors in proliferative diabetic retinopathy

Angiogenesis is regulated by the counterbalancing of angiogenic stimulators and angiogenic inhibitors (Figure 66.2).

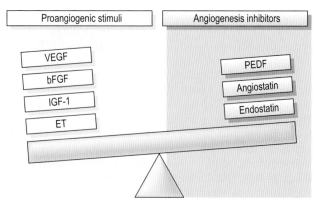

Figure 66.2 Angiogenic factors in proliferative diabetic retinopathy. VEGF, vascular endothelial growth factor; bFGF, basic fibroblast growth factor, IGF-1, insulin-like growth factor-1; ET, endothelin; PEDF, pigment epithelium-derived factor.

> **Box 66.3 Vascular endothelial growth factor**
>
> - Induced by hypoxia
> - Stimulates vascular proliferation
> - Increases vascular permeability
> - Elevated in diabetic retinopathy (proliferative diabetic retinopathy > nonproliferative diabetic retinopathy)

In the normal adult retina, angiogenic inhibitors predominate, maintaining relative quiescence of the retinal vasculature. In pathologic conditions such as diabetic retinopathy, the balance swings in favor of proangiogenic stimuli leading to the development of retinal neovascularization. Proangiogenic factors include VEGF, basic fibroblast growth factor (bFGF), IGF-1, and ET, all of which have been implicated in diabetic retinopathy.[29] Alternatively, decreased levels of angiogenic inhibitors, such as pigment epithelium-derived factor (PEDF), angiostatin, and endostatin, likely contribute to the formation of new vessels in diabetic retinopathy. Angiogenic factors and angiogenic inhibitors are discussed further in Chapter 70.

Vascular endothelial growth factor

VEGF is possibly the most important biochemical agent in the development of PDR. VEGF is produced by numerous retinal cells and is induced by hypoxia (Box 66.3). VEGF acts to produce both vascular proliferation and increased vascular permeability.[30] Studies have confirmed that VEGF levels are increased in the retina and vitreous in patients with diabetic retinopathy.[31] Furthermore, as expected, VEGF levels are higher in patients with PDR than with NPDR.[32] Laser photocoagulation has been associated with a 75% decrease in VEGF levels in patients with PDR, suggesting that the formation and regression of new vessels are correlated with VEGF levels.[31] Elevated VEGF levels have been confirmed in animal models of diabetic retinopathy as well. In the oxygen-induced retinopathy model, retinal VEGF levels are elevated and correlate with progression of retinal neovascularization.[33] In a primate model, induction of retinal ischemia via laser occlusion of retinal veins resulted in increased levels of VEGF in the aqueous and was associated with NVI.[34] Furthermore, intravitreal injection of VEGF in monkeys has been shown to induce the development of NVI and neovascular glaucoma, similar to that seen in humans with advanced PDR.[35]

Pigment epithelium-derived factor

PEDF inhibits endothelial cell proliferation and migration and to date appears to be the most potent endogenous angiogenic inhibitor in the eye.[36] PEDF levels are decreased by hypoxia. Animal studies have demonstrated that decreased levels of PEDF are associated with the development of retinal neovascularization,[33] and laser photocoagulation produces increased levels of PEDF.[37] In humans, PEDF levels in the vitreous have been found to be significantly lower in patients with PDR as compared to individuals without diabetes.[38] Also, lower levels of PEDF have been found to be predictive of progression of diabetic retinopathy.[39] These studies demonstrate that PEDF likely plays a significant role in the pathogenesis of PDR. Ongoing studies are examining the potential utility of exogenous PEDF in the treatment of neovascular disease.

Endostatin

Endostatin also acts to inhibit proliferation of vascular endothelial cells. Patients with diabetic retinopathy have been demonstrated to have decreased levels of endostatin in the aqueous and vitreous.[40] Lower levels of endostatin have been found to be predictive of a higher risk of progression of PDR after vitreous surgery as compared to patients with high endostatin levels.[41] Recent animal studies using adenoviral vectors for delivery of endostatin into the eye have demonstrated reduction and/or inhibition of neovascularization.[42] Ongoing studies will further evaluate the potential uses for endostatin in the treatment of neovascular disease.

Treatment

Treatment for early stages of diabetic retinopathy has been covered in previous chapters. The gold standard of treatment for PDR is panretinal photocoagulation (PRP). The utility of PRP was demonstrated in the Diabetic Retinopathy Study which determined that PRP for high-risk PDR, defined as neovascularization of the disc greater than one-third disc diameters, neovascularization elsewhere plus vitreous hemorrhage, or any neovascularization of the disc plus vitreous hemorrhage, reduces the risk of severe vision loss by 50%.[43] The role of vitrectomy in the management of PDR was first evaluated by the Diabetic Retinopathy Vitrectomy Study (DRVS).[44] The study proved a role for vitrectomy in the management of vitreous hemorrhage in individuals with type 1 diabetes or in all cases if there is significant fibrovascular proliferation and/or incomplete PRP. Vitreoretinal surgical techniques advanced rapidly immediately after the DRVS, and with even more recent progress, most surgeons currently maintain much broader indications for surgery. Vitrectomy will be considered in all cases of nonclearing vitreous hemorrhage persisting longer than 3 months,

---

Box 66.4 Treatment considerations

- Laser photocoagulation
- Vitrectomy
- Needs further study:
  - Antivascular endothelial growth factor agents
  - Aldose reductase inhibitors
  - Protein kinase C inhibitors
  - Antioxidants

---

tractional retinal detachment, and select cases of cystoid macular edema.

Recent research has focused on developing therapeutic modalities which target the biochemical alterations which precipitate diabetic retinopathy (Box 66.4). These new agents, including aldose reductase inhibitors, PKC inhibitors, and antioxidants have the potential to prevent the biochemical sequela of hyperglycemia. Furthermore, angiogenesis inhibitors appear to have a role in the treatment of diabetic retinopathy. Although no angiogenesis inhibitor is yet approved for the treatment of diabetic retinopathy, many agents are currently in clinical trials. Several nonrandomized trials have demonstrated a role for anti-VEGF agents in the management of both DME and PDR, and these agents are being used off-label in select cases. See Chapter 65 for a discussion of the uses of these agents with respect to DME. Specific to PDR, anti-VEGF agents have been used as a preoperative adjunct to vitrectomy for vitreous hemorrhage and appear to facilitate surgery and reduce the rate of intraoperative and postoperative hemorrhage.[45] Anti-VEGF agents may also obviate the need for vitrectomy in PDR with vitreous hemorrhage by inducing closure of active vessels and clearance of hemorrhage, and allowing PRP to be performed.[46] Furthermore, anti-VEGF agents cause quicker regression of active vessels when compared to PRP.[47] Expedient resolution of vessels has shown particular importance in the management of neovascular glaucoma. One study demonstrated complete resolution of NVI in 82% of treated cases, and all cases showed decreased leakage on fluorescein within 24 hours of injection.[48]

Conclusions

The role of hyperglycemia in the pathogenesis of diabetic retinopathy has been well described. However, the underlying biochemical mechanisms which precipitate this visually devastating disease are complex. Recent studies have revealed that an altered balance between angiogenic stimuli and inhibitors contributes to the development of diabetic retinopathy. Laser photocoagulation, although beneficial, is most useful only in the late stages of disease, after irreversible pathology has already occurred. Similarly, surgery is primarily useful in the treatment of late complications of disease. Research investigating the mechanisms of diabetic retinopathy has led to the development of many new potential therapeutic options. The gold standard of laser photocoagulation in the treatment of diabetic retinopathy is now supplemented and may ultimately be supplanted by the availability and utility of vasoactive pharmaceuticals. Anti-VEGF agents are already being used in the management of select cases of both DME and proliferative retinopathy. Ongoing studies will clarify their particular indications and optimal regimens. Future work will further elucidate the mechanisms of diabetic retinopathy, allowing for the development of new therapeutic options. By targeting the specific metabolic byproducts that produce vascular injury and hypoxia, it may ultimately be possible to curb the disease at a preproliferative state.

Key references

A complete list of chapter references is available online at www.expertconsult.com. See inside cover for registration details.

7. Aiello LP, Bursell SE, Clermont A, et al. Vascular endothelial growth factor-induced retinal permeability is mediated by protein kinase C in vivo and suppressed by an orally effective beta-isoform-selective inhibitor. Diabetes 1997;46:1473–1480.

10. Kamiuchi K, Hasegawa G, Obayashi H, et al. Intercellular adhesion molecule-1 (ICAM-1) polymorphism is associated with diabetic retinopathy in type 2 diabetes mellitus. Diabetic Med 2002;19: 371–376.

11. Beranek M, Kankova K, Benes P, et al. Polymorphism R25P in the gene encoding transforming growth factor-beta is a newly identified risk factor for proliferative diabetic retinopathy. Am J Med Genet 2002;109:278–283.

19. Joussen AM, Murata T, Tsujikawa A, et al. Leukocyte-mediated endothelial cell injury and death in the diabetic retina. Am J Pathol 2001;158:147–152.

27. Tripathi RC, Li J, Tripathi BJ, et al. Increased level of vascular endothelial growth factor in aqueous humor of patients with neovascular glaucoma. Ophthalmology 1998;105:232–237.

30. Dvorak HF, Brown LF, Detmar M, et al. Vascular permeability factor/vascular endothelial growth factor, microvascular hyperpermeability, and angiogenesis. Am J Pathol 1995;146:1029–1039.

31. Aiello LP, Avery RL, Arrigg PG, et al. Vascular endothelial growth factor in ocular fluid of patients with diabetic retinopathy and other retinal disorders. N Engl J Med 1994;331:1480–1487.

32. Adamis AP, Miller JW, Bernal MT, et al. Increased vascular endothelial growth factor levels in the vitreous of eyes with proliferative diabetic retinopathy. Am J Ophthalmol 1994;118:445–450.

34. Miller JW, Adamis AP, Shima DT, et al. Vascular endothelial growth factor/vascular permeability factor is temporally and spatially correlated with ocular angiogenesis in a primate model. Am J Pathol 1994;145:574–584.

35. Tolentino MJ, Miller JW, Gragoudas ES, et al. Vascular endothelial growth factor is sufficient to produce iris neovascularization and neovascular glaucoma in a nonhuman primate. Arch Ophthalmol 1996;114:964–970.

40. Noma H, Funatsu H, Yamashita H, et al. Regulation of angiogenesis in diabetic retinopathy: possible balance between vascular endothelial growth factor and endostatin. Arch Ophthalmol 2002;120: 1075–1080.

42. Auricchio A, Behling KC, Maguire AM, et al. Inhibition of retinal neovascularization by intraocular viral-mediated delivery of anti-angiogenic agents. Mol Ther: J Am Soc Gene Ther 2002;6:490–494.

45. Rizzo S, Genovesi-Ebert F, DiBartolo E, et al. Injection of intravitreal bevacizumab as a preoperative adjunct before vitrectomy surgery in the treatment of severe proliferative diabetic retinopathy (PDR). Graefes Arch Clin Exp Ophthalmol 2008;246:837–842

46. Minnella AM, Savastano CM, Ziccardi L, et al. Intravitreal bevacizumab in proliferative diabetic retinopathy. Acta Ophthalmol Scand 2007;86:683–687.

48. Avery RL, Pearlman J, Pieramici DJ, et al. Intravitreal bevacizumab in the treatment of proliferative diabetic retinopathy. Ophthalmology 2006;113:1695.e1–1695. e15.

CHAPTER 67

Diabetic macular edema

Pascale Massin, Michel Paques, and Jean-Antoine Pournaras

Overview

Diabetic macular edema (DME) can cause structural retinal changes severe enough to make it the most common cause of visual loss in patients with diabetes. DME is defined by retinal thickening involving or threatening the center of the macula, secondary to the intraretinal accumulation of fluid in the macular area. Although the pathogenesis of DME is still not fully understood, it is mainly caused by the breakdown of the inner blood–retinal barrier. DME can develop at all stages of diabetic retinopathy (DR), but appears to occur more frequently as the severity of DR increases. Risk factors for DME include duration of diabetes, poor glycemic control, hypertension, proteinuria, and hypercholesterolemia. Combined with laser photocoagulation, therapy is therefore directed at controlling these factors. However, other therapies directed at the causative mechanisms of DME are currently being investigated in clinical trials.

Clinical background

Key symptoms and signs

DME is usually diagnosed by stereoscopic slit-lamp biomicroscopy, which may reveal signs such as intraretinal cysts (defining cystoid macular edema) and/or retinal hard exudates (Figures 67.1 and 67.2). Hard exudates are intraretinal lipid deposits that usually accumulate at the border of the thickened retina. They probably result from lipid precipitation due to a differential reabsorption of water-soluble molecules and lipids.

Visual deterioration due to macular edema is usually slow, and only occurs when retinal thickening involves the center of the fovea. In the Early Treatment Diabetic Retinopathy Study (ETDRS), the 3-year risk of moderate visual loss was 33% when thickening initially involved the center of the fovea, and 22% when it did not.[1] Severe visual loss usually results from longstanding DME resulting in degeneration of the photoreceptor–retinal pigment epithelial (RPE) complex and/or combined severe macular capillary closure. Lastly, retinal degeneration may also result from the presence of large plaque of hard exudates under the central fovea. Spontaneous fluctuations of DME during the day as well as long-term variations have been reported in several studies.[2-4]

Classifications of diabetic maculopathy (Table 67.1)

Several classifications of diabetic maculopathy have been proposed, based on the risk of vision loss.

In 1983, focal and diffuse DME was distinguished, as well as ischemic maculopathy.[5] Focal DME is defined by localized retinal thickening, often surrounded by exudate rings, resulting from leakage from microaneurysms, and/or intraretinal microvascular abnormalities. The prognosis of focal DME is generally good, as it responds well to laser photocoagulation. Diffuse DME consists of generalized thickening of the central macula caused by widespread leakage from dilated capillaries in this area. The effect of laser treatment on diffuse DME is limited. Finally ischemic maculopathy is secondary to extended occlusion of macular capillaries. Frequently, there is combined pathology of focal and diffuse edema as well as ischemia. Nevertheless, classifying the maculopathy according to its predominant features is useful from a therapeutic and prognostic point of view.

In the ETDRS classification, the severity of DME is based according to its distance from the center of the macula. Clinically significant macular edema (CSME) is defined as retinal thickening and/or adjacent hard exudates that either involve or threaten the center of the macula to spread into it.[1] Patients with CSME should be considered for focal laser photocoagulation.

In an attempt to improve communication worldwide between ophthalmologists and primary care physicians caring for patients with diabetes, an international clinical disease severity scale was developed for DR and macular edema.[6]

Epidemiology (Box 67.1)

Diabetic maculopathy is the main cause of vision loss in diabetic patients, occurring in 7–10% of the diabetic population.[7,8]

Macular edema incidence has been studied in the Wisconsin Epidemiologic Diabetic Retinopathy Study.[9,10] The results of this study demonstrated a higher 4- and 10-year DME incidence in diabetic patients with early onset (8.2% and 20% respectively) and in those with late onset and

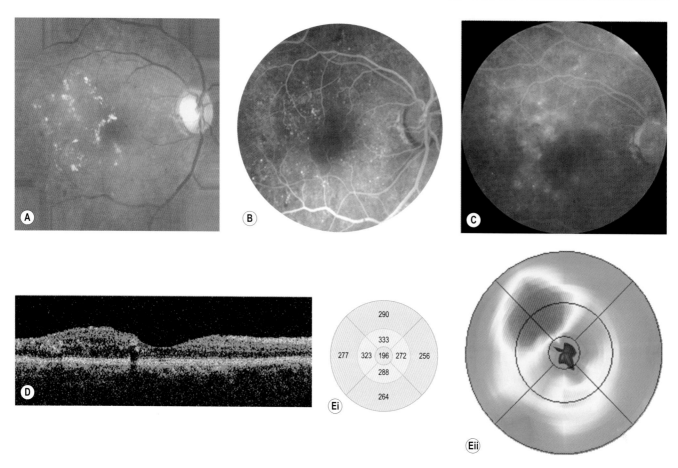

Figure 67.1 Focal diabetic macular edema. (A) Color fundus photography shows clinically significant macular edema with a ring of hard exudates temporal to the fovea. (B and C) Early and late phases of angiography show microaneurysms temporal to the macula, and fluorescein leakage from them. (D) Optical coherence tomography 3 horizontal scan shows increased retinal thickness temporal to the fovea with low reflective spaces consistent with intraretinal fluid accumulation and highly reflective intraretinal dots corresponding to hard lipid retinal exudates. (E) The retinal false-color map disclosed areas of increased retinal thickness. (Gaudric and Haouchine, Atlas d'Ophtalmologie. OCT de la Macula. Elsevier Masson, France, 2007.)

Table 67.1 Classifications of diabetic macular edema (DME)

Bresnick classification of DME	
Focal DME	Localized retinal thickening often surrounded by exudates
Diffuse DME	Generalized thickening of the central macula
Ischemc maculopathy	Extended macular capillary occlusion
ETDRS classification of DME	
Macular edema	Retinal thickening and/or exudates within one disc diameter of the center of the macula
Clinically significant DME	Any of the following features:
	Thickening of the retina at or within 500 μm of the center of the macula
	Hard exudates at or within 500 μm of the center of the macula
	A zone or zones of retinal thickening one disc area or larger, any part of which is within one disc diameter of the center of the macula
International classification	
Macular edema	Any apparent retinal thickening or exudates in posterior pole
Mild DME	Some retinal thickening or exudates in posterior pole, but distant from the center of the macula
Moderate DME	Retinal thickening or exudates approaching the center of the macula, but not involving the center
Severe DME	Retinal thickening or exudates involving the center of the macula

ETDRS, Early Treatment Diabetic Retinopathy Study.

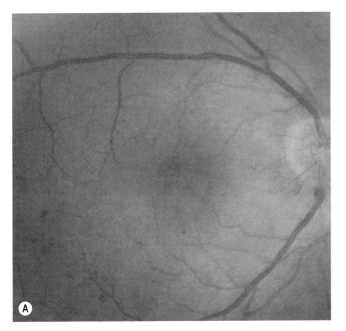

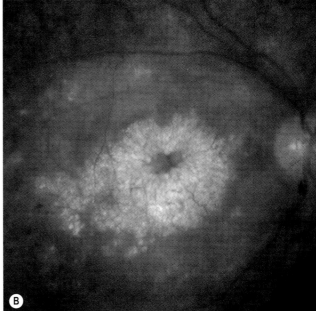

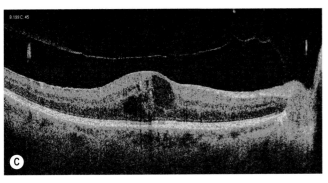

Figure 67.2 Diffuse macular edema. (A) Color fundus photography shows no hard exudates. (B) Late-phase angiogram shows cystoid macular edema. (C) Optical coherence tomography horizontal scan shows macular thickening with loss of the normal foveal contour and low reflective spaces consistent with intraretinal fluid accumulation and macular cysts. The posterior hyaloid is detached from the fovea.

Box 67.1 Risk factors for diabetic macular edema

- Duration of diabetes
- Diabetic retinopathy severity level
- Hyperglycemia
- Hypertension
- Dyslipidemia
- Nephropathy

Box 67.2 Diagnosis and follow-up of diabetic macular edema

Diagnosis
- Slit-lamp biomicroscopy
- Stereoscopic photography
- Fluorescein angiography
- Optical coherence tomography (OCT)

Follow-up
- Slit-lamp biomicroscopy
- Stereoscopic photography
- OCT

---

taking insulin (8.4% and 26% respectively) compared to those not taking insulin (2.9% and 14% respectively). Risk factors that contribute to the progression of DME include increasing levels of hyperglycemia, diabetes duration, severity of DR at baseline, diastolic blood pressure, and the presence of gross proteinuria.[7,9–12] The UK Prospective Diabetes Study Group clearly demonstrated the beneficial effect of tight blood pressure control on DME in type 2 diabetic patients as it showed, at 9 years of follow-up, a 47% reduced risk of visual loss due to reduced incidence of macular edema.[13] Lastly, several studies found a correlation between elevated rate of serum lipids and the amount of lipid exudates.[7,14,15]

Diagnostic workup (Box 67.2)

Until recently, the clinical detection and evaluation methods currently used have been limited to slit-lamp biomicroscopy

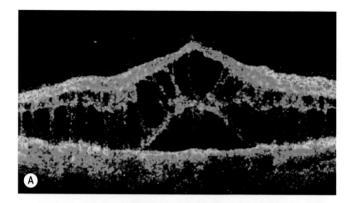

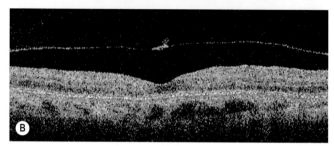

Figure 67.3 Evolution after intravitreal injection of triamcinolone acetonide. (A) Diffuse cystoid diabetic macular edema with serous detachment of the fovea, which appears as an optically clear space between the retina and the retinal pigment epithelium. (B) Four weeks after triamcinolone injection, diabetic macular edema has completely resolved. The posterior hyaloid is detached from the macula.

> **Box 67.3 Contribution of optical coherence tomography to the management of diabetic macular edema (DME)**
>
> - Accurate measurement of macular thickness
> - Detection of intraretinal cysts and serous retinal detachment
> - Analysis of the vitreomacular relationship:
>   - Tractional DME with thickening of the posterior hyaloid
>   - Early posterior vitreous detachment
> - Neuronal remodeling, including loss of outer-segment reflectance

and stereoscopic photography. However, both methods are subjective and insensitive to small changes in retinal thickness.

Fluorescein angiography facilitates the visualization of the breakdown of the inner blood–retinal barrier, demonstrating leakage of fluorescein from the macular capillaries or microaneurysms into the retinal tissue; it may also show its accumulation within cystoid spaces. However, fluorescein leakage alone does not necessarily indicate the presence of macular edema. Fluorescein angiography is also useful to identify macular capillary nonperfusion, which may be combined with DME.

Profound change in the diagnosis and management of DME has occurred since the advent of OCT in the late 1990s (Box 67.3). OCT was first described by Huang et al in 1991.[16] Since it became commercially available in 1995, there has been tremendous progress in this technology. OCT provides both cross-sectional imaging of the retina and reliable quantitative measurement of macular thickness. First OCT devices were based on the principle of low-coherence interferometry, which measures the time-of-flight delay of light reflected from ocular structures. To date, time domain OCT using the Stratus OCT instrument (Carl Zeiss Meditec, Dublin, CA) has been the most widely used tool. This instrument acquires images at a rate of 400 axial scans per second, with an axial resolution of 10 μm. Recently, a new class of OCT instruments employing spectral (Fourier) domain technology has been developed, with a scan rate of at least 20 000 axial scans per second and an improved axial resolution of 5 μm.

In the case of DME, OCT demonstrates increased retinal thickness with areas of low intraretinal reflectivity prevailing in the outer retinal layers, and loss of foveal depression. Hard exudates are detected as spots of high reflectivity, and are found primarily in the outer retinal layers (Figure 67.1); intraretinal cysts appear as small round intraretinal hyporeflective lacunae (Figure 67.2). OCT seems particularly useful to detect a feature combined with macular edema that is not easily seen on biomicroscopy – serous retinal detachment (Figure 67.3). It is seen in 15% of eyes with DME.[17] The pathogenesis and prognostic value of serous retinal detachment are not clearly established, but it does not appear to have any negative prognostic value.[18,19] OCT may also show a disruption in the line of the inner/outer-segment photoreceptors, which is an indicator of poor visual prognosis (Figure 67.4).

OCT seems particularly relevant to analyze the vitreomacular relationship. Perifoveal detachment of the posterior hyaloid, which appears slightly reflective, is quite common, and corresponds to early posterior vitreous detachment.[20] But, in some cases of DME, the posterior hyaloid on OCT is thick and hyperreflective, and is partially detached from the posterior pole, but remains attached to the disk and to the top of the raised macular surface, on which it exerts traction (Figure 67.5). In these cases, vitrectomy is beneficial.[21,22]

One major advantage of OCT is that it allows measurement of retinal thickness from tomograms by means of computer image-processing techniques. Several studies have shown the reliability and good reproducibility of such measurements.[23–25] OCT is thus an accurate tool to follow the spontaneous evolution of DME, as well as its response to treatments.

Treatment (Table 67.2)

It is now widely accepted that control of systemic factors, which may worsen DME, is essential. These factors include glycemic and blood pressure control, as well as anemia, hyperlipidemia, and all causes of intravascular fluid overload (congestive heart failure, renal failure, hypoalbuminemia).[26]

Randomized studies have clearly demonstrated the efficacy of laser photocoagulation to prevent vision loss from DME.[1,27,28] In the ETDRS, eyes with nonproliferative DR and macular edema were randomly assigned to early focal/grid photocoagulation or nonphotocoagulation. After 3 years of follow-up, 24% of the control group lost three lines of the ETDRS visual acuity chart compared with 12% of the treated

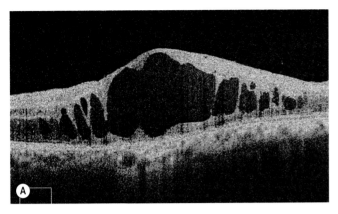
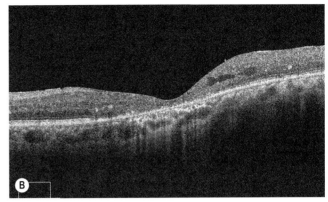

Figure 67.4 Break in the inner/outer-segment line of the photoreceptors. (A) Optical coherence tomography (OCT): cystoid macular edema, with large central hyporeflective cavity. (B) After triamcinolone injection, diabetic macular edema has completely resolved. There is macular atrophy. A break in the inner/outer-segment line of the photoreceptors is visible on OCT, explaining bad visual recovery.

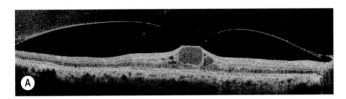

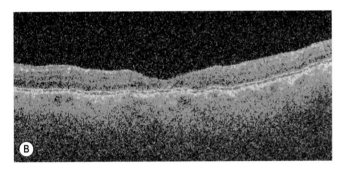

Figure 67.5 Tractional diabetic macular edema (DME). (A) Before vitrectomy: diffuse DME with a thickened and highly reflective posterior hyaloid which is partially detached from the posterior pole, but remains attached to the top the fovea, on which it exerts traction. (B) DME has completely resolved after vitrectomy.

Table 67.2 Treatment for diabetic macular edema (DME)

Control of systemic factors	Glycemia, blood pressure, and lipids
Laser photocoagulation	Indicated in cases of clinically significant DME (moderate or severe DME)
	More effective on focal than on diffuse DME
Alternative treatments for diffuse DME	Vitrectomy for tractional DME
	Intravitreal steroids
	Antivascular endothelial growth factor therapy is under investigation

eye. However, this beneficial effect was only observed in eyes with clinically significant DME, for which prompt photocoagulation is thus highly recommended. In addition, laser photocoagulation was more effective for focal than diffuse DME. In eyes with diffuse DME, more than 15% of patients go on losing vision despite previous laser photocoagulation.[29] Laser photocoagulation may also be associated with severe side-effects such as laser burns to the fovea, enlargement of laser scars over time, choroidal neovascularization, and subretinal fibrosis.

The exact mechanism of action of laser photocoagulation is not known. It may be due to an enhanced proliferation of RPE and endothelial cells, leading to a restoration of the blood–retinal barrier,[30,31] or a better oxygenation of the inner retina from the choriocapillary after destruction of oxygen-consuming photoreceptors.[32] A retinal vasoconstriction has indeed been observed after grid laser photocoagulation for DME.[33]

The drawbacks and side-effects of laser photocoagulation have led to the search for alternative treatments for DME. They include vitrectomy and intravitreal injection of steroids or anti-vascular endothelial growth factor (VEGF) drugs.

A beneficial effect of vitrectomy to reduce DME and improve visual acuity has been demonstrated in eyes with DME associated with a taut and thickened posterior hyaloid exerting macular traction[21,22,34,35] (Figure 67.5). In cases of DME without any vitreomacular traction, the effect of vitrectomy remains unclear.[36–38]

Several studies have shown the efficacy of intravitreal injections of triamcinolone acetonide (IVTA) to reduce DME temporarily and increase visual acuity (Figure 67.5).[3,39–41] The mean reduction in macular thickening reaches 85% 3 months after injection with a mean two lines of improvement of visual acuity.[4,41] However, recurrence of DME occurs 3–6 months after injection. Side-effects of IVTA include ocular hypertension in up to 50% of patients, glaucoma requiring surgery in 2%, and cataract surgery in 54% within 2 years of injection.[4] Recently, the Diabetic Retinopathy Clinical Research network (DRCR.net), comparing the efficacy and safety of 1-mg and 4-mg doses of preservative-free intravitreal triamcinolone in comparison with focal/grid laser photocoagulation in patients with DME, showed that, over a 2-year period, focal/grid laser photocoagulation is more effective and has fewer side-effects than triamcinolone.[42]

Steroids act by reducing vascular permeability: indeed, steroids stabilize endothelial tight junctions and increase their numbers. They may also inhibit production of

VEGF.[43–45] Steroids also suppress inflammation and inhibit the migration of leukocytes.

Extensive data have established that VEGF is involved in the vascular permeability observed in DR.[46,47] These data support the use of anti-VEGF therapy for diffuse DME. Pegaptanib is an anti-VEGF aptamer, binds to VEGF$_{165}$, sequestering it and preventing VEGF receptor activation. A phase II trial evaluating the efficacy and safety of injections of three doses (0.3, 1, and 3 mg) of pegaptanib versus placebo every 6 weeks has shown interesting results, with better median visual acuity at 6 months in the group treated with 0.3 mg as compared with sham. Phase III trial is under way.[48] Ranibizumab, which is a recombinant humanized monoclonal antibody fragment with specificity for all iso-forms of human VEGF, is also under investigation for DME. A phase II trial investigating the efficacy and safety of two concentrations of intravitral ranibizumab (0.3 and 0.5 mg) in patients with DME with center involvement, compared with sham, showed a significant improvement of visual acuity in patients who received ranibizumab, with a mean average change in visual acuity from baseline to month 1 through month 12 of 7.6 letters, versus 1.2 letters in the sham group. Treatment with both doses of ranibizumab was associated with a significant decrease in central retinal thickness on OCT (Massin P and the RESOLVE Study Group, presented at the American Academy of Ophthalmology, Atlanta, 2008). Encouraging results were also observed in the phase II READ II trial (Nguyen, presented at the American Academy of Ophthalmology, 2008). Finally, comparing the results of intravitreal bevacizumab injection alone or in combination with intravitreal triamcinolone acetonide versus macular photocoagulation as a primary treatment for DME, Soheilian et al[49] found that intravitreal bevacizumab injection in patients with DME yielded a better visual outcome at 24 weeks compared with macular photocoagulation, although its effect on decreasing retinal edema was transient.

Pathophysiology

The breakdown of the inner blood–retinal barrier is the most important mechanism leading to visual loss, but capillary nonperfusion and possibly direct neuronal damage are also major actors. Macular edema thus represents the result of multiple processes affecting a number of interdependent cell populations. The dominant paradigm attributes a major role to the interaction of a variety of factors, including overproduction of VEGF, inflammation, and endothelial dysfunction. Yet, because of its complexity and the lack of a convenient animal model, the pathophysiology of the onset and complications of DME remains still largely uncertain.

Inner blood–retinal barrier dysfunction (Box 67.4)

The blood–retinal barrier isolates the neural elements of the retina from the circulation in order to facilitate the control of the extracellular milieu. The inner blood–retinal barrier schematically comprises intercellular barrier (tight junctions between adjacent endothelial cells) and transcellular barrier (as shown by the relative paucity of intracellular vesicles).[50] Plasma may flow between endothelial cells, suggesting opening of tight junctions, or through endothelial cells, due to increased membrane permeability or vesicular trans-

> **Box 67.4 Factors possibly involved in blood–retinal barrier breakdown during diabetic retinopathy**
>
> - Vascular endothelial growth factor overproduction
> - Activation of protein kinase C
> - Hepatocyte growth factor
> - Histamine
> - Activation of bradykinin by carbon anhydrase released by erythrocytes
> - Impaired vascular autoregulation
> - Endothelial dysfunction
> - Inflammation, including leukostasis

port.[51,52] Dysfunctional blood–retinal barrier is always present in visible manifestations of microvascular remodeling such as microaneurysms, but normal-appearing capillaries may also leak fluorescein, suggesting that barrier dysfunction precedes morphological changes of capillaries.

Tight junctions are made of a complex aggregate of proteins, among them occludin claudins, zonula occludens-1 (ZO-1), zonula occludens (ZO-2), and zonula occludens-3 (ZO-3). Experimental diabetes causes disorganization of the tight junction proteins, as shown by the reduction of occludin content in retinal endothelial cells,[53,54] resulting in reversibly increased permeability. Both VEGF and hepatocyte growth factor administration in vitro reduce occludin content and lead to tight junction complex internalization in vascular endothelial cells.[47,55–57] The effect of VEGF on tight junction is partly mediated by occludin phosphorylation, and indeed activation of protein kinase C (PKC) participates in the mechanism of VEGF-induced vascular permeability.[46,58]

In vivo, it is likely that macular edema results at least in part from the action of VEGF on vascular endothelial tight junction proteins and transcellular flow. Increased expression of VEGF in the retina is indeed an early change observed in experimental diabetes. It may result from local tissue ischemia due to microcapillary occlusions, or may be due to an inflammatory response, possibly through activation of the receptor for advanced glycation end-products.[59] There is evidence that VEGF exerts neuroprotective effects on neurons and thus may be a response of neurons and glia to physiological stresses imposed by chronic hyperglycemia.[53] Yet, as clinical experience shows, the effect of specific anti-VEGF therapy is often partial, suggesting the involvement of other crucial partners in the maintenance of DME. Other biochemical pathways may be involved in the breakdown of the blood–retinal barrier, such as PKC activation.[46] The effect of ruboxistaurine, a tissue-specific PKC-ß inhibitor, has now been evaluated in several trials.[60] The PKC-Diabetic Retinopathy Study evaluated the effects of three different doses of oral ruboxistaurin versus a placebo on the progression of DR, while the PKC-Diabetic Macular Edema Study evaluated the effect of the same doses of ruboxistaurine versus a placebo on the progression of macular edema.[60,61] Neither of these studies demonstrated any significant changes in primary endpoint. However, in the PKC-DRS, compared to placebo, 32 mg/day ruboxistaurine was associated with a delayed occurrence of vision loss, probably due to less progression of macular edema. And in the PKC-DME Study, a subgroup analysis showed a slower progression of DME in patients treated with 32mg ruboxistaurine compared to placebo. Further trials focusing on the effect of ruboxistaurine on DME are underway.

It is known that cells surrounding retinal capillaries, especially astrocytes, play a critical role in induction and maintenance of the blood–retinal barrier function. To what extent primary neuroglial dysfunction plays a role in BRB breakdown remains to be determined.

More recently, it has been suggested that retinal hemorrhages are involved in the onset and/or maintenance of macular edema. This hypothesis states that an enzymatic cascade initiated by carbon anhydrase released by erythrocytes may increase local levels of bradykinin, a potent vasodilator.[62] This enzymatic cascade involves decreased local pH due to the release of HCO_3^-, subsequent activation of factor XII, increase in kallicrein levels, and finally transformation of kininogen into bradykinin. Since several of these actors have pharmacological inhibitors, these findings may be of therapeutic interest. However, the involvement of this mechanism in humans remains to be demonstrated.

Water homeostasis in the retina (Figure 67.6)

As blood–barrier breakdown affects vision only in presence of retinal thickening, elucidating the cause of fluid accumulation itself may provide novel therapeutic clues for macular edema. A poorly understood phenomenon is retinal distension, which implies impaired circulation of water within the retina. The Müller cells actively pump out the extracellular milieu of the retina in the vitreous, as do the RPE cells in the choroid. There are many substances that are known to flow easily through the retina, even large molecules such as antibodies.

Such accumulation is intriguing in the presence of a large potential reservoir (the vitreous) and of actively pumping cells closely apposed to the retina (Müller cells and the RPE). Thus, it seems that the inner and/or outer limiting membranes are a mechanical barrier to the diffusion of fluids.

Fluid accumulation during macular edema is generally assumed to be located in the extracellular space (so-called vasogenic edema), as suggested by fluorescein leakage during angiography. However, there are experimental and clinical arguments for the participation of an inflation of intracellular compartment, mainly Müller cells.[63] Indeed, in many cases of macular edema there is no detectable leakage of fluorescein, and Müller cells are known to increase their cytoplasmic volume in response to some stimuli such as ischemia–reperfusion. Thus, cytotoxic edema from ischemia may participate in retinal thickening. Increased volume of Müller cells may also be a consequence of their role in the water homeostasis of the retina; they are indeed known to express AQP4 aquaporine channels.[64] Dysfunction or death of Müller cells is also a likely explanation for the formation of large cystoid spaces, which are similar to some extent to the cyst seen in retinoschisis. It may also cause impairment of outflow from the retina, but experimental demonstrations of such a phenomenon are as yet lacking.

It is likely that there is dysfunction of the outer blood–retinal barrier in diabetic retinopathy, although there have been few investigations of it; it seems that in response to inner blood–retinal barrier rupture, the RPE cells increase their pumping activity, but this increase cannot ensure complete clearing of plasma molecules beyond a certain point.

The cause of the preferential accumulation of fluid in the fovea may be due to its specific architecture, especially the absence of astrocytes and of a dense vascular bead; thus, the fovea is a weak point mechanistically speaking, and fluid easily accumulates there because there is less restriction to retinal distension than elsewhere in the retina.

Vascular dysfunction and inflammation

The retina controls its own blood flow in response to local and systemic influences by means of a variety of cellular and chemical factors. Such autoregulation is crucial for the maintenance of a constant blood flow despite strong, minute-to-minute changes in perfusion pressure and metabolic needs. Diabetic patients have an impaired endothelial function that occurs very early in the course of the disease. Recent experiments have shown that the vasodilatory effect of flicker light is impaired before the onset of clinically detectable DR.[65] Diabetic patients are also known to have chronically dilated retinal vessels, possibly due to chronic ischemia.[66] This may locally increase hydrostatic pressure and hence aggravate retinal edema. Interestingly, steroids, which are known to reduce macular edema, are also potent vasoconstrictors of retinal vessels,[67] as well as anti-VEGF molecules. The therapeutic effect of oxygen on macular edema has also been attributed to vasoconstriction.[68]

Endothelial dysfunction also provides a basis for the chronic, low-grade inflammation observed in experimental and clinical diabetes. Increased leukocyte adherence, or leukostasis, has been shown to occur early in DR, and may account for both capillary closure and blood–retinal barrier rupture.[69] Another aspect of chronic inflammation is related to microglial cells, which are chronically activated during diabetes.[70] Because activated microglia release proinflammatory cytokines and chemokines, such as VEGF and tumor necrosis factor, it is likely that they further exacerbate retinal vascular permeability in diabetes.

Role of systemic factors (Box 67.5)

When the blood–retinal barrier is open, Starling's laws influence the net movement of water and solutes out of capillaries, leading to macular edema formation.[71] Starling's law

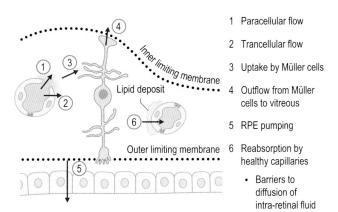

1	Paracellular flow
2	Trancellular flow
3	Uptake by Müller cells
4	Outflow from Müller cells to vitreous
5	RPE pumping
6	Reabsorption by healthy capillaries
•	Barriers to diffusion of intra-retinal fluid

Figure 67.6 Flow of plasma components during diabetic macular edema.

Box 67.5 Aggravating factors of diabetic macular edema

Systemic factors

- Hypertension
- Intravascular fluid overload (congestive heart failure, renal failure, hypoalbuminemia)

Mechanical factors

- Vitreomacular traction
- Epiretinal membrane

states that the net movement of fluid out of capillaries is determined by the sum of hydrostatic and oncotic pressures. Therefore, changes in accumulation of water and solutes in the retina may be due either to changes in hydrostatic (e.g., arterial pressure) or oncotic (e.g., protein content) pressure. Thus, systemic mechanisms leading to increased hydrostatic pressure such as hypertension, or intravascular fluid overload, as observed in cases of congestive heart failure, or renal failure, as well as decreased oncotic pressure (hypoalbuminemia) may worsen DME, and should be actively managed.

Mechanical factors (Box 67.5)

Several observations have suggested that the vitreous may play a role in the pathogenesis of DME. Indeed, Hikichi et al

observed a more frequent spontaneous resolution of DME when the posterior hyaloid was completely detached from the posterior pole.[72] Sebag observed increased levels of early glycation products, as well as advanced glycation end-products in the vitreous of diabetic patients compared to controls.[73] These alterations may lead to liquefaction and destabilization of the vitreous gel. Furthermore, the vitreoretinal adhesion often remains strong despite gel liquefaction.[74] Destabilization of the central vitreous cortex together with the persistent attachment of the vitreous cortex to the retina may thus lead to traction on the macula, and contribute to the development of DME. Such mechanism is obvious in cases of diffuse DME combined with a taut and thickened posterior hyaloid, for which the beneficial effect of vitrectomy has been demonstrated.[21] Mechanical traction by epiretinal membranes may also aggravate edema, which is relieved by surgical ablation.

Conclusion

If the treatment of DME is still mainly based on laser photocoagulation, the control of systemic factors seems crucial to prevent its worsening. Pharmacological approaches, including anti-VEGF therapy and steroids, are under investigation. The increased understanding of the complex mechanisms which are involved in the pathogenesis of DME will further enhance our therapeutic possibilities.

Key references

A complete list of chapter references is available online at www.expertconsult.com. See inside cover for registration details.

1. Early Treatment Diabetic Retinopathy Study research group. Photocoagulation for diabetic macular edema. ETDRS report number 1. Arch Ophthalmol 1985;103:1796–1806.

4. Gillies MC, Sutter FK, Simpson JM, et al. Intravitreal triamcinolone for refractory diabetic macular edema: two-year results of a double-masked, placebo-controlled, randomized clinical trial. Ophthalmology 2006;113:1533–1538.

6. Wilkinson CP, Ferris FL 3rd, Klein RE, et al. Proposed international clinical diabetic retinopathy and diabetic macular edema disease severity scales. Ophthalmology 2003;110:1677–1682.

9. Klein R, Klein BE, Moss SE, et al. The Wisconsin Epidemiologic Study of Diabetic Retinopathy. XV. The long-term incidence of macular edema. Ophthalmology 1995;102:7–16.

13. UK Prospective Diabetes Study Group. Tight blood pressure control and risk of macrovascular and microvascular complications in type 2 diabetes: UKPDS 38. Br Med J 1998;317:703–713.

26. Gardner TW, Antonetti DA, Barber AJ, et al. Diabetic retinopathy: more than meets the eye. Surv Ophthalmol 2002;47(Suppl. 2):S253–S262.

32. Bresnick GH. Diabetic macular edema. A review. Ophthalmology 1986;93:989–997.

42. A randomized trial comparing intravitreal triamcinolone acetonide and focal/grid photocoagulation for diabetic macular edema. Ophthalmology 2008;115:1447–1449, e1441–1410.

46. Aiello LP, Bursell SE, Clermont A, et al. Vascular endothelial growth factor-induced retinal permeability is mediated by protein kinase C in vivo and suppressed by an orally effective beta-isoform-selective inhibitor. Diabetes 1997;46:1473–1480.

53. Antonetti DA, Barber AJ, Khin S, et al. Vascular permeability in experimental diabetes is associated with reduced endothelial occludin content: vascular endothelial growth factor decreases occludin in retinal endothelial cells. Penn State Retina Research Group. Diabetes 1998;47:1953–1959.

57. Jiang WG, Martin TA, Matsumoto K, et al. Hepatocyte growth factor/scatter factor decreases the expression of occludin and transendothelial resistance (TER) and increases paracellular permeability in human vascular endothelial cells. J Cell Physiol 1999; 181:319–329.

62. Gao BB, Clermont A, Rook S, et al. Extracellular carbonic anhydrase mediates hemorrhagic retinal and cerebral vascular permeability through prekallikrein activation. Nat Med 2007;13:181–188.

69. Joussen AM, Murata T, Tsujikawa A, et al. Leukocyte-mediated endothelial cell injury and death in the diabetic retina. Am J Pathol 2001;158:147–152.

70. Rungger-Brandle E, Dosso AA, Leuenberger PM. Glial reactivity, an early feature of diabetic retinopathy. Invest Ophthalmol Vis Sci 2000;41:1971–1980.

71. Stefansson E. Ocular oxygenation and the treatment of diabetic retinopathy. Surv Ophthalmol 2006;51:364–380.

CHAPTER 68

Dry age-related macular degeneration and age-related macular degeneration pathogenesis

Marco Zarbin and Janet S Sunness

Clinical background

Clinical manifestations of dry age-related macular degeneration (AMD) include drusen, retinal pigment epithelium (RPE) hyperplasia, RPE depigmentation, and geographic atrophy (GA) (Box 68.1). The prevalence of early AMD is 18% in the population aged 65–74 years and 30% in those older than 74 years.[1] GA is the advanced atrophic form of dry AMD. Approximately 3.5% of people aged 75 and older have GA,[2] and its prevalence is greater than 20% among persons aged 90 and older.[3] In the 70s and 80s, choroidal new vessels (CNVs) are approximately twice as common as GA, but GA is more common in the oldest group.

In many patients, small areas of GA develop near the fovea, often in areas of resorbed drusen or mottled hypo- and hyperpigmentation (Figure 68.1). Over time these areas enlarge, creating multifocal GA surrounding the fovea. The areas may then coalesce, first into a horseshoe-shaped area of atrophy and later into a ring of atrophy, still sparing the foveal center. Finally, the fovea becomes atrophic, and the patient must use eccentric vision for all visual tasks.[4–7] When the fovea is surrounded by atrophy, the patient may be able to read single small letters on a visual acuity chart but may have great difficulty reading because the surrounding scotomata block off parts of words and sentences. Similarly, these patients may have difficulty recognizing faces, because parts of the face are obscured by the scotomata. In addition, these small spared areas pose a great challenge for low-vision rehabilitation, in that too much magnification will put more of the word in the blind area and may actually make reading more difficult. Patients often use two areas for fixation, a central one for small print and an eccentric one to see the larger picture.[8,9] This pattern of disease progression can lead one to underestimate the severity of visual impairment associated with GA if one measures central visual acuity solely.

GA is an important cause of moderate and severe visual loss among AMD patients. In a large natural history study, 40% of the patients with GA and vision of 20/50 or better

worsened by 3 or more lines on an Early Treatment of Diabetic Retinopathy visual acuity chart over a 2-year follow-up period. A total of 27% of the patients with this good baseline visual acuity worsened to 20/200 or less by 4 years of follow-up.[10] The degree of impairment in dim environments at baseline is predictive of subsequent visual acuity loss.[11] Thus, there is very significant decline in visual acuity during a 2-year period among patients with GA.

The appearance and rate of enlargement of atrophy are very symmetric between eyes in patients with bilateral GA, who constitute the majority of GA patients. The enlargement rate appears to be characteristic of the individual, and this between-subjects factor is more significant than is the size of the GA in estimating the subsequent rate of GA enlargement.[7]

Choroidal neovascularization is relatively uncommon in patients with bilateral GA without CNVs in either eye at baseline. In contrast, patients with CNVs in one eye and GA without CNVs in the fellow eye have a much higher rate of developing CNVs in the eye with GA.[12,13] It is not yet understood why some patients are more likely to develop CNVs, and others are more likely to develop GA.

The differential diagnosis of dry AMD includes Stargardt disease, central areolar choroidal atrophy, Doyne honeycomb dystrophy, drug toxicity, Best disease, adult vitelliform dystrophy, and some forms of retinitis pigmentosa (Box 68.2). Membranoproliferative glomerulonephritis type II (MPGN II) can be associated with drusen, GA, and CNVs.[14–19]

Pathology

The abnormal extracellular matrix (ECM) of AMD eyes includes basal laminar deposit, basal linear deposit, and their clinically evident manifestation, soft drusen. The RPE deposits cytoplasmic material into Bruch's membrane throughout life, possibly to eliminate cytoplasmic debris or as a response to chronic inflammation (see Pathophysiology, below).[20–23] Histologically, AMD eyes exhibit abnormal extracellular material in two locations: (1) between the RPE plasmalemma and the RPE basement membrane (basal laminar deposit); and (2) external to the RPE basement membrane within the collagenous layers of Bruch's membrane (basal linear deposit).[24] Although basal laminar deposit persists in areas of GA, basal linear deposit disappears, which is consistent with the notion that basal linear deposit arises mostly from the RPE–photoreceptor complex.[25] Basal linear deposit may be more specific to AMD than basal laminar deposit.[26] Soft drusen can represent focal accentua-

tions of basal linear deposit in the presence or absence of diffuse basal linear deposit-associated thickening of the inner aspects of Bruch's membrane.[24,27] Soft drusen can also represent a localized accumulation of basal laminar deposit in an eye with diffuse basal laminar deposit.[27]

Drusen represent the earliest clinical finding in AMD (Box 68.3). Drusen composition and origin have been analyzed

---

Box 68.1 Clinical findings in dry age-related macular degeneration

- Drusen
- Retinal pigment epithelium (RPE) hyperplasia
- RPE depigmentation
- Geographic atrophy

Box 68.2 Conditions mimicking dry age-related macular degeneration

- Stargardt disease
- Central areolar choroidal atrophy
- Doyne honeycomb dystrophy
- Drug toxicity
- Best disease
- Adult vitelliform dystrophy
- Membranoproliferative glomerulonephritis type II
- Some forms of retinitis pigmentosa

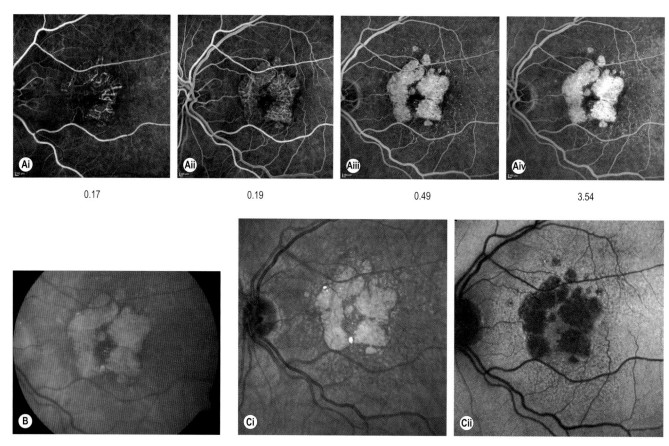

0.17   0.19   0.49   3.54

Figure 68.1 Imaging geographic atrophy. This patient has multifocal geographic atrophy, which has coalesced to form almost a ring around the fovea. Although there is foveal sparing, there are small regions of atrophy within the spared area as well. There are two small areas of calcific drusen, at 11 o'clock and 6 o'clock. (Ai–iv) Fluorescein angiogram. There is a loss of the choriocapillaris, so that the larger choroidal vessels are seen early in the angiogram. In the late frames, there is hyperfluorescence without leakage, corresponding to the area of geographic atrophy. (B) Color fundus photo. The atrophy is well delineated by its lighter color and the increased visibility of underlying choroidal vessels. (C) Infrared imaging. The atrophy is well visualized using infrared imaging, which emphasizes deep retinal structure. (D) Autofluorescence imaging. Retinal autofluorescence is typically produced by lipofuscin within retinal pigment epithelium (RPE) cells. In geographic atrophy, the RPE cells are no longer present, and the area is dark on autofluorescence imaging. There is some increased autofluorescence immediately surrounding the geographic atrophy, which may reflect lipofuscin-laden RPE at risk for atrophy. (Courtesy of Dr. Frank Holz.)

Box 68.3 Histopathology of age-related macular degeneration

- Accumulation of abnormal extracellular material (basal laminar and basal linear deposit)
- Geographic atrophy (loss of photoreceptors and subjacent retinal pigment epithelium and choriocapillaris)
- Choroidal neovascularization

Table 68.1 Some molecular constituents of drusen

α_1-Antichymotrypsin
α_1-Antitrypsin
Alzheimer's amyloid β peptide
Advanced glycation end products
Amyloid P component
Apolipoprotein B and E
Carbohydrate moieties recognized by wheatgerm agglutinin, *Limax flavus* agglutinin, concanavalin A, *Arachea hypogea* agglutinin, and *Ricinis communis* agglutinin
Cholesterol esters
Clusterin
Complement factors (C1q, C3c, C4, C5, C5b-9 complex)
Cluster differentiation antigen
Complement receptor 1
Factor X
Heparan sulfate proteoglycan
Human leukocyte antigen-DR
Immunoglobulin light chains
Major histocompatibility antigen class II
Membrane cofactor protein
Peroxidized lipids (derived from long-chain polyunsaturated fatty acids, i.e., linolenic acid and docosahexanoic acid, which are normally found in photoreceptor outer segments)
Phospholipids and neutral lipids
Tissue inhibitor of matrix metalloproteinases-3
Transthyretin (major carrier of vitamin A in the blood)
Ubiquitin
Vitronectin

extensively.[28-38] Small (i.e., 63-μm-diameter) drusen generally do not signify the presence of AMD.[1,24,39,40] Excessive numbers of small hard drusen, however, can predispose to RPE atrophy at a relatively young age.[41] Soft drusen are usually pale yellow and large with poorly demarcated boundaries. Many different molecules have been identified in drusen, most of which seem to be the product of oxidative and inflammatory processes (Table 68.1). Many of the molecular constituents of drusen are synthesized by RPE, neural retina, or choroidal cells, but some are derived from extraocular sources.

Areas of GA have a loss of RPE cells as well as overlying photoreceptors and subjacent choriocapillaris atrophy.[39,42] Choriocapillaris may be lost as a result of RPE loss,[43,44] and assessment of the region immediately outside the area of GA indicates that the RPE cells are lost first.[45] In many patients with GA, there is increased fundus autofluorescence in the area surrounding the GA, termed the junctional zone.[46] This autofluorescence is a product of RPE cells laden with lipofuscin.[47] Lipofuscin, particularly the *N*-retinylidene-*N*-retinylethanolamine component (A2E: see Pathophysiology, below), is harmful to RPE cells[48] and may be partly responsible for GA progression. Using a scanning laser ophthalmoscope (such as the Heidelberg retinal analyzer, HRA) with argon blue light and a barrier filter and with image averaging techniques, one can obtain a high-resolution fundus autofluorescence image (Figure 68.1). Areas that are dark have lost autofluorescence because there is RPE atrophy or attenuation. Areas that are bright have increased lipofuscin deposition. The pattern of increased autofluorescence may be useful in predicting the rate of enlargement of areas of GA.[49]

Etiology

The prevalence of both CNVs and GA is much higher in white populations as compared with black populations.[50-53] Smoking increases the risk of developing GA and may also increase its rate of progression.[54,55] The presence of drusen measuring 250 μm or greater and pigmentary abnormalities are risk factors for the development of GA.[56] The way that inflammatory and immunologic factors relate to the development of AMD is not yet clear, but is an active area of investigation.

Pathophysiology

Aging–AMD overlap

Some of the biochemical and histopathological features of AMD seem to occur as a normal part of aging (e.g., lipofus-

cin accumulation in RPE cells and oxidative damage).[57] Up to 65% of the proteins identified in drusen are present in drusen derived from AMD as well as healthy age-matched donors.[58] Approximately 33% of the drusen-derived proteins from AMD donors, however, are not observed in healthy donor drusen. Thus, despite the fact there is some degree of continuity between aging changes in the photoreceptor–RPE–Bruch's membrane–choriocapillaris complex and aging changes associated with AMD, aging and AMD seem to be distinct conditions (Box 68.4).

It is hypothesized that the photoreceptor–RPE–Bruch's membrane–choriocapillaris complex is a site of chronic oxidative damage, which is most pronounced in the macula (Figure 68.2). This damage incites inflammation, mediated via complement activation, at the level of RPE–Bruch's membrane–choriocapillaris. Patients with mutations in components of the complement system are less able to modulate the inflammatory response, resulting in excessive cellular damage and accumulation of extracellular debris. These changes, which involve modification of the ECM, cause additional inflammation and cell damage. This chronic inflammatory response involves cellular components of the immune system as well as the classical and alternate pathways of the complement system. Accumulation of abnormal extracellular material (including membranous debris, oxidized molecules, ECM molecules, and components of the complement system) is thus a sign of chronic inflammatory damage, is manifest in part as drusen and pigmentary abnormalities, and fosters the development of the late sequelae of AMD in susceptible individuals, i.e., GA and/or CNVs. Many treatments for AMD under investigation are based on concepts related to this hypothesis of pathogenesis. Evidence regarding this hypothesis is considered below.

Lipofuscin increases the risk of oxidative damage to RPE cells and possibly to photoreceptors and choroidal capillaries

Lipofuscin comprises a group of autofluorescent lipid–protein aggregates present in nonneuronal and neuronal tissues. Undegradable products of photoreceptor outer-segment metabolism are the major source of RPE lipofuscin.[59] Lipofuscin accumulates in RPE cells as they age,

increases the risk of oxidative damage to RPE cells, reduces RPE phagocytic capacity, and can cause RPE death.[59–63]

The reaction product of ethanolamine and two retinaldehyde molecules, A2E, is the major photosensitizing chromophore in lipofuscin that causes reactive oxygen species (ROS) production. A2E interferes with lysosomal enzyme activity, reduces lysosomal protein and glycosaminoglycan degradation, and inhibits RPE phagolysosomal degradation of photoreceptor phospholipid.[64–66] RPE cells with excessive A2E exhibit membrane blebbing and extrusion of cytoplasmic material into Bruch's membrane. Excessive RPE lipofuscin (and A2) accumulation may play a critical role in the pathogenesis of GA.[49]

AMD is associated with oxidative damage

Aging is associated with increased oxidative damage and impaired function of antioxidant systems (see Zarbin[57] for references). RPE susceptibility to oxidative damage increases with aging.[67,68] Epidemiological studies, AMD histochemistry, and drusen biochemistry indicate that oxidative reactions play a central role in AMD pathophysiology. Each of these areas will be considered briefly.

Epidemiology

Age, smoking, and race are associated with at least a twofold increased risk of AMD.[51,53,69] The effect of age on risk may indicate that oxidative damage must be gradual and cumulative for AMD to develop. Also, it may be a sign that mitochondrial DNA damage plays a role in AMD pathogenesis (please see below).[70] Smoking depresses antioxidants (e.g., decreases plasma vitamin C and carotenoids), induces hypoxia and ROS, and alters choroidal blood flow.[71]

White individuals have a relatively higher risk of large drusen, pigmentary abnormalities, and exudative AMD complications compared with blacks.[50,52] Differences in melanin content may underlie, in part, the racial differences in the risk of advanced AMD. Melanin reduces lipofuscin accumulation in RPE cells, possibly by interacting with transition metals and scavenging radicals to function as an antioxidant.[72] However, the role of ethnicity may reflect the importance of other genetic differences among races. Different ethnic groups may have different genetic mutations underly-

---

Box 68.4 Pathophysiology of age-related macular degeneration (AMD)

- AMD is associated with chronic oxidative damage to the outer retina, retinal pigment epithelium, Bruch's membrane, and choriocapillaris, and impaired function of antioxidant systems
- AMD is associated with chronic inflammation
- Increased risk of drusen, geographic atrophy, and choroidal new vessels is associated with mutations in components of the complement pathway, which is part of the innate immune system
- Oxidative damage can activate the complement pathway
- AMD risk-enhancing mutations not directly involving the complement pathway are also linked to inflammation and/or oxidative damage

---

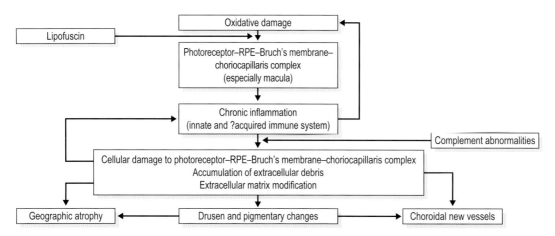

Figure 68.2 Proposed model of age-related macular degeneration pathogenesis. RPE, retinal pigment epithelium. See text for details.

ing the risk of developing AMD.[73] This notion is consistent with the different clinical manifestations of AMD in different ethnic groups. In contrast to whites, for example, soft drusen are only a moderate risk indicator for developing CNVs among Japanese patients, and the 5-year risk of developing CNVs in the second eye is relatively low among Japanese patients.[74]

The Age-Related Eye Disease Study (AREDS)[75] demonstrated that, among patients with extensive intermediate drusen, at least one large druse, noncentral GA in one or both eyes, advanced AMD in one eye, or vision loss in one eye due to AMD, supplementation with ascorbic acid, vitamin E, beta-carotene, zinc oxide, and cupric oxide reduced the risk of developing advanced AMD from 28% to 20% and the rate of at least moderate vision loss from 29% to 23%. The AREDS data may mean that oxidative damage plays a role in the progression of AMD in its clinically evident intermediate and late stages and that disease progression can be altered with antioxidant supplementation. However, zinc also affects the complement system (e.g., inhibits C3 convertase activity),[76] and C3a des Arg (a cleavage product of C3a that reflects complement activation) levels are higher in patients with AMD versus controls.[77]

AMD histochemistry

Using biomarkers of oxidative damage in postmortem eyes from AMD patients, Shen and coworkers found that many eyes with advanced GA showed evidence of widespread oxidative retinal damage, primarily in the inner and outer nuclear layers.[78] The authors posited that a subpopulation of patients with GA have a major deficiency in their oxidative defense system.

Iron is an essential element for enzymes involved in the phototransduction cascade, in outer-segment disc membrane synthesis, and in the conversion of all-*trans*-retinyl ester to 11-*cis*-retinol in the RPE (see He et al[79] for references). Free Fe^{2+} catalyzes the conversion of hydrogen peroxide to hydroxyl radical, which causes oxidative damage (e.g., lipid peroxidation, DNA strand breaks). Iron accumulation in the RPE and Bruch's membrane is greater in AMD eyes than in controls, including cases with early AMD, GA, and/or CNVs.[80] Some of this iron is chelatable.[80] One patient with GA also had iron accumulation in the photoreceptors and internal limiting membrane as well as increased ferritin (which sequesters intracellular iron) and ferroportin (an iron export protein that transports unutilized/unstored intracellular iron).[81] Increased intracellular iron causes oxidative photoreceptor damage.[82] Although iron overload is a feature of AMD pathobiology, it is not clear that iron overload is a cause of AMD.[79]

Drusen biochemistry

Advanced glycation end products occur in soft drusen, in basal laminar and basal linear deposits, and in the cytoplasm of RPE cells associated with CNVs.[30,58] Advanced glycation end products induce increased expression of cytokines known to occur in CNVs.[30] Carboxymethyl lysine, a product of lipoprotein peroxidation or sequential oxidation and glycation, is present in drusen and CNVs.[58,83] One study of drusen protein composition reported oxidative protein modifications in tissue inhibitor of matrix

metalloproteinases-3 and vitronectin.[58] Also, carboxyethyl pyrrole (CEP) protein adducts, which are uniquely generated from the oxidation of docosahexaenoate-containing lipids, were present and were much more abundant in drusen from AMD versus age-matched control donors.[58] (Docosahexaenoic acid is abundant in the outer retina, where it is readily susceptible to oxidation.[84]) Gu and coworkers[85] found that the mean level of anti-CEP immunoreactivity in AMD human plasma was 1.5-fold higher than in age-matched controls. Sera from AMD patients demonstrated mean titers of anti-CEP autoantibody 2.3-fold higher than controls.[85] In addition to being consistent with the notions that AMD is associated with oxidative damage and that CEP immunoreactivity and autoantibody titer may predict AMD susceptibility, these results indicate that the immune system may play a role in AMD pathogenesis.

AMD is associated with chronic inflammation

Anatomic studies provided initial evidence for the role of inflammation in the early and late stages of AMD (see Zarbin[57] for references). In addition to membranous debris that is probably derived from RPE cells,[42,57,86] drusen contain complement components C3 and C5, components of the membrane attack complex (C5b-9), complement factor H (CFH), and C-reactive protein (CRP) (Table 68.1).[32,33,35,87,88] Bioactive fragments of C3 (C3a) and C5 (C5a) are present in drusen and induce vascular endothelial growth factor expression in RPE cells.[89] These findings provide a mechanistic explanation for the fact that confluent soft drusen are a risk factor for CNVs in AMD eyes. In fact, CNVs cannot be induced by laser photocoagulation in C3-deficient mice.[90] Thus, the presence of proinflammatory molecules in drusen creates a stimulus for chronic inflammation in the RPE–Bruch's membrane–choriocapillaris complex that can result in some features of late AMD.

Drusen, GA, and CNVs are associated with mutations in components of the complement pathway, which is part of the innate immune system[92]

Three enzyme cascades comprise the complement system (Figure 68.3): the classical pathway (activated by antigen–antibody complexes and surface-bound CRP), the alternative pathway (activated by surface-bound C3b, microbial pathogens, or cellular debris), and the lectin pathway (activated by mannose, a typical component of microbial cell walls, and oxidative stress).

Mutations in the CFH gene (*CFH*), as well as in the closely related genes *CFHR1*, *CFHR2*, *CFHR3*, *CFHR4*, and *CFHR5*, are strongly associated with both increased and decreased risk for AMD.[88,93–97] The *CFH* Y402H variant (in which tyrosine is replaced with histidine at amino acid 402) is located within a binding site for CRP and is associated with increased risk for drusen, GA, and CNVs.[98–101] Individuals homozygous for the *CFH* Y402H variant have a 48% risk of developing GA or CNVs by age 95 years versus a risk of 22% in noncarriers.[101] Nonetheless, one study reported that no single polymorphism (including Y402H) could account for the contribution of the *CFH* locus to disease susceptibility.[102]

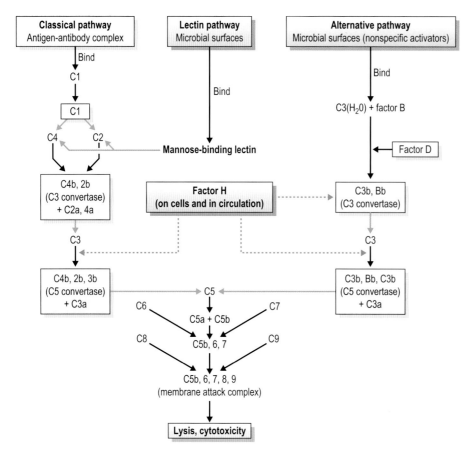

Figure 68.3 The complement pathway. Alternative pathway C3 convertase (C3bBb) cleaves C3 into C3a and C3b, which fosters the cleavage of C5 and, ultimately, the formation of a membrane attack complex (C5b, 6, 7, 8, 9) that causes cell lysis.[91,92] The alternative pathway is indiscriminate, with the propensity to damage host and foreign surfaces equally. Host cells use membrane-integrated and surface-attached plasma regulators to control complement activation at the cell surface.[153] Regulators expressed on the host cell surface include CD35 (complement receptor 1), CD46 (membrane cofactor protein), CD55 (decay-accelerating factor), C8-binding protein, and CD59. Soluble regulators include complement factor H (CFH), factor H-like protein 1 (FHL-1), which is an alternative splice product of the *CFH* gene, complement factor I, C1 inhibitor, C4 binding protein, clusterin, and vitronectin.[91,153] CFH binds and inactivates C3b bound to intact host cells, accelerates the decay of C3 convertase, and is a cofactor for complement factor I (a serine protease that inactivates C3b bound to the host cell), thus protecting intact host cells and permitting destruction of foreign or damaged host cells (see Donoso et al[92] and Oppermann et al[161] for references). C-reactive protein (CRP) binding to CFH increases its affinity for C3b, which results in downregulation of complement activity. (CRP can activate the classical pathway, however, through its interaction with C1q.[162]) The classical, the lectin, and the alternative pathways all generate membrane attack complexes via C3 cleavage.[92] Thus, CFH can inhibit cell lysis and cytotoxicity arising from all three pathways. The presence of multiple, redundantly acting regulators allows host cells to remain protected, even if any single regulator is defective/missing.[153] In the setting of inactive/absent CFH, the lack of cell surface complement regulators may lead to tissue-specific damage.[163] C3 is the most abundant complement component in plasma, and C3 mRNA is present in the retina, retinal pigment epithelium (RPE), and choroid.[35] The ocular distribution of CFH, factor B, C2, and C3 protein is similar, involving mainly the RPE, Bruch's membrane, and drusen.[104] (Redrawn with permission from Donoso LA, Kim D, Frost A, et al. The role of inflammation in the pathogenesis of age-related macular degeneration. Surv Ophthalmol 2006;51:137–152.)

Altered interactions of CRP and CFH may lead to changes in C3b activation. Homozygotes with the 402HH genotype have a 2.5-fold increase in CRP in the RPE and choroid compared with 402YY controls, independent of AMD disease status.[103] CFH and FHL-1 with the Y402H mutation display reduced binding to CRP, heparin, and RPE cells, which can cause inefficient complement regulation at the cell surface, particularly when CRP is recruited to sites of injury.[97]

Mutations in factor B (BF) and complement component 2 (C2) alter the risk of AMD.[104] Both risk and protective BF and C2 haplotypes exist. These effects may be independent of *CFH* mutations.[105] C2 is involved in C3 cleavage via the classical pathway, and BF is involved in C3 cleavage via the alternative pathway (Figure 68.3).[92]

A single nucleotide polymorphism in the C3 gene (R80G) was strongly associated with AMD in both an English and a Scottish group of patients.[106] The estimated population-attributable risk was 22%.

Oxidative damage can activate the complement system

Cultured immortalized RPE cells that have accumulated A2E and are irradiated to induce A2E photo-oxidation form C3 split products in overlying serum.[107] Thus, products of the photo-oxidation of bis-retinoid lipofuscin pigments in RPE cells may serve as a trigger for the complement system.[107]

Given the relative abundance of lipofuscin in the submacular RPE, this trigger could predispose the macula to chronic inflammation and AMD. These experiments link RPE lipofuscin, oxidative damage, drusen, and inflammation, all of which have been implicated in AMD pathogenesis.[57,92,107]

Oxidative stress reduces the ability of interferon-γ to increase *CFH* expression in RPE cells.[108] Interferon-γ-induced increase in *CFH* is mediated by transcriptional activation by STAT1, and its suppression by oxidative stress is mediated by acetylation of FOXO3, which enhances FOXO3 binding to the *CFH* promoter and inhibits STAT1 interaction with the *CFH* promoter.

Hollyfield and coworkers described an animal model that links oxidative damage and complement activation to AMD.[109] Mice were immunized with mouse serum albumin adducted with CEP, a unique oxidation fragment of docosahexaenoic acid that is present in drusen of AMD eyes.[58] Immunized mice developed antibodies to the hapten, fixed C3 in Bruch's membrane, accumulated drusen, and developed lesions resembling GA. Choroidal neovascularization was not observed. An intact immune system is required for these events, which may mean that both the adaptive and innate components of the immune system are required for the development of GA.

Among patients with defective complement regulation and MPGN II, drusen tend to occur in the macular region (as do GA and CNVs).[14,17] One may speculate that oxidative damage is more pronounced in the macular region, and, as a result, chronic inflammatory damage is more concentrated in the macula.

AMD risk-enhancing mutations not directly involving the complement pathway are also linked to inflammation and/or oxidative damage (Table 68.2)

An AMD susceptibility locus on chromosome 10 (10q26) seems to play a major role in AMD pathogenesis.[110-115] The protein encoded by the hypothetical gene *LOC387715* (with an alanine-serine polymorphism as the likely disease-causing variant) in 10q26 may be involved in AMD pathogenesis and is flanked by *PLEKHA1* and high-temperature requirement factor A1 (*HTRA1*). Although two groups found that mutations in *HTRA1* are associated with increased risk of AMD (Table 68.2), another group found that this gene was only indirectly associated with AMD.[116] Mutations in *CFH, BF, C2,* and *HTRA1* seem to confer risk in an independent, log-additive fashion.[111,114,117]

Mitochondrial haplogroup H is associated with a reduced prevalence of any AMD.[118] Haplogroup J is associated with a higher prevalence of large, soft distinct drusen, and haplogroup U is associated with an increased prevalence of RPE abnormalities.

In contrast to mutations affecting the complement system, mutations in *Fibulin5,*[119] *Fibulin6,*[120,121] apolipoprotein E (APOE),[122-125] and possibly *ABCA4*[126-131] may cause AMD but only in a relatively small number of patients. Some of these (or related) mutations seem to enhance complement activation either through alterations in the ECM or through increased lipofuscin accumulation.[132]

Mutations causing nonexudative versus exudative complications of AMD

The TLR3 412Phe variant of the Toll-like receptor 3 gene (*TLR3*) seems to confer protection against GA among Americans of European descent with AMD, possibly by suppressing RPE apoptosis.[133] This association was only evident if controls were limited to patients with fewer than five small drusen. Since *TLR3* encodes a viral sensor that supports innate immunity, these results may mean that viral double-stranded DNA plays a role in the development of GA.[134]

Currently identified AMD-associated mutations in *CFH, TLR4, LCO387715/HTRA1, C2-BF,* and *C3* do not predispose to the development of GA versus CNVs to any significant degree.[99,101,106,111,135,136] These observations are consistent with the notion that GA and CNVs have a common pathogenesis at least with regard to the involvement of the complement system. Perhaps these genes play a critical role in the relatively early stages of AMD pathogenesis. Even among whites, for example, only a minority of patients with soft drusen progress to advanced AMD, which may mean that the main risk loci identified so far (1q32 and 10q26) are associated with development of the early manifestations of AMD and that the late manifestations are under the control of different genes and/or are a consequence of processes that are initiated relatively early in the disease. One study demonstrated that loci on chromosomes 5 (5p13) and 6 (6q21-23) seem to influence the rate of pigmentary abnormalities and GA progression.[137] These findings may indicate that separate genes modulate the risk of developing soft drusen versus pigmentary abnormalities and GA.[138] Other investigators have not reported identical results, but different methodologies were used.[139,140]

Data on gene–environment interactions seem to be inconclusive.[101,111,113,114,141-145] Nonetheless, it is interesting to note that cigarette smoking decreases plasma CHF levels,[146] and smoke-modified C3 has diminished binding to CFH.[147] Decreased levels or activity of CFH may result in uncontrolled complement-mediated tissue damage to the RPE–Bruch's membrane–choriocapillaris complex.

Table 68.2 Some age-related macular degeneration risk-enhancing mutations not directly involving the complement pathway

Locus/gene	Comment
HTRA1[117,164]	HTRA1 is a serine protease that is a member of the heat shock proteases and is expressed in retina
9q32-33/*TLR4* (Toll-like receptor 4)[135]	Mediates proinflammatory signaling, involved in outer-segment phagocytosis
LOC387715/ARMS2[116]	Localizes to mitochondrial outer membrane when expressed in mammalian cells
Fibulin5	
Fibulin6	
Apolipoprotein E	
ABCA4	

> ### Box 68.5 Treatment strategies for age-related macular degeneration
>
> - Reduce lipofuscin formation
> - Manage abnormalities of the complement system
> - Inhibit oxidative chemical reactions
> - Neuroprotection
> - Cell-based therapy

Treatment strategies

Antioxidants do not seem to be effective in the prevention of early AMD (i.e., drusen, retinal pigmentary changes: Box 68.5).[148] AREDS[75] did not show a statistically significant benefit of the AREDS formulation for either the development of new GA or for involvement of the fovea in eyes with pre-existing GA. In part, this result may be due to the paucity of GA patients in the study. The AREDS 2 study (http://www.clinicaltrials.gov/ct2/show/NCT00345176?term=AREDS&rank=1) will likely include more GA patients and provide more information about GA and its progression, and whether the proposed treatment benefits eyes with GA. Some additional strategies for dry AMD treatment are considered below.

Reduce lipofuscin formation

The fenretinide study aims at reducing lipofuscin accumulation, using an oral agent. Fenretinide binds serum retinol binding protein, displaces all-*trans*-retinol from RBP, and thus induces a loss of complex formation with transthyretin.[149] The result is impaired RPE uptake of all-*trans*-retinol, slowing of the visual cycle, and reduced lipofuscin deposition in a mouse model of Stargardt disease.[150] This molecule may reduce lipofuscin accumulation in GA and may slow the enlargement rate of GA (http://www.clinicaltrials.gov/ct2/show/NCT00429936?term=fenretinide&rank=28). Another approach is to inhibit the conversion of all-*trans*-retinyl ester to 11-*cis*-retinol by blocking RPE65 using nontoxic small molecules.[151]

Manage abnormalities of the complement system

Rheopheresis is under study for the treatment of dry AMD (http://www.clinicaltrials.gov/ct2/show/NCT00078221?cond=%22Dry+AMD%22&rank=4).[152] Perhaps this approach could remove chelatable pro-oxidants (e.g., iron) from Bruch's membrane or remove inhibitors of the regulators of the complement system. (The renal abnormalities in patients with MPGN and complement deregulation have been managed with plasma infusion and/or exchange,[153] and plasma exchange has been effective in treating neuroimmunological disorders.[154] However, chronic plasma infusion may not be a successful long-term therapy.[155])

In a preclinical model, Nozaki and coworkers[89] have shown that genetic ablation of receptors for C3a or C5a reduces CNV formation after laser injury and that antibody-mediated neutralization of C3a or C5a or pharmacological blockade of their receptors also reduces CNV formation. It is not clear whether this approach would also be helpful in the prevention of GA, but there is an animal model in which the approach may be tested.[109]

Gene therapy to silence genes by preventing mRNA expression is under clinical study for treatment of CNVs. This approach may be useful for prevention of nonexudative manifestations of AMD since deletion of genes closely related to CFH (i.e., *CFHR1* and *CFHR3*) seems to be strongly protective against AMD.[96] However, since the Leu-Leu genotype of *TLR3* is associated with increased apoptosis in RPE compared to the Leu-Phe genotype and since the TLR3 412Leu variant is associated with a relative increased risk of GA, short-interfering RNA therapies in the eye may be toxic.[134]

Inhibit oxidative chemical reactions

The OMEGA study uses an eyedrop with a prodrug, OT 551, to treat GA.[156] This prodrug penetrates the eye well and is converted in the eye to the active drug, which has an antioxidant effect and may reduce angiogenesis (http://www.clinicaltrials.gov/ct2/show/NCT00485394?term=Othera&rank=1).

Elucidation of the mechanism of suppression of interferon-γ-induced expression of *CFH* by oxidative stress provides targets for therapeutic intervention. Wu and coworkers suggested that local administration of acetylase inhibitors could help to blunt the oxidative stress-induced suppression of *CFH* expression in RPE cells.[108] Sustained increased expression of SIRT1 by gene transfer would accomplish the same goal. Ultimately, one could envision combination therapy in patients at risk for, or who show early signs of, AMD aimed at direct reduction of oxidative stress with antioxidants, suppression of acetylation of FOXO3, and use of other inhibitors of complement activation.

Cell-based therapy

Transplanted cells can secrete numerous molecules that may exert a beneficial effect on the host retina (i.e., neuroprotection), choroid, or both, even if they do not cure the underlying disease.[157] In the case of nonexudative AMD, cell transplants may prevent progression of GA (through replacement of dysfunctional or dead RPE) and may even bring about some visual improvement in selected patients (through rescue of photoreceptors that are dying but not dead).[158,159] The Ciliary Neurotrophic Factor (CNTF) study capitalizes on the ability of CNTF to slow degeneration and protect photoreceptors.[160] Encapsulated cells are implanted into the eye. These cells are genetically engineered to produce CNTF. The capsule allows CNTF to diffuse into the eye but does not allow the cells to migrate out of the capsule (http://www.clinicaltrials.gov/ct2/show/NCT00277134?term=CNTF&rank=2).

Conclusion

Dry AMD is a major cause of visual loss in industrialized societies. Pathological features include the accumulation of an abnormal ECM and photoreceptor, RPE, and choriocapillaris atrophy. One hypothesis of AMD pathophysiology is that oxidative damage incites inflammation at the level of RPE–Bruch's membrane–choriocapillaris, which is mediated via complement activation. Some patients with mutations in the complement system are less able to modulate the inflammatory response, resulting in excessive cellular damage and accumulation of extracellular debris. This chronic inflammatory response involves cellular components of the immune system as well as the classical and alternate pathways of the complement system. Accumulation of abnormal extracellular material, manifest in part as drusen and pigmentary abnormalities, fosters the development of the late sequelae of AMD in susceptible individuals. Many treatments for dry AMD are under investigation (e.g., antioxidant therapy, reduction of lipofuscin formation, management of complement system abnormalities, cell-based therapy) and are based on concepts related to this hypothesis of pathogenesis.

Key references

A complete list of chapter references is available online at www.expertconsult.com. See inside cover for registration details.

5. Sarks JP, Sarks SH, Killingsworth MC. Evolution of geographic atrophy of the retinal pigment epithelium. Eye 1988;2:552–577.

7. Sunness JS, Margalit E, Srikumaran D, et al. The long-term natural history of geographic atrophy from age-related macular degeneration: enlargement of atrophy and implications for interventional clinical trials. Ophthalmology 2007;114:271–277.

32. Anderson DH, Mullins RF, Hageman GS, et al. A role for local inflammation in the formation of drusen in the aging eye. Am J Ophthalmol 2002;134:411–431.

44. Korte GE, Burns MS, Bellhorn RW. Epithelium–capillary interactions in the eye: the retinal pigment epithelium and the choriocapillaris. Int Rev Cytol 1989;114:221–248.

49. Holz FG, Bindewald-Wittich A, Fleckenstein M, et al. Progression of geographic atrophy and impact of fundus autofluorescence patterns in age-related macular degeneration. Am J Ophthalmol 2007;143:463–472.

57. Zarbin MA. Current concepts in the pathogenesis of age-related macular degeneration. Arch Ophthalmol 2004;122:598–614.

78. Shen JK, Dong A, Hackett SF, et al. Oxidative damage in age-related macular degeneration. Histol Histopathol 2007;22:1301–1308.

88. Hageman GS, Anderson DH, Johnson LV, et al. A common haplotype in the complement regulatory gene factor H (HF1/CFH) predisposes individuals to age-related macular degeneration. Proc Natl Acad Sci USA 2005;102:7227–7232.

89. Nozaki M, Raisler BJ, Sakurai E, et al. Drusen complement components C3a and C5a promote choroidal neovascularization. Proc Natl Acad Sci USA 2006;103:2328–2333.

92. Donoso LA, Kim D, Frost A, et al. The role of inflammation in the pathogenesis of age-related macular degeneration. Surv Ophthalmol 2006;51:137–152.

93. Klein RJ, Zeiss C, Chew EY, et al. Complement factor H polymorphism in age-related macular degeneration. Science 2005;308:385–389.

94. Edwards AO, Ritter R 3rd, Abel KJ, et al. Complement factor H polymorphism and age-related macular degeneration. Science 2005;308:421–424.

95. Haines JL, Hauser MA, Schmidt S, et al. Complement factor H variant increases the risk of age-related macular degeneration. Science 2005;308:419–421.

109. Hollyfield JG, Bonilha VL, Rayborn ME, et al. Oxidative damage-induced inflammation initiates age-related macular degeneration. Nat Med 2008;14:194–198.

150. Radu RA, Han Y, Bui TV, et al. Reductions in serum vitamin A arrest accumulation of toxic retinal fluorophores: a potential therapy for treatment of lipofuscin-based retinal diseases. Invest Ophthalmol Vis Sci 2005;46:4393–4401.

Neovascular age-related macular degeneration

David E Lederer, Scott W Cousins, and Karl G Csaky

Age-related macular degeneration (AMD) is a disease associated with a deterioration of central vision. As AMD is the leading cause of blindness in persons aged 75 and older in the USA and other countries worldwide, its importance cannot be underestimated.[1,2]

AMD is a spectrum of disease that is diagnosed based on clinical examination. It can be divided into nonneovascular, also known as dry or nonexudative disease, and neovascular, also known as wet or exudative disease. Advanced AMD is a term used to describe the most severe forms of AMD, namely geographic atrophy involving the center of macula, the fovea, or features of choroidal neovascularization (CNV). CNV is the growth of new blood vessels from the choroid toward the retina. They breach Bruch's membrane and proliferate under the retinal pigment epithelium (RPE) and/or the retina.

Treatment of CNV has blossomed recently with the advent of anti-vascular endothelial growth factor (VEGF) therapy, yet a cure still remains elusive. A thorough understanding of the pathogenesis of neovascular AMD is important both for treating patients with AMD and for exploring new modes of therapy.

Clinical background

AMD involves the photoreceptors responsible for central vision, thus explaining the most common clinical presentation. Patients with neovascular AMD will typically note decreased or distorted vision. However other typical complaints include scotomas, micropsia or, occasionally, the patient may be asymptomatic.[3] Symptoms are secondary to fluid and/or blood within or under the retina that results in disruption of the retinal architecture. Clinical examination combined with ancillary testing will confirm the presence of CNV, the hallmark of neovascular AMD (see diagnostic workup, below). As the disease progresses, complications such as RPE tears, breakthrough vitreous hemorrhage, or disciform scarring may result.

Historical development

Natural history data of neovascular AMD have been evaluated in a meta-analysis providing a sound basis for treatment. Using 53 trials a comprehensive study concluded that vision loss of 0–3 lines occurred in 76% of untreated patients at 3 months. Severe visual loss (> 6 lines) was seen in 10% of untreated patients at 3 months, 28% at 1 year, and 43% at 3 years.[4]

Interestingly, while AMD was described as early as 1885, most of the current concepts of neovascular disease are attributed to J Donald M Gass and his work starting as early as the late 1960s. However, it was not until the early 1990s and the publication of the Macular Photocoagulation Study (MPS) that a documented effective treatment was achieved from a randomized controlled clinical trial (Figure 69.1). Yet, the MPS only demonstrated a favorable treatment benefit for patients with extra- or juxtafoveal CNV due to the immediate visual loss associated with thermal laser performed to the foveal center.[5,6] The next major breakthrough came in the late 1990s with the advent of photodynamic therapy (PDT). This opened the door to treating more patients using angiographic-based categories. Major clinical trials demonstrated a beneficial effect in treating subfoveal CNV in the reduction of moderate (3 or more lines) and severe (6 or more lines) visual loss in patients treated with PDT therapy versus placebo at 1 and 2 years. However, even the most efficacious subgroup analysis still demonstrated a 23% chance of moderate visual loss by 1 year despite treatment.[7,8]

Basic research into understanding the pathophysiology of neovascular AMD identified angiogenic growth factors as key regulators of CNV. This, in turn, led to the development of pharmacotherapy aimed at inhibiting angiogenic factors. In 2004 pegaptanib (Macugen) emerged as the first drug selectively to block the angiogenic factor VEGF-A, specifically targeting the 165 isoform. Treatment of CNV regardless of angiographic characteristics was proven in the VEGF Inhibition Study in Ocular Neovascularization (VISION) trial. It was ascertained that 71% of treated patients lost less than 3 lines of vision versus 55% for the control groups.[9] In 2005, off-label bevacizumab (Avastin) began to be used to treat patients with neovascular AMD, with anecdotal reports indicating excellent results. In particular, some patients noted an improvement in visual acuity.[10,11]

Stabilization and improvement of visual acuity were further categorized in the clinical trials surrounding ranibizumab (Lucentis) therapy. Ranibizumab is an intravitreal injectable medication approved by the Food and Drug Administration that, like bevacizumab, binds all isoforms of

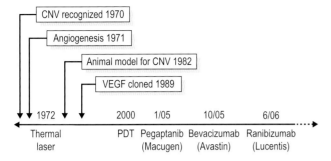

Figure 69.1 Timeline of discovery of therapy for neovascular age-related macular degeneration. CNV, choroidal neovascularization; VEGF, vascular endothelial growth factor; PDT, photodynamic therapy.

VEGF-A. Compared to bevacizumab it is smaller and has a greater affinity for VEGF.[12] Two phase III clinical trials proved the efficacy of intravitreal ranibizumab as approximately 95% of patients lost less than 3 lines of vision in the treated groups versus nearly 65% in the controls. Perhaps even more surprising was that these trials represented the first prospective, randomized, controlled clinical trials to show a gain in visual acuity in neovascular AMD, with approximately 35% of treated patients gaining 3 or more lines of vision versus 5% in the control groups.[13,14]

Treatment of neovascular AMD is an area of blossoming growth. From initial treatment with thermal laser to modern approaches of VEGF blockade, the treatment of neovascular AMD is now aimed at early diagnosis and visual improvement rather than slowing the natural history. As we continue to understand more of the pathophysiology behind neovascular AMD, we will see a proliferation of new therapies and a combination of existing treatment options.

Epidemiology

AMD is a common disease that predominantly affects the elderly white population. Epidemiologic studies have provided estimates of disease prevalence in a variety of countries across the world. A large meta-analysis was performed providing pooled data on the prevalence of neovascular AMD by age, gender, and race.[15] Selected data are presented in Table 69.1 and the reader is referred to the original studies for further details.

Diagnostic workup

The diagnosis of neovascular AMD is ascertained based on clinical symptoms and signs. Metamorphopsia and decreased visual acuity are the most common symptoms. Clinical examination by slit-lamp biomicroscopy may show a grayish-green membrane under the retina, hemorrhage under or within the retina, and/or RPE detachments. However, ancillary testing is an important adjunct to diagnosis in many cases and serves as confirmatory evidence prior to initiating treatment (Box 69.1).

Traditionally, ancillary testing and diagnostic confirmation were based on fluorescein angiography (Figure 69.2). With the development of optical coherence tomography

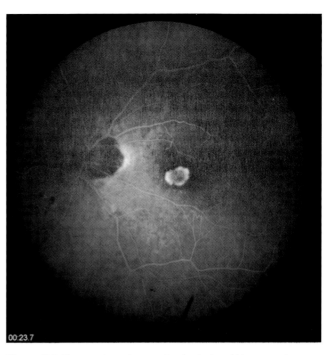

Figure 69.2 Fluorescein angiogram of a classic choroidal neovascular membrane.

Table 69.1 Prevalence rates for wet age-related macular degeneration

Age (years)	White females	White males	Black females	Black males
55–59	0.16	0.28	0.60	0.30
60–64	0.26	0.42	0.73	0.37
65–69	0.51	0.73	0.89	0.45
70–74	1.09	1.33	1.08	0.55
75–79	2.40	2.49	1.31	0.67
≥80	11.07	8.29	1.78	0.92

Modified from The Eye Diseases Prevalence Research Group. Prevalence of age-related macular degeneration in the United States. Arch Ophthalmol 2004;122:564–572.
Data are presented as prevalence per 100 individuals.

Box 69.1 Diagnostic workup for neovascular age-related macular degeneration includes many ancillary testing techniques

- Fluorescein angiography assesses leakage from incompetent neovascular vessels imaging the area of choroidal neovascularization
- Optical coherence tomography uses reflected light to create an optical cross-section of the retina enhancing morphometric evaluation
- Dynamic indocyanine green angiography assesses flow within the choroidal vasculature enabling visualization of the following vascular patterns:
  - Capillary-dominated lesions
  - Arteriolar-dominated lesions
  - Mixed capillary–arteriolar lesions

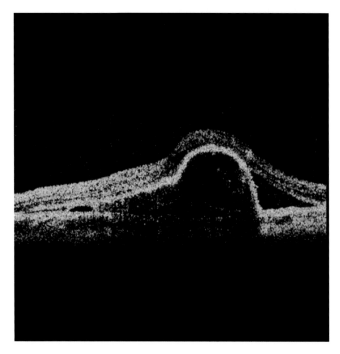

Figure 69.3 Optical coherence tomography of a patient with neovascular age-related macular degeneration showing evidence of both a pigment epithelial detachment and subretinal fluid.

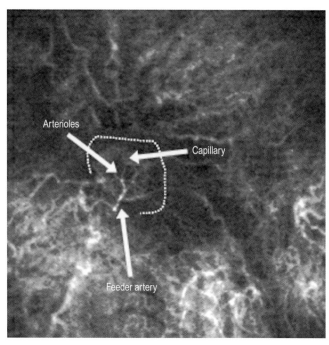

Figure 69.4 Single frame from a dynamic indocyanine green angiography of a choroidal neovascular lesion demonstrating a mixed capillary–arteriolar lesion.

(OCT), this serves as a critical adjunctive tool (Figure 69.3). More recently, dynamic indocyanine green (ICG) angiography has allowed visualization of the neovascular complex and morphologic determination (Figure 69.4). Finally, the role of fundus autofluorescence is being evaluated for a complementary role in determining RPE health.[16]

Due to the biochemical properties of fluorescein dye, 15% is nonprotein-bound in the blood stream after injection. This allows fluorescein to leak out of incompetent neovascular vessels imaging the area of CNV. Fluorescein angiographic patterns can be subdivided into classic and occult based on the pattern of leakage. OCT has further helped diagnose and follow CNV lesions. In this imaging modality, reflected light is used to create an optical cross-section of the retina. Typical findings include any combination of the following: subretinal fluid, RPE detachments, diffuse retinal thickening, cystic changes within the retina, and hyperreflectivity corresponding to the neovascular lesion. Dynamic ICG angiography has been another area of recent development in defining morphologic patterns of CNV. Due to the near-infrared range of light absorption (~805 nm) and emission spectrum (~835 nm) and protein-bound affinity (98%) of ICG dye, visualization of the choroidal vasculature is possible. Furthermore, with the advent of confocal scanning lasers and rapid computer-processing algorithms, the sequence can be viewed as a dynamic movie (16 frames per second) versus static images (maximum 1 frame per second). This allows dynamic ICG to evaluate flow within the vasculature and not merely leakage, as traditional fluorescein and static ICG angiography have done in the past. The authors have evaluated hundreds of cases and determined the following patterns of pathophysiologic sig-

---

Box 69.2 Subtypes of neovascular age-related macular degeneration

- Traditional choroidal neovascularization is a process where new blood vessels grow from the choroid, breach Bruch's membrane, and proliferate under the retinal pigment epithelium and/or retina
- Polypoidal choroidal neovascularization is defined as aneurysmal, or polypoidal, dilations of the inner choroidal vasculature
- Retinal angiomatous proliferation is defined as a neovascular process commencing with an angiomatous proliferation within the retina

---

nificance: capillary-dominated lesions, arteriolar-dominated lesions, and mixed subtypes of the two. Ongoing research into this modality will help to define the role of dynamic ICG angiography in prognosticating therapeutic responsiveness.

Differential diagnosis

The differential diagnosis of neovascular AMD can be viewed from three separate perspectives. First, as our understanding has developed surrounding neovascular AMD, three main subtypes have been delineated: polypoidal CNV, retinal angiomatous proliferation (RAP), and traditional CNV (Box 69.2).

Polypoidal CNV is defined as aneurysmal, or polypoidal, dilations of the inner choroidal vasculature and is best imaged with ICG angiography.[17] RAP is defined as a neovascular process commencing with an angiomatous proliferation within the retina that subsequently invades subretinally and eventually progresses to develop a chorioretinal anastomosis.[18] Both polypoidal CNV and RAP are subtypes of the occult type of CNV and have been clinically detected using ICG angiography. Traditional CNV is a process where new blood vessels grow from the choroid, breach Bruch's membrane, and proliferate under the RPE and/or retina.

The second perspective to view the differential diagnosis of neovascular AMD is other causes of CNV besides AMD. While the list is extensive, common diseases include high myopia, angioid streaks, choroidal rupture posttrauma, and intraocular inflammatory disease.

Finally, the differential diagnosis of neovascular AMD may be viewed from the perspective of other diseases that simulate CNV but are not true CNV. Diseases such as central serous chorioretinopathy and adult-onset foveovitelliform macular dystrophy can be difficult to distinguish from true CNV. To confound matters, both diseases can also be complicated by true CNV. However, typical history and ancillary testing will allow differentiation in challenging cases.

Pathology

The clinical hallmark of AMD in general is the presence of soft drusen and pigmentary changes in the macula. Pathologically this has correlated with basal laminar deposits. Basal laminar deposits represent material accumulation between the basal aspect of the RPE and its underlying basement membrane. As basal laminar deposits continue to enlarge, and eventually become continuous, a correlation with basal linear deposits is noted. Meanwhile, basal linear deposits represent accumulation of material between the basement membrane of the RPE and the inner collagenous zone of Bruch's membrane. The combination of continuous basal laminar deposits and basal linear deposits represents the earliest pathological changes seen in AMD.[19] The clinical manifestations of the advanced stages of theses pathologic changes are noted as drusen deposits under the neurosensory retina.

As AMD develops, morphologic changes in the macular region are noted. Eyes with neovascular AMD are noted to have increased degrees of calcification and fragmentation of Bruch's membrane when compared to age-matched controls. These morphologic changes in Bruch's membrane are not noted in subjects with nonneovascular AMD. However, the fellow eyes of subjects with unilateral neovascular AMD do have increased amounts of Bruch's membrane calcification and fragmentation (Figure 69.5).[20]

Histopathology of excised choroidal neovascular membranes from human eyes with AMD has demonstrated a variety of structural and cellular components. Variability in the degree of fibrosis versus inflammatory nature of the membrane has been noted and may reflect activity and chronicity.[21] Cellular components have included RPE cells, myofibroblasts, vascular endothelial cells, and inflammatory cells. In particular, while leukocytes were noted focally within the core of the membrane, macrophages were seen diffusely scattered. It is interesting to note that polymorphonuclear cells are rarely seen[22] (Box 69.3).

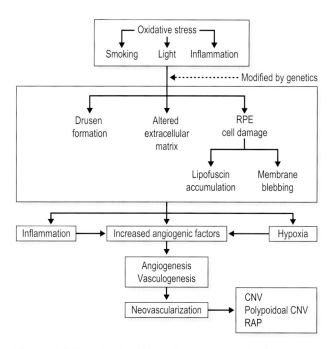

Figure 69.5 Normal and pathologic changes associated with aging in neovascular age-related macular degeneration. RPE, retinal pigment epithelium; CNV, choroidal neovascularization; RAP, retinal angiomatous proliferation.

Box 69.3 Key pathologic features of neovascular age-related macular degeneration

- Bruch's membrane calcification
- Bruch's membrane fragmentation
- Important cellular components of neovascular membranes

Inflammatory

- Macrophages: microglia and bone marrow-derived
- Leukocytes

Fibrosis

- Myofibroblasts

Other

- Vascular endothelial cells: local resident cells and vascular progenitor cell precursors
- Retinal pigment epithelium cells

Pathophysiology

A variety of etiologic components contribute to the pathophysiology of neovascular AMD. These include pathologic changes associated with aging, genetic polymorphisms, aberrant tissue response to injury from oxidative stress, and biochemical modulators of neovascularization (Figure 69.6). We will review each etiology and its accompanying pathophysiologic derangements in turn.

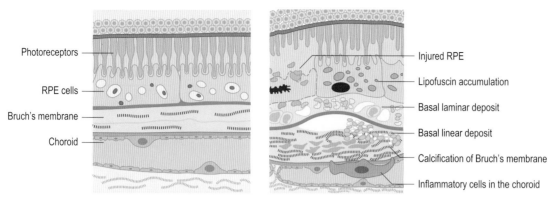

Photoreceptors

RPE cells

Bruch's membrane

Choroid

Injured RPE

Lipofuscin accumulation

Basal laminar deposit

Basal linear deposit

Calcification of Bruch's membrane

Inflammatory cells in the choroid

Figure 69.6 Proposed sequence of events leading to the development of neovascular age-related macular degeneration. RPE, retinal pigment epithelium.

Pathologic changes associated with aging

As previously noted, neovascular AMD is accompanied by several morphologic changes in the choroid and Bruch's membrane. Bruch's membrane is actually a representation of several layers, including the basement membrane of the RPE, an inner collagenous zone, an elastic layer, an outer collagenous zone, and finally the basement membrane of the choriocapillaris. The compositions of basal laminar and basal linear deposits that accumulate in AMD speak to the mechanisms responsible for the development of this disease. Specifically, these deposits are comprised of lipids, proteins, cellular structures from RPE cells and choroidal dendritic cells, and a smaller amount of carbohydrates at their core.[23] As proposed by Hageman et al,[23] the biogenesis of drusen begins with RPE injury from a variety of factors, including genetic mutations and oxidative injury from light and systemic factors such as smoking, lipofuscin accumulation, and ischemia. This leads to RPE cell death and the release of stimulatory molecules (for example, cytokines) that recruit dendritic cells from the choroidal circulation. The dendritic cells send cellular processes through Bruch's membrane and undergo local maturation to form the core of the drusen. Further amplification of this local inflammatory response may result in complement activation, extracellular matrix (ECM) proteolysis, and macrophage recruitment.

Other morphologic changes associated with aging include an age-related accumulation of lipofuscin in the RPE cytoplasm from 1% by volume in the first decade of life to 19% in the ninth decade, thickening of Bruch's membrane from 2 μm at birth to 4–6 μm by the 10th decade of life, and decreased permeability of substances across Bruch's membrane.[24–26] It is likely that this combination of aging in conjunction with genetic predispositions, drusen accumulation, oxidative stress, and inflammatory changes contributes to the neovascularization seen in neovascular AMD.

Genetics

Genetics is a well-established risk factor for the development of AMD. Epidemiologic evidence in twin studies has demonstrated a higher concordance among monozygotic versus dizygotic twins.[27] As genetic testing has evolved several genes have been isolated that portend a high risk for the develop-

ment of AMD. In an excellent review by Montezuma et al[28] the authors note the most commonly implicated gene is complement factor H (*CFH*) on chromosome 1q. Additionally, the genetic polymorphisms seen in the genes *PLEKHA1/LOC387715/HTRA1* on chromosome 10q appear to be important. The genetic polymorphisms associated with these genes account for, approximately, a 2–10-fold increased risk of developing AMD independent of, but modified by, other risk factors such as ethnicity, environmental exposures (e.g., smoking), and systemic health (e.g., body mass index). CFH gene polymorphisms may cause loss of inhibition of the complement system thus allowing complement-mediated damage of the RPE. Meanwhile, *HTRA1* overexpression may disrupt Bruch's membrane through the degradation of the ECM, which may permit vascular remodeling. Of the three proposed genes on chromosome 10q this is the most attractive based on biologic plausibility. Other genes identified in AMD linkage and association studies include adenosine triphosphate-binding cassette rim protein (ABCR), apolipoprotein E (ApoE), and specifically the e2 genotype, the HLA genes, and polymorphisms in the gene for vascular endothelial growth factor, to name a few.[28]

While these candidate genes have not all been evaluated in a population with only neovascular AMD, the genetic polymorphisms in *CFH* and *LOC387715/HTRA1* have been assessed and shown to account for, on average, up to a four-fold and 33-fold increased risk of developing neovascular AMD, respectively.[29]

Response to injury

Injury to the RPE cells is believed to play a key role in the pathogenesis of neovascular AMD (Box 69.4). Injury comes from a variety of sources, including oxidative stress from the environment, systemic risk factors, and aberrant immunity. As noted above, injury to the RPE cells incites a cascade of events leading to drusen formation. Additionally, there is a strong inflammatory component to neovascular membranes (see Pathology). It is interesting to note the findings from the Age Related Eye Disease Study (AREDS)[30] showing a statistically significant benefit (odds ratio 0.62, 99% confidence interval 0.43–0.90) in preventing the development of neovascular AMD in subjects at highest risk. This suggests a putative role of oxidative stress in the development of neo-

Box 69.4 Response to injury hypothesis

Enciting events

Oxidative stress

- Smoking
- Free radicals: generated from light exposure, retinal oxygen demands, and photopigment recycling

Accumulation of basal laminar and basal linear drusen

Effects on tissue

- Nonlethal cell membrane blebbing
- Dysregulated turnover of the extracellular matrix
- Inflammation

vascular AMD as the constituents of the vitamin supplementation under investigation are thought to exert their effect by acting as antioxidants. These findings highlight the importance of zinc and vitamins A, C, and E and epidemiologic data support the role of lutein, zeaxanthin, and omega-3 long-chain polyunsaturated fatty acids.[31]

Oxidative stressors

Oxidative stress via smoking is a well-established risk factor for AMD and may confer, on average, a two- to threefold risk of developing neovascular disease.[32]

Light exposure is another source of oxidative stress and may be involved in the production of free radicals. Free radicals are not merely produced due to the high irradiation levels of the retina but also due to the retina's high oxygen demands and photopigment recycling with its incumbent induction of oxidative stress.[33]

The RPE and retinal tissue are also affected by basal laminar, basal linear, and clinically observable drusen. This abnormal accumulation of extracellular material under the RPE and within Bruch's membrane leads to not merely a compositional change in the tissue but also to alteration in permeability to molecular flow to and from RPE cells.[26] These findings imply a deranged tissue response that may contribute to further damage when under conditions of oxidative stress.

Effect of oxidative stress on tissues

While oxidative stress may lead to lethal responses, i.e., cell death, it may also lead to nonlethal responses that induce a functional change from baseline compatible with continued life but leading to tissue, and ultimately organ, dysfunction. The pathogenesis of this dysfunction can come from multiple etiologies, including cell membrane blebbing and dysregulated turnover of the ECM.

Nonlethal cell membrane blebbing is the process by which a cell can pinch off part of its plasma membrane and cytosol in an attempt to discard damaged cellular organelles, molecules, and lipid membranes. Importantly, nuclear fragmentation and cellular death do not occur.[34]

Dysregulated production and breakdown of the ECM may also contribute to the pathogenesis of AMD. This is because the normal anatomy and physiology of the ECM in most tissue require continuous turnover of collagen and other matrix components in a tightly regulated manner with rela-

tively small dysregulation producing profound changes in the ECM. This is evidenced by in vitro studies demonstrating RPE cellular dysfunction from oxidative stress and noting an abnormal increase in ECM with the accumulation of collagen and altered matrix metalloproteinase activity.[35]

Inflammatory response and tissue injury

The inflammatory response to oxidative injury is also an area of intense investigation. CNV membranes are known to have many cellular components, including inflammatory cells composed of a significant macrophage presence.[21] It is interesting to note that macrophage depletion in animal models decreases the severity of CNV lesions.[36] Additionally, patients with activated macrophages, defined as higher levels of tumor necrosis factor-α mRNA, demonstrated a fivefold increased prevalence of CNV secondary to AMD.[37] Furthermore, many of the macrophages in CNV lesions have been shown to be composed of bone marrow-derived versus resident microglia (specialized tissue-resident macrophages within neuronal tissues), macrophages. This indicates a role of bone marrow-derived cellular constituents that may contribute to CNV.

Importance of extracellular matrix

The ECM is important to allow vascular remodeling. Specifically, the matrix metalloproteinases are a family of proteolytic enzymes that function to degrade the ECM. The tissue inhibitors of metalloproteinases serve to modulate this proteolytic activity and a pathological balance between the two is present in neovascular AMD.[38]

The inciting event is likely a combination of genetics, oxidative stress, and hypoxia and upregulation of proangiogenic molecules that ultimately leads to ECM breakdown, allowing vascular remodeling and neovascularization under the control of angiogenic mediators.

Neovascularization: angiogenesis and vasculogenesis

Changes in the local environment of the retina arise from a variety of etiologic sources, including genetics, aging, oxidative damage, and response to injury. Ongoing research indicates that these local changes combine to result in abnormal neovascularization typically arising from the choroid and growing toward the retina. As with all vascular growth, these vessels may arise as endothelial sprouts from pre-existing capillary channels (termed angiogenesis) or de novo from circulating bone marrow-derived cells (termed vasculogenesis) (Figure 69.7).[39,40] It is helpful to look at each concept in turn to understand their contribution to what we have generically termed CNV in neovascular AMD.

Angiogenesis is an area of significant research. While many etiologic factors exist, the upregulation of angiogenic factors is at the heart of the concept and the RPE serves as an important modulator of this activity.[41] In brief, proangiogenic molecules serve as a stimulus for the resident endothelial cells of the choriocapillaris to undergo proliferation.[42] VEGF-A is known to be a key molecular component of this process. Yet, angiogenic molecules in general are

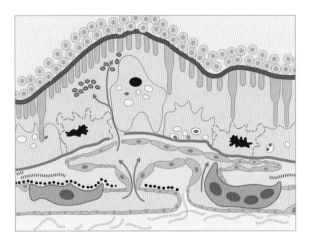

Angiogenesis: CNV arising from preexisting choriocapillaris vasculature

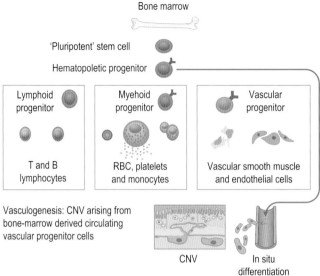

Figure 69.7 Two paradigms for choroidal neovascularization (CNV).

represented by pro- and antiangiogenic types. However these interactions are complex and some molecules regulate vascular proliferation differently in vivo compared to in vitro. In general, well-characterized proangiogenic molecules include VEGF and fibroblast growth factor with more complex roles for angiopoietins. Meanwhile, the best-characterized antiangiogenic molecule is pigment epithelium-derived growth factor.[43] In the angiogenesis theory of neovascularization, proangiogenic factors regulate, in a multistep process, the proteolysis of the surrounding ECM, allowing endothelial cell migration, proliferation, and capillary tube formation.

In contrast, vasculogenesis refers to the formation of blood vessels de novo from circulating vascular progenitor cells (VPCs), which home to the site of future neovascularization and differentiate to become endothelial cells and vascular smooth-muscle cells (Box 69.5). The stimulus for recruitment of these cells may come from oxidative stress, hypoxia, or upregulation of angiogenic molecules, similar to the concept of angiogenesis.[44] Yet, the distinguishing factor of the vasculogenesis theory is based on circulating VPCs rather than a simple proliferation of endogenous endothelial cells. Recent research into the role of vasculogenesis in CNV has begun to solidify this concept as a contributor to CNV in neovascular AMD.[40,45] Specifically, identification of bone marrow-derived endothelial cells, vascular smooth-muscle cells, and macrophages from animal models of CNV has been demonstrated.[46] Furthermore, approximately 50% of endothelial cells in neovascular membranes are noted to be derived from bone marrow sources, reiterating the importance of vasculogenesis in neovascularization.[47]

Conclusion

Understanding the pathophysiology of neovascular AMD is crucial to improving diagnosis and therapies for this disease.

First, we need to refine our understanding of pathologic changes associated with aging and their relationship to genetic polymorphisms. Combined with tissue response to injury from oxidative stress and hypoxia we will unravel the association with angiogenic factor modulation. Finally, understanding the role of both angiogenesis and vasculogenesis in neovascular formation will allow further therapeutic intervention. By combining traditional examination techniques with imaging modalities such as dynamic ICG angiography we will be able to study in vivo these neovascular changes. With these pathophysiologic advancements new treatment modalities to control and finally cure this prominent disease will be developed.

Key references

A complete list of chapter references is available online at www.expertconsult.com. See inside cover for registration details.

6. Macular Photocoagulation Study Group. Visual outcome after laser photocoagulation for subfoveal choroidal neovascularization secondary to age-related macular degeneration. The influence of initial lesion size and initial visual acuity [see comment]. Arch Ophthalmol 1994;112:480–488.

7. Treatment of age-related macular degeneration with photodynamic therapy (TAP) study group. Photodynamic therapy of subfoveal choroidal neovascularization in age-related macular degeneration with verteporfin: one-year results of 2 randomized clinical trials – TAP report [see comment] [erratum appears in Arch Ophthalmol 2000;118:488]. Arch Ophthalmol 1999;117:1329–1345.

13. Brown DM, Kaiser PK, Michels M, et al. Ranibizumab versus verteporfin for neovascular age-related macular degeneration [see comment]. N Engl J Med 2006;355:1432–1444.

14. Rosenfeld PJ, Brown DM, Heier JS, et al. Ranibizumab for neovascular age-related macular degeneration [see comment]. N Engl J Med 2006;355:1419–1431.

15. Friedman DS, O'Colmain BJ, Munoz B, et al. Prevalence of age-related macular degeneration in the United States [see

comment]. Arch Ophthalmol 2004;122:564–572.

17. Yannuzzi LA, Wong DW, Sforzolini BS, et al. Polypoidal choroidal vasculopathy and neovascularized age-related macular degeneration. Arch Ophthalmol 1999;117:1503–1510.

18. Yannuzzi LA, Negrao S, Iida T, et al. Retinal angiomatous proliferation in age-related macular degeneration [see comment]. Retina 2001;21:416–434.

23. Hageman GS, Luthert PJ, Victor Chong NH, et al. An integrated hypothesis that considers drusen as biomarkers of immune-mediated processes at the RPE–Bruch's membrane interface in aging and age-related macular degeneration. Prog Retin Eye Res 2001;20:705–732.

24. Feeney-Burns L, Hilderbrand ES, Eldridge S. Aging human RPE: morphometric analysis of macular, equatorial, and peripheral cells. Invest Ophthalmol Vis Sci 1984;25:195–200.

29. Hughes AE, Orr N, Patterson C, et al. Neovascular age-related macular degeneration risk based on CFH, LOC387715/HTRA1, and smoking. PLoS Med 2007;4:e355.

30. Age-Related Eye Disease Study Research G. A randomized, placebo-controlled,

clinical trial of high-dose supplementation with vitamins C and E, beta carotene, and zinc for age-related macular degeneration and vision loss: AREDS report no. 8 [see comment]. Arch Ophthalmol 2001;119:1417–1436.

37. Cousins SW, Espinosa-Heidmann DG, Csaky KG. Monocyte activation in patients with age-related macular degeneration: a biomarker of risk for choroidal neovascularization? Arch Ophthalmol 2004;122:1013–1018.

39. Killingsworth MC. Angiogenesis in early choroidal neovascularization secondary to age-related macular degeneration. Graefes Arch Clin Exp Ophthalmol 1995;233:313–323.

45. Csaky KG, Baffi JZ, Byrnes GA, et al. Recruitment of marrow-derived endothelial cells to experimental choroidal neovascularization by local expression of vascular endothelial growth factor. Exp Eye Res 2004;78:1107–1116.

46. Espinosa-Heidmann DG, Caicedo A, Hernandez EP, et al. Bone marrow-derived progenitor cells contribute to experimental choroidal neovascularization. Invest Ophthalmol Vis Sci 2003;44:4914–4919.

CHAPTER 70

Inhibition of angiogenesis

Anthony P Adamis and Adrienne J Berman

Clinical background

Ocular angiogenesis can be physiological or pathological, with physiological ocular angiogenesis occurring primarily during embryonic development (reviewed by Gariano[1]). Ocular angiogenesis in adults is usually pathological and is a major cause of vision loss and blindness due to conditions such as choroidal neovascularization (CNV) related to age-related macular degeneration (AMD), diabetic retinopathy, neovascular glaucoma, corneal neovascularization, and retinopathy of prematurity. Each of these is discussed in at length elsewhere in this volume.

Research into mechanisms of physiological and pathological angiogenesis has led to a deeper understanding of molecular and cellular mechanisms involved in angiogenesis, with a principal focus of research efforts being the identification of molecules involved in promotion and inhibition of ocular neovascular disease. This chapter will focus on the molecules for which the role in ocular angiogenesis is best characterized, especially those that have led to the development of new drugs, and will present an overview of existing and developing therapies derived from this work.

Pathophysiology

The pathogenesis of ocular neovascularization involves a complex interaction between proangiogenic and antiangiogenic factors and molecules. There is also accumulating evidence supporting the inflammatory nature of both AMD and diabetic retinopathy. The depletion of monocytes inhibited pathologic (but not physiologic) retinal neovascularization in experimental models, strongly supporting a role for inflammation in ocular neovascular disease (Figure 70.1).[2] Certain haplotypes of factor H, a regulatory component of the complement cascade, are associated with an increased risk of developing AMD (reviewed by Donoso et al[3]). In addition, complement factors C3a and C5a[4] and C5b–9 (the membrane attack complex, or MAC)[5] were identified in drusen of patients with AMD. Extensive deposits of C3d and C5b–9 have also been identified in the choriocapillaris of human eyes with clinically evident diabetic retinopathy, but not in the vast majority of control eyes,[6] and elevated levels of assorted complement factors have been found in the vitreous of patients undergoing surgery for proliferative diabetic retinopathy.[7] Since complement is involved in opsonization, chemotaxis, and activation of leukocytes (reviewed by Rus et al[8]), the presence of complement in AMD and diabetic retinopathy lesions together with the co-localization of immune cells is evidence of active inflammation.

The final stage of angiogenesis involves stabilization of nascent vasculature by a process known as maturation, which involves selective pruning (remodeling) and recruitment of mural cells (pericytes and smooth-muscle cells). Leukocytes are believed to contribute actively to vascular pruning (Figure 70.2) through Fas/FasL-mediated endothelial cell apoptosis.[9] Maturation is tightly regulated by levels of vascular endothelial growth factor (VEGF),[10] with new vessels becoming refractory to VEGF withdrawal over time.[11] In other studies, maturation corresponded with the expression of angiopoietin 1 (Ang1) and platelet-derived growth factor-B (PDGF-B)[12] and prevention of mural cell binding to the endothelium by PDGF-B blockade resulted in disorganized retinal vasculature; normalization was restored by the administration of Ang1.[13]

The complexity of the pathogenesis of ocular neovascularization suggests numerous potential targets for intervention in the treatment of ocular neovascular diseases; yet this same complexity suggests that different interventions may be needed, either alone or in combination, to provide optimal benefits to all patients.

Endogenous promoters of angiogenesis

There are many molecules known to promote angiogenesis for which there is evidence supporting a role in the etiology of ocular neovascular disease (Box 70.1).

Vascular endothelial growth factor

A major research effort has identified VEGF as a master regulator in both physiologic and pathologic angiogenesis and a major contribution to ocular neovascular diseases. Elevated levels of VEGF have been shown to accompany the development of neovascularization in conditions such as retinal vein occlusion,[14] neovascular glaucoma,[15] retinopathy of prematurity,[16] and proliferative diabetic retinopathy.[14] VEGF has also been found to be overexpressed in the retinal pigment epithelium (RPE) in surgically excised CNV membranes of patients with AMD.[17]

A number of approaches have demonstrated that VEGF is both necessary and sufficient for the development of

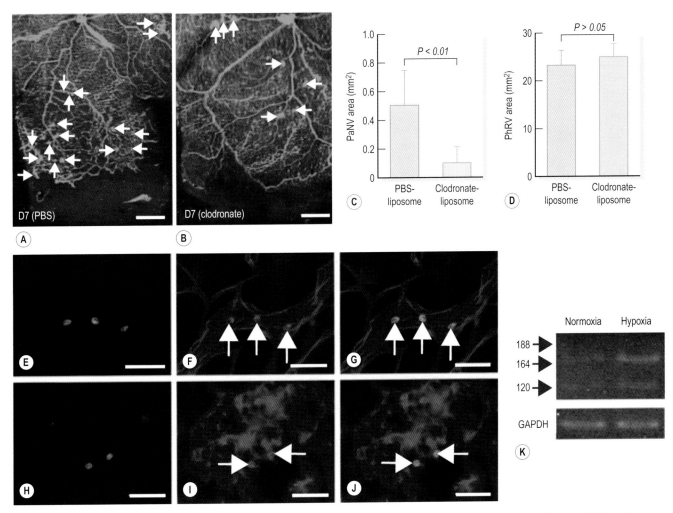

Figure 70.1 The role of monocytes in pathologic retinal neovascularization. At day 7 (D7), pathologic neovascularization (arrows) was not inhibited in mice (*n* = 8) treated with phosphate-buffered saline (PBS; control) liposomes (A); but was inhibited in mice (*n* = 8) treated with clodronate liposomes (B). Notably, the area of pathologic neovascularization (PaNV) was significantly reduced in mice treated with clodronate liposomes (C), whereas the area of physiologic revascularization (phRV) was not (D). (E–J) Monocyte adhesion was observed just before and during pathologic neovascularization (H–J). Green fluorescence from the anti-CD13 antibody (E and H) and red fluorescence from the rhodamine-coupled Con A (F and I) identified the Con A-stained cells as being CD13-positive leukocytes (arrows) when the images were superimposed (G and J). (K) Monocyte vascular endothelial growth factor (VEGF) mRNA expression in normoxia (21% oxygen) and hypoxia (1% oxygen). VEGF levels were markedly increased in response to hypoxic stimulation. Bars: (E–J) 50 μm; (A and B) 0.5 mm. (Modified from Ishida S, Yamashiro K, Usui T, et al. Leukocytes mediate retinal vascular remodeling during development and vaso-obliteration in disease. Nat Med 2003;9:781–788.)

Box 70.1 Promoters of angiogenesis relevant to ocular neovascularization

- Angiopoietins
- Delta/Notch
- Ephrins
- Erythropoietin
- Fibroblast growth factor-2
- Integrins
- Matrix metalloproteinases
- Platelet-derived growth factor-B
- Tumor necrosis factor-α
- Vascular endothelial growth factor

ocular neovascularization. Experimentally induced ocular elevations of VEGF achieved by various means have led to pathological ocular neovascularization[18-20] while inactivation of VEGF resulted in inhibition of ocular neovascularization.[2,21,22] VEGF is produced by many cell types in the retina, including neurons, glia, and RPE cells.[23-25] Hypoxia strongly induces the expression of VEGF through stabilization of hypoxia-inducible factor-1 alpha, a transcriptional regulator.[26]

Alternative splicing of the VEGF gene results in six major isoforms.[27] Evidence from rodent models suggests that $VEGF_{164/165}$ ($VEGF_{164}$ is the rodent equivalent of human $VEGF_{165}$) was preferentially upregulated in ischemia-induced pathological neovascularization and was significantly more potent at inducing inflammation.[28]

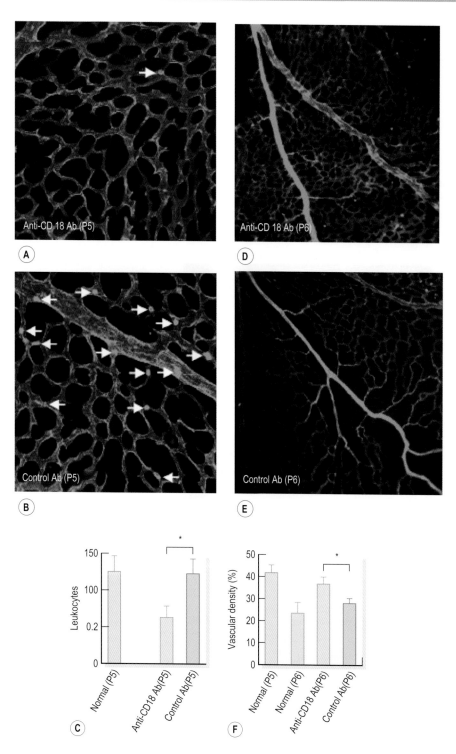

Figure 70.2 Vascular pruning is dependent on leukocyte adhesion. (A, B) Systemic administration of an antibody (Ab) against CD18, a molecule involved in leukocyte adhesion, reduced the number of adherent leukocytes in the normal rat retina on postnatal day 5, whereas a control antibody did not. (C) There was a significant reduction in the number of adherent leukocytes in rats treated with the anti-CD18 antibody ($n = 12$; 59.9 ± 15.6) versus those treated with a control antibody ($n = 10$; 119.2 ± 21.9, $P < 0.01$). (D, E) CD18 blockade led to suppression of vascular pruning on postnatal day 6, when compared with those treated with a control antibody. (F) There was a significant reduction in the vascular density within five disc diameters of the optic disc between rats treated with the anti-CD18 antibody ($n = 10$; $36.7 \pm 3.3\%$) and control rats ($n = 8$; $27.3 \pm 2.7\%$, $P < 0.01$). (Modified from Ishida S, Yamashiro K, Usui T, et al. Leukocytes mediate retinal vascular remodeling during development and vaso-obliteration in disease. Nat Med 2003;9:781–788.)

Platelet-derived growth factor-B

The PDGF group of dimeric proteins is composed of combinations of four different polypeptide chains (PDGF A–D) with a cellular distribution that includes fibroblasts, vascular smooth-muscle cells, endothelial cells, RPE cells, and macrophages. PDGFs interact with two related tyrosine kinases, PDGF receptor (PDGFR)-α and PDGFR-β, leading to receptor dimerization and autophosphorylation (reviewed by Heldin and Westermark[29]).

During angiogenesis, the homodimeric PDGF-B has been found to play a particularly important role in the recruitment of PDGFR-β-expressing mural cells (pericytes and vascular smooth-muscle cells) to the developing vasculature (Figure 70.3).[30] Jo et al[11] employed three different murine models to study the contributions of signaling induced by VEGF and PDGF-B in ocular neovascularization. Physiologic development of neonatal retinal vasculature was significantly inhibited by blockade of signaling induced by PDGF-B but not by VEGF164; simultaneous blockade of both factors

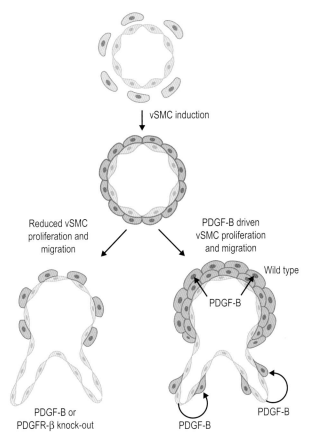

↓ vSMC induction

Reduced vSMC proliferation and migration

PDGF-B driven vSMC proliferation and migration

Wild type

PDGF-B

PDGF-B or PDGFR-β knock-out

PDGF-B

PDGF-B

Figure 70.3 The role of platelet-derived growth factor (PDGF)-B in the development of vessel walls. Undifferentiated mesenchymal cells (gray) surrounding the newly formed endothelial tube (yellow) are induced to become vascular smooth-muscle cells (vSMC) and to assemble into a vascular wall (red). During vessel growth and sprouting, PDGF is released by the endothelium to drive vSMC proliferation and migration. In mice lacking PDGF-B or PDGFR-ß, there is reduced vSMC proliferation and migration, which results in vSMC hypoplasia of larger vessels and pericyte deficiency in capillaries. (Reproduced with permission from Hellstrom M, Kalen M, Lindahl P, et al. Role of PDGF-B and PDGFR-beta in recruitment of vascular smooth muscle cells and pericytes during embryonic blood vessel formation in the mouse. Development 1999;126:3047–3055.)

led to additional reductions. In contrast, blocking PDGF-B had little effect on developing or established neovascularization in a model of CNV, whereas VEGF inhibition significantly reduced the growth of new vessels; the most potent inhibition was again observed when both factors were inhibited. Finally, PDGF-B blockade of established corneal neovascularization between days 10 and 20 postinjury led to detachment of mural cells from corneal neovessels (Figure 70.4A) while PDGR-B blockade immediately following corneal injury did not significantly reduce neovascularization; in contrast, blocking VEGF led to a significant inhibition in the growth of new vessels. In established vessels, the combination led to the regression of pathological vessels. When both factors were blocked there was a significantly greater reduction than with VEGF inhibition alone (Figure 70.4B).[11] In these models, inhibition of PDGF-B signaling led to pericyte depletion in retinal and corneal vessels, but not in quiescent adult limbal vessels,[11] suggesting that therapies which block both VEGF and PDGF-B are more likely to achieve regression of both established and developing ocular neovascular lesions.

Fibroblast growth factor 2

Experimental models have not clearly defined the role of fibroblast growth factor 2 (FGF2; also known as basic FGF) in ocular neovascular disease. While studies have demonstrated the presence of FGF2 in surgically removed CNV membranes,[31] other studies suggest that FGF overexpression is insufficient in itself to provoke CNV in the absence of an additional stimulus such as cell injury.[32,33]

Tumor necrosis factor-α

The role of tumor necrosis factor-α (TNF-α) in ocular neovascularization is not fully understood; it may contribute to angiogenesis indirectly by promoting leukostasis in neovascular tissues[34] and by inducing expression factors such as VEGF, Ang1, and Ang2.[35] Although intravitreal administration of infliximab, an anti-TNF-α monoclonal antibody, reduced the formation of laser-induced CNV in a rat model,[36] findings with ischemia-induced retinopathy models in knockout mice were inconclusive. In mice lacking TNF-α expression there was no reduction in neovascularization with respect to wild-type mice,[34] while mice lacking TNF-receptor p55 had a reduction in ischemia-induced neovascularization.[37] These apparent contradictions in results may reflect differences in experimental methodology.

Angiopoietins 1 and 2

Ang1 and Ang2 are factors that act as ligands for Tie2, a receptor tyrosine kinase. Ang1 binds to and induces the phosphorylation of Tie2 whereas Ang2 usually behaves as an antagonist of Ang1 and Tie2 (reviewed by Eklund and Olsen[38]). Both Ang1 and Ang2 have been found to co-localize with VEGF in neovascular proliferative membranes of patient eyes.[39]

Ang1 is produced by vascular smooth-muscle cells.[40] Experimentally induced elevations in Ang1 in rodents caused reductions in retinal vascular leukocyte adhesion, endothelial cell damage, and blood–retinal barrier breakdown in a diabetic retinopathy model,[41] suppressed the development of CNV following laser wounding, and inhibited VEGF-mediated breakdown of the blood–retinal barrier in response to ischemia[42]; however, Ang1 had no effect on established neovascularization.[43]

Ang 2, which is produced by endothelial cells and is prominently expressed at sites of vascular remodeling,[38] is believed to serve primarily as an antagonist to Ang1/Tie2 during angiogenesis.[44] Studies suggest that Ang2 functions as a promoter of angiogenesis, mainly in combination with VEGF,[45] and induces vascular regression when VEGF levels are low.[46] Thus, the bulk of evidence suggests that Ang1 acts largely to inhibit the development of neovascularization whereas Ang2 acts to destabilize the vascular endothelium, making it more responsive to factors such as VEGF (Figure 70.5).[47]

Notch

Notch (named for a mutant fruit fly with notched wings) is a 300kDa transmembrane receptor that is involved in the development of a wide range of tissues; it is cleaved on activation, releasing an intracellular domain that activates

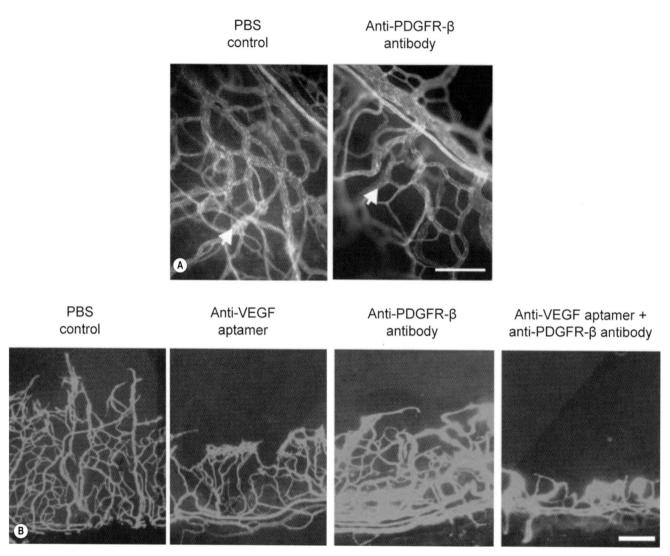

PBS
control

Anti-PDGFR-β
antibody

PBS
control

Anti-VEGF
aptamer

Anti-PDGFR-β
antibody

Anti-VEGF aptamer +
anti-PDGFR-β antibody

Figure 70.4 The effects of platelet-derived growth factor (PDGF)-B blockade on mural cells and vascular growth in a corneal neovascularization model. (A) Mice were injected with anti-PDGFR-ß antibody or phosphate-buffered saline (PBS) every day starting at 10 days postinjury and sacrificed at 20 days postinjury. Neovasculature from mice treated with the anti-PDGF-ß antibody demonstrated reduced mural cell coverage when compared with PBS-treated mice. Scale bar = 20 µm. (B) Corneal injury was induced in mice, followed immediately by daily treatment with one of the following: PBS, a pegylated anti-vascular endothelial growth factor (VEGF) aptamer, an anti-PDGFR-ß antibody, or a combination of the anti-VEGF aptamer and the anti-PDGFR-ß antibody. Neovasculature is shown in green. Scale bar = 100 µm. Quantitative analysis demonstrated that the anti-VEGF aptamer significantly reduced neovascularization when compared with PBS or the anti-PEGFR-ß antibody ($P < 0.01$), while the combination significantly reduced neovascularization when compared with the aptamer alone ($P < 0.05$). (Modified from Jo N, Mailhos C, Ju M, et al. Inhibition of platelet-derived growth factor B signaling enhances the efficacy of anti-vascular endothelial growth factor therapy in multiple models of ocular neovascularization. Am J Pathol 2006;168:2036–2053.)

Notch-targeted genes (reviewed by Lai[48]). Angiogenesis occurs when specialized endothelial cells known as tip cells lead the migration of vascular sprouts in response to a concentration gradient of VEGF; tip cells express high levels of VEGF receptor-2 (VEGFR-2) and PDGF-B.[49] Activation of Notch signaling upon interaction with the delta-like ligand-4 (Dll-4) restricts tip cell formation, thus establishing correct sprouting and branching patterns.[50] Consistent with these findings, overexpression of Dll4 in endothelial cells was found to reduce their expression of VEGFR-2 and inhibit their migratory and proliferative responses to VEGF.[51] There is little information available at present regarding a potential role for Notch in ocular neovascularization, however.

Ephrins

The ephrins and their ligands, the Eph receptor kinases, regulate vessel patterning during angiogenesis.[52] There are two subclasses, ephrinA/ephrinB, and EphA/EphB, each with many members (reviewed by Zhang and Hughes[53]). All ephrins are membrane-bound proteins; ephrinBs, but not ephrinAs, possess a cytoplasmic signaling domain that mediates forward or reverse signaling (Figure 70.6) (reviewed by Dodelet and Pasquale[54]). A role for EphrinA/EphA interactions in ocular neovascularization is unclear at present so this section will focus on the role of EphrinB/EphB interactions in angiogenesis.

Quiescent/resting vasculature

Ang-1 / Ang-2

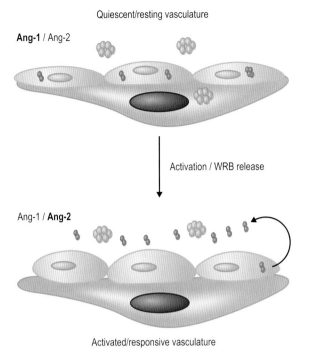

Activation / WRB release

Ang-1 / **Ang-2**

Activated/responsive vasculature

Figure 70.5 Ang-Tie functions in the regulation of quiescent and activated vasculature. The quiescent, resting endothelium (upper) has an antithrombotic and antiadhesive luminal cell surface. Ang1 (shown as multimeric: white), is secreted by periendothelial cells at a constitutive low level. By acting on the endothelium to maintain low-level Tie2 phosphorylation, Ang1contributes to maintaining the vascular endothelium in the resting state. Ang2 (dimeric: gray) is stored in endothelial cell Weibel–Palade body (WPB) of the quiescent vasculature. Endothelial cell activation (lower) involves the release of the endothelial cell WPBs, and concomitant liberation of a variety of stored factors, including Ang2. The resultant Ang1/Ang2 ratio is now biased more in favor of Ang2, leading to endothelial destabilization, and making the endothelial cell layer more responsive to other stimuli, including proinflammatory cytokines. (Reproduced with permission from Pfaff D, Fiedler U, Augustin HG. Emerging roles of the Angiopoietin-Tie and the ephrin-Eph systems as regulators of cell trafficking. J Leukoc Biol 2006;80:719–726.)

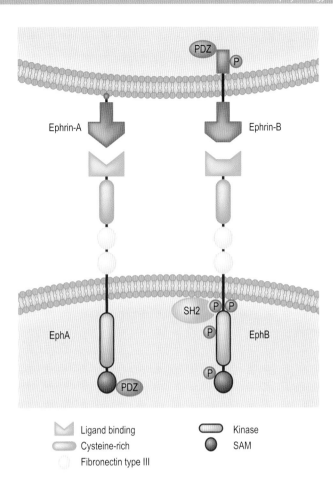

Figure 70.6 The structure of ephrins and Eph receptors. Both ephrins and Eph receptors are membrane-bound proteins. However, ephrinAs are tethered to the cellular membrane while ephrinBs have transmembrane and cytoplasmic signaling domains. Binding of ephrins to Eph receptors leads to clustering of receptors, which in turn leads to autophosphorylation of multiple tyrosine residues and provides docking sites for *src*-homology domain-containing downstream effectors. The carboxyl terminus of both Eph receptors contains a sterile alpha motif (SAM) and a PDZ domain (shown here for EphA, but these also apply to EphB), which promote receptor clustering subsequent to ligand binding. (Reproduced with permission from Dodelet VC, Pasquale EB. Eph receptors and ephrin ligands: embryogenesis to tumorigenesis. Oncogene 2000;19:5614–5619.)

EphrinB2 is preferentially expressed on arteries,[55] whereas the receptor EphB4 is preferentially expressed on veins[56]; this expression pattern is believed to be a key determinant of venous and arterial identity. Forward signaling following binding of ephrin B2 to EphB4 usually leads to reduced proliferation and migration of EphB4-expressing cells, while reverse signaling promotes increased proliferation and migration of ephrinB2-expressing cells.[57] In patients with proliferative diabetic retinopathy or retinopathy of prematurity, ephrinB2, EphB2, and EphB3 were all expressed on fibroproliferative membranes, but not EphB4.[58] The lack of EphB4 expression in these tissues may be a factor contributing to the disorganized neovasculature characteristic of proliferative membranes.[58]

Erythropoietin

Erythropoietin is best known as an inducer of erythropoiesis in response to hypoxia,[59] and has been proposed to contribute to ocular neovascular disease based on studies demonstrating elevated vitreous levels of erythropoietin in patients with diabetic retinopathy[60,61] and diabetic macular edema (DME).[62] In a murine ischemia-induced retinopathy model, blockade of erythropoietin caused a dose-dependent reduction in retinal neovascularization to levels comparable to those obtained with VEGF blockade.[60] Recent work suggests that the timing of erythropoietin supplementation versus blockade may also determine if angiogenesis is enhanced or suppressed.[63]

Integrins

Integrins are a family of heterodimeric transmembrane proteins that mediate adhesion to the extracellular matrix as well as between cells. They have roles in modulating signaling kinases and are involved in cell survival, proliferation, and migration. Integrins $\alpha_v\beta_3$ and $\alpha_v\beta_5$ are preferentially expressed on proliferating endothelial cells; their binding to matrix proteins such as fibronectin and vitronectin regulates endothelial cell migration, proliferation, and survival.[64] Vasculature in neovascular AMD (NV-AMD) expressed only $\alpha_v\beta_3$, whereas $\alpha_v\beta_3$ and $\alpha_v\beta_5$ were expressed in proliferative diabetic retinopathy; mature vasculature expressed neither integrin.[64] Inhibition of $\alpha_v\beta_3$ and/or $\alpha_v\beta_5$ was found to inhibit pathological retinal neovascularization in rodent models,[65,66] but did not inhibit CNV.[67]

Integrin $\alpha_5\beta_1$, the fibronectin receptor, is expressed at low levels on mature vessels but at high levels on angiogenic sprouts[67] and is highly upregulated on activated endothelial cells and tumor blood vessels.[68] It has been identified in surgical specimens from NV-AMD (KU Loeffler, unpublished data), proliferative vitreoretinopathy, and proliferative diabetic retinopathy.[69] Inhibition of $\alpha_5\beta_1$ suppresses pathological corneal, retinal, and CNV in multiple rodent and primate models.[70-72]

Matrix metalloproteinases

Matrix metalloproteinases (MMPs) have been shown to contribute to ocular neovascularization in studies with mice lacking expression of MMP-2 and/or MMP-9.[73] MMPs may also contribute to angiogenesis by regulating the bioavailability of VEGF by proteolytic release of the receptor-binding domain of $VEGF_{165}$ from the matrix-binding domain[74] and by inducing proteolysis, pigment epithelium-derived factor (PEDF), an inhibitor of angiogenesis.[75]

Endogenous inhibitors of angiogenesis

A variety of inhibitors of angiogenesis have been proposed to be involved in ocular neovascularization (Box 70.2).

Soluble VEGFR-1

Soluble VEGF receptor-1 (sVEGFR-1) is a secreted form of the receptor that inhibits VEGF.[76] Evidence in mice suggests that corneal avascularity is maintained in large measure due to sVEGFR-1 binding to VEGF in the cornea.[77] Thus, sVEGFR-1 is a potent, naturally occurring inhibitor of VEGF in the eye.

$VEGF_{xxx}b$

$VEGF_{xxx}b$ isoforms comprise a family of differentially spliced, potentially antiangiogenic VEGF isoforms that have been found to be underexpressed in eyes with diabetic retinopathy compared to eyes from nondiabetic patients.[78] These findings suggest that diabetic retinopathy may be associated with a switch in splicing from antiangiogenic to proangiogenic isoforms.[78]

Box 70.2 Inhibitors of angiogenesis involved in ocular neovascularization

- Soluble vascular endothelial growth factor (VEGF) receptor-1
- $VEGF_{xxx}b$ proteins
- Cryptic collagen IV epitope
- Other inhibitors

Cryptic collagen IV epitope

The cryptic epitope of collagen type IV, a component of the basement membrane of blood vessels, contributes to angiogenesis by mediating a shift in integrin binding from $\alpha_v\beta_3$ to $\alpha_v\beta_1$.[79] Blocking this epitope inhibited corneal[79] and CNV[80] in murine models. MMP-2 localization at the site of the lesion preceded that of the cryptic epitope, suggesting that MMP proteolysis was responsible for exposure of the epitope.[80]

Other inhibitors

Other endogenous factors for which evidence supports an inhibitory role in angiogenesis include pigment epithelium-derived factor (PEDF), angiostatin, endostatin, plasminogen kringle 5, kallistatin, and thrombospondin-1. It is suggested that readers interested in more information about these factors refer to the excellent recent review by Zhang and Ma.[81]

Antiangiogenic therapies for ocular neovascular disease

Antiangiogenic therapies for ocular neovascular disease include anti-VEGF agents, the only approved therapies to date, and multiple other agents under investigation (Box 70.3).

Agents targeting VEGF

Pegaptanib sodium

Pegaptanib sodium (Macugen (OSI), Eyetech/Pfizer) is a pegylated oligonucleotide that selectively binds $VEGF_{165}$ and is administered every 6 weeks by intravitreal injection.[82] Pegaptanib was evaluated for treatment of NV-AMD in two randomized, controlled trials (VEGF Inhibition Study In Ocular Neovascularization trials) involving three different doses of pegaptanib and sham.[82] In a combined analysis, the 0.3-mg dose of pegaptanib sodium demonstrated efficacy at 2 years resulting in stabilization of vision (59% versus 45% for controls having a ≤3-line loss); subgroup analysis demonstrated similar efficacy for all angiogenic subtypes. The chance of having a 3-line gain was relatively low (10% towards 4% for the control group after 2 years),[83] although in a subsequent analysis of patients with early lesions (i.e., >54 letters and lesion size <2 disk areas at baseline), 76% with pegaptanib versus 50% in the usual care group lost ≤3 lines.[84] The long-term ocular and systemic safety of pegaptanib in treatment of NV-AMD is excellent.[85] Pegaptanib was also effective in diabetic patients with retinal neovascularization.[86]

Ranibizumab

Ranibizumab (Lucentis, Genentech) is a humanized monoclonal antibody antigen-binding fragment (Fab) that binds all isoforms of VEGF. In a randomized, controlled phase III trial (MARINA), patients with minimally classic or purely occult CNV received monthly injections of 0.3 or 0.5 mg ranibizumab or sham treatment for 24 months; at 12 months, 95% versus 62% of eyes (ranibizumab versus sham)

Box 70.3 Approved and investigational antiangiogenic therapies for ocular neovascular disease

Approved
- Pegaptanib sodium (anti-vascular endothelial growth factor (VEGF))
- Ranibizumab (anti-VEGF)

Investigational (a partial list of compounds in or entering human clinical trials)
- Other anti-VEGF agents
  - Bevacizumab
  - VEGF-Trap-Eye
  - Small interfering RNAs
    - Bevasiranib
    - AGN211745
- Corticosteroids
  - Triamcinolone acetonide
  - Anecortave acetate
  - Dexamethasone
  - Fluocinolone
- Complement antagonists
  - Anticomplement factor D antibody
  - ARC1905
  - Eculizumab
  - JPE1375
  - PMX53
  - POT-4
  - TA106
  - TT30
- Integrin antagonists
  - JNJ-26076713
  - JSM6427
  - Volociximab
- Other therapeutic approaches
  - AdGVPEDF.11D versus pigment epithelium-derived factor
  - Tumor necrosis factor-α
  - E10030 versus platelet-derived growth factor
  - Sirolimus
  - Mecamylamine
  - RTP801i-14
  - iCo-007
  - Palomid 529
  - Radiation brachytherapy
  - Tyrosine kinase inhibitors
    - TG100801
    - Pazopanib
  - Vascular disrupting agents
    - Combretastatin A4P (Zybrestat)
    - OC-10X

lost <15 letters and 34% of eyes receiving the 0.5-mg dose had gains of 15 letters. At 24 months, 90% of eyes in the 0.5-mg group lost <15 letters compared to 53% in the control group; the mean gain in the 0.5-mg group was 7 letters.[87] Efficacy was independent of baseline vision and lesion size/composition. In the ANCHOR trial, ranibizumab was found to be superior to photodynamic therapy (PDT) with verteporfin for treatment of AMD.[88] The drug was well tolerated overall.[87]

Bevacizumab
Bevacizumab (Avastin, Genentech) is a humanized anti-VEGF monoclonal antibody related to ranibizumab that is approved for intravenous administration in the treatment of colorectal cancer[89] and is being used off-label as an intravitreal treatment for ocular neovascular disease. Since the safety of intravitreal bevacizumab has not been evaluated in randomized, controlled trials and the long-term effects of intravitreal bevacizumab are unknown, a multicenter trial sponsored by the National Eye Institute to assess the relative safety and efficacy of bevacizumab with respect to ranibizumab is ongoing.[90]

Other anti-VEGF agents
VEGF-Trap-Eye (Regeneron Pharmaceuticals) is a VEGFR-Fc fusion protein administered via intravitreal injection that prevents the binding of all isoforms of VEGF isoforms and placental growth factor (which is related to VEGF) to their cellular receptors. Results of a phase II, dose-ranging trial involving 157 patients with NV-AMD showed significant reductions in mean retinal thickness and improvements in visual acuity from baseline after 12 weeks of treatment.[91] The current phase III trial is comparing every-4 versus every-8-week VEGF Trap dosing versus monthly ranibizumab for NV AMD.[92]

Bevasiranib (formerly known as Cand5, Okpo Health) is a small interfering RNA that inactivates VEGF messenger RNA (mRNA), inhibiting the production of all isoforms of VEGF. A phase III trial has been terminated in which intravitreal bevasiranib was evaluated as a maintenance agent in NV-AMD every 8 or 12 weeks following monthly induction with ranabizumab.[93] AGN211745 (formerly known as Sirna 027, Allergan) is a small interfering RNA that blocks the VEGFR-1 receptor. It is administered by intravitreal injection and was in phase II trials that have been terminated.[94]

Corticosteroids

Triamcinolone acetonide, dexamethasone, and fluocinolone
Triamcinolone acetonide, a potent anti-inflammatory corticosteroid with prolonged activity, is being used off-label as an intravitreal treatment for ocular neovascular diseases (reviewed by Jonas[95]). Although triamcinolone may be used in an adjuvant setting (such as with concurrent PDT), there are insufficient data to support the use of triamcinolone as monotherapy for NV-AMD. Triamcinolone is also associated with a high risk of adverse effects such as increased intraocular pressure and cataract development.

Dexamethasone, an even more potent anti-inflammatory corticosteroid, is also being used intravitreally off-label in combination with PDT and anti-VEGF therapy for NV-AMD.[96] An extended-release formulation of dexamethasone (Posurdex, Allergan) is being evaluated in phase II clinical trials in combination with ranibizumab for the treatment of NV-AMD.[97]

Fluocinolone acetonide was studied in high-dose extended-release formulation as monotherapy for non-AMD

CNV, but had high rates of complications.[98] It is currently entering phase II clinical trials at a lower dose, administered as an extended-release formulation by the Medidur intravitreal device, in combination with ranibizumab for patients who have reached a plateau after ranibizumab monotherapy for NV-AMD.[99]

Anecortave acetate

Anecortave acetate (Retaane, Alcon) is an angiostatic corticosteroid that blocks the migration of proliferating endothelial cells by inhibiting MMPs; it is administered every 6 months by posterior juxtascleral injection. A phase III randomized study comparing anecortave acetate with PDT in patients with NV-AMD found comparable efficacy in terms of < 3-line loss between groups at 12 months.[100]

Complement antagonists

The complement pathway offers numerous potential targets for inhibition of angiogenesis; however, it is too early to know which target or targets will be the most effective. Compstatin, a small peptide inhibitor of C3 convertase currently being evaluated in clinical trials for eye disease, is being tested in phase I trials for treatment of NV-AMD as the intravitreally injected drug POT-4 (Potentia Pharmaceuticals).[101] Eculizumab (Soliris, Alexion Pharmaceuticals) is a monoclonal antibody that binds C5 and prevents cleavage into C5a (an inflammatory anaphylotoxin) and C5b (part of the C5b–C9 membrane attack complex). It is the first Food and Drug Administration-approved complement inhibitor, indicated for intravenous administration in paroxysmal nocturnal hemoglobinuria, and is in preclinical development as an intravitreal agent for NV-AMD (JP Springhorn, unpublished data). ARC1905 (Ophthotech), an anti-C5 aptamer, is in phase I clinical trials for NV-AMD alone and in combination with ranibizumab.[102]

Approaches that target the C5a–C5aR pathway are being investigated (Jerini Ophthalmic; Arana Therapeutics) which may offer the potential for clinical efficacy while allowing the production of the C5b–C9 membrane attack complex; deficiencies in C5, C5b, and C6–9 are known to lead to increased bacterial infections and, in particular, meningococcal disease.[103] A monoclonal antibody against complement factor D is in preclinical development for both dry AMD and NV-AMD (J Le Coulter, unpublished data). In addition, Taligen Therapeutics has two agents in preclinical development for treating NV-AMD: TA106, a monoclonal antibody Fab that blocks complement factor B, and TT30, targeting complement factor H.[104]

Integrin antagonists

JSM6427 (Jerini Ophthalmic), a specific small-molecule inhibitor of $\alpha_5\beta_1$ that showed antiangiogenic, antifibrotic, antiproliferative, and anti-inflammatory effects in preclinical models,[70–72] is currently in phase I safety and pharmacokinetic testing with single and repeat intravitreal injections for advanced NV-AMD.[105] Volociximab, a monoclonal antibody against $\alpha_5\beta_1$ currently in phase II trials for several types of cancer, was recently licensed for ophthalmic use (Ophthotech) and is in phase I clinical trials for NV-AMD.[106] Finally, an oral $\alpha_v\beta_3/\alpha_v\beta_5$ antagonist is in preclinical development for the treatment of diabetic retinopathy (Johnson and Johnson JNJ-26076713).[107]

Other therapeutic approaches based on modulating angiogenic factors

Other therapeutic approaches may prove useful in treating ocular neovascular disease. In one approach, an adenoviral vector expressing PEDF was administered intravitreally to 28 patients with NV-AMD in a phase I study, with most patients experiencing stable vision at 6 months postinjection.[108] Another approach is suggested by the previously described preclinical data in which the anti-TNF-α antibody infliximab reduced the formation of CNV[36]; these findings have gained validation from a small study in which three patients experienced regression of NV-AMD while receiving intravenous infliximab for treatment of arthritis.[109] In addition, an intravitreally injected anti-PDGF aptamer (E10030; Ophthotech) that showed potential in inducing regression of established CNV in preclinical studies when used in combination with anti-VEGF therapy has recently entered phase I safety trials in NV-AMD in combination with ranibizumab.[110]

Sirolimus, an mTOR kinase inhibitor that suppresses cytokine-driven T-cell proliferation, is used systemically for preventing organ transplant rejection and cardiac stent stenosis; it has immunosuppressive, antipermeability, antifibrotic, antiangiogenic, antimigratory, and antiproliferative properties. It is currently in phase I/II clinical trials for NV-AMD and DME as a subconjunctival or intravitreal injection (MacuSight).[111] Another agent in phase I clinical trials as an intravitreal injection is RTP801i-14/REDD14NP (Quark Pharmaceuticals), an siRNA against the hypoxia-inducible gene *RTP801* that demonstrated anti-inflammatory, antiapoptotic, and antiangiogenic effects in preclinical models.[112] Another agent, iCO-007 (iCo Therapeutics), is a second-generation antisense inhibitor targeting C-raf kinase mRNA and is thought have utility in the treatment of retinal neovascular diseases such as diabetic retinopathy; it is currently in phase I clinical trials as an intravitreal agent for treatment of diffuse DME.[113] Palomid 529 is a small molecule that inhibits bFGF- and VEGF-stimulated endothelial cells[114] and has been shown to be effective in preclinical models of CNV and retinal neovascularization[114,115]; it is anticipated to enter human clinical trials at the end of 2009 as an intravitreal injection.[116]

Since radiation preferentially affects dividing cells, many studies have looked at external-beam radiation for NV-AMD, with inconclusive results. In a slightly different approach, strontium-90 beta irradiation applied directly over the macula during vitrectomy using a brachytherapy device (EpiRad 90, Neovista) is currently in phase III clinical trials for NV-AMD in combination with ranibizumab.[117]

Several topically administered compounds are in clinical trials for NV-AMD, including TG100801 (TargeGen), a prodrug that inhibits the VEGFR and src tyrosine kinases[118]; pazopanib (GlaxoSmithKline),[119] a small-molecule tyrosine kinase inhibitor against VEGFR-1, -2, and -3, c-kit, and PDGFR, is also under study. Zybrestat (OXiGENE), a small-molecule endothelium-targeting vascular disrupting agent in phase III clinical trials for oncology, is being formulated for topical delivery after being administered intravenously for myopic CNV.[120] Finally, OC-10X (OcuCure Therapeutics), a vascular disruptor that binds the β-tubulin subunit, is in development for topical treatment of NV-AMD and diabetic retinopathy after animal studies showed suppression and regression of neovascularization.[121]

Conclusions

A greater understanding of the factors involved in promoting and inhibiting angiogenesis has led to the development of new therapies for treating ocular neovascular diseases such as AMD and diabetic retinopathy. While the only approved therapies are those targeting VEGF, there are new investigational agents in development that may provide additional options, either alone or in combination with anti-VEGF therapy, for the treatment of ocular neovascular diseases.

Key references

A complete list of chapter references is available online at www.expertconsult.com. See inside cover for registration details.

2. Ishida S, Usui T, Yamashiro K, et al. VEGF164-mediated inflammation is required for pathological, but not physiological, ischemia-induced retinal neovascularization. J Exp Med 2003;198: 483–489.

3. Donoso LA, Kim D, Frost A, et al. The role of inflammation in the pathogenesis of age-related macular degeneration. Surv Ophthalmol 2006;51:137–152.

4. Nozaki M, Raisler BJ, Sakurai E, et al. Drusen complement components C3a and C5a promote choroidal neovascularization. Proc Natl Acad Sci USA 2006;103:2328–2333.

9. Ishida S, Yamashiro K, Usui T, et al. Leukocytes mediate retinal vascular remodeling during development and vaso-obliteration in disease. Nat Med 2003;9:781–788.

11. Jo N, Mailhos C, Ju M, et al. Inhibition of platelet-derived growth factor B signaling enhances the efficacy of anti-vascular endothelial growth factor therapy in multiple models of ocular neovascularization. Am J Pathol 2006;168:2036–2053.

14. Aiello LP, Avery RL, Arrigg PG, et al. Vascular endothelial growth factor in ocular fluid of patients with diabetic retinopathy and other retinal disorders. N Engl J Med 1994;331:1480–1487.

18. Tolentino MJ, McLeod DS, Taomoto M, et al. Pathologic features of vascular endothelial growth factor-induced retinopathy in the nonhuman primate. Am J Ophthalmol 2002;133:373–385.

22. Krzystolik MG, Afshari MA, Adamis AP, et al. Prevention of experimental choroidal neovascularization with intravitreal anti-vascular endothelial growth factor antibody fragment. Arch Ophthalmol 2002;120:338–346.

23. Adamis AP, Shima DT, Yeo KT, et al. Synthesis and secretion of vascular permeability factor/vascular endothelial growth factor by human retinal pigment epithelial cells. Biochem Biophys Res Commun 1993;193:631–638.

24. Aiello LP, Northrup JM, Keyt BA, et al. Hypoxic regulation of vascular endothelial growth factor in retinal cells. Arch Ophthalmol 1995;113:1538–1544.

31. Frank RN, Amin RH, Eliott D, et al. Basic fibroblast growth factor and vascular endothelial growth factor are present in epiretinal and choroidal neovascular membranes. Am J Ophthalmol 1996;122: 393–403.

41. Joussen AM, Poulaki V, Tsujikawa A, et al. Suppression of diabetic retinopathy with angiopoietin-1. Am J Pathol 2002;160:1683–1693.

77. Ambati BK, Nozaki M, Singh N, et al. Corneal avascularity is due to soluble VEGF receptor-1. Nature 2006;443:993–997.

82. Gragoudas ES, Adamis AP, Cunningham ET Jr, et al. Pegaptanib for neovascular age-related macular degeneration. N Engl J Med 2004;351:2805–2816.

86. Adamis AP, Altaweel M, Bressler NM, et al. Changes in retinal neovascularization after pegaptanib (Macugen) therapy in diabetic individuals. Ophthalmology 2006;113: 23–28.

CHAPTER 71

Retinal detachment

Steven K Fisher and Geoffrey P Lewis

Clinical background

Retinal detachment (RD) is a physical separation of the neural retina from the retinal pigmented epithelium (RPE). An important physiological ramification of the creation of a detachment is an increase in the physical distance between the photoreceptor cells and their blood supply, the choroicapillaris. Detachment recreates a space that disappears during early embryonic development.

Definitions: types of retinal detachment

Detachment occurs in three categories: exudative (or serous), traction, and rhegmatogenous (Box 71.1).

Serous detachment

Serous detachment occurs as fluid accumulates between the neural retina and RPE, but the retina remains physically intact.[1] Serous detachments may be idiopathic or occur as part of inflammatory reaction, or as a result of neoplastic ocular tumors (Box 71.2).

Tractional detachment

Tractional detachment occurs as a result of "vitreoretinal adhesions" or the growth of cells in the vitreous that attach to the surface of the retina and contract, mechanically creating an RD.

Rhegmatogenous detachment

This is the commonest form of RD and the focus of this chapter. It results from a tear across the retina, creating a physical continuity between the vitreous and RPE–photoreceptor interface and thus resulting in the accumulation of "foreign" fluid beneath the retina and a subsequent detachment (Figure 71.1).

Tractional detachments can also be rhegmatogenous, i.e., a complex form of RD (Figure 71.2).[2] These often result from fibrotic or scar tissue that forms on either surface of the retina after reattachment. Contraction of this scar tissue can cause traction on the retina with wrinkling and redetachment and often retearing of a previous break or creation of new ones. This is a visually devastating condition and its prevalence has remained discouragingly static over the years.

Symptoms, signs of retinal detachment, and diagnostics

All RDs are accompanied by some loss of visual function but this will vary depending upon the type of detachment, its size, and retinal location, making it difficult to ascribe one set of symptoms to the condition (Box 71.3). Diagnosing RD is complex, with many qualifications.

Abnormal vision is the only reliable symptom of RD. But the types of abnormal vision are large and varied: light flashes, floaters, changes in the peripheral visual field, decreased acuity, defective color vision, distorted vision (metamorphopsia), or even unilateral double vision (diplopia). Patients often remain unaware of large peripheral detachments until they approach the macula and begin to produce a visual field defect. Many times they are discovered during an ocular examination. Foveal detachment always involves loss of central visual acuity. Indeed, the duration of a foveal rhegmatogenous RD is based upon the time of patient-observed decrease in visual acuity.[3] A macular rhegmatogenous RD will generally produce visual acuity loss that cannot be corrected, while blurred vision produced by a centrally located serous detachment (central serous retinopathy, or CSR) can often be corrected by shifting the focal plane of the image to a more forward location. The book series *Retina* includes much information relevant to diagnosing detachments.[4]

History

Greg Joseph Beer provided what is generally described as the earliest description of detachment in the early 18th century[3,5]; his observations were done without benefit of an ophthalmoscope (an instrument with magnifying lenses that allows examination of the inside of the eye). After Hermann von Helmholtz recognized the importance of the ophthalmoscope in about 1850, detailed descriptions of detachments and accompanying breaks or tears proliferated rapidly.

The first treatment of rhegmatogenous RD by sealing the retinal break with a red-hot probe occurred in 1889, and was revived as a standard treatment by Jules Gonin. Gonin was also the first to suggest a relationship between detachment duration and successful visual recovery. His technique is

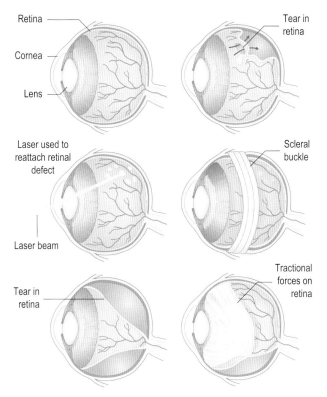

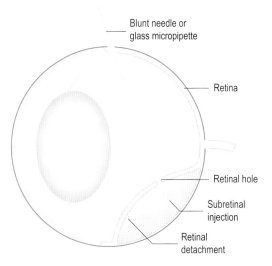

Figure 71.2 Rhegmatogenous detachments can be created in animal models by the injection of fluid between the neural retina and underlying retinal pigmented epithelium. The pipette or needle will leave a hole in the retina that will remain open and even expand, creating the retinal break characteristic of this type of detachment.

Figure 71.1 In a rhegmatogenous detachment a tear or break forms in the retina, allowing fluid from the vitreous cavity to enter, and creating a space between the neural retina and retinal pigmented epithelium (RPE). A laser can be used to "seal" the retinal tear and encircling bands of material (scleral buckle) can be used to indent the wall of the eye so that the retina is reapposed to RPE. Natural adhesion forces will allow reattachment to occur. A rhegmatogenous detachment may detach the whole retina. A serious complication of reattachment is the formation and attachment of scar tissue on the vitreal surface of the retina, which can become contractile and subsequently create a traction detachment.

Box 71.3

A monograph, *Retinal Detachment*, prepared in 1979 for the American Academy of Ophthalmology,[3] is a valuable resource describing much of the history associated with the diagnosis, symptoms, and treatment of detachment. It is referenced here although out of print, because copies exist in libraries and used copies presumably can be found for sale. Much of the historical information presented here is derived from that source

---

Box 71.1

Rhegma, derived from Greek, refers to a break in continuity

Box 71.4

A scleral buckle consists primarily of a band or bands of material, now usually silicone rubber and/or silicone sponges in a variety of configurations surgically placed to encircle the globe and to indent the wall of the eye in the region of the detachment.[6] A scleral buckle is used in conjunction with cyrotherapy or laser treatment to seal the retinal break

---

Box 71.2

Central serous retinopathy (CSR) or central serous choreoretinopathy results from serous detachment of the macula. It occurs most commonly in middle-aged males. The mechanisms are poorly understood. These detachments usually, but not always, resolve spontaneously. Even those that do resolve can have lasting effects on vision[1]

Box 71.5

The gases sulfur hexafluoride (SF_6) and perfluoropropane (C_3F_8) are commonly used in pneumatic retinopexy

---

credited with moving an inevitably blinding condition into a treatable one. The next major advance occurred 70 years later when Custodis described the "scleral buckle"[6] (Box 71.4).

This technique achieved a success rate of between 75 and 88%.[7] In the early 1970s Norton[8] described the use of "pneumatic retinopexy," or injection of an expanding gas bubble into the vitreous cavity (Box 71.5) to reappose the retina and RPE (once these tissues are moved into close physical proximity, natural adhesive forces will usually cause them to

reattach[9]). There is still much ongoing discussion on the use of scleral buckling, primary vitrectomy, and pneumatic retinopexy[6,7,10–12] to treat rhegmatogenous RD.

The success rate for rhegmatogenous RD after one surgical procedure is now cited as in the range of 80–95%.[7] That number rises closer to 95% if a second reattachment procedure is performed.

Surgical success refers to a reapposition of the sensory retina and RPE and does not refer specifically to the return of vision. Redetachment by traction on the retina and imperfect vision can both occur after successful reattachment. The goal of experimental detachment in animal models is gaining an understanding of underlying cellular mechanisms that will presumably aid in developing improvements in the treatment of the primary detachment as well as the means for preventing the occurrence of secondary tractional RD.

Epidemiology

The incidence of rhegmatogenous RD is described as anywhere from 1 in 10 000 to 1 in 15 000 in the general population. This translates to a prevalence of about 0.3% or approximately 1 in 300 patients over the course of the average patient lifetime. The risk levels for RD vary slightly among different studies but there is general agreement that if ocular trauma is factored out, the prevalence among men and women is about equivalent.

Prognosis and complications

Rhegmatogenous RD is still the condition most frequently treated by retinal surgeons (H. Heimann, personal communication). About 5% of reattachments fail for unknown reasons. Traction detachment caused by proliferative vitreoretinopathy (PVR: the growth of cellular "membranes" on the retinal surface) remains the most common reason for failure, with a rate of 7–10% in primary surgeries and even higher when a second procedure is necessary.[2,13,14] Many studies have shown significant effects of rhegmatogenous RD on functional vision after successful repair. Burton[15] and Tani et al[16] estimated that 30–40% of reattachment patients do not achieve reading ability. A variety of studies estimate that 50% require low-vision aids in order to achieve reading ability (H. Heimann, personal communication). While functional recovery after reattachment is remarkable, it is also true that there is room for improvement.

The development of PVR or subretinal fibrosis (growth of cellular membranes in the subretinal space, i.e., on the photoreceptor surface) is probably the most ominous complication of reattachment. The incidence of PVR is well documented, but that of subretinal fibrosis is not because of the difficulty of resolving these fine cellular membranes by ophthalmic exam. The cellular membranes that form are complex, consisting of at least glial cells, macrophages, and RPE cells. Their attachment to the retina (whether on the vitreal or photoreceptor surface) and contraction can cause wrinkling and redetachment (Figure 71.1). Subretinal fibrosis also effectively blocks the regeneration of outer segments in animal models.[17] PVR was named without a clear link to the actual process of cell division. Indeed, this link is suggested by a variety of data, but not proven. Both cell growth (hypertrophy) and actual proliferation probably play a role (see below). The demonstration that detachment stimulates intraretinal proliferation of all nonneuronal cell types,[18,19] coupled with the assumption that proliferation is generally a part of scar formation, makes antiproliferative agents attractive prospects for preventing or controlling these conditions. Clinical trials with the common antiproliferative drug, 5-fluorouracil (5-FU), proved disappointing,[20] but other antiproliferative agents are providing more encouraging results in animal models.[21] Evidence in mice lacking the

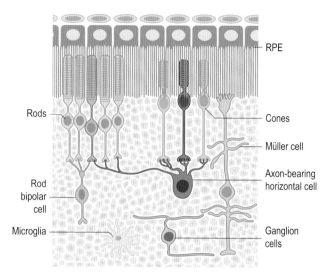

Figure 71.3 Cell types that have been shown to respond to retinal detachment include the retinal pigmented epithelium, rod and cone photoreceptors, rod bipolar cells, axon-bearing horizontal cells, ganglion cells, Müller cells, and microglia.

expression of glial fibrillary acidic protein (GFAP) and vimentin demonstrates that inhibitors of these intermediate filament proteins may lead to better treatment of the proliferative diseases because subretinal scars do not form in these animals.[22] There are currently no such agents available for medical use. The only therapy for PVR or subretinal fibrosis is surgical removal of the cellular membranes, but even successful removal may lead to disappointing results and carries its own risk. PVR is covered at greater length in Chapter 78.

Pathology

For many years the degeneration of photoreceptor outer segments was recognized as the main cellular pathology of RD. The migration of RPE cells from the monolayer and glial cell expansion to form fibrotic lesions or scars on the retina was also recognized in early pathological studies. More detailed studies by electron microscopy and especially the use of immunohistochemical labeling and confocal imaging have revealed many complex cellular responses to detachment extending through all retinal layers (Figure 71.3).

Reattachment was assumed to return the retina to its "normal" state based on early observations of outer-segment regeneration ("After surgical reattachment the receptor cell outer segments regenerate, the discs assume a normal pattern, and the phagosomes again return to the retinal pigment epithelial cells"[3]). Reattachment instead results in what has been referred to as a "patchwork"[17,23] of recovery across the RPE–photoreceptor interface (Figures 12 and 13 in Fisher et al[24]).

Etiology

Aging, myopia, local retinal atrophy (i.e., lattice degeneration), and cataract surgery are all well-recognized factors that increase risk of detachment. Less common factors include congenital eye disease, retinoschisis, uveitis, diabetic retinopathy, premature birth, inflammation, or a family history of detachments[25] (http://www.nei.nih.gov/health/retinaldetach/index.asp#5). In some cases there is a clear association with inherited diseases (Norrie disease, Stickler's syndrome, X-linked retinoschisis) while in other cases a role for inheritance may be suggested but poorly understood. The database, Online Mendelian Inheritance in Man (http://www.ncbi.nlm.nih.gov/sites/entrez?db=omim), provides information suggesting many potential roles for inheritance in RD. Predicting risk in an individual is complex because of the number of interacting factors that can come into play. Although there have been major improvements in cataract surgery this procedure still produces a significant increase in risk for rhegmatogenous RD.[26] Vitreous liquefaction and posterior vitreous detachment (PVD), which produces traction on the retina, are key pathogenic mechanisms in rhegmatogenous RD.[25,27] Before the age of 60, about 10% of patients experience PVD, while this number rises to about 25% between the ages of 60 and 70 and to slightly over 60% in patients over the age of 80. Epidemiological data suggest that the incidence of detachment begins to rise in the fourth decade of life. There is presently no method for preventing vitreous liquification and subsequent PVD. Prophylactic vitrectomy or scleral buckle is rarely performed. Laser photocoagulation or cryotherapy is used around retinal breaks or sites of obvious viteroretinal adhesion to increase chorioretinal adhesion and prevent subsequent detachment but the results are not unequivocal.[27] The prevention of detachment in eyes at risk is a worthy research goal.[27]

Pathophysiology

In recent years it has been recognized that effects of RD occur well beyond the RPE–photoreceptor interface and range from rapid changes in gene expression and protein phosphorylation to neuronal remodeling.[28–32] Many changes described in animal models (Figure 71.4) have been validated in data from human detachment specimens.[33]

The retinal pigmented epithelium

The responses of the RPE monolayer to detachment have not been extensively studied. Its two most prominent responses are proliferation and loss of specialized apical microvilli.[9,34,35] Proliferation begins within a day of RD. A combination of proliferation and migration of the cells can result in complex layers or assemblies in the subretinal space. These do not appear to hinder outer-segment regeneration after reattachment if their orientation is correct.[17] The RPE regenerates de novo its apical microvilli after reattachment, including those highly specialized to ensheath cones. The nature of the signal that induces regeneration is unknown.

Photoreceptors

Until recently, photoreceptors received the most attention in experimental studies of detachment. It is their regenerative capacity that allows the recovery of vision after reattachment. Outer-segment regeneration is a manifestation of the ongoing outer-segment renewal process.[36] In the detached retina the outer segments of both rods and cones degenerate

relatively rapidly, within a day, but the two cell types react differently in other ways. For example, rods continue synthesizing proteins specific to their outer segments, while cones appear to shut down this process.[37] Detachment evokes a series of events in photoreceptors that has been described as "deconstruction"[38] (Figure 71.1) to reflect the fact that the whole cell is affected, often resulting in apoptotic death[39] mediated by caspase activation.[40]

The accumulation of opsin in the plasma membrane is a sensitive indicator of outer-segment damage[41] (Figure 71.1). It also provides a good comparison of rods and cones. Rods show the presence of opsin in their plasma membrane in detachments of a month or more in duration. Cones, however, show the presence for a short period of time, usually 3–7 days.[24,37] Photoreceptors lose the distinct compartmentalization of organelles in their inner segments and show a decrease in their mitochondrial population.[39] Many rod synapses are withdrawn into the outer nuclear layer and their ultrastructural organization is distinctly altered, suggesting almost certain changes in the flow of information from rods to second-order neurons[41,42] (Figure 71.5).

After reattachment rod terminals begin repopulating the outer plexiform layer. This regrowth appears to be imperfect after 28 days of reattachment and perhaps accounts for lingering visual deficits in some reattachment patients. Some rod axons regrow beyond their target layer and into the inner retina in both experimental and human RD. This event also occurs in the early development of mammalian retina, suggesting that reattachment reinitiates some developmental programs.

Second- and third-order neurons

The withdrawal of rod synaptic endings raises the question of the response by cells that connect to them: rod bipolar and axon-bearing horizontal cells. There is no evidence for cell death among inner retinal neurons; however, confocal imaging shows clearly that these cells remodel the processes that connect them to rod photoreceptors. Rod bipolar cells show rapid neurite sprouting with fine thread-like processes extending deep into the outer nuclear layer, usually terminating near withdrawn rod terminals.[43] Dendrites are probably pruned from these cells as well. Axon-bearing horizontal cells in feline retina rapidly upregulate their expression of neurofilament protein and the axon terminal portion of the cell sprouts neurites that grow into the outer nuclear layer (Figure 71.6). Many of these terminate near withdrawn rod terminals. Others, however, grow along reactive Müller's glia into the subretinal space where they can extend for great lengths along subretinal glial scars.[24]

A subpopulation of ganglion cells, those with the largest cell bodies, undergo dramatic changes that mirror the responses of horizontal cells. They upregulate the expression of two proteins, GAP 43 and neurofilament protein, both of which are expressed at low levels in adult ganglion cell bodies and dendrites[30] (Figure 71.6). The same population sprouts neurites as they structurally remodel. These neurites are extensive and may grow from the cell base into the vitreous, or across the retina and into the subretinal space. In all cases the aberrant processes that grow out of the neural retina are structurally associated with gliotic Müller cell scars.

Thus the detachment of the neural retina from the RPE initiates a series of events in neurons throughout the retina,

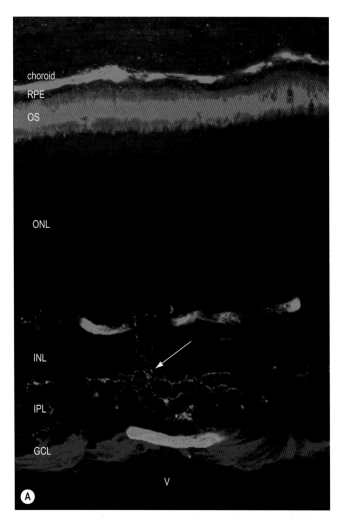 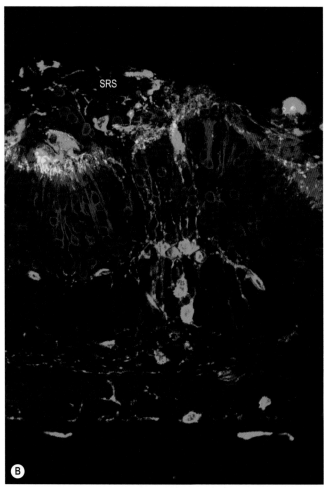

Figure 71.4 Laser scanning confocal microscope images of immunocyotochemical labeling demonstrating reactions of the retina to experimental detachment. Sections of normal (A) and detached (B) feline retina labeled with antibodies to rod opsin (red) and glial fibrillary acidic protein (GFAP, blue), and the isolectin, B4 (green). In the normal retina labeling with the rod opsin antibody is limited to the outer-segment (OS) layer which is apposed to the retinal pigmented epithelium (RPE). Anti-GFAP labels only the astrocytes among the optic axon and ganglion cell (GCL) layers. Isolectin B4 labels the stellate microglia (arrow) in the inner retina. In a retina detached for 28 days, rod outer segments have degenerated, and rod opsin is now found distributed in the plasma membrane around the rod cell bodies in the outer nuclear layer (ONL). Müller cells (the radial blue processes) are now heavily labeled with the anti-GFAP. These cells hypertrophy in response to injury and can grow into the subretinal space (SRS) where they form a glial scar. Microglia become reactive and migrate into the outer retina. Macrophages (which also label with the isolectin) enter the SRS. Note that some rod photoreceptors (red) have moved into the SRS in the region of the large glial scar. v, vitreous cavity; IPL, inner plexiform layer; INL, inner nuclear layer. Scale bar = 20 μm.

not just among photoreceptors. Ensuing changes in synaptic circuitry could have a profound effect on retinal function and there is evidence that the activity of ganglion cells is abnormal in the detached feline retina (Minglian Pu, personal communication). The reorganization of synaptic circuitry after reattachment may underlie the long-term changes in vision that are known to occur in many reattachment patients.

Müller cells

Müller cells are the complex radial glia of the retina (Figure 71.3). In simplest terms, Müller cells can be thought of as monitoring and regulating the retinal environment, and thus playing a critical role in normal retinal function.[44] They also become highly reactive to detachment, showing changes in early-response genes within hours,[29,31] and changes in structure and protein expression within a day. They proliferate,

with a peak response reached 3–4 days after detachment, but continuing at a low level thereafter (Figure 71.7). These cells also undergo a stereotypical structural remodeling that results in the formation of glial scars on both surfaces of the retina, thus contributing to (and perhaps initiating) the diseases subretinal fibrosis and PVR (see Fisher et al[24] for a review).

Müller cells alter their expression pattern for many proteins, including the enzymes glutamine synthetase and carbonic anhydrase, the retinoid-binding protein CRALBP, and the cytoskeletal proteins tubulin, GFAP, and vimentin. An accumulation of the latter two is a hallmark response of these cells to retinal injury (Figures 71.4, 71.6, and 71.7). While intermediate filaments are often regarded as scaffold proteins, there is increasing evidence that they do more. Mice lacking the expression of both (vim[-/-]GFAP[-/-]) show less photoreceptor cell death after detachment.[45] The same knockout strain does not form subretinal scars after detach-

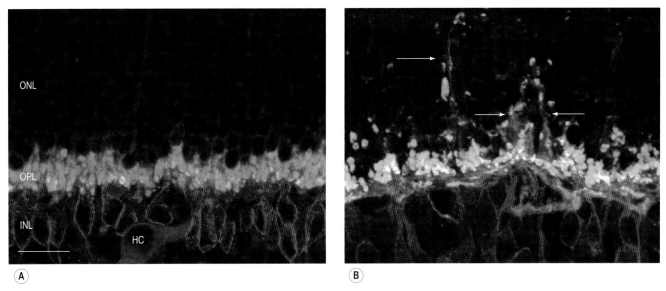

Figure 71.5 Laser scanning confocal microscope images demonstrating additional reactions to experimental detachment. Normal (A) and detached (B) feline retina. Photoreceptor synaptic terminals labeled with an antibody to synaptobrevin (green) form a distinct layer on the border of the outer plexiform layer (OPL). Rod bipolar cells, labeled with an antibody to protein kinase C (red) have their dendrites extending into the synaptic invaginations of the rod synaptic terminals. Axon-bearing horizontal cells (HC), labeled with an antibody to calbindin (blue), are also postsynaptic to rods. After detachment there is a rapid retraction of many rod axons so that their terminals now lie in the outer nuclear layer (ONL), disrupting the layering of the OPL. As rod terminals withdraw, fine neurites grow from both rod bipolar (arrows) and horizontal cells (double arrow) into the ONL (other examples shown in Figure 71.6), demonstrating the remodeling of rods and second-order neurons in response to detachment. INL, inner nuclear layer. Scale bar = 20 μm.

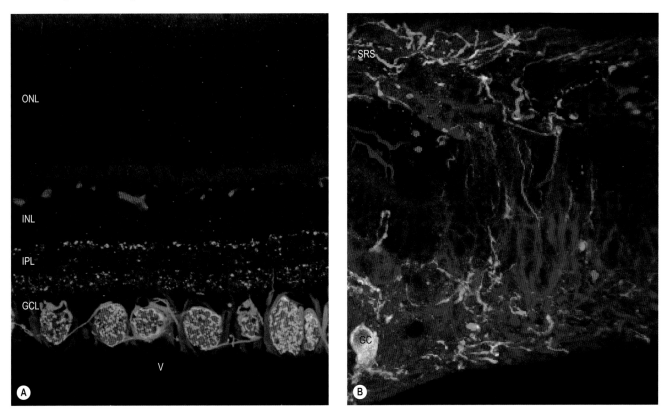

Figure 71.6 Reactions of various cell types to experimental detachment. In a normal feline retina (a) antineurofilament antibody (red) labels ganglion cell axons between the ganglion cell layer (GCL) and vitreous cavity (v), a subset of horizontal cell processes on the border of the inner nuclear layer (INL) and a few fine ganglion cell dendrites in the inner plexiform layer (IPL). An antibody to GAP43 labels sparsely arrayed dendrites of ganglion cells in the IPL. Anti-glial fibrillary acidic protein (GFAP, blue) heavily labels the astrocytes among the ganglion cell axons. After 1 month of detachment, Müller cells have upregulated GFAP expression and in some areas undergone hypertrophy and grown into the subretinal space (SRS) to form glial scars. Many GAP43-positive processes are found throughout the retina and in the subretinal scar. These neurites arise from ganglion cell bodies that re-express GAP43 in response to detachment. These cells, like the horizontal cells, also begin to express neurofilament protein heavily. The yellow ganglion cell (GC) is labeled with antibodies to both GAP43 and neurofilament protein. Neurites from both ganglion cells and horizontal cells course through the area of increased GFAP expression and into the glial scar in the SRS. IPL, inner plexiform layer; ONL, outer nuclear layer. Scale bar = 20 μm.

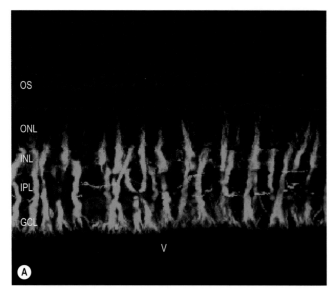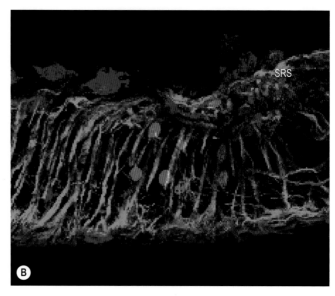

Figure 71.7 Laser scanning confocal microscope images demonstrating the proliferative response to detachment. Normal (A) and 7-day detached (B) rabbit retina are labeled with antibodies to vimentin (green), and bromodeoxyuridine (BrdU, red) as well as with the isolectin B4 (blue). BrdU labels the nuclei of cells undergoing division. In normal retina (A), BrdU-labeled cells are almost never encountered, vimentin extends throughout the cytoplasm of Müller cells, and microglia (blue) are limited to the inner retina. In the detached retina, BrdU labels the nuclei of many cells with some remaining in the inner nuclear layer (INL) while others have migrated into the outer nuclear layer (ONL) and into the large glial scar formed by hypertrophic Müller cell processes (green) in the subretinal space (SRS). A relationship between Müller cell proliferation and glial scar formation is suggested by data of this type. Reactive microglia migrate throughout the retina while macrophages, which also label with the isolectin, enter the SRS. v, vitreous cavity; GCL, ganglion cell layer; IPL, inner plexiform layer. Scale bar = 20 μm.

ment.[22] An association between the upregulation of these proteins and expansion of the Müller cells seems obvious when observing the changes by immunocytochemistry (Figures 71.4, 71.6, and 71.7). There are also data suggesting that the predominant intermediate filament protein expressed in a Müller cell will determine whether they grow into the vitreous cavity or subretinal space.[25]

Proliferation, intermediate filaments, subretinal fibrosis, and PVR

Both PVR and subretinal fibrosis are considered "proliferative diseases," and yet the link between the diseases and the actual proliferation of any cell type is weak. Bromodeoxyuridine (BrdU) labeling studies show that nuclei of Müller cells synthesizing DNA on the third day after detachment have migrated into subretinal membranes by day 7 (Figure 71.7). It seems logical that this correlation could be extrapolated to Müller cells forming membranes on the vitreal surface, but there are no actual experimental data. Thus, as mentioned earlier, agents that prevent proliferation or those that reduce intermediate filament synthesis may reduce the risk for these complications or even cause their regression, thus reducing the need for secondary surgical procedures.

Microglia and the immune response

Microglial cells are immune cells that in their unactivated state reside in the inner retina. After detachment they proliferate, assume a rounded shape, and migrate into the photoreceptor layer where they scavenge dead or dying cells.[46] Microglia may cause or prevent photoreceptor cell death by modulating the release of trophic factors from Müller cells.[47] Macrophages from the circulation enter the subretinal space, where they also scavenge debris from degenerated outer segments (Figures 71.4, 71.6, and 71.7). Microarray analysis of mRNA expression in porcine retinas detached for 24 hours identified significant increases in the expression of many genes involved in the immune and inflammatory responses.[32] In reattached retina the presence of microglia correlates strongly with the degree of photoreceptor recovery.[42] The immune system's role in detachment is only beginning to be appreciated.

In summary, rhegmatogenous RD remains a serious retinal problem that can result in long-lasting visual deficits. The study of animal models and comparisons to data from human tissue are providing new information at the cellular and molecular levels that may help understand why successful anatomical reattachment can still leave a patient with imperfect vision,[48] or why some detachments lead to PVR while others do not.

Key references

A complete list of chapter references is available online at www.expertconsult.com. See inside cover for registration details.

2. Bradbury MJ, Landers MB III. Pathogenetic mechanisms of retinal detachment. In: Ryan S (ed.) Retina, 4th edn. Philadelphia, PA: Elsevier Mosby, 2006:1987–1993.

6. Williams GA, Aaberg TM. Techniques of scleral buckling. In: Ryan S (ed.) Retina, 4th edn. Philadelphia, PA: Elsevier Mosby, 2006:2010–2046.

9. Marmor MF. Mechanism of normal retinal adhesion. In: Ryan S (ed.) Retina, 4th edn. Philadelphia, PA: Elsevier Mosby, 2006:1849–1869.

14. Joeres S, Kirchhof B, Joussen AM. PVR as a complication of rhegmatogeneous retinal detachment: a solved problem? Br J Ophthalmol 2006;90:796–797.

15. Burton TC. Recovery of visual acuity after retinal detachment involving the macula. Trans Am Ophthalmol Soc 1982;80:475–497.

16. Tani P, Robertson DM, Langworthy A. 1981. Prognosis for central vision and anatomic reattachment in rhegmatogenous retinal detachment with macula detached. Am J Ophthalmol 1981;92:611–620.

18. Fisher SK, Erickson PA, Lewis GP, et al. Intraretinal proliferation induced by retinal detachment. Invest Ophthalmol Vis Sci 1991;32:1739–1748.

24. Fisher SK, Lewis GP, Linberg KA, et al. Cellular remodeling in mammalian retina: results from studies of experimental retinal detachment. Prog Retina Eye Res 2005;24:395–431.

28. Geller SF, Lewis GP, Fisher SK. FGFR1, signaling, and AP-1 expression following retinal detachment: reactive Müller and RPE cells. Invest Ophthalmol Vis Sci 2001;42:1363–1369.

30. Zacks DN, Han Y, Zeng Y, et al. Activation of signaling pathways and stress-response genes in an experimental model of retinal detachment. Invest Ophthalmol Vis Sci 2006;47:1691–1695.

33. Sethi CS, Lewis GP, Fisher SK, et al. Glial remodeling and neural plasticity in human retinal detachment with proliferative vitreoretinopathy. Invest Ophthalmol Vis Sci 2005;46:329–342.

38. Lewis GP, Mervin K, Valter K, et al. Limiting the proliferation and reactivity of retinal Müller cells during detachment: the value of oxygen supplementation. Am J Ophthalmol 1999;128:165–172.

41. Lewis GP, Sethi CS, Charteris DG, et al. The ability of rapid retinal reattachment to stop or reverse the cellular and molecular events initiated by detachment. Invest Ophthalmol Vis Sci 2002;43:2412–2420.

46. Lewis GP, Sethi CS, Carter KM, et al. Microglial cell activation following retinal detachment: a comparison between species. Mol Vis 2005;11;491–500.

CHAPTER 72

Retinopathy of prematurity

Mary Elizabeth Hartnett and Cynthia A Toth

Clinical background

Retinopathy of prematurity (ROP) is a leading cause of childhood blindness worldwide and develops after birth in preterm infants, especially those born at less than 1500 g birth weight or younger than 32 weeks' gestational age. There are no symptoms or obvious signs of ROP. Therefore, longitudinal dilated examinations of the retinas of infants at risk are necessary to determine when treatment is needed, or that retinal vascular development is complete and the risk of ROP is no longer present. The goal of examinations is to detect and treat severe ROP in order to prevent progressive retinal detachment, in which poor vision occurs even when successful retinal surgery can be performed.

Based on the International Classification of ROP (ICROP),[1] ROP is characterized by several parameters: zone, stage, extent of stage, and the presence or absence of plus disease. At any examination, the risk of a bad outcome depends on the presence of plus disease or stage 3 ROP (both defined below and important features of severe ROP) as well as the postgestational age of the infant (i.e., the gestational age + chronologic age from birth in weeks).

The zone of ROP is the retinal area supplied by retinal vessels and is an indicator of the extent of retinal vascular development (Figure 72.1). Zone I is the smallest, having the largest area of avascular retina. Zone III is the most vascularized (except for complete vascularization) and has a very low risk of a poor outcome. There are five stages of ROP. Stages 1 through 3 are the acute forms of ROP and are characterized by the appearance of the retina at the junction of vascular and avascular retina. A line (stage 1) or ridge (stage 2 (Figure 72.2A) can often regress without developing into severe ROP. Stage 3 ROP has intravitreous neovascularization, a feature of severe ROP (Figure 72.2B). Stages 4 (Figure 72.2C) and 5 (Figure 72.2D) describe partial or complete retinal detachment, respectively, and are associated with vitreous and fibrovascular changes. The extent of ROP indicates the number of clock hours of a stage. Plus disease is the presence of dilated and tortuous retinal vessels and is a feature of severe ROP (Figure 72.3).

One point of clarification is the difference between retinal drawings and images of dissected retinal flat mounts. The retina covers the inner sphere of the eyeball, and when dissected, must be cut with relaxing incisions in order to flatten it on to a microscope slide. The result is a clover-leaf appearance (Figure 72.4). However, clinicians and surgeons represent the retina as a round clock face and use clock hours to describe the location of pathologic features on the retina.

Severe ROP portends an increased risk of developing retinal detachment and poor vision (Box 72.1). Therefore treatment, preferably with laser,[2,3] is strongly considered at certain levels of severe ROP, threshold disease and type 1 prethreshold ROP[2] (Table 72.1). A form of severe ROP is aggressive posterior ROP (APROP), which appears at young postgestational ages in preterm infants, who have immature retinal vascular development and large avascular retinal areas (Box 72.2). Neovascularization in stage 3 appears broad and flat in APROP (Figure 72.5). Despite standard of care treatment, these eyes often have poor outcomes.[4,5]

Historical development

In the 1940s, ROP manifested as a white pupil and was termed retrolental fibroplasia (RLF).[6] Most RLF was stage 5 ROP with a retrolental membrane and occurred in older and larger infants. Michaelson,[7] Ashton and Cook,[8] and Patz[9] described the hypothesis of hyperoxia-induced vaso-obliteration followed by relative hypoxia and the release of an "angiogenesis" or "vasoproliferative" factor. Further validation from studies with animal models (see below) led to improved monitoring of oxygen to preterm infants in neonatal intensive care units (NICUs). ROP virtually disappeared, because hyperoxia at birth was avoided. (Standard of care today is maintenance of infant oxygen saturation in the mid 80 and low 90 percentages.) But as infants of younger gestational ages and of lower birth weights have survived, ROP has re-emerged.[10] Besides absolute oxygen level, now fluctuations in oxygen also are recognized as important in the pathogenesis of severe ROP (Box 72.3).[11-15]

Xenon photocoagulation was reported as a treatment for ROP in 1976 by Nagata.[16] The initial observations of Folkman et al[17] of a tumor angiogenesis factor were described in the Friedenwald lecture presented by Arnall Patz in 1980.[9] In 1984, ICROP[1] described and characterized stages of ROP earlier than stage 5. The Multicenter Clinical Trial for Cryotherapy for Retinopathy of Prematurity (CRYO-ROP) found

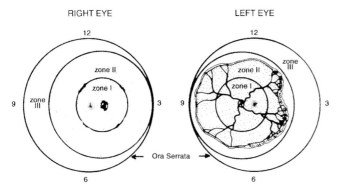

RIGHT EYE   LEFT EYE

Figure 72.1 Drawing showing zones used in classifying retinopathy of prematurity. Zone I represents the least mature retina, being a circle centered on the optic nerve with a radius twice the distance from the optic nerve to the macula. Zone II is a circle centered on the optic nerve with a radius equal to the distance from the optic nerve to the nasal ora serrata. Zone III is the most mature, with the lowest risk of a bad outcome, and represents the temporal crescent.

Box 72.1 Screening and care for acute severe retinopathy of prematurity (ROP)

- Definitions of severe ROP have changed from the Multicenter Clinical Trial for Cryotherapy for Retinopathy of Prematurity (CRYO ROP) study to the Early Treatment for ROP (ETROP) study
- CRYO ROP study termed severe ROP as threshold disease: the presence of zone I or II, stage 3 (5 contiguous or 8 total clock hours with plus disease)
- ETROP defined type 1 prethreshold ROP as zone I, any stage with plus disease, or stage 3, without plus disease, or zone II, stage 2 or 3 with plus disease
- Treatment, preferably with laser, is now considered when the risk of a poor outcome approaches 15% (ETROP) whereas with threshold ROP the risk is 50%
- Cryotherapy has been reported to be associated with more inflammation and with subretinal plaques. Laser is currently preferred
- Consideration of other pharmacologic therapies is under way

---

Table 72.1 Definitions of threshold and type 1 prethreshold retinopathy of prematurity (ROP)

Threshold ROP (CRYO-ROP) (risk of unfavorable outcome approaches 50%)[148]	Type 1 prethreshold ROP (ETROP) (risk of unfavorable outcome is ≥ 15%)[149]
Zone I or II: stage 3 (5 contiguous or 8 total clock hours with plus disease)	Zone I: any stage with plus disease
	Zone I: stage 3 without plus disease
	Zone II: stage 2 or 3 with plus disease

The ETROP recognized plus disease as two quadrants of dilated and tortuous vessels[149] whereas CRYO-ROP[148,150] defined it as four quadrants.
CRYO-ROP, Multicenter Clinical Trial for Cryotherapy for Retinopathy of Prematurity; ETROP, Early Treatment for ROP.

Box 72.2 Aggressive posterior retinopathy of prematurity (APROP)

- APROP presents early with plus disease and often zone I vascularization
- Outcomes have been poor both based on laser treatment for acute early ROP and later treatment for stage 4 fibrovascular ROP
- Stage 3 ROP has a different appearance than in most severe ROP. The neovascularization is flat and can be easily misidentified as intraretinal vessels at the junction with the avascular zone. Therefore, it is important to follow carefully after laser. Skip lesions will seem to appear when flat neovascularization regresses. More laser should be applied

---

that obliteration of the avascular retina in ROP with cryotherapy at a certain threshold of severity (Table 72.1) significantly reduced blindness and retinal detachment.[18] The CRYO-ROP study group reported on the natural history of ROP (for review, see McColm and Hartnett[19]). Since the development of laser via indirect delivery, treatment of acute ROP has been preferentially performed using laser (Figure 72.6), which is less destructive and causes less inflammation than cryotherapy (Box 72.4).[2,3] The Early Treatment for ROP Study (ETROP) found that treatment of eyes with type 1 prethreshold ROP (Table 72.1) further reduced the risk of a bad outcome. ETROP also emphasized plus disease and reduced the importance of extent of stage in defining high-risk eyes.

Epidemiology

The Institute of Medicine reported preterm births up 30% from 1981 (www.iom.edu/Object.File/Master/35/975/pretermbirth.pdf), now accounting for 12.5% of all births in the USA. With increases in prematurity,[20,21] ROP has also become a leading cause of childhood blindness worldwide.[21] A report from a national registry of children in the USA (Babies Count) indicated that ROP was the earliest cause of visual impairment and one of the three most prevalent visual conditions along with cortical visual impairment and optic nerve hypoplasia.[22] ROP of any stage affects approximately 16 000 infants each year in the USA. Most early stages of ROP resolve and about 1100 infants require treatment. Even with treatment, blindness occurs in 550 infants/year (National Eye Institute statement on ROP, October 2007: http://www.nei.nih.gov/health/rop/). In the USA, ROP is seen more commonly in Caucasians than African Americans but once severe ROP occurs, the outcomes appear similar.[23] Asians also have an increased risk of ROP.[24] ROP in developing nations is seen in infants of larger birth weight and older gestational ages than in the USA,[25] possibly because of variations in ethnic groups, regulation and monitoring of oxygen delivery, and the availability of prenatal care.

Genetics

A genetic component to ROP appears to be present, although the understanding of the contribution of genetic polymorphisms to the risk of ROP is incomplete. Based on a retrospective analysis in monozygotic and dizygotic twins, a 70%

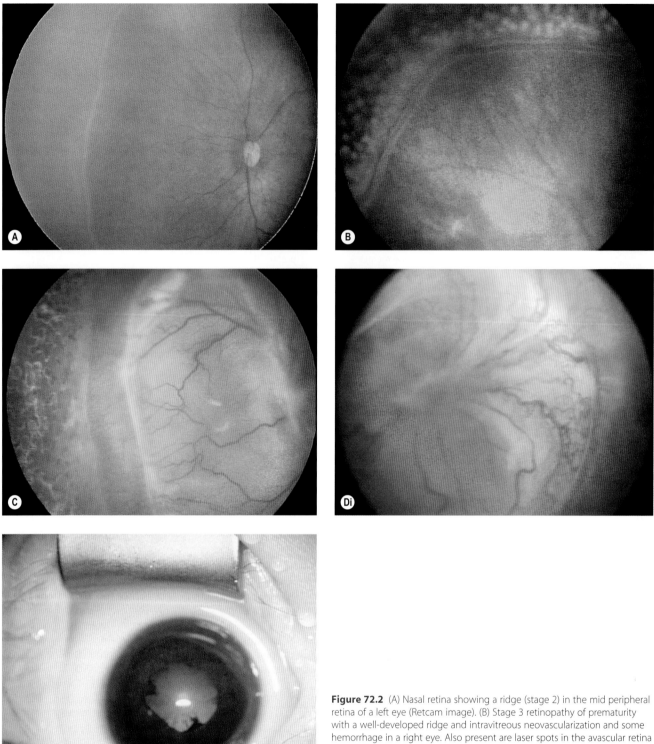

Figure 72.2 (A) Nasal retina showing a ridge (stage 2) in the mid peripheral retina of a left eye (Retcam image). (B) Stage 3 retinopathy of prematurity with a well-developed ridge and intravitreous neovascularization and some hemorrhage in a right eye. Also present are laser spots in the avascular retina temporal to the neovascularization. (C) Temporal retinal detachment involving the macula in stage 4 retinopathy of prematurity with overlying fibrovascular proliferation in a right eye. Pigmented laser spots are present in the avascular retina. (D) Early stage 5 retinopathy of prematurity (1); retrolental fibroplasia causing leukocoria (2).

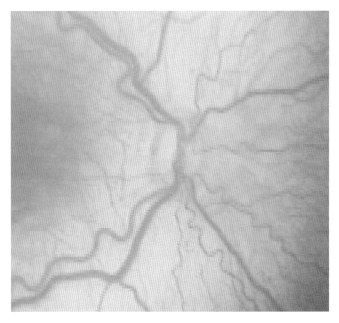

Figure 72.3 Example of dilated and tortuous vessels in plus disease.

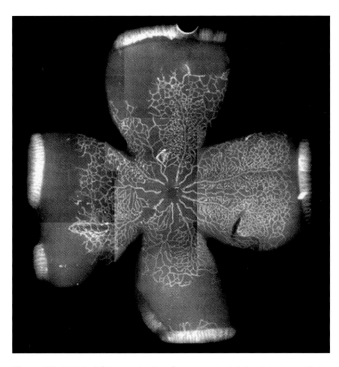

Figure 72.4 Retinal flat mount taken from a postnatal day-14 rat pup that was exposed to oxygen-induced retinopathy, demonstrating a peripheral avascular retina. Vessels are visualized with lectin staining. In the rodent the optic nerve is central and no macula is present. The ora serrata appears as fringe in the periphery of the image. To flatten the retina, four radial cuts are made and the result is a clover-leaf.

variance in the susceptibility of ROP was found to be from genetic factors.[26]

The Norrie disease gene produces the gene product, norrin, which is also a downstream ligand for receptors in the Wnt pathway. The Wnt pathway and norrin are important in retinal and vascular development[27,28] and abnormalities are present in patients with Norrie disease. Genetic mutations in the Norrie disease gene [Xp11.2-11.3] were reported to account for 3% of cases of advanced ROP,[29] but another study having racially diverse populations reported no significant increase in the prevalence of polymorphisms in infants with severe ROP compared to control premature infants with no or minimal ROP.[30] One study reported on samples from 109 patients with diverse pediatric vitreoretinopathies including ROP and 54 controls. Mutations within the cysteine knot configuration of the Norrie disease gene were associated with severe retinal dysplasia whereas other polymorphisms within the gene had less severe vitreoretinopathies.[31] This study suggested that, within severe ROP, polymorphisms in the Norrie disease gene may account for a subgroup with severe retinal dysplasia. Controversy in the association of mutations in the Norrie disease gene may also reflect differences based on ethnic variability.[32]

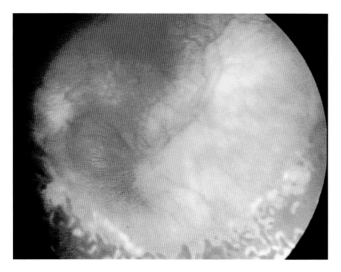

Figure 72.5 Aggressive posterior retinopathy of prematurity with broad lacy neovascularization in an eye that had previous laser treatment.

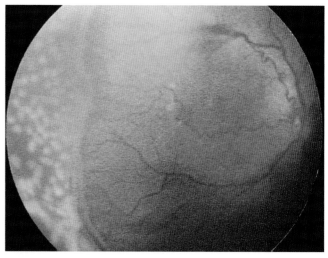

Figure 72.6 Laser treatment in avascular retina temporal to intravitreous neovascularization. There is evidence of an area where laser is not sufficiently confluent ("skip lesion").

One study found an association of severe ROP with certain polymorphisms in the gene of vascular endothelial growth factor (VEGF),[33] whereas another study found different associations.[34] Overexpression of VEGF was reported in an unusual case of ROP.[35] Some polymorphisms in VEGF may be linked differentially to others and the effects of these may differ among ethnic groups.[32] Despite the finding that low serum systemic insulin-like growth factor-1 (IGF-1) was associated with more severe ROP,[36] one study failed to show a relationship between a prevalent polymorphism in the IGF-1 receptor and the presence of ROP.[37] The role of genetics requires greater study and will continue to be elucidated along with the effect of environmental factors on gene function.

Diagnostic workup and treatment

The published guidelines from the American Academy of Pediatrics, American Academy of Ophthalmology, and American Association for Pediatric Ophthalmology and Strabismus are:

> infants with a birth weight of less than 1500 g or gestational age of 30 weeks or less and selected infants between 1500 and 2000 g or gestational age of more than 30 weeks with an unstable clinical course

should have retinal screening with pupil dilation and indirect ophthalmoscopy.[38,39] The first examination is recommended at 4–6 weeks after birth or at 31 weeks' postgestational age (whichever is later) and prior to discharge from the hospital. Examinations are performed approximately every 2 weeks if there is incomplete retinal vascular development without ROP or weekly with evidence of ROP until treatment is recommended (Table 72.1) or until regression of ROP occurs and retinal vascular development is completed.

The use of wide-angle photography or quantification of plus disease to detect high-risk ROP is being studied.[40–42] Images would be obtained at a remote facility and transmitted for review to a reading center. The center would detect "clinically significant ROP" and notify the remote facility that the infant requires an examination and possible treatment by a qualified ophthalmologist. A successful system requires careful coordination to avoid missing any infant with severe ROP.

For eyes that progress to stage 4 ROP (partial retinal detachment), the vitreous appears to play an important role. Both changes at the junction and fibrovascular organization within the vitreous have been associated with and are predictive of progressive stage 4 ROP.[43,44] The severity of the retinal detachment depends on the total area of the fibrovascular proliferation that grows and interacts with the vitreous collagen. The vitreous provides a scaffold for invading cells. Cell contraction on the vitreous collagen is believed to lead to tractional retinal detachments.[43,44] Whereas most stage 4 ROP begins as a retinal detachment at the junction of vascular and avascular retina, APROP may produce more severe detachments because of extensive cell invasion into broad sheets of vitreous in the posterior retina, i.e. usually within zone I. From optical coherence tomography (OCT), changes at the vitreoretinal interface of the posterior retina are recognized (Figure 72.7).[45] The role of transforming growth factor-β (TGF-β) in wound healing and the changes in concentrations of TGF-β and VEGF in the developing preterm infant have been proposed. Study of the mechanisms of stages 4 and 5 ROP is difficult because of lack of ideal animal models and the difficulty in studying human infants.[46,47] Once progressive stage 4 ROP is diagnosed, surgery is performed to release vitreous tractional forces that detach the retina.[43,44,48]

Differential diagnosis

Several conditions can manifest as either early or late stages of ROP based on the progression of the disease. Examples include familial exudative vitreoretinopathy (FEVR), Norrie disease, and incontinentia pigmenti. Other conditions cause media opacity from diseased cornea, lens, vitreous, or retina and produce a white pupil or leukocoria mimicking stage 5 ROP. Notable examples include persistent fetal vasculature,

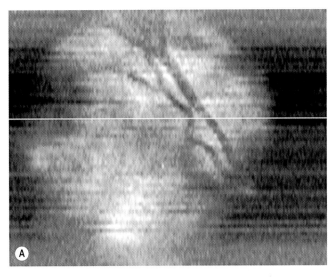

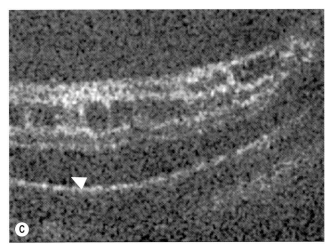

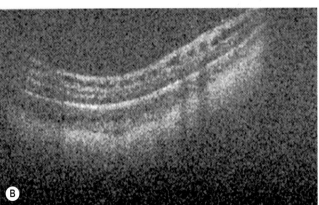

Figure 72.7 Spectral domain optical coherence tomogram (SDOCT) images of a 14-week-old infant born at 24 weeks. The infant has a 4A traction retinal detachment and had previous laser treatment for stage 3, zone 1 ROP. (A) The image is not a photograph of the retina, but an axial summation of the stack of 100 SDOCT images. (B) B-scan SDOCT image is taken at the site of the white line and shows inner retinal cysts which are more confluent in (C), obtained from the periphery within the area of traction detachment (white arrow in subretinal space). These images suggest retinal schisis from traction from the vitreous with cellular infiltration and attachment to the retinal surface. The SDOCT B-scans were denoised and the left image created from these denoised images was adaptively enhanced for contrast by Sina Farsiu, PhD.

a typically unilateral developmental abnormality; chronic vitreous hemorrhage; retinoblastoma, a childhood cancer; Coats disease, a retinovascular condition that can lead to exudative retinal detachment; and infectious endophthalmitis, that can occur from systemic infection or conjunctivitis, as in the case of *Pseudomonas*,[49] or after surgery. It should be noted that endophthalmitis can occur in preterm infants, whereas other conditions usually occur in full-term infants or children.

Pathology

In ROP, the peripheral avascular retina lacks retinal vascularization. At the junction of vascular and avascular retina, aberrant angiogenesis (stage 3 ROP) grows into the vitreous. The avascular retina that forms after hyperoxia-induced vaso-obliteration in the cat or mouse or after fluctuations in oxygen in the rat (see below) is hypoxic.[50,51] The hypoxia is believed to occur because of reduced oxygen supply from an incompletely developed retinal vasculature in the face of a regressing hyaloid vasculature,[52] increased metabolic and oxygen demand of maturing photoreceptors,[53,54] and the possible inability of the choroid to adjust its oxygen concentration in the young animal even with increases in inspired oxygen level.[51,55] Although several growth factors, including

erythropoietin, IGF-1, and hypoxia-inducible factor-1α (HIF-1α), have been reported to be involved in the pathomechanisms of ROP models,[56–58] VEGF has also been shown to be consistently important in other human diseases with intravitreous neovascularization.[59–61] The avascular retina has been shown to express VEGF in animal models.[60,62] Also VEGF was overexpressed in the avascular retina of a human infant with stage 3 ROP.[63] The junction of vascular and avascular retina was described as a proliferation of primitive vascular mesenchyme (possibly describing angioblasts) in a vanguard of advancing vasculature with an intraretinal band of endothelial cells in the rearguard, and extraretinal neovascularization extending into vitreous.[64,65] With the change from a vascularly active process (stage 3 ROP) to a fibrovascular one (stage 4 ROP), there is often mesenchymal tissue that will fold upon itself to form a retinal detachment[64,65] (Figure 72.8).

Etiology

Environmental risk factors

Although genetics plays a role, outside stimuli, such as nutrition and oxygen, are important in the development of ROP. Arginyl-glutamine and omega-3 fatty acids have been shown

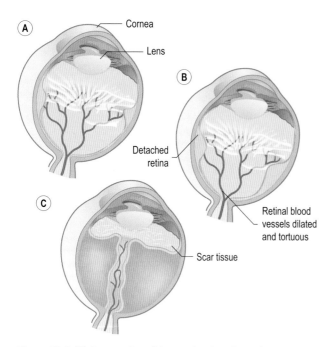

Figure 72.8 (A) Cross-section of the eye showing elevated intravitreous neovascularization at the junction of vascular and avascular retina (stage 3 ROP). (B) Interactions with the vitreous collagen lead to fibrovascular contraction and elevation of the retina (stage 4 ROP). (C) Continued contraction leads to total retinal detachment and a retrolental fibrovascular membrane (stage 5 ROP).

to reduce intravitreous neovascularization or avascular retina, respectively, in the mouse oxygen-induced retinopathy (OIR) model.[66,67]

Role of oxygen: animal models of oxygen-induced retinopathy

After the initial appearance of ROP/RLF in the 1940s, the importance of high oxygen at birth was appreciated and animal models of OIR were developed. Most of these models exposed animals to high constant oxygen, which has been found both to cause capillary obliteration[68] and to inhibit the differentiation of precursor cells into endothelial cells.[69] Now, high oxygen at birth is avoided in NICUs in the USA. However, these models continue to provide important data in understanding the role of oxygen exposure in retinal vascular development and in pathologic angiogenesis. The cat model was used in initial observations of hyperoxia-induced vaso-obliteration[9,70] and in describing the role of astrocytes in retinal vascular development.[71,72] The mouse OIR model permits the study of mechanisms of hyperoxia-induced vaso-obliteration and relative hypoxia by permitting the use of genetically manipulable animals.[68] No model reproduces stage 4 or 5 ROP. However, the beagle OIR model develops retinal folds similar to those reported in human fibrovascular ROP[64] at the junction of vascular and avascular retina.[73]

The rat 50/10 OIR model[74] provides the most relevant model of acute ROP in the USA today. Inspired oxygen extremes in the rat 50/10 OIR model led to rat arterial oxygen levels[75] similar to the transcutaneous oxygen levels measured in a preterm infant who developed severe ROP.[12] Also, rather than constant oxygen used in other models,[50,68,76,77] the 50/10 OIR model exposes pups to repeated fluctuations in oxygen, which increase the risk of severe ROP.[12,14,78] The 50/10 OIR model reproducibly and consistently develops first avascular retina (analogous to zone of human ROP),[75,79] then vessel tortuosity[80] (analogous to plus disease in ROP), and later intravitreous neovascularization (analogous to stage 3 ROP).[79,81]

Other retinopathy models mimic conditions that occur in the preterm infant, including hypercarbia[82] and metabolic acidosis.[83] Newborn pups exposed to minute-to-minute oxygen fluctuations similar in extremes to what human preterm infants experience develop vascular abnormalities in the peripheral retinas,[84] particularly if the fluctuations are performed around a hyperoxic rather than hypoxic mean.[11]

Similar in all animal models is the creation of avascular retina associated with intravitreous neovascularization at junctions of vascular and avascular retina at a time during development when oxygen supply is limited because of insufficiently developed retinal vascularization and a regressing hyaloidal vasculature while oxygen demand is increased from maturing photoreceptors.

The role of supplemental oxygen

As discussed above, high constant oxygen caused vaso-obliteration through apoptosis, resulting in hypoxic avascular areas of retina,[50] and subsequent intravitreous neovascularization (see above). Likewise, fluctuations in oxygen caused apoptosis of endothelial cells, in part causing larger avascular retinal areas in the 50/10 OIR model.[85]

Some studies showed that supplemental oxygen reduced the severity of OIR.[86] Mice raised in sustained hyperoxia beyond postnatal day (p)12 had less vaso-obliteration and neovascularization compared to mice exposed to the standard OIR model.[87] Rats exposed to oxygen fluctuations and recovered in supplemental oxygen (28%) rather than room air had reduced intravitreous neovascularization at some time points.[88] Despite these data, the Supplemental Therapeutic Oxygen for Prethreshold ROP (STOP-ROP) multicenter clinical trial did not find an overall significant benefit from supplemental oxygen given to infants with prethreshold ROP.[89]

In the 50/10 OIR model, supplemental oxygen increased nicotinamide adenine dinucleotide phosphate (NADPH) oxidase activation, accounting partly for pathologic intravitreous neovascularization, even though it also reduced neurosensory retinal VEGF.[51] Furthermore, hypoxic retina, quantified by insoluble retinal pimonidazole (Hypoxyprobe), was not reduced with supplemental oxygen. These results show that increased oxygen in the retinal vasculature reduces the stimulus for VEGF production but does not overcome overall retinal hypoxia that may occur with increased metabolic demand of developing photoreceptors. Furthermore, the retinal hypoxia appears unmet by the choroid. It was previously found that, unlike in the adult rat, the choroid in the p15 rat was unable to support increased oxygen tension with supplemental oxygen.[55] Therefore, supplemental oxygen may not have as beneficial an effect as hoped in the retina and it can also lead to greater complications of pulmonary disease.[89]

Pathophysiology

ROP is complex. Many changes occur from the in utero environment to that after birth, including oxygen concentration, growth factor relationships, and nutrition. The effects of prematurity and environmental factors necessary to keep premature infants alive on the pathophysiology of ROP are incompletely understood. Below is evidence of growth factor signaling in retinal vascular development and in the pathogenesis of ROP.

Signaling through VEGFA in development, as a survival factor, and in disease

VEGFA has emerged as one of the most important angiogenic factors in the development of human intravitreous neovascularization.[59,61] (VEGFA is the most widely studied ligand of the VEGF family and will be referred to as VEGF in this chapter). Besides its role in pathology, however, it is important in retinal vascular development,[71,72] and is also an endothelial and neuronal survival factor.[90–92]

To understand ROP, it is important first to understand the known processes in human retinal vascular development. It is believed that vasculogenesis or de novo development of central vasculature around the optic nerve occurs from angioblasts, endothelial cell precursors.[93] Angioblasts do not have markers commonly thought to be present on endothelial cells like CD31, CD34, and von Willebrand's factor but do express CD39 and CXCR4.[94,95] Retinal vascular development is believed to be completed mainly through a process of angiogenesis,[96] but the role of circulating endothelial precursors is being appreciated more.[94] During angiogenesis, a front of migrating cells, e.g., astrocytes in cat[72] or angioblasts in dog,[97] sense physiologic hypoxia and express VEGF. The ensuing endothelial cells are attracted to VEGF and migrate to create blood vessels.[72] The VEGF signaling pathway has been found to regulate and integrate several cell processes that are important during sprouting angiogenesis. Whereas VEGF concentration is thought to regulate endothelial cell division rate,[98,99] the presentation of VEGF, as in a gradient, may regulate filopodia formation of endothelial tip cells at the migrating front and direct the growth of endothelial cells.[100] The delta-like ligand 4/Notch1 (Dll4/Notch1) signaling pathway regulates VEGF-induced endothelial tip/stalk cells at the junction of vascular and avascular retina and permits ordered angiogenesis.[101]

VEGF signaling is also important in preventing hyperoxia-induced vaso-obliteration. Exogenous VEGF injected into the vitreous prior to hyperoxia reduced vaso-obliteration.[102] Stimulation of VEGF receptor 1 (VEGFR1) with the specific ligand placental growth factor (PlGF-1), prior to hyperoxia, reduced vaso-obliteration,[103] whereas stimulation of VEGFR2 with the specific ligand VEGFE did not. VEGFR1 has a higher affinity for VEGF than does VEGFR2, but its receptor tyrosine kinase is less active.[104] In mouse development, expression of VEGFR1 RNA increased significantly more than did the expression of VEGFR2 RNA. In addition, VEGFR1 RNA was localized to the developing vasculature, thus supporting its role in vascular development, whereas VEGFR2 RNA was localized to the neuronal retina.[105–107] VEGFR1 is believed to limit excessive VEGF signaling through VEGFR2 during development[98] and permit ordered angiogenesis.[108]

The hypoxic, avascular retina that occurs from hyperoxia-induced vaso-obliteration in the mouse OIR or from repeated oxygen fluctuations in the rat 50/10 OIR expresses excess VEGF[62,109] and is causally related to pathologic intravitreous neovascularization,[110,111] in part through the src kinase pathway.[112] Compared to hypoxia alone, repeated fluctuations in oxygen, a risk factor for ROP,[12–15] were shown to increase RNA expression of $VEGF_{164}$, an isoform created through alternative splicing of the parent VEGF mRNA.[109] $VEGF_{164/165}$ was also reported to increase leukostasis, endothelial apoptosis, and avascular retina in the mouse OIR model.[113] An intravitreous neutralizing antibody made against $VEGF_{164}$ at a dose that inhibited signaling through VEGFR2, but not VEGFR1, significantly reduced intravitreous neovascularization in the retina in the 50/10 OIR model.[111] In addition, numerous studies have shown that inhibiting VEGF through other mechanisms reduced intravitreous neovascularization.[114]

Although inhibition of VEGF alone does not inhibit intravitreous neovascularization completely, combinations of inhibitors that affect multiple receptors do.[115,116] However, in the case of ROP in which development of the vasculature and retina is ongoing, complete inhibition of angiogenesis or removal of survival aspects of growth factors is not desirable. VEGF is important in development, survival, and also in the pathogenesis of ROP. Thus, data suggest that the amount, presentation, isoform expression, and timing of VEGF are important. Below are studies providing evidence of the role of other growth factors (Box 72.5).

HIF-1alpha

Stabilization of HIF-1α occurs under hypoxic conditions or secondary to reactive oxygen species (ROS) generated from NADPH oxidase, nitric oxide, mitochondria, and other enzymes.[117] HIF-1α binds to the hypoxia response elements to cause transcription of several genes, including angiogenic factors, VEGF, and erythropoietin.[117] A knockout to HIF-1α is lethal but a knockout to the HIF-1α-like factor (HLF)/HIF-2α provided evidence that erythropoietin was a major gene involved in intravitreous neovascularization after relative hypoxia from hyperoxia-induced vaso-obliteration.[56]

Box 72.5 Vascular endothelial growth factor (VEGF)

- VEGF is present in human retinopathy of prematurity (ROP) and in animal models of oxygen-induced retinopathy
- Inhibition of VEGF with a neutralizing antibody reduces both tortuosity and dilation of vessels in animal models (analogous to plus disease) and intravitreous neovascularization (analogous to stage 3 ROP)
- Dose of antibody is important in animal models, with low doses having apparent rebound effects
- VEGF is important as a survival factor for neurons, endothelial cells, and retinal pigment epithelium
- VEGF is important in maintenance of adult tissues and in vascular homeostasis
- Intravitreous doses in the infant eye result in higher systemic concentrations in blood than in the adult

Erythropoietin

Erythropoietin is angiogenic, erythropoietic, and neuroprotective. It is upregulated after stabilization of HIF-1α in response to hypoxia.[117] Besides being a target for oxygen-induced retinopathy in the mouse model,[56] clinical studies have shown an association between the number of administrations of erythropoietin for anemia of prematurity and the prevalence of severe ROP.[118,119] These studies link erythropoietin use in preterm infants and the experimental findings from HLF/HIF-2α knockout mice.[56]

IGF-1 and IGF-BP3

IGF-1 is important in physical growth and influences birth weight. IGF-1 levels that occur in utero are not maintained upon birth in preterm infants.[120] Low serum IGF-1 correlated with increased avascular retina in human ROP.[36] Furthermore, transgenic mice expressing a growth hormone antagonist gene, or wild-type mice treated with an inhibitor to growth hormone, had reduced retinal neovascularization in the mouse OIR model of hyperoxia induced vaso-obliteration and angiogenesis.[57,58] IGF-1 was also found to be important for maximal signaling through the mitogen-activated protein (MAP) kinase pathway, which is important in cell proliferation. In addition, VEGF and IGF-1 synergistically triggered Akt, which is important in cell survival.[36] Based on these findings, it is theorized that IGF-1, which is low in the preterm infant, is necessary for early retinal vascular survival and growth, but can result in later intravitreous neovascularization in ROP. However, timing and dose appear critical.

A hypoxia-regulated binding protein of IGF-1, IGF-1BP3, was shown to be important in reducing hyperoxia-induced vaso-obliteration and in promoting vascular regrowth into the retina.[121,122] IGF-BP3 was shown to promote differentiation of endothelial precursor cells into endothelial cells and in promoting angiogenic processes, such as cell migration and tube formation.[122]

Mechanisms of avascular retina

The size of the avascular zone of retina is directly associated with poor outcomes from severe ROP.[18,123] As discussed earlier, both hyperoxia-induced vaso-obliteration and fluctuating oxygen can lead to increased avascular retina in OIR models.[81] The ischemic microenvironment created by avascular regions[50,51] produces angiogenic factors, like VEGF,[7,124] that cause intravitreous neovascularization.[110,111] Studies support the concept that increased apoptosis leads to increased avascular areas; for example, through inflammatory leukostasis[125,126] or, in bcl-2 knockout mice, through a defect in protection against apoptosis.[127] Furthermore, growth factors, including VEGF, IGF-1, IGF-1BP3,[102,103,121,122] and nutritional supplements, including omega 3 fatty acids,[66,67] can reduce the apoptosis of endothelial cells from newly formed capillaries if given prior to the hyperoxic insult in the mouse OIR model. Finally, the use of antioxidants has shown benefit in reducing the size of the avascular areas of retina in animal models.[85,128–130]

Reactive oxygen species

Oxidative stress has been proposed to be important in the development of ROP,[131,132] because the retina is susceptible to oxidative damage given its high metabolic rate and rapid rate of oxygen consumption.[133] In addition, the premature infant has a reduced ability to scavenge ROS,[134] increasing its vulnerability to oxidative stress. End-products of ROS, lipid hydroperoxides (LHP), were significantly increased in the 50/10 OIR model at time points corresponding to intravitreous neovascularization.[85] When injected into the vitreous, LHP caused intravitreous neovascularization in the rabbit.[135] Also, ROS can trigger signaling pathways relevant to apoptosis[136] or angiogenesis,[137] both important in the pathogenesis of ROP.

Treatment of pups in the 50/10 OIR model or humans with ROP using a broad antioxidant, *n*-acetylcysteine,[138,139] failed to show reduction in clock hours of intravitreous neovascularization, or avascular retinal area.[85,140] In a clinical trial in preterm infants, there was no difference in the incidence in ROP between those receiving *n*-acetylcysteine or control.[140] However, reduction in ROS with preparations of vitamin E[128,129] or liposomes containing the antioxidant enzyme, manganese superoxide dismutase (MnSOD), reduced OIR severity.[130] Also, a meta-analysis of infants treated with vitamin E showed a significant reduction in severity of ROP. Reducing the activation of NADPH oxidase, an enzyme that produces ROS, can also reduce the size of the avascular areas[85] and subsequent intravitreous neovascularization in certain OIR models.[51]

Light was proposed to be important in ROP development through photo-oxidation of polyunsaturated fatty acids within photoreceptor outer segments. On the other hand, during the dark, photoreceptors are more metabolically active. A clinical trial testing the effect of light or shade on the development of ROP showed no significant difference.[141]

Inflammatory aspects

Resident macrophages and microglia are necessary for retinal vascular development[142] and in remodeling of the retinal vasculature,[126] but can also be involved in pathologic angiogenesis and photoreceptor apoptosis.[126,143,144] Macrophages produce ROS from activated NADPH oxidase, oxidoreductases, or nonenzymatically as side products of reactions utilizing electron transfer.[136] Macrophages can produce nitric oxide, which is involved in angiogenic signaling,[136,145] and can express inflammatory cytokines in response to hypoxia[146] and release VEGF.[147] Furthermore, VEGF$_{164}$ is upregulated by fluctuations in oxygen in the 50/10 OIR model[109] and was found to be proinflammatory by increasing adhesion molecules in vessels and by attracting monocytes in vivo.[113,148]

Summary

The role of VEGFA and its receptors, as well as the effects and interactions with other factors, is complex when considering the pathogenesis of ROP. The concentration, presentation, isoform expression, and coordination in development are important. Also the effect and type of oxygen stress appear important. Since fluctuations in oxygen as well as absolute oxygen concentration are important, growth factors and signaling pathways that are involved in the relative hypoxia-induced angiogenesis following hyperoxia require further study. Broad inhibition of VEGF, use of antioxidants, or reduction in inspired oxygen concentration may be detri-mental to the developing preterm infant. Also the systemic concentration from intravitreous drugs is greater in infants than adults because of an approximate 10-fold difference in the vitreous/blood volumes. New treatments for ROP are on the horizon but these issues must be considered in the devel-oping preterm infant.

Key references

A complete list of chapter references is available online at www.expertconsult.com. See inside cover for registration details.

1. International Committee. An international classification of retinopathy of prematurity. Br J Ophthalmol 1984;68:690–697.

2. Early Treatment for Retinopathy of Prematurity Cooperative Group. Revised indications for the treatment of retinopathy of prematurity: results of the early treatment for retinopathy of prematurity randomized trial. Arch Ophthalmol 2003;121:1684–1694.

3. Cryotherapy for Retinopathy of Prematurity Cooperative Group. Multicenter trial of cryotherapy for retinopathy of prematurity: Snellen visual acuity and structural outcome at 5½ years after randomization. Arch Ophthalmol 1996;114:417–424.

12. Cunningham S, Fleck BW, Elton RA, et al. Transcutaneous oxygen levels in retinopathy of prematurity. Lancet 1995;346:1464–1465.

19. McColm JR, Hartnett ME. Retinopathy of prematurity: current understanding based on clinical trials and animal models. In: Hartnett ME (ed.) Pediatric Retina. Philadelphia, PA: Lippincott Williams & Wilkins, 2005:387–409.

36. Hellstrom A, Peruzzu C, Ju M, et al. Low IGF-1 suppresses VEGF-survival signaling in retinal endothelial cells: direct correlation with clinical retinopathy of prematurity. Proc Natl Acad Sci USA 2001;98:5804–5808.

43. Coats DK. Retinopathy of prematurity: involution, factors predisposing to retinal detachment, and expected utility of preemptive surgical reintervention. Trans Am Ophthalmol Soc 2005;103:281–312.

44. Hartnett ME, McColm JR. Retinal features predictive of progression to stage 4 ROP. Retina 2004;24:237–241.

47. Trese MT, Capone A. Retinopathy of prematurity: evolution of stages 4 and 5 ROP and management. A. Evolution to retinal detachment and physiologically based management. In: Hartnett ME (ed.) Pediatric Retina. Philadelphia, PA: Lippincott Williams & Wilkins, 2005:387–409.

48. Capone A Jr, Hartnett ME, Trese MT. Treatment of retinopathy of prematurity: peripheral retinal ablation and vitreoretinal surgery. In: Hartnett ME (ed.) Pediatric Retina. Philadelphia, PA: Lippincott Williams & Wilkins, 2005:387–409.

54. Berkowitz BA, Roberts R, Penn JS, et al. High-resolution manganese-enhanced MRI of experimental retinopathy of prematurity. Invest Ophthalmol Vis Sci 2007;48:4733–4740.

55. Cringle SJ, Yu PK, Su EN, et al. Oxygen distribution and consumption in the developing rat retina. Invest Ophthalmol Vis Sci 2006;47:4072–4076.

68. Smith LEH, Wesolowski E, McLellan A, et al. Oxygen induced retinopathy in the mouse. Invest Ophthalmol Vis Sci 1994;35:101–111.

75. Penn JS, Henry MM, Tolman BL. Exposure to alternating hypoxia and hyperoxia causes severe proliferative retinopathy in the newborn rat. Pediatr Res 1994;36:724–731.

82. Holmes JM, Zhang S, Leske DA, et al. Carbon-dioxide induced retinopathy in the neonatal rat. Curr Eye Res 1998;17:608–616.

88. Berkowitz BA, Zhang W. Significant reduction of the panretinal oxygenation response after 28% supplemental oxygen recovery in experimental ROP. Invest Ophthalmol Vis Sci 2000;41:1925–1931.

111. Geisen P, Peterson L, Martiniuk D, et al. Neutralizing antibody to VEGF reduces intravitreous neovascularization and does not interfere with vascularization of avascular retina in an ROP model. Mol Vis 2008;14:345–357.

CHAPTER 73

Retinal energy metabolism

Robert A Linsenmeier

Clinical background (Box 73.1)

Altered retinal oxygenation plays a central role in the pathogenesis of many retinal diseases and a hypothesized role in others.[1] Unfortunately, despite decades of work in some cases, the precise role of oxygen in certain complex diseases remains elusive.

There are three different categories of situations in which oxygen can play a critical role in disease. First, and most obvious, are situations involving ischemia. Because oxygen is usually the limiting substrate for metabolism, and cannot be stored, even a short-term loss of oxygen leads to devastating consequences in conditions such as central or branch retinal artery occlusion (Chapter 63). Ischemia is certainly involved in other cases, such as after capillary dropout in diabetes (Chapters 65 and 66). These conditions involve anoxia, because there is essentially no redundancy or safety factor in the retinal circulation where one arteriole or capillary can take over oxygenation of a region ordinarily supplied by another vessel. The choroidal circulation is usually not affected in the same diseases, but cannot compensate for the loss of retinal circulation when an individual is breathing air.[2-5]

The extent to which substrates other than oxygen are involved in ischemic diseases is not generally clear. During retinal artery or capillary occlusion, one might expect that glucose from the choroid could diffuse into the inner retina to allow glycolytic metabolism, but this is uncertain. Purely glycolytic metabolism also leads to acidosis, which is observed in animal models of retinal artery occlusion.[6] Interestingly, in primates and cats, retinal function does return to a large extent if circulation is restored within about 1.5 hours,[7,8] which is far longer than the brain could survive. The long survival time probably does not reflect an inherent difference in retinal and brain neurons, but rather the small reservoir of glucose in the vitreous and the remaining supply from the choroid, neither of which has an analog in the brain. Elevating glucose prior to ischemia in rats prolongs the survival of the electroretinogram during ischemia, providing some support for this idea.[9]

Some investigators believe that less severe reductions in blood flow through the retinal or choroidal circulation, which produce milder hypoxia, play a role in diabetes,[10,11] glaucoma,[12,13] and age-related macular degeneration.[14,15] In diabetes, for example, hypoxia could be caused by the upregulation of adhesion molecules and leukostasis that is known to occur.[10,16] In many tissues, hypoxia leads to a dramatic elevation in the level of the transcription factor hypoxia-inducible factor 1α (HIF-1α), not because synthesis is increased, but because degradation is prevented during hypoxia. HIF-1α increases in the retina in many situations.[17] HIF-1α has multiple downstream effects, including the upregulation of vascular endothelial growth factor (VEGF), which is a hallmark of diabetic retinopathy and wet macular degeneration. Complicating the picture, however, are findings that VEGF and HIF-1α can increase as a result of factors other than hypoxia.[18,19]

The second role for oxygen in disease is the situation where there is nothing wrong with the circulation per se, but there is a mismatch between oxygen supply and metabolic demand. An important and underappreciated example of this is in retinal detachment (Chapter 71), where the choroid is functional, but is too far from the photoreceptors to supply their needs fully.[20,21] Theoretically, metabolic starvation of the inner-segment mitochondria would occur with even very small separations between the choroid and photoreceptors,[20] as would occur in the presence of large drusen, so it is possible that a supply–demand mismatch contributes to the loss of photoreceptors in dry age-related macular degeneration, which occurs directly over drusen.[22] In these cases the mismatch is caused by insufficient supply. Only one case is known at present where the mismatch is caused by increased metabolic rate. This is the situation that leads to the loss of photoreceptors in some hereditary degenerations (Chapter 76). In rd mice[23] and in some cases of human retinitis pigmentosa,[24] phosphodiesterase (PDE) activity is reduced. This is expected to lead to increased cyclic guanosine monophosphate (cGMP) levels, which in turn would lead to increased numbers of open channels in the photoreceptors, increased influx of Na^+ and Ca^{2+}, and a greater demand for adenosine triphosphate (ATP) to operate Na^+ and Ca^{2+} pumps than the cell can meet. Whether metabolic overload causes loss of photoreceptors or other retinal neurons in other situations is not known.

The third situation is one in which there is too much oxygen. This has long been recognized as a fundamental problem in retinopathy of prematurity[25] (Chapter 72), preventing the growth of retinal blood vessels in the neonate, and more recently it has been recognized to be the reason why retinal blood vessels ultimately disappear or are seriously attenuated in all forms of retinitis pigmentosa.[26,27] Oxidative damage is also thought to play a role in reperfusion injury in the retina.[28]

The presence of the choroidal circulation offers possibilties for therapy, because it is rarely compromised at the same time as the retinal circulation. The leading hypothesis for the success of panretinal photocoagulation in proliferative diabetic retinopathy is that laser destruction of the photoreceptors removes their oxygen demand, allowing choroidal oxygen to reach the inner retina. This relieves hypoxia and reduces angiogenesis.[11] Intraretinal Po_2 measurements show that O_2 levels do increase after photocoagulation.[29] Choroidal oxygen is probably also responsible for the benefit of hyperbaric oxygen in cystoid macular edema.[30] We and others have also argued that treatment with hyperoxia would be beneficial in arterial occlusion[7] and retinal detachment,[21,31] and that attempts at using hyperoxia previously have misunderstood some of the key features of retinal oxygenation outlined below.

This chapter gives an overview of retinal energy metabolism and substrate supply, providing a basis for understanding the potential roles of these topics in the etiology of the diseases covered in more detail elsewhere.

Pathology

There are many studies showing detrimental effects of reduced oxygen and substrates in acute experiments, but only a few studies investigating whether reduced supply of substrates, in the absence of any disease, can cause retinal pathology, because chronic, moderate changes that would mimic disease are more difficult in an experimental setting. However, the experiments that have been done reveal aspects of pathology similar to those that would be observed in disease. For example, in birds, it has been shown that reduced choroidal blood flow can cause photoreceptor loss and upregulation of GFAP,[32] as well as decreased acuity.[33] In rat retina, chronic systemic hypoxia (10% inspired oxygen) leads to apoptosis of photoreceptors.[34] Hypoxia can also itself lead to neovascularization.[35]

Etiology

Apart from the comments under clinical background, consideration of oxygen in the etiology of different diseases is left to the chapters on individual diseases.

Pathophysiology

A number of properties make the retina unique, in terms of: (1) the supply of oxygen and glucose to the retina by its circulations; (2) the utilization of the substrates to provide ATP; and (3) the relative importance of the cellular processes that use the ATP. A great deal is known about the first two topics. The third has been more difficult to investigate and our knowledge is mainly about photoreceptors.

Supply of oxygen and glucose from the circulation (Box 73.2)

The retina of humans and many other mammals is supplied by two circulations, both of which are essential (Figure 73.1). The choroidal circulation lies behind the retinal pigment epithelium and the retinal circulation lies within the inner half of the retina, except in the central part of the fovea, where the retinal circulation is absent. Because the two circulations have such different physiological properties, they must be treated separately. The retinal circulation is like the circulation of the brain in most respects. The flow rate is modest, on the order of 25 µl/min, or 20–25 ml/(100 g-min) of retina if normalized to the whole retinal weight,[36–44] or about 40–50 ml/(100 g-min) if normalized by the inner retinal weight (half the total retinal weight), which is what the retinal circulation normally supplies. This is called the "nutrient flow rate" below. The retinal blood flow rate is controlled by tissue oxygen and metabolite levels, with hypoxia and hypercapnia increasing flow, and hyperoxia

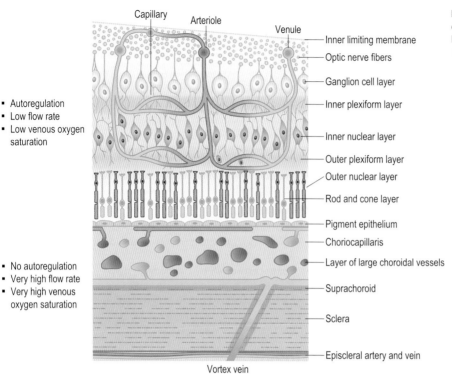

- Autoregulation
- Low flow rate
- Low venous oxygen saturation

Capillary
Arteriole
Venule

Inner limiting membrane
Optic nerve fibers
Ganglion cell layer
Inner plexiform layer
Inner nuclear layer
Outer plexiform layer
Outer nuclear layer
Rod and cone layer
Pigment epithelium
Choriocapillaris
Layer of large choroidal vessels
Suprachoroid
Sclera
Episcleral artery and vein

- No autoregulation
- Very high flow rate
- Very high venous oxygen saturation

Vortex vein

Figure 73.1 Schematic of the retinal and choroidal circulations. (Modified from Kaufman P, Alm A (eds) Alder's Physiology of the Eye, 10th edn. St. Louis, MO: Mosby, 2003.)

decreasing flow.[37,45–49] Increased activity of retinal neurons caused by visual stimuli can increase retinal blood flow,[50] but the blood flow in steady illumination is only transiently increased relative to the flow in the dark.[51] There is no autonomic control of the retinal vessels after the retinal artery enters the eye at the center of the optic nerve.[52]

In contrast, the choroidal circulation has a flow rate of 700–900 μl/min,[37,38,43,44] or 1200–1500 ml/(100 g-min) if normalized by choroidal weight,[37,39,42,43] or still slightly higher if normalized by the outer retinal weight. The choroidal flow rate changes little in response to hypoxia or hyperoxia, although it does increase in hypercapnia.[37,53–55] Instead, autonomic control is very strong,[52,56,57] with sympathetic influences decreasing flow, and facial nerve stimulation increasing flow.[58,59] Flow rate increases somewhat in response to illumination,[60] but this is when the photoreceptors need less oxygen, so it cannot be a metabolically dependent effect.

Oxygen supply

The retina is critically dependent upon a continuous supply of oxygen, with loss of vision occuring only 5–10 seconds after intraocular pressure is raised to a level that occludes all circulation to the retina.[61,62] It is known that oxygen is the important factor, because vision can be slightly, but not usefully, prolonged if an individual breathes oxygen before the occlusion.[61,62] Levels of oxygen in the retina have been measured by a variety of techniques,[1,63] including optical and magnetic resonance measurements that are valuable because they are noninvasive,[64–66] but here we focus on microelectrode measurements within the retina and measurements of oxygen in the two circulations, which yield information useful for determining metabolic rate.[67]

The choroidal circulation is normally responsible for most of the oxygen needed by the photoreceptors, while the retinal circulation provides most or all of the oxygen needed

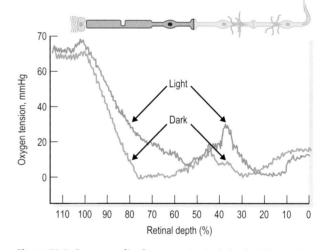

Figure 73.2 Oxygen profiles from cat retina in dark adaptation and at a steady illumination sufficient to saturate the rod system, and a schematic diagram of retinal structure. Retinal depth is defined to be zero at the vitreal–retinal border, and 100% at the choriocapillaris. (Modified from Wangsa-Wirawan ND, Linsenmeier RA. Retinal oxygen: fundamental and clinical aspects. Arch Ophthalmol 2003;121:547–557.)

by the inner retina. Both circulations are required, and neither can compensate for the loss of the other under ordinary conditions. One might expect that there would be a minimum PO_2 at the depth where the supply from the two circulations meets. There is such a location, but it varies with illumination, and may be different in different animals. In darkness in cat,[67] monkey,[68] and presumably human retina, the minimum PO_2 is not at the middle of the retina, but is far distal, in the photoreceptor inner-segment layer, about 35 μm from the choroid (Figure 73.2). Despite the distal location of this minimum, the retinal circulation only provides about 10% of the oxygen used by the photoreceptors.[67,68] During strong illumination, in cat[67] and rat,[69] the oxygen gradient extends further toward the inner retina, and generally provides all of the oxygen for the photoreceptors, and possibly a little for the outer plexiform layer. However, in monkey, the change in the shape of the gradient is less dramatic,[69] and the choroid does not provide all the oxygen for the photoreceptors during illumination.

One of the often confusing aspects of retinal oxygenation is why choroidal blood flow should be so high. By employing the Fick principle, a mass balance on oxygen, it is possible to calculate the total amount of oxygen extracted from each circulation:

$$QO_2c = Fc\left(SaO_2 - SvcO_2\right) \text{ for the choroidal circulation, and}$$

$$QO_2r = Fr\left(SaO_2 - SvrO_2\right) \text{ for the retinal circulation.}$$

where QO_2 is the oxygen utilization of the tissues supplied by the choroidal (c) and retinal (r) circulations, F is the nutrient flow rate discussed above, SaO_2 is arterial oxygen saturation (about 20 vol% or 0.2 ml O_2/ml blood), and SvO_2 is venous saturation. Because of the technical difficulty of measuring flow rates and choroidal venous saturation, wide variations in Fc, Fr, and $SvcO_2$ have been reported. Nevertheless, it is instructive to use reasonable in vivo values, which come from monkeys, cats, pigs, and humans: Fc = 1400 ml/(100 g-min),[37,39,42-44,58] Fr = 45 ml/(100 g-min),[36] $SvcO_2$ = 0.19–0.195 ml O_2/ml blood,[44,70] and $SvrO_2$ = 0.13 ml O_2/ml blood.[71-73]

$$Qo_2c = 1400 \times \left(0.2 - 0.195\right) = 7.00\,ml\,O_2/(100g\text{-}min)$$

$$Qo_2r = 45 \times \left(0.2 - 0.13\right) = 3.15\,ml\,O_2/(100g\text{-}min)$$

These averaged values do not account for regional variation across the retina, and would be slightly different if all the values were from a single animal (e.g., Figure 73.3).[74] No matter how the calculation is done, however, both circulations contribute substantially to the oxygen supply of the retina. In addition, these equations reflect clearly that there can be a tradeoff between flow rate and arteriovenous difference to achieve a particular metabolic rate. Moreover they make clear why the high choroidal flow rate is required. The high flow rate allows a low oxygen extraction, and in turn, the high choriocapillaris and venous PO_2, seen in oxygen profiles.[20] A high PO_2 at the choroid is essential in providing a large driving force for oxygen diffusion to the photoreceptor inner segments, which begin about 30 μm from the choroid and have an unusually high oxygen demand. High choroidal blood flow may also assist in heat removal.

Glucose supply

Aside from oxygen, the most critical substrate for the retina is glucose, which can also be analyzed by the Fick principle. About one-sixth as much glucose as oxygen is needed for oxidative metabolism on a molar basis, but much larger quantities of glucose are used whenever glycolysis ends with lactate production. Using the Fick principle to investigate glucose utilization is difficult, because the arteriovenous differences of glucose and lactate are small, and because they require blood collection from a retinal vein or vortex vein,

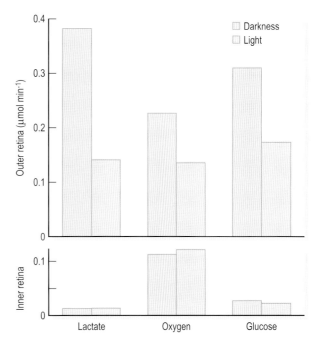

Figure 73.3 Production of lactate and consumption of oxygen and glucose in pig inner and outer retina. Orange (lefthand) bars are for dark adaptation; lavender (righthand) bars are for light adaptation. (Modified from Wang L, Tornquist P, Bill A. Glucose metabolism of the inner retina in pigs in darkness and light. Acta Physiol Scand 1997;160:71–74.)

but this has been done for both circulations in pig[44,73] and for the choroidal circulation in cat.[43] Results for pig are shown in Figure 73.3. Both circulations deliver glucose. There is a separation of inner and outer retina in terms of glucose supply, as there is in oxygen supply, and it appears that the retinal circulation provides almost all the glucose needed in the inner half of the retina. A small amount of lactate appears in the retinal circulation, but it is not clear that any of it is produced in the inner retina. It may instead diffuse to the inner retina from the large amount of lactate that is normally produced in the outer retina. As Figure 73.3 illustrates, glucose consumption in the outer retina is greater than oxygen consumption, especially in darkness, which implies that a great deal is used for aerobic glycolysis, e.g., lactate production. Depending on how the computation is done, the values in Figure 73.3 for dark adaptation imply that 60–85% of the outer retinal glucose is used for lactate production. In vitro experiments on rat and rabbit support the conclusion that a large percentage of glucose is used for lactate production in the outer retina.[75,76]

Localization and mechanisms of ATP generation

Oxidative metabolism (Box 73.3)

Oxidative metabolism is not uniform throughout the retina, as one can appreciate from the distribution of mitochondria.[77] The retinal pigment epithelial cells are located in a region with high PO_2, and have numerous mitochondria, but exhibit lactate production rates similar to[78] or higher than[79] their oxygen consumption rates. The outer segments and outer nuclear layer have no mitochondria, but the inner seg-

Box 73.3 Retinal oxygenation

- Inner and outer retina both consume large amounts of O_2 (3–5 ml O_2/100g/min)
- Outer retinal Qo_2 confined to the inner segments and synaptic regions of photoreceptors
- Inner retinal Qo_2 probably highest in inner plexiform layer, but more uniform than in outer retina
- High local Qo_2 of inner segments keeps their Po_2 at just a few mmHg in darkness
- Light reduces photoreceptor oxygen utilization by 30–50%
- Inner retinal Po_2 is slightly below 20 mmHg on average
- Steady light does not influence inner retinal metabolism, but flashing light probably increases metabolism

Box 73.4 Retinal lactate production

- Photoreceptors generate a substantial amount of lactate, even when the retina is well oxygenated
- As much as 90% of the glucose used by the photoreceptors goes to lactate production
- Lactate production by photoreceptors increases further during hypoxia or anoxia (Pasteur effect), compensating for the loss of oxidative metabolism
- Lactic acid production makes the outer retina acidic (pH about 7.2 at the lowest)
- Lactate production in the inner retina of humans and animals with a retinal circulation is very low

Table 73.1 Comparison of macaque and cat retinal oxygenation

	Macaque perifovea	Cat area centralis
Minimum Po_2 in dark (mmHg)	3.8 ± 1.9	5.2 ± 5.1
Choroidal Po_2 (mmHg)	48 ± 13	54 ± 12, 41.2 ± 16.2
Fraction of O_2 supplied to photoreceptors by choroid	0.85 (dark), 0.89 (light)	0.91 (dark), 0.93 (dark), 1.0 (light)
Q_{av}, dark (ml/100 g/min)	4.9*	4.1*± 3.8*, 4.9 ± 1.9, 4.4
Q_{av}, light/Q_{av}, dark	0.72, 0.75	0.33, 0.51, 0.61
Inner retinal Po_2, dark (mmHg)	20.4 ± 7.7 (cynomolgus), 10.6 ± 4.6 (rhesus)	18.5 ± 1.8, 12.1 ± 4.4, 15.5
Inner retinal Po_2 in light, (mmHg)	24.9 ± 7.4 (cynomolgus) 5.8 ± 2.9 (rhesus)	12.6 ± 0.8 at Pao_2 of 85 mmHg, 18.5

Values are means ± SD. Where more than one value is given, they are from different original studies. Qo_2, oxygen utilization; Q_{av} is Qo_2 averaged over outer retina; P_aO_2, arterial partial pressure of O_2; Pc, average choroidal Po_2.
*Values from regression of Q_{av} on PC at PC = 50 mmHg.
Data from Birol G, Wang S, Budzynski E, et al. Oxygen distribution and consumption in the macaque retina. Am J Physiol 2007;293:H1696–H1704.

ments have many. Mitochondria occupy 54–66% of the inner-segment volume in primate rods and 74–85% of inner-segment volume in primate cones.[80] The Qo_2 of the inner segments of rods is extremely high, about 20 ml/(100 g-min) in darkness, based on microelectrode measurements and a mathematical model of oxygen diffusion in cats and monkeys.[67,68] Inner segments comprise only about 20–25% of the outer half of the retina, so if the high value of Qo_2 in the inner segments is averaged together with the lack of any oxygen consumption over the other 75–80% of the outer retina, the total photoreceptor Qo_2 is 4–5 ml/(100 g-min),[68] similar to the value obtained from the Fick principle above. A summary of the parameters of cat and monkey retinal oxygenation, showing their fundamental similarity, is given in Table 73.1.

At a particular retinal eccentricity, the inner segments of cones have a total mitochondrial amount that can be 10 times greater than that in rods.[80] The foveal cones, although

thin, are also richer in mitochondria than rods. While it has not been possible to measure individual cone oxygen consumption, it is highly unlikely that their metabolic rate is 200 ml/(100 g-min), as the relative amounts of mitochondria alone might suggest. Further, recent measurements show that foveal Qo_2 is lower than Qo_2 of parafoveal retina,[68,81] even though the total mitochondrial density is higher in the fovea. Thus, it seems that mitochondrial amounts in the retina cannot be taken alone as an index of metabolic rate, and it has been argued that cone mitochondria may serve an optical function as well as a metabolic one.[80]

In the inner retina, the plexiform layers are richer in mitochondria than the nuclear layers.[77] These layers also tend to be the location of the capillaries, and Po_2 profiles (Figure 73.2) often have peaks in these regions that reflect those oxygen sources. Measurements in cat[82] and rat[83] by different techniques reinforce the conclusion that the inner and outer retina have similar overall rates of oxygen utilization. In most cases it has not been possible to tease apart Qo_2 of different layers of the inner retina, but one group has attempted to analyze the Qo_2 of just the oxygen-consuming layers in rat.[84,85]

For many years it has been clear that photoreceptor metabolism decreases during illumination (Figure 73.3), which is seen in oxygen profiles as an increase in the Po_2 of the distal retina during illumination (Figure 73.2). The magnitude of the change is dependent on the level of illumination and on the species, with the maximum change being about a factor of two. This has been best studied in rod-dominated animals and rod-dominated regions of the retina, but clearly also occurs in cones.[68] The decrease in metabolism with light is relatively rapid, occurring with a time constant of about 25 seconds in primates.[86] The metabolism of the inner retina is independent of the level of steady illumination,[73,74,82] but deoxyglucose measurements suggest that it probably increases in response to time-varying illumination.[74]

Aerobic and anaerobic glycolysis (Box 73.4)

Unfortunately, no technique is available to measure gradients of glucose within the retina, which would reveal local glucose utilization in the way that oxygen measurements reveal local oxidative metabolism. However, other lines of evidence point to the photoreceptors as the most active site of glycolysis. In addition to the measurements of Figure 73.3,[73] and in vitro work to isolate the site or sites of glycolysis,[75,76] two types of study have provided further localization.

First, lactate dehydrogenase activity was shown to be high in the inner segments, outer nuclear layer, and outer plexiform layer of monkey retina, and about half as great in the inner retina.[87] The inner retina relies much more on glycolysis in animals such as rabbits, which have little retinal circulation[87] and very low levels of oxygen and oxidative metabolism.[88,89] Second, because lactate production is correlated with H^+ production, pH gradients across the retina have also been used as a surrogate measure of glycolysis. In cat, the highest $[H^+]$ is in the outer nuclear layer,[90,91] and mathematical modeling indicates that both the outer nuclear layer and inner segments produce H^+.[90] It should be noted that the H^+ measurements actually reveal the layers in which H^+ is extruded from cells, i.e., where the transporters are, and not necessarily the layers with the highest intracellular production of H^+.

The rate of photoreceptor glycolysis, like the rate of oxidative metabolism, decreases with illumination, by less than 10% in rat,[76] and about 50% in cat[43,90] and pig.[44] Presumably the reason for high glycolysis in darkness is that there is not enough oxygen available to produce the required ATP oxidatively, and the very low P_{O_2} observed in the distal retina of cat and monkey supports this – a small part of the retina is normally almost anoxic. However, extremely low intraretinal P_{O_2} has not been observed in rat retina[84,85] where glycolysis is still pronounced in dark adaptation, and glycolysis is not reduced to zero during illumination, a condition in which oxygen is not limiting in any species. Consequently, the reason for the constitutively high level of aerobic glycolysis is not completely clear.

Effects of hypoxia

Decreases in blood P_{O_2} affect the inner and outer retina differently (Figure 73.4). Inner retinal P_{O_2} is well protected by the metabolic regulation of the retinal circulation discussed above, and P_aO_2 must fall to 40 mmHg or less before inner retinal P_{O_2} is affected in cats. It should be emphasized that this result is for the normal retina, and it is expected that diseases that affect retinal vascular autoregulation may be more detrimental to inner retinal P_{O_2}. Unlike the retinal circulation, and as also shown in Figure 73.4, choroidal P_{O_2} decreases in even relatively mild episodes of hypoxia, decreasing the flux of oxygen to the photoreceptors in the dark, and reducing their oxygen consumption.[67]

Compensating at least to some extent for the loss of oxidative metabolism in the outer retina in hypoxia is a strong Pasteur effect, a dramatic increase in glycolytic activity that occurs in all species studied.[76,88,92,93] The changes in retinal function resulting from hypoxia are complex[94,95] and will not be considered here. While the Pasteur effect is very strong in the photoreceptors, it cannot completely compensate when there is no oxygen, so ATP levels fall[76] and the electroretinogram cannot be sustained during anoxia. Lactate production is low in the inner retina (Figure 73.3), and there is little information on whether there is a Pasteur effect of any consequence in the inner retina.

Processes that use ATP

Photoreceptors

It is instructive to evaluate how ATP is used by the retina. Photoreceptors appear to use the largest fraction of their ATP for the Na^+/K^+ ATPase that is localized to the inner segments.[88,96,97] This requires more ATP than in many cells, because many cyclic nucleotide-gated light-dependent channels are open in the dark, giving photoreceptors an unusually high conductance to Na^+ and Ca^{2+}. The substantial Ca^{2+} influx is handled by an electrogenic transporter in the outer segment that moves one K^+ and one Ca^{2+} out for every 4 Na^+ that enter.[98] The Na^+ influx through the Ca^{2+} exchanger, plus the influx through the light-dependent channels, both have to be handled by the Na^+/K^+ ATPase. In the dark this process alone is estimated to require half of the ATP used by the photoreceptor.[88] This ATP requirement decreases substantially during illumination, but only approaches zero if all the light-dependent channels close.

The only other component of ATP utilization that appears to be strongly light-dependent is the turnover of cGMP. In the dark, guanylate cyclase catalyzes a constant production of cGMP from guanosine triphosphate (GTP), and there is a constant breakdown of cGMP by PDE. A pulse of light causes a transient increase in PDE activity, lowering cGMP and closing channels, as is well known.[99,100] A longer episode of illumination leads not only to activation of PDE but also to activation of guanylate cyclase, because channel closure reduces intracellular Ca^{2+}, and Ca^{2+} negatively regulates guanylate cyclase. Thus, during illumination, the concentration of cGMP decreases, but the rates of formation and degradation of cGMP increase. This increased turnover requires more GTP, and in turn, more ATP. Thus there is expected to be a component of photoreceptor metabolic rate that increases during illumination, and such a component has been demonstrated in several studies.[88,97,101] It can be isolated by eliminating the larger Na^+ pumping component pharmacologically.

Transduction requires smaller amounts of ATP and GTP for rhodopsin phosphorylation, activation of the G protein transducin, and possibly other events,[96] but most are early in the transduction cascade, so they precede the amplification steps that cause cGMP turnover and Na^+ pumping to have large metabolic requirements.

In addition to the above events, all of which are dependent on processes in the outer segment, the photoreceptor

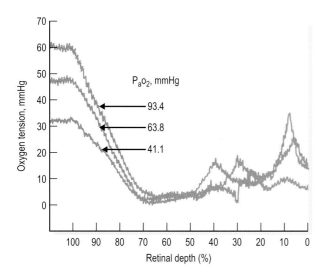

Figure 73.4 Oxygen profiles in hypoxia in the dark-adapted cat retina. Arterial P_{O_2} in the three profiles was 93.4, 63.8, and 41.1 mmHg from top to bottom. (Modified from Linsenmeier RA, Braun RD. Oxygen distribution and consumption in the cat retina during normoxia and hypoxemia. J Gen Physiol 1992;99:177–197.)

may have other transport functions, notably H^+ extrusion in exchange for Na^+, and possibly rebalancing gradients that are altered by the operation of voltage-dependent conductances in the rest of the cell. The relative importance of these processes has recently been analyzed.[102] Synthesis of membranes, particularly the synthesis of new disks, and of other lipids, proteins, and RNA is also believed to require relatively little energy,[96] but some of these estimates are based on parameters from other tissues and need to be revisited.

The photoreceptor synaptic terminals in the outer plexiform layer, at the border between the inner and outer retina, are far from the main metabolic engine of the photoreceptors, and have their own mitochondria.[103] There is no direct information on whether the ATP they produce is all utilized in the synapse, but this seems likely. Recycling of glutamate, filling and moving vesicles, and pumping of Na^+ and Ca^+ require this ATP. Because the photoreceptor releases more glutamate in darkness, all of these processes are likely to require more ATP in darkness than in light, but there are no data on this point.

Inner retina

As noted above, the inner retina in animals that have a retinal circulation uses about the same amount of oxygen as the inner retina, but the processes that require this energy have been difficult to investigate. Working in rabbit, which as noted above uses largely glycolytically derived energy for the inner retina, Ames and Li showed that pharmacologically induced changes in glutamatergic transmission produced changes in glycolysis of up to 50%.[104] Neurons in the off pathway of the retina are expected to be relatively depolarized in darkness, and would therefore have high Na^+ conductance, although probably not as high as rods. They would then have relatively high oxygen demand. Neurotransmitter synthesis and recycling and, for some cells, recovery of Na^+ gradients after spike generation would be expected to be the other consumers of ATP.

Conclusion

A great deal is known about retinal energy metabolism under normal and experimentally altered conditions. A number of cases can also be identified where changes in metabolism or in substrate supply play some role in disease. The remaining challenges are to sort out whether changes in metabolism in diseases are primary or secondary, and whether the knowledge about retinal energy metabolism can be used to devise therapies.

Key references

A complete list of chapter references is available online at www.expertconsult.com. See inside cover for registration details.

2. Alder VA, Ben-Nun J, Cringle SJ. PO_2 profiles and oxygen consumption in cat retina with an occluded retinal circulation. Invest Ophthalmol Vis Sci 1990;31:1029–1034.

11. Stefansson E. Ocular oxygenation and the treatment of diabetic retinopathy. Surv Ophthalmol 2006;51:364–380.

17. Arjamaa O, Nikinmaa M. Oxygen-dependent diseases in the retina: role of hypoxia-inducible factors. Exp Eye Res 2006;83:473–483.

27. Penn JS, Li S, Naash MI. Ambient hypoxia reverses retinal vascular attenuation in a transgenic mouse model of autosomal dominant retinitis pigmentosa. Invest Ophthalmol Vis Sci 2000;41:4007–4013.

29. Budzynski E, Smith JH, Bryar P, et al. Effects of photocoagulation on intraretinal PO_2 in cat. Invest Ophthalmol Vis Sci 2008;49:380–389.

31. Mervin K, Valter K, Maslim J, et al. Limiting photoreceptor death and deconstruction during experimental retinal detachment: the value of oxygen supplementation. Am J Ophthalmol 1999;128:155–164.

67. Linsenmeier RA, Braun RD. Oxygen distribution and consumption in the cat retina during normoxia and hypoxemia. J Gen Physiol 1992;99:177–197.

68. Birol G, Wang S, Budzynski E, et al. Oxygen distribution and consumption in the macaque retina. Am J Physiol 2007;293:H1696–H1704.

73. Wang L, Tornquist P, Bill A. Glucose metabolism of the inner retina in pigs in darkness and light. Acta Physiol Scand 1997;160:71–74.

74. Bill A, Sperber GO. Aspects of oxygen and glucose consumption in the retina: effects of high intraocular pressure and light. Graefes Arch Clin Exp Ophthalmol 1990;228:124–127.

76. Winkler BS. A quantitative assessment of glucose metabolism in the isolated rat retina. In: Christen Y, Doly M, Droy-Lefaix M, et al. (eds) Les Séminaires ophthalmologiques d'IPSEN. Vision et adaptation. Paris: Elsevier, 1995.

81. Yu DY, Cringle SJ, Su EN. Intraretinal oxygen distribution in the monkey retina and the response to systemic hyperoxia. Invest Ophthalmol Vis Sci 2005;46:4728–4733.

83. Medrano CJ, Fox DA. Oxygen consumption in the rat outer and inner retina: light- and pharmacologically induced inhibition. Exp Eye Res 1995;61:273–284.

88. Ames A, Li YY, Heher EG, et al. Energy metabolism of rabbit retina as related to function: high cost of Na transport. J Neurosci 1992;12:840–853.

91. Yamamoto F, Borgula GA, Steinberg RH. Effects of light and darkness on pH outside rod photoreceptors in the cat retina. Exp Eye Res 1992;54:685–697.

CHAPTER 74

Retinitis pigmentosa and related disorders

Eric A Pierce

Clinical background

The term retinitis pigmentosa (RP) is used to describe a group of inherited disorders in which vision loss is caused by degeneration of the rod and cone photoreceptor cells of the retina. RP occurs in nonsyndromic and syndromic forms. It has recently been recognized that in many of the syndromic disorders of which RP is a part, the common link between the affected tissues is cilia, as the light-sensitive outer segments of photoreceptor cells are specialized sensory cilia (Figure 74.1).

Symptoms and signs

In all types of RP, nyctalopia (night blindness) is often the first symptom noticed. This is due to dysfunction and death of rod photoreceptor cells, which mediate vision under conditions of dim illumination. This symptom is often noticed in adolescence, but the age of onset can be variable, ranging from early childhood to adulthood. Loss of peripheral visual field follows, and is progressive, resulting in constriction of visual fields. Central vision, mediated predominantly by cone photoreceptor cells, is ultimately lost in many cases as well, often in later adulthood.[1]

The progression of visual symptoms is associated with dysfunction and death of photoreceptor cells and consequent changes in the retinal pigment epithelium, which is visible on fundus exam. For example, in childhood, the fundus may appear relatively healthy, or small regions of depigmentation may be noted prior to the detection of the typical bone spicule pigmentation in the midperiphery (Figure 74.2A). As more photoreceptor cells die, and visual field is lost, fundus abnormalities become more notable, with more prominent bone spicule pigmentation and associated retinal atrophy (Figure 74.2B). Eventually, attenuation of retinal blood vessels and optic atrophy are evident, as further loss of photoreceptor cells and secondary loss of retinal ganglion cells occurs (Box 74.1).

Other degenerations

In addition to RP, many other inherited retinal degenerations have been described. These have been classified clini-cally by their age of onset, the types of photoreceptor cells affected, the region of the retina involved, and rates of progression. Leber congenital amaurosis (LCA) is a severe early-onset form of retinal degeneration, in which poor vision associated with nystagmus is evident early in childhood. Cone and cone–rod dystrophies are characterized by early-onset cone dysfunction, in contrast to RP, in which rods are typically affected first. Congenital stationary night blindness is characterized by early-onset night -blindness like RP, but has a more stable clinical course.[2,3]

Epidemiology

The prevalence of RP in the USA, Europe, and Japan is approximately 1 in 4000.[3] This translates into ~1.5 million individuals affected with RP worldwide. Data from the Beijing Eye Study suggest that the prevalence in China may be higher, at approximately 1 in 1000. These data predict approximately 1.3 million people affected with RP in China alone, although this estimate is based on a relatively small sample size compared to the total Chinese population.[4] Data from studies in Japan and Denmark and Kuwait indicate that RP is among the leading causes of blindness or visual impairment, especially in working-aged people, accounting for 25–29% cases in that age group (21–60 years).[3]

Diagnostic workup

Clinical evaluation of a patient with symptoms of RP, such as nyctalopia and decreased visual fields, involves thorough ophthalmic examination, testing of visual function, consideration of systemic evaluations, and genetic testing. Visual acuity may remain normal even in later stages of classic RP, in which rod photoreceptors are affected first. Early loss of central acuity suggests the possibility of early cone photoreceptor dysfunction. Anterior-segment exam is important to rule out other causes of vision loss, and to look for posterior subcapsular cataracts, which develop in up to 50% of patients with RP.[5]

Visual field testing is important both for detecting field loss for diagnostic purposes, and for following disease status over time. Full-field evaluations using a Goldmann perimeter or Humphrey field analyzer are useful for detecting the midperipheral scotomas typically observed in patients with

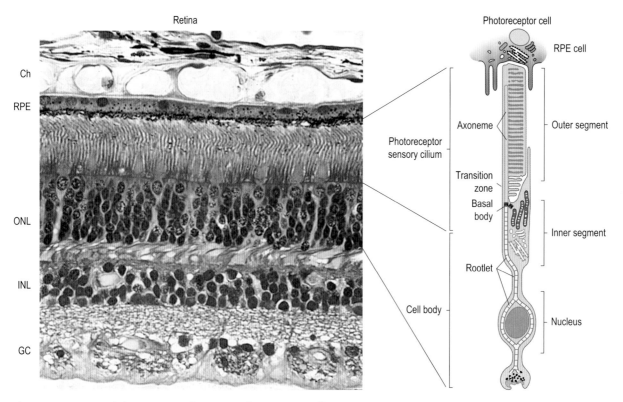

Figure 74.1 Retina and photoreceptor cell structure. Left, cross-section of human retina, showing retinal layers. Right, drawing of rod photoreceptor cell, showing different portions of the cell. The photoreceptor sensory cilium is indicated. Ch, choroid; GC, ganglion cell layer; INL, inner nuclear layer; ONL, outer nuclear layer; RPE, retinal pigment epithelium.

Box 74.1 Retinitis pigmentosa – clinical features

Symptoms
- Nyctalopia
- Peripheral field loss
- Progressive loss of central vision later in disease

Exam findings
- Diminished electroretinograms, rod greater than cone
- Bone spicule pigmentation
- Vascular attenuation
- Optic atrophy

RP. Progression of field loss is associated with loss of rod and cone photoreceptor function, resulting in small residual islands of vision.[6]

Electroretinography

Electroretinogram (ERG) testing is an important diagnostic tool for patients with RP. The ERG measures the function of rod and cone photoreceptors. It is a measure of the field potential generated by the circulating ion currents in photoreceptor cells.[7] Standards for the performance of ERGs have been established by the International Society for Clinical Electrophysiology of Vision (ISCEV).[8] In the ISCEV standard ERG evaluation, five steps are used to evaluate rod and then cone function: the rod ERG, the combined rod–cone ERG, oscillatory potentials, single flash cone ERG, and

30-Hz flicker ERG.[8] Responses to low levels of white or blue light in dark-adapted subjects are used to evaluate rod photoreceptor function. A brighter standard flash of white light is then used to elicit a maximal or combined response from both the rod and cone photoreceptors. A typical response includes a negatively deflected a-wave, followed by a positive b-wave (Figure 74.3). The a-wave is a measure of the photoreceptor response; the b-wave is thought to be generated by cells in the inner retina.[9]

Following light adaptation, cone responses to a single white flash are recorded in the presence of background illumination. Finally, flicker ERGs recorded at approximately 30 flashes per second (30 Hz) are used to measure responses from cones; rod photoreceptors cannot recover rapidly enough to respond to the rapid flashes[8] (Figure 74.4).

In patients with RP, ERG responses are decreased. Indeed, decreased photoreceptor function can be detected by ERG in children who remain asymptomatic until young adulthood.[1] In RP, decreased rod photoreceptor responses are typically noted first, followed by decreases in cone responses. A typical young adult with RP will have reduced amplitudes of both rod and cone responses, and delays in the response times (Figures 74.3 and 74.4). Patients with more severe retinal degeneration, such as early-onset forms of RP or LCA, may have nondetectable ERG responses (Figures 74.3 and 74.4).

ERG amplitudes can provide objective measures of retinal function, and thus are useful for accurate diagnosis and for tracking the course of disease.[1,3] It has also been suggested that the amplitudes of the 30-Hz cone response can be used to provide information about visual prognosis.[10] The dark

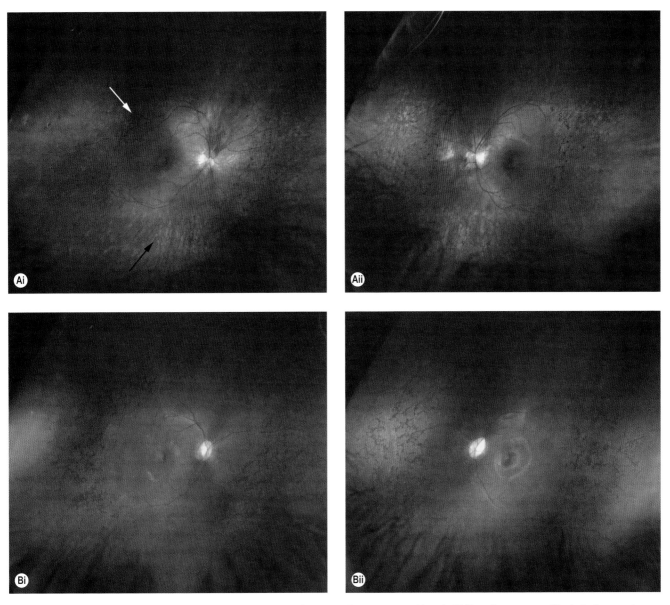

Figure 74.2 Fundus appearance in retinitis pigmentosa (RP). (A) Fundus images from a patient with early RP. Note the presence of both depigmented areas (black arrow) and early bone spicule pigment (white arrow). (B) Fundus images from a patient with more advanced RP. Note increased bone spicule pigmentation in the midperiphery, attenuation of retinal blood vessels, and early pallor of the optic nerves. Note: these fundus photos were taken with the Optos fundus imaging system, which provides a wide-angle view of the fundus. This scanning laser ophthalmoscope system uses red and green lasers, and thus produces images with slightly different colors than standard fundus cameras.

adaptation threshold can also be a useful assessment of rod photoreceptor function. This test measures the lowest intensity of white light that can be perceived in a dark-adapted state.[11] Optical coherence tomography (OCT) can be useful for monitoring the thickness of the retina in patients with RP.[12]

Genetic testing

Genetic testing to identify the mutations which cause an individual patient's disease has become an important part of clinical care of patients with RP and related disorders. This is important because it can help confirm the diagnosis, assist with family planning, and provide more detailed information about the prognosis of the specific form of RP identified. Genetic diagnoses will also be increasingly important as genetic treatments for RP and related disorders are developed.

Clinical genetic testing for RP is improving, and several clinical labs now provide relevant testing. An up-to-date list can be found at www.genetests.org. Identification of pathogenic mutations in patients with RP can be challenging, due in part to the polygenic nature of these disorders (see below).[13] New developments with high-throughput mutation detection and sequencing will hopefully simplify this process in the relatively near future.[14,15]

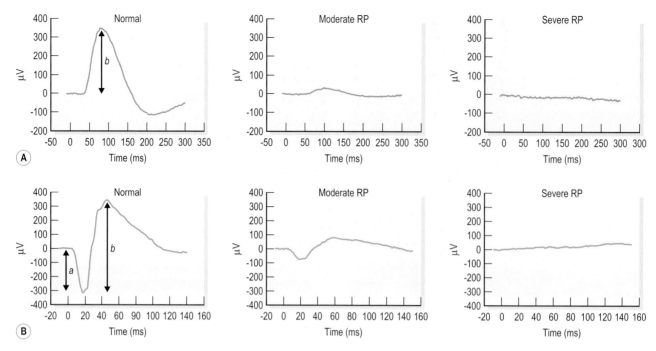

Figure 74.3 Standard scotopic electroretinograms (ERGs). Example traces of ERG results from a normal subject, a patient with moderate retinitis pigmentosa (RP), and a patient with severe RP. (A) Rod ERGs generated response to dim flashes of white light. (B) Combined rod–cone ERGs generated in response to a brighter flash of white light. The negatively deflected *a*-wave, and positive *b*-wave are indicated. The time to peak (implicit time) and amplitude of the responses are decreased.

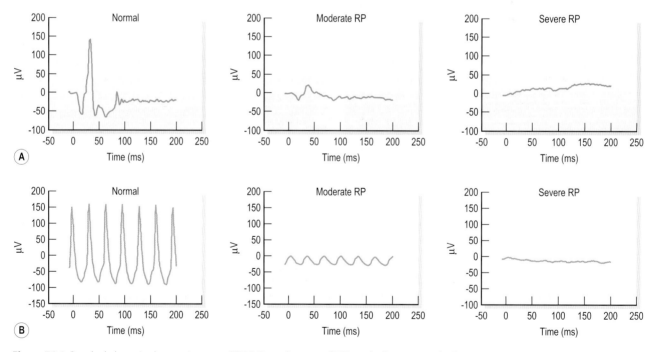

Figure 74.4 Standard photopic electroretinograms (ERGs). Example traces of ERG results from a normal subject, a patient with moderate retinitis pigmentosa (RP) and a patient with severe RP. (A) Cone ERGs generated response to a single flash of white light. (B) 30-Hz flicker cone ERGs.

Systemic evaluation

As discussed below, RP and related retinal degenerations are often associated with systemic disorders. It is therefore important to consider potential disease associations when evaluating patients with RP. This is especially true for children. Common systemic associations include defects in other sensory or primary cilia, such as hearing loss in Usher syndrome, cystic renal disease in Alstrom, Bardet–Biedl, Joubert, and Senior Loken syndromes. Retinal degeneration can also occur in the setting of mitochondrial disease, and metabolic disorders. Three specific forms of RP that are important to consider in children are Refsum's disease (phytanic acid oxidase deficiency), Bassen–Kornzweig syndrome (abetalipoproteinemia), and RP with ataxia caused by α-tocopherol transport protein deficiency, as early intervention can be beneficial in these disorders.[16]

Differential diagnosis

Other retinal degenerative disorders can present with visual symptoms like those caused by RP. The fundus appearance in gyrate atrophy is distinct from that of RP, with patches of choroidal and retinal atrophy in the midperiphery. Plasma ornithine levels are elevated in this disease, which is caused by deficiency of the ornithine aminotransferase (OAT) gene. Fundus appearance is also helpful for distinguishing choroideremia from RP. In this X-linked condition, RPE and choroidal atrophy are evident on fundus exam.[17]

Treatment

Several studies have been performed to assess the value of nutritional supplements for patients with RP. A randomized clinical trial demonstrated that vitamin A supplementation slowed the decline of photoreceptor cell loss as measured by 30-Hz cone ERG amplitude in patients with RP.[18] Vitamin A supplementation was also associated with slower loss of visual field in the subset of trial patients who performed the visual field tests with the greatest precision.[19] Studies of dietary supplementation with the omega-3 fatty acid docosahexaenoic acid (DHA), which is present at relatively high levels in photoreceptor outer-segment membranes, did not show a clear benefit.[20,21]

Several promising treatments for RP and related disorders are nearing or in clinical trials. The value of sustained intraocular release of the neurotrophic factor ciliary neurotrophic factor (CNTF) is being evaluated in a phase II trial, after being found to be safe in a small phase I study.[22] Gene augmentation therapy for specific forms of RP, LCA, and related disorders has shown promise in preclinical and early phase I research studies.[23–26] Based on these results, further clinical trials of gene therapy for LCA2, caused by mutations in the RPE65 gene, are currently in progress in England and the USA. RNA interference-mediated knockdown of mutant alleles that cause disease via dominant negative mechanisms is also being evaluated.[27] Several approaches to using stem cells for the treatment of inherited retinal degenerations have also shown promise, including the use of RPE-like cells derived from human embryonic stem cells.[28]

Pathology

Several clinicopathologic studies of the pathology of RP have been reported. These studies show that loss of vision in end-stage RP correlates with widespread loss of photoreceptors. In samples from patients with retained vision, a single layer of cones with shortened outer segments was observed in the macula, reflecting the slower loss in cones in most types of RP. Bone spicule pigmentation is caused by migration of RPE cells into the retina, where they cluster around blood vessels.[29] Pathologic studies also show that the neural retina undergoes significant remodeling in human RP.[30,31] Loss of

photoreceptors, especially cones, appears to trigger retinal remodeling, with changes in cell organization and connections. These include neuronal and glial migration, rewiring of retinal circuits with elaboration of new neurites and synapses, and glial hypertrophy.[29,32] These remodeling changes may affect the success of potential therapeutic strategies for RP and related disorders.

Etiology

Genetics of RP and related disorders

Nonsyndromic RP

RP and related disorders are caused by mutations in genes which encode proteins that are required for photoreceptor cell function. These disorders are genetically heterogeneous, with over 80 disease genes identified to date (Tables 74.1–74.3). Indeed, it has recently been pointed out that photoreceptor cells are subject to more genetic diseases than any other cell type.[33] The website RetNet provides a curated listing of disease genes and loci for retinal degenerative disorders.[34]

It is has been estimated that 65% of RP cases are nonsyndromic.[35] Of these, autosomal-recessive RP is the most common form, accounting for 50–60% of cases. This includes simplex cases of RP, which are assumed to be primarily recessive, although dominant mutations have been detected in patients with simplex disease.[36,37] Autosomal-dominant forms of RP are estimated to account for 30–40% of cases, and X-linked RP for 5–15% of cases.[3,35] Other less common modes of inheritance have also been reported, including digenic RP requiring mutations in two genes (PRPH2 and ROM1) and RP due to mutations in mitochondrial genes.[38–40]

In aggregate, the mutations in the identified genes account for approximately 56% of patients with autosomal RP, 30% of patients with autosomal-recessive RP, and nearly 90% of patients with X-linked RP.[3,35] This suggests that many additional disease genes remain to be identified, especially for recessive forms of RP. Consistent with this suggestion, new disease loci continue to be identified; an additional 19 genetic loci for RP and related disorders are listed in RetNet.

Syndromic RP

Approximately 25–30% of individuals with RP have associated nonocular disease. As described in more detail below, the majority of these syndromic forms of RP are cilia-related disorders, including Alstrom, Bardet–Biedl, Joubert, Senior Loken/nephronophthisis and Usher syndromes.[3,35,41,42] The most common syndromic form of RP is Usher syndrome, accounting for approximately 10% of RP cases. Mutations in the USH2A gene also cause a significant proportion of recessive RP without hearing loss (Table 74.3 and Box 74.2).[3]

In Bardet–Biedl syndrome (BBS), RP is found in association with multiple cilia-related disorders, including cystic renal disease, polydactyly, mental retardation, obesity and gonadal malformations, diabetes, and situs inversus.[41] To date, mutations in 12 genes have been identified to cause BBS, which is estimated to account for 5% of cases of RP.[3,35] In addition to autosomal-recessive inheritance, oligogenic

Table 74.1 Summary of disease genes and loci

Disease category	Inheritance pattern	Total number of genes and loci	Number of identified genes
Nonsyndromic			
Cone–rod dystrophy	AD	7	5
Cone–rod dystrophy	AR	5	3
Leber congenital amaurosis	AR	15	14
Retinitis pigmentosa	AD	16	15
Retinitis pigmentosa	AR	18	13
Retinitis pigmentosa	XL	6	2
Ciliopathy syndromes			
Alstrom syndrome	AR	1	1
Bardet–Biedl syndrome	AR	12	12
Nephronophthisis-associated	AR	9	8
Usher syndrome	AR	11	9
Other syndromic disorders			
Lipofuscinoses		2	2
Mitochondrial disorders		4	4
Refsum disease		4	4

AR, autosomal recessive; AD, autosomal dominant; XL, X-linked.

Table 74.2 Genetics of nonsyndromic retinitis pigmentosa (RP)

	Gene symbol	Protein name	%[1]	Function/mechanism of disease[2]
adRP				
	RHO	Rhodopsin	25	Phototransduction, cilia structure
	RP1	Retinitis pigmentosa 1	5.5	Cilia structure
	PRPF31	Pre-mRNA processing factor 31	5	RNA splicing
	PRPF3	Pre-mRNA processing factor 3	4	RNA splicing
	PRPH2	Peripherin 2	2.5	Cilia structure
	PRPF8	Pre-mRNA processing factor 8	2	RNA splicing
	IMPDH1	Inosine monophosphate dehydrogenase 1	2	Nucleotide biosynthesis
	NRL	Neural retina leucine zipper	1	Overexpression of rhodopsin
	CRX	Cone–rod homeobox protein	1	Cilia structure – transcription factor
	CA4	Carbonic anhydrase IV		pH balance
	FSCN2	Fascin 2		Cilia structure
	GUCA1B	Guanylate cyclase activator 1B		Phototransduction
	SEMA4A	Semaphorin B		Cilia structure
	TOPORS	Topoisomerase I binding, arginine/serine-rich		RNA splicing
	RP9	Retinitis pigmentosa 9		RNA splicing
	NR2E3	Photoreceptor-specific nuclear receptor		Cilia structure – transcription factor
	Unknown		45	
arRP				
	USH2A	Usherin	8	Cilia structure
	ABCA4	ATP-binding cassette, subfamily A member 4	5.6	Visual cycle
	CNGB1	Cyclic nucleotide gated channel beta 1	4	Phototransduction

Table 74.2 Summary of disease genes and loci—cont'd

	Gene symbol	Protein name	%[1]	Function/mechanism of disease[2]
	PDE6B	Phosphodiesterase 6B, cGMP-specific, rod, beta	3.5	Phototransduction
	PDE6A	Phosphodiesterase 6A, alpha subunit	3.5	Phototransduction
	RPE65	Retinal pigment epithelium-specific protein 65 kDa	2	Visual cycle
	CNGA1	Cyclic nucleotide gated channel alpha 1	1	Phototransduction
	CRB1	Crumbs homolog 1	1	Retinal organization
	LRAT	Lecithin retinol acyltransferase	1	Visual cycle
	MERTK	MER receptor tyrosine kinase	1	Retinal pigment epithelium function
	TULP1	Tubby-like protein 1	1	Cilia structure
	RHO	Rhodopsin	1	Phototransduction, cilia structure
	RLBP1	Retinaldehyde binding protein 1	1	Visual cycle
	CERKL	Ceramide kinase-like	1	Sphingolipid metabolism
	RGR	Retinal G-protein-coupled receptor	0.5	Visual cycle
	NR2E3	Photoreceptor-specific nuclear receptor	0.25	Cilia structure – transcription factor
	SAG	S-arrestin		Phototransduction
	NRL	Neural retina leucine zipper		Overexpression of rhodopsin
	RP1	Retinitis pigmentosa 1		Cilia structure
	PRCD	Progressive rod–cone degeneration		
	PROM1	Prominin 1		Cilia structure
	Unknown		60–70	
X-linked RP				
	RPGR	Retinitis pigmentosa GTPase regulator		Cilia structure
	RP2	XRP2 protein		
	Unknown		10–20	
LCA				
	CEP290	Centrosomal protein 290 kDa	15	Cilia structure
	GUCY2D	Guanylate cyclase 2D, membrane (retina-specific)	12	Phototransduction failure
	CRB1	Crumbs homolog 1	10	Retinal organization
	IMPDH1	Inosine monophosphate dehydrogenase 1	8	Nucleotide biosynthesis
	RPE65	Retinal pigment epithelium-specific protein 65 kDa	6	Visual cycle
	AIPL1	Aryl hydrocarbon receptor interacting protein-like 1	5	Cilia structure – chaperone
	RPGRIP1	Retinitis pigmentosa GTPase regulator interacting protein 1	4	Cilia structure
	RDH12	Retinol dehydrogenase 12 (all-trans and 9-cis)	3	Visual cycle
	LCA5	Leber congenital amaurosis 5	2	Cilia structure
	CRX	Cone–rod homeobox protein	1	Cilia structure – transcription factor
	TULP1	Tubby-like protein 1	1	Cilia structure
	MERTK	MER receptor tyrosine kinase		RPE function
	LRAT	Lecithin retinol acyltransferase		Visual cycle
	RD3	Retinal degeneration 3		
	Unknown		20–30	

[1]Estimated percentage of patients with subtype of retinitis pigmentosa with mutations in indicated gene. Data regarding LCA from den Hollander AI, Roepman R, Koenekoop RK, Cremers FP. Leber congenital amaurosis: genes, proteins and disease mechanisms. *Prog Retin Eye Res* 2008;27:391–419.
[2]Broad categories of proposed protein function and/or mechanism by which mutations cause disease.
adRP, autosomal-dominant RP; arRP, autosomal-recessive RP.

Table 74.3 Genetics of syndromic retinitis pigmentosa

	Gene symbol	Protein name
Bardet–Biedl syndrome		
	BBS1	Bardet–Biedl syndrome 1
	BBS2	Bardet–Biedl syndrome 2 protein
	ARL6	ADP-ribosylation factor-like 6
	BBS4	Bardet–Biedl syndrome 4
	BBS5	Bardet–Biedl syndrome 5
	MKKS	McKusick–Kaufman syndrome protein
	BBS7	Bardet–Biedl syndrome 7 protein
	TTC8	Tetratricopeptide repeat domain 8
	BBS9	Parathyroid hormone-responsive B1
	BBS10	Bardet–Biedl syndrome 10
	TRIM32	TAT-interactive protein, 72 kDa
	BBS12	Bardet–Biedl syndrome 12
Alstrom	ALMS1	Alms1
Nephronophthisis-associated (Joubert, Senior Loken)		
	NPHP1	Nephrocystin
	INVS	Inversin
	NPHP3	Nephronophthisis 3
	NPHP4	Nephroretinin
	IQCB1	IQ motif containing B1
	CEP290	Centrosomal protein 290 kDa
	AHI1	Abelson helper integration site 1
	RPGRIP1L	RPGRIP1-like
Usher syndrome		
Usher 1	MYO7A	Myosin VIIA
	CDH23	Cadherin-related 23
	PCDH15	Protocadherin 15
	USH1G	Usher syndrome 1G protein
	USH1C	Harmonin
Usher 2	USH2A	Usherin
	GPR98	G protein-coupled receptor 98
	DFNB31	CASK-interacting protein CIP98
Usher 3	CLRN1	Clarin 1
Other syndromic disorders		
Batten disease	CLN3	Ceroid-lipofuscinosis, neuronal 3
HARP	PANK2	Pantothenate kinase 2
Refsum disease	PEX1	Peroxin1
	PEX7	Peroxisomal biogenesis factor 7
	PHYH	Phytanoyl-CoA 2-hydroxylase
	PXMP3	Peroxin 2
Ataxia with retinitis pigmentosa	TTPA	Tocopherol (alpha) transfer protein
Abetalipoproteinemia	MTTP	Microsomal triglyceride transfer protein large subunit
Mitochondrial	MT-ATP6	ATPase subunit 6
	MT-TH	Mitochondrially encoded tRNA histidine
	MT-TS2	Mitochondrially encoded tRNA serine 2
	(KSS)	(multiple mitochrondrial deletions)

inheritance of BBS has also been reported. In these cases, disease is caused by mutations in two distinct BBS genes, with two mutations in one gene (which are not sufficient to cause disease alone) and a single mutation in the second.[41,43] These and other recent findings have led to the suggestion that the severity of disease in ciliopathies such as BBS and RP may be due to the total mutational load on ciliary function.[44] This concept is especially pertinent for RP, as it has long been recognized that the severity of disease can vary significantly among patients with RP caused by the same identified mutation.[3,45] In these situations, it is likely that mutations in genes other than the identified disease gene may modify the disease severity.

Pathophysiology

Photoreceptor sensory cilia

Photoreceptor cells are sensory neurons that elaborate a highly specialized, light-sensitive organelle, the outer segment. It has recently been recognized that photoreceptor outer segments are specialized sensory cilia (Figure 74.1). This has come as part of the recognition of the importance of primary and sensory cilia in biology and disease.[46] It is now evident that primary cilia are present on most cells in the human body. All cilia are composed of a microtubule-based axoneme surrounded by a distinct domain of the plasma membrane. The axonemes are derived from and anchored to the cell via basal bodies.[47] These structures are typically sensory organelles, and are involved in many critical aspects of cell biology.[48,49] For example, sensation of flow by primary cilia is required for maintenance of renal nephron structure and body axis determination. Recent evidence has also revealed that primary cilia play important roles in various aspects of development, such as planar cell polarity and hedgehog signaling.[46,50]

The sensory cilia elaborated rod and cone photoreceptors are among the largest of mammalian cilia.[49,51] Like other cilia, the outer segments contain an axoneme, which begins at the basal bodies and passes through a transition zone (the so-called "connecting cilium") and into the outer segment (Figure 74.1). The basal bodies also nucleate the ciliary

rootlet, which extends into the inner segment.[51] The photoreceptor sensory cilium (PSC) complex comprises the outer segment and its cytoskeleton, including the rootlet, basal body, and axoneme (Figure 74.1). The outer-segment membrane domain of the PSC complex is highly specialized, with discs stacked in tight order at 30 per micron along the axoneme. The proteins required for phototransduction are located in or associated with these discs.

PSC dysfunction and photoreceptor cell death

The value of recognizing photoreceptor outer segments as cilia is that it connects retinal degenerative disorders such as RP to other cilia disorders. In addition, recognition of RP as a cilia disorder (ciliopathy) can also help with understanding disease pathogenesis. That is, many of the mutations identified to cause RP and related disorders exert their pathogenic effects by causing cilia dysfunction, which in turn leads to photoreceptor cell death. If the affected genes are expressed exclusively or predominantly in the retina, then nonsyndromic RP results. More widespread expression of the disease genes may result in systemic disorders reflecting the locations of gene expression.[41,42]

Defective signaling in photoreceptor cilia

One general mechanism by which disease-causing mutations damage photoreceptors is by causing defects in phototransduction. In a general way, this is similar to defective signaling that is thought to underlie other ciliopathies, such as polycystic kidney disease, in which cilia defects result in dysfunction of the ion channel formed by the polycystin proteins, alterations in Wnt signaling, and changes in cell cycle regulation.[42]

Disruption of the phototransduction cascade at any point can lead to defects in signaling, and thus in vision (Figure 74.5). Indeed, mutations in genes that encode many of the proteins involved in phototransduction have been found to cause RP and related disorders (Tables 74.2 and 74.3). For example, mutations in PDE6A and PDE6B, which encode the α- and ß-subunits of the phosphodiesterase, lead to recessive RP.[52,53] They also cause photoreceptor degeneration in rd mice, rcd1 dogs.[54–56] Study of these animal models shows that loss of phosphodiesterase activity leads to persistent elevation of cGMP levels, and chronically open cGMP-gated channels. It is hypothesized that the chronically open cGMP-gated channels in patients and animals with PDE6A and PDE6B mutations result in metabolic overload, by demanding continuous activity of the Na⁺/K⁺-ATPase exchanger to maintain electrochemical gradients in photoreceptor cells. Mutations in rhodopsin can also disrupt phototransduction, and are a common cause of RP.[3,35]

Defective photoreceptor function can also result from mutations in the genes that encode the proteins which regulate the phototransduction cascade. For example, patients with mutations in the genes that encode rhodopsin kinase and arrestin have a form of congenital stationary night blindness called Oguchi disease.[57,58] These mutations are thought to lead to continuous activation of phototransduction, since the negative regulators of the process are missing. It is hypothesized that the photoreceptor degeneration which occurs in these patients and animals is similar to the

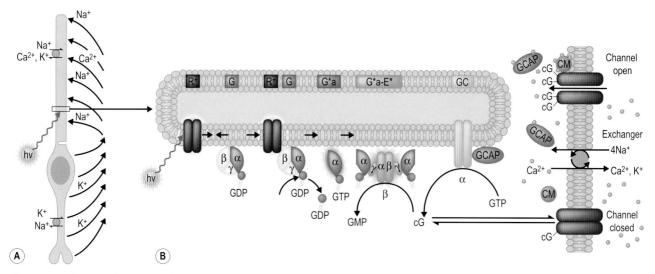

Figure 74.5 Phototransduction cascade. Phototransduction is mediated rhodopsin and cone opsins, which are G-protein-coupled receptors. (A) Image of rod photoreceptor cell with circulating current of ions indicated. (B) Magnified depiction of the phototransduction cascade. In the dark, cGMP generated by guanylate cyclase (GC) keeps the cGMP-gated channels in the outer-segment plasma membrane open, allowing for influx of sodium and calcium. Detection of light by opsins leads to a conformational change of the 11-*cis*-retinal chromophore to all-*trans*-retinal. The resulting change in the conformation of the opsin protein (R*) activates a signal amplification cascade, which begins with activation of transducin (G). Activated transducin in turn activates the multisubunit photoreceptor phosphodiesterase (E), encoded by the *PDE6* group of genes. Activated phosphodiesterase breaks down cGMP (cG), and decreased levels of cGMP result in closure of the cGMP-gated membrane channels. Closure of the channels leads to hyperpolarization of the photoreceptor cell, altering the neurotransmission to the bipolar cells, and ultimately creating the sensation of vision. This phototransduction system, which greatly amplifies the opsin response, is tightly regulated, with a series of proteins that function to shut down the signal, including recoverin, rhodopsin kinase, and arrestin. Guanylate cyclase activity is also regulated, by the guanylate cyclase activator proteins (GCAP1). CM, calmodulin. (Redrawn from illustrations courtesy of Dr. Edward Pugh.)

retinal degeneration that occurs in animals following continuous exposure to light. Support for this "equivalent light" hypothesis has recently been provided from studies of mice with deletions of genes that encode components of the retinoid cycle and the phototransduction cascade.[59]

RPE proteins/visual cycle defects

Another class of mutations that lead to defects in phototransduction are those that disrupt the recycling of the opsin chromophore from all-*trans* to 11-*cis*-retinal. This visual cycle involves reduction of all-*trans*-retinal to the retinol form, transport from the photoreceptor cilia to the RPE, where the 11-*cis* form is regenerated via a series of enzymatic reactions prior to transport back to the photoreceptor outer segments.[60] The classic example of retinal degeneration caused by a visual cycle defect is mutations in the *RPE65* gene, which cause LCA. The RPE65 protein has recently been identified to be the retinal isomerohydrolase.[61,62] Lack of this protein leads to failure of phototransduction due to lack of 11-*cis* retinal. A similar situation is hypothesized to occur secondary to mutations in the *LRAT* gene.[63] Mutations in RPE proteins can also lead to retinal degeneration via defects in phagocytosis of shed photoreceptor outer segments.[64]

Defective photoreceptor cilia formation

Another important cause of photoreceptor cilia dysfunction is defects in cilia structure.[65] Since photoreceptor outer segments turn over every 10 days, they are susceptible to errors in formation and in maintenance.[66] In the most basic form of disease in this category, photoreceptor outer segments do

not form. This has been observed in rhodopsin knockout mice, and is hypothesized to occur in patients with recessive RP caused by null mutations in rhodopsin.[67,68] Lack of photoreceptor outer-segment formation has also been observed in mice with targeted deletion of the cone–rod homeobox (*Crx*) gene.[69] CRX is a transcription factor which stimulates expression of photoreceptor-specific genes. Mutations in *CRX* cause LCA, as well as other retinal degenerations, possibly via disruption of photoreceptor outer-segment formation due to alterations in expression of photoreceptor cilia genes.[70]

Photoreceptor outer segments also fail to form in rds mice, which have a mutant peripherin 2 (*Prph2*) gene.[71] Mutations in the human *PRPH2* gene cause dominant retinal degenerations, including RP.[72,73] As heterozygous *rds* mice have defects in outer-segment formation, it is hypothesized that this is also the mechanism of human disease.[74] Severe defects in outer-segment formation were observed in semaphorin 4a (*Sema4a*) knockout mice.[75] Mutations in this gene cause dominant RP, possibly by altering outer-segment organization.[76]

A number of proteins produced by retinal degeneration disease genes have been identified to be components of the basal body, transition zone (connecting cilium), and axoneme of photoreceptor sensory cilia. Mutations in many of these genes are thought to cause disease by resulting in production of disorganized photoreceptor outer segments. The retinitis pigmentosa 1 (RP1) protein has been observed to be part of the axoneme of photoreceptor sensory cilia.[77,78] Targeted alterations in the mouse retinitis pigmentosa 1 homolog (*Rp1h*) gene gene also lead to production of disorganized outer segments, with failure of discs to align along the axoneme.[79] Based on these data, it is hypothesized that mutations in the human *RP1* gene, which have been identified to cause dominant and recessive RP, cause disease by disruption of photoreceptor cilia structure.[78] The retinitis pigmentosa GTPase regulator (RPGR) protein and its interacting protein RPGRIP1 localize to the transition zone/connecting cilia of photoreceptor cells. Mutations in these genes cause LCA and X-linked RP. Disruption of these genes in mice also leads to production of disorganized outer segments.[80,81]

As described above, RP occurs in the setting of other cilia disorders, including BBS, Alstrom syndrome, Joubert syndrome and Senior Loken syndrome/nephronophthisis. Many of the proteins produced by the BBS, Alstrom syndrome 1 (ALMS1), Joubert, and nephronophthisis genes have been localized to cilia and basal bodies.[41,42] Animal models for several of these disorders have been generated or identified, and demonstrate that defects in or lack of these cilia proteins lead to production of disorganized photoreceptor outer segments. For example, *Bbs1* M390R knockin mice and *Bbs2* null mice have disorganized outer segments. Photoreceptor degeneration and defects in photoreceptor protein transport were detected in the *Bbs4* knockout mice. All three mouse models also demonstrate other cilia defects, including lack of flagella on sperm.[82–85]

Other widely expressed proteins

In addition to the cilia proteins described above, mutations in genes that encode several other widely expressed proteins have been found to harbor mutations which cause nonsyndromic RP. Several hypotheses have been suggested to explain how the identified mutations lead to photoreceptor-specific disease. In the case of mutations in the inosine monophosphate dehydrogenase 1 (*IMPDH1*) gene, whose mutations cause dominant RP, it has been suggested that retina-specific disease may be related to the relatively high level of IMPDH1 protein in the retina, and unique retinal isoforms of the protein, which may perform retina-specific function(s).[86] Mutations in several components of the spliceosome, which is responsible for splicing pre-mRNA transcripts into mature mRNAs, have also been found to cause dominant RP. These genes include pre-mRNA-processing factors 3, 8, and 31 (*PRPF3*, *PRPF8*, *PRPF31*) and retinitis pigmentosa 9 (*RP9*).[87–90] It has been suggested that mutations in these RNA-splicing factors could cause RP by disrupting the splicing of retina-specific genes. Alternatively, global defects in splicing could result in retina-specific disease due to the high biosynthetic demand of photoreceptor cells.[87]

Programmed cell death

As for many neurodegenerative diseases, it has been suggested that programmed cell death (PCD) is the final common pathway to photoreceptor cell death in retinal degenerations. Evidence from studies of animal models indicates that at least some forms of inherited retinal degeneration photoreceptor cells die via the type of PCD called apoptosis.[91–93] Apoptosis is characterized by specific morphologic changes which are generated by a cascade of biochemical events that are mediated in part by caspases.[94] For several other animal models of retinal degeneration, however, it is evident that PCD occurs in a caspase-independent fashion. In these models, it appears that increased intracellular calcium levels lead to activation of calpains and cathepsins, which can be associated with a distinct form of PCD called necrosis.[95,96] These findings highlight the point that the specific mechanisms by which mutations in retinal degeneration disease genes lead to PSC dysfunction and ultimately death of rods and cones remain to be defined.[65,97]

It is hoped that, as additional information about the mechanisms by which mutations in retinal degeneration disease genes cause photoreceptor cell death is gained from research, it will be applied to the development of therapies to prevent loss of vision from these disorders.

Key references

A complete list of chapter references is available online at www.expertconsult.com. See inside cover for registration details.

1. Berson EL. Retinitis pigmentosa. The Friedenwald lecture. Invest Ophthalmol Vis Sci 1993;34:1659–1676.

2. Weleber RG. Infantile and childhood retinal blindness: a molecular perspective (the Franceschetti lecture). Ophthalm Genet 2002;23:71–97.

3. Hartong DT, Berson EL, Dryja TP. Retinitis pigmentosa. Lancet 2006;368:1795–1809.

7. Lamb TD, Pugh EN Jr. Phototransduction, dark adaptation, and rhodopsin regeneration the proctor lecture. Invest Ophthalmol Vis Sci 2006;47:5137–5152.

8. Marmor MF, Holder GE, Seeliger MW, et al. Standard for clinical electroretinography (2004 update). Doc Ophthalmol 2004;108:107–114.

10. Berson EL. Long-term visual prognoses in patients with retinitis pigmentosa: the Ludwig von Sallmann lecture. Exp Eye Res 2007;85:7–14.

14. Stone EM. Genetic testing for inherited eye disease. Arch Ophthalmol 2007;125:205–212.

19. Berson EL, Rosner B, Sandberg MA, et al. Vitamin A supplementation for retinitis pigmentosa. Arch Ophthalmol 1993;111:1456–1459.

22. Sieving PA, Caruso RC, Tao W, et al. Ciliary neurotrophic factor (CNTF) for human retinal degeneration: phase I trial of CNTF delivered by encapsulated cell intraocular implants. Proc Natl Acad Sci USA 2006;103:3896–3901.

25. Maguire AM, Simonelli F, Pierce EA, et al. Safety and efficacy of gene transfer for Leber's congenital amaurosis. N Engl J Med 2008;358:2240–2248.

34. RetNet website address. 2008. http://www.sph.uth.tmc.edu/Retnet/.

35. Daiger SP, Bowne SJ, Sullivan LS. Perspective on genes and mutations causing retinitis pigmentosa. Arch Ophthalmol 2007;125:151–158.

41. Badano JL, Mitsuma N, Beales PL, et al. The ciliopathies: an emerging class of human genetic disorders. Annu Rev Genomics Hum Genet 2006;7:125–148.

42. Hildebrandt F, Zhou W. Nephronophthisis-associated ciliopathies. J Am Soc Nephrol 2007;18:1855–1871.

60. Saari JC. Biochemistry of visual pigment regeneration: the Friedenwald lecture. Invest Ophthalmol Vis Sci 2000;41:337–348.

CHAPTER 75

Visual prostheses and other assistive devices

Muhammad Ali Memon and Joseph F Rizzo III

The field of retinal prosthetics began about 20 years ago, largely because of advances in microelectronic technology[1,2] which permitted the development of electronically sophisticated devices that were small enough to be implanted into the eyeball. The remarkable success of cochlear implants, which has been achieved without a large number of electrodes or very advanced electronic technology, served as a beacon for the emerging field of visual prosthetics. This chapter provides an overview of the challenges and achievements in the development of visual prostheses, which have the potential to provide vision to patients for whom there is otherwise little opportunity for significant rehabilitation. Potential sites for implementation of a visual prosthesis include the subretinal space, epiretinal surface, optic nerve, lateral geniculate nucleus (LGN), and visual cortex (Figure 75.1).

Clinical background

Blindness is one of the most common forms of disability, and in industrialized countries retinal disease accounts for the majority of blind patients. Age-related macular degeneration (AMD) and retinitis pigmentosa (RP) are the two retinal diseases causing blindness that are considered to be potentially treatable with a retinal prosthesis. There are roughly 2 million Americans with AMD, and the percentage of affected individuals is expected to increase by 50% by the year 2020.[3,4] RP is the leading cause of inherited blindness in the world, affecting roughly 1.7 million patients. The cost to the US government to provide support services for the blind is enormous, reaching $4 billion annually.[5]

Pathology

AMD and RP cause blindness because of grossly similar pathologies (Figure 75.2), although the mechanisms of injury are different. Both diseases cause blindness because of a loss of the rods and cones (i.e., the photoreceptors),[6,7] which are the only cells in the retina that can convert incoming light into neural signals that create conscious visual perception. The neural signals are propogated to retinal ganglion cells (RGC) in the inner retina, which connect the eye to the brain and remain relatively healthy in AMD and RP.[7–11] A prosthesis can potentially restore vision to patients with these diseases by providing electrical stimulation to the RGCs, which will then conduct the visual information to the brain. Diseases that damage the inner retina or optic nerve, like diabetic retinopathy and glaucoma, would not be amenable to the use of a retinal prosthesis.

The belief that there was "sparing" of RGCs was based upon the interpretation of standard histopathology of the retinas of affected patients (Figure 75.2: upper right and lower). More careful study of such retinas, however, showed the "sparing" to be relative.[9–11] For RP, there is a loss of 30–70% of the RGCs; there is greater loss of RGCs in the peripheral retina, and cell loss is greatest in more advanced cases, especially in the X-linked and recessive forms of RP.[10,11] The loss of RGCs is the result of anterograde transsynaptic degeneration, invasion of inwardly migrating retinal pigment epithelial cells into the blood vessels of the inner retina, and perhaps compression of axons due to altered anatomy of the inner retina.[12–14] In patients with severe RP, only about 300,000 of the average 1.2 million RGCs in normally sighted humans survive. This degree of survival would still seem to be adequate to support the delivery of a substantial amount of visual information to the brain. By comparison, the auditory nerve contains roughly 30,000 cells,[15] and stimulating some fraction of these cells has been sufficient to provide useful hearing for deaf patients, although admittedly the more complex visual sense will require more detailed information transfer.

Robert Marc has described in detail a predictable and orderly "reorganization" of molecules, synapses, cells, and networks in retinas following degeneration of photoreceptors.[16–19] The neural retina initially responds to loss of photoreceptors by showing subtle changes in neuronal structure, like neuronal swelling and disruption of microtubular structure (i.e., phase I changes). In phase II, there is death of photoreceptors – first rods, then cones. The loss of cones is followed by whole-scale reorganization of retinal cell layers and interconnections. Prior to their death, the metabolically stressed photoreceptors sprout neurites that extend, quite anomalously, up to the inner plexiform layer and ganglion cell layers. As the photoreceptors die, the bipolar cells retract their dendrites; the horizontal cells retract their dendrites within the outer plexiform layer while (anomalously) extending axonal processes and dendrites toward the inner plexiform layer. The Müller cells increase synthesis of their

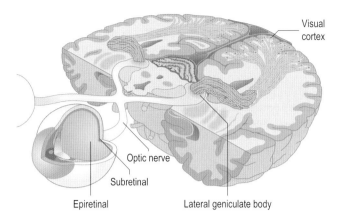

Figure 75.1 Potential sites for implantation of a visual prosthesis.

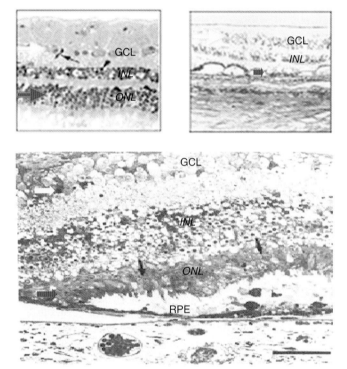

Figure 75.2 Photomicrographs of normal retina (upper left) with its normal complement of three cellular layers, and two retinas with degeneration of the photoreceptors (upper right and lower). Upper right: histology of the retina from a human with age-related macular degeneration. Lower: histology from the nasal foveal region from a human patient with retinitis pigmentosa. Both of the degenerated retinas show a dramatic loss of photoreceptors from the normal 6+ layers of cells that are present in the central retina of humans (compare appearance at red arrows in the normal versus diseased retinas). Both degenerated retinas also show a moderate presence of many cell bodies in the retinal ganglion cell layer (yellow arrows). Most of the neurons in this layer send axons to form the optic nerve.

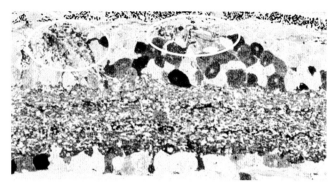

Figure 75.3 Retinal histology obtained by fusion of computational molecular phenotyping data sets with conventional electron microscopy showing GABAergic amacrine cells forming multiple, focal microneuromas (circled). Each microneuroma receives processes from nearby amacrine cells that appear to have migrated distally in the retina. (Reproduced with permission from Jones BW, Marc RE. Retinal remodeling during retinal degeneration. Exp Eye Res 2005;81:123–137.)

locations, development of new and aberrant synapses, creation of reciprocal synapses, "synaptic microneuromas" (Figure 75.3), and widespread death of all neuronal cell types in the retina.

Furthermore, the degeneration of photoreceptors alters the physiology of the surviving RGCs, which develop an increased spontaneous firing rate.[20] The increased spontaneous activity might produce "noise" within the signal transduction pathway, which could complicate the attempt to create a useful visual image. As such, a new body of research is being pursued within the field of retinal prosthetics to define the response properties of degenerating retinas, with special emphasis on the response characteristics of retinal neurons following electrical stimulation.[21-27]

More specific rationale for treatment of retinal blindness with a retinal prosthesis

Guidelines for considering the use of a retinal prosthesis should require that a patient had normal vision at some point in life. This provides assurance that the complex series of interconnections between the photoreceptors and the primary visual cortex had at one time been properly established.

RP is widely considered to be the primary target for a retinal prosthesis because affected patients often become more severely blind than patients with AMD. Thus, the Food and Drug Administration would almost certainly require a greater demonstration of safety and efficacy for any proposal to use a retinal prosthesis for AMD, since these patients generally have better vision and therefore would be taking a greater risk than patients with RP.

The hope that vision with spatial detail can be achieved is based upon the presence of a predictable topographic order along the afferent visual pathway between the photoreceptors and the visual cortex. It therefore seems reasonable to assume that direct electrical stimulation of bipolar cells or RGCs (but not their overlying axons) might generate percepts at locations within the visual field similar to those which would have been obtained by photic stimulation in

intermediate filament proteins and extend processes beneath the retina that form a dense fibrotic layer within the subretinal space,[16,17] which would presumably complicate attempts to stimulate the surviving cells of the outer retina from the subretinal space.

In phase 3, the reorganizing retina displays widespread sprouting of new neurites, migration of neurons into ectopic

Box 75.1 Conceptual foundation for development of retinal prosthesis

- In patients with photoreceptor loss, a retinal prosthesis has the potential to improve vision by delivering electrical stimulation to retinal nerve cells that survive the degeneration of photoreceptors
- The rationale for use of a retinal prosthesis is based on the premise of a predictable topographic order extending from cells of the retina, especially the retinal ganglion cells (RGCs), to the visual cortex, such that electrical stimulation of the retina in a specific geometric pattern could yield percepts of a similar geometry
- Successful candidates for a prosthesis should have had normal vision at some point in their lives and a substantial survival of RGCs to make it possible to deliver electrical input to the brain by electrically stimulating the retina
- There is relative preservation of RGCs in age-related macular degeneration, but in retinitis pigmentosa there is significant "reorganization" of the retinal neurons and glia of the middle and inner retina, including sprouting of new neuritis by neural cells, development of aberrant synapses, and significant cell death (including in the RGC layer), which complicates the goal of creating useful vision for blind patients with a retinal prosthesis
- Diseases that cause significant damage to the optic nerve, like glaucoma, could not be treated with a retinal prosthesis

the same area (Box 75.1). Indeed, human patients who have been severely blind for decades from RP have seen photopsias of varying degrees of detail (and more, see below) following electrical stimulation of the retina by numerous groups.[28–34]

More detailed considerations of prosthetic intervention in AMD

Visual loss with AMD is limited to central vision, and although patients can be significantly handicapped for tasks like reading, retention of peripheral vision provides them with some degree of independence. A prosthesis for patients with AMD would only be helpful if it could improve central vision, which is a much more demanding goal than helping patients with RP by providing relatively coarse visual input to help with navigation.

The same rationale of relative preservation of RGCs for use of a retinal prosthesis has been offered for AMD as for RP, although the story is more complex. In the aging retina, photoreceptor loss begins in the parafoveal region (initially inferiorly) and is dominated by loss of rods. Early on, this cell loss can occur without RPE abnormalities, although in many cases RPE abnormalities, mostly drusen, are evident and constitute perhaps the most important clinical signs of dry AMD.[35,36] For wet AMD, the pathology is much more severe, with marked loss of photoreceptors and moderately severe (50% loss) of RGCs overlying the areas of photoreceptor degeneration, although, in some cases, the inner retina can be relatively spared.[37] For dry AMD, these surviving photoreceptors also may not have normal synaptic connections[38]; and unlike RP, there is only scant physiological

evidence that RGCs can be stimulated to produce vision in patients with AMD.[39] There are also a number of other anatomical features of the central macula that will likely complicate efforts to obtain vision in the range of 20/400 or better for patients with AMD. First, the anticipation that patients might see a geometrically similar (pattern to the stimulus) pattern is confounded by the fact that the RGCs are stacked upon one another within the parafovea. Thus, there may be a lack of topographical order for the central-most RGCs such that adjacent RGCs might not correspond to adjacent points in the visual field.[40]

For patients with wet AMD, the scarring that follows the hemorrhages can severely distort the retinal contour (Figure 75.4), which to some extent would complicate surgical positioning or attachment of the prosthesis to the inner retinal surface.[41] As such, the anatomy of each patient with AMD will have to be considered individually, and it must be assumed that some severely blind patients with AMD will not be good candidates for a prosthesis.

Etiology of outer retinal degenerations

The etiologies of AMD and RP are discussed in Chapters 68, 69, and 74.

Management

Attempts to assist patients with AMD or RP have included use of optical and electro-optical devices, such as telescopes, closed-circuit monitors and mobility training, primarily to learn how to use a cane for walking. These strategies can be beneficial but are limited in the functional gains that can be made. Newer rehabilitation strategies are also being explored, including sensory substitution; transplantation of stem cells, embryonic, or adult cells; and molecular genetic approaches, which may offer the best long-term treatment option. A prosthesis also has the significant advantage that restoration of function could be achieved by stimulation of nerve fibers that had been properly established during development – no new connections would have to be developed, as would be the case for transplanted cells.

The relative merits and disadvantages of various alternative strategies that could potentially be used in lieu of a retinal prosthesis are briefly compared below.

Sensory substitution

In sensory substitution therapy, a sensory modality is used to provide spatial information about the environment that cannot be appreciated by the compromised visual system. A customized device captures visual information and relays it to a nonvisual sense, like the tactile or the auditory system, to provide input about the spatial detail of the patient's local environment. The late Paul Bach-y-Rita, a pioneer in this field, advocated the introduction of visual information (captured with a camera) through tactile input to the skin or tongue. His subjects were (to some extent) able to recreate an impression of their environment, experience a sense of

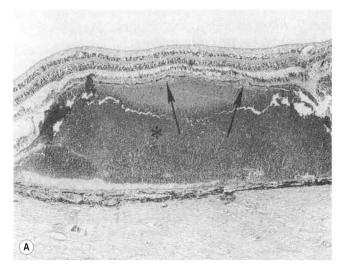 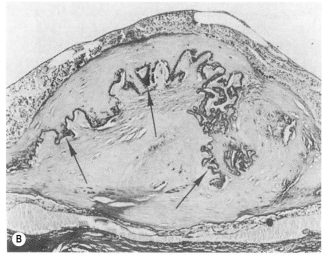

Figure 75.4 Left: hemorrhagic detachment of retinal pigment epithelium (RPE) (asterisk). Drusen are detached (arrows) along with RPE. Ganglion cell and inner nuclear layers are relatively spared over this large lesion. The irregular contour of the surface of the retina would complicate surgical attachment of the prosthesis (hematoxylin and eosin stain, ×40). Right: a very large disciform lesion, the larger portion of which is located between two layers of the Bruch's membrane and smaller portion between the inner layer of the Bruch's membrane and the degenerated retina. The inner layer of Bruch's membrane is considerably thickened and redundant (arrows). There is significant destruction of inner retinal architecture over most of the lesion with some sparing of the ganglion cell layer seen to the far right. (Reproduced with permission from Spencer WH. Ophthalmic Pathology: An Atlas and Textbook, 3rd edn, vol. 2. Philadelphia: WB Saunders, 1985.)

objects in space, and perform "eye"–hand coordination tasks.[42]

A more recent device uses a camera to capture visual images, which are then electronically modified (by configuring the loudness, frequency, and inter-ear disparity) to provide a "soundscape" that represents the visual landscape.[43] Some completely blind patients have navigated through unfamiliar environments and even found their way through a maze on a computer screen using only the auditory cues provided by this vOICe device (Figure 75.5 and Box 75.2).

Gene therapy

The efforts to treat blindness by transferring healthy genes to repair genetic mutations achieved a major milestone in 2001 when Acland et al[44] demonstrated that blind dogs (suffering from a retinal disease caused by the same mutation that causes Leber congenital amaurosis in humans) were able to regain lost sight. Within 3 months, the dogs were able to navigate within a dimly lit room.[44] More recently, modifications of their packaging techniques have produced a 90% reduction of the amplitude of nystagmus.[45] Additional studies on blind large animals[46,47] and rodent models of retinal degeneration have provided substantial evidence that gene replacement therapy, or gene silencing therapy, represents a scientifically sound strategy potentially to treat certain forms of retinal blindness.[48–50] Gene therapy trials to treat early-onset retinal degeneration have taken place in the USA and England, and have shown modest but encouraging visual results.[51]

Transplantation

Human transplantation studies, following earlier animal studies,[52–54] have been performed using RPE, retinal neurons,

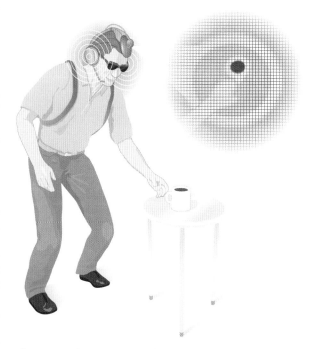

Figure 75.5 The vOICe system allows a visually impaired person to "see" by using the ears for visual input. Software that can be run by laptop computer carried in a backpack translates images captured by a video camera into sounds that the brain can use to create crude mental renderings.

partial-thickness sections of retina, and stem cells. These studies have ranged from a single patient to 56 patients, and most report relatively short follow-up of the patients. Generally, the transplants have been well tolerated and immune rejections and surgical complications have been uncommon.

Box 75.2 Approaches to treatment of age-related macular degeneration (AMD) and retinitis pigmentosa (RP)

- Historically, patients with severe visual loss from RP have benefited from use of a white cane, which provides important assistance for navigation. Patients with severe loss of central vision, from either RP or AMD, can benefit from use of optical or electronic devices such as telescopes and closed-circuit monitors
- Molecular genetic approaches for treatment of one form of RP have recently provided some benefit to blind humans
- Transplantation of stem cells, retinal pigment epithelium (RPE), or retinal neurons has been generally well tolerated in animals and humans, and in some cases has provided some benefit to blind patients
- Human trials with ciliary neurotrophic factor administration have shown enhancement of RPE survival and a delay in visual loss in some human patients
- Sensory substitution recreates an impression of the environment using sensation to a nonvisual sense such as touch or hearing. This approach can assist in navigation but could not restore "sight"

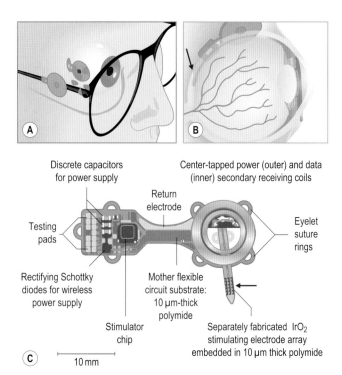

Figure 75.6 Minimally invasive, subretinal prosthetic system designed, built, and tested by the Boston Retinal Implant Project. (A and B) An illustration of our device, as seen from the front of a patient (A) and in a sagittal projection of the eye (B). The visual image is obtained by an external camera on a pair of spectacles and is translated into an electromagnetic signal that is transmitted wirelessly to the implanted components of the device, which are sutured to the sclera. Electrical power is also transmitted similarly from the primary to the secondary coil. The sagittal view reveals that only the electrode array (arrow) penetrates the wall of the eye. (C) An illustration of our first-generation device that we have used for animal tests. The secondary coils for power and data transmission (shown on the right) and the integrated circuit and discrete electronic components (shown on the left) are all mounted on a flexible, polyimide substrate. Only the stimulating electrode array (red arrow) enters the eye, where it is positioned within the subretinal space. Calibration bar (lower left).

Many studies have reported improvement in visual acuity in some patients, occasionally up to four lines on a Snellen chart. In general, patients with wet AMD generally fared worse than dry AMD or RP patients, and worse pretreatment vision correlated with decreased chance of benefit from transplantation.[54–63]

Neurotrophic factors

Ciliary neurotrophic factor (CNTF), a chemical which may be released normally by the RPE in response to cellular injury, has demonstrated significant retinal protection in animal models of RP where a delay in photoreceptor cell loss and enhancement of RPE survival in a rat model were demonstrated.[64,65] A company called Neurotech USA has created an encapsulated vehicle containing RPE cells that have been modified using viral vectors to secrete CNTF continuously.[66] Neurotech has conducted a phase I trial on 10 RP patients, 7 of whom demonstrated improved visual acuity, which was maintained in 3 patients 6 months after the removal of implant. However, one patient suffered a complete choroidal detachment.[67] Other neurotrophic factors, like brain-derived neurotrophic factor and nerve growth factor, have also shown some neuroprotective benefit in animal experiments[68] and may be other options for future human tests.

What is a visual prosthesis?

A retinal prosthesis is a complex device that functions by: (1) capturing visual images; (2) communicating the images to electronic components that interface with the retina; and (3) selectively delivering electrical pulses to the retina to create vision (Figure 75.6). The neurons can also be stimulated by some nonelectrical means using neurotransmitters or cations.[69–72] Although such nonelectrical strategies offer the potential for being less toxic to the host tissue, development lags substantially behind the efforts to use electrical stimulation.

Attempts to develop visual cortical prostheses began in the 1970s,[73,74] and have been advanced by Drs. Normann (University of Utah) and separately by Philip Troyk (Illinois Institute of Technology).[75] Advancements in microtechnology roughly 20 years ago allowed our group and another at Duke University to begin efforts to develop a retinal prosthesis. Since then, the field has enjoyed enormous growth and now includes 22 retinal prosthetic research groups in six countries. There is not yet enough evidence to know which approach(es) might be preferable, and it is possible different diseases might be treated differently.

Comparison of different types of visual prosthetic devices

Each of the locations being considered as a site for a visual prosthesis (Figure 75.1) has certain advantages and disadvantages, and each approach has merit (Box 75.3). In general,

Box 75.3 Potential sites for implantable visual prostheses

- A retinal prosthesis functions by capturing visual images and communicating them to electronics that interface with the retina to deliver electrical stimulation to the retina for creation of a visual percept. Location of the prosthesis at the level of the eye has the advantage of being the most surgically accessible site of the visual system but this approach cannot treat diseases of the optic nerve

- An optic nerve prosthesis cannot treat glaucoma, but the surgical approach at the level of the orbit permits placement of a relatively small number of electrodes with a surgery that is more straightforward compared to an intraocular surgery. However, the optic nerve within the orbit is invested by the full complement of meninges, which complicates placement of a large number of electrodes at this level. By comparison, the intracranial optic nerve segment has the advantage of not being covered with the outer meningeal layers, but the surgical approach is much more invasive

- A lateral geniculate body (LGB) prosthesis has the potential psychophysical benefit of segregation of visual stream into different physiological pathways (e.g., for spatial and motion detection) and afferent fibers from both eyes intermingle at that level. However, interfacing with LGB requires a "deep brain" neurosurgical procedure, but with modern stereotactic surgical methods this approach is becoming relatively straightforward for physicians and patients

- Visual cortical prostheses, like the LGB prosthesis, can potentially treat all of the most common causes of blindness. Implantation of a cortical prosthesis, however, requires an extensive "open" neurosurgical procedure

the more central the placement of a prosthesis, the greater the range of diseases it can treat. For instance, a retinal prosthesis could not be used to treat glaucomatous blindness (because of damage to the optic nerve), but a LGN or cortical approach could potentially provide some vision. By comparison, the convoluted topography of the visual cortex and the need for a substantial neurosurgical procedure to implant a cortical device impose challenges on the widespread use of visual cortical prosthetic devices (Figure 75.1). On the other hand, the eye is prone to develop chronic inflammations whereas the brain seems to respond fairly indolently to long-term implantation of foreign material.[76,77] A cuff electrode array can be easily placed around the optic nerve in the orbit, but in this location the nerve is invested by all three meningeal sheaths and requires greater charge density for stimulation. Conversely, placing electrodes on the meninges-free, intracranial part of the optic nerve would require a large craniotomy. At the level of the LGN, it would be very challenging to implant a large number (i.e., hundreds) of electrodes that might ultimately be needed to create spatially detailed vision there.[78] The recent use of small craniotomies for placement of deep brain implants in the treatment of patients with Parkinson's and other neurological diseases has been well tolerated, and it is possible that some similar technique can be adapted for visual cortical implants in the future. Each potential site for a visual prosthesis has its advantages and drawbacks.

What has been achieved to date?

The following is a brief discussion of the results of testing for each type of visual prosthetic device. An example of some psychophysical tests used by one group to test patients who have received a retinal prosthesis is shown in Figure 75.7. At the end, a summary of results across all of these studies will be provided.

Visual cortical prosthesis

Brindley produced crude perceptions by implanting an electronically primitive device into the visual cortex of a patient who was completely blind from glaucoma.[73,79] Later, Dobelle and Mladejovsky[74] showed that multiple phosphenes could be perceived simultaneously following stimulation of multiple cortical electrodes, and that there was a perceptual alignment of the phosphenes that roughly correlated with the spatial organization of the visual cortex.[79] These experiments were conducted by delivering stimulation to the surface of the cortex, which required high charge levels and produced only coarse two-point discrimination of phosphenes. In efforts to address these shortcomings, Hambrecht's group (at the National Institutes of Health) reported the perception in a patient of multiple phosphenes that formed a straight line.[80] Normann and colleagues (University of Utah) worked toward improving electrode design and techniques for surgical implantation of their device in the brain,[81,82] and this has contributed significantly to the development of a motor prosthesis that has recently shown promising results in paralyzed patients.[83-85] Phil Troyk and coworkers at the Illinois Institute of Technology have implanted 128 electrodes into the visual cortex of monkeys and have demonstrated the ability of the monkeys to learn to direct their eyes accurately toward specific points in space in relation to which electrodes were driven.[86] Interestingly, there was a "learning effect" such that the psychophysical performance of the monkeys was initially quite poor but then after some months improved substantially over a very short period of time.

Retinal and optic nerve prostheses

The following is a brief summary of all projects that have performed psychophysical experiments after chronic implantation of a prosthetic device in humans (Box 75.4). In general, none of the retinal groups has yet published the results of a large number of psychophysical experiments with multiple trials and statistics of accuracy and reproducibility. In part, some of the lack of information may be related to the fact that the more recent (and potentially better-performing) devices have been implanted only recently. The fact that some of these data are considered proprietary by some companies is also limiting the flow of results in scientific journals. This review is at best an approximation of the results that can be gleaned from published results, scientific presentations, or information available on the official websites of some of these companies. Without a similar degree of published information from each company, it is possible that the following summary inaccurately portrays the achievements of some groups. Any such seeming biases are unintentional.

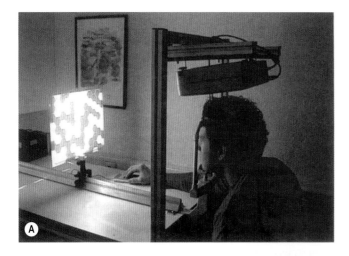

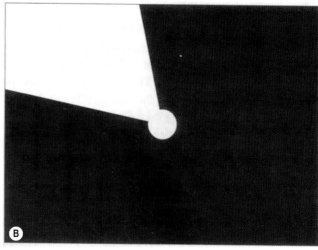

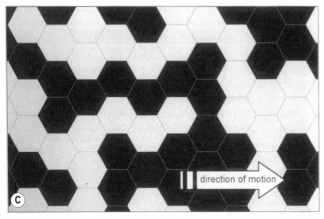

direction of motion

Figure 75.7 Photograph of the technical setup for testing some aspects of visual function following receipt of a retinal prosthesis, as developed by Retina Implant AG. Top: an LCD projector is mounted upside-down over the patient's head and projects on a screen 60 cm ahead of the patient. The patient uses a key pad to enter responses. Lower left: example of image localization test. A fixation spot is positioned in the middle of the screen. After a few seconds, a wedge-shaped bright stimulus appears at one of eight orientations (in this example, across the upper left side of the visual field). Lower right: example image of the motion test in which random patterns of white and black hexagons move across the screen, in this case to the right.

Box 75.4 Results of chronic human implantation of retinal prostheses

- Several groups worldwide have conducted chronic implantation of retinal prostheses in humans. In general, patients have tolerated the implants well

- In general, patients who have been blind from retinitis pigmentosa can see phosphenes of light in response to electrical stimulation of the retina. The appearance of the percepts generally varies as the particular type of electrical stimulation is varied, which offers the hope of being able to customize stimulus patterns to create useful vision for some blind patients

- None of the results to date has convincingly shown, by standard scientific methods, that blind patients can utilize a retinal prosthesis to improve their quality of life, although there is significant preliminary evidence to suggest that such benefits will be realized by some patients

of information has been published at this time are briefly discussed below.

The most fundamental achievement of these studies is the determination of psychophysical threshold. These thresholds have varied widely but tend to be in the range of 1–3 mC/cm^2 range, which is near or above the acceptable safe charge limits for the metal electrodes that were used.[31,87,88] Some thresholds, especially after long-term implantation, have been substantially below 1 mC/cm^2, which is a more encouraging number for chronic stimulation.[31,89] In general, the psychophysical thresholds have been at least four times higher for patients with RP compared to normally sighted patients,[90,91] and, as described above, this may partly be the result of pathology that develops in degenerated retinas, among other factors. Thus far, the only strategy to reduce electrical stimulation thresholds in degenerate retinas has been achieved by infusion of CNTF into the vitreous cavity of rats.[71]

Retinal prosthesis

Five companies (two from the USA, three from Germany) have performed chronic implants of retinal prosthetic devices in humans. Three of the groups have used an epiretinal approach, the other two a subretinal approach. The results of four of the companies for which the most amount

Optobionics

The first to perform chronic human testing was Optobionics (Wheaton, IL), which implanted a photodiode array into the eyes of 12 RP patients. This device was designed to operate only from the power of incident light reaching the retina, and this was widely considered to be insufficient to drive retinal neurons.[92] The intensity of light needed to drive the retinal neurons was in fact similar to the brightness of the summer sun at noon.[93] Most subjects reported improvement in acuity, sensitivity, visual field size, or motion perception. Chow's group then reported that the visual benefits experienced by their patients resulted from a "trophic" effect that was unrelated to point-to-point electrical stimulation.[94] The trophic effect might be similar to that originally discovered in experiments on retinal transplantation, that is believed to be related to a soluble factor produced by the RPE.[95–98] Perhaps any type of subretinal implant might benefit from some tropism that might occur secondary to the surgery to introduce the device.

Second Sight Medical Products

This company is now in a second phase I trial of their second-generation device, which utilizes modified electronics from a cochlear prosthesis.

Second Sight has performed two types of psychophysical experiment on their chronically implanted patients. The first type of experiment used stimuli unrelated to the environment but allowed the researchers to study the relationship between stimulus parameters and visual perception. The second type of experiment assessed the degree to which patients could appreciate the presence of objects imaged by a camera within their environment. With the first set of studies, electrical stimulation of the retina allowed patients to identify: (1) which of the two electrodes had been activated in a two-point discrimination task; (2) the direction of "movement" when electrodes were activated sequentially; and (3) whether electrodes were activated in rows or columns.[31,89,99,100] With the second type of experiment, the subjects failed to perform better than chance when they had to keep their head stationary while a bright object was moved across the visual field. However, when allowed to scan the visual field, the subjects could variably: (1) identify which quadrant the object was in; (2) count the number of objects presented on a screen; (3) identify the orientation of the long limb of the letter "L"; and (4) choose between a knife, cup, and plate that were randomly presented on a flat surface.[31,89,99,100]

Patients are now being allowed to use the second-generation device outside the laboratory. Scientific data have not yet been presented on this device, although nonscientific statements by some of the patients are clearly very positive.

Intelligent Medical Implants

Intelligent Medical Implants (IMI, based in Zug, Switzerland) utilizes a microfilm epiretinal implant introduced through the pars plana.[101] Their first-generation electrode array included 19 electrodes; the current array includes 49 electrodes. The initial publication of their human studies reported that the patients were able to ascertain different impressions of their brightness, shape, color, and duration of stimuli, and with practice, the patients could differentiate the relative localization of stimuli, recognize basic patterns such as lines and spots, and detect motion. In their acute trial consisting of 20 RP patients, visual percepts appeared like little stars, circles, triangles, rectangles, half-moons, and solar eclipses in white, yellow, and blue colors, and had the brightness of candle light or lamp.[88] IMI is conducting a multicenter trial across Europe.

Retina Implant AG

This company emerged from research led by E. Zrenner, based in Tübingen, Germany. Their implant contains 1500 light-sensitive elements that are designed to act as a photo-detecting array *and* a 4 × 4 array of hard-wired electrodes. Like the Second Sight device, hard-wired electrodes are connected to the electronic elements positioned behind the ear. The surgical group, led by Helmut Sachs, has been successful in (at least) 7 of 7 patients using a transchoroidal approach to the subretinal space. This surgical approach is more challenging (but potentially more advantageous) compared to the pars plana approach in which foreign elements are left in position toward the front of the eye, as this latter technique can predispose to extrusion of the devices through the conjunctiva and possibly an infection. One patient has elected to keep his device long-term and has provided very useful psychophysical information.

Psychophysical results have mostly been obtained from the 16 hard-wired electrodes. Four of the 7 patients reported some degree of pattern recognition and 2 of these patients reported the perception of pea-sized objects with single-electrode stimulation.[102] Patients were able to report variation of brightness and sizes of percepts with varying strength of stimulation, orientation of horizontal and vertical lines, the relative position of electrodes, and the direction of movement following sequential activation of the electrodes.[87,103,104]

Experiments conducted by photic activation of the photodiode array allowed 3 patients to perceive light in certain shapes and patterns. Some patients detected single spots of light of only 100–400 µm diameter. One patient was able to locate white dinner plates on a dark tablecloth.[103]

Optic nerve prostheses

Veraart and coworkers have performed implants of a cuff with four electrodes around the optic nerves of two RP patients. Using a camera-based system, their patients reported some characteristics of the electrically induced phosphenes such as their shape, size, basic structure, location, and brightness. These researchers reported an 87% success rate with pattern recognition of basic forms, but with a relatively long time delay of 53 seconds for patients to discern the perception of objects. With training, the subjects learned to scan more effectively, discriminate objects on a table (e.g., cup, eating utensil) more quickly, and were able to reach out and grasp them. The appearance of the phosphenes could be modified by varying the strength of the electrical pulses and one patient reported being able to generate a letter "C" by stimulating in a particular way through three electrodes.[30,105,106] More recently, a Chinese program was formed under the direction of Drs. Lee (surgeon) and Q. Ren (engineer) to develop an optic nerve prosthesis with penetrating electrodes.

Summary of human implantation with retinal prosthetic devices

The collective outcome of human testing for visual prosthetic devices has demonstrated that: (1) patients who have been legally blind for decades can reliably see phosphenes in response to electrical stimulation; and (2) modulation of electrical stimulation can create multiple images that are geometrically similar to the pattern of electrical stimulation. Although the induced percepts have generally been crude, the more recent chronic experiments have shown that blind patients can detect large moving objects, identify large letters by scanning, and report the orientation of lines generated by electrical stimulation. These outcomes, which have been found to a similar degree by multiple groups, are one of the most encouraging aspects of the psychophysical results obtained to date. It is also notable, however, that no retinal group has yet provided a sufficiently detailed description of their tests (including number of raw trials, standard errors, false-positive and false-negative responses across a reasonably large number of trials) to allow an independent researcher the opportunity to assess the validity of the conclusions of their published works.

The variability in testing methods also makes it difficult to draw comparisons of the qualitative differences in results across groups. One less encouraging result from the collective body of work is the general lack of very obvious improvements in the spatial quality of perception over the last couple of years. Perhaps this is just the result of the normal delay in reporting, or perhaps the field has hit a psychophysical plateau.

The challenge of creating "useful" and spatially more detailed visual perceptions at least partly relates to the need to develop substantially better knowledge about improved methods for stimulating the afferent visual pathway. In this regard, the status of the visual prosthetic projects is not unlike the history of cochlear implants, which required many years of work to discover methods that ultimately produced great success in helping many deaf patients. Overall, the results of human testing to date support the hope that artificial stimulation will one day provide "useful" vision for the blind. It should be remembered that, for severely blind patients, even crude visual assistance that would help patients navigate more safely in an unfamiliar environment would be a substantial improvement in their quality of life.

Key references

A complete list of chapter references is available online at www.expertconsult.com. See inside cover for registration details.

1. Rizzo JF 3rd, Wyatt J, Humayun M, et al. Retinal prosthesis: an encouraging first decade with major challenges ahead. Ophthalmology 2001;108:13.

3. Congdon N, O'Colmain B, Klaver CC, et al. Causes and prevalence of visual impairment among adults in the United States. Arch Ophthalmol 2004;122:477–485.

7. Adler R, Curcio C, Hicks D, et al. Cell death in age-related macular degeneration. Mol Vision 1999;5:31.

17. Jones BW, Marc RE. Retinal remodeling during retinal degeneration. Exp Eye Res 2005;81:123–137.

29. Rizzo JF 3rd, Wyatt J, Loewenstein J, et al. Methods and perceptual thresholds for short-term electrical stimulation of human retina with microelectrode arrays. Invest Ophthalmol Vis Sci 2003;44:5355–5361.

30. Veraart C, Wanet-Defalque MC, Gerard B, et al. Pattern recognition with the optic nerve visual prosthesis. Artif Organs 2003;27:996–1004.

31. Mahadevappa M, Weiland JD, Yanai D, et al. Perceptual thresholds and electrode impedance in three retinal prosthesis subjects. IEEE Trans Neural Syst Rehabil Eng 2005;13:201–206.

41. Rizzo JF, Wyatt JL. Retinal prosthesis. In: Berger J, Fine S, Maguire M (eds) Age-Related Macular Degeneration. St. Louis, MO: Mosby, 1999;429–430.

51. Bainbridge JW, Smith AJ, Barker SS, et al. Effect of gene therapy on visual function in Leber's congenital amaurosis. N Engl J Med 2008;358:2231–2239.

65. LaVail MM, Unoki K, Yasumura D, et al. Multiple growth factors, cytokines, and neurotrophins rescue photoreceptors from the damaging effects of constant light. Proc Natl Acad Sci USA 1992;89:11249–11253.

74. Dobelle WH, Mladejovsky MG. Phosphenes produced by electrical stimulation of human occipital cortex, and their application to the development of a prosthesis for the blind. J Physiol 1974;243:553–576.

78. Rizzo J. Embryology, anatomy and physiology of the afferent visual pathway. In: Miller NR, Newman NJ, Kerrison JB, et al (eds) Walsh and Hoyt's Clinical Neuro-Ophthalmology. Philadelphia, PA: Lippincott Williams and Wilkins, 2005:3–82.

88. Hornig R, Zehnder T, Velikay-Parel M, et al. The IMI retinal implant system. In: Humayun MS, Weiland JD, Chader G, et al (eds) Artificial Sight Basic Research, Biomedical Engineering, and Clinical Advances. New York: Springer, 2007:111–128.

89. Yanai D, Weiland J, Mahadevappa M, et al. Visual performance using a retinal prosthesis in three subjects with retinitis pigmentosa. Am J Ophthalmol 2007;5:820–827.

103. Zrenner E. Restoring neuroretinal function: new potentials. Doc Ophthalmol 2007;115:56–59.

CHAPTER 76

Paraneoplastic retinal degeneration

Grazyna Adamus

Overview

Paraneoplastic retinopathies (PRs) represent visual dysfunctions and retinal degeneration associated with known or suspect malignancies, without direct involvement of the eye. PRs are believed to originate from an autoimmune process involving circulating autoantibodies elicited against cancer antigens that also recognize retinal antigens. PRs include cancer-associated retinopathy, melanoma-associated retinopathy, and bilateral diffuse uveal melanocytic proliferation syndrome (Table 76.1).

Clinical background

Key symptoms and signs

Cancer-associated retinopathy (CAR) syndrome

CAR was first recognized as a paraneoplastic disorder, in association with small cell lung cancer (SCCL) and retinal dysfunction and degeneration. Besides SCCL, CAR occurs with other associated tumors, mostly carcinomas of the breast, endometrium, ovary, colon, bladder, and prostate,[1] as well as lymphomas and thymoma.

In CAR, the progression of retinal degeneration is examined by electroretinogram (ERG), visual field, and fundus examination.[2] Patients frequently describe the sudden onset of a sensation of flickering or shimmering lights and night blindness, with additional visual loss over weeks to several months. Rod dysfunction is characterized by night blindness and prolonged dark adaptation. Cone degeneration features include decreased visual acuity, sensitivity to light and glare, reduced color vision, and central and ring scotomas. The fundus can initially appear normal, but narrowed retinal arteries, retinal pigment epithelial mottling, and optic nerve pallor can be observed on ophthalmic examination. Vision loss is associated with decreased responses of cone and rod responses. Ocular symptoms may precede the diagnosis of cancer by months to years; thus, recognition of CAR facilitates early diagnosis of malignancy.

Antiretinal CAR autoantibodies are detected in blood by Western blotting (Figure 76.1).[1] The most recognized autoantibodies are against recoverin and α-enolase, but autoantibodies with other specificities can also be detected (Table 76.2). Patients with different antiretinal autoantibodies may have different clinical manifestations (Box 76.1). Antirecoverin CAR presents with symptoms of night blindness, photopsias, loss of peripheral or pericentral visual field, reduced central acuity, and widespread rod and cone dysfunction.[2] Anti-α-enolase CAR presents with varying degrees of central or pericentral visual field loss, shimmering photopsias, loss of color vision, reduced vision in bright light, and night blindness.[3] Thus, autoantibodies can serve as a biomarker for the prognosis and management of CAR.

Melanoma-associated retinopathy (MAR) syndrome

MAR is associated with visual loss, antiretinal autoantibodies, and diagnosed cutaneous malignant melanoma, often at the end-stage of metastasis.[4] MAR was first described in 1988 by Berson and Lessell.[5] Patients with MAR have nearly normal vision but develop night blindness, shimmering light, photopsia, and loss of peripheral vision that appear months to years after diagnosis of a tumor. The average time from the diagnosis of cancer to diagnosis of MAR averages 3.6 years.[4] The typical ERG pattern in MAR shows a slight reduction in scotopic a-wave, and a marked reduction or absence of dark-adapted b wave (Box 76.2).[6] Autoantibodies against bipolar cells were first reported in patients with MAR,[7] and recently, autoantibodies against other retinal proteins have also been found in these patients (Table 76.2).

Autoimmune retinopathy (AR)

Patients can have symptoms resembling CAR or MAR, and antiretinal autoantibodies, but have no tumor at the time of initial evaluation. AR is the preferred term for this acquired autoimmune-mediated condition (Table 76.1). The presence of autoantibodies without known malignancy leads to several speculations on the origin of autoimmune responses. Most likely, they originate from a very small tumor, too small to be detected by conventional methods, but the immune system detects it. The tumor might be detected clinically in the subsequent years. The length of the diagnostic follow-up period necessary to detect the tumor in clinical PR is under investigation. Thus far, it ranges from months up to 5 years, but it can be longer.[1] Antirecoverin antibodies are typically associated with CAR and have rarely been reported in AR patients. In such cases, antiretinal autoanti-

Table 76.1 Types of autoimmune retinopathy associated with the presence of circulating autoantibodies

Symptoms and signs	Paraneoplastic		Nonparaneoplastic	
	CAR syndrome	MAR syndrome	Autoimmune retinopathy	Retinal dystrophy
Visual loss	Bilateral	Bilateral	Initially unilateral/asymmetric	Bilateral/symmetric
Age at onset (years)	60+	30+	~40	Variable
Time course	Weeks/months	Years	Months/years	Months/years
Symptoms	Photopsia, progressive vision loss	Photopsia, night blindness	Photopsia, vision loss	Variable symptoms
Exam	Normal	Normal	Normal	Vascular leakage/exudates
Visual fields	Ring scotomas	Normal/central loss	Ring scotomas	Variable
Electroretinogram	Flat/severe loss	Loss of b-wave	Loss of b-wave/diffuse loss/flat	Variable
Systemic diseases	Carcinomas, lymphomas, thymoma	Cutaneous metastatic melanoma	Autoimmune disease with familiar history	None
Histopathology	Photoreceptor degeneration	Bipolar cells, unknown	Unknown	Unknown
Circulating antibodies	Recoverin, enolase, others	Bipolar cells, others	Enolase, CAII, p35, p40, others	Various

CAR, cancer-associated retinopathy; MAR, melanoma-associated retinopathy.

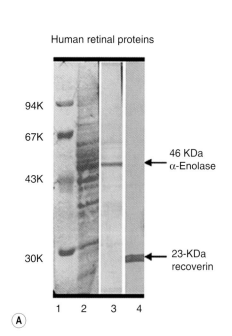

Human retinal proteins

94K
67K
43K
30K

46 KDa
α-Enolase

23-KDa
recoverin

1 2 3 4

(A)

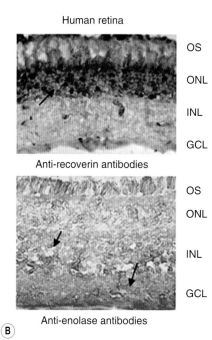

Human retina

OS
ONL
INL
GCL

Anti-recoverin antibodies

OS
ONL
INL
GCL

Anti-enolase antibodies

(B)

Figure 76.1 Autoantibody testing by Western blotting and immunocytochemistry. (A) Western blotting showing immunostaining of human retinal proteins by patient's serum: 1, molecular standards; 2, retinal proteins; 3, human serum recognizing α-enolase; 4, human serum recognizing recoverin on the blot. (B) Immunohistochemistry: antirecoverin serum antibodies bind to photoreceptor cell layer (outer retina), and anti-α-enolase serum binds to the inner and ganglion cell layers, and also stains neuronal fibers. OS, outer segments; ONL, outer nuclear layer; INL, inner nuclear layer; GCL, ganglion cell layer.

Box 76.1 Anti-retinal autoantibodies

Different autoantibodies, such as antirecoverin and anti-α-enolase, can be associated with different clinical presentations, phenotypic findings, and electroretinogram patterns

Box 76.2 Paraneoplastic retinopathies

Electroretinograms, visual field analysis, and autoantibody detection, in combination with an evaluation for a systemic malignancy, are essential for diagnosing cancer- and melanoma-associated retinopathy

bodies may be involved in tumor regression. This "new class" of retinopathies with autoantibodies cannot be ignored and needs to be followed up in ophthalmic examination. The condition can be classified as CAR or AR (= probable PR), based on clinical symptoms, the presence or absence of autoantibodies, and the presence or absence of cancer (Box 76.3).

Bilateral diffuse uveal melanocytic proliferation (BDUMP)

BDUMP is a rare syndrome that involves painless, bilateral vision loss, serous retinal detachment, and a systemic malignant neoplasm. Visual loss is due to the proliferation of

Table 76.2 Target autoantigens in paraneoplastic retinal degeneration

Autoantigen	Molecular weight	Binding in the retina	Molecular function	Presence in cancer	First described
Recoverin	23 kDa	Photoreceptor cells, ONL, BCL	Calcium-binding protein, phototransduction	SCCL, endometrial, others	Thirkill et al 1987[11] Polans et al 1991[13]
Neurofilament proteins	70, 145 200 kDa	Ganglion cells	Structural proteins	SCCL	Kornguth et al 1986[55]
α-enolase	46 kDa	GCL and diffuse staining of all layers	Glycolysis	Endocrine cancers	Adamus et al 1993[56]
Photoreceptor cell nuclear receptor (PNR)	46.5 kDa	ONL, INL, and photoreceptor cells	Photoreceptor cell development or maintenance	Lung, poorly differentiated carcinoma	Eichen et al 2001[57]
Bipolar cell antigen	?	Bipolar cells	?	Cutaneous melanoma, colon	Milam et al 1993[7]; Jacobson and Adamus 2001[58]
P60	60 kDa	?	?	SCCL	Murphy et al 1997[21]
P35	35 kDa	Miller cells	?	None	Peek et al 1998[59]
P22	22 kDa	Retina; optic nerve	?	Melanoma	Keltner and Thirkill 1999[60]
Hsc 70	70 kDa	?	Heat shock protein chaperone cytosolic peptides	SCCL	Ohguro et al 1999[61]
P45	45 kDa	?	?	Ovarian	Yoon et al 1999[62]
Tubby-like protein 1 (TULP1)	78 kDa	OPL, INL, ONL at the myoid to the synaptic terminal of rods and cones	Transcription factor or rhodopsin transport	Endometrial	Kikuchi et al 2000[63]
PTB-like protein (PTBLP)	58 kDa	Nuclei of GCL	RNA-binding protein	Endometrial	Kikuchi et al 2000[64]
P65	65 kDa	ONL	?	Lymphoma	To et al 2002[65]
P75/LEDGF	75 kDa	?	A survival factor	None	Chin et al 2006[66]
P40	40 kDa	Outer segments	Cone-specific	Laryngeal carcinoma	Parc et al 2006[67]
Arrestin	48 kDa	Photoreceptor cells	Phototransduction	Breast	Jacobson 1996[68]; Misiuk-Hojlo et al 2007[69]
Carbonic anhydrase II	30 kDa	GCL and photoreceptor cells	pH control	Colon, rectal	Adamus 2009[70]
120 kDa	120 kDa	Photoreceptor cells	Phototransduction	Melanoma	Sotodeh et al 2005[71]
Transducin-β	35 kDa	Photoreceptor cells	Phototransduction	Melanoma	Potter et al 2002[72]
Transducin-α	40 kDa	Photoreceptor cells	Phototransduction	Breast, lung, prostate, uterine	Adamus et al 2008[73]

? unknown; ONL, outer nuclear layer; BCL, bipolar cell layer; SCCL, small cell lung cancer; GCL, ganglion cell layer; INL, inner nuclear layer; OPL, outer plexiform layer.

uveal melanocytes occurring throughout the uvea without metastasis outside the eye.[8] The most common tumors are ovary and uterus in women and the lung in men. Most patients die from metastasis of their primary tumor within a year of BDUMP diagnosis. Autoantibodies against retinal or uveal antigens are not usually tested.

Historical development

In 1976, Sawyer et al[9] first described PR as the progressive loss of vision with ring scotomas and nearly absent ERG in 3 women with SCCL. Interestingly, visual symptoms preceded the cancer diagnosis, leading them to postulate that

Box 76.3 Autoimmune retinopathy

Patients can have symptoms resembling cancer- or melanoma-associated retinopathy and antiretinal autoantibodies, but without diagnosed tumor

Box 76.4 Diagnostic autoantibodies

Various antiretinal autoantibodies can be found in sera from patients with paraneoplastic retinopathies; thus, the absence of autoantibodies against recoverin (23 kDa) does not exclude a paraneoplastic retinopathy diagnosis

Table 76.3 Clinical criteria for paraneoplastic retinopathy

1. Unexplained, painless, and progressive retinal dysfunction
2. Abnormal electroretinogram
3. Patients may have the following clinical symptoms (these symptoms may be restricted or multifocal):
   a. Photopsia
   b. Blurred vision
   c. Progressive worsening of visual acuity and visual fields
   d. Ring scotomas
4. Suspected or diagnosed cancer
5. Exclusion criteria
   a. No known genetic (familial) causes
   b. No ocular infection
   c. No ocular trauma
   d. No intraocular surgery (other than cataract surgery)
   e. No drug toxicity
   f. No retinal detachment
   g. No typical age-related macular degeneration
   h. No active ocular inflammation

Table 76.4 Enolase in disease

1. Autoantibodies against α-enolase reported in inflammatory, degenerative, and psychiatric disorders
2. Anti-α-enolase antibodies associated with systemic and invasive autoimmune disorders
3. High incidence of autoantibodies in autoimmune diseases:
   a. Cancer-associated retinopathy (68.8%, 11 of 16)
   b. Polyglandular syndrome type 1 (80%, 35 of 44)
   c. Primary (69%, 60 of 87) and secondary (58%, 14 of 24) membranous nephropathy
   d. Autoimmune hepatitis type 1 (60%, 12 of 20)
   e. Mixed cryoglobulinemia with renal involvement (63.6%, 7 of 11)
   f. Cystoid macular edema (60%, 6 of 10)
   g. Endometriosis (50%, 21 of 41)
   h. Rheumatoid arthritis (25%, 36 of 145)
4. Healthy subjects have autoantibodies ranging from 0% (0 of 91) to 11.7% (7 of 60)

photoreceptor degeneration was caused by remote effects from the cancer. In later years, circulating antibodies against retinal proteins were reported in sera from cancer patients with visual problems, suggesting that antiretinal autoantibodies may play a role in PR pathogenicity.[10,11] Immunostaining of the outer retina with CAR antibodies further supported the autoimmune nature of the syndrome, as did beneficial effects of steroids on vision. The hypothesis was that vision loss was due to serum autoantibodies, originating from the immune response against tumor antigens and cross-reacting with retinal proteins, which led to rod and cone dysfunction. The syndrome was named "cancer-associated retinopathy," and the associated 23-kDa reactive protein was called "the CAR antigen."[11] The CAR antigen has since been sequenced and identified as "recoverin."[12-14] However, 50% of symptomatic patients have high titers of autoantibodies against proteins other than recoverin (Table 76.2).[1] Therefore, the absence of antibodies to recoverin does not exclude a diagnosis of PR (Box 76.4).

Epidemiology

PRs are rare. It is estimated that paraneoplastic diseases occur in fewer than 1% of cancer patients.[15] Although more PR cases have been reported in recent years and the number is growing, the incidence of CAR and MAR remains unknown. Moreover, most patients with cancers, including melanoma, may not consider their vision symptoms due to their malignancy, and consequently, they do not report vision problems. The average age of a CAR patient is 63 years, with women affected more than men at a ratio of 2 : 1.[1] At an average age of 57.5 years, males with melanoma appear to have a higher risk of developing MAR than women, even though cutaneous malignant melanoma affects men and women equally.[4,16] AR affects twice as many women as men, at an average age of 55. BDUMP is very rare and also affects more women than men, at a ratio of 2 at an average of 63 years.[8] Thus far, there is no known genetic involvement in CAR and MAR development.

Diagnostic workup

Diagnosis of PRs is difficult (Table 76.3), and patients are frequently misdiagnosed. Ocular symptoms may develop

Box 76.5 Diagnostic criteria

Based on clinical presentation and findings, and on the presence or absence of antibodies and cancer, patients can be classified as having a paraneoplastic retinopathy or autoimmune retinopathy (= possible paraneoplastic retinopathy)

before diagnosis of cancer, and CAR and MAR can occur in patients without tumors (Table 76.1). About 50% of patients have retinopathy symptoms as the first manifestation.[17] Nearly 50% of symptomatic patients initially have negative antibody tests, and few of the seropositive patients have antirecoverin antibodies.[1] Importantly, the presence of antirecoverin autoantibodies indicates a high likelihood of associated neoplasm, particularly SCCL and gynecological cancers in women (Box 76.5). Anti-α-enolase CAR occurs predominantly with cancers with endocrine features, and visual symptoms typically develop months to years after discovery of the malignancy. Antienolase autoantibodies have also been reported in a diverse range of inflammatory, degenerative, and psychiatric disorders (Table 76.4), and in

~10% of normal subjects (0–11%).[18,19] The production of MAR autoantibodies has rarely been linked to the remission or stabilization of melanoma, indicating that an antibody response is usually insufficient to protect against spreading. If ophthalmologic findings, including ERG and antibodies, are indicative of CAR and MAR, a cancer workup is recommended. A worsening of symptoms may precede a recurrence or metastasis.

Treatment

There is no established protocol for PR treatment. Without treatment, antirecoverin CAR almost always progresses rapidly to severe vision loss, often to no light perception. Management of CAR is generally ineffective, although some patients benefit from systemic corticosteroids, plasmapheresis, or intravenous immunoglobulins (IVIg).[20–22] Recently, a beneficial effect from alemtuzumab (anti-CD52 monoclonal antibody) has been reported.[23] In MAR patients, prednisone seems not to improve ocular symptoms, and plasmapheresis reduces antibody titer without improving vision.[4] Clinical trials evaluating the benefits of IVIg therapy, alone or with corticosteroids, are needed to manage PRs and AR better.

Prognosis and complications

Prognosis depends on the type of serum autoantibodies present, the underlying tumor, and its stage of development. Patients with antirecoverin antibodies have the worst prognosis because their disease is typically progressive and advances to complete loss of vision. However, there are patients with antirecoverin autoantibodies whose retinal degeneration follows a slow course. Unlike antirecoverin CAR, which often precedes a cancer diagnosis by months to over a year, PR associated with anti-α-enolase autoantibodies usually develops months to years after the discovery of the malignancy and accompanies a slower vision loss with bouts of stable vision.[3] MAR patients have the worst survival prognosis[24] because MAR presents after the melanoma is diagnosed, often at the metastatic stage.

Pathology

In histopathological studies of CAR, postmortem eyes revealed extensive rod and cone degeneration.[10,25,26] The striking disappearance of photoreceptor cells and of the outer nuclear layer (ONL) in the retina was evident, but the inner retina was preserved (Figure 76.2). No or very low inflammation in the uvea, retina, and vitreous was found, suggesting a noninflammatory aspect to retinal degeneration. The molecular mechanism by which cell loss occurs in the retina will be described later in this chapter. Histopathological examination of postmortem MAR eyes showed a marked reduction in the density of bipolar neurons in the inner nuclear layer (INL), but photoreceptor cell neurons in the ONL were normal. Retinal ganglion cells were present, although many showed evidence of transsynaptic atrophy. These histopathological changes were consistent with clinical, immunologic, and electrophysiologic findings that implicate photoreceptor or bipolar cells as the site of the paraneoplastic process in PRs.[27]

Etiology

PR etiology and the source of antigenic stimulation are largely unknown. The first cases of CAR were associated with SCCL. Since recoverin is a photoreceptor-specific, calcium-binding protein, there was a question as to whether autoantibodies that bind to the photoreceptor recoverin bind to a "cross-reactive antigen" in tumor tissue. Indeed, unaltered recoverin was expressed in malignant cells of SCCL in a CAR patient who had circulating antirecoverin autoantibodies.[28] This study strongly implicated an immune mechanism initiated by antitumor recoverin responses in a subset of patients.[29] Recoverin is expressed in ~70% of lung cancer tissue, not only in tumors of CAR patients but also in tumors of patients without ocular symptoms.[30–32] Serum autoantibodies were present in 20% of lung cancer patients, and CAR occurred in only 1% of these patients, suggesting that recoverin expression is not strongly coupled with cancer cell differentiation.[29] Recoverin can be found in tumors during neoplastic development, and this might be related to the

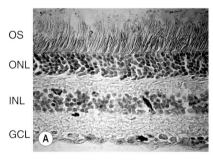
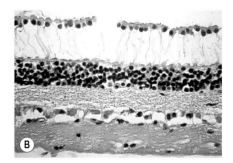
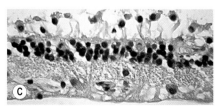

OS
ONL
INL
GCL

(A)   (B)   (C)

Normal Retina   CAR Retina

Figure 76.2 Pathology of cancer-associated retinopathy (CAR). Photograph of a retina from a CAR patient with small cell carcinoma of the lung, showing loss of the photoreceptor cell layer in comparison to the normal retina. OS, outer segments; ONL, outer nuclear layer; INL, inner nuclear layer; GCL, ganglion cell layer.

location of the recoverin gene at chromosome 17p13.1, in proximity to the tumor suppressor gene p53.[33] A single mutation may activate the recoverin gene and deactivate the p53 gene, in effect causing the aberrant expression of recoverin in tumor cells. During tumor turnover, the immune system could elicit antirecoverin immune responses. Thus, autoantibodies originating against tumor recoverin may cross-react with the photoreceptor recoverin, causing immune-mediated photoreceptor degeneration. Identification of immunogenic, tumor-associated molecules is not only a crucial step in understanding molecular mechanisms of CAR, but also in understanding the role of these molecules in clinical diagnosis or therapy.

α-Enolase is a common autoantigen found in the retina and in malignant cells in lung cancer.[34] Autoantibodies against α-enolase have been found in 13.8–65% of patients with different subtypes of lung cancer. Such a high enolase overexpression and high autoantibody levels usually correlate with a poor prognosis.[34,35] Moreover, the triggering of distinct immune responses by tumor antigens emerging during the course of disease has been observed in a CAR patient.[36] Initially, the serum showed antiretinal 35-kDa autoantibodies before SCCL surgery, antiretinal 35-kDa and 46-kDa (α-enolase) autoantibodies 1 week after surgery, and only antienolase 1 month after surgery. These findings suggest "epitope spreading," which refers to the development of an immune response to epitopes, distinct from and noncross-reactive with the initial disease-causing epitope.[37] Epitope spreading enhances the heterogeneity and pathogenicity of CAR antibodies and can only be discovered in follow-up examination.

Antibipolar cell autoantibodies were originally demonstrated in MAR,[7] but an autoantigen in the bipolar cell was not identified. In addition, MAR autoantibodies against photoreceptor proteins were detected in a subset of melanoma patients (Table 76.2). Photoreceptor proteins – such as rhodopsin, transducin, cGMP-phosphodiesterase 6, cGMP-dependent channels, guanylyl cyclase, rhodopsin kinase, recoverin, and arrestin – can be expressed in melanoma cells, which can potentially induce autoantibody responses in melanoma patients, leading to an immune attack on the retina.[38] Taken together, these findings provide a sound foundation for immunological mechanisms of PRs (Box 76.6).

Pathophysiology

In the last several years, studies of PR pathological mechanisms have been undertaken by several groups. Based on clinical presentation, presence of autoantibodies and extraocular tumors, a possible mechanism causing retinal degeneration has been proposed, in which serum autoantibodies against recoverin and other retinal antigens play a

central role in pathogenicity. The molecular pathology of CAR caused by autoantibody occurs in two steps (Figure 76.3): (1) antitumor response, involving an immune response that is elicited against aberrantly expressed antigens in tumor, during which the autoantibodies, when they reach high titers, gain access to the retina through the blood–retina barrier; and (2) antiretinal response, involving autoantibodies penetrating retinal layers and being taken up into target cells, where they block the target antigen metabolic function, which in effect induces apoptosis and cell death. Because recoverin and α-enolase have been initially linked to CAR,

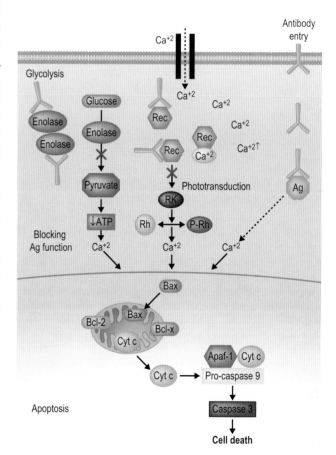

Figure 76.3 Illustration depicting molecular aspects of apoptosis in retinal cells induced by autoantibodies. Antibody entry is necessary to start the apoptotic process in retinal cells. After antirecoverin and anti-α-enolase antibodies translocate to the cytoplasm by endocytosis, they bind to the appropriate autoantigen in the cytoplasm and block the target antigen metabolic function, in effect leading to an increase in intracellular Ca²⁺. Blocking of the α-enolase function decreases glycolytic adenosine triphosphate (ATP) production and increases intracellular Ca²⁺. Antirecoverin antibodies inhibit recoverin function, which leads to higher levels of rhodopsin phosphorylation and the continuous opening of cGMP-gated channels, resulting in the accumulation of intracellular Ca²⁺ within cells. Blocking of other antigen (Ag) function may also lead to intracellular Ca²⁺. The rise in Ca²⁺ induces an increase in proapoptotic Bcl-x$_s$ and Bax proteins and a decrease in antiapoptotic Bcl-x$_L$ and Bcl-2, which is followed by the release of cytochrome c from the mitochondria and the downregulation of apaf-1. Cytochrome c initiates apoptosis by inducing formation of the caspase 9–apaf-1 complex. All of these events correlate with the sequential activation of caspase 9 and caspase 3, as well as the degradation of the caspase substrate poly (ADP-ribose) polymerase (PARP) and the fragmentation of DNA, a hallmark of apoptosis.

Box 76.6 Cancer and retinopathy

Paraneoplastic retinopathies are autoimmune-mediated disorders triggered by aberrant expression of retinal antigens in distant tumors

Table 76.5 Recoverin as an autoantigen

1. A 23-kDa calcium-binding protein
2. Present in the cytoplasm of photoreceptor and bipolar cells of the retina
3. Regulates (inhibits) rhodopsin phosphorylation in a calcium-dependent manner
4. Also found in various tumors (cancer-associated retinopathy (CAR) and ~50% non-CAR tumors)
5. Regulates cell proliferations of the tumors (?)
6. A potent antigen and pathogen
7. Induces experimental uveitis in rats
8. The sequence 64–70 in proximity of the first calcium-binding motif EF-hand 2 is highly antigenic and pathogenic

Table 76.6 Enolase – multifunctional protein

1. A 46-kDa protein
2. Has glycolytic (metabolic sensor) and nonglycolytic functions (transcriptional regulation)
3. Belongs to a novel class of surface proteins without classical machinery for surface transport
4. Forms three heterodimeric forms with tissue-specific distributions
   a. α-enolase, the embryonic form, all tissues (nonneuronal enolase)
   b. β-enolase is expressed in skeletal and cardiac muscle
   c. γ-enolase in nervous tissue (neuronal-specific enolase)
5. Has multiple locations in the cell (cytosolic, membrane, nuclear)
6. Has 100% homology with myc promoter-binding protein (MBP-1)
7. Serves as a plasminogen receptor on the surface of a variety of hematopoetic, epithelial, and endothelial cells
8. Stimulates immunoglobulin production
9. Functions as a heat shock protein
10. Binds cytoskeletal and chromatin structures

most mechanistic studies have focused on them.[39–41] Below we discuss in vitro and in vivo evidence underlying the molecular mechanism of retinal degeneration associated with autoantibodies against recoverin and α-enolase.

Recoverin

Recoverin is a 23-kDa, calcium-binding protein present mostly in photoreceptor cells: it regulates rhodopsin phosphorylation in visual transduction (Table 76.5). Recoverin is highly immunogenic and pathogenic. Two linear stretches of amino acids within the human recoverin sequence form the major epitopes for autoantibodies: residues 48–52 (QFQSI) and residues 64–70 (KAYAQHV) in proximity to the calcium-binding domain EF-hand 2.[42] The binding of autoantibodies has been found to be dependent on recoverin calcium-binding properties since conformational changes induced by the bound calcium enhance antibody binding. Moreover, the sequence 64–70 has been found to be a major pathogenic site, causing intraocular inflammation and the degeneration of photoreceptor cells in Lewis rats immunized with recoverin or its peptides.[28,43] In addition, this immunogenic sequence induces peptide-specific Th and cytotoxic T-lymphocyte responses.[28,44]

α-Enolase

Enolase plays a role in glycolysis (Table 76.6). About 40% of retinopathy patients have anti-α-enolase autoantibodies, and half of seropositive patients are cancer survivors.[1,18] Anti-α-enolase autoantibodies can also be found in a number of inflammatory, degenerative, and neurologic diseases, and in healthy subjects (Table 76.4).[45] Because of such a wide prevalence of antienolase autoantibodies, fine epitope maps were studied in human α-enolase to determine their role in pathogenicity. Epitope mapping revealed three epitopes within the residues 31–38 (FRAAVPSG), 176–183 (ANFREAMR), and 421–428 (AKFAGRNF) for all CAR autoantibodies tested.[46] However, 70% of CAR patients, particularly those with breast or bladder cancer, recognized a unique epitope sequence 56–63 (RYMGKGVS).[47] The epitope sequences are located in proximity to external loops of the enolase molecule: loop 1: 37–43, the catalytic site; loop 2: 153–166; and loop 3: 251–276, the plasminogen-binding site.[45] Depending on specificity, anti-α-enolase autoantibod-

ies may label several layers and cell types within the retina, whereas antirecoverin autoantibodies bind exclusively to rods and cones and to some bipolar cells (Figure 76.2).

Apoptosis of retinal cells

Antiretinal autoantibodies, including recoverin, are cytotoxic to E1A.NR3 retinal cells.[48] When living cells are grown with these antibodies, destruction of these cells in a dose- and time-dependent manner occurs only in cells expressing the autoantigen.[48] Antirecoverin IgG, as well as its Fab fragments, penetrates retinal cells by an active process of endocytosis.[39] This antibody-mediated destruction of retinal cells is independent of complement and IgG from normal subjects is not cytotoxic. Importantly, the antibodies induce morphological changes in cells that are characteristic of apoptosis. Moreover, antibodies injected intravenously into Lewis rats penetrated the blood–ocular barrier, reached the retina, and caused the death of some photoreceptors.[40] Direct intravitreal injection of antirecoverin autoantibodies into the vitreous of rat eyes caused apoptotic cell death within the outer and bipolar cell layers, as evidenced by DNA fragmentation, nuclear chromatin condensation, and increased vacuolization of photoreceptor outer segments.[49] Rats receiving antirecoverin antibodies lost 25–30% of nuclei in the ONL and INL, whereas all controls had unchanged numbers of nuclei. Antibodies against α-enolase that specifically labeled the ganglion cell layer and INL, when injected into the vitreous, penetrated these target layers and, consequently, cell death was induced through an apoptotic process.[50] The apoptotic nuclei detected by a DNA fragmentation assay and caspase 3-positive cells were co-localized in these layers. Additional studies showed that when antirecoverin and anti-α-enolase antibodies translocated to the cytoplasm, they induced an increase in proapoptotic Bcl-x$_S$ and Bax proteins, and decreased antiapoptotic Bcl-x$_L$ which was followed by the release of cytochrome c from mitochondria and the downregulation of apaf-1.[39,51] These events correlated with the sequential activation of caspase 9 and caspase 3, as well as the degradation of the

Box 76.7 Apoptosis

Antiretinal autoantibodies are inducers of apoptosis in retinal cells through the mitochondrial pathway involving caspases 9 and 3

Box 76.8 Calcium and retinopathy

An increase in intracellular free Ca^{2+} may constitute a common mechanism in photoreceptor cell death induced by different antiretinal autoantibodies

caspase substrate poly (ADP-ribose) polymerase (PARP) and the fragmentation of DNA, a hallmark of apoptosis (Box 76.7).[39] Thus, autoantibodies are inducers of apoptosis through the mitochondrial pathway involving caspases 9 and 3 (Figure 76.3).

Once antirecoverin antibodies access rod photoreceptor cells, they block recoverin function, which leads to an increase in intracellular free Ca^{2+}.[52] This increase and the inhibition of rhodopsin phosphorylation activate caspase-dependent apoptotic pathways.[41,53] In vivo studies showed that Ca^{2+}-dependent suppression of rhodopsin phosphorylation was abolished, and the level of rhodopsin phosphorylation was significantly enhanced in the presence of antirecoverin IgG, but not in the presence of normal IgG.[41] These effects likely occur from the inhibition of recoverin function, leading to higher levels of rhodopsin phosphorylation and continuous opening of cGMP-gated channels, in turn resulting in an accumulation of intracellular Ca^{2+} within photoreceptor cells. Therefore, uncontrolled states of the phototransduction pathway and the rise in free Ca^{2+} by blocking the recoverin function with autoantibodies may be an important, mechanistic step in the degeneration of photoreceptor cells. Also, antienolase antibodies penetrate retinal cells and cause apoptosis through the inhibition of the enolase catalytic function, resulting in the depletion of glycolytic adenosine triphosphate and leading to an increase in intracellular Ca^{2+}.[50,51] L-type voltage-gated Ca^{2+} channel blockers (nifedipine, d-cis-diltiazem, and verapamil) are effective in blocking the antibody-induced intracellular Ca^{2+} rise and in suppressing proapoptotic Bax. Thus, chronic access of autoantibodies to the retina may result in inhibition of the antigen function and elevation of intracellular

Ca^{2+}, leading to the activation of apoptosis pathways and subsequent cell death.[51] Since the increase in intracellular Ca^{2+} appears to be a key element in the induction of apoptosis, this increase likely constitutes a common mechanism in photoreceptor cell death that is induced by antiretinal autoantibodies (Box 76.8).

In MAR, evidence of autoantibody involvement in bipolar cell inactivation is supported by results obtained from injecting MAR autoantibodies into the vitreous of monkeys, resulting in a transient alteration of ERG patterns, similar to those of MAR.[54] The proposed mechanism involves an autoantibody response against yet-to-be-identified melanoma antigens that cross-react with specific antigens in the retina. This immunological reaction causes the depolarization of bipolar cells of rod and cone systems of the ON pathway.[7] Immunohistochemistry showed positive staining of the outer plexiform and nerve fiber layers, but the significance of such reactivity in pathogenesis was not explained.[4] Also, the aberrant expression of MAR antigens in melanoma may underlie a similar mechanism, as in CAR. The heterogeneity in autoantibody specificity may explain the variation and complexity of clinical symptoms in retinopathy patients.

Acknowledgments

This study was supported by a grant EY13053 from the National Institutes of Health, by an unrestricted grant to the OHSU Casey Eye Institute from Research to Prevent Blindness, New York, NY, and by the Foundation Fighting Blindness.

Key references

A complete list of chapter references is available online at www.expertconsult.com. See inside cover for registration details.

1. Adamus G, Ren G, Weleber RG. Autoantibodies against retinal proteins in paraneoplastic and autoimmune retinopathy. BMC Ophthalmol 2004;4:5.

2. Jacobson DM, Thirkill CE, Tipping SJ. A clinical triad to diagnose paraneoplastic retinopathy. Ann Neurol 1990;28:162–167.

3. Weleber RG, Watzke RC, Shults WT, et al. Clinical and electrophysiologic characterization of paraneoplastic and autoimmune retinopathies associated with antienolase antibodies. Am J Ophthalmol 2005;139:780–794.

4. Keltner JL, Thirkill CE, Yip PT. Clinical and immunologic characteristics of melanoma-associated retinopathy syndrome: eleven new cases and a review of 51 previously published cases. J Neuroophthalmol 2001;21:173–187.

7. Milam AH, Saari JC, Jacobson SG, et al. Autoantibodies against retinal bipolar cells in cutaneous melanoma-associated retinopathy. Invest Ophthalmol Vis Sci 1993;34:91–100.

38. Bazhin AV, Schadendorf D, Willner N, et al. Photoreceptor proteins as cancer-retina antigens. Int J Cancer 2007;120:1268–1276.

39. Shiraga S, Adamus G. Mechanism of CAR syndrome: anti-recoverin antibodies are the inducers of retinal cell apoptotic death via the caspase 9- and caspase 3-dependent pathway. J Neuroimmunol 2002;132:72–82.

41. Maeda T, Maeda A, Maruyama I, et al. Mechanisms of photoreceptor cell death in cancer-associated retinopathy. Invest Ophthalmol Vis Sci 2001;42:705–712.

49. Adamus G, Machnicki M, Elerding H, et al. Antibodies to recoverin induce apoptosis of photoreceptor and bipolar cells in vivo. J Autoimmun 1998;11:523–533.

51. Magrys A, Anekonda T, Ren G, et al. The role of anti-alpha-enolase autoantibodies in pathogenicity of autoimmune-mediated retinopathy. J Clin Immunol 2007;27:181–192.

61. Ohguro H, Ogawa K, Nakagawa T. Recoverin and Hsc 70 are found as autoantigens in patients with cancer-associated retinopathy. Invest Ophthalmol Vis Sci 1999;40:82–89.

70. Adamus G. Autoantibody targets and their cancer relationship in the pathogenicity of paraneoplastic retinopathy. Autoimmun Rev 2009;8:410–414.

CHAPTER 77

Cellular repopulation of the retina

Budd AL Tucker, Michael J Young, and Henry J Klassen

Clinical background

Advances in the treatment of diseases involving the ocular anterior segment, particularly the lens and cornea, have greatly decreased the prevalence of visual impairment caused by dysfunction of these structures. Unfortunately, treatment of diseases impacting structures of the posterior segment, particularly the retina and optic nerve, have not advanced to the same extent and as a consequence these conditions are now the major source of incurable blindness in the developed world (Box 77.1). The reasons for this are not hard to discern in that both the retina and optic nerve are components of the central nervous system (CNS) and it has long been appreciated that the mammalian CNS exhibits a very restricted capacity for endogenous regeneration. Furthermore, what little capacity exists diminishes further with postnatal maturation. Additional barriers to the development of effective restorative treatments for the retina and its central projections are numerous and include the complex phenotypes of retinal cells, particularly photoreceptors and ganglion cells, as well as the need for an unusually precise cytoarchitecture. This is true both in terms of outer segment packing and the topographic organization of output fibers projecting to the visual centers of the brain.

As a consequence of the many challenges involved, there are at present no restorative treatments for retinal cell loss. This situation may change; however, a growing body of experimental data suggests that many of the barriers to retinal repair in mammals are not insurmountable. In particular, stem cell transplantation and tissue engineering have recently emerged as promising strategies for repopulating the cellular constituents of the retina.[1] Alternatively, it is conceivable that an electronic prosthesis could bypass the damaged components of the retina and convey visual information directly to downstream visual neurons, although this fascinating strategy will need to overcome difficulties faced when attempting to use artificial constructs to stimulate high-resolution visual acuity. For now, it appears that the most straightforward method of restoring retinal function resulting from cell loss is to replace those cells through transplantation.

Etiology

Work in animal models and limited studies in human subjects have shown that a number of different tissues and cell types can survive as allografts in the ocular posterior segment, in either the vitreous cavity or subretinal space.[2-11] The general facility of graft survival seen likely results in part from the degree of immune privilege afforded in these locations.[12-16] Vitreal delivery may be adequate for some applications and cell types; however, subretinal placement is preferable for restoration of photoreceptors and the retinal pigment epithelium (RPE), as is needed in retinitis pigmentosa (RP) and to varying extents in retinal detachment and age-related macular degeneration. In terms of relevant cell types for outer retinal repopulation, both photoreceptors[17] and RPE cells[18] survive transplantation beneath the retina; however, the reluctance of donor photoreceptors to make functional connections with the surviving host circuitry[19] and failure of donor RPE cells to reform a polarized monolayer on Bruch's membrane[20-22] have frustrated attempts to achieve functional repair of the outer retina using grafts of freshly isolated cells alone. Here we will focus on the challenges facing photoreceptor replacement and consider the advantages of using cultured allogeneic retinal progenitor cells (RPCs) as donor material.

To repopulate the outer nuclear layer with functional photoreceptors, there is a fundamental problem to overcome. This is the physical barrier to neurite outgrowth presented by hypertrophy of the outer limiting membrane (OLM) following photoreceptor loss. The OLM is not in fact a membrane per se but rather is an emergent structural element formed by the joined outer ends of retinal Müller cells. In the setting of photoreceptor degeneration, the OLM undergoes thickening in association with upregulation of the markers neurocan and CD44. Regenerating neurites originating from either above or below have great difficulty crossing this barrier.[23] In fact, the phenomena of glial hypertrophy and scar formation are common in the setting of CNS disease and injury and have frequently been implicated in the failure of endogenous regenerative mechanisms to bridge a lesion.[24]

Box 77.1 Impact of retinal degenerative disease

- Degenerative diseases impacting structures of the posterior segment of the eye, particularly the retina and optic nerve, are currently the major source of incurable blindness in the developed world
- There is an urgent need to reconstruct, via cellular replacement, the damaged or lost layers of the retina

Box 77.2 Strategies for retinal transplantation

- Two promising approaches for targeted repopulation of the retina following injury/disease include transplantation of stem/progenitor cells and transplantation of intact retinal sheets

We have shown that grafted CNS progenitor cells are not impeded by a hypertrophied OLM and can migrate across this barrier in large numbers.[10,11] The ability to migrate into the mature, diseased retina is one remarkable characteristic of CNS progenitor cells that recommends them as a potential tool for use in retinal repopulation. Moreover, these cells not only migrate into the retina, but also exhibit widespread integration into the local cytoarchitecture, with tropism for regions of injury or disease. In the case of RPCs, there is also the potential to differentiate into cells with morphological features and marker expression characteristic of photoreceptors.

Retinal transplantation

To achieve functional repair in patients afflicted with retinal degenerative disorders, there is an urgent need to reconstruct, via cellular replacement, the damaged or lost layers of the retina. While restorative repair of the retina is a daunting challenge, a range of data suggests that such a goal is now feasible. Two approaches for targeted repopulation of the retina are considered below and include stem/progenitor cell transplantation and retinal sheet transplantation, both of which pose a variety of advantages and disadvantages (Box 77.2).

Stem/progenitor cell transplantation

Over the past decade, stem/progenitor cell transplantation as a means of inducing tissue reconstruction and functional regeneration has garnered extensive interest in the field of regenerative medicine. Within the retina in particular, many exciting advances have been made. One significant achievement came in 2004 when we were able to show that a subset of transplanted RPCs developed into a variety of mature retinal neurons, including retinal ganglion and photoreceptor cells.[10] Since then, numerous studies reporting varying degrees of success have utilized an assortment of different cell types ranging from the fate-restricted photoreceptor precursor to the pluripotent embryonic stem (ES) cell.[25–28] ES cells are of particular interest due to their ability to undergo unlimited expansion and subsequent tissue-specific differentiation. These inherent properties may allow one to generate

a sufficiently large number of cells in order to perform clinical transplantation from single isolations rather than requiring multiple new donations, as is potentially the problem when using more terminally differentiated cell types. However, as cited above, these cells are pluripotent, meaning they can be induced to generate cell types for each of the three germ layers and as such, are not retina-specific. Thus, protocols for retina/cell type-specific differentiation are required. In light of this, many labs have been aggressively searching for the proper method of retinal cell induction. One of the first published reports of RPC, and subsequent retinal cell generation, from human ES cells came from Lamba and colleues in 2006.[27] In this publication, the group was able to show that they could reliably produce healthy functioning photoreceptors, albeit at low levels, using a relatively simple induction protocol.[27] Since then, similar studies using variations of Reh's methods have reported an increased generation of retina-specific cell types, photoreceptor cells in particular, in a range of organisms including primate and human.[25]

Retinal sheet transplantation

Like stem cells, retinal sheets, including full-thickness and photoreceptor only, have also been used in an attempt to achieve retinal reconstruction and visual restoration following injury and disease. The goal of these techniques is to deliver retinal tissue with proper laminar structure and cellular organization directly to the site of injury in an attempt to form new functional connections between remaining host tissue and healthy donor material. Although extensive connections and subsequent visual restoration have not yet been achieved by using this technique, significant progress, particularly when using developing tissue, has been made.[2,29–34] For instance, when embryonic rat retina was transplanted into the subretinal space of degenerating animals, the tissue was shown to survive without immune rejection, develop normally, continue to respond to light for up to 3 months after transplantation, and form limited functional connections with the host.[31] Apart from functional integration, similar results have also been reported in a pig model of RP. For example, Ghosh et al[35] have shown that transplanted retinal tissue isolated from healthy fetal donors can survive and maintain proper laminar structure and cellular organization within the subretinal space of the host for up 6 months post-transplantation. However, an issue that remains when using full-thickness retinal grafts is the introduction of redundancy into the system. For instance, in diseases such as RP where there is a progressive loss of photoreceptor cells with sparing of the inner retinal circuitry (albeit temporarily), full-thickness transplants would result in replication of a majority of the retinal cell types. Thus, in a situation such as this, transplantation and subsequent integration of photoreceptor sheets, void of all other retinal structures, would be beneficial. Although extensive research has yet to be carried out using this approach, studies with promising findings have been reported. For instance, as with full-thickness retinal grafts, transplantation of photoreceptor sheets has enjoyed prolonged survival and structural preservation.[36,37]

As promising as the abovementioned studies may be, issues such as inadequate cellular/axonal integration following stem/progenitor cell and retinal sheet transplantation remain. Modest functional integration may be accounted for by a variety of factors, including the lack of cellular support and survival following bolus stem cell injection, and inadequate growth responses of retinal tissue transplantation. Most important, however, is the presence of a postinjury inhibitory extracellular CNS environment.

Pathophysiology

Glial scar formation

Unlike the peripheral nervous system (PNS), the regenerative capacity of the CNS following injury is extremely limited. Amongst other reasons, the paucity of regeneration can be attributed to the presence of an inhospitable extracellular environment (Box 77.3). Unlike the PNS, the CNS is plagued by an abundance of myelin-associated extracellular matrix (ECM) proteins such as myelin-associated glycoprotein (MAG), Nogo, and Omgp that are well known for their ability to inhibit axonal extension and cellular migration.[38–40] For instance, in 1988, Caroni and Schwab identified the first of these myelin-associated molecules, later termed Nogo, as being a potent inhibitor of fibroblast cell migration and neurite extension.[38]

The abovementioned ECM molecules typically exert their action by binding a common complex of cell surface receptors, in the case of Nogo consisting of the Nogo receptor (NgR) in conjunction with p75 (low-affinity neurotrophin receptor), Lingo, and TROY. Collectively, the binding of these molecules stimulates an inhibitory intracellular signaling cascade which utilizes the small GTPase-dependent enzyme RhoA.[41–45] Activation of RhoA and its downstream effectors ultimately stimulates growth cone collapse, axon retraction, and cellular repulsion by negative regulation of the actin cytoskeleton.[46–49] Thus, chemical and/or enzymatic inhibition/neutralization of these ECM molecules or their downstream targets has been shown to alleviate inhibitory myelin-associated growth inhibition in a variety of CNS compartments, including the optic nerve. For instance, in the absence of Nogo-induced RhoA activation, by using either AAV-induced dominant negative NgR expression or NgR-null mice, significantly enhanced retinal ganglion cell axon extension was observed.[50,51] Similarly, animals vaccinated with spinal cord homogenates rich in myelin-associated proteins could extend axons significantly further than control animals following optic nerve injury.[52] Likewise, when serum from vaccinated animals was used to treat purified cultures of retinal ganglion cells in vitro, it was found that MAG-induced growth cone collapse and axon retraction were alleviated.[52] In light of these findings, regen-

eration of the retinal ganglion cell layer following injury could potentially benefit from negative regulation of the aforementioned molecules.

As initially suggested, retinal degenerative diseases such as age-related macular degeneration and RP predominantly affect the photoreceptor layer of the retina which, unlike most other CNS tissues, is void of myelin and the associated oligodendrocytes. Thus, the environmental inhibitors mentioned above which impede ganglion cell and optic nerve regeneration are not a factor. Why then are attempts at stimulating retinal regeneration via photoreceptor or stem cell transplantation still largely unsuccessful? The lack of functional integration following transplantation is in large part due to the presence of injury-induced glial scar formation. The retina, like other nervous system compartments, undergoes a process known as reactive gliosis. This is an injury-initiated event that involves the infiltration of a variety of cell types, with the most prominent being activated astroglia. Activation, a process that results in the upregulation of the intermediate filament proteins glial fibrillary acidic protein and vimentin, is crucial for glial scar formation.[53]

In the retina, the major glial cell type responsible for reactive scarring following disease-induced retinal degeneration is the Müller glial cell. During retinal reactive gliosis, hypertrophic Müller glia undergo the activation and upregulation of the above-mentioned intermediate filament proteins (Figure 77.1A), after which they respond by extending projections from their original location (forming the OLM) into the subretinal space.[54,55] Here, these projections proceed to form a dense fibrotic barrier that contains a variety of growth-inhibitory extracellular matrix/adhesion molecules, including the chondroitin sulfate proteoglycan (CSPG) Neurocan and the hyaluronan-binding glycoprotein CD44 (Figure 77.1B and C). Both Neurocan and CD44 have previously been shown to function as chemical inhibitors to axon growth and cellular migration, thus preventing regeneration and functional synapse formation.[1,56–61] For instance, we have previously shown that an abundance of these molecules, deposited by reactive glial cells at the outer limits of the degenerative mouse retina, prevent neurite extension and subsequent integration following retinal transplantation (Box 77.4).[1]

Although the exact cell surface receptors for these inhibitory glial scar-related proteins are not well characterized (as with the myelin inhibitors), their actions are exerted via activation of the RhoA signaling pathway.[62–64] Thus, RhoA inhibition or the removal of the inhibitory glial scar-related proteins could potentially act to enhance axonal extension and cellular migration following retinal transplantation. A variety of approaches have been taken in an attempt to remove these inhibitory ECM molecules, including enzymatic degradation of the proteins themselves. Two enzymes that have been utilized for such a purpose are chondroitinase ABC and the matrix metalloproteinase MMP2. Chondroitinase ABC, which takes advantage of the native structure of CSPGs by cleaving the glycosaminoglycan (GAG) side chains from the CSPG protein core, has been shown to enhance the integration of grafted Müller stem cells into the degenerating retina following transplantation.[65] A drawback when using chondroitinase is that it only reduces CSPG activity related with GAG side chain removal. Thus, the remaining inhibitory core proteins, such as that of Neuro-

---

Box 77.3 The inhibitory CNS extracellular environment

- The inability of the injured central nervous system to regenerate can in part be attributed to the presence of an inhospitable extracellular environment, predominated by the presence of inhibitory glial scar/myelin-related extracellular matrix proteins that prevent axon extension and transplant integration

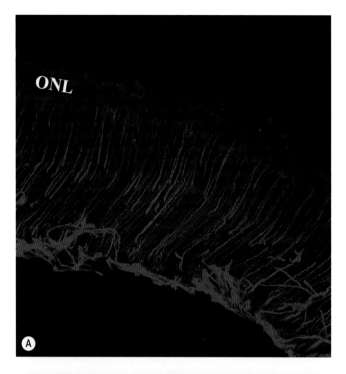

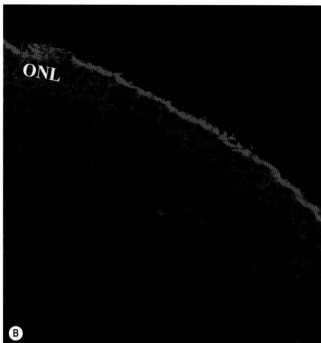

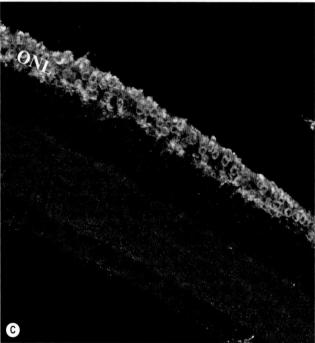

Figure 77.1　Injury-induced Müller cell activation stimulates inhibitory extracellular matrix molecule deposition and glial barrier formation. Eyes from adult retinal degenerative mice (Rho-/-) were enucleated, fixed, cryoprotected, sectioned, and immunostained for glial fibrillary acidic protein, CD44, Neurocan, and recoverin. (A) Representative micrographs illustrating CD44 (blue) and GFAP (red) expression in the adult degenerative Rho-/- mouse retina. Activated Müller cells extend processes through the degenerating photoreceptor layer (outer nuclear layer) into the subretinal space and deposit CD44 at the outer limits of the retina. (B) Representative micrographs illustrating CD44 (red) and Neurocan (blue) expression in the adult Rho-/- mouse retina. Inhibitory glial barrier-associated proteins, CD44, and Neurocan, deposited at the outer limits of the degenerating retina. (C) Representative micrograph illustrating CD44 (red), Neurocan (blue), and Recoverin (green) expression in the adult Rho-/- mouse retina. Inhibitory CD44 and Neurocan molecules are intertwined within the degenerating photoreceptor layer, preventing cellular/axonal integration following subretinal transplantation.

Box 77.4　Injury-induced glial cell reaction

- Retinal injury/degeneration stimulates reactive gliosis, a process characterized by Muller glia hypertrophy, increased intermediate filament expression, and process extension
- Reactive gliosis leads to the formation of a dense fibrotic barrier at the outer part of the injured/degenerating retina that contains, amongst other things, the growth-inhibitory extracellular matrix/adhesion molecules Neurocan and CD44

can, can still function to inhibit axonal regeneration and cellular migration.[66] Similarly, chondroitinase functions on the CSPG family of proteins only and therefore the inhibitory CD44 component of the glial barrier would remain even after chondroitinase treatment. MMPs, unlike chondroitinases, do not confer their function via GAG side-chain removal and, as such, are not restricted to CSPG degradation. Rather, this family of molecules are well known for their ability to degrade a variety of ECM and cell adhesion proteins, including CD44, the CSPGs and the aforemen-

Box 77.5 Combating inhibitory ECM molecules

- Matrix metalloproteinase 2 (MMP2) has the ability to degrade the inhibitory glial barrier-associated proteins CD44 and Neurocan, thus abrogating their inhibitory influence on the scarred retina. This in turn allows for integration and synapse formation following transplantation

tioned myelin-associated inhibitors.[67–69] MMP2 in particular has been shown to cleave both CD44 and Neurocan, thus releasing their negative hold on axonal extension and cellular migration.[1,70–73] For instance, in a recent study, we discovered that endogenous MMP2 induction resulted in glial barrier-associated CD44 and Neurocan degradation at the outer limits of heavily scarred degenerating retina, subsequently stimulating integration and synapse formation between the host and healthy transplanted tissue grafts.[1] Conversely, chemical and/or genetic inhibition/removal of MMP2 was shown to abolish cellular migration and axonal extension completely in this model (Box 77.5).[1,72] As a result, there now exists a strategy of removing inhibitory

barriers in the degenerated retina, permitting the establishment of new connections from retinal transplants, be they of stem cell origin, sheets of retinal tissue, or other yet-to-be-developed techniques.

Conclusions

Here we have described several approaches to repopulating the mature, diseased retina with new cells. The goal of all of these studies is the functional reconstruction of the CNS, restoring sight to the blinded eye. At present, this remains a dream. It is, however, a dream shared by many talented scientists and clinicians, not to mention millions of patients and their families throughout the world. Difficult challenges such as these must be solved one step at a time. It is heartening to realize that we have made tremendous progress in the last 10 years in this field. While much remains to be done, we are now on the brink of achieving significant restoration of function in large-animal models of retinal degeneration. Although the precise pathway to clinical application is not yet clear, the present rate of progress bodes well for the ultimate success of retinal repopulation.

Key references

A complete list of chapter references is available online at www.expertconsult.com. See inside cover for registration details.

1. Zhang Y, Klassen HJ, Tucker BA, et al. CNS progenitor cells promote a permissive environment for neurite outgrowth via a matrix metalloproteinase-2-dependent mechanism. J Neurosci 2007;27:4499–4506.

4. Klassen H, Kiilgaard JF, Zahir T, et al. Progenitor cells from the porcine neural retina express photoreceptor markers after transplantation to the subretinal space of allorecipients. Stem Cells 2007;25:1222–1230.

7. Tao S, Young C, Redenti S, et al. Survival, migration and differentiation of retinal progenitor cells transplanted on micro-machined poly(methyl methacrylate) scaffolds to the subretinal space. Lab Chip 2007;7:695–701.

8. Tomita M, Lavik E, Klassen H, et al. Biodegradable polymer composite grafts promote the survival and differentiation of retinal progenitor cells. Stem Cells 2005;23:1579–1588.

10. Klassen HJ, Ng TF, Kurimoto Y, et al. Multipotent retinal progenitors express developmental markers, differentiate into retinal neurons, and preserve light-mediated behavior. Invest Ophthalmol Vis Sci 2004;45:4167–4173.

11. Young MJ, Ray J, Whiteley SJ, et al. Neuronal differentiation and morphological integration of hippocampal progenitor cells transplanted to the retina of immature and mature dystrophic rats. Mol Cell Neurosci 2000;16:197–205.

12. Streilein JW, Ma N, Wenkel H, et al. Immunobiology and privilege of neuronal retina and pigment epithelium transplants. Vision Res 2002;42:487–495.

23. Zhang Y, Kardaszewska AK, van Veen T, et al. Integration between abutting retinas: role of glial structures and associated molecules at the interface. Invest Ophthalmol Vis Sci 2004;45: 4440–4449.

24. Silver J, Miller JH. Regeneration beyond the glial scar. Nat Rev Neurosci 2004;5: 146–156.

26. MacLaren RE, Pearson RA, MacNeil A, et al. Retinal repair by transplantation of photoreceptor precursors. Nature 2006;444:203–207.

27. Lamba DA, Karl MO, Ware CB, et al. Efficient generation of retinal progenitor cells from human embryonic stem cells. Proc Natl Acad Sci USA 2006;103: 12769–12774.

35. Ghosh F, Engelsberg K, English RV, et al. Long-term neuroretinal full-thickness transplants in a large animal model of severe retinitis pigmentosa. Graefes Arch Clin Exp Ophthalmol 2007;245:835–846.

56. Busch SA, Silver J. The role of extracellular matrix in CNS regeneration. Curr Opin Neurobiol 2007;17:120–127.

69. Yong VW. Metalloproteinases: mediators of pathology and regeneration in the CNS. Nat Rev Neurosci 2005;6:931–944.

73. Tucker B, Klassen H, Yang L, et al. Elevated MMP expression in the MRL mouse retina creates a permissive environment for retinal regeneration. Invest Ophthalmol Vis Sci 2008;49: 1686–1695.

CHAPTER 78

Proliferative vitreoretinopathy

Clyde Guidry

Clinical background

Proliferative vitreoretinopathy (PVR) is defined as the "growth of membranes on both surfaces of the detached retina and on the posterior surface of the detached vitreous gel." The name was introduced in 1983 by the Retina Society Terminology Committee[1] as part of a classification scheme for a group of intraocular complications previously known by more descriptive terms, including "massive vitreous retraction," "massive preretinal retraction," and "massive periretinal proliferation." PVR is not a distinct disease per se, but is instead a complication common to a variety of clinical disorders. It is most prevalent as a clinical complication of surgical procedures to correct rhegmatogenous retinal detachments, which are detachments that follow formation of a retinal tear or hole. Tractional forces generated within the scar tissue-like PVR membranes can be transmitted to the retina and cause complete retinal detachment, retinal degeneration, and permanent blindness.

Pathology

Studies of PVR chronology report average development times between the initial symptoms and retinal detachment ranging between 1 and 2 months and which vary with the type of initiating event and disease severity.[2] Tissue changes associated with PVR can vary widely in both severity and location at initial diagnosis. The classification scheme used to describe these two features was suggested by the Retina Society Terminology Committee[1] in 1983. Stage A PVR refers to minimal or earliest signs of potential disease, including vitreous haze, protein flare, or the presence of pigmented cell clumps thought to be derived from the retinal pigmented epithelium (RPE: Figure 78.1A). PVR stage B describes moderate, but nonetheless overt, signs of PVR, including traction or wrinkling of the retinal surface, rolled edges of a retinal break, or blood vessel distortion (Figure 78.1B). PVR stage C was originally proposed to describe marked and then massive, full-thickness retinal folds that involved one to three quadrants of the eye (Figure 78.1C) and stage D indicates complete retinal detachment into a funnel shape. However, this portion of the classification scheme was later modified to include a single stage C that was subdivided into

six categories providing specific information about the severity and location of advanced PVR (Table 78.1).[3]

Etiology

PVR development is most often associated with the formation of retinal holes or tears and its prevalence under these circumstances correlates with the size and/or number of retinal defects. The ultimate success rate of surgical procedures to close retinal defects and correct the rhegmatogenous retinal detachments is now extremely high, exceeding 90%.[4] However, PVR develops in 5–10% of these cases and remains the leading cause of surgical failure.[1] Depending on the severity or location, penetrating ocular injuries and other ocular trauma also have a high risk of developing PVR.[5] This is also true for conditions that lead to retinal or vitreous hemorrhage.[6] PVR is also associated with seemingly unrelated conditions such as aphakia, which is the absence of the natural crystalline lens, and pseudophakia, which indicates the presence of a synthetic lens. Genetic predisposition per se does not appear to be a major factor in the development of PVR. However, PVR may be more common in genetic diseases in which risk factors such as the formation of retinal holes, tears, and detachments are more prevalent, such as severe myopia and connective tissue disorders such as Stickler and Marfan syndromes.[7]

Treatment

Treatments for PVR vary according to disease severity and the perceived risk of developing more aggressive disease.[6,8] Early PVR that does not involve new retinal holes or tears or otherwise alter visual acuity might be monitored in the hope that it will remain asymptomatic. Light to moderate PVR might be treated with an encircling scleral band designed to close the retinal break through external deformation of the globe. More severe disease may require vitrectomy which involves surgical removal of the vitreous gel and replacement with a buffered saline solution. It may also be necessary to dissect and peel the epiretinal scar tissues off to lessen traction on the retina. Severe cases involving large expanses of retinal detachment under traction may require even more aggressive procedures such as temporary replacement of vitreous fluid with gas or silicone oil to encourage retinal reattachment and tamponade the retinal defects. In the most advanced cases it may be necessary to remove retinal tissue in relaxing retinectomies. The extraordinary skill with which these techniques are applied has resulted in a surprisingly high rate of surgical success. Anatomic correction, defined by successful retinal reattachment, is accomplished in 60–80% of PVR cases. This is somewhat lower in cases of extremely severe or advanced disease. Unfortunately, high surgical success rates are not necessarily indicative of visual success. The risk of developing recurrent PVR is extremely high (approximately 40%) and often requires revision surgeries. Also, the more aggressive treatment options like gas or silicone oil tamponade, while essential to a successful surgical outcome, can lead to other unrelated complications

such as cataractous changes or glaucomatous increases in intraocular pressure. Finally, and perhaps most importantly, even relatively brief periods of retinal detachment can lead to significant loss of retinal function. Successful, uncomplicated surgical correction of retinal detachments within 7 days allows more than 80% of patients to recover ambulatory vision of 20/200 or better.[9] However, when recurrent disease and other complications are considered, these percentages fall to between 40 and 80%.[6]

Pathophysiology

While the initiating events and disease course can be highly variable, PVR is ultimately a cellular disorder in that it is dependent upon the combined actions of individual cells.[10] Minimally, the intravitreal form of PVR requires that the pathogenic cells gain access to the vitreal space through avenues which vary according to cell type. The pathogenic cells must then proliferate to achieve the required critical mass and generate the tractional forces that ultimately cause traction retinal detachment. The ability to arrest any of these critical activities would result in control of PVR and prevent its recurrence. As a result, much of the research into PVR pathogenic mechanisms has focused on identifying the cells involved (Box 78.1) and on the critical pathogenic activities (Box 78.2).

Pathogenic cells

Cells derived from the RPE have long been considered key players in the pathogenesis of PVR.[11] The RPE is a monolayer of darkly pigmented cells that underlies and provides physiologic support to the attached neural retina (Figure 78.2). Studies of PVR epiretinal tissues originally identified RPE based on pigment content and ultrastructural morphology. With the advent of immunochemical labeling techniques for microscopy, RPE have since been positively identified in

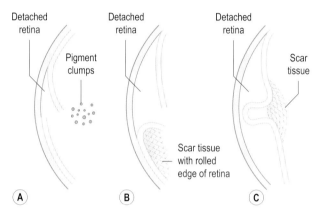

Figure 78.1 An illustration of the three stages of proliferative vitreoretinopathy-related change in the retina. (A) A moderate-sized retinal detachment with a break and clumps of pigmented cells dispersed/suspended within the vitreous gel. (B) A larger area of retinal detachment with fibrous scar tissue rolling one of the edges of the retinal break. (C) An extensive retinal detachment with the retina held in a full-thickness fold by scar tissue.

Table 78.1 Classification of proliferative vitreoretinopathy

Grade	Type of contraction	Location	Summary
A			Retinal pigment epithelium clumps in vitreous and on retina, protein flare
B			Surface wrinkling, rolled edges of tears, vascular tortuosity
C			Full-thickness retinal folds
	1	Posterior	Star-fold
	2	Posterior	Confluent irregular folds in posterior retina, remainder of retina drawn posteriorly, optic disc may not be visible
	3	Anterior	Subretinal napkin ring or irregular elevation of the retina
	4	Posterior	Irregular folds in anterior retina, series of radial folds more posteriorly, irregular circumferential retinal fold in coronal plane
	5	Anterior	Smooth circumferential retinal fold in coronal plane
	6	Anterior	Circumferential fold of retina at insertion of posterior hyaloid pulled forward; trough of peripheral retinal, ciliary processes under traction with possible hypotony; iris may be retracted

Reproduced with permission from Lean JS, Stern WH, Irvine AR, et al. Classification of proliferative vitreoretinopathy used in the silicone study. The Silicone Study Group. Ophthalmology 1989;96:765–771.

Box 78.1 Cell types associated with proliferative vitreoretinopathy

- Retinal pigmented epithelial cells
- Müller glia
- Retinal astrocytes
- Immune cells (macrophages, lymphocytes, hyalocytes)
- Fibroblasts of unknown origin

Box 78.2 Pathogenic cellular activities in proliferative vitreoretinopathy

- Cell migration or dispersion into vitreous
- Cell proliferation
- Tractional force generation

these tissues using antibodies raised against cytokeratins present in normal RPE and other proteins with limited ocular distribution such as cellular retinaldehyde-binding protein. RPE can be detected in nearly all PVR epiretinal membranes.[12–14] However, in studies in which cell populations were actually quantified, RPE usually represents less than 25% of the total population.[12,14] Under normal conditions RPE cells are not in direct physical contact with the vitreous and so their involvement in PVR is thought to require the creation of a retinal defect such as a hole or tear. In addition to migration through retinal defects, there is evidence that RPE can be physically dispersed into the vitreous if attached to a large, horseshoe-shaped retinal tear or even during retinal detachment surgeries that involve physical manipulation of the external globe wall.

Evidence of glial involvement in the pathogenesis of PVR is similar to RPE except that the glia are potentially derived from two retinal cell types. Retinal astrocytes are derived from the nerve fiber layer near the vitreoretinal interface (Figure 78.3). Müller cells are radially oriented, transretinal glia whose broad endfeet join and comprise the vitreoretinal interface (Figure 78.4). Early light microscopic studies of PVR scar tissues tentatively identified glia in these tissues by size and morphology. The immunochemical studies that followed confirmed these findings by detecting cells positive for glial fibrillary acid protein (GFAP) in most of the PVR epiretinal membranes examined.[12–16] However, when quantified, glia detected using this antigen consistently represented a minority of the overall cell population.[14,16] At least two studies distinguished between astrocytes and Müller glia using proteins specific to the latter cell type, including cellular retinaldehyde-binding protein, carbonic anhydrase, and glutamine synthetase. Cells positive for these antigens were detected, indicating that some of the glia present in PVR epiretinal membranes are derived from Müller cells.[15,17] Recent studies have now provided direct evidence of retinal glial cell migration on to the retinal surface in human and animal studies.[18] In this case, vitreal Müller cell migration was induced by retinal detachment and then reattachment.

There are also reports identifying other cell types in epiretinal membranes including lymphocytes,[19,20] macrophages,[19,21] and hyalocytes,[22] a vitreous cell with macrophage-like characteristics[23] leading to speculation

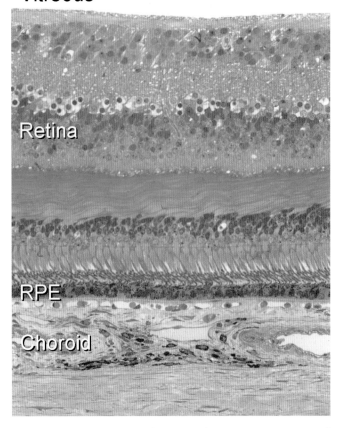

Figure 78.2 Light micrograph of posterior pole section pointing out retinal pigmented epithelium monolayer beneath retina. (Courtesy of Dr. Christine Curcio, University of Alabama School of Medicine.)

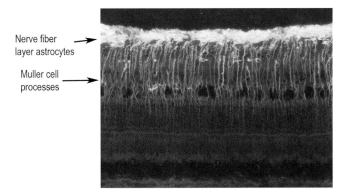

Figure 78.3 Glial fibrillary acid protein localization to astrocytes and Müller glia in porcine retina.

about the role of inflammation as an associated process in PVR. Other important cell types consistently reported in epiretinal membranes are fibroblast-like cells, also described as fibrocytes or myofibroblasts.[12–14] In addition to cell morphology, immunochemical identification of these cells is primarily based on the absence of other ocular cell marker proteins and the presence of the myoid protein α-smooth-muscle actin.[24] As with RPE cells, fibroblasts are reported in virtually all PVR epiretinal membranes examined and, when

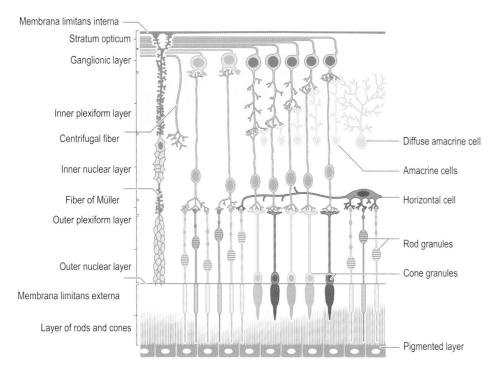

Membrana limitans interna
Stratum opticum
Ganglionic layer

Inner plexiform layer
Centrifugal fiber
Inner nuclear layer
Fiber of Müller
Outer plexiform layer

Outer nuclear layer

Membrana limitans externa

Layer of rods and cones

Diffuse amacrine cell
Amacrine cells
Horizontal cell
Rod granules
Cone granules
Pigmented layer

Figure 78.4 Retinal cell types. Representative schematic to illustrate transretinal Müller cell morphology.

quantified, represent the most abundant cell population in these tissues. The origins of fibroblasts in PVR epiretinal membranes are uncertain and, while it has been suggested that they originate from local connective tissues, there is no direct evidence of fibroblast translocation into the vitreal space. There is, however, evidence suggesting that fibroblast-like cells can arise from local ocular populations. Within days of isolation and introduction into tissue culture, RPE and Müller cells express α-smooth-muscle actin de novo and reduce expression of their respective marker proteins (cytokeratin 18 and GFAP), yielding a cell type that is immunochemically indistinguishable from the fibroblasts detected in epiretinal membranes.[25-27]

Cell proliferation and apoptosis

Of the pathogenic activities associated with PVR, cell proliferation has received the most attention. Cell division as a pathogenic mechanism in PVR epiretinal membranes has been confirmed directly in studies using antibodies against the Ki67 nuclear protein, which is detectable throughout the mitotic cell cycle and absent in G_0, and the proliferation cell nuclear antigen (PCNA), which is abundant during early S-phase.[28-31] With this approach, evidence of proliferation can be detected in the majority of PVR specimens examined. Interestingly, in two studies in which the positive populations were quantified, the percentages varied widely from as low as 0% to as high as 99%.[28,31] Surprisingly, in neither study did the percentage of actively proliferating cells correlate with disease duration or stage, suggesting that the variance is a reflection of the heterogeneous origins and pathogenesis of this disorder. On the opposite end of the proliferation spectrum, there is also compelling evidence of cell apoptosis in PVR epiretinal membranes. Two of the Ki67

studies mentioned above also quantified apoptotic cells in the same specimens using terminal uridine deoxynucleotidyl transferase dUTP nick end labeling (TUNEL).[28,31] In this case, the results were more consistent in that the majority of the samples examined were positive for apoptosis and the proportions of positive cells were consistently lower, ranging from 0 to 10% in one study. Dual-label immunochemical experiments to identify the apoptotic cell types revealed that many were derived from RPE rather than glia. Finally, both studies reported a correlation with disease duration in that the proportion of apoptotic cells increases with long-term detachments.

Nearly two decades of immunochemical studies performed on PVR vitreous fluids and epiretinal membranes have implicated a relatively long list of growth factors, cytokines, and chemokines as potentially involved in modulating cell growth in PVR.[32,33] The list of growth factors includes, but is not limited to, members of the transforming growth factor,[28,34,35] platelet- derived growth factor,[36-39] epidermal growth factor,[37,40-44] fibroblast growth factor,[45-47] insulin-like growth factor,[44,48,49] tumor necrosis factor,[50,51] hepatocyte growth factor,[52-55] and connective tissue growth factor families.[56-58] In most cases there is also evidence of production by local cells, most often RPE or Müller cells. These growth factor families have also been demonstrated to modulate RPE or glial cell growth, migration, or apoptosis in tissue culture models, providing some indirect evidence of their potential effects in PVR. Unfortunately, there is limited direct evidence about which mitogens actually drive RPE or glial cell proliferation in situ. In light of the complex effects on cell behavior and growth factor interactions reported, it seems likely that the causal growth factors, like the disease, will also vary with the inductive events and disease stage.

Another important area in PVR research is the potential use of antineoplastic agents to control cell growth. The list of drugs tested is extensive, with 5-fluorouracil, a cell cycle-dependent pyrimidine analog, successfully used to control scarring in glaucoma filtration surgeries, probably being the most extensively studied drug of this type.[59] Studies using tissue culture models demonstrated the capacity of this drug to control cell growth and traction retinal detachment in simplified animal models designed to mimic key features of PVR. However, the outcomes in clinical trials dating back more than 25 years have been mixed. As a result, antineoplastic drugs are not routinely used as adjunctive therapies in retinal detachment surgery. The major hurdles seem to be the relatively short half-life of the drugs following introduction into the vitreal cavity and an understandable reluctance to perform repeated intraocular injections which in and of themselves are an added risk factor for PVR development. Investigators are currently exploring alternative drug delivery systems designed to maintain therapeutic drug levels for longer periods[60] and antineoplasmic agents as combined therapies[4] to improve drug effectiveness when applied at the time of surgery.

Tractional force generation

Cell-generated tractional forces applied to the vitreous matrix or retinal surface cause retinal detachment and represent another potential target for intervention. While research in this field is less abundant, our understanding of this activity in PVR is comparable to that of cell proliferation. The capacity for significant tractional force generation is present in a minority of cell types and is mechanistically limited to cells expressing α-smooth-muscle actin[61] and the necessary collagen-binding integrin receptors.[62,63] In PVR epiretinal membranes, α-smooth-muscle actin expression is detected in the fibroblast-like cells mentioned previously.[24] As also mentioned previously, both RPE and Müller cells express α-smooth-muscle actin de novo following isolation and, with expression, acquire the capacity to generate tractional forces on collagen matrices in vitro.[25,64] With these observations in mind, it seems most likely that fibroblast-like cells derived from RPE and/or Müller cells are the sources of tractional forces generated in PVR. Tractional force generation, like cell proliferation, is not a constitutive behavior but is instead stimulated by exogenous growth factors. Thus far, the list of growth factors capable of stimulating RPE and Müller cell tractional force generation is fairly short, and includes members of the transforming growth factor-β, platelet-derived growth factor, and insulin-like growth factor families.[25,64–66] PVR vitreous is able to stimulate tractional force generation in tissue culture models in vitro and neutralizing antibodies against insulin-like growth factors and platelet-derived growth factors are able to attenuate the majority of this activity, suggesting that these growth factor families represent the major stimuli in PVR.[49]

Conclusions

PVR is a cellular disorder that develops in response to several types of retinal defects and results in the introduction or migration of extravitreal cells into the vitreal cavity. Untreated, PVR can result in traction retinal detachment and blindness. The principal effector cells in PVR are most likely derived from the RPE and retinal glia and the major pathogenic activities, cell growth and extracellular matrix contraction, are potentially driven by multiple growth factors produced by local cells and/or derived from blood. At present, the most successful treatments for PVR involve surgical correction of the retinal defect and removal of the proliferating tissues. The major challenge is to find more effective avenues through which these essential pathogenic activities can be arrested in the early stages to prevent disease progression and/or recurrence.

Acknowledgments

The author is indebted to John O Mason III, MD and Sudipto Mukherjee, MD, PhD for their helpful comments during manuscript preparation.

Key references

A complete list of chapter references is available online at www.expertconsult.com. See inside cover for registration details.

1. The classification of retinal detachment with proliferative vitreoretinopathy. Ophthalmology 1983;90:121–125.

2. Mietz H, Heimann K. Onset and recurrence of proliferative vitreoretinopathy in various vitreoretinal disease. Br J Ophthalmol 1995;79:874–877.

3. Lean JS, Stern WH, Irvine AR, et al. Classification of proliferative vitreoretinopathy used in the silicone study. The Silicone Study Group. Ophthalmology 1989;96:765–771.

6. Pastor JC, de la Rua ER, Martin F. Proliferative vitreoretinopathy: risk factors and pathobiology. Prog Retin Eye Res 2002;21:127–144.

8. Pastor JC. Proliferative vitreoretinopathy: an overview. Surv Ophthalmol 1998;43:3–18.

9. Ross WH. Visual recovery after macula-off retinal detachment. Eye 2002;16:440–446.

11. Machemer R, van Horn D, Aaberg TM. Pigment epithelial proliferation in human retinal detachment with massive periretinal proliferation. Am J Ophthalmol 1978;85:181–191.

12. Hiscott PS, Grierson I, McLeod D. Retinal pigment epithelial cells in epiretinal membranes: an immunohistochemical study. Br J Ophthalmol 1984;68:708–715.

17. Guerin CJ, Wolfshagen RW, Eifrig DE, et al. Immunocytochemical identification of Muller's glia as a component of human epiretinal membranes. Invest Ophthalmol Vis Sci 1990;31:1483–1491.

18. Fisher SK, Lewis GP. Muller cell and neuronal remodeling in retinal detachment and reattachment and their potential consequences for visual recovery: a review and reconsideration of recent data. Vis Res 2003;43:887–897.

24. Walshe R, Esser P, Wiedemann P, et al. Proliferative retinal diseases: myofibroblasts cause chronic vitreoretinal traction. Br J Ophthalmol 1992;76:550–552.

25. Grisanti S, Guidry C. Transdifferentiation of retinal pigment epithelial cells from epithelial to mesenchymal phenotype. Invest Ophthalmol Vis Sci 1995;36:391–405.

29. Heidenkummer HP, Kampik A, Petrovski B. Proliferative activity in epiretinal membranes. The use of the monoclonal antibody Ki-67 in proliferative vitreoretinal diseases. Retina 1992;12:52–58.

64. Guidry C. Tractional force generation by porcine Muller cells: development and differential stimulation by growth factors. Invest Ophthalmol Vis Sci 1997;38:456–468.

Immunologic mechanisms of uveitis

Steven Yeh, Zhuqing Li, and Robert B Nussenblatt

Overview

A deeper appreciation of the pathogenic mechanisms underlying uveitis, or intraocular inflammation involving the uveal tract (i.e., iris, ciliary body, choroid), has contributed to our abilities to treat these potentially vision-threatening conditions. The spectrum of uveitis ranges from acute, self-limited episodes of anterior uveitis to severe, progressive panuveitis syndromes, which may lead to blindness if not properly managed with immunosuppressive treatment regimens.

This chapter highlights our current knowledge regarding the pathogenic immune mechanisms underlying uveitic conditions. Topics discussed include pathologic features and etiologies of common clinical uveitic conditions, animal models of uveitis, the contribution of immunogenetics to uveitis, the cellular immune response described in patients with uveitic disease, and soluble mediators of inflammation (i.e., cytokines and chemokines). We also discuss the key principle of immune tolerance, which is thought to be compromised in uveitic disease. Specific disease entities are mentioned as related to these central concepts; however, a full discussion of the broad range of uveitic diseases is beyond the scope of this chapter and several excellent reviews regarding specific disease entities are available.[1,2]

Clinical background

The anatomic classification of uveitis using the Standardization of Uveitis Nomenclature (SUN) Working Group scheme is the preferred method of classifying disease for both patient care and research purposes (Table 79.1). The goals of the SUN classification scheme included improving clinical research across centers, permitting the meta-analyses of data, and improving our understanding of the varied therapeutic responses of patients to different disease processes.[3] Ocular inflammatory disease is termed "anterior uveitis" when inflammation involves the iris and ciliary body (Figure 79.1), "intermediate uveitis" with inflammation primarily found in the vitreous cavity (Figure 79.2), and "posterior uveitis" in conditions involving the retina and choroid. The term "panuveitis" refers to inflammation in all three anatomic locations, including the iris/ciliary body, vitreous

cavity, and retina and/or choroid (Figure 79.3). Because the literature differs with respect to uveitis classification prior to implementation of the SUN criteria, some of the literature referenced in this chapter classifies disease by systemic entity (e.g., Behçet's disease-associated uveitis). In the future, it will be important to understand the pathogenesis of specific disease entities (e.g., sarcoidosis-associated intermediate uveitis) in addition to a more general understanding of disease pathogenesis according to anatomic classification (e.g., acute anterior uveitis).

Pathology

Pathologic examination of ocular specimens has provided valuable information about the cellular mediators (discussed below), tissue injury, and healing mechanisms that are observed in patients with uveitis. Immune cells identified in pathologic specimens have included T- and B-cell lymphocytes, macrophages, and epithelioid cells.

For example, in sarcoidosis-associated uveitis, CD4+ T cells predominate, although CD8+ T cells and B cells have also been observed.[4,5] Granulomas consisting of multinucleated giant cells (macrophage aggregates) and epithelioid cells are also seen; however, granulomas have also been identified in other uveitic processes, including ocular tuberculosis and sympathetic ophthalmia.

Following the infiltration of ocular tissue by inflammatory cells, the release of cytokines (discussed below) and the recruitment of additional leukocytes lead to further tissue injury and resultant scarring and fibrosis. These processes are exemplified by the late phase of Vogt–Koyanagi–Harada's (VKH) disease, in which subretinal fibrosis and choroidal neovascularization are observed in a significant percentage of patients with chronic VKH disease.[6]

Etiology

Determining the etiology of a particular uveitic syndrome may be a difficult task because of the wide array of diagnostic considerations. However, correct identification of the predominant anatomic location of a disease entity is helpful in narrowing the differential diagnosis. The SUN Working Group criteria were valuable in describing the four major

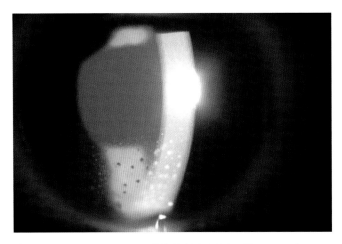

Figure 79.1 Keratic precipitates (KP). Multiple inferior KP on corneal endothelium may be observed in anterior uveitis. Numerous granulomatous KP are found on the inferior corneal endothelium.

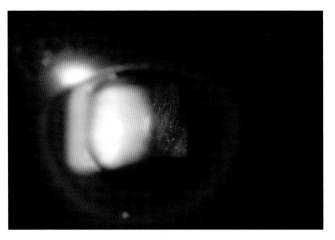

Figure 79.2 Intermediate uveitis. Diffuse vitritis in an elderly patient. Primary intraocular lymphoma may masquerade as an intermediate uveitis and should be considered in the differential diagnosis in elderly patients.

Table 79.1 The Standardization of Uveitis Nomenclature (SUN) working group anatomic classification of uveitis

Type	Primary site of inflammation*	Includes
Anterior uveitis	Anterior chamber	Iritis Iridocyclitis Anterior cyclitis
Intermediate uveitis	Vitreous	Pars planitis Posterior cyclitis Hyalitis
Posterior uveitis	Retina or choroid	Focal, multifocal, or diffuse choroiditis Chorioretinitis Retinochoroiditis Retinitis Neuroretinitis
Panuveitis	Anterior chamber, vitreous, and retina or choroid	

*As determined clinically.
Reproduced with permission from Jabs DA, Nussenblatt RB, Rosenbaum JT, et al. Standardization of uveitis nomenclature for reporting clinical data. Results of the first international workshop. Am J Ophthalmol 2005;140:509–516.

classes of uveitis: (1) anterior uveitis; (2) intermediate uveitis; (3) posterior uveitis; and (4) panuveitis.

Etiologies of anterior uveitis include sarcoidosis, human leukocyte antigen (HLA)-B27-associated uveitis, syphilis, tuberculosis, and Lyme disease. Causes of intermediate uveitis also include sarcoidosis, syphilis, Lyme disease, and tuberculosis. However, entities more commonly associated with intermediate uveitis (cf. anterior uveitis) include multiple sclerosis (MS), human T-cell lymphotrophic virus-1 (HTLV-1), and primary intraocular lymphoma, which may masquerade as a chronic vitritis in an elderly patient (i.e., masquerade syndrome). Posterior uveitis may be caused by systemic conditions, including sarcoidosis, syphilis, tuberculosis, and Lyme disease. Some causes of posterior uveitis

isolated to the eye include serpiginous choroidopathy, birdshot retinochoroidopathy, and multiple evanescent whitedot syndrome (Box 79.1). Panuveitis, which includes anterior-chamber, vitreous, retina, and choroidal inflammation, may be observed in sarcoidosis, syphilis, tuberculosis, VKH disease, and sympathetic ophthalmia. Endophthalmitis may also manifest as a panuveitis, and infectious etiologies of ocular inflammation (e.g., bacterial, fungal, viral) should also be considered in certain clinical situations. For example, in immunosuppressed patients (e.g., cancer patients on chemotherapy, patients with indwelling catheters and lines), fungal and bacterial endophthalmitis should be considered in cases of panuveitis. In other clinical settings (e.g., African-American patients with hilar adenopathy) other considerations such as sarcoidosis should be higher on the differential diagnosis of panuveitis.

Pathophysiology

Animal models of uveitis

Experimental models of uveitis have contributed greatly to our understanding of uveitis. Each of these models involves the activation of the immune system against specific retinal or uveal tract antigens (Box 79.2).[7] During induction of experimental autoimmune uveitis or uveoretinitis (EAU), animals are sensitized to known retinal antigens such as retinal S-antigen, RPE65,[8] or interphotoreceptor-binding protein (IRBP),[9,10] which are emulsified in complete Freund's adjuvant to augment the immune response. A second agent such as pertussis toxin is also used to activate the immune response further. Using this technique, inflammation of the iris, ciliary body, retina, and choroid is consistently observed. With this reproducible technique, it is possible to study the cellular components, soluble mediators and their receptors, therapies, and drug delivery systems targeted against the inflammatory response.[11]

Endotoxin-induced uveitis (EIU) has also been a useful animal model of uveitis. In this animal model, lipopolysaccharide (endotoxin) is administered to the animal, leading

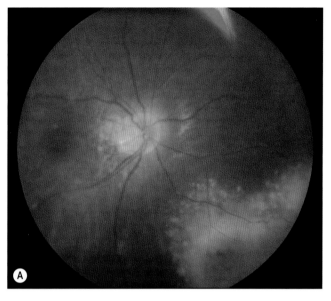
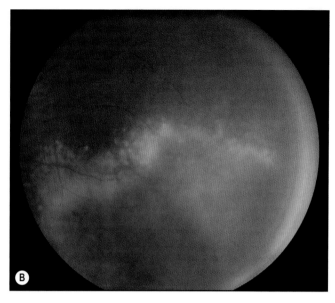

Figure 79.3 Panuveitis due to presumed sarcoidosis. Inferonasal region (A, B) of chorioretinal inflammatory infiltrates in a patient with panuveitis and an elevated angiotensin-converting enzyme level. High-resolution chest computed tomography scan revealed mediastinal adenopathy.

Box 79.1 Anatomic classification of uveitis and disease considerations

- The anatomic classification of uveitis based on the Standardization of Uveitis Nomenclature Working Group criteria is currently the preferred method of describing uveitis for patient care and research purposes
- The four major classes of uveitis include anterior, intermediate, posterior uveitis, and panuveitis, which may be useful in narrowing the differential diagnosis of a uveitic syndrome
- CD4+ T cells play a key role in mediating ocular inflammation in uveitis; however, CD8+ T cells, B lymphocytes, and macrophages have also been implicated
- Systemic autoimmune conditions such as sarcoidosis and Vogt–Koyanagi–Harada's disease may cause uveitis. Infectious causes include syphilis, tuberculosis, and Lyme disease
- Etiologies of posterior uveitis with localized ocular inflammation include birdshot retinochoroidopathy, serpiginous choroidopathy, and multiple evanescent white-dot syndrome

---

Box 79.2 Cellular and soluble mediators of inflammation in uveitis

- Animal models of uveitis, particularly experimental autoimmune uveitis, have been important in characterizing the pathogenesis of uveitis, as well as in studying immunosuppressive agents for the treatment of disease
- The relationship between immunogenetics and the clinical expression of uveitis remains under investigation; however, the recent identification of the NOD2 gene mutation in patients with ocular and systemic granulomatous inflammation is supportive of the importance of genetics in uveitis
- Immune cells implicated in uveitis include CD4+ T-helper cells, cytotoxic CD8+ T cells, B cells, macrophages, and natural killer cells
- Subtypes of CD4+ T-helper cells include Th1 and Th17 cells, which are thought to be proinflammatory. Other CD4+ T-helper cell subtypes may play an immunoregulatory role
- Interleukin-1, interleukin-6, and tumor necrosis factor-α are key proinflammatory cytokines seen in uveitis
- Mechanisms of immunoregulation include peripheral tolerance (active suppression and immune ignorance) and central tolerance (thymic-negative selection). Loss of these control mechanisms may be relevant to the clinical expression of uveitis

---

to an acute inflammatory response in the uveal tract that occurs 6 hours after endotoxin injection and peaks within 24 hours. Iris hyperemia, miosis, increased aqueous humor protein, and infiltration of the anterior chamber and uvea by inflammatory cells are observed following EIU induction.[12]

A model of experimental autoimmune anterior uveitis (EAAU) has also been described previously. EAAU is induced in animal models via injection of a number of peptides, including myelin basic protein,[13] melanin-bound antigens of the retinal pigment epithelium,[14] or melanin-associated antigen.[15] Experimental models have also been described for specific uveitic syndromes, including VKH disease in dogs[16] and rats,[17] ocular histoplasmosis,[18] and ocular toxoplasmosis.[19] Because much of our knowledge stems from studies in animal models, some of these studies are referenced in the discussion of clinical uveitis throughout this chapter. Table

79.2 highlights various details of the animal models used in the study of uveitis.

Immunogenetics and uveitis

The relationship between immunogenetics and the clinical manifestation of ocular inflammatory disease has been the subject of several recent reviews.[20,21] Genes may influence individual susceptibility to an inflammatory disease; however, the mechanisms leading from a specific genetic profile to the disease phenotype may also involve environ-

Table 79.2 Experimental models of uveitis

Experimental model	Inciting antigen(s)	Animals studied	Anatomic/histologic localization of uveitis
Experimental autoimmune uveitis	Retinal S-antigen, IRBP, recoverin (antigens emulsified with complete Freund's adjuvant)*	Mouse, rat, rabbit, guinea pig, nonhuman primates	Anterior chamber, iris, ciliary body, vitreous infiltrates, retina, subretinal space
Endotoxin-induced uveitis	Lipopolysaccharide/endotoxin	Mouse, rat	Anterior chamber, iris, ciliary body, vitreous
Experimental autoimmune encephalomyelitis	Myelin basic protein	Mouse, rat	Anterior uveitis, retinal vasculitis
Vogt–Koyanagi–Harada model	Tyrosinase related protein 1 (TRP1)	Dogs	Anterior-chamber infiltrates, vitreous infiltrates, choroidal and retinal inflammation, exudative retinal detachments

IRBP, interphotoreceptor-binding protein.
*Pertussin toxin is also administered in some models of experimental autoimmune uveitis.
Modified from Yeh S, Nussenblatt RB, Levy-Clarke GA. Emerging biologics in the treatment of uveitis. Exp Rev Clin Immunol 2007;3:781–796.

mental triggers, loss of regulatory elements preventing ocular autoimmunity, and other yet undefined mechanisms.

The HLA genes, which are located on chromosome 6, are responsible for expression of major histocompatibility complex (MHC) class I and II antigens. MHC class I antigens are found on almost all cells in the human body, whereas MHC class II antigens are located primarily on cells involved in antigen presentation, such as lymphocytes and dendritic cells (tissue macrophages). Both HLA class I MHC and class II MHC associations with uveitis have been reported in a number of uveitic syndromes. Specifically, the association of HLA-B27 with acute anterior uveitis and a variety of associated systemic diseases, including the seronegative spondyloarthropathies, has been observed.[22] A class I MHC association with uveitis has been observed in the posterior uveitic syndrome birdshot retinochoroidopathy; greater than 90% of individuals diagnosed with this syndrome carry a copy of the HLA-A29 allele.[23,24] Behçet's disease, which may present with panuveitis, retinal vasculitis, or acute anterior uveitis, has been associated previously with HLA-B51.[25,26] Class II MHC associations have been identified in patients with VKH disease[27] (HLA-DR1 and -DR4) and in pars planitis[28] (HLA-DR2). Table 79.3 summarizes the known HLA-associations of various uveitic syndromes.

Single-nucleotide polymorphisms (SNPs) that may predispose individuals to a certain disease phenotype have also been studied recently. El-Shabrawi et al reported an association of specific SNPs within the tumor necrosis factor-α (TNF-α) promoter that may increase the susceptibility of HLA-B27-positive individuals towards the development of intraocular inflammation.[29] A correlation of clinical phenotype in patients with anterior uveitis and SNPs within the cytokine genes interleukin (IL)-1R, IL-6, IL-10, and TNF has also been reported.[30,31]

Besides examining single-nucleotide changes in DNA, other investigators have examined the role of differential gene expression in producing various ocular inflammatory phenotypes. In a recent study by Li et al, gene expression profiling using cDNA microarray analysis of peripheral

Table 79.3 Selected ocular diseases and their human leukocyte antigen (HLA) associations

Disease	Antigen
Acute anterior uveitis	HLA-B27 (W) HLA-B8 (AA)
Anklyosing spondylitis	HLA-B27 (W) HLA-B7 (AA)
Behçet's disease	HLA-B51 (O)
Birdshot retinochoroidopathy	HLA-A29
Ocular cicatricial pemphigoid	HLA-B12 (W)
Presumed ocular histoplasmosis	HLA-B7 (W)
Reiter's syndrome	HLA-B27 (W)
Rheumatoid arthritis	HLA-DR4 (W)
Sympathetic ophthalmia	HLA-A11 (M)
Vogt–Koyanagi–Harada disease	MT-3 (O)

AA, African-American; M; mixed ethnic study; O, oriental; W, white.
Modified from Nussenblatt RB. Elements of the immune system and concepts of intraocular inflammatory disease pathogenesis. In: Nussenblatt R (ed.) Uveitis: Fundamentals and Clinical Practice. Philadelphia, PA: Mosby, 2004.

blood samples in patients with noninfectious uveitis revealed increased expression of several cytokine, chemokine, and chemokine receptor genes when compared to normal controls.[32] The examination of local gene expression in EAU demonstrated a local upregulation of inflammatory cytokines and chemokines with a bias towards a T-helper cell type 1 (Th1)-immune response (see below); specifically, upregulation of interferon-γ (IFN-γ), RANTES/CCL5, and MIG/CXCL9 with low levels of the T-helper cell type 2 (Th2) cytokines IL-4 and IL-5 was observed.[33] Further analysis of differential gene expression may help to identify inflammatory mediators responsible for specific disease phenotypes in the future.

In 2001, a single gene mutation in the nucleotide oligomerization domain (NOD2) gene was identified as a cause of the familial form of uveitis known as familial juvenile systemic granulomatosis (Blau syndrome or Jabs disease).[34] Blau syndrome consists of a triad of uveitis, arthritis, and skin inflammation. The uveitis has been previously characterized in 16 patients from eight families. In this series, 15 of 16 patients presented with multifocal choroiditis and panuveitis whereas only one patient presented with anterior uveitis.[35] The NOD2 gene mutation causes structural changes in an intracellular protein named CARD15, which is thought to be involved in the recognition of intracellular bacteria via recognition peptide motifs in microbial cell walls. The precise pathways that result in uveitis clinically are under investigation.

Cellular mediators of uveitis

Immune cellular mediators of uveitis have been studied extensively in animal models of uveitis, as well as from the peripheral blood, aqueous, and vitreous samples from patients with uveitis.

Macrophages play a significant role in the ocular immune response, serving at least three major functions. These include the direct killing of foreign pathogens and clearing of diseased tissue, the activation of the immune system via antigen presentation, and the secretion of potent inflammatory cytokines IFN-γ, TNF-α, and IL-1 that augment the immune response.[36]

The T-cell response is thought to be the arm of the immune system primarily responsible for the majority of uveitic syndromes, with CD4+ T-helper (Th) cells being the subset of immune cells most commonly implicated.[37] The successful use of a humanized monoclonal blocking antibody against T-cell growth factor IL-2 receptor (CD25) in treating uveitis further supported the critical role of T cells in the pathogenesis of human uveitis.[38] T-cell receptors recognize specific antigen epitopes presented in the context of MHC by antigen-presenting cells (e.g., macrophages, dendritic cells). CD8+ T cells recognize antigen presented in the context of class I MHC molecules, whereas CD4+ T cells recognize antigen presented by class II MHC molecules. A second signal, or costimulatory signal, via the interaction of CD28 (T-cell surface antigen) and B7 antigen (antigen-presenting cell), is required for T-cell activation. Ophthalmic inflammatory diseases thought to be CD4+ T-helper cell-mediated include sarcoidosis,[39] VKH disease,[40,41] and intermediate uveitis.[42] Pathologic evidence from patients with sarcoidosis has demonstrated a predominantly CD4+ T-cell population.[5] However, other disease entities such as Behçet's disease have been associated with a cytotoxic CD8+ T-cell population.[43]

The Th cell response is divided into Th1, Th2, and recently described Th17 subtypes, all of which are associated with specific cytokine profiles and cellular responses. The Th1 cellular response is thought to be proinflammatory and is most commonly associated with proinflammatory cytokines, including IFN-γ, IL-12, IL-1, IL-6, and TNF-α. The Th2 cellular response is more commonly associated with atopic disease, and often an anti-inflammatory response. Its associated cytokines include IL-4, IL-5, and IL-10. Recently, Th17 cells, associated with IL-17 and the IL-23 family of cytokines, have been implicated in the pathogenesis of uveitis and scleritis.[44] One report described an elevation of IL-23p19 mRNA, IL-23 levels, and increased IL-17 by stimulated peripheral blood mononuclear cells and CD4+ T cells in patients with VKH disease.[45] Recent evidence has also suggested that the presence of Th17 cells in inflamed tissue may contribute to chronicity of ocular inflammation; further studies are underway to characterize this pathway better.

The role of a population of regulatory T cells has been characterized in EAU but regulatory T cells have been difficult to isolate and characterize in patients with uveitis. In EAU mice immunized with IRBP, adoptively transferred CD4+CD25+ regulatory T cells (obtained from naïve mice) resulted in decreased clinical severity and histopathologic scores. In addition, EAU mice that received CD4+CD25+ cells demonstrated reduced proliferation of uveitogenic T cells isolated from their cervical lymph nodes and spleens.[46] In another study by Silver et al, vaccination of naked DNA encoding IRBP protected mice from the development of EAU following immunization with IRBP at least 10 weeks after vaccination. In addition, IRBP-specific CD4+CD25(high) T cells derived from vaccinated mice conferred protection to EAU-challenged recipients and were found in vitro to be FoxP3-positive and antigen-specific.[47]

While T cells are thought to be the immune cell most intimately associated with the pathogenesis of the majority of uveitic syndromes, B cells may also play a limited role in some forms of uveitis. For example, in the subretinal fibrosis and uveitis syndrome, histopathologic investigation has revealed a markedly inflamed choroid with a predominance of plasma cells and B cells.[48] The deposition of complement and IgG within Bruch's membrane was reported in this syndrome; another report of this syndrome implicated the involvement of T cells, as similar proportions of T and B cells were found in areas of choroid with infiltrating immune cells.[49] Several other ocular inflammatory diseases in which B cells have been identified in limited numbers in pathologic specimens include VKH,[50] ocular sarcoidosis,[5] and sympathetic ophthalmia[51,52]; however, these conditions are thought to be primarily T-cell-mediated conditions.

Recent interest in the precise role of natural killer (NK) cells in patients with autoimmune disease has arisen from several studies suggesting that a distinct population of immunoregulatory NK cells arises during the treatment of active uveitis or MS with humanized monoclonal antibody (mAb) against IL-2 receptor (daclizumab, Zenapax).[53,54] In both MS and in active uveitis, the administration of daclizumab was associated with an increase in a population of CD56[bright] NK cells. In MS patients, daclizumab therapy was associated with a decrease in T-cell populations and an increase in CD56[bright] NK cells, which correlated with clinical treatment response. Furthermore, in vitro studies demonstrated that NK cells inhibited T-cell survival via a contact-dependent mechanism.[53] In patients with active uveitis, a smaller population of CD56[bright] cells was observed when compared to patients with inactive uveitis following treatment with daclizumab. Additionally, CD56[bright] cells were able to secrete IL-10 in large amounts, whereas CD56[dim] cells were unable to do so, suggesting a possible mechanism by which CD56[bright] cells could potentially serve an immunoregulatory function.[54]

Soluble mediators of uveitis and cell adhesion molecules

Cytokines

The most well-characterized group of soluble mediators of inflammation in uveitis are cytokines, chemical mediators involved in the recruitment of ocular immune cells, augmentation of the immune response, and tissue damage in some cases. A number of soluble inflammatory mediators of uveitis have been characterized in both peripheral blood serum samples and ocular fluids (i.e., aqueous and vitreous), as well as in experimental models of uveitis.

In EAU, the Th1-mediated cellular immune response and its associated cytokines predominate. Foxman et al observed an elevation of Th1-associated cytokines and chemokines, including IL-1α, IL-1ß, IL-1R antagonist, IL-6, TNF-α, and IFN-γ in the EAU model.[55] IL-1 and TNF-α receptor-deficient mice show decreased inflammation in an immune complex model of uveitis, suggesting a role for these cytokines in this animal model of uveitis[56] (Figure 79.4). Antagonists of cytokines and chemokines associated with Th1-mediated ocular inflammation have demonstrated some efficacy in the treatment of uveitis (see below), and further exploration of therapeutic agents targeting these soluble mediators of inflammation is warranted.

In patients with noninfectious intermediate and posterior uveitis, serum levels of IL-2 receptor and soluble TNF-α receptor were elevated compared to normal controls.[57] Besides TNF-α receptor levels, aqueous and serum levels of

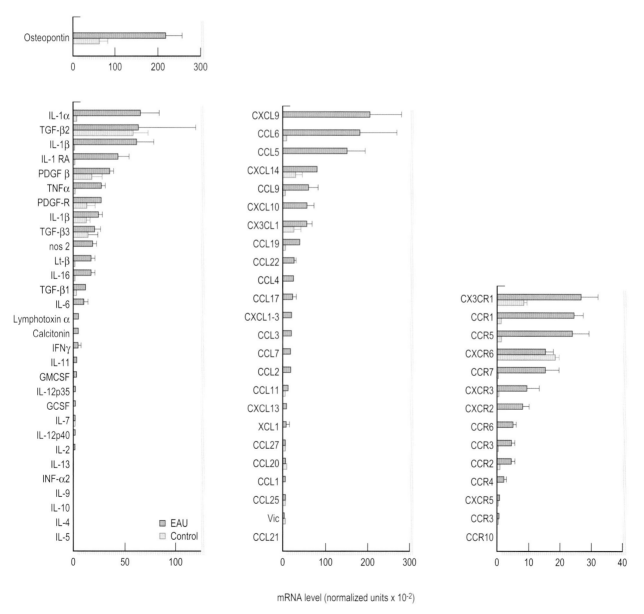

Figure 79.4 Upregulation of cytokines, chemokines, and chemokine receptor mRNA transcripts in eyes with interphotoreceptor-binding protein-immunized experimental autoimmune uveitis animals. (Adapted from Foxman EF, Zhang M, Hurst SD, et al. Inflammatory mediators in uveitis: differential induction of cytokines and chemokines in Th1- versus Th2-mediated ocular inflammation. J Immunol 2002;168:2483–2492.)

TNF-α have also been elevated in uveitis patients.[58] Lacomba et al reported an elevation in IL-2 and IFN-γ in both the aqueous and sera of patients with uveitis when compared to controls.[59]

Cytokine profiles likely differ between specific disease entities, and this has been studied in several reports. For example, levels of TNF-α were observed to be elevated in the aqueous humor in HLA-B27 patients with uveitis.[60] This may explain, in part, the disease-specific efficacy reported on infliximab for the use of HLA-B27-associated uveitis.[61] In one patient with uveitis associated with the chronic infantile neurological cutaneous articular (CINCA) syndrome, which is thought to be an IL-1-mediated inflammatory process, the successful use of the IL-1 receptor antagonist anakinra has been reported.[62] In patients with active Behçet's disease, elevated levels of serum TNF-α receptor have been identified, as well as an increase in IL-10 and IL-12[63]; studies in Behçet's disease-associated uveitis treated with the TNF-α antagonist infliximab have demonstrated an ability to reduce the number of uveitis relapses,[64,65] a reduction in daily immunosuppressive requirement,[63,64] and improved visual acuity in some cases.[66]

Chemokines, growth factors, and other mediators of inflammation

Patterns of chemokines, or chemoattractant cytokines, have also been identified in both patients and in animal models of uveitis. In one report of patients with acute idiopathic anterior uveitis, levels of the chemokines IL-8, interferon-inducible protein-10 (IP-10), MCP-1, RANTES and macrophage inflammatory protein-1β (MIP-1β) were increased and correlated with disease severity.[67] In another study examining aqueous humor samples in patients with active uveitis, IL-6, IL-10, IFN-γ, soluble vascular cell adhesion molecule (sVCAM), regulated on activation, normal T cell was expressed and secreted (RANTES), and IP-10 was elevated when compared to uveitis patients with quiescent disease. In studies in EAU, elevations of Th1-associated chemokine receptors (CCR5, CXCR3,) have been described.[55] An elevation in fractalkine (CX3CL1) and fractalkine receptor (CX3CR1) has also been described in EAAU.[68] Abu El-Asrar et al reported an increased level of the chemoattractant IP-10, gelatinase A, and gelatinase B in the aqueous humor of patients with active uveitis.[69]

The role of vascular permeability in the pathogenesis of uveitis and uveitis-associated cystoid macular edema (CME) has received some attention in the literature that warrants further investigation. Fine et al observed a significant increase in levels of vascular endothelial growth factor (VEGF) in aqueous specimens from uveitis patients with CME when compared to those patients without CME.[70] A recent retrospective review evaluated the efficacy of the anti-VEGF agent bevacizumab for uveitic CME. In this study, 6 of 13 patients treated with bevacizumab experienced a significant reduction in foveal thickness over a median follow-up period of 91 days; however, the logMAR visual acuity change over the follow-up period was not significant.[71] It is possible that, while VEGF may play a role in the pathogenesis of uveitic CME, the blockade of underlying, persistent inflammation also needs to be addressed to prevent the cycle of inflammation and subsequent breakdown of retinal vascular permeability.

Cellular adhesion molecules

Cellular adhesion molecules expressed in the eye direct leukocyte trafficking during episodes of ocular inflammation. In pathologic specimens of enucleated eyes from uveitis patients, intercellular adhesion molecule-1 (ICAM-1) was observed on endothelial cells of retinal and choroidal blood vessels. Lymphocyte function-associated antigen-1 (LFA-1) has also been identified on lymphocytes infiltrating ocular tissues.[72] In a murine model of EAU, ICAM-1 (CD54) and LFA-1 (CD11a/CD18) have been observed on endothelial cells and lymphocytes; in this study, ICAM-1 appeared before histological evidence of inflammation. Treatment with monoclonal antibody to both molecules reduced ocular inflammation clinically and histologically.[73] Efalizumab, humanized IgG1 anti-CD11a has been utilized for the treatment of psoriasis[74] and more recently has been used in a phase I/II trial for renal transplantation,[75] but further clinical studies are needed in uveitis before implementation into clinical practice.

The role of tolerance in uveitis

Self-tolerance, the ability to distinguish self from foreign antigens, is critical to the prevention of ocular autoimmunity.[76] Central tolerance involves the elimination of self-reactive T-cell clones during thymic maturation of lymphocytes, whereas peripheral tolerance involves regulatory elements that prevent the expression of autoimmunity once immunoreactivity against self-antigen has been established. During thymic T-cell maturation, the positive selection of T cells capable of reacting against foreign antigen presented by antigen-presenting cells first occurs; in negative selection, T cells reactive against self-antigen are clonally deleted to mediate central tolerance. Animal studies by Egwuagu et al demonstrated that thymic expression of retinal antigens was correlated to resistance to EAU. In their study, murine, rat, and primate strains in which thymic expression of the retinal antigen IRBP was not observed were susceptible to the development of EAU when immunized with IRBP.[77] In contrast, animal species with thymic expression of S-antigen and IRBP were less susceptible to EAU induction. Negative selection appears to be disrupted in the monogenic disease autoimmune polyendocrinopathy–candidiasis–ectodermal dystrophy (APECED), which features autoimmunity involving multiple organs, including ophthalmic structures. Disease features are caused by a mutation in the autoimmune regulatory gene (Aire) whose gene product plays a role in the thymic expression of peripheral self-antigens.[78] In a murine model of APECED, Aire-deficient mice demonstrated reduced thymic transcription of peripheral antigens resulting in widespread systemic and retinal autoimmunity.[79] Interestingly, loss of thymic expression of a single retinal antigen IRBP has been demonstrated to cause spontaneous retinal autoimmunity, even in the presence of functional AIRE gene.[80]

The two major mechanisms implicated in peripheral tolerance to self-antigens are active suppression and immune ignorance (Figure 79.5). CD4+ T-lymphocyte subsets thought to play a role in active suppression are composed of natural T-regulatory cells and adaptive T-regulatory cells. Natural T-regulatory cells are believed to be antigen-specific and

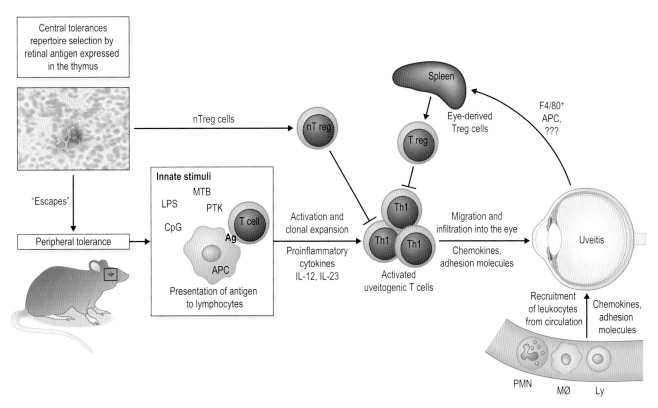

Figure 79.5 Schematic representation of critical checkpoints in ocular autoimmunity. (Adapted from Caspi RR. Ocular autoimmunity: the price of privilege? Immunol Rev 2006;213:23–35.)

exhibit in vitro suppression of target immune cells.[81] Other CD4+ T-lymphocyte populations, termed adaptive Tr1 and Th3 cells, are generated against self and foreign antigens, and appear to mediate immunosuppression via the immunoregulatory cytokines IL-10 and TGF-ß.[82] The proinflammatory cytokines IL-1 and IL-6 may disrupt natural T-regulatory cell-mediated immunosuppression and monoclonal antibodies targeting these cytokines may mediate immunosuppressive effects via restoration of natural T-regulatory cell function.[82] Immune ignorance involves the failure of effector T cells to recognize peripheral antigen, and consequently, failure of T-cell activation.

Attempts to induce peripheral tolerance have been made with a number of both experimental and clinical protocols. The induction of peripheral tolerance via the oral administration of retinal antigen was initially characterized in EAU. When Lewis rats were fed with retinal S-antigen, the clinical expression of EAU via retinal S-antigen immunization was markedly suppressed. Splenocytes harvested from mice who exhibited this form of tolerance were able to suppress the activation of CD4+ S-antigen-specific T-cell culture line when exposed to S-antigen. Interestingly, this antigen-specific in vitro suppression was blocked by administration of anti-CD8 antibody, indicating that the suppression mechanism was a CD8+ T-cell-dependent process.[83] In a phase I/II randomized masked trial of the oral administration of a mixture of retinal antigens, retinal S antigen alone or placebo was given orally to patients to induce peripheral tolerance. Patients who were fed purified S antigen appeared more likely to be tapered off immunosuppressive medications than patients receiving placebo, with a trend towards statisti-

cal significance.[84] Further studies to understand and potentially utilize this mechanism of immunosuppression are warranted.

Therapeutic advances in uveitis

Although corticosteroids are effective in the management of acute uveitic conditions, their numerous side-effects (e.g., hypertension, osteoporosis, weight gain, hyperglycemia, cushingoid body habitus) warrant consideration of other corticosteroid-sparing agents including the antimetabolites (methotrexate, azathioprine, mycophenolate mofetil), T-cell calcineurin inhibitors (ciclosporin, tacrolimus), and alkylating agents (cyclophosphamide, chlorambucil).[85,86] The majority of these medications target T-cell processes to curb ocular and systemic inflammation. Specifically, the antimetabolites affect immune cell production while calcineurin inhibitors modulate T-cell function. The alkylating agents, which cross-link DNA and prevent cell replication, have been successful in the treatment of severe, refractory ocular inflammatory diseases such as Wegener's granulomatosis-associated scleritis, but they are associated with significant side-effects, including secondary malignancies (e.g., bladder carcinoma in patients on cyclophosphamide) and opportunistic infections.

Recently, more specific biologic agents targeting soluble cytokine mediators and their receptors have been used to target specific arms of the immune response (e.g., TNF-α antagonists, anti-IL-2 receptor daclizumab) (Box 79.3). Currently, three available TNF-α antagonists are infliximab,

daclizumab was able to prevent the expression of sight-threatening inflammatory disease in 8 of 10 patients treated over 1 year.[98] The etiologies of uveitis treated in this study included a number of Th1-mediated conditions, including sarcoidosis, VKH, idiopathic intermediate uveitis, and multifocal choroiditis.

While these biologic therapies have demonstrated efficacy for a variety of uveitic conditions, our increasing understanding of the pathogenic immunologic pathways mediating ocular inflammation will likely result in more targeted therapies against specific uveitic disease processes.

Conclusion

As we continue to reach a better understanding of the pathogenic mechanisms underlying uveitis, the number of therapeutic alternatives will likely continue to expand for the benefit of our patients. While immunogenetics may predispose certain individuals to the development of ocular inflammatory disease, a myriad of posttranscriptional factors are undoubtedly at play. Experimental models of uveitis including EAU have played an important role in our understanding of uveitis; other disease-specific models of uveitis will likely aid in the development of therapy for known targets. Knowledge of immune cell interactions, including Th1/Th2, Th17, regulatory T cells, NK cells, cytokines, chemokines, growth factors, and cellular adhesion molecules, will allow us to design therapies to disrupt pathogenic interactions in the future. In addition, we have learned that disruption of central or peripheral tolerance may lead to autoimmune consequences; the re-establishment of peripheral tolerance to self-reactive T-cell clones is a therapeutic avenue that requires further study. A number of biologic agents targeting cytokines, cytokine receptors, and other soluble mediators of inflammation (e.g., daclizumab, infliximab, adalimumab, anakinra) have been utilized for the successful treatment of uveitis. Their efficacy in specific inflammatory diseases and their long-term side-effect profiles surely warrant further investigation, but this class of medications appears to be promising for the treatment of ocular inflammatory disease.

adalimumab, and etanercept. Infliximab has demonstrated efficacy in the treatment of a number of uveitic conditions including Behçet's disease,[87,88] HLA-B27-associated uveitis,[89] juvenile idiopathic arthritis-associated uveitis,[90] and other forms of pediatric uveitis.[91] Adalimumab has similarly demonstrated efficacy in the treatment of pediatric uveitis and Behçet's disease.[92,93] Etanercept, however, has shown limited efficacy in the treatment of uveitis when compared with infliximab[94] and has reportedly been associated with uveitis exacerbations in some cases.[95]

Daclizumab, a humanized monoclonal antibody targeting the IL-2 receptor found on activated T cells, has been previously used for the successful prevention of renal allograft rejection[96] and for the treatment of subsets of T-cell leukemia/lymphoma, which express high levels of IL-2 receptor.[97] Several prospective studies[98,99] and retrospective reviews[100,101] have also reported the efficacy of daclizumab as a corticosteroid-sparing agent in patients with intermediate, posterior, and panuveitis. In one prospective study,

Key references

A complete list of chapter references is available online at www.expertconsult.com. See inside cover for registration details.

1. Boyd SR, Young S, Lightman S. Immunopathology of the noninfectious posterior and intermediate uveitides. Surv Ophthalmol 2001;46:209–233.
2. Whitcup SM, Nussenblatt RB. Immunologic mechanisms of uveitis. New targets for immunomodulation. Arch Ophthalmol 1997;115:520–525.
3. Jabs DA, Nussenblatt RB, Rosenbaum JT. Standardization of Uveitis Nomenclature (SUN) working group. Standardization of uveitis nomenclature for reporting clinical data. Results of the First International Workshop. Am J Ophthalmol 2005;140:509–516.
5. Chan CC, Wetzig RP, Palestine AG, et al. Immunohistopathology of ocular sarcoidosis. Report of a case and discussion of immunopathogenesis. Arch Ophthalmol 1987;105:1398–1402.
20. Martin TM, Rosenbaum JT. Genetics in uveitis. Int Ophthalmol Clin 2005;45:15–30.
23. Nussenblatt RB, Mittal KK, Ryan S, et al. Birdshot retinochoroidopathy associated with HLA-A29 antigen and immune responsiveness to retinal S-antigen. Am J Ophthalmol 1982;94:147–158.
32. Li Z, Liu B, Maminishkis A, et al. Gene expression profiling of autoimmune noninfectious uveitis disease. J Immunol 2008;181:5147–5157.
34. Miceli-Richard C, Lesage S, Rybojad M, et al. CARD15 mutations in Blau syndrome. Nat Genet 2001;29:19–20.
40. Sugita S, Takase H, Taguchi C, et al. Ocular infiltrating CD4+ T cells from patients with Vogt–Koyanagi–Harada

disease recognize human melanocyte antigens. Invest Ophthalmol Vis Sci 2006;47:2547–2554.

44. Amadi-Obi A, Yu CR, Liu X, et al. TH17 cells contribute to uveitis and scleritis and are expanded by IL-2 and inhibited by IL-27/STAT1. Nat Med 2007;13:711–718.

47. Silver PB, Agarwal RK, Su SB, et al. Hydrodynamic vaccination with DNA encoding an immunologically privileged retinal antigen protects from autoimmunity through induction of

regulatory T cells. J Immunol 2007;179:5146–5158.

55. Foxman EF, Zhang M, Hurst SD, et al. Inflammatory mediators in uveitis: differential induction of cytokines and chemokines in Th1- versus Th2-mediated ocular inflammation. J Immunol 2002;168:2483–2492.

70. Fine HF, Baffi J, Reed GF, et al. Aqueous humor and plasma vascular endothelial growth factor in uveitis-associated cystoid macular edema. Am J Ophthalmol 2001;132:794–796.

86. Jabs DA, Rosenbaum JT, Foster CS, et al. Guidelines for the use of immunosuppressive drugs in patients with ocular inflammatory disorders: recommendations of an expert panel. Am J Ophthalmol 2000;130:492–513.

94. Galor A, Perez VL, Hammel JP, et al. Differential effectiveness of etanercept and infliximab in the treatment of ocular inflammation. Ophthalmology 2006;113:2317–2323.

CHAPTER 80

Herpesvirus retinitis

Sally S Atherton and Mei Zheng

Clinical background

Acute retinal necrosis (ARN), which was first reported by Urayama and colleagues, occurs rarely but is a potentially blinding disorder.[1] Most cases of ARN are unilateral, although approximately one-third of patients develop bilateral disease which may occur either coincident with involvement of the presenting eye, or weeks, months, or years later.[2] ARN is observed most commonly in the immunocompetent host but occasionally occurs when there is immunocompromise. Although varicella-zoster virus (VZV) was associated with the initial description of ARN, subsequently herpes simplex virus (HSV) type 1 (HSV-1), HSV type 2 (HSV-2), Epstein–Barr virus (EBV), and, very rarely, cytomegalovirus (CMV) were also implicated in its pathogenesis (Box 80.1).[3-8] A member of the herpesvirus family is presumed to be the pathogenic agent in cases in which a close (usually) temporal relationship between clinical herpetic infection and the onset of the retinal infection is observed.

Patients with herpesvirus retinitis will commonly present with blurred vision caused by inflammatory debris in the vitreous humor. Some patients may also have ocular pain which is indicative of inflammation of the anterior segment of the eye. HSV retinitis is characterized by marked retinal edema, exudate, hemorrhage, and vascular occlusion (Figures 80.1 and 80.2). The disease may start in the posterior pole, equator, or periphery and is commonly associated with swelling of the optic disc and rhegmatogenous retinal detachment that usually occurs after a period of several weeks.[9] Unless recognized quickly, retinitis may progress to ARN.

As defined by the American Uveitis Society (AUS), the features of ARN are not disease-specific or immune status-specific but are rather determined by the clinical characteristics of the disease and its course. These features include: (1) one or more discrete foci of necrosis in the periphery of the retina; (2) rapid progression in the absence of treatment; (3) circumferential spread; (4) occlusive arteriolar vasculopathy; and (5) inflammation in the anterior chamber and/or in the vitreous (Box 80.2). Additional features may include optic neuropathy, scleritis, and pain.[10] ARN is commonly seen in those with normal to mildly depressed immune status. Another syndrome involving herpesvirus infection of the retina is progressive outer retinal necrosis (PORN), which is characterized by decreased vision, floaters, and loss of peripheral vision. However, in contrast to ARN, there are cottonwool spots and multifocal areas of retinal whitening with confluent necrosis are observed, but retinal vasculitis and intraretinal hemorrhages are rare. PORN is usually observed in patients with moderate-to-severe immunosuppression, such as those with acquired immunodeficiency syndrome (AIDS).[11] The original definition of ARN included the requirement that patients be immunocompetent; however, as noted above, the immune status of the patient is not an important clinical criterion, so ARN may also be observed in immunosuppressed patients.

ARN is rare. A study to assess the incidence of ARN in the UK revealed an incidence of approximately 1 case per 1.6–2.0 million people per year (Box 80.3).[12] Because of the small number of individuals who develop ARN, large-scale genetic studies to determine whether there are genetic predilections toward ARN have not been done. However, in a study of 27 patients with ARN, the frequency of the HLA-DQw7 antigen was significantly increased in ARN patients compared with controls (55% versus 19%) and the BW62, DR4 was also more common in ARN patients (16% versus 2.6%).[13] In another study, HLA-DR9 was associated with more severe ARN and 50% of the patients with fulminant ARN had the HLA-DR9 genotypes compared with none of the patients with milder disease.[14] It has also been suggested that impaired control of latent HSV-1 is attributable to defects in the ability of plasmacytoid dendritic cells to produce type 1 interferons in response to herpesvirus infection.[15] Therefore, in addition to the possibility of increased risk of ARN in patients with certain HLA phenotypes, other non-HLA-associated factors such as the ability of certain cells to produce interferon may also play a role in predisposition to development of ARN and/or its severity.

There appears to be a difference in age distribution between ARN caused by HSV-1 or VZV and ARN caused by HSV-2, but this distribution is not absolute. A review of 28 patients (30 eyes) with ARN suggested that patients with ARN resulting from HSV-1 or VZV are usually older (median age 47 and 57 years, respectively) whereas those patients with ARN resulting from HSV-2 are often younger (median age, 20 years). ARN is occasionally observed in patients coincident with or following encephalitis or meningitis; in the former, ARN is usually due to HSV-1 while in the latter, ARN is usually caused by HSV-2.[5,16,17]

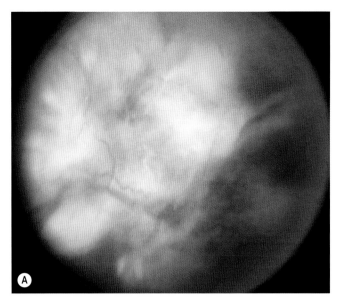 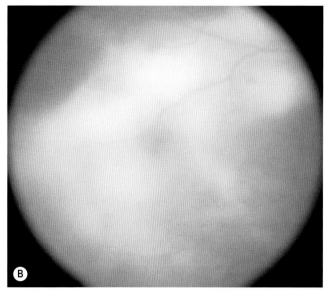

Figure 80.1 Fundus photographs of acute retinal necrosis in a human patient showing active necrosis, hemorrhage, and an area of scarring (A) and a retinal vessel in an area of necrosis (B). (Courtesy of the Department of Ophthalmology, Medical College of Georgia, Augusta, Georgia.)

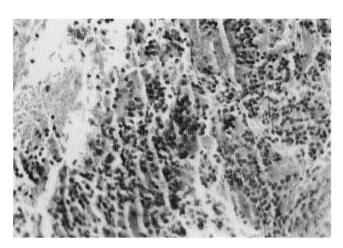

Figure 80.2 Photomicrograph of hematoxylin and eosin-stained section of a retinal biopsy from a human patient with acute retinal necrosis. There is loss of the retinal architecture and extensive inflammation. (Courtesy of the Department of Ophthalmology, Medical College of Georgia, Augusta, Georgia.)

Box 80.2 Clinical characteristics of acute retinal necrosis

- Characteristics are defined clinically, not disease- or immune status-specific
- One or more discrete foci of necrosis in the periphery of the retina
- Rapid progression in the absence of treatment
- Circumferential spread
- Occlusive arteriolar vasculopathy
- Inflammation in the anterior chamber and/or in the vitreous
- Optic neuropathy, scleritis, and pain may also be present

Box 80.3 Patient-specific factors in development of acute retinal necrosis

- Human leukocyte antigen (HLA) type
- Ability to produce type 1 interferons in response to infection
- Age
- Prior infection
- Triggering event (trauma, surgery, corticosteroid treatment, others?)

Box 80.1 Causes of acute retinal necrosis

- Varicella-zoster virus (VZV) – most common
- Herpes simplex virus type 1 (HSV-1)
- Herpes simplex virus type 2 (HSV-2)
- Epstein–Barr virus (EBV)
- Cytomegalovirus (CMV) – rarely in immunocompetent patients

Diagnosis

The diagnosis of viral retinitis depends on the ocular and systemic manifestations as well as the clinical examination of the fundus of the eye. While comparison of local and systemic antiviral antibody titers as well as virus isolation have been used to diagnose the disease, the current standard for diagnosis of viral infection of the retina is polymerase chain reaction (PCR) of aqueous humor and/or vitreous samples to detect viral DNA.[18,19] PCR is exquisitely sensitive and specific; for example, the sensitivity and specificity of PCR for diagnosis of VZV infection are 100% and 97%, respectively.[20]

A number of diseases may result in retinitis and, even if viral, not all of these diseases are caused by a member of the herpesvirus family.[21,22] The differential diagnosis of herpesvirus retinitis should include Behçet's disease, CMV retinitis, HSV-1 and 2 retinitis, lymphocytic choriomeningitis virus

Box 80.4 Differential diagnosis of acute retinal necrosis

- Varicella-zoster virus retinitis
- Herpes simplex virus type 1 retinitis
- Herpes simplex virus type 2 retinitis
- Epstein–Barr virus retinitis
- Cytomegalovirus retinitis
- Behçet's disease
- Lymphocytic choriomeningitis virus retinitis
- Primary intraocular lymphoma
- Sarcoidosis
- Syphilis
- Toxoplasmosis

retinitis, primary intraocular lymphoma, sarcoidosis, syphilis, toxoplasmosis, and VZV-induced retinitis (Box 80.4). In infants with apparent congenital chorioretinitis, the diagnostic workup should include lymphocytic choriomeningitis virus serology, especially if antibody titers for *Toxoplasma gondii*, rubella virus, CMV, and HSV are negative.[23]

Treatment

The usual treatment of ARN is intravenous aciclovir, corticosteroids, and aspirin, followed by oral aciclovir. Intravitreal injections of foscarnet and oral aciclovir have been used in mild cases that have been detected early. VZV has also been successfully treated with brivudine (not currently available in the USA) and valganciclovir.[24–26] In general, retinal necrosis which progresses rapidly to the posterior pole is associated with a poor visual outcome. Eyes with less than grade II necrosis extension are good candidates for prophylactic peripheral retinal photocoagulation. Not surprisingly, early detection, prompt treatment with aciclovir, and rapid repair of retinal detachments seem to improve the final visual outcome.[27] The issue of long-term prophylactic antiviral therapy to prevent ARN in an uninvolved fellow eye or to prevent ARN in a patient with a history of meningitis or encephalitis caused by a member of the herpesvirus family has not been resolved.[28] However, since there is currently no way to predict who among patients with unilateral ARN will develop ARN in the fellow eye, long-term prophylactic antiviral therapy appears to be warranted.

If the diagnosis of ARN is not made quickly or if appropriate antiviral and anti-inflammatory therapies are delayed, retinitis caused by any of the three neurotropic herpesviruses (i.e., HSV-1, HSV-2, VZV) will usually progress quickly to ARN. Therefore, the prognosis for many patients with herpesvirus infections of the retina is poor because of the rapid and destructive nature of the disease.[29] Although there are several antiviral agents that can be administered intravenously, intraocularly, and/or orally, many patients still experience significant vision loss because of optic neuritis, necrosis of the retina in or near the macula, or rhegmatogenous retinal detachment.[30,31] Therefore, preventing/reducing vision loss in patients with ARN requires early detection (usually by PCR of aqueous or vitreous samples) and prompt treatment with the appropriate therapeutic regimen.

Pathology

The characteristics of ARN are focal, well-demarcated areas of retinal necrosis in the peripheral retina, circumferential progression of necrosis (which occurs rapidly in the absence of antiviral therapy), occlusive vasculopathy, and inflammation in both the anterior chamber and the vitreous humor. Optic neuritis and late retinal detachments are also observed in association with the disease, and, as noted above, even with treatment, severe visual impairment and/or blindness may result.[5,29]

Etiology

Although bacteria, fungi, and parasites may all infect the posterior segment of the eye, members of the herpesvirus family are among the most common causes of infection involving the eye. The ubiquitous nature of the human herpesviruses together with the permissiveness in the human neuronal system for herpesvirus infection and transmission have conspired to make several of the herpesviruses the most common agents of chorioretinitis. Five of the eight members of the human herpesvirus family have the ability to cause retinitis. The first herpesvirus virus to be identified as a cause of ARN was VZV, and this virus remains the most common cause of ARN (accounting for 50–80% of cases) followed by HSV-1 and HSV-2. Rare cases of ARN caused by EBV and CMV (in immunocompetent patients) have been reported. However, given the ubiquitous nature of the human herpesviruses and the constant development of increasingly sensitive identification methodology, perhaps it would not be too surprising if other members of the herpesviruses are also identified as causative agents of retinal infections.

In infants, herpes simplex retinitis can result from congenital infection or from acute infection acquired during passage through an infected birth canal. Congenital HSV retinitis is defined as disease transmitted during gestation, before initiation of labor and delivery. In most cases of congenital HSV retinitis, the mothers have a history of newly acquired genital herpes infection which usually occurs during the second trimester.[32] Active genital infection in the mothers at delivery is extremely rare compared with the neonatal acquired herpes retinitis, but sometimes it is difficult to differentiate congenital HSV retinitis from neonatally acquired HSV retinitis. Neonatal ocular infection with HSV is usually bilateral and is observed in infants from 2 days to several weeks of age; however, retinal findings may not be apparent until 3 weeks of age or after. Most cases of neonatal HSV retinitis occur concomitantly with HSV infection of the central nervous system (CNS) with only about 20% of cases of HSV retinitis associated with HSV conjunctivitis, keratitis, or disseminated dermatitis. ARN has also been described in children, and HSV-2 is the most common cause of ARN in children.

In adults, herpesvirus retinitis may result from acute virus infection or from reactivation of latent virus. A history of neonatal herpes infection is a risk factor for HSV-2 retinitis, as is a history of viral meningitis. The fact that HSV-2 retinitis has been observed following triggering events such as neurosurgery, periocular trauma, and administration of high-dose corticosteroids supports the idea that, at least for HSV-2 retinitis, most cases in adults are due to reactivation rather than acute infection.

In summary, ARN is most commonly caused by VZV, followed by HSV-1 and HSV-2 with only rare cases of ARN attributable to EBV or to CMV. Management of patients with ARN should include prompt diagnosis as well as prompt initiation of appropriate antiviral therapy. Prophylactic laser barrier treatment has been shown to lower the incidence of retinal detachment and administration of systemic corticosteroids (in addition to antiviral therapy) helps to limit damage caused by the severe inflammation associated with ARN. Retinal detachment may occur acutely or several months after onset of symptoms; vitrectomy and prompt repair of retinal detachments may result in improved acuity.

Pathophysiology

The pathogenesis of ARN in humans remains unclear but, as with most viral infections in immunocompetent hosts, is likely to result from a combination of virus replication and factors of both the innate and adaptive immune responses. Uncertainty about the pathogenesis in humans is mainly because of the very few samples available for study and because many of the samples that have been available for study represent only the end-stage of the disease with little evidence of active viral replication and considerable amounts of necrotic/scarred retinal tissue. Furthermore, most of the clinical reports of ARN are focused on the etiology of the infection and the clinical presentation in order to guide treatment, rather than on the pathogenesis of the disease. Another drawback to deciphering the pathogenesis of ARN in human patients is that, in most cases, sequential samples of ocular fluids or of retina tissues are not available and extensive testing at nonocular sites is not usually performed (for example, imaging studies of the CNS).

Route of infection

There are three possible routes by which virus might enter the retina: (1) hematogenously; (2) direct spread from an infected anterior segment of the eye to the posterior segment; and (3) spread from the CNS to the retina. If the blood–retinal barrier is breached, free virus in the circulation (or circulating virus-infected cells) might enter and infect the retina. Since one phase of VZV infection involves systemic spread of the virus, this might occur in patients with VZV ARN. However, since HSV-1 and HSV-2 do not usually spread via the hematogenous route, hematogenous spread of these viruses to the retina appears to be unlikely. Since many patients with retinitis also have anterior uveitis, direct spread of virus from the front of the eye to the back of the eye is a possibility. However, even though ARN is caused by the same members of the herpesvirus family that also cause keratitis, association of herpetic keratitis/herpes uveitis with ARN syndrome in one eye is uncommon and there have been few reports of herpes keratitis immediately antecedent or coincident to ARN.

Although the route by which HSV spreads to the retina to cause ARN in human patients has not been elucidated, reports of encephalitis or meningitis preceding symptoms of ARN in some human patients suggest that, at least in some cases, the virus spreads from the brain to the eye.[30,31] The observation that several patients with ARN had optic neuropathy coincident with or immediately preceding their infection further suggests that, in humans, one route by which the neurotropic herpesviruses reach the retina is via the optic nerve.

Therefore with the caveat that animal models of disease generally do not have 100% fidelity to their human counterpart, animal models may provide a way to gain insight into the pathogenesis of ARN caused by the neurotropic herpesviruses. Acute retinitis which evolves to ARN that shares some clinical and histopathologic similarities with ARN in humans is observed in rabbits and euthymic mice following uniocular anterior-chamber inoculation of HSV-1.[33,34] In the mouse model, the retina of the uninoculated contralateral eye is virus-infected, and acute retinitis that progresses to necrosis is observed beginning around 7 days postinoculation and continuing thereafter (Figure 80.3). Although the route by which viruses gain access to the body may differ in animal models (HSV is injected to the anterior chamber of one eye) from those of human patients (skin, eye infection, encephalitis, meningitis, pharyngitis), the outcome is similar retinal pathology in both animal model and human patients.

Although virus tracing experiments cannot be performed in humans, a variety of methods can be used to trace the route of spread of neurotropic virus in animals. Using a LacZ-containing recombinant of HSV-1, Vann and Atherton showed that, in the mouse model of ARN, virus spreads from the anterior chamber of the injected eye to the retina of the uninoculated eye via synaptically connected neurons.[35] Sequentially, this pathway involves the ipsilateral ciliary ganglion (day 2 postinoculation), the ipsilateral Edinger–Westphal nucleus (day 3 postinoculation), the ipsilateral suprachiasmatic nucleus (SCN) (day 5 postinoculation), and the contralateral optic nerve and retina (on and after day 6–7 postinoculation). Paradoxically, although the anterior segment of the injected eye is virus-infected and there is extensive inflammation, in immunocompetent mice, the retina of the injected eye does not become virus-infected. Also, although the contralateral SCN becomes infected with virus on day 7 postinoculation, virus does not spread from this site to infect the optic nerve and retina of the ipsilateral injected eye, suggesting that virus cannot spread to the retina of the injected eye either directly or indirectly (by retrograde spread from the CNS).

Role of the immune cells

In addition to identification of sites of virus infection and of sequential spread, a number of factors have been identified that play a role in the pathogenesis of the disease in the mouse that may be applicable to increasing our understanding of the infectious process in humans. In the mouse, virus does not spread directly from the anterior segment to the retina and in humans, direct spread from an infected anterior segment to the posterior segment is observed rarely, if at all. While the reason for this is not immediately apparent, especially since there is not a physical anatomic barrier to prevent such spread, studies using the mouse suggest that the early responders of the innate immune system (includ-

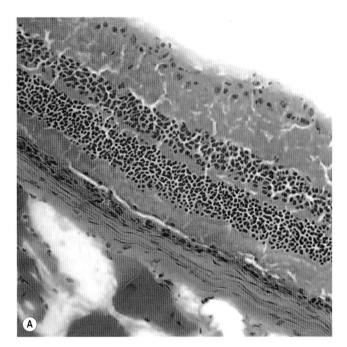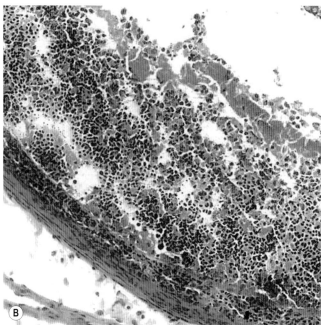

Figure 80.3 Photomicrographs of hematoxylin and eosin-stained sections of the retina of a normal mouse (A) and of a mouse with acute retinal necrosis following uniocular anterior-chamber inoculation of herpes simplex virus type 1 (B). The architecture of the retina with acute retinal necrosis is disorganized; there is extensive inflammation in the retina and choroid and debris from retinal cells.

ing natural killer (NK) cells and polymorphonuclear leukocytes (PMN)) participate in limiting direct virus spread and, by extension, perhaps also in limiting virus replication.

NK cells have been identified in the aqueous of an ARN patient.[36] In the mouse, NK cell activity is increased in the virus-infected eye compared with mock injected controls and depletion of NK cells correlates with spread of HSV-1 from the infected anterior segment to the retina.[37] Additional studies in the mouse in which PMNs were depleted by treatment with Gr-1 antibody (specific for PMN) indicate that PMNs also play a role.[38] The mechanism by which these cells either separately or together with NK cells (since NK cells are not depleted by Gr-1 antibody treatment) limit virus spread from the anterior segment of the eye to the posterior segment are currently being investigated and preliminary studies suggest that interferons are likely to be involved.

While limitation of virus spread from the anterior to the posterior part of the eye appears to be due to modulators of the innate immune response, results from studies using the mouse model together with those from human patients suggest that the contributors to destruction of a virus-infected retina are more complicated. Replicating virus is almost certainly required. In sequential studies in the mouse, a direct correlation was observed between the amount of virus and the extent of retinal destruction.[39] However, since the pace of retinal destruction proceeds more slowly in athymic or in T-cell-depleted mice, it is likely that T cells along with other components of the innate and adaptive immune responses contribute to the process in mice and by extrapolation, most likely in humans.[40]

Involvement of T cells in human patients with ARN is supported by the studies of Verjans and colleagues who reported that intraocular T cells of patients with HSV-induced ARN recognize HSV tegument proteins VP11/12 and VP13/14.[41] However, although T cells may play a cytotoxic role and kill virus-infected retinal cells, they may also be protective and their presence may explain why so few of the many individuals who are seropositive for one or more of the neurotropic herpesviruses (HSV-1, HSV-2, VZV) develop ARN. In the mouse model of ARN, T cells play a role in limiting virus spread in the CNS and both CD4+and CD8+ T cells have been implicated in the prevention of retrograde virus spread from the contralateral SCN of the hypothalamus into the optic nerve and retina of the injected eye.[42] Furthermore, the presence of T cells in the contralateral SCN correlates with protection of the ipsilateral retina.[43] However, how T cells limit virus in the CNS and perhaps within the eye remains to be elucidated.

In addition to T cells, studies using the mouse model indicate that macrophages may also play a role in the pathogenesis of virus infection after uniocular anterior chamber or intravitreal inoculation.[44,45] Systemic depletion of microphages by treatment with clodronate-containing liposomes correlated with increased titers of virus in the SCN following anterior-chamber inoculation of HSV-1. When the levels of tumor necrosis factor-α (TNF-α), a product of macrophages, were measured, the amount of TNF-α was significantly reduced in the SCN of macrophage-depleted mice. However, while these results implicate macrophages and TNF-α in protection, the mechanism by which such protection occurs has not been determined. Moreover, merely increasing the amount of TNF-α at sites of virus infection was not protective. When mice were infected with a recombinant of HSV-1 that produces TNF-α constitutively, neither the timing of virus spread nor the path of virus spread from the injected eye to the contralateral optic nerve and retina was affected. However, in the uninoculated eye, the titer of virus was significantly higher and the speed of retinal destruction was more rapid.[46] Thus, production of TNF-α and infiltration of macrophages seem to play an important role in limiting virus spread and/or virus replication in the CNS but whether the role of TNF-α during virus infection is protective, destructive, or both remains to be determined.

The response of different types of cells to virus infection is just beginning to be studied. For example, Toll-like receptors (TLR), an important component of the innate immune response to many pathogens, function by activation of NF-κB followed by production of proinflammatory cytokines.[47] Expression of TLRs in the retina of the uninoculated eye in response to virus infection is dynamic and different TLRs are expressed on retinal cells at different times during the course of the infection. For example, expression of TLR3 is increased in the retina of the uninoculated eye shortly before the onset of acute retinitis and decreases gradually during the course of the infection. TLR7 increases steadily during the course of the infection, while TLR9 is maximal at the peak of the acute disease coincident with the highest titers of virus (Zheng and Atherton, unpublished data). Such temporal expression suggests that TLRs are involved in the infectious process but the mechanism of their involvement is not understood.

Since many cases of ARN in human patients result from infection from reactivated virus, these individuals will have virus-specific immune cells, including memory T cells as well as antibody to the virus (Box 80.5). The role of antiviral antibody in ARN has not been explored but such antibody could facilitate destruction of the virus-infected retinal cells by antibody-dependent cellular cytotoxicity or it could help to limit virus by neutralizing extracellular virus.

Following uniocular anterior-chamber injection of HSV-1, mice develop anterior-chamber associated immune deviation which is characterized by downregulation of virus-specific delayed-type hypersensitivity with preservation of virus-specific antibody responsiveness.[48] Results of studies by Kezuka and colleagues have suggested that a similar downregulation of VZV-specific T-cell immunity occurs in some ARN patients.[49,50] Therefore, it may be postulated that a failure of T-cell immunity to control virus spread from a site of virus reactivation into neurons synaptically connected to the optic nerve and retina, and/or within the retina may play a role in the pathogenesis of ARN.

Box 80.5 Contributors to the pathogenesis of acute retinal necrosis

- Spread of virus from a primary or reactivated infection into the eye
- Virus replication in the retina
- Cells of the innate immune response (natural killer cells, macrophages, polymorphonuclear leukocytes), cytokine production, upregulation of Toll-like receptors on ocular cells in response to infection (?)
- Virus-specific cytotoxic T cells
- Induction of anterior-chamber-associated immune deviation (ACAID)
- Role of antiviral antibody (in latently infected individuals) unknown

---

Summary

Observations and laboratory studies of human patients together with virologic and immunologic studies using the mouse model underscore the idea that the pathogenesis of ARN caused by neurotropic members of the herpesvirus family is complex. While virus infection must occur, the roles of virus type-specific factors and of viral genetics have not yet been investigated. It is likely that both innate and adaptive immune responses play a role in the destruction of virus-infected retinal cells. However, irrespective of how these factors contribute, given the usually poor visual outcome in human patients with ARN, the most important question to be addressed is whether there are specific parameters that can be used to predict who among the very large number of individuals who are seropositive for one or more of the neurotropic herpesviruses is at the highest risk of developing viral retinitis and ARN and to monitor and treat these individuals appropriately. Until this question is answered, early identification of the infection along with prompt initiation of antiviral therapy remain the best options for preservation of sight.

Key references

A complete list of chapter references is available online at www.expertconsult.com. See inside cover for registration details.

1. Urayama A, Yamada N, Sasaki T, et al. Unilateral acute uveitis with retinal periarteritis and detachment. Jpn J Clin Ophthalmol 1971;25:607–619.

10. Holland GN. Standard diagnostic criteria for the acute retinal necrosis syndrome. Executive Committee of the American Uveitis Society. Am J Ophthalmol 1994;117:663–667.

11. Holland GN. The progressive outer retinal necrosis syndrome. Int Ophthalmol 1994;18:163–165.

13. Holland GN, Cornell PJ, Park MS, et al. An association between acute retinal necrosis syndrome and HLA-DQw7 and phenotype Bw62, DR4. Am J Ophthalmol 1989;108:370–374.

15. Kittan NA, Bergua A, Haupt S, et al. Impaired plasmacytoid dendritic cell innate immune responses in patients with herpes virus-associated acute retinal necrosis. J Immunol 2007;179:4219–4230.

20. Knox CM, Chandler D, Short GA, et al. Polymerase chain reaction-based assays of vitreous samples for the diagnosis of viral retinitis. Use in diagnostic dilemmas. Ophthalmology 1998;105:37–44.

23. Balansard B, Bodaghi B, Cassoux N, et al. Necrotising retinopathies simulating acute retinal necrosis syndrome. Br J Ophthalmol 2005;89:96–101.

25. Aizman A, Johnson MW, Elner SG. Treatment of acute retinal necrosis

syndrome with oral antiviral medications. Ophthalmology 2007;114:307–312.

28. Cordero-Coma M, Anzaar F, Yilmaz T, et al. Herpetic retinitis. Herpes 2007;14:4–10.

33. Whittum JA, McCulley JP, Niederkorn JY, et al. Ocular disease induced in mice by anterior chamber inoculation of herpes simplex virus. Invest Ophthalmol Vis Sci 1984;25:1065–1073.

35. Vann VR, Atherton SS. Neural spread of herpes simplex virus after anterior chamber inoculation. Invest Ophthalmol Vis Sci 1991;32:2462–2472.

41. Verjans GM, Feron EJ, Dings ME, et al. T cells specific for the triggering virus infiltrate the eye in patients with herpes simplex virus-mediated acute retinal necrosis. J Infect Dis 1998;178:27–33.

49. Kezuka T, Sakai J, Minoda H, et al. A relationship between varicella-zoster virus-specific delayed hypersensitivity and varicella-zoster virus-induced anterior uveitis. Arch Ophthalmol 2002;120:1183–1188.

CHAPTER 81

Sympathetic ophthalmia

Mirunalini Kumaradas and Narsing A Rao

Clinical background

Sympathetic ophthalmia (SO) is a rare intraocular inflammation that presents as a bilateral diffuse granulomatous uveitis following penetrating trauma or ocular surgery involving one eye. Following trauma to one globe (the exciting eye), intraocular inflammation develops in the fellow eye (the sympathizing eye) after a variable period of time ranging from a few days to decades. Although the pathophysiology of this disease is not clearly understood, an autoimmune process against peptides of melanocytes has been proposed. In 1830 Mackenzie gave a detailed clinical description of SO,[1] and Fuchs established the pathological features of this disease in 1905.[2]

SO is a potentially devastating disease with many exacerbations, and long-term follow-up is essential. A high index of suspicion, early diagnosis, advances in surgical procedures, and the use of immunomodulatory agents have improved the visual outcome of SO.

Symptoms and signs

SO can present with diverse clinical presentations, and any bilateral uveitis following ocular surgery or trauma to an eye should alert the ophthalmologist to the possibility of this entity.

The onset of inflammation in the sympathizing eye has been reported to appear any time between 5 days and 66 years after the initial trauma.[1,3] However, 80% of patients manifest with symptoms and signs of intraocular inflammation within 3 months, and 90% show evidence of inflammation within 1 year of the time of the initial insult.[1]

Patients usually present with mild ocular pain, photophobia, epiphora, and blurring of vision. Their near vision may sometimes be compromised. The clinical signs may vary from a mild anterior uveitis to severe granulomatous panuveitis associated with moderate to severe vitritis.

Posterior-segment findings include papillitis, generalized retinal edema, and diffuse choroiditis. Small yellow-white lesions may be seen in the mid periphery of the retina and these are recognized as Dalen–Fuchs nodules (Box 81.1). The fundus examination might also show evidence of multiple choroidal granulomas and exudative retinal detachment. Although patients with SO develop signs of panuveitis, they may initially present with clinical features of posterior uveitis in the sympathizing eye.

Inadequately treated SO will run a complicated course of chronic recurrent uveitis. This, in turn, could cause secondary glaucoma, cataract, choroidal neovascularization, subretinal fibrosis, chorioretinal and optic atropy, and finally phthisis bulbi.

Historical development

Duke-Elder and Perkins state that the first reference in the literature to the concept of SO is from Agathias in the anthology compiled from Constantius Cephalis in 1000 AD.[1] Though many references to this disease entity were reported during the seventeenth and eighteenth centuries, the first comprehensive description of SO was written by William Mackenzie in 1830. He described many cases of SO and concluded with a complete discussion of this entity. Prichard, in 1851, was the first to practice enucleation of the injured eye as a therapeutic measure to save the opposite eye. But Critchett, in 1863, showed that enucleation was ineffective once the inflammation develops in the sympathizing eye. Knowledge of SO further increased after Schirmer's (1905) critical survey and Fuchs' (1905) classical histological studies of this disease.

Epidemiology

There is a disparity in the reported incidence of SO, and the reliability of the reported figures is questionable because the suspected diagnosis was confirmed histopathologically in less than one-third of cases and 15% of the pathologically diagnosed cases were not identified clinically.[4] Liddy and Stuart estimated the incidence of SO as 0.19% following penetrating injuries and 0.007% following ocular surgery.[5] In 2000 Kilmartin et al estimated an incidence of 0.03/100 000 for the general population of the UK.[6]

Although SO was once considered a disappearing disease, recent incidence figures, particularly for postsurgical cases, suggest an increasing trend. Advances in surgical training and the use of microsurgical instrumentation have enabled better management of traumatized eyes that would other-

---

Box 81.1 Posterior-segment findings in sympathetic ophthalmia

- Vitritis
- Papillitis
- Choroiditis
- Exudative retinal detachment
- Dalen–Fuchs nodules

Box 81.2 Differential diagnosis of sympathetic ophthalmia

- Vogt–Koyanagi–Harada disease
- Phacoanaphylaxis
- Sarcoidosis
- Posterior scleritis
- Uveal lymphoid infiltration

---

wise have been enucleated in the past. In 1982, Gass reported an incidence of 0.06% after vitrectomy and 0.01% incidence when vitrectomy was the only operative procedure causing the penetrating wound.[7]

Chan et al, in their retrospective study from 1982 to 1992, reported that 28% of patients with SO developed it following intraocular surgical procedures.[8] Kilmartin et al reported in 2000 that ocular surgery, especially retinal surgery, accounted for 56% of all cases of SO.[6] A report by Su and Chee stated that the proportion of SO caused by ocular surgery is 70%.[9] All of these studies indicate that ocular surgery as a precipitating factor is gaining importance.

Previous studies indicate that SO is more prevalent in males and in children.[2,10] But recent reports show no gender predominance and a smaller number of cases occurring in children.[6] Elderly patients appear to be at an increased risk, probably because of the increased frequency in ocular surgery performed in this age group.[6]

Diagnostic workup

The clinical diagnosis of SO is based on history and clinical examination. There are no specific laboratory studies to establish the diagnosis. However, fluorescein angiography (FA) and indocyanine green (ICG) angiography are helpful in supporting the diagnosis.

The characteristic features of SO as seen on FA are multiple tiny foci of leakage at the level of retinal pigment epithelium (RPE) with late coalescence if there are areas of exudative detachment. Another, less common, angiographic appearance is similar to that seen in acute posterior multifocal placoid pigment epitheliopathy. Here the lesions appear as early focal obscuration of background choroidal fluorescence with late staining.[11]

Since the disease predominantly involves the choroid, use of ICG could help support the diagnosis of SO.[12] Two ICG patterns have been observed. In the first type, the hypofluorescent dark dot appearing during the intermediate phase persisted throughout the late phase; in the second type, the dots faded away during late phase. The first pattern was thought to represent chorioretinal atropic areas, and the second was thought to correspond to active choroidal space-occupying lesions. Hence, some believe that ICG provides additional information about choroidal involvement and subsequent evolution of the lesion.[12] However, the enucleated SO globes reveal no histopathologic evidence of chorioretinal atropy. Moreover, the retina is typically spared from the inflammatory cell infiltration.

Ultrasound scans help to establish choroidal thickening, predominantly in the posterior choroid, and optical coherence tomography is believed to aid in monitoring the therapeutic response in patients with shallow retinal detachment.

Differential diagnosis

When considering the differential diagnosis of SO, it is important to rule out intraocular infections that could cause severe endophthalmitis. Posttraumatic iridocyclitis may also cause an inflammatory reaction, but neither endophthalmitis nor iridocyclitis involves the fellow eye.

The differential diagnosis also includes any other cause of granulomatous uveitis, especially phacoanaphylaxis, Vogt–Koyanagi–Harada disease (VKH), sarcoidosis, or posterior scleritis (Box 81.2).

Phacoanaphylaxis is a chronic granulomatous inflammation that occurs following traumatic or surgical lens capsule disruption and could closely simulate the clinical signs of SO. It typically manifests as a granulomatous anterior uveitis. The choroid, retina, and optic nerve are not usually involved in the disease process. Studies have shown that phacoanaphylaxis can coexist with SO (4–25%), and even though phacoanaphylaxis is normally a unilateral inflammation, bilateral occurrence has been reported in the absence of SO changes.[13] In such cases, the posterior choroid is not thickened with inflammatory cellular infiltration, as seen in SO, and thus, no evidence of a thickened choroid is shown by ultrasonography. In bilateral phacoanaphylaxis, the first eye involved is usually quiet by the time the inflammation begins in the second eye. In contrast, in SO the exciting eye is usually severely inflamed at the time the sympathizing eye becomes involved.

VKH disease is a bilateral, diffuse, granulomatous uveitis with clinical, histopathological, immunohistochemical, and FA manifestations that are strikingly similar to those of SO. These associations suggest that the two conditions may involve closely related antigens and similar immune mechanisms. Shindo et al reported similar genetic backgrounds in patients with SO and VKH.[14] Moorthy et al showed virtually identical histopathological changes in SO and VKH, including preservation of the choriocapillaris in acute VKH cases.[15] Both entities have been associated with headache, tinnitus, alopecia, poliosis, and vitiligo.[16] In most instances, a history of penetrating trauma would be the most helpful factor in making the diagnosis of SO.

Ocular sarcoidosis is another disease with a clinical resemblance to SO. However, systemic manifestations of sarcoidosis, if present, might help in the diagnosis. In the absence of such manifestations, the characteristic findings of SO seen in FA and ultrasound scan would help differentiate these two entities.

Both posterior scleritis and SO may present with exudative retinal detachment and disc edema. However, SO is typically a bilateral disease, whereas posterior scleritis most commonly presents as a unilateral inflammation. Although ultrasound scans may reveal diffuse choroidal thickening and exudative retinal detachment in both of these entities, choroidal thickening in posterior scleritis shows high internal reflectivity with evidence of retrobulbar edema.

Treatment

The successful control of inflammation in patients with SO depends on early and aggressive treatment with large doses of corticosteroids until the inflammation is resolved. Before the use of corticosteroids, the prognosis for SO was considered very poor. Makley and Azar reported in 1978 that patients treated with corticosteroids had a favorable visual outcome, with 64% attaining a final visual acuity of 20/60 or better.[17] Lubin et al in 1980 supported these data and demonstrated that corticosteroid therapy changed both the character and the severity of the inflammatory process.[10] In 1983, Reynard et al stated that corticosteroid therapy prevented severe visual loss.[18]

Some patients may be refractory to corticosteroid therapy or may experience unacceptable side-effects during treatment. Such patients have been shown to benefit from steroid-sparing immunosuppressive drug therapy, including methotrexate, cyclophosphamide, ciclosporin A, chlorambucil, and mycophenolate mofetil. Enucleation of the injured globe within 2 weeks of penetrating trauma is generally believed to prevent the development of SO. But with the advances in surgical techniques, many eyes once considered nonviable may have a fair prognosis and the injured eye might eventually have the better vision. Hence, the decision to perform primary enucleation should be made cautiously. Enucleation should be considered in those cases where the traumatized eye has no light perception, has a total afferent pupillary defect, and is severely disorganized, making it impossible to repair surgically. In such situations it is important to discuss with the patient the possibility of developing SO in the nontraumatized eye, and enucleation should be carried out within 2 weeks of trauma.

The advantage of enucleating the exciting eye once the disease has started in the sympathizing eye is a controversial issue. Review of the literature shows conflicting results with regard to the benefits of enucleation after the onset of inflammation. It is therefore important to try saving the injured eye, especially if any potential for useful vision exists in the exciting eye.

Prognosis and prevention

Before the use of corticosteroids, the visual prognosis of SO was generally considered to be poor. The aggressive use of corticosteroids in combination with immunosuppressive therapy has improved the visual prognosis. However, the relapsing nature of the disease demands careful long-term follow-up to prevent serious complications associated with recurrences.

It is interesting to analyze a few studies which stated prognostic factors based on histopathological findings. Lubin et al reported a direct correlation between the severity of inflammation in the exciting eye and the final visual acuity of the sympathizing eye.[10] However, Winter[19] and Reynard et al[18] observed no direct correlation.

Makley and Azar[17] reported on the long-term follow-up of patients with SO in 1978. In their series, they observed that relapses and complications such as secondary glaucoma, cataract, exudative retinal detachment, and choroidal scarring were common among patients with SO. Many patients treated with steroids retained a favorable visual acuity. The duration of such corticosteroid therapy was variable and ranged from a few months to 6 years.

The only suggested prevention for SO is early enucleation of the injured globe. In 2006, Su and Chee stated that industrial safety laws that mandate the use of personal protective equipment while working would reduce the incidence of work-related trauma and help reduce the incidence of SO.[9] Advances in surgical techniques have enabled ophthalmologists to operate successfully on severely traumatized eyes and achieve good wound closure of penetrating eye injuries. This would, in turn, prevent the escape of uveal antigen to the regional lymphatic system, thereby reducing the incidence of SO. It is also important to remember the association of SO with intraocular surgical procedures, especially in patients with a previous history of penetrating trauma or repeated surgery. Such patients should be closely monitored, and appropriate levels of anti-inflammatory drug therapy should be introduced with any early evidence of inflammation.

Pathology

SO has a broad histolopathologic presentation. The classic description represents a diffuse nonnecrotizing granulomatous inflammation made up of lymphocytic infiltration of the choroid with nests of epitheliod cells and a few multinucleated giant cells (Figure 81.1). These epithelioid and giant cells often contain melanin pigment. Similar inflammatory infiltrate could be seen in the iris, ciliary body, and pars plana region. Absence of necrosis is a characteristic feature. The retina and choriocapillaris are not usually involved in the inflammatory process.

The cytologic composition of the infiltrating cells was demonstrated by immunohistochemistry. Jakobiec et al reported that the choroidal infiltration was predominantly T lymphocytes of cytotoxic subset.[20] They demonstrated that the epithelioid cells and phagocytic cells in the choroid harbor antigenic determinants specific to cells originating from the reticuloendothelial system. However, the identity and origin of these epithelioid cells have not been clearly elucidated.[20] Chan et al in 1985 found that the predominant T-cell subtype within the choroid was the helper variety.[21] The specimen used for this analysis was obtained at a relatively earlier stage in the disease process than the one studied by Jakobiec et al. Hence it was postulated that T-helper cells predominate at an earlier stage of the disease and T-cytotoxic cells at the latter part of the disease process. Plasma cells

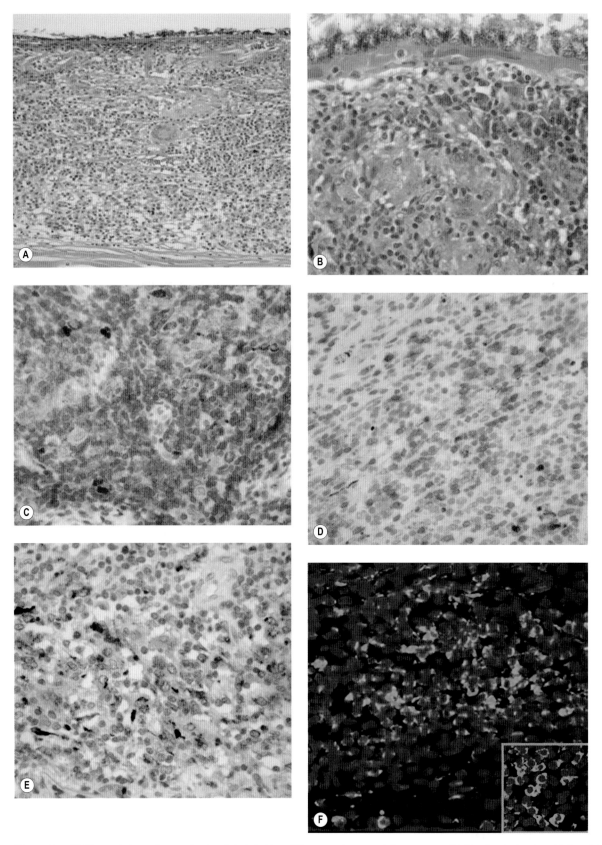

Figure 81.1 (A) Histopathology of sympathetic ophthalmia. Note diffuse granulomatous inflammatory cell infiltration in the choroid. A multinucleated giant cell is present. Hematoxylin and eosin × 100. (B) Histopathology of sympathetic ophthalmia. Higher magnification shows preserved choriocapillaris. Choroid reveals granulomatous inflammation. Hematoxylin and eosin × 100. (C) Immunohistochemistry of sympathetic ophthalmia. CD 4-positive cells are distributed throughout the choroidal inflammatory infiltration. (D) Immunohistochemistry of sympathetic ophthalmia. Note CD 8-positive cells in the choroidal infiltration. (E) Immunohistochemistry of sympathetic ophthalmia. Several CD 68-positive cells are present in the uveal inflammatory infiltration. (F) Immunofluorescent preparation of sympathetic ophthalmia. Tumor necrosis factor-alpha-positive cells are present within choroidal inflammatory infiltration. Insert shows interleukin-1-beta-positive cells in the choroidal infiltration.

were believed to represent an altered cellular infiltrate in the uvea due to corticosteroid therapy. Eosinophils were thought to infiltrate at an early stage in the disease process.[10]

Nodular clusters, referred to as Dalen–Fuchs nodules, were often seen lying between the RPE and Bruch's membrane. These nodules were made up of focal collections of epithelioid cells, modified RPE cells, and lymphocytes. Jakobiec et al believed that these epithelioid cells were similar in origin to the choroidal infiltrate and were derived from bone marrow monocytes.[20] In contrast, a few reports suggested that the epithelioid cells of the Dalen–Fuchs nodules could be altered RPE cells.[22,23]

The small depigmented lesions seen in the peripheral fundus in chronic VKH and SO patients clinically were thought to represent Dalen–Fuchs nodules. But Inomata and Rao reported that these lesions represented the focal disappearance of RPE cells and the presence of chorioretinal adhesions; they found no histologic confirmation that these were Dalen–Fuchs nodules.[24]

Croxatto et al described atypical histopathologic features of SO.[25] They showed that choriocapillaris was focally involved rather frequently (40%) and that retinal perivasculitis was seen in many patients (50%). These findings were associated with severe choroidal inflammation.

The sclera could be involved, with infiltration especially around the emissary veins, and there could be a granulomatous process extending from the juxtapapillary choroid into the optic nerve and surrounding meningeal sheaths.[4,10,24]

Many studies have described an association between the degree of pigmentation and the intensity of uveal inflammation in SO. Marak and Ikui reported in 1980 that the severity of inflammation and the proportion of epithelioid cell response in the choroid were related to the degree of pigmentation. Hence, they stated, choroidal thickening was more marked in eyes removed from heavily pigmented patients than in those removed from white patients.[26]

Etiology

Although a penetrating wound appears to be a predisposing and required condition for the development of SO, not all patients who have an ocular injury develop SO. This suggests a possible genetic predisposition to the development of SO.

Genetic risk factors

There may be a possible genetic predisposition to the development of SO. Human leukocyte antigen (HLA) types reported in SO include HLA-11,[4] HLA-DR4/DRw53, HLA-DR4/DQw3,[27] HLA-DRB1*O4, -DQA1*03, and -DQB1*04.[14] In addition, the HLA-DRB1*04-DQA1*3 haplotype is a marker of a more severe clinical phenotype in SO, with increased disease susceptibility in British and Irish patients.[28] Recent evidence has shown that cytokine gene polymorphisms are markers for disease severity in SO.[29] Polymorphisms that result in the upregulation of proinflammatory cytokines are predicted to create a proinflammatory environment in the eye and worsen the severity of inflammation. These markers were also associated with disease recurrence. Analyzing cytokine gene polymorphism before starting treatment with biological agents (e.g., antitumor

necrosis factor drugs) might help us to identify patients who will benefit most from such therapies.

Other risk factors

The most important risk factor for the development of SO is a history of penetrating ocular injury. An overwhelming number of SO patients show evidence of such an injury in the exciting eye.

The importance of penetrating ocular trauma in the pathogenesis of SO was explained by Rao et al, who demonstrated that bilateral panuveitis developed after a subconjunctival injection of retinal antigen in one eye.[30] They postulated that the penetrating injury exposed the regional lymphatics to intraocular antigens, initiating an immune reaction.

SO following nonpenetrating injury is rare. Only a few cases of SO following cyclocryotherapy and Nd:YAG cyclotherapy without prior history of trauma or surgery have been reported. Nonetheless, one should always be careful in recommending such therapy for patients with glaucoma, especially if there is a past history of surgery or trauma. It is also important to monitor patients after cyclodestructive procedures to detect early evidence of SO. It is advisable to titrate carefully the amount of Nd:YAG cyclotherapy to prevent excessive treatment.

Although rare, there have been case reports of SO following diode laser cyclophotocoagulation,[9] ruthenium plaque brachytherapy,[31] and irradiation for ocular melanoma.[32] However, a microperforation of the globe in such cases cannot be excluded completely.

In contrast to previous literature, recent incidence data showed an increase in SO following surgical procedures.[6,9] Advances in surgical training and surgical instrumentation have enabled ophthalmologists to operate on complicated, severely damaged eyes that, in the past, would have been enucleated. These developments could conceivably contribute to the recent increasing trend of ocular surgery being an important cause of SO. Many surgical procedures have been associated with SO. Examples include cataract surgery, glaucoma filtering procedure, and retinal surgery evisceration.

The role of vitrectomy in inducing SO is still unclear. While several cases have been reported, the majority of these cases had a history of either penetrating trauma or repeated surgical procedure in the past. In 1982, Gass[7] reported a 0.06% incidence of SO after vitrectomy and stated that, if vitrectomy was considered as the only surgical procedure causing a penetrating wound, the incidence would be 0.01%. Kilmartin et al, in 2000,[33] stated that there is a significant risk of developing SO following vitrectomy and stressed the importance of counseling patients about this possibility before performing vitrectomy. It was postulated that the breakdown of the blood–retinal barrier and the subclinical incarceration of uveal tissue at the wound site could contribute to the development of SO. These uveal tissue antigens can also be released during cryoretinopexy and subretinal fluid drainage. The development of signs of uveitis in the opposite eye after vitrectomy, especially in patients with repeated surgeries, should alert the surgeon to the possibility of SO.

It is thought that removal of the exciting eye by enucleation rather than by evisceration is a safer procedure, because evisceration is believed to leave behind uveal tissue that could cause an immune response leading to SO. However, there is a general consensus that prosthetic motility and long-term socket stability are better in patients who undergo evisceration rather than enucleation. The scleral shell is also thought to provide a barrier for orbital spread of infection. In contrast to these advantages it is reported that evisceration could cause possible dissemination of an unsuspected tumor or can lead to inadequate volume if the eye is phthisical.

Although cases of SO following evisceration have been reported, the majority of these eyes had a history of previous trauma or surgical procedure. Therefore, it is unclear whether the initial injury or surgery was responsible for the occurrence of SO.[34-37] SO has a very low incidence and a large number of cases would need to be studied to arrive at a conclusive statistical proof of the association between evisceration and SO.

Pathophysiology

Several studies have proposed a T-cell-mediated autoimmune reaction to antigenic protein from the uvea–retina as the pathogenic mechanism for the development of SO.[20,21,24,38] Wong et al reported enhanced transformation of peripheral lymphocytes from patients with SO exposed to uveal–retinal extracts in tissue culture, suggesting that these patients have lymphocytes that are sensitized to components of uveal–retinal antigen.[39] Various ocular antigens such as uveal melanin, uveal melanocytes, RPE, and retinal S-antigen have been implicated in the pathogenesis of SO in the past. In the animal model of uveitis, Rao et al showed that guinea pigs injected with retinal S-antigen developed an ocular inflammatory reaction similar to that of SO, including granulomatous panuveitis and focal collections of inflammatory cells at the level of RPE similar to Dalen–Fuchs nodules.[40] Furthermore, experimental observations noted that intraocular injection with retinal S-antigen produced a mild inflammation in the injected eye, with no sympathetic inflammation in the fellow eye. In contrast, subconjunctival injection produced a marked intraocular inflammation in both the injected eye and the fellow eye.[30] These observations could be explained by the phenomenon of "immune privilege." This phenomenon is believed to be due to features such as the presence of a tight blood–ocular barrier, lack of intraocular lymphatic system, and an intraocular microenvironment that is immunosuppressive. Hence, antigens experimentally placed in the eye would fail to reach the lymphatic system directly and would first encounter immunologic surveillance in the spleen via the blood stream. This, in turn, would fail to produce an immunopathologic response in the host. In contrast, subconjunctival injection of the retinal S-antigen would provide antigen access to the regional lymph nodes via the conjunctival lymphatics, leading to an immunopathologic reaction in the form of bilateral intraocular inflammation.

It is hypothesized that ocular trauma would cause an enhanced release of sequestered self antigens, which would stimulate the local antigen-presenting cells (APC). These, in turn, would carry the antigen to draining lymph nodes via the conjunctival lymphatics, where T-cell activation would then take place. Once activated, T cells would enter the eye

tissue and be exposed to target antigens leading to the initiation of an inflammatory process.

The possibility of a cell-mediated immune reaction in the pathogenesis of SO has been supported by many immunohistochemical studies. SO includes a cellular infiltrate of predominantly T lymphocytes in the choroid. Immunohistochemical studies have demonstrated that these cells predominantly exhibit markers of CD4 (helper) variety. The CD4-positive T cells respond to peptides (antigens) when presented with major histocompatibility complex (MHC) class II molecules (HLA complex). These molecules are expressed by the bone marrow-derived APC cells within the uvea. Antigens are processed by these cells via a complex intracellular system and then bound to HLA molecules on the surface of APC.

Polymorphism in the HLA genes is believed to influence the initial presentation of disease-inducing peptides (antigens) to the T cells through their effect on HLA peptides, binding affinity. These strong binding sites form a stable complex with antigens and influence the selection and activation of T cells, thereby leading to disease susceptibility.

Various ocular antigens, have been hypothesized to be involved in the pathogenesis of SO. Yamaki et al,[41] in 2000, demonstrated that lymphocytes from patients with VKH disease were reactive to peptides derived from tyrosinase family proteins and that pigmented rats immunized with these peptides developed a disease similar to human VKH disease. Tyrosinase family proteins are enzymes needed for melanin formation and are expressed on melanocytes. It was suggested that SO, which resembles VKH clinically as well as histopathologically, was an autoimmune process against tyrosinase family protein. Furthermore these peptides were reported to contain HLADRB1*0405 binding sites, which are associated with antigen presentation to T lymphocytes in patients with SO. Once the T cells recognize these surface antigens, they trigger the inflammatory process by releasing cytokines that initiate a sequence of events leading to the recruitment of additional inflammatory cells to the site of inflammation. Finally, all of these activated inflammatory cells would cause tissue damage by releasing various secretory products, such as proteases and free radicals (Figure 81.2).

Studies have investigated the role of RPE in the downregulation of inflammation.[42,43] These cells were believed to synthesize and release a protein called "retinal pigment epithelial protective protein" that provides protection against extracellular superoxide formation in uveitis. These findings could explain the constant histopathological feature observed in SO, wherein the choriocapillaris layer and the retina are preserved despite extensive uveal infiltration by inflammatory cells. But it should be noted that severe choroidal inflammation could cause disruption of the RPE and allow T lymphocytes to migrate into the retina, leading to retinal autoimmunity caused by altered tolerance to the retinal protein(s). In 2002 Wang et al reported a case of progressive subretinal fibrosis with multifocal granulomatous chorioretinitis after intraocular surgery and proposed that this was a variant of SO based on histopathologic and immunohistochemical findings. Furthermore, Wang et al demonstrated the presence of antibodies directed against retinal photoreceptors and pigment epithelium. Based on their findings,

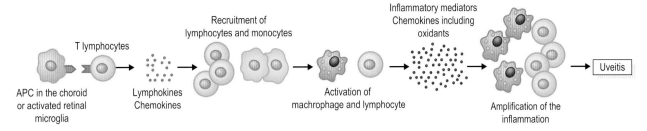

Figure 81.2 Diagrammatic representation of T-cell-mediated uveitis. CD4+ (helper) T lymphocytes recognize antigens on the surface of antigen-presenting cell (APC) when presented with major histocompatibility complex (MHC) class II molecules. This antigen recognition results in the generation of cytokines that causes recruitment and activation of lymphocytes and monocytes. These activated cells in turn release inflammatory mediators and oxidants, leading to amplification of the inflammatory process and resulting in clinically recognizable uveitis.

they postulated that altered tolerance to retinal protein played a role in the pathogenesis of SO.[44]

Summary

SO is a T-cell-mediated autoimmune disease that is directed against antigenic peptides of the uveal melanocytes or retina or RPE. Clinical history of penetrating ocular injury with subsequent development of bilateral intraocular inflammation is a distinguishing feature of this entity. It is essential to begin aggressive treatment promptly with corticosteroids, and if necessary, to introduce immunomodulatory therapy once the possibility of infection and malignancy is carefully ruled out. As relapses are common, these patients should have long-term follow-ups to prevent the development of complications associated with chronic intraocular inflammation.

Key references

A complete list of chapter references is available online at www.expertconsult.com. See inside cover for registration details.

4. Marak GE Jr. Recent advances in sympathetic ophthalmia. Surv Ophthalmol 1979;24:141–156.

6. Kilmartin DJ, Dick AD, Forrester JV. Prospective surveillance of sympathetic ophthalmia in the UK and Republic of Ireland. Br J Ophthalmol 2000;84:259–263.

10. Lubin JR, Albert DM, Weinstein M. Sixty-five years of sympathetic ophthalmia. A clinicopathologic review of 105 cases (1913–1978). Ophthalmology 1980;87:109–121.

13. Easom H, Zimmerman LE. Sympathetic ophthalmia and bilateral phacoanaphylaxis. A clinicopathologic correlation of the sympathogenic and sympathizing eyes. Arch Ophthalmol 1964;72:9–15.

16. Rao NA, Marak GE. Sympathetic ophthalmia simulating Vogt–Koyanagi–Harada's disease: a clinico-pathologic study of four cases. Jpn J Ophthalmol 1983;27:506–511.

19. Winter FC. Sympathetic uveitis; a clinical and pathologic study of visual result. Am J Ophthalmol 1955;39:340–347.

25. Croxatto JO, Rao NA, McLean IW, et al. Atypical histopathologic features in sympathetic ophthalmia. A study of a hundred cases. Int Ophthalmol 1982;4:129–135.

30. Rao NA, Robin J, Hartmann D, et al. The role of the penetrating wound in the development of sympathetic ophthalmia: experimental observations. Arch Ophthalmol 1983;101:102–104.

36. Levine MR, Pou CR, Lash RH. The 1998 Wendell Hughes lecture. Evisceration: is sympathetic ophthalmia a concern in the new millennium? Ophthalm Plast Reconstr Surg 1999;15:4–8.

44. Wang RC, Zamir E, Dugel PU, et al. Progressive subretinal fibrosis and blindness associated with multifocal granulomatous chorioretinitis:a variant of sympathetic ophthalmia. Ophthalmology 2002;22:109–111.

CHAPTER 82

Scleritis

Srilakshmi M Sharma and James T Rosenbaum

Introduction

Scleritis is a rare inflammatory disease which affects the sclera and its adjacent structures such as the episclera, uvea, and cornea. Scleritis can cause severe, disabling pain, destruction of scleral tissue, and the risk of significant visual loss.

The pathophysiology of scleritis is complex, incompletely understood, and complicated by the heterogeneity of the disease as well as the dearth of studies into the immunopathology.

Clinical background

Classification of scleritis

Scleritis may be classified anatomically and by histopathology. The most widely accepted method of classification of scleritis is that described by Watson et al in the 1960s (Table 82.1).[1]

Historical development and demographic data

Scleritis was described in 1702.[2] An early description of scleritis distinguishing it from episcleritis was made in 1830, as reported by Watson and Hayreh in 1976.[3] The prevalence of scleritis has been estimated at 8 cases in 100 000 and the incidence at 1.3 cases per 100 000 person-years.[4] There are no described racial or geographic differences. Females are affected slightly more frequently by scleritis (1.6 : 1).[5,6] It can affect any age but is rarely observed in children. The mean age of onset of scleritis is 45–60 years.

Clinical features of scleritis

Key ocular signs and symptoms

- Pain in scleritis is the main symptom. It can be severe, gnawing, or boring in nature and can affect sleep.
- Scleritis is often painless in chronic rheumatoid arthritis when the presentation is scleromalacia perforans,

which is an extra-articular manifestation of rheumatoid arthritis.
- Redness of the sclera due to dilation and hypervascularity of scleral and episcleral vessels gives the eye a bloodshot appearance (Figure 82.1). Redness of the sclera may be:
  - Localized to one or more sectors of the sclera
  - Diffuse.
- Scleral thinning and reorganization of scleral collagen fibrils cause translucency of the sclera and a bluish appearance (Figure 82.1).
- Posterior scleritis is typically painful at rest and on eye movement. Redness may not be visible. Occasionally posterior scleritis may be painless.
- Risk factors for an underlying systemic disease include bilateral disease, necrotizing scleritis, scleromalacia perforans, a positive rheumatoid factor, or antineutrophil cytoplasmic antibody (ANCA) test.[7]
- An episodic nature of disease may suggest a diagnosis such as relapsing polychondritis or inflammatory bowel disease.
- Corneal changes may also occur in scleritis, causing a sclerokeratitis.
- Scleritis may accompany other ocular signs such as an orbital inflammatory mass in Wegener's granulomatosis.

Diagnostic workup

Nearly 50% of patients with scleritis have an underlying systemic disease identifiable on medical examination (Box 82.1).[8] The systemic associations with scleritis are summarized in Table 82.2 along with appropriate tests for each condition.

Tests and investigations in scleritis

Making a diagnosis of scleritis is usually done on clinical grounds, with the exception of the B scan in posterior

Table 82.1 Classification of scleritis[1,3]

	Anatomical classification	Histological description	Clinical features of scleritis
Episcleritis	Anterior	Nodular	
		Simple	
Scleritis	Anterior	Nodular	A nodule is a localized edematous area, giving the sclera an elevated smooth, rounded appearance. A scleral nodule is usually very tender and can accompany a diffuse scleritis. It can be single or multiple
		Diffuse	Margins of scleral involvement are ill defined, may be localized to an area of sclera, or may be extensive. Anterior scleritis is bilateral in 50% of cases.[23] During an episode of scleritis the area of redness can migrate to occupy different areas or recur in different areas
		Necrotizing with inflammation	All of the above features may be present. There is an avascular area in acute inflammation which is white in appearance. This leads to necrosis, thinning of the cornea, and sometimes perforation
		Necrotizing without inflammation	Scleromalacia perforans. This is seen most frequently in rheumatoid arthritis. Despite the degree of thinning of the sclera, perforation rarely occurs
	Posterior	Nodular Diffuse Necrotizing (seen on histopathology)	Accounts for 7% of cases of scleritis. It usually presents with periorbital pain, worse with eye movement or headache. The pain is often exacerbated with eye movement. One-third present with visual loss.[5] If an anterior scleritis also exists then the likelihood of there being a systemic disease also increases.[5] Other features include serous retinal detachment, swollen optic disc, and optic atrophy, subretinal granulomas, macular edema, choroidal folds at the macula and elsewhere, and choroidal effusions[5,54]

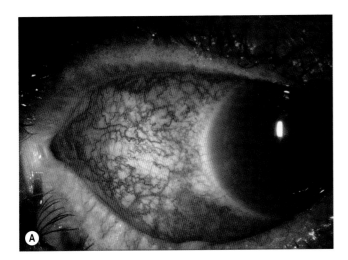

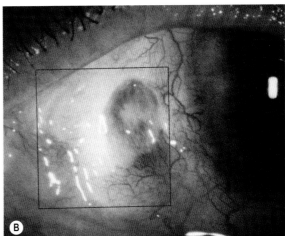

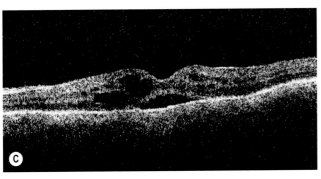

Figure 82.1 (A) Nonnecrotizing anterior scleritis. (B) Necrotizing anterior scleritis (note white area of necrosis and scleral thinning (box)). (C) Ocular coherence tomography showing macular edema and retinal pigment epithelium detachment in posterior scleritis.

Table 82.2 Systemic associations with scleritis

Systemic disease association with scleritis	Frequency of scleritis occurring in the systemic disease	Associated ocular features	Main manifestations of systemic disease	Serological markers which may be associated with systemic disease
Rheumatoid arthritis[32,55]	0.6%	Nodular or diffuse scleritis Rare presentation with scleromalacia perforans Peripheral ulcerative keratitis	Usually a polyarthritis affecting hands and wrists Subcutaneous rheumatoid nodules	RhF+ in nodular scleritis or scleromalacia perforans
Inflammatory bowel disease[56,57]	18%	Nodular anterior uveitis	History of colitis, weight loss Spondyloarthropathy	Colonoscopy + biopsy
Wegener's granulomatosis[58]	<10%	Orbital pseudotumor Peripheral ulcerative keratitis	Sinusitis, dacroadenitis Epistaxis Cranial nerve lesions Renal disease	cANCA or pANCA+ve Urine analysis Orbital biopsy
Relapsing polychondritis[59]	40%	Episcleritis	Recurrent episodes of cartilage inflammation Deformation of nose, auricle, trachea. stridor, hoarse voice Tinnitus, hearing loss	Clinical diagnosis Biopsy can be supportive
Spondyloarthropathy (psoriatic, reactive arthritis, AS)*	0.04%[†]	Anterior uveitis	Spondyloarthropathy	HLA B27+ Sacroiliac films Biopsy for psoriasis
Systemic lupus erythematosus	<2%	Keratoconjunctivitis sicca Sjögren's syndrome Episcleritis Retinopathy	Photosensitive, malar rash Serositis Polyarthropathy Vasculitis Scleritis usually indicates active disease	ANA+ dsDNA+ ESR
Polyarteritis nodosa	Rare	Peripheral ulcerative keratitis		Abdominal arteriogram
Cogan's disease	Rare	Interstitial keratitis	Hypertension Hearing loss	Biopsy
Microscopic polyarteritis	Rare		Pulmonary vasculitis	pANCA
Churg–Strauss syndrome	Rare		Pulmonary vasculitis	pANCA
Takayasu arteritis	Rare		Hypertension Aortitis	MRA ± arteriogram
Giant cell arteritis*	Very rare		Bitemporal headache, weight loss, polymyalgia	High ESR. Temporal artery biopsy
Tophaceous gout	Very rare			Uric acid

*Causes an anterior ischemia which may cause scleritis.
[†]Prevalence of spondyloarthropathies in the population is approximately 2 in 1000.[60] If 2% of scleritis is caused by spondyloarthropathy then the frequency at which scleritis occurs in this disease may be approximated to 0.04%.
RhF, rheumatoid factor; cANCA, cytoplasmic-staining antineutrophil cytoplasmic antibodies; pANCA, perinuclear-staining antineutrophil cytoplasmic antibodies; HLA, human leukocyte antigen; ANA, antinuclear antibody; dsDNA, double-stranded DNA; ESR, erythrocyte sedimentation rate; MRA, magnetic resonance angiography.

scleritis (Figure 82.2). There are a few tests that would be recommended as screening tests for all patients without an established cause (Table 82.2). Other tests should be guided by systemic symptoms, clinical course, and/or exposure to infective agents.

In general, the typical panel of blood tests that all patients with scleritis should have is summarized in Table 82.3. A recent study has proposed that a rheumatoid factor should also be obtained as a screening test.[7]

Significance of antineutrophil cytoplasmic antibodies

Antineutrophil antibodies (ANCA) are used as clinical markers of disease for a number of vasculitides. The most relevant disease associations in the context of scleritis are Wegener's granulomatosis, polyarteritis nodosa, microscopic polyarteritis, and Churg–Strauss syndrome (Box 82.2). ANCA is the recommended screening test as:

Table 82.3 Screening tests in scleritis

Test	Description of test	Comments
ANCA	Indirect immunofluorescence for presence and titer of antibodies in the cytoplasm of neutrophils	If this is positive, this may indicate presence of a vasculitis, indicating further workup and medical consultation
FTA	Immunoassay to diagnose syphilis. This is a rare cause of scleritis but it may have long latency and many presentations. It can be easily treated	A positive test may indicate untreated syphilis, previously treated syphilis, or a false-positive result
ESR	Indicator of nonspecific inflammation	If elevated it suggests the presence of active systemic disease
Chest X-ray (optional depending on risk factors for tuberculosis/lung disease)	X-ray imaging of the lung parenchyma and hilae	Hilar adenopathy in sarcoidosis. An apical calcified scar suggests previous tuberculosis. Parenchymal changes may indicate areas of vasculitis, fibrosis, or interstitial lung disease (seen in vasculites or rheumatoid arthritis)

ANCA, antineutrophil cytoplasmic antibodies; FTA, fluorescent treponemal antibody; ESR, erythrocyte sedimentation rate.

- A positive ANCA may be the presenting symptom of a systemic vasculitis.[9,10]
- In a proportion of cases who present with apparently idiopathic scleritis, a positive ANCA may predict development of Wegener's disease in some patients.[7]

Box 82.1

- Most cases of scleritis that are associated with disease have symptoms of systemic disease at the time of presentation
- In the vasculitides scleritis may be the presenting feature

---

Box 82.2

- Antineutrophil cytoplasmic antibody (ANCA)-positive scleritis – patients have more serious ocular disease, especially visually significant corneal complications[8]
- ANCA-positive cases of scleritis are more likely to be associated with a systemic disease than ANCA-negative cases of scleritis
- Most ANCA-positive scleritis patients do not have a past history of immune-mediated disease[9]

Perinuclear-staining ANCA (pANCA) tends to be linked with renal vasculitis and microscopic polyarteritis. Cytoplasmic-staining ANCA (cANCA) positivity is highly associated with Wegener's granulomatosis.[11] Sensitivity is 67% for patients with active systemic disease and specificity is 96%.[12] There is sometimes clinical overlap in phenotypes of cANCA and pANCA systemic vasculitis; therefore the pANCA may be positive in a Wegener's-like vasculitic picture.

Role of rheumatoid factor testing

In the general population (without rheumatoid arthritis) the prevalence of rheumatoid factor is around 15%. However, it has been suggested that, even in the absence of joint symptoms, a positive rheumatoid factor is an independent risk factor for developing rheumatoid arthritis.[7] Anticitrullinated peptides are highly specific for RA. Their role in evaluating scleritis has not been studied.

Antinuclear antibodies (ANA) should be tested if scleritis secondary to systemic lupus erythematosus is in the differential diagnosis.[13] In the general population 30% of females are ANA-positive so a positive ANA is not diagnostic of this condition.

Differential diagnosis

The most common differential diagnosis is episcleritis (Tables 82.4 and 82.5, Box 82.3).

Other differentials of scleritis

- Conjunctivitis
- Keratoconjunctivitis sicca
- Anterior uveitis
- Vascular abnormalities of the conjunctiva, e.g., hemangioma
- Malignant infiltration, e.g., lymphomatous or leukemic[14]
- Scleral hyaline plaque: these can be confused with scleromalacia perforans. These are small translucent wedge or circular-shaped areas of sclera. The sclera at the center of the lesions is thin and the underlying uvea is visible through it. It is sometimes seen with calcification. These lesions occur mostly in the population over 60. The plaque can be bilateral and requires no treatment
- Anterior scleral staphyloma (Figure 82.3).

This unusual condition can be due to progressive myopia, severe chronic glaucoma, or rarely in children after a trabeculectomy. The appearance is similar to that of scleromalacia perforans. In chronic glaucoma the pressure has to be chronically and significantly raised to cause this appearance.

Treatment of scleritis

Usually active disease requires therapy. Deciding whether scleritis is active is usually according to the degree of pain,

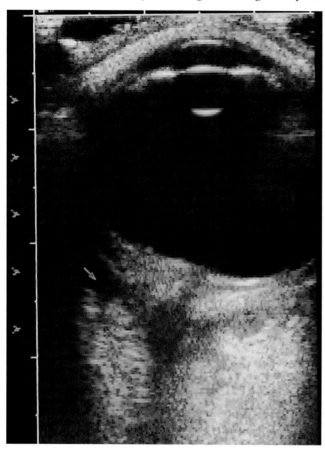

Figure 82.2 B-scan ultrasound of posterior scleritis showing thickening of posterior sclera and the T-sign reflecting edema along the optic nerve and within the subtenon space. (Reproduced with permission from Watson P et al (eds) Sclera and Systemic Disorders, 2nd edn. Butterworth and Heinemann, 2004.)

difficulty on eye movement, redness, and presence of necrosis. Optic nerve swelling, serous detachments, or demonstration of sclera thickening and edema on B-mode ultrasonography are all features of active posterior scleritis.

About 25% of cases with scleritis overall will require immunosuppressive therapy but the proportion is 70% or more in those with necrotizing disease.

Selection of a particular drug may depend on knowledge of how the underlying disease responds and is tailored to knowledge of the patient's medical and social history.

Box 82.3 Episcleritis

- Episcleritis is a more benign condition than scleritis, which affects the episclera
- It has a milder course than scleritis and does not affect vision
- Treatment of episcleritis rarely requires little more than topical treatment with steroids or nonsteroidal anti-inflammatory agents

---

Table 82.5 Differentiation between episcleritis and scleritis

Episcleritis	Scleritis
Discomfort rather than severe pain	Pain usually severe. May be severe enough to disturb or prevent sleep. May cause pain on moving the eye
Redness of the episclera tends to be mild. Superficial phenylephrine 2.5% will blanch superficial episcleral vessels within 10 minutes	Deep "brick-red" injection of vessels involving the sclera Phenylephrine 2.5% blanches episcleral vessels within 10 minutes
Responds to topical treatment or nonsteroidal anti-inflammatory	May additionally require systemic immunosuppression
Will not cause necrotization/ scleral thinning	May cause a necrotizing process involving sclera and associated structures

Table 82.4 Clinical imaging in scleritis

Imaging test	Indication for use	Features if test is abnormal
B-mode ultrasonography (10 Mz) (B scan)	Diagnosis of posterior scleritis	T sign indicating posterior scleral edema
Ultrasound biomicroscopy	Diagnosis of anterior scleritis and scleral necrosis	Scleral thickening and focal hyporeflectivity
Anterior-segment fluorescein angiography	Diagnosis of scleritis and necrosis	Hyperfluorescence and leakage from episcleral vessels. Areas of capillary shutdown
Posterior-segment fluorescein angiography	Investigate the differential of posterior scleritis or unexplained visual loss	Can assist in differential diagnosis of a fundal mass, and diagnose serous detachments, cystoid macular edema
Ocular coherence tomography	Posterior scleritis or unexplained visual loss	Cystoid macular edema and serous detachment
Computed tomography orbits	Additional test for posterior scleritis or where an inflammatory orbital mass is suspected	This can detect scleritis or inflammation of tissue within the orbit and orbital masses CT can also be used to detect sinusitis
Magnetic resonance imaging orbits	If additional high-resolution information about the soft tissue is required	Generally not used to diagnose scleritis. May reveal orbital massor myositis

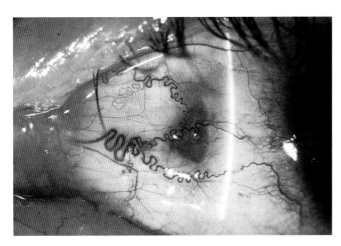

Figure 82.3 Image of scleral hyaline plaque. They may be calcified or without calcification. They are of no pathological significance. (Reproduced with permission from Watson P et al (eds) Sclera and Systemic Disorders, 2nd edn. Butterworth and Heinemann, 2004.)

Treatment of infectious scleritis is directed at the underlying cause. Steroid should be avoided in the initial stage of therapy of a possible infection. In herpes zoster, the treatment of choice is aciclovir or valaciclovir acutely and this may be continued prophylactically.

Drugs used in scleritis

Nonimmunosuppressive drugs

Nonsteroidal anti-inflammatory drugs can be very effective therapy with full resolution of symptoms in about one-third of patients with scleritis.[15]

Immunosuppressives used in scleritis

Corticosteroids

• Oral corticosteroids are highly effective at suppressing inflammation in the short term. Severe inflammation can be treated with 1 mg/kg at the outset with a subsequent tapering regimen. If chronic therapy with corticosteroids is required, a steroid-sparing agent should be considered.

• Subconjunctival steroid depot may be successful for noninfectious cases of anterior, nonnecrotizing scleritis.[16] This route should be chosen with caution due to a risk of inducing scleral necrosis.

Cyclophosphamide is an alkylating drug and is a potent immunosuppressant with a side-effect profile which includes a risk of malignancy, hemorrhagic cystitis, and neutropenia. It is the treatment of choice for scleritis associated with systemic vasculitides, such as Wegener's granulomatosis or polyarteritis nodosa. It can also be used when scleritis is refractory to other forms of therapy.

Methotrexate, mycophenolate mofetil, and ciclosporin have been used successfully to treat scleritis.[17-19]

Biologic therapy for scleritis

Inhibitors of tumor necrosis factor-α (TNF-α) are increasingly used in the treatment of uveitis, although they have been less well studied in scleritis. Three agents are used in clinical practice: infliximab, humira, and etanercept. Etanercept is not as effective as others in treating eye disease.[20] Small series and case reports demonstrate some success with infliximab in scleritis with and without associated systemic disease.[21]

Rituximab is a genetically engineered, chimeric, murine/human monoclonal IgG1 antibody directed against the CD20 antigen found on the surface of pre-B and mature B cells. Rituximab has been shown to be successful in the treatment of ANCA-positive vasculitides and preliminary success has been reported in the treatment of scleritis.[22]

Prognosis

A diagnosis of necrotizing scleritis carries a 60% chance of developing ocular or systemic complications and up to 30% of patients have a loss in visual acuity.[10,23]

Studies of rheumatoid arthritis show that development of necrotizing scleritis, as well as other extra-articular manifestations, has been associated with reduced life expectancy and poor prognosis. The explanation is most likely to be that presence of extra-articular complications of rheumatoid arthritis reflects a more severe disease, and may accompany complications of therapy and other comorbidities such as cardiovascular health.[24,25]

Newer data suggest that the subset of patients who are either pANCA- or cANCA-positive have a more aggressive course with increased risk of visual loss and ocular complications. They are also more likely to require immunosuppressive therapy.[26]

Complications of scleritis

About 60% of patients with scleritis develop complications[10,23]:

• Roughly 15–30% of patients with scleritis develop visual loss.
• Visual loss is more strongly associated with systemic disease.
• Anterior uveitis occurs in approximately one-third of cases.
• Peripheral ulcerative keratitis (PUK) occurs in up to 15% (Figure 82.5).
• Cataract occurs in about 15% of cases.
• Some fundus abnormalities are present in 6% overall.

Posterior-segment complications tend to be associated with posterior scleritis. Exudative retinal detachments may cause visual loss. Cystoid macular edema may occur in posterior scleritis but rarely does so in necrotizing anterior scleritis. Vitritis rarely occurs in scleritis.[5]

Glaucoma occurs in roughly 9–13% of cases of scleritis.[23,27] Raised intraocular pressure or glaucoma may be an acute presenting feature of anterior scleritis due to raised episcleral pressure reducing aqueous outflow or it may complicate scleritis chronically. In posterior scleritis, a large serous retinal detachment can be rarely complicated by angle closure glaucoma due to anterior displacement and rotation of the ciliary body.[28]

Corneal complications of scleritis[29] (Box 82.4)

Some corneal change has been found in 29% of patients with scleritis.

Corneal change in scleritis is described broadly as sclerokeratitis. Two main types of sclerokeratitis occur, infiltrative or destructive, and these are summarized in Table 82.6. Visual loss may occur when the optical axis is obscured by opacities or when destructive changes occur.

The presence of corneal thinning in sclerokeratitis is a sign of destruction of the cornea and frequently represents veno-occlusive disease. Early detection of destructive keratitis in scleritis is important as some types can be rapidly visually threatening and may cause corneal perforation. Sometimes, peripheral corneal thinning or Terriens-like change can occur with little inflammation.

The presence of infiltrates in the cornea does not usually signify destructive vaso-occlusive disease.

Peripheral ulcerative keratitis

This is a visually threatening clinical presentation of a sclerokeratitis (Figure 82.5). It is very rare and has an estimated incidence of 3 per 1 million people per year.[10,27,30] The systemic diseases associated with PUK include rheumatoid arthritis (34–42%), ANCA-associated vasculitides, poly-arteritis nodosa, and systemic lupus erythematosus.[27,31] Approximately one-fourth of cases have an undiagnosed systemic disease at the time of presentation. The main differential diagnosis for PUK is microbial keratitis. The workup is otherwise identical to that for scleritis. Treatment is usually high-dose steroids and immunosuppression.

PUK can progress to a corneal melt syndrome where the stroma becomes involved, and ultimately corneal perforation. It may be painless in rheumatoid arthritis.

Etiology

Disease associations in scleritis

- 50% of patients with scleritis have an underlying systemic disease (Table 82.7).[8]
- 5–10% of these cases are associated with infection.

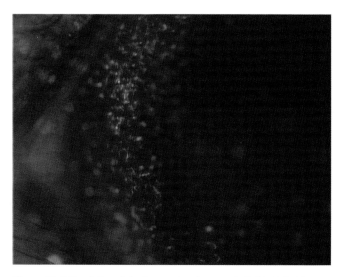

Figure 82.4 Dendritic cells in the peripheral cornea (cells labeled with fluorescent marker). (Courtesy of Dr. Ellen Lee, Casey Eye Institute.)

Table 82.6 Summary of corneal changes in scleritis (sclerokeratitis)

Infiltrative		Type of scleral inflammation	Location of corneal change
Stromal keratitis			
	Localized	Usually nonnecrotizing	Next to area of scleral inflammation
	Acute	Necrotizing	Stromal Central cornea
	Deep	Nonnecrotizing and necrotizing	Deep stromal. Similar to interstitial keratitis seen in infections. Anywhere on cornea
	Diffuse	Nonnecrotizing and necrotizing	Midstromal. Central cornea
Destructive	Peripheral corneal thinning*	Nonnecrotizing or necrotizing	Corneal gutter forms at limbal cornea. Terriens-like change forms 2–3 mm from limbal edge
	Peripheral ulcerative keratitis	Necrotizing disease	Peripheral cornea Involves outer layers of cornea
	Keratolysis/corneal melt syndrome	Necrotizing disease	Central or peripheral

*Very mild or no inflammation.

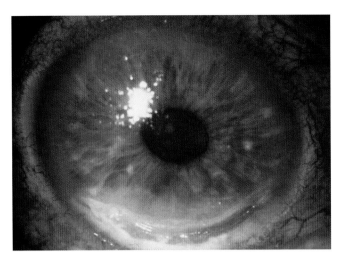

Figure 82.5 Peripheral ulcerative keratitis. Fluorescein stains the area of keratitis in this image.

Box 82.5 Special features of rheumatoid scleritis

- Nodular rheumatoid arthritis can cause a nodular anterior scleritis or chronic, frequently painless, scleral thinning called scleromalacia perforans
- The rheumatoid nodule, the scleral nodule found in rheumatoid scleritis, and the scleral lesion in scleromalacia perforans are histologically similar
- In all three there is a granulomatous, inflammatory infiltrate with neutrophils, epitheloid giant cells, and plasma cells
- Scleromalacia perforans is extremely rare due to improved therapies for rheumatoid arthritis

---

Rheumatoid arthritis-associated scleritis is frequently bilateral and tends to appear after symptoms of rheumatoid arthritis have become established. The majority of cases of scleritis occur in the presence of seropositive rheumatoid arthritis with subcutaneous nodules (Box 82.5).[32]

The vasculitides constitute 7% of all scleritis cases.[23] Although any vasculitis can cause a scleritis, Wegener's granulomatosis is the most common. The majority of patients with a systemic etiology will present with symptoms of systemic disease that precede onset of scleritis, but vasculitis is frequently an exception to this rule.

Relapsing polychondritis is a rare disease which can present at any age. The hallmark of the disease is inflammation of cartilaginous structures such as the pinna of the ear, the cartilage of the nose, and the tracheal cartilage.

Inflammatory bowel disease is a relatively common group of systemic illnesses. A minority of patients with inflammatory bowel disease may present with ocular manifestations preceding systemic onset.[33] Usually the patient will have symptoms of active bowel disease on history.

Systemic lupus erythematosus is a systemic autoimmune disease. It has a number of other ocular manifestations, including keratoconjuctivitis sicca and retinopathy, especially in the form of cottonwool spots.

Table 82.7 Etiology of scleritis (where there is no frequency noted, the condition is rare and there are no representative data regarding frequency of occurrence)

	Disease	Approximate frequency of disease among patients with scleritis (%)
Systemic disease	Rheumatoid arthritis	15
	Wegener's granulomatosis	6
	Relapsing polychondritis	4
	Systemic lupus erythematosus	3
	Inflammatory bowel disease	3
	Seronegative spondyloarthropathy	2
	Polyarteritis nodosa	0.6
Infection	Herpes zoster (varicella-zoster)	5
	Herpes simplex	2
	Syphilis	2
	Coxsackie B5	
	Lyme (*Borrelia burgdorferi*)	
	Human immunodeficiency virus (HIV)	
	Toxoplasma	
	Mycobacterial species (*M. tuberculosis, M. leprae, M. chelonae*)	
	*Pseudomonas aeruginosa**	
	*Staphylococcus**	
	*Streptococcus**	
	Acanthamoeba†	
	Haemophilus	
	*Aspergillus**	
	*Corynebacterium**	
	Serratia	
	*Nocardia**	
Drugs	Bisphosphonates Mitomycin	
Malignancy	Primary, e.g., choroidal melanoma Secondary malignancy	
Surgically induced following:	Cataract surgery Vitreoretinal surgery Scleral buckle Trabeculectomy	

*Associated with surgery/trauma.
†Usually associated with contact lens keratitis.

Rare associations with scleritis include Takayasu's arteritis, cryoglobulinemic vasculitis (associated with hepatitis C), Churg–Strauss syndrome, giant cell arteritis, and Cogan's disease, all of which are vasculitides. Behçet's is another rare cause.

Other causes of scleritis

Infectious scleritis

Many infections can cause scleritis but varicella-zoster causing herpes zoster ophthalmicus is most common. Scleritis is a feature in 8% of cases of herpes zoster ophthalmicus.[34,35]

An infectious cause of scleritis should be suspected in cases that occur after trauma or surgery. Other features of bacterial or fungal infections in the sclera are an indolent course of scleral destruction and abscess formation or suppuration.

In bacterial or fungal cases (suppurative), surgical debridement as well as antimicrobial therapy is sometimes required as the penetration of systemic antimicrobials into the sclera is poor.

Surgically induced necrotizing scleritis (SINS)

SINS usually arises within 9 months of surgery but it can be activated long after.

Common precipitants of SINS are pterygial surgery, trabeculectomy, and cataract surgery. In rare cases treatment with an anti TNF-α agent (infliximab) has been used to control the necrotizing process but generally systemic steroids are adequate.[36]

Trauma/other injury

Trauma and chemical injury can cause a localized scleritis. Control of the inflammatory response is indicated for symptom relief and prevention of complications. Treatment is with an oral nonsteroidal anti-inflammatory or with oral/topical corticosteroids.

Drug-induced scleritis

Two agents which have been described as causing scleritis are:

- Mitomycin C, usually in glaucoma or pterygium surgery[37]
- Bisphosphonates (Box 82.6).

The bisphosphonates are potent inhibitors of osteoclasts used in the prevention and treatment of osteoporosis.They cause scleritis, but so rarely that they can still be prescribed safely in people with ocular inflammatory disease.

Malignancy

Occasionally primary intraocular tumors and secondary tumors can precipitate an acute inflammatory scleritis.

Box 82.6 Episcleritis and Bisphosphonates

- Episcleritis due to bisphosphonates does not require cessation of the drug. It can be treated with nonsteroidal anti-inflammatories. In scleritis associated with bisphosphonates, the drug may have to be discontinued

---

Sometimes a malignant deposit such as lymphomatous infiltration or a metastatic deposit such as that from squamous carcinoma can mimic a scleritis. Melanoma is the most reported intraocular malignancy associated with scleritis.[38,39]

Genetics

There is no recognized inheritance pattern for scleritis and most cases present de novo or in the context of systemic disease. There is no strong association with human leukocyte antigens (HLA) in scleritis.[40,41]

Pathology

Scleral structure

Scleral anatomy

The sclera forms the fibrous coat of the eye and has a white, opaque appearance due to the dense, irregular arrangement of collagen fibrils. The sclera provides a tough housing for intraocular contents and maintains the shape of the eye. The sclera comes to an end anteriorly where it attaches to the limbus of the cornea. Posteriorly the sclera fuses with the sheath of the optic nerve.

Types I, III, V, and VI collagen are present in sclera. Type I is found in the highest proportion. Elastic fibers constitute a small part of the fibrillar scaffold of the scleral substance. Collagen and elastic fibers confer mechanical properties, including viscoelasticity and limited distension of the sclera. The extracellular matrix of the sclera also consists of proteoglycan.

Episcleral anatomy

The episclera is a thin, highly vascular tissue which consists of a uniform arrangement of collagen bundles which are attached tightly to blood vessels. The episclera blends with the stroma of the sclera which lies underneath it.

Blood supply to the sclera and episclera

The sclera is relatively avascular and there is no direct blood supply to the scleral stroma. Blood vessels and nerves pass

---

Table 82.8 Cases of scleritis and episcleritis attributed to bisphosphonates reported until 2008 worldwide

	Cases of scleritis	Cases of episcleritis
Pamidronate	11	1
Alendronate	9	1
Risedronate	4	1
Ibandronate	No data	1

No data at time of writing in 2008 for zolendronate, etidronate, tiludronate, or clodronate.
Sources: World Health Organization adverse drug events database. World Health Organization Uppsala Monitoring Center, Uppsala, Sweden. Data with kind permission of National Registry of Drug-Induced Ocular Side Effects, USA.

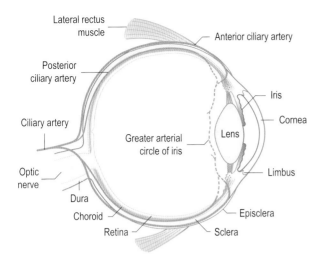

Figure 82.6 Blood supply to the sclera and episclera. (Modified from Watson P et al (eds) Sclera and Systemic Disorders, 2nd edn. Butterworth and Heinemann, 2004.)

through the sclera, including the long and short posterior ciliary arteries, their associated nerves, and the vortex veins. The sclera derives its nutrition from choroidal and episcleral vascular networks.[42]

There are three main vascular layers of the episclera. It is the deeper plexus that is involved in scleritis.[1]

1. Conjunctival plexus: the most superficial plexus of fine vessels movable over underlying structures.
2. Superficial episcleral plexus: a radially arranged plexus lying in the episcleral tissues.
3. Deep episcleral plexus: a network which penetrates the sclera.

Nerve supply

The severe pain in scleritis may be explained by the fact that its sensory nerve supply is very rich. Pain arises due to direct stimulation of nerve roots or by distension of the scleral tissue when scleral edema occurs.

The sensory nerve supply arises from the branches of the nasociliary branch of the trigeminal nerve. The nerve supply to the anterior sclera is from the long posterior ciliary nerves and the posterior sclera is supplied from the short ciliary nerves.

Histopathology

It is widely accepted that noninfectious scleritis is an immune-mediated disease (Figure 82.4). In support of this, highly magnified dynamic images using intravital microscopy show the presence of numerous leukocytes involved in rolling and arresting in the endothelium of active scleritis[43] (Figure 82.7).

Scleritis has been histopathologically divided into necrotizing and nonnecrotizing types of inflammation (Table 82.8). The necrotizing type has been further classified into three main groups, summarized in Table 82.3. There is an additional fourth group which consists of patients with sarcoidosis.

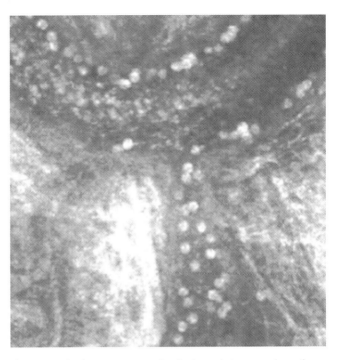

Figure 82.7 Leukocyte movement in scleral vessels. Large numbers of rolling and arrested leukocytes are evident along the wall of the vessels. (Image taken with Heidelberg confocal laser microscope; HRTII, Heidelberg Engineering, Heidelberg, Germany.) (Reproduced with permission from Lim LL, Hoang L, Wong T et al. Intravital microscopy of leukocyte-endothelial dynamics using the Heidelberg confocal laser microscope in scleritis and allergic conjunctivitis. Mol Vis 2006;12:1302–1305.)

1. Necrotizing scleritis consists of rheumatoid and rheumatoid-like necrotizing scleritis, including systemic vasculitides or connective tissue diseases.[44]
2. Postinfection scleral inflammation.
3. Idiopathic necrotizing scleral inflammation.

Pathophysiology

The pathophysiology of scleritis is incompletely understood and there are probably diverse mechanisms depending on the etiology of the scleritis. In autoimmune diseases, immune complexes circulate and can deposit in and around episcleral vessels, inciting an immune response. In many cases, however, there is no immune complex deposition and scleritis is thought to be T-cell-driven. Patients respond to different types of therapy, suggesting that differential response to treatment can further classify patients.

Immune response in scleritis

Understanding the pathogenesis of scleritis is daunting because: (1) the disease is relatively rare; (2) biopsy is rarely obtained; (3) the disease is clinically diverse; and (4) there are no ideal animal models. Much remains to be done to clarify the pathophysiology.

Role of T cells in scleritis

In studies of nodular scleritis the cellular infiltrate seems to be composed of macrophages, CD4+ T cells, and CD8+

Table 82.9 Histopathological features of necrotizing scleritis[44,61]

	Necrotizing scleritis in rheumatoid and rheumatoid-like vasculitis	Necrotizing scleritis in idiopathic scleritis	Postinfective scleritis, e.g., herpes zoster
Location of inflammatory infiltrate	Anterior in rheumatoid. Also involves the choroid in aggressive forms of nonrheumatoid disease such as Wegener's	Anterior and posterior	Mainly anterior
Presence of vasculitis and ischemia	Vasculitis and ischemia	No vasculitis or ischemia	Some vasculitis
Types of inflammatory infiltrate	Neutrophils as well as lymphocytes, plasma cells, and histiocytes. Giant cells and epithelioid cells at the site of granulomas	Mainly lymphocytes, fibroblasts, histiocytes. Giant cells are rare	Lymphoctes Neutrophils
Principal histopathological feature	Zonal granulomatous inflammation around central necrosis	Nonzonal distribution of inflammation	Focal granulomatous inflammation around necrotic sclera

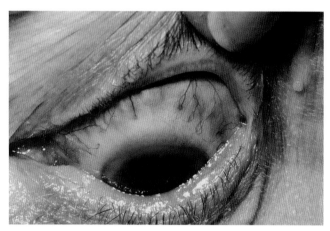

Figure 82.8 Scleromalacia perforans. (Reproduced with permission from Watson P et al (eds) Sclera and Systemic Disorders, 2nd edn. Butterworth and Heinemann, 2004.)

T cells, indicating a dominant T-cell-mediated immune response.

The infiltrate in necrotizing scleritis has been reported to consist predominantly of CD4+ T cells, a mixture of plasma cells, some CD20-positive B cells and macrophages (Table 82.9). Unlike nonnecrotizing forms, in necrotizing scleritis activated macrophages organize themselves into granulomas. The T-cell infiltrate is often perivascular but has also been inconsistently seen within the vessel, supporting the theory that there is a vasculitic process underlying the pathogenesis.[40,41]

Recently a newly described Th17 subset of CD4+ T cells and its secreted product, the cytokine interleukin (IL)-17, have been localized to the eye in active scleritis and uveitis of humans.[45] Antibodies to IL-17 also dampen inflammation of experimental autoimmune uveoretinitis (EAU). The Th17 subset has been recognized to play a role in diverse autoimmune diseases.[46,47]

Role of TNF-α

TNF-α is a potent cytokine which has a central role in the inflammation of chronic autoimmune diseases. TNF-α has been localized to tissue specimens of necrotizing scleritis.[48,49] Blockade of TNF-α using infliximab, a humanized mouse,

chimeric monoclonal antibody in patients with scleritis, both idiopathic and associated with underlying systemic disease, has proved very effective clinically.[21]

Role of B cells and autoantibodies in autoimmune scleritis

Scleritis has traditionally been considered a T-cell disease but there is probably a greater role for the B cell in the pathogenesis of scleritis than conventionally understood. There is also some evidence for a role for ANCA antibodies in mediating vasculitis.[21,50] A heavy infiltrate of B cells may be seen in autoimmune scleritis.[51] In autoimmune vasculitis, for example Wegener's granulomatosis, the B cell has become a promising treatment target.[52] There have also been early reports of the utility of rituximab, a potent B-cell-depleting agent, in scleritis.

Role of matrix metalloproteinases

Matrix metalloproteinases (MMPs) are important in normal connective tissue turnover, wound healing, and angiogenesis. There is overproduction of MMP-9, stromelysin and, to a lesser extent, tissue inhibitor of metalloproteinases-1 (TIMP-1) in biopsy specimens of necrotizing scleritis.[48,53] MMPs degrade collagen and other extracellular matrix components. An imbalance of the local TIMP:MMP ratio results in scleral destruction.

Conclusion

Scleritis is a rare but serious and potentially vision-threatening condition with a variety of ocular manifestations. The strong association with systemic disease means that the ophthalmologist needs to have an understanding of systemic disease, prognostic factors, and natural history in order to determine the diagnosis effectively and institute therapy. The prognosis for scleritis is good, with a wide range of immunosuppressives available for therapy.

The pathogenesis of scleritis is complex with multiple components of the immune response implicated in the evolution of scleritis. Advances in understanding of the immunology of autoimmune disease are also enabling us to understand ocular inflammation better. This increased knowledge is directly translated into clinical practice, as seen in the development of new, exciting therapies for scleritis.

Key references

A complete list of chapter references is available online at www.expertconsult.com. See inside cover for registration details.

1. Watson PG, Hayreh SS, Awdry PN. Episcleritis and scleritis. I. Br J Ophthalmol 1968;52:278–279.

5. McCluskey PJ, Watson PG, Lightman S, et al. Posterior scleritis: clinical features, systemic associations, and outcome in a large series of patients. Ophthalmology 1999;106:2380–2386.

7. Lin P, Bhullar SS, Tessler HH, et al. Immunologic markers as potential predictors of systemic autoimmune disease in patients with idiopathic scleritis. Am J Ophthalmol 2008;145:463–471.

8. Watson PG. The diagnosis and management of scleritis. Ophthalmology 1980;87:716–720.

9. Akpek EK, Thorne JE, Qazi FA, et al. Evaluation of patients with scleritis for systemic disease. Ophthalmology 2004;111:501–506.

10. Sainz de la Maza M, Foster CS, Jabbur NS. Scleritis associated with systemic vasculitic diseases. Ophthalmology 1995;102:687–692.

19. Sen HN, Suhler EB, Al-Khatib SQ, et al. Mycophenolate mofetil for the treatment of scleritis. Ophthalmology 2003;110:1750–1755.

23. Jabs DA, Mudun A, Dunn JP, et al. Episcleritis and scleritis: clinical features and treatment results. Am J Ophthalmol 2000;130:469–476.

24. Lachmann SM, Hazleman BL, Watson PG. Scleritis and associated disease. Br Med J 1978;1:88–90.

26. Hoang LT, Lim LL, Vaillant B, et al. Antineutrophil cytoplasmic antibody-associated active scleritis. Arch Ophthalmol 2008;126:651–655.

27. Sainz de la Maza M, Foster CS, Jabbur NS, et al. Ocular characteristics and disease associations in scleritis-associated peripheral keratopathy. Arch Ophthalmol 2002;120:15–19.

30. McKibbin M, Isaacs JD, Morrell AJ. Incidence of corneal melting in association with systemic disease in the Yorkshire region, 1995–7. Br J Ophthalmol 1999;83:941–943.

61. Rao NA, Marak GE, Hidayat AA. Necrotizing scleritis. A clinico-pathologic study of 41 cases. Ophthalmology 1985;92:1542–1549.

CHAPTER 83

Infectious uveitis

Pooja Bhat, Allen Tony Jackson, and C Stephen Foster

Overview

Uveitis can be infectious or noninfectious in origin. Although the most common etiology of uveitis is considered to be immune-mediated in developed countries, there remain many cases of uveitis caused by infectious agents. Infectious uveitis can become latent, smoldering, and chronic and mimic autoimmune uveitis. While autoimmune uveitis responds to corticosteroids or immunosuppressive chemotherapy, such treatment may worsen infectious uveitis. It is, therefore, essential to identify cases of chronic uveitis caused by microbes in order to initiate specific and appropriate antimicrobial therapy. The diagnosis of infectious uveitis can be established in most cases based on patient demographics, mode of onset of and morphology of the lesions, and the association with other systemic infectious diseases. Laboratory testing and imaging techniques are important tools that help refine the diagnosis. In this chapter, some of the major bacterial, viral, and parasitic infections leading to uveitis are discussed.

HERPESVIRUSES

Herpes group of viruses are ubiquitous in nature and can be found in nearly all animal species. Several different herpesviruses have been described so far and eight of them are found in humans: herpes simplex virus-1 (HSV-1), herpes simplex virus-2 (HSV-2), varicella-zoster virus (VZV), human cytomegalovirus (CMV), Epstein–Barr virus (EBV) and human herpesviruses 6, 7, and 8 (HHV-6, HHV-7, and HHV-8).[1]

Herpes simplex retinitis has been discussed in Chapter 80. This section therefore covers CMV, EBV, and VZV.

CYTOMEGALOVIRUS

Clinical background

Key symptoms and signs

CMV retinitis commonly affects the peripheral retina and symptoms of early disease may be minimal or absent. Blur-ring, floaters and central scotomas may develop with the affection of the central retina.[2]

Historical development

CMV eye disease was first reported in 1947,[3] being a rare clinical entity mostly seen in adults under medical immunosuppression. In the 1980s, with the acquired immunodeficiency syndrome (AIDS) pandemic, CMV became a frequent form of posterior uveitis.[4] In the mid-1990s, before the introduction of highly active antiretroviral therapy (HAART), about 30% of patients with AIDS developed CMV retinitis during their lifetime. However, the introduction of HAART achieved a 75% reduction in the incidence of CMV retinitis.[2]

Epidemiology

About half of the normal population has antibodies against CMV.[1] However, CMV infection in immunocompetent hosts does not usually produce symptomatic disease. The mode of transmission is by direct person-to-person contact and the virus is shed predominantly in urine, saliva, and semen. Most of the CMV retinitis cases result from reactivation of previously acquired disease. In patients with AIDS, CMV is one of the most common opportunistic infection. CMV retinitis usually presents in an advanced disease stage and is strongly associated with a low CD4+ T-cell count below 50 cells/mm^3.[2,5]

Diagnostic workup

The diagnosis is principally based clinically, with the typical clinical features in an immunocompromised patient. Detection of anti-CMV antibody from the vitreous and/or aqueous humor (and comparing it with the serum levels using the Goldmann–Witmer coefficient) can be helpful in selected cases. Viral culture and polymerase chain reaction (PCR) from ocular tissue (if other malignant entities are suspected) or fluid can demonstrate the existence of viral DNA, but it is important to remember that this does not directly confirm the diagnosis of CMV retinitis, because CMV can persist in the tissue without causing disease.[1,2]

Differential diagnosis

CMV retinitis must be differentiated from retinitis due to HSV or VZV, syphilitic retinitis, toxoplasma retinochoroiditis, intraocular lymphomas and fungal infections.[1]

Treatment

The first step is to improve, if possible, the immune status of the patient. In AIDS, HAART therapy has demonstrated immune reconstruction and is beneficial not only for prevention, but also for treating CMV retinitis.[6] Systemic and local anti-CMV drugs are needed in almost all AIDS patients. The most common include ganciclovir, foscarnet, and cidofovir. Others approved for treatment include fomivirsen and valganciclovir. These drugs are usually administered systemically, but in patients with intolerance or progression, intravitreal (injections or implants) ganciclovir or foscarnet can also be considered. The size of the lesion will be the main sign to evaluate the response to the treatment. In chronic immunocompromised patients, the anti-CMV therapy must be maintained indefinitely.[6-8]

Prognosis and complications

Rhegmatogenous retinal detachment (RD) is a common complication of CMV retinitis. This is usually associated with retinal necrosis and multiple retinal breaks. A vitrectomy with silicone oil tamponade has been shown to be an effective treatment for patients who have an RD caused by CMV retinitis.[9,10]

The course of CMV retinitis in the HAART era shows that the rate of retinitis progression is decreased compared with the pre-HAART era, even among those with low CD4+ T-cell counts. The incidence of visual impairment during follow-up after CMV retinitis is substantially lower among patients who receive HAART, especially those observed to have immune recovery. However, among patients with CD4+ T-cell counts less than 50 cells/mm³, while on HAART, the rates were more similar to those from the pre-HAART era.[6-8]

Pathology

CMV retinitis is a slowly expanding lesion, usually beginning as a small, white, retinal infiltrate (Figure 83.1). Initially, it can simulate a cottonwool spot, commonly present in human immunodeficiency virus (HIV) retinopathy. The clinical features, representing distinct manifestations of the same entity, are mainly:

1. Granular, white, multifocal satellite lesions of patchy retinitis (may represent infection of a terminal vessel) with limited or no retinal hemorrhage. This variant often shows a central atrophic zone.
2. Arc-shaped solitary expanding patch of retinitis, usually concurrent with multiple retinal hemorrhages and no atrophic zone in the center of the lesion. This variant is normally referred to as "fulminant" retinitis and is probably caused by infection of the major vascular arcades.

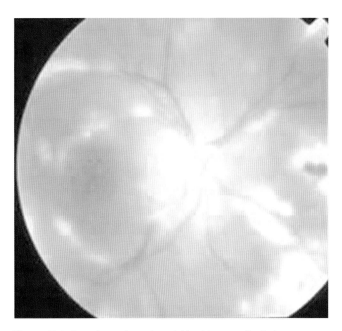

Figure 83.1 Extensive perivascular retinitis with areas of retinal hemorrhages and whitening secondary to cytomegalovirus infection.

3. Sometimes, in CMV retinitis, the perivasculitis may be predominant with some retinal necrosis. This variant is called "frosted-branch angiitis CMV retinitis." The degree of vitritis in these patients is typically low because of the extreme immunosuppression.[1,2,6,7]

Etiology

CMV, a human herpesvirus, is an omnipresent microbe in the general population, but it seldom causes clinically apparent disease in an immunocompetent individual. Neonates and immunocompromised patients are the main groups at risk for CMV retinitis, which is the most frequent cause of blindness among patients with AIDS.[6,7]

Pathophysiology

After primary infection, CMV remains in its host, establishing a latent infection typical for all herpesviruses. CMV generally reactivates from latency associated with T-cell impairment. In most cases, the retina is infected via hematogenous spread. Damage of capillary endothelial cells caused by HIV infection probably facilitates the passage of CMV-infected cells through the blood–retinal barrier.[1,2]

EPSTEIN–BARR VIRUS

Clinical background

Key symptoms and signs

EBV may affect the eye in many different ways, usually as conjunctivitis or uveitis, and often occurs in primary infections in the context of infectious mononucleosis. Follicular conjunctivitis is the most frequent ocular feature. Severe bilateral iritis and iridocyclitis have also been reported. Almost all structures of the posterior segment can be affected. Macular edema, retinal hemorrhages, punctate outer retinitis with secondary subretinal neovascularization, and subretinal fibrosis may occur. Multifocal choroiditis and other posterior-segment pathologies are uncommon and have been described in patients with infectious mononucleosis and, more recently, in patients suffering from X-linked lymphoproliferative disorder, AIDS, or even in otherwise healthy individuals.[11-14]

Historical development

EBV was first isolated in 1964 from a cultured Burkitt's lymphoma cell line. During recent decades, EBV has been implicated in a broad spectrum of human diseases like infectious mononucleosis, anaplastic nasopharyngeal carcinoma, and B-cell lymphomas, among others.[15]

Epidemiology

EBV infection is distributed worldwide. Antibodies against EBV can be detected in approximately 90% of the population but only a few suffer from ocular disease.[1,16]

Transmission requires contact with body fluids, primarily saliva, but also through blood transfusions. Primary infection is usually subclinical or leads to mild symptoms typical of a nonspecific viral illness, but in some cases it takes the clinical picture of infectious mononucleosis, especially when it affects adolescents.[16,17]

Diagnostic workup

Serum antibody titers against EBV may be helpful, especially if the initial high levels are followed by a subsequent decrease coinciding with the resolution of the acute phase. Other techniques like PCR or biopsy of the affected tissues may also be helpful in selected cases.[13,14]

Differential diagnosis

Posterior-segment findings may appear similar to those caused by tuberculosis, syphilis, or sarcoidosis. Retinal and choroidal infiltrations may be confused with acute phases of toxoplasmosis, histoplasmosis, or white-dot syndromes.[1]

Treatment

Ocular disease is commonly self-limiting and no treatment is indicated. Uveitis sometimes requires corticosteroid therapy. Severe cases, especially those rare instances where the posterior segment is affected, may require similar antiviral agents as those used in acute retinal necrosis syndrome: intravenous aciclovir, ganciclovir, brivudine, valganciclovir, and foscarnet.[16]

Prognosis and complications

The panuveitis and choroiditis in patients with EBV infection can be complicated by macular edema and cataract forma-

tion. Visual prognosis is usually poor in patients with chronic smoldering chorioretinitis leading to subretinal neovascularization or cystoid macular edema.[1,16]

Pathophysiology

EBV shows B-cell tropism. However, the precise role of this virus in associated diseases is not well understood, but defective immunosurveillance against the virus may permit an uncontrolled proliferation of EBV-infected cells.[1]

EBV belongs to the gamma herpesvirus family.

VARICELLA-ZOSTER VIRUS

Clinical background

Key symptoms and signs

Systemic manifestations

Systemic manifestations consist of general malaise, fever, and headache. Subsequently, the characteristic papules, macules, vesicles, and, later, crusting occur with VZV.

Ocular manifestations

Ocular manifestations include trabeculitis, iridocyclitis, acute retinal necrosis (Figure 83.2), and variants of necrotizing herpetic retinopathy. Inflammation of the endothelium occurs relatively early in the course of disease and leads to stromal and epithelial edema. Endotheliitis is typically accompanied by signs of mild anterior-chamber inflammation. Keratic precipitates often appear under affected regions of the cornea and they can be either small or large (mutton fat). Iridocyclitis tends to occur within 1–2 weeks of disease onset, but can appear many months later. Later, inflammation is mediated by an immune reaction against persistent viral antigen presence in the corneal stroma. Sectoral occlu-

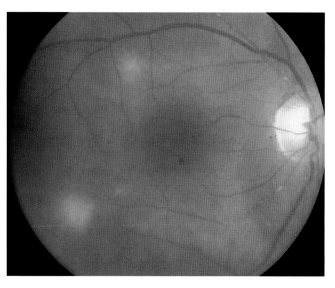

Figure 83.2 Foci of retinitis in acute retinal necrosis. Note the perivascular infiltrates along the arteries.

sion of the iris vasculature leads to atrophic sectoral patches in approximately 20% of cases and can produce hypopigmentation or, infrequently, hyperpigmentation, and iris sphincter damage.[18,19]

Historical development

Giovanni Filippo provided the first description of the varicella virus. Herpesvirus infections of the uvea were characterized in the late 1970s and Culbertson and associates proved the pathogenic connection of herpesviruses in 1982.[1]

Epidemiology

Ninety percent of the population demonstrates serologic evidence of exposure to VZV by age 60, but only 20% will have experienced an episode of viral reactivation.[18,19]

Diagnostic workup

The diagnosis is based on a typical clinical picture of unilateral involvement, corneal hypoesthesia, and pattern of keratic precipitates, mild flare and cells in the anterior chamber with foci of iris stromal sectorial atrophy. Aqueous humor aspirates can be analyzed for antibodies directed against VZV by enzyme-linked immunosorbent assay (ELISA). Viral DNA within the aqueous can be detected by PCR technology.[18,20]

Differential diagnosis

Other viruses of the herpes family, like CMV, EBV, and HSV, can mimic iridocyclitis caused by VZV. Syphilis, tuberculosis, leprosy, lymphogranuloma venereum, and chronic myelomonocytic leukemia can also be considered.[1,18,19,21]

Treatment

Systemic antivirals are the mainstay management of VZV uveitis – usually oral aciclovir but also famciclovir and valaciclovir (a prodrug of aciclovir). Topical corticosteroids are used to control iridocyclitis and the inflammatory manifestations of corneal disease, including disciform keratitis, endotheliitis, and keratouveitis. In the acute stages, cycloplegic agents are used to relieve the discomfort of photophobia and prevent the formation of synechiae.[18,19,22]

Prognosis and complications

The most frequent ocular complication is secondary glaucoma. Posterior pole complications can develop and these include cystoid macular edema, epiretinal membrane, papillitis, retinal fibrosis, and detachment. VZV uveitis typically runs a chronic course and visual prognosis is dependent on the severity of complications and its treatment.[19,22]

Pathology

Histologic reports on VZV uveitis have revealed perineuritis and perivasculitis with infiltration by chronic inflammatory cells consisting of plasma cells and lymphocytes. Occlusive vasculitis plays an important role in sectoral iris atrophy.[1]

Etiology

Primary infection with VZV causes varicella disease ("chickenpox") and reactivation of the virus leads to zoster ("shingles").

Pathophysiology

VZV establishes its latent phase in the satellite cells of sensory ganglia; the thoracic and lumbar dermatomes are most frequently involved clinically. The trigeminal ganglion is often also infected. In the pathogenesis of persistent or recrudescent viral ocular disease, immune reactions against viral antigens and against tissue autoantigens produced from viral damage play a major role.[18]

HSV-1, HSV-2, VZV, and HHV-8 belong to the subfamily of alpha herpesviruses. The clinical picture of various forms of intraocular inflammation caused by alpha herpesviruses is similar and therefore it may be difficult to distinguish VZV from HSV. Nevertheless, HSV as a cause of iridocyclitis and trabeculitis is often overlooked. Corneal lesions (Figure 83.3) or a history of herpetic keratitis in an eye with iritis must be considered herpetic in origin unless proven otherwise. A high degree of suspicion for HSV anterior uveitis must be maintained in unilateral involvement diminished corneal sensation and typical iris stromal atrophy. This condition responds promptly to aciclovir therapy, which may be required chronically. Diagnosis of HSV can be confirmed by PCR testing of the aqueous humor for herpetic DNA (Box 83.1).

Other viruses causing uveitis are summarized in Table 83.1.

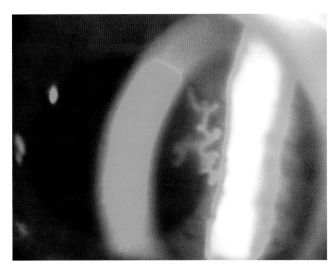

Figure 83.3 Dendrites with anterior stromal haze in herpes simplex virus-associated keratouveitis.

BARTONELLA

Clinical background

Key symptoms and signs

Systemic manifestations include myalgia, malaise, fatigue, low-grade fever, and lymphadenopathy. Ocular manifestations are typically unilateral and can present in both immunocompetent and immunocompromised patients. Neuroretinitis appears to be most common and is usually unilateral, with optic disc edema (Figure 83.4) and a macular star.[23,24] A multifocal retinitis and/or choroiditis can also develop, as can chorioretinitis, serous macular detachments, intraretinal hemorrhages, cottonwool spots, Parinaud's oculoglandular syndrome, conjunctivitis, anterior and posterior uveitis, and vascular lesions of the optic nerve.

Historical development

Barton described the first human *Bartonella* infection in 1909.[25] Foshay created the term "cat-scratch fever" in 1932.[26]

Box 83.1 Ocular manifestations of herpesviruses

- Cytomegalovirus retinitis: slowly expanding white infiltrate in the peripheral retina
  - Granular, white, multifocal satellite lesions of patchy retinitis with limited or no retinal hemorrhages
  - Arc-shaped solitary expanding patch of retinitis with multiple retinal hemorrhages
  - Extensive perivasculitis with "frosted-branch angiitis" appearance
- Epstein–Barr virus: follicular conjunctivitis is the most frequent ocular feature
  - Anterior and posterior uveitis may occur
- Varicella-zoster virus: anterior/posterior-segment findings
  - Keratitis
  - Iritis/iridocyclitis
  - Trabeculitis
  - Acute retinal necrosis
- Herpes simplex virus: spectrum of ocular signs similar to varicella-zoster virus; high degree of suspicion if:
  - Corneal hypoesthesia
  - Iris stromal atrophy and transillumination defects

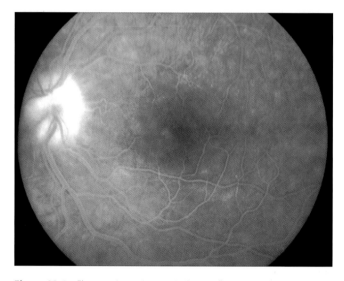

Figure 83.4 Fluorescein angiogram in *Bartonella*-associated panuveitis with papilledema and cystoid macular edema.

Table 83.1 Infectious uveitis caused by viruses

Disease	Organism	Ocular signs and symptoms	Transmission	Treatment
Rift Valley fever	Plebovirus	Anterior uveitis Vitritis Macular exudative lesions Retinal edema Retinal hemorrhage Retinal vasculitis	Mosquito *Culex* *Aedes*	Ribavirin* RVF MP-12 vaccine*
Measles	Morbillivirus	Retinopathy Retinitis Retinochoroidal atrophy Macular star Papillitis Arteriolar attenuation	Respiratory secretions	Self-limiting Gamma-globulin IFN-alpha Inosiplex IVIg + Inosiplex Vitamin A
Rubella	Rubella virus	Pigmentary retinopathy Retinitis Subretinal neovascularization Subretinal hemorrhages Disciform scarring Optic neuritis Retinal detachments	Transplacental Transcervical Respiratory secretions	Self-limiting Systemic steroids

*Experimental use.
RVF MP-12, Rift valley fever vaccine; IFN, interferon; IVIg, intravenous immunoglobulin.

Sweeny and Drance made the correlation between intraocular inflammation and cat-scratch disease (CSD) in 1970.[27]

Epidemiology

CSD has been shown to be a worldwide zoonotic infection with the reservoir for *Bartonella henselae* in domestic cats.[23] CSD is the leading cause of regional lymphadenopathy in children and young adults worldwide. Prevalence of neuroretinitis in the context of CSD is approximately 1–2%.[28,29] The infection is not known to be transmitted from human to human. The prevalence of CSD in the USA is approximately 22 000 cases per year.[30]

Diagnostic workup

The diagnosis of CSD is primarily based on clinical features supported by laboratory testing with detection of DNA of *B. henselae* by PCR technology using a very small sample of serum or other body fluids. Other tests include enzyme immunoassay (EIA) and Western blot test.[24,25]

Differential diagnosis

Other causes of regional lymphadenopathy and conjunctivitis include tularemia, sporotrichosis, tuberculosis, syphilis, lymphogranuloma venereum, leprosy, and *Yersinia*. Neuroretinitis may be seen in syphilis, tuberculosis, toxoplasmosis, varicella, herpes simplex, toxocariasis, leptospirosis, and infectious mononucleosis. A macular star with vitritis can be seen in toxoplasmosis and vascular disorders such as anterior ischemic optic neuropathy, acute systemic hypertension, and increased intracranial pressures.[1,24,25]

Treatment

There are no formalized guidelines which one can follow to treat the ocular complications associated with *B. henselae*. Despite this, several groups have used oral ciprofloxacin, prednisone, and doxycycline, with favorable responses.[31,32] Elevated immunoglobulin (Ig) M or IgG titers for *B. henselae* can be suggestive of current or past infection.

Prognosis and complications

CSD typically runs a self-limiting course in immunocompetent hosts. Antimicrobial therapy in immunocompromised hosts results in a dramatic response and hence these have been recommended for severe ocular or systemic complications of CSD. Visual prognosis of most patients with CSD-associated neuroretinitis is therefore excellent.[23]

Etiology

B. henselae, one of the four human species of *Bartonella*, has been implicated as the cause of CSD. This species predominantly causes neuroretinitis, while the three others cause endocarditis (*B. elizabethae*), Carrion's disease (*B. bacilliformis*), and trench fever (*B. quintana*).[25] Regnery et al[33] showed that 86% of patients with CSD had *B. henselae* antibodies as compared to 6% of those who were healthy

---

Box 83.2 *Bartonella*

- Zoonosis
- Reservoir of *B. henselae* in cats
- Affects children and young adults
- Presents with oculoglandular syndrome
- Neuroretinitis may be the foremost ocular manifestation
- Oral antibiotics (tetracyclines) and oral corticosteroids may be used for treatment

---

patients. PCR assays have shown that infected cats harbor fleas infected by *B. henselae*. Transmission from cat to cat occurs via the cat flea *Ctenocephalides felis*. It is thought to be central to the pathogenesis of CSD in human beings, perhaps by dropping contaminated feces on to the fur and dander of infested cats. The predominant mode of transmission of *B. henselae* is through a cat bite or scratch.[1,23,24]

Pathophysiology

The exact pathophysiology of CSD-associated neuroretinitis is not completely understood. Intraocular infection or direct involvement of the optic nerve by *B. henselae* has been implicated (Box 83.2). The ocular findings may also represent a parainfectious inflammatory response.[1,23]

SYPHILIS

Clinical background

Key symptoms and signs

Systemic manifestations

Primary syphilis is characterized by a chancre at the inoculation site that appears 2–6 weeks after infection and resolves about 4 weeks after its appearance. If untreated, the disease progresses to secondary syphilis, with generalized maculopapular rash and lymphadenopathy. The rash typically affects the palms and soles, and can be accompanied by fever, malaise, headache, nausea, hair loss, mouth ulcers, and joint pain. At this stage, the eyes are affected in 10% of cases.[34] Then, during the latent stage, there are no evident systemic disease manifestations, and the infection is not contagious. This stage can last for the patient's lifetime. Tertiary syphilis can affect any system, but mainly the cardiovascular (aortitis, aortic aneurysm, aortic valve insufficiency) and neurologic system (meningovascular syphilis, tabes dorsalis). The typical lesion in this stage is the gumma, which is a granuloma, and can be found anywhere in the body.

Ocular manifestations

Most patients with syphilitic uveitis develop it during the latent stage of the infection. Anterior uveitis may be unilateral or bilateral, granulomatous, or nongranulomatous. It can present with iris nodules or atrophy, anterior-chamber cells with or without anterior vitritis, dilated iris vessels, interstitial keratitis, and lens dislocation. Syphilis can affect

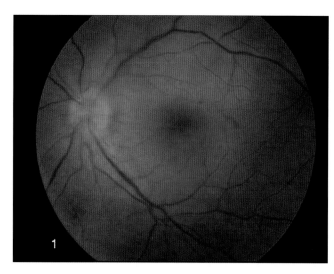

Figure 83.5 Syphilitic panuveitis with vitritis, vitreous hemorrhage, and papillitis.

Box 83.3 Syphilis

- Great masquerader
- Stages are primary, secondary, latent, and tertiary
  - No uveitis in primary stage
  - Uveitis may present in the remaining stages but most commonly in the latent stage
- Anterior uveitis, diffuse chorioretinitis, and necrotizing retinitis may be seen
- Diagnostic tests include:
  - Rapid plasma reagin (RPR)/Venereal Disease Research Laboratory (VDRL)
  - Fluorescent treponemal antibody absorption test (FTA-ABS)
  - Microhemagglutionation assay for *Treponema pallidum* (MHA-TP)
  - *Treponema pallidum* immobilization (TPI) test
  - *Treponema pallidum* particle agglutination (TP-PA)
  - Dark-field microscopy
  - Polymerase chain reaction (PCR)
- Treatment: benzathine penicillin or penicillin V

---

the posterior segment (Figure 83.5), most commonly causing chorioretinitis. The fundus lesions are usually grayish yellow in color. Other manifestations include disc edema, arterial or venous vasculitis, vitritis, intermediate uveitis, serous RD, neuroretinitis, and necrotizing retinitis. Complications include glaucoma, cataracts, macular edema, and choroidal neovascular membranes.[34-38]

Historical development

Schaudin and Hoffman isolated the spirochete in 1905 from the skin lesions of infected patients.[39]

Epidemiology

Although it was the second leading cause of uveitis before the 1940s, currently it comprises about 1–2% of all uveitis cases.[40]

Diagnostic workup

Available nonspecific serological tests that quantify the amount of serum anticardiolipin antibody are the rapid plasma reagin (RPR) and the Venereal Disease Research Laboratory (VDRL). The results depend on the status of infection and treatment. Titers are usually high in active infection, but drop when the disease is not active (latent infection or after successful treatment). Specific tests measure the amount of serum antibody against treponemal antigens. The fluorescent treponemal antigen absorption test (FTA-ABS) is the one mostly used. This test becomes positive during the secondary stage of syphilis and remains positive for the patient's lifetime. This test is more sensitive during the latent stage, which is when uveitis usually develops. With the microhemagglutination assay for *T. pallidum* (MHA-TP) test, treponemes can be visualized by incubating infected body fluid (from chancre or skin pustule) with fluorescent-tagged antibody and visualizing it under dark-field microscopy. The *T. pallidum* particle agglutination test (TP-PA) is used to confirm a positive FTA-ABS. Patients with uveitis who are diagnosed with syphilis must have examination of the cerebrospinal fluid.[41-43]

Differential diagnosis

Syphilitic uveitis must be differentiated from other causes of granulomatous uveitis like tuberculosis, leprosy, sarcoidosis, and herpes. It is also in the differential diagnosis of intermediate uveitis and therefore may be confused with Lyme disease or sarcoidosis.[41]

Treatment

Penicillin is the treatment of choice in syphilis, either intramuscular or intravenous. As syphilitic uveitis is considered a form of neurosyphilis, the intravenous regimen is favored. Alternative treatments for penicillin-allergic patients include doxycycline or tetracycline. Penicillin desensitization is another option for these patients.[44]

Prognosis and complications

Complications from syphilitic uveitis include cataracts, glaucoma, macular edema, epiretinal membranes, RD, chorioretinitis, and neovascular memebranes. Complications secondary to treatment include Jarisch–Herxheimer reaction manifesting as fever, myalgia, malaise, and headache.

Syphilis, if recognized early and treated appropriately, can result in a cure. If untreated, prolonged syphilitic disease can permanently damage the eye and can result in significant morbidity and mortality due to cardiovascular complications.[42]

Etiology

Syphilis is an infection caused by the spirochete *Treponema pallidum*. It can mimic many different diseases throughout its course, for which is has been called the "great imitator" (Box 83.3). It can persist in the affected person for a lifetime, and if left untreated can progress through four stages. It is a sexually transmitted disease, which enters the body through the genitals, mouth, or skin breaks.

Pathophysiology

The inflammatory response against the spirochete causes the damage and destruction of ocular tissue. The host immune response role in syphilitic infection is being investigated. The difficulty in culturing *T. pallidum* in vivo has been an impediment in the study and of its pathogenic mechanisms. Long-term immunity against syphilis is not conferred after initial infection and reinfection can occur in previously treated individuals. A switch from Th1-mediated process (during the first infection) to a Th2-mediated process with subsequent infections has been implicated.[1,43]

Other bacteria causing uveitis are summarized in Table 83.2.

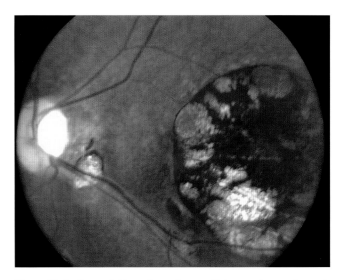

Figure 83.6 Congenital toxoplasmosis scar with temporal excavation and atrophy of the optic nerve with juxtapapillary scar along the inferior arcade.

TOXOPLASMOSIS

Clinical background

Key symptoms and signs

Congenital toxoplasmosis involves the central nervous system and it may present several months or even years after infection, with several features characteristic of the disease, such as paralysis, encephalomyelitis, seizures, hydrocephalus, microcephaly, and intracranial calcifications. In the acquired form of the infection, lymphadenopathy is the most common finding. However, the disease is typically self-limiting in the immunocompetent patient.

Ocular manifestations vary. In the congenital form, the most common finding is retinochoroiditis, occurring in 70–90% of the cases. Associated ocular sequelae include cataracts, nystagmus, optic atrophy, and strabismus. In the posterior segment, *T. gondii* has a strong predilection for invading the macula and optic nerve, with a tendency to recur. A yellow, elevated, fluffy lesion is seen in the hallmark "headlight in the fog" appearance of the active *Toxoplasma* lesion. In the active form of the disease, vitritis is almost always present in all cases. Vasculitis, choroiditis, neuroretinitis, papillitis, and necrotizing retinitis may present as well.[45,46] Retinochoroidal scars (Figure 83.6) are typically found in both the acquired and congenital forms and can be solitary or multiple.

In the anterior segment, mutton-fat keratic precipitates, anterior-chamber reaction, and posterior synechiae may be present in the active part of the disease.

Historical development

In 1940, Pinkerton and Weinman described the first case of acquired toxoplasmosis with ocular manifestations.[47] However, the initial case of congenital toxoplasmosis was reported by Janku in 1923.[48]

Epidemiology

Toxoplasmosis is the leading cause of posterior uveitis in the world in otherwise healthy individuals. Toxoplasmosis is a very widely distributed zoonosis. Seropositive individuals typically live in countries with tropical climates. In certain countries like France, by the fourth decade of life, 90% of the French population is seropositive for toxoplasmosis. In the USA, 70% of the population over 50 shows seropositivity. The incidence of congenital toxoplasmosis in the USA is approximately 0.2–1%.[49-51]

Diagnostic workup

The Sabin and Feldman dye, hemagglutination, ELISA, complement fixation, and immunofluorescence antibody tests may be used to detect for presence of toxoplasmosis.[52,53] PCR of samples of the aqueous or vitreous humor can confirm the presence of *T. gondii* with high specificity and selectivity.

Fluorescein angiogram (FA) and indocyanine green angiography (ICGA)

During the early phase of an FA study, there is hypofluorescence of the lesion which then leaks dye in late phase. In ICGA, active retinochoroiditis may reveal areas of hypofluorescence or hyperfluorescence in the early phases and, in the later phase, hyperfluorescence predominates.

Differential diagnosis

Congenital toxoplasmosis must be differentiated from other infectious diseases of the TORCH group (rubella, CMV, and herpes) as well as tuberculosis, syphilis, and AIDS. Recurrent toxoplasma lesions adjacent to the older ones may resemble serpiginous choroiditis. Necrotizing retinitis caused by other agents must be considered, such as herpes viridae, fungal retinitis, septic retinitis, and toxocariasis. Atypical forms of toxoplasmosis may resemble white-dot syndromes.[52-54]

Table 83.2   Infectious uveitis caused by bacteria

Disease	Organism	Ocular signs and symptoms	Transmission	Treatment
Tuberculosis	*Mycobacterium tuberculosis*	Disseminated choroiditis Focal choroiditis Anterior tuberculosis Uveitis Panophthalmitis	Direct entry Hematogenous	INH Rifampicin Pyrazinamide Ethambutol
Lyme borreliosis	*Borrelia burgdorferei*	Anterior, intermediate, panuveitis Neuroretinitis Retinal vasculitis Choroiditis Optic neuritis Papilledema Papillitis	*Ixodes ricinus*	Doxycycline Amoxicillin Cefuroxime
Leptospirosis (zoonosis)	*Leptospira interrogans*	Anterior uveitis Vitritis Choroiditis Papillitis Panuveitis Retinal vasculitis	Contaminated water and soil Transplacental	Doxycycline Cephalosporins
Brucellosis (zoonosis)	*Brucella melitensis* *Brucella abortus* *Brucella suis* *Brucella neotomae* *Brucella ovis* *Brucella canis* *Brucella maris*	Iridocyclitis: granulomatous nongranulomatous Vitritis Panuveitis Multifocal choroiditis Retinitis and vasculitis Endophthalmitis	Unpasteurized milk and cheese Contaminated meat	 Combination of tetracycline + streptomycin Doxycycline + gentamicin
Whipple's disease	*Tropheryma whippelii*	Vitritis Vitreous and retinal hemorrhages Retinitis Choroiditis Optic atrophy Retrobulbar neuritis	Unknown	Chloramphenicol Penicillin Ampicillin TMP–SMX Doxycycline
Rickettsioses (zoonosis)	*Rickettsia rickettsii* *Rickettsia conorii* *Rickettsia africae*	Anterior nongranulomatous uveitis Iris nodules Hypopyon uveitis	*Ixodes* tick Mite Arthropod bite	
Spotted fever gp	*Rickettsia australis* *Rickettsia sibirica* *Rickettsia japonica* *Rickettsia akari*	Papillitis Cottonwool spots Intraretinal hemorrhages Tortuous retinal vein		
Typhus gp	*Rickettsia prowazekii* *Rickettsia typhi* *Rickettsia tsutsugamushi*	Vasculitis Retinal vessel occlusion Capillary nonperfusion	Louse Flea Mite	
Q fever	*Coxiella burnetii*	Retinal infiltrates	Tick	
Sennetsu	*Ehrlichia sennetsu*			
Ehrlichiosis	*E. chaffeensis*			
Leprosy	*Mycobacterium leprae*	Early diminished pupillary reaction Reduced accommodation Early presbyopia Iridocyclitis: granulomatous nongranulomatous Iris pearls Choroiditis: peripheral nonspecific disseminated	Airborne Skin lesions Transplacental Breast milk	Dapsone Rifampicin Clofazimine Quinolones Minocycline Clarithromycin

INH, isonicotinic hydrazide, TMP-SMX, trimethoprim sulfamethoxazole.

Table 83.3 Infectious uveitis caused by parasites

Disease	Organism	Ocular signs and symptoms	Transmission	Treatment
Free-living amebas and amebiasis	*Acanthamoeba*	Anterior uveitis	Contaminated water	Biguanide
	Naegleria	Hypopyon	Inhalation of cysts	Diamidine
		Chorioretinitis		Imidazoles
		Keratitis and scleritis		Aminoglycosides
Giardiasis	*Giardia lamblia*	Anterior uveitis	Contaminated water	Mepacrine HCl
		Choroiditis		Metronidazole
		Salt-and-pepper alterations		
		Vitelliform macular lesions		
		Retinal vasculitis		
Trypanosomiasis	*Trypanosoma* species	Toxic amblyopia		Pentamidine
African	*Trypanosoma rhodesiense*	Retinal lesions	Tsetse fly	Suramin
	Trypanosoma gambiense	Periorbital edema		Melarsoprol
American	*Trypanosoma cruzi*	RPE defects	Reduviid insect	
Pneumocytosis	*Pneumocytis carinii*	Choroiditis	IC states	TMP-SMX
		Choroidal infiltrates	Respiratory secretion	IV pentamidine
		Vitritis		
Toxocariasis (zoonosis)	*Toxocara canis*	Anterior uveitis	Oral ingestion	Corticosteroids
	Toxocara cati	Posterior synechiae	Contaminated soil	Local
		Granulomas	Contact with infected dogs	systemic
		Chronic endopthalmitis		Thiabendazole
		Cyclitic membranes	infected cats	Vitrectomy
		Papilltis		Cryopexy
		Retrolental masses		Photocoagulation
Ascariasis	*Ascaris lumbricoides*	Iridocyclitis:	Ingestion of eggs	Mebendazole
		granulomatous		Albendazole
		nongranulomatous		Pamoate
		Papillitis		Pyrantel
		Periphlebitis		
		Vitreous hemorrhages		
Onchocerchiasis	*Onchocerca volvulus*	Anterior uveitis:	*Simulium* fly	Ivermectin
		granulomatous		
		nongranulomatous		
		Optic atrophy		
		Chorioretinitis		
		RPE atrophy		
Loiasis	*Loa loa*	Anterior uveitis	Chrysops fly	DEC
		Choroidal lesions		
		Retinal edema		
Cysticercosis	*Taenia solium*	Anterior uveitis	Ingestion of larvae	Vitrectomy
	Cysticercus cellulosae	Vitritis		Retinotomy
		Retinal edema		Worm removal
		Papilledema		
		Retinal vascular sheathing		
		Pthisis bulbi		
Schistosomiasis	*Schistosoma haematobium*	Anterior uveitis	Contaminated water	Praziquantel
	Schistosoma japonicum	Choroiditis		Corticosteroids
	Schistosoma mansoni	RPE inflammation		
		Retinitis, vasculitis		
		Optic atrophy		

IC, immunocompromised; RPE, retinal pigment epithelium; TMP-SMX, trimethoprim sulfamethoxazole; IV, intravenous; DEC, diethylcarbamazine.

Table 83.4 Infectious uveitis caused by fungi

Disease	Organism	Ocular signs and symptoms	Transmission	Treatment
Presumed ocular histoplasmosis syndrome (POHS)	*Histoplasma capsulatum*	Disseminated choroiditis Maculopathy Peripapillary changes Vitritis absent	Inhalation of spores	Photocoagulation Systemic steroids Periocular steroids
Candidiasis	*Candida* species	Chorioretinitis Endophthalmitis Vitreal exudates Retinal necrosis Cyclitic membranes Phthisis bulbi	IC states Hematogenous Ocular surgery Ocular trauma	Amphotericin B* Vitrectomy Flucytosine Ketoconazole Fluconazole
Coccidiodomycosis	*Coccidiodes immitis*	Iridocyclitis: granulomatous Choroiditis Chorioretinitis Vitritis Perivascular sheathing	Inhalation of spores Hematogenous	Amphotericin B Fluconazole Iatraconazole
Cryptococcosis	*Cryptococcus neoformans*	Papilledema Optic neuropathy Chiasmal involvement Optic atrophy Choroiditis Retinitis	IC states Inhalation Pigeon feces Contaminated soil Hematogenous Iris masses	Fluconazole Oral flucytosine + IV amphotericin B Vitrectomy IV amphotericin B
Sporotrichosis	*Sporothrix schenckii*	Choroiditis Vitritis Retinitis Panuveitis Endophthalmitis	Inoculation Inhalation Hematogenous	SSKI Amphotericin B Flucytosine Iatraconazole

*Intravenous and intravitreal.
IC, immunocompromised; IV, intravenous; Iv, intravitreal; SSKI, saturated solution of potassium iodide.

Treatment

Medical treatment of toxoplasmosis employs corticosteroids and various antimicrobial agents. The use of pyrimethamine, sulfadiazine, and corticosteroids is the gold standard since Eyles and Coleman advocated this triad of treatment in 1953.[55] Folinic acid is used as adjuvant therapy to pyrimethamine, which has antifolate properties. Other agents used include clindamycin, spiramycin, atovaquone, tetracycline, minocycline, clarithromycin, azithromycin, trimethoprim, sulfamethoxazole, and trovafloxacin. Laser photocoagulation and pars plana vitrectomy have had limited success.

Prognosis and complications

Complications like granulomatous iritis, secondary glaucoma, retinal vasculitis, vascular occlusions, rhegmatogenous and serous RD, and secondary pigmentary retinopathies might disguise the original toxoplasmic lesion and make the correct diagnosis difficult. Prognosis of this disease depends on the presence of macular involvement as the active disease is typically self-limiting. Factors responsible for a poor visual prognosis include proximity to the fovea, large lesions, and duration of the disease. Early diagnosis and appropriate treatment are essential to minimize complications and loss of vision.[53,56]

Pathology

T. gondii is found in the host's saliva, urine, semen, and peritoneal fluid. The organism presents in three forms: tachyzoite, bradyzoite, and sporozoite. Tachyzoites are responsible for the acute form of the disease. Tachyzoites stain with Giemsa and have a bluish cytoplasm and a reddish ovoid nucleus. Cysts have eosinophilic walls with the bradyzoites inside and are periodic acid–Schiff-positive.[53]

Etiology

Toxoplasma gondii is an intracellular obligate protozoan, which causes ocular toxoplasmosis by the release of actively proliferating tachyzoites. It is transmitted to humans via ingestion of tissue cysts in raw or undercooked meat or through contact with the fecal matter of cats, which contains *T. gondii* oocysts. The disease may be congenital, acquired, and ocular (Box 83.4).[53,54]

Box 83.4 Toxoplasmosis

- Leading cause of posterior uveitis
- Congenital form presents with retinochoroiditis, cataracts, nystagmus, strabismus with or without systemic central nervous signs and symptoms
- Acquired form may present with focal retinitis, retinochoroiditis, and scarring
- Predilection for the macula and optic nerve with tendency to recur
- Gold standard for therapy is pyrimethamine, sulfadiazine, and corticosteroids

Pathophysiology

Cell-mediated immunity is the major mechanism involved in resolution of active disease. It is characterized by activation of macrophages, natural killer cells, and release of cytokines. The local ocular responses tend to be suppressed to limit tissue damage as the eye is an immune-privileged tissue. Another strategy developed by the organism to evade host defense mechanism is encystment. Tissue cysts become invisible to the immune system, thereby allowing the cysts to remain dormant for extended periods of time.[56]

Other parasites and fungi causing uveitis are summarized in Tables 83.3 and 83.4.

Key references

A complete list of chapter references is available online at www.expertconsult.com. See inside cover for registration details.

1. Heilingenhaus A, Helbig H, Fiedler M. Herpesviruses. In: Foster CS, Vitale AT (eds) Diagnosis and Treatment of Uveitis. Philadelphia: Saunders, 2002:315–332.

6. Jabs DA, Van Natta ML, Thorne JE, et al. Studies of Ocular Complications of AIDS Research Group. Course of cytomegalovirus retinitis in the era of highly active antiretroviral therapy: 1. Retinitis progression. Ophthalmology 2004;111:2224–2231.

11. Raymond LA, Wilson CA, Linnemann CC. Punctate outer retinitis in acute EBV infection. Am J Ophthalmol 1987;104:424–426.

20. Chan CC, Shen D, Tuo J. Polymerase chain reaction in the diagnosis of uveitis.

Int Ophthalmol Clin 2005;45:41–55.

21. Baltatzis S, Romero-Rangel T, Foster CS. Sectorial keratitis and uveitis: differential diagnosis. Graefes Arch Clin Exp Ophthalmol 2003;241:2–7.

22. Miserocchi E, Waheed NK, Dios E, et al. Visual outcome in herpes simplex virus and varicella zoster virus uveitis: a clinical evaluation and comparison. Ophthalmology 2002;109:1532–1537.

23. Cunningham ET, Koehler JE. Ocular bartonellosis. Am J Ophthalmol 2000;130:340–349.

34. Crouch ER, Goldberg MF. Retinal periarteritis secondar to syphilis. Arch Ophthalmol 1975;93:384–387.

35. Tamesis R, Foster CS. Ocular syphilis. Ophthalmology 1990;97:1281–1287.

45. Park SS, To KW, Friedman AH, et al. Infectious causes of posterior uveitis. In: Albert DM, Jakobiec FA (eds) Principles and Practice of Ophthalmology. Philadelphia: WB Saunders, 1994:460–461.

52. Holland GN. Ocular toxoplasmosis: a global reassessment. Part II: disease manifestations and management. Am J Ophthalmol 2004;137:1–17.

56. Holland GN. Reconsidering the pathogenesis of ocular toxoplasmosis. Am J Ophthalmol 1999;128:502–505.

CHAPTER 84

Ocular sarcoidosis

Russell N Van Gelder and Suzanne M Dintzis

Overview

Sarcoidosis (from the Greek, meaning "tumor-like") is a systemic inflammatory condition that may affect many organs. Its hallmark is the noncaseating granuloma, a non-specific but highly suggestive pathologic finding. Although sarcoidosis most commonly affects the lungs and lymph nodes, the eyes are frequently affected. Because the ocular manifestations of sarcoidosis may be protean, this condition is considered in the differential diagnosis in nearly every case of ocular inflammatory disease. Significant progress has been made in the past several years in understanding the pathogenesis of sarcoidosis.

Clinical background

Historical development

Sarcoidosis was first recognized by the London physician, Dr. Jonathan Hutchinson, who in 1877 described a series of patients with purple skin plaques on the hands and feet. Twelve years later, Dr. Cesar Boeck gave the name "sarcoid" to a disease process featuring multiple benign skin lesions. The first description of sarcoidosis affecting the eye was in 1909 with the description of Heerfordt syndrome, featuring parotid inflammation, uveitis, facial nerve palsy, and fever.

Key symptoms and signs

Sarcoidosis most often presents in the eye as uveitis. Uveitis is a general term referring to inflammation of the iris (iritis), vitreous body (intermediate uveitis), or retina and choroid (retinitis and choroiditis; retinal vasculitis may also accompany these findings). Typical symptoms of anterior uveitis are redness, pain, and aversion to bright lights (photophobia). Intermediate uveitis typically presents as new "floaters" in the patient's vision. Posterior uveitis may present with loss of central visual acuity, new visual field defects, or generalized blurring of the vision (often macular edema).

Ocular sarcoidosis can present with many different signs (Box 84.1). The conjunctiva may contain macroscopic granulomas that can be observed at the slit lamp. The lacrimal glands may be enlarged from granulomas, which may con-

tribute to dry eye. The classic intraocular presentation of sarcoidosis is of an anterior or panuveitis, featuring large clumps of white blood cells adherent to the corneal endothelium, known as "mutton fat keratic precipitates" (Figure 84.1). The anterior chamber frequently contains free-floating leukocytes. These are quantified on a standardized scale by the clinician, with 1+ cells corresponding to 6–15 visible cells in a 1×1 mm slit beam, to 4+ cells which are too numerous to count. The clinician may also observe flare in the anterior chamber as visible diffusion of the slit-lamp beam. This phenomenon arises from increased protein concentration in the aqueous humor due to compromise of the blood–aqueous barrier. The iris can develop adhesions to the lens, called posterior synechiae. Intraocular pressure may be elevated from trabecular meshwork inflammation or anterior synechiae from the iris to the peripheral cornea, blocking the trabecular meshwork. The pressure may also be reduced from ciliary body inflammation. The vitreous cavity often features white blood cell infiltration, which can be diffuse in the liquid anterior vitreous, or more clumped in the formed vitreous. The clumped cells are sometimes referred to as "snowballs." Posteriorly, the most common manifestation of sarcoidosis is the choroidal granuloma (Figure 84.2). These may be solitary or numerous, and may range from whitish in color to yellow. The vasculitis associated with sarcoidosis is most often seen on the veins. An unusual form of periphlebitis, called "tache de bougie" (candle wax drippings) occurs in patients with sarcoidosis. In a small proportion of cases sarcoid optic nerve head granulomas may be observed. Because of its protean ocular manifestations, sarcoidosis is often considered one of the "great masquerade" conditions, along with syphilis and tuberculosis.

Outside the eye, sarcoidosis typically presents in the lungs, where it may present as chronic cough or shortness of breath; approximately one-third of cases are found as an incidental finding on chest X-ray. Pulmonary sarcoidosis is staged based on the radiographic findings. The first stage is visible hilar adenopathy. In the second stage, pulmonary infiltrate is seen along with the hilar lymphadenopathy. In the third stage, the adenopathy is resolved but the infiltrates remain. Stage 4 sarcoidosis features pulmonary fibrosis; the prognosis for this stage of sarcoidosis is poor. Sarcoidosis may present in almost any other organ system. It is associated with liver granulomas, diffuse lymphadenopathy, deep

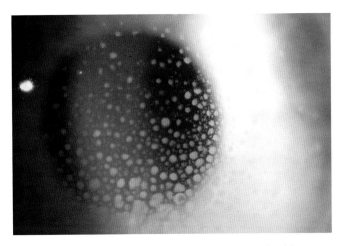

Figure 84.1 Mutton fat keratic precipitates from uveitis attributable to sarcoidosis.

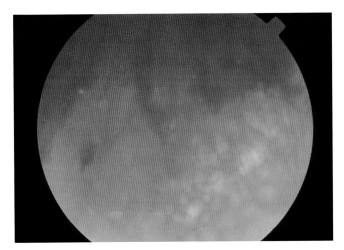

Figure 84.2 Multiple small choroidal granulomas in peripheral retina secondary to sarcoidosis.

Box 84.1 Clinical features of ocular sarcoidosis

Anterior inflammation
- White blood cells in anterior chamber
- Keratic precipitates (clumped cells on corneal endothelium)
- Posterior synechiae (adhesions between iris and lens)

Intermediate inflammation
- White blood cells in vitreous cavity, diffuse or clumped

Posterior inflammation
- Choroidal granulomas
- Retinal periphlebitis (taches de bougie)
- Cystoid macular edema

---

brain granulomas, and skin findings, including erythema nodosum.

Epidemiology

The incidence and prevalence of sarcoidosis vary markedly with geographic locale and patient population. The inci-

dence in African-Americans and in the USA has been estimated at approximately 40–80 per 100 000 person-years, compared with 4–8 per 100 000 person-years in the Caucasian population.[1,2] Hispanic individuals appear to be affected more commonly than Caucasians. The disease is also seen in Europe, with an incidence approximately 20 per 100 000 in the UK, and 24 per 100 000 in Sweden.[3] There has been a suggestion of female preponderance in some studies, although this has not been observed consistently.

Genetics

While sarcoidosis is not transmitted according to Mendelian genetics, there have been suggestions of familial aggregation and racial differences which support the notion that sarcoidosis may occur preferentially in genetically susceptible hosts. For example, siblings of those affected with sarcoid have a modestly increased disease risk with an odds ratio of about 5.[4,5] A genome-wide scan performed in German families with sarcoidosis has yielded a possible susceptibility gene on chromosome 6, called BTL2, which is a B7-family costimulatory molecule involved in immune regulation.[6,7] Chromosome 5 has also been identified as potentially harboring candidate genes.[8,9]

Differential diagnosis

The differential diagnosis of sarcoidosis in the eye is broad. It nearly always includes other granulomas and inflammatory conditions such as tuberculosis and syphilis. Other etiologies, including atypical mycobacterial infection, endophthalmitis, herpetic eye disease, and autoimmune conditions such as Vogt–Koyanagi–Harada syndrome, may appear very similar to sarcoidosis clinically.

Diagnostic workup

Definitive diagnosis of sarcoidosis requires pathologic examination of biopsy tissue. The source of this tissue is rarely the eye; frequently, bronchoscopy will be used to generate diagnostic material. Mediastinoscopy may also be used for the biopsy of the hilar lymph nodes. Surface lymphadenopathy may be biopsied transcutaneously. Nondirected conjunctival biopsy has a very low yield in sarcoidosis,[10] but biopsy of visible conjunctiva granulomas may be an expeditious way for the ophthalmologist to make this diagnosis. Lacking tissue diagnosis, several laboratory tests may provide supportive (but not definitive) evidence for this diagnosis. Historically, the Kveim–Siltzbach test was used in the diagnosis of sarcoidosis.[11] In this test, a standardized extract from the spleen of a patient with sarcoidosis was injected subcutaneously into an individual suspected of having sarcoidosis. Several days later, formation of a granuloma at the site of injection is suggestive of the recipient patient having sarcoidosis. This test is no longer used clinically, but has important implications for the pathophysiology of sarcoidosis (see below). The serum angiotensin-converting enzyme (ACE) level is frequently elevated in patients with sarcoidosis. The positive and negative predictive values of this test for the disease, however, are relatively low, of the order of 83% and 58%, respectively.[12] Gallium-67 uptake scanning has been utilized in a number of studies and may be relatively specific for sarcoidosis, particularly if the "panda sign" is seen. This sign refers to the take-up of gallium by the lacrimose glands, parotid glands, and sinuses, resulting in an image of the face resembling a panda. The combination of elevated ACE level and positive gallium scan is thought to have a positive predictive value in excess of 95%.[13,14] Elevated serum calcium and serum lysozyme have also been suggested as markers for systemic sarcoidosis but have low positive and negative predictive values. Definitive diagnosis of sarcoidosis always requires tissue biopsy.

Treatment

Ocular sarcoidosis is typically treated with corticosteroids. Anterior disease is often responsive to topical or periocular medication alone. Posterior-segment disease frequently requires oral corticosteroids. As sarcoidosis may be chronic, this may require substitution of steroid-sparing medications for corticosteroids after several weeks. Methotrexate has been used in a number of studies and appears efficacious for this task.[15] Additionally, tumor necrosis factor-α inhibitors may have good efficacy for the treatment of sarcoidosis.[16,17]

Prognosis

Few data exist on the overall prognosis of patients with ocular sarcoidosis. Most cases are relatively easily treated, but a subset of patients may permanently lose vision from either the sarcoid granulomas themselves (i.e., optic nerve head granulomas or submacular granulomas), or complications secondary to chronic uveitis, such as a cystoid macular edema.[18]

Pathology

Granulomatous inflammation is a distinctive pattern of chronic inflammatory infiltrate in which the predominant cell type is an activated macrophage. A granuloma is a microscopic focus of inflammation characterized by a collection of modified epithelial-like (epithelioid) macrophages (Figure 84.3). The epithelioid macrophage contains pale pink granular cytoplasm with indistinct cell membranes. Frequently epithelioid macrophages may fuse to form giant cells (40–50 μm) with multiple nuclei (Figure 84.4). The pathologic diagnosis of sarcoidosis requires the histologic identification of epithelioid granulomas within involved tissue and the exclusion of known causes of granulomatous disease, especially those of infectious etiology. Granulomatous inflammation is encountered in association with a variety of infectious and noninfectious agents, including mycobacterial and some mycotic, bacterial and parasitic infections, berylliosis, some types of vasculitis, and as a reaction to poorly soluble particulate matter. Even after extensive workup many granulomatous lesions remain unclassified.

Although there is no reliable method to distinguish sarcoidal granulomas from those of other disease processes, there are some characteristics of sarcoidal granulomas which may be useful. The granulomas of sarcoidosis are well formed in that the epithelioid and giant cells are compact with sharp circumscription from the surrounding tissue. The granulomas usually exhibit a uniform appearance suggesting

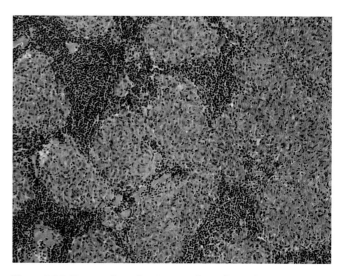

Figure 84.3 Hematoxylin and eosin stain of a mediastinal lymph node demonstrating noncaseating granulomas typical of sarcoidosis.

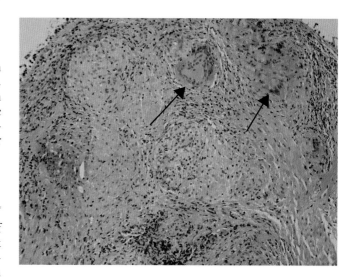

Figure 84.4 Multinucleated giant cell in sarcoidosis (arrow).

formation at a single point in time. Early, cellular granulomas become replaced by more fibrotic, hyalinized lesions as the disease progresses. Small central foci of amorphous granular debris (necrosis) may be seen in up to one-third of open lung biopsies in patients with sarcoidosis. Collections of neutrophils (suppuration) and confluent foci of necrosis are usually absent. Abundant necrosis is very unusual for typical sarcoidosis and should alert the clinician to exclude infection. The terms "caseating" and "noncaseating" are often used to describe granulomatous inflammation. Caseation refers to the white, cheesy gross appearance of tissue necrosis most commonly seen in foci of tuberculous infection. Caseation has been used interchangeably with the microscopic description of necrosis and, as described above, should be absent in sarcoidosis.

A variety of nonspecific intracellular inclusions may be seen in the granulomas of sarcoidosis. Schaumann bodies, or conchoidal bodies, consisting of a concentric laminated concretion of calcium salts and iron with a mucopolysac-

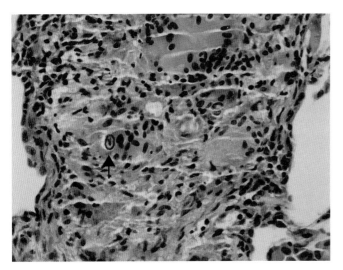

Figure 84.5 Schaumann body associated with sarcoid granulomas (arrow).

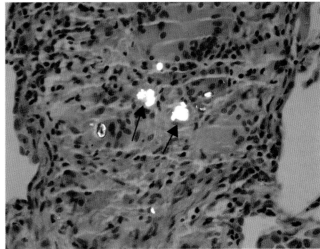

Figure 84.6 Birefringent calcium oxalate crystals associated with sarcoid granulomas (arrows).

Box 84.2 Key pathologic features of sarcoidosis

- Granulomatous inflammation featuring epithelioid histiocytes
- Inflammation is noncaseating (i.e., not necrotic)
- Multinucleated giant cells
- Schaumann bodies (concretions of calcium salts, iron, and mucopolysaccharides)
- Birefringent calcium oxalate crystals
- Disease progression is associated with fibrosis

---

charide matrix, occur in up to 70% of cases (Figure 84.5 and Box 84.2). Birefringent calcium oxalate crystals are seen within giant cells almost as frequently (60%) (Figure 84.6). Less frequently seen is the star-shaped densely eosinophilic asteroid body. Hamazaki–Wesenberg bodies are yellow-brown oval or spindle-shaped structures which are believed to represent large lysosomes. They are often found in the subcapsular sinuses of lymph nodes involved with sarcoidosis. These various inclusions can be very prominent and are important to recognize in order not to mistake them for causative foreign material or infection.

Because pulmonary involvement is almost universal, the histologic diagnosis of sarcoidosis is often rendered on material obtained by lung or bronchial biopsy. In lung tissue, granulomatous inflammation may be found in the bronchial or bronchiolar submucosa accounting for the over 90% diagnostic yield of bronchoscopic biopsy. Studies of bronchoalveolar lavage and bronchoscopic biopsy material in patients with sarcoidosis have demonstrated a predominance of CD4+ T cells, which is helpful in diagnosis. The combination of a CD4-to-CD8 ratio greater than 4 : 1, a lymphocyte percentage greater than 16%, and a biopsy demonstrating granulomas is associated with a 100% positive predictive value for distinguishing sarcoidosis from other interstitial lung diseases, and an 81% positive predictive value for distinguishing sarcoidosis from all other diseases.[19]

The early sarcoid granuloma consists predominately of CD4+ T cells and monocytes. The monocytes mature into macrophages and occasional multinucleated giant cells. It is generally assumed that sarcoidal granulomas are initiated when macrophages phagocytose an inciting antigen in a classic major histocompatibility complex (MHC) II restricted pathway. The antigen-presenting cells stimulate the proliferation of the CD4+ T cells and macrophages which in turn secrete inflammatory mediators such as interferon-γ, tumor necrosis factor-α and interleukin-2, believed to be important for granuloma formation.

Factors altering the immune response influence the development of sarcoidosis and help to define the immunologic features required for granulomas to form. In studies of human immunodeficiency virus (HIV)-infected patients, sarcoidal granulomas disappear when patient's T-cell counts drop below 200/μl.[20] Implementation of effective antiviral therapy can result in sarcoid recrudescence. Cytokine therapy used for cancer or HIV treatment has also been associated with the clinical development of sarcoidosis.[21] Interferon-α used in the treatment of hepatitis C can trigger or exacerbate sarcoidosis.[22] Sarcoidosis is also known to occur in association with a variety of autoimmune diseases.

Etiology

A number of environmental risk factors have been identified for sarcoidosis. In the Isle of Man study, the predominant risk factor for sarcoidosis was living within 100 meters of another individual with sarcoidosis, suggesting some transmissible agent.[23,24] Older literature suggested that nurses have a sevenfold higher lifetime risk of sarcoidosis than the average population.[25] Certain environmental triggers have been suggested in outbreaks of sarcoidosis. Most recently, it is suspected that the dust fallout from the twin towers collapse in 2001 led to a small epidemic of new sarcoidosis cases in the ensuing several years in New York city.[1]

Transplant studies also suggest a transmissible agent. These are based mostly on small case studies. In one study, an individual with a known history of sarcoidosis served as a bone marrow donor for his brother, who did not have disease at time of engraftment. Despite aggressive immunomodulation postimplantation, the sibling developed sarcoidosis within several weeks of the transplant.[26] Similar transmission from affected donor to naïve host has been associated with cardiac transplantation.[27] Conversely, sarcoid-positive recipients typically redeveloped disease in naïve organs. The estimated rate of redevelopment of pulmonary sarcoidosis in lung transplantation is close to 80%.

As noted above, it is not thought that sarcoidosis is a genetic disease per se. However, there are diseases that are nearly identical in clinical appearances to sarcoidosis that clearly have a genetic basis. Blau syndrome is also a multi-organ-system granulomatous inflammation, typically affecting children. It is transmitted as an autosomal-recessive trait. The disease is due to mutations in the NOD2/CARD15 gene.[28] This gene has been implicated in Toll-like receptor (TLR) signaling, suggesting that aberrant innate immunity to bacterial pathogens may underlie sarcoidosis. Similarly, linkage has been reported between TLR polymorphisms and sarcoidosis.[29] Human leukocyte antigen (HLA) DRB1*1101 has also been associated with sarcoidosis.[30]

Pathophysiology

The data suggesting a transmissible agent as a trigger for sarcoidosis have led to many studies examining pathology specimens for the presence of possible microbial infection. Among the earlier hypotheses for this pathogen was "L-form" mycobacteria. These are thought to be mycobacterial species that lack cell walls, and are therefore not amenable to staining with standard reagents. Molecular biologic studies have suggested a high rate of detection of mycobacterial DNA in the lymph nodes of patients with sarcoidosis.[31] Although some studies have suggested a high rate of human herpesvirus-8 infection in sarcoid lymph nodes, this result has not been replicated across multiple populations.[32,33]

Research groups in Japan have found a high rate of propionibacteria in lymph nodes of patients with sarcoidosis.[34] In particular, *Propionibacterium acnes* has been identified in bronchoalveolar lavage washings of a high proportion (~70%) of sarcoid patients.[35] The same bacteria have also been identified in vitreous samples from patients with sarcoidosis.[36] Animal studies have suggested that *Propionibacterium* is able to prime the host in the development of sarcoid-like pulmonary granulomatosis in mice.[37,38] However, the finding of propionibacteria in granulomas of non-Asian sarcoidosis patients has been limited to date.

The Kveim–Siltzbach reagent was an obvious place to look for a microbial pathogen in sarcoidosis. However,

detailed examination of this reagent for bacterial DNA by polymerase chain reaction yielded no evidence of infection.[39] Kveim–Siltzbach reagent has long been noted to be resistant to protease treatment. Song and colleagues digested the reagent with a cocktail of proteases, and separated the resulting degraded proteins on one-dimensional gel electrophoresis. They then probed this protein by Western blot using sera from patients with and without sarcoidosis. This analysis revealed a single band of protein that was both protease-resistant and an antigenic target in patients affected with sarcoidosis. Mass spectroscopy analysis of this band revealed that it was the catalase gene of *Mycobacterium tuberculosis*.[40] Subsequent work challenging T cells of patients with sarcoidosis with peptides derived from bacterial catalase has revealed that a high proportion of sarcoidosis patients do indeed have reactivity to mycobacterial antigens.[41] Interestingly, the majority of these patients do not show skin responses to purified protein derivative (PPD), suggesting that either this represents a variant of *M. tuberculosis* that does not feature reactivity to the antigens found in the PPD reagent, or that sarcoidosis may be due to a related mycobacterial species with a very similar catalase gene.

Summary

Sarcoidosis is a multisystem granulomatous inflammatory disease of unknown etiology. It frequently affects the eyes, typically causing intraocular inflammation. Recent work has suggested a coherent model for the genesis of sarcoidosis. Disseminated infection with a relatively indolent bacterial species such as a nontuberculous mycobacterium or *Propionibacterium* results in a mild inflammatory response. The bacterium is cleared by the innate and adaptive immune systems, but protease-resistant antigens cannot be effectively processed. These antigens than become a nidus for chronic inflammatory disease, particularly in genetically susceptible individuals (i.e., those with impaired innate immune responses as the result of specific polymorphisms). Thus, the pathology of sarcoidosis resembles conditions of inflammation due to other nonclearable antigens, such as silicosis or berylliosis.

These insights into pathophysiology portend the possibility of improved diagnostic tests for sarcoidosis; if a small subset of bacterial pathogens are found to incite sarcoidosis, T-cell reactivity to the specific protease-resistant antigens may provide very specific and rapid noninvasive diagnostic tests. At present it is unclear how specific intervention could be engineered for clearance of protease-resistant antigens, as is suggested by this model. Thus, we will likely be treating ocular sarcoidosis with general immunomodulatory treatments for the foreseeable future.

Key references

A complete list of chapter references is available online at www.expertconsult.com. See inside cover for registration details.

2. Prezant DJ, Dhala A, Goldstein A, et al. The incidence, prevalence, and severity of sarcoidosis in New York City firefighters. Chest 1999;116:1183–1193.

3. Hosoda Y, Yamaguchi M, Hiraga Y. Global epidemiology of sarcoidosis. What story do prevalence and incidence tell us? Clin Chest Med 1997;18:681–694.

4. Rybicki BA, Sinha R, Iyengar S, et al. Genetic linkage analysis of sarcoidosis phenotypes: the sarcoidosis genetic analysis (SAGA) study. Genes Immun 2007;8:379–386.

10. Dios E, Saornil MA, Herreras JM. Conjunctival biopsy in the diagnosis of ocular sarcoidosis. Ocul Immunol Inflamm 2001;9:59–64.

18. Edelsten C, Pearson A, Joynes E, et al. The ocular and systemic prognosis of patients presenting with sarcoid uveitis. Eye 1999;13:748–753.

23. Hills SE, Parkes SA, Baker SB. Epidemiology of sarcoidosis in the Isle of Man – 2: evidence for space-time clustering. Thorax 1987;42:427–430.

26. Heyll A, Meckenstock G, Aul C, et al. Possible transmission of sarcoidosis via allogeneic bone marrow transplantation. Bone Marrow Transplant 1994;14:161–164.

28. Miceli-Richard C, Lesage S, Rybojad M, et al. CARD15 mutations in Blau syndrome. Nat Genet 2001;29:19–20.

40. Song Z, Marzilli L, Greenlee BM, et al. Mycobacterial catalase-peroxidase is a tissue antigen and target of the adaptive immune response in systemic sarcoidosis. J Exp Med 2001;201:755–767.

Index

NB: Page numbers in **bold** refer to boxes, figures and tables

E